Become PRACTICE READY using PEARSON RESOURCES

Simplify your study time by using the resources included with this textbook at **http://nursing.pearsonhighered.com**.

This book includes the following materials for you to use:

- Learning Outcomes
- NCLEX-PN® Review Questions
- Animations and Videos
- Case Studies
- and More...

Enhance your SUCCESS with the additional resources below.
For more information and purchasing options visit **www.mypearsonstore.com**.

For Your Classroom Success
Companion workbook that helps you succeed in practical/vocational nursing Includes learning outcomes, NCLEX-PN®-style review questions, critical thinking case studies, and more!

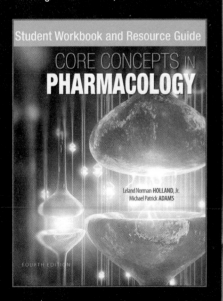

Student Workbook and Resource Guide

CORE CONCEPTS in PHARMACOLOGY

Leland Norman HOLLAND, Jr.
Michael Patrick ADAMS

FOURTH EDITION

For Your Clinical Success
My Nursing App™

www.mynursingapp.com

Clinical references across the nursing curriculum available!

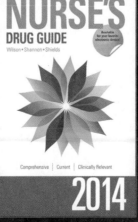

PEARSON
NURSE'S
DRUG GUIDE
Wilson • Shannon • Shields

Available for your favorite electronic device

Comprehensive | Current | Clinically Relevant
2014

For Your
NCLEX-PN® Success

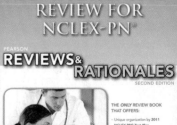

MARYANN HOGAN

COMPREHENSIVE REVIEW FOR NCLEX-PN®

PEARSON
REVIEWS& RATIONALES
SECOND EDITION

THE ONLY REVIEW BOOK THAT OFFERS:
- Unique organization by 2011 NCLEX-PN® Test Plan
- More than 1,500 NCLEX-style questions, comprehensive rationales & strategies in the book
- Online Nursing Reviews & Rationales with additional 3,800 practice questions & eText
- Nursing Notes guide to the 2011 NCLEX-PN® Test Plan

WITH JULIE SKRABAL, MSN, RN

ALWAYS LEARNING

PEARSON

Become Practice-Ready with Pearson Custom Library

Design your nursing textbooks to be as unique as you (and your students) are.

www.pearsoncustomlibrary.com

Comprehensive Nursing Care
Revised 2e, Ramont, Niedringhaus, Towle

Medical-Surgical Nursing Care
4e, Burke, Mohn-Brown, Eby

Fundamental Nursing Care
2e, Ramont, Niedringhaus

Maternal-Child Nursing Care
Towle, Adams

Maternal-Newborn Nursing Care
Towle

Pediatric Nursing Care
Adams, Towle

Mental Health Nursing Care
2e, Eby, Brown

Each book in the series shares a similar design and contains similar features to enhance the student's learning experience. It gives students more time to focus on content and less on "learning the book". Books in the series share a consistent reading level and dedicated focus on what the LPN/LVN needs to know and do and priorities for action.

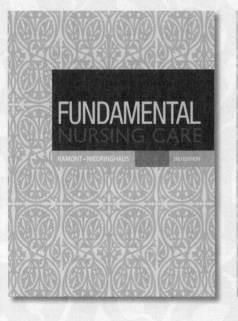

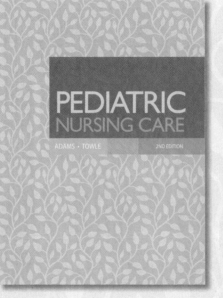

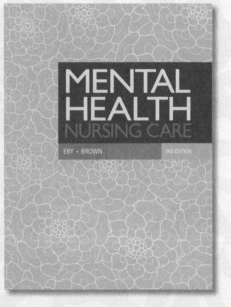

BRIEF CONTENTS

UNIT I
Basic Concepts in Pharmacology   1

CHAPTER 1   Introduction to Pharmacology: Drug Regulation and Approval   2

CHAPTER 2   Drug Classes, Schedules, and Categories   12

CHAPTER 3   Methods of Drug Administration   20

CHAPTER 4   What Happens After a Drug Has Been Administered   41

CHAPTER 5   The Nursing Process in Pharmacology   51

CHAPTER 6   The Role of Complementary and Alternative Therapies in Pharmacology   59

CHAPTER 7   Substance Abuse   69

UNIT II
The Nervous System   85

CHAPTER 8   Drugs Affecting Functions of the Autonomic Nervous System   86

CHAPTER 9   Drugs for Anxiety and Insomnia   105

CHAPTER 10   Drugs for Emotional, Mood, and Behavioral Disorders   122

CHAPTER 11   Drugs for Psychoses   142

CHAPTER 12   Drugs for Degenerative Diseases and Muscles   157

CHAPTER 13   Drugs for Seizures   180

CHAPTER 14   Drugs for Pain Management   197

CHAPTER 15   Drugs for Anesthesia   217

UNIT III
The Cardiovascular and Urinary Systems   233

CHAPTER 16   Drugs for Lipid Disorders   234

CHAPTER 17   Diuretics and Drugs for Electrolyte and Acid–Base Disorders   248

CHAPTER 18   Drugs for Hypertension   265

CHAPTER 19   Drugs for Heart Failure   287

CHAPTER 20   Drugs for Angina Pectoris, Myocardial Infarction, and Stroke   301

CHAPTER 21   Drugs for Shock and Anaphylaxis   319

CHAPTER 22   Drugs for Dysrhythmias   331

CHAPTER 23   Drugs for Coagulation Disorders   346

UNIT IV
The Immune System   361

CHAPTER 24   Drugs for Inflammation and Fever   362

CHAPTER 25   Drugs for Immune System Modulation   373

CHAPTER 26   Drugs for Bacterial Infections   387

CHAPTER 27   Drugs for Fungal, Viral, and Parasitic Diseases   412

CHAPTER 28   Drugs for Neoplasia   430

UNIT V
The Respiratory and Digestive Systems   453

CHAPTER 29   Drugs for Respiratory Disorders   454

CHAPTER 30   Drugs for Gastrointestinal Disorders   476

CHAPTER 31   Vitamins, Minerals, and Nutritional Supplements   496

UNIT VI
The Endocrine and Reproductive Systems   509

CHAPTER 32   Drugs for Endocrine Disorders   510

CHAPTER 33   Drugs for Diabetes Mellitus   528

CHAPTER 34   Drugs for Disorders and Conditions of the Reproductive System   542

UNIT VII
The Skeletal System, Integumentary System, and Eyes and Ears   563

CHAPTER 35   Drugs for Bone and Joint Disorders   564

CHAPTER 36   Drugs for Skin Disorders   582

CHAPTER 37   Drugs for Eye and Ear Disorders   598

APPENDIX A	References	**611**
APPENDIX B	Brief Answers to NCLEX-PN® and Case Study Questions	**621**
APPENDIX C	Calculating Dosages	**624**

| INDEX | **626** |
| GUIDE TO SPECIAL FEATURES | **657** |

***APPENDIX D** (Complete Answers and Rationales for NCLEX-PN® Review and Case Study Questions) and the **GLOSSARY** appear on the textbook's website.

CORE CONCEPTS IN
PHARMACOLOGY

FOURTH EDITION

Leland Norman Holland, Jr., PhD
Program Manager
Hillsborough Community College, Brandon Campus, Tampa, Florida

Michael Patrick Adams, PhD, RT(R)
Professor, Anatomy and Physiology
Saint Petersburg College, Saint Petersburg, Florida
Formerly Dean, Health Professions
Pasco-Hernando Community College, New Port Richey, Florida

Jeanine Lynn Brice, RN, MSN
Nursing Tutor
Saint Petersburg College, Saint Petersburg, Florida
Formerly Professor of Nursing
Pasco-Hernando Community College, New Port Richey, Florida

PEARSON

Boston Columbus Indianapolis New York San Francisco Upper Saddle River
Amsterdam Cape Town Dubai London Madrid Milan Munich Paris Montréal Toronto
Delhi Mexico City São Paulo Sydney Hong Kong Seoul Singapore Taipei Tokyo

Library of Congress Cataloging-in-Publication Data

Holland, Leland Norman.
  Core concepts in pharmacology / Leland Norman Holland, Jr., Michael Patrick Adams, Jeanine Brice. — Fourth edition.
      p. ; cm.
  Includes bibliographical references and index.
  ISBN-13: 978-0-13-344981-5
  ISBN-10: 0-13-344981-5
  I. Adams, Michael, (date) author.   II. Brice, Jeanine, author.   III. Title.
  [DNLM: 1. Pharmacological Phenomena. 2. Drug Therapy. QV 37]
  RM301.14
  615'.1—dc23   2013042150

Publisher: Julie Levin Alexander
Assistant to the Publisher: Regina Bruno
Development Editor: Rachel Bedard
Editorial Assistant: Erin Sullivan
Program Manager: Erin Rafferty
Project Manager: Michael Giacobbe
Production Editor: Andrea Stefanowicz, PreMediaGlobal
Creative Director: Andrea Nix
Cover and Interior Designer: Mary Siener
Media Product Manager: Karen Bretz & Tanika Henderson
Director of Marketing: David Gesell
Marketing Coordinator: Michael Sirinides
Composition: PreMediaGlobal
Cover Printer: Lehigh Phoenix Color
Printer/Binder: Courier/Kendallville

Notice: The authors and the publisher of this volume have taken care to make certain that the doses of drugs and schedules of treatment are correct and compatible with the standards generally accepted at the time of publication. Nevertheless, as new information becomes available, changes in treatment and in the use of drugs become necessary. The reader is advised to carefully consult the instruction and information material included in the package insert of each drug or therapeutic agent before administration. This advice is especially important when using, administering, or recommending new and infrequently used drugs. The authors and publisher disclaim all responsibility for any liability, loss, injury, or damage incurred as a consequence, directly or indirectly, of the use and application of any of the contents of this volume.

PEARSON

10 9 8 7 6 5 4 3 2 1
ISBN 10: 0-13-344981-5
ISBN 13: 978-0-13-3449815

PREFACE

Pharmacology is one of the most challenging subjects for those embarking on careers in the health sciences. By its very nature, pharmacology is an interdisciplinary subject, borrowing concepts from a wide variety of the natural and applied sciences. Prediction of drug action, the ultimate goal in the study of pharmacology, requires a thorough knowledge of anatomy, physiology, chemistry, and pathology as well as of the social sciences of psychology and sociology. It is the interdisciplinary nature of pharmacology that makes the subject difficult to learn, but fascinating to study.

This text presents pharmacology from an interdisciplinary perspective. The text draws upon core concepts of anatomy, physiology, and pathology to make drug therapy understandable. The text does not assume that the student comes to the course with a strong background in the natural or applied sciences. Instead, the prerequisite science knowledge necessary for understanding drug therapy is reviewed in each chapter that presents the core concepts in pharmacology.

ORGANIZATION

The authors use numbered core concepts, a concise means of communicating to the student the most important pharmacologic information. These core concepts are stated at the beginning of each chapter, so that the student can get an overview of what is to be learned. They are repeated at the end of the chapter, with a brief summary of each important concept.

Disease and Body System Approach

Core Concepts in Pharmacology is organized according to body systems and diseases. The framework places the drugs in the context of how they are used therapeutically. This makes it easy for the student to locate all relevant anatomy, physiology, pathology, and pharmacology in the same chapter in which the drugs are discussed.

Prototype Approach to Drug Therapy

The vast number of drugs taught in a pharmacology course is staggering. To facilitate learning, this text highlights one or two most representative drugs in each classification as prototypes and introduces them in detail. **Drug Prototype** boxes showcase these important medications.

Focused Nursing Content

This text provides focused nursing content, allowing students quick access to essential content for safe, effective drug therapy. **Nursing Process Focus** charts provide a succinct, easy-to-read view of the most commonly prescribed drug classes. Need-to-know nursing actions are presented in a format that reflects the "flow" of the Nursing Process: nursing assessment, potential nursing diagnoses, planning, interventions (including patient education and discharge planning), and evaluation. Rationales for interventions are included in parentheses. The Nursing Process Focus charts clearly identify what nursing actions are most important.

NEW TO THIS EDITION

- *2 New Chapters!* Because of the expansion in pharmacologic development in immune modulation and diabetes management, these topics are presented in new chapters.
- *Updated and Revised!* All drugs updated and prototypes adjusted to reflect modern drug usage.
- *Updated and Revised! Safety Alert* features throughout the text call attention to medication errors and The Joint Commission safety guidelines.
- *Drug Prototype* boxes include both therapeutic and pharmacological drug classifications.
- *Added! Black Box Warnings* for the drugs designated as special risk.
- *Updated and Revised!* End of chapter **NCLEX-PN® questions completely revised**. Full rationales and NCLEX tagging are provided in an online appendix.
- *Updated! Glossary* provided with definitions of all key terms.
- *Addition of off-label uses of drugs* and adverse effects to drug tables as appropriate.
- *Completely Revised!* The Nursing Process Focus charts reflecting current nursing practice.

DESIGN AND FEATURES

Focus on Core Information

The numbered **Core Concepts** identify ideas and provide an overview of the chapter.

The **Drug Snapshot** provides an at-a-glance list of the drug classes and related drug prototypes covered in each chapter.

Key Terms with page numbers help students review important vocabulary terms.

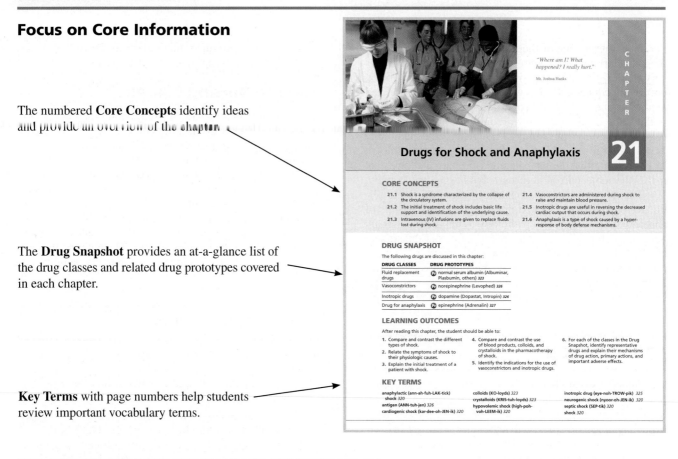

Concept Reviews are questions placed strategically throughout the chapter to stimulate student comprehension and retention as they read.

Concept Review   13.1

■ What is epilepsy? What is the difference between a seizure and a convulsion? Name and identify signs of the more common types of seizures.

Prototype Approach

The prototype approach introduces the one or two most representative drugs in each classification in detail. **Drug Prototype** boxes highlight these important drugs. This edition includes both therapeutic and pharmacologic drug classifications.

The new **Black Box Warning** element identifies extremely adverse drug reactions associated with use of a particular drug.

Drug tables provide the most important information for each drug in a user-friendly format. Drugs profiled within that chapter are also identified with a **Prototype icon**.

TABLE 13.4 Succinimides		
Drug	**Route and Adult Dose**	**Remarks**
ethosuximide (Zarontin)	PO; 250 mg bid, increased every 4–7 days (max: 1.5 g/day)	For absence seizures, myoclonic seizures, and akinetic epilepsy; may cause nausea, anorexia, abdominal pain, vomiting, gum overgrowth, blood disord behavioral changes, rash (Stevens–Johnson syndrome)
methsuximide (Celontin)	PO; 300 mg/day, may increase every 4–7 days (max: 1.2 g/day in divided doses)	For absence seizures; may be used in combination with other anticonvulsan in mixed types of seizure activity; may cause dizziness, drowsiness, blurred vision, increased risk for suicidal thoughts, fetal toxicity

HIGHLIGHTS KEY INFORMATION FOR SAFE, EFFECTIVE NURSING CARE

NURSING PROCESS FOCUS Patients Receiving Atypical Antipsychotic Therapy

ASSESSMENT	POTENTIAL NURSING DIAGNOSES
Prior to administration: ■ Obtain a complete health history including cardiovascular, renal and liver conditions, allergies, drug history, and possible drug interactions. ■ Acquire baseline vital signs and ECG, laboratory blood levels (CBC, chemistry, drug screening, renal and liver function studies) and urine specimens for laboratory analysis. ■ Determine neurological status. (altered thought processes, hallucinations, level of consciousness [LOC], mental status, and identification of recent mood and behavior patterns). ■ Identify patient support system(s).	■ *Risk for Injury* related to adverse effects of drug therapy, and thought processes ■ *Ineffective Therapeutic Regimen Management* related to noncompliance with medication regimen, presence of adverse effects, and need for long-term medication use ■ *Anxiety* related to symptoms of psychosis ■ *Noncompliance* related to length of time before drug reaches therapeutic levels, desire to use alcohol or illegal drugs ■ *Deficient Knowledge* related to a lack of information about disease process and drug therapy

PLANNING: PATIENT GOALS AND EXPECTED OUTCOMES
The patient will: ■ Experience therapeutic effects (reduction of psychotic symptoms). ■ Be free from or experience minimal adverse effects from drug therapy. ■ Verbalize an understanding of the drug's use, adverse effects and required precautions. ■ Adhere to recommended treatment regimen.

IMPLEMENTATION	
Interventions and (Rationales)	**Patient Education/Discharge Planning**
■ Administer medication correctly and evaluate the patient's knowledge of proper administration. (Ensuring proper administration helps to avoid unnecessary adverse effects and interactions with other medications while determining effectiveness.)	Instruct the patient: ■ Not to take any other medication or herbal therapies unless approved by the healthcare provider. ■ That it may take up to six weeks for full therapeutic effects to be seen.
■ Monitor RBC and WBC counts. (Agranulocytosis [WBCs below 3,500] can be a life-threatening adverse effect of these medications, which may also suppress bone marrow and lower infection-fighting ability.)	Instruct the patient to: ■ Keep appointments for laboratory testing. ■ Report any sore throat, signs of infection, fatigue without apparent cause, or bruising to the healthcare provider.
■ Observe for adverse effects. (These drugs may affect blood pressure, heart rate, and other autonomic functions.)	Instruct the patient to report any adverse effect such as drowsiness, dizziness, depression, anxiety, tachycardia, hypotension, nausea/vomiting, excessive salivation, changes in urinary frequency or urgency, incontinence, weight gain, muscle pain or weakness, rash, and fever to the healthcare provider.
■ Monitor for anticholinergic adverse effects. (These medications may cause mouth dryness, constipation, or urinary retention.)	Instruct the patient to: ■ Increase dietary fiber, fluids, and exercise to prevent constipation. ■ Relieve symptoms of dry mouth with sugar-free hard candy or chewing gum and frequent drinks of water. ■ Immediately notify the healthcare provider if urinary retention occurs. Possible catheter placement may be necessary.
■ Monitor for therapeutic effects, e.g., decrease of psychotic symptoms. (Decreased symptoms indicate an effective dose and type of medication.)	Instruct the patient to: ■ Notice increases or decreases of symptoms of psychosis, including hallucinations, abnormal sleep patterns, social withdrawal, delusions, or paranoia. ■ Contact the healthcare provider if symptoms do not decrease over a six-week period.
■ Monitor for alcohol or illegal drug use. (Used concurrently, these will cause increased CNS depression. The patient may decide to use alcohol or illegal drugs as a means of coping with symptoms of psychosis and may stop taking the drug.)	Instruct the patient to avoid alcohol or illegal drug use. Refer the patient to AA, NA, or other support group as appropriate.
■ Monitor caffeine use. (Use of caffeine-containing substances inhibits the effects of antipsychotics.)	Instruct the patient about: ■ Common caffeine-containing products. ■ Acceptable substitutes, including decaffeinated coffee and tea, and caffeine-free soda.
■ Monitor for smoking. (Heavy smoking may decrease blood levels of the drug.)	Instruct the patient to stop or decrease smoking. Refer to smoking cessation programs if indicated.
■ Monitor older adult patients closely. (Older patients may be more sensitive to anticholinergic adverse effects.)	Instruct older adult patients on ways to counteract anticholinergic effects of the medication while taking into account any other existing medical problems.

EVALUATION OF OUTCOME CRITERIA
Evaluate the effectiveness of drug therapy by confirming that patient goals and expected outcomes have been met (see "Planning"). *See Table 11.4 for a list of drugs to which these nursing actions apply.*

Nursing Process Focus charts provide a succinct, easy-to-read view of the most important nursing actions for the commonly prescribed drug classes. Need-to-know nursing actions are presented in the charts; they also include patient education and discharge planning.

The nursing student needs to learn how to teach drug administration to patients and families. To help the student, each drug chapter contains concise **Patients Need to Know** boxes that help students teach patients and families about drug information and administration.

PATIENTS NEED TO KNOW

Patients taking antiseizure medications need to know the following:

In General

1. Never abruptly stop taking antiseizure medication; doing so can cause seizures to return.
2. Avoid alcohol and other CNS depressants because they can increase sedation.
3. Antiseizure medications may cause drowsiness; avoid driving and the use of machinery that could lead to injury.
4. It may require several dosage adjustments over many months to find the dosage that allows performance of normal daily activities while controlling seizures.
5. It is important to keep laboratory appointments because many antiseizure medications require blood testing to ensure that the drug is at a safe and effective level in the blood.
6. Consult a healthcare provider before trying to become pregnant; some antiseizure medications are not safe to use during pregnancy.
7. Report excess fatigue, drowsiness, agitation, confusion, or suicidal thoughts to a healthcare provider.

Regarding Hydantoins and Related Medications

8. Report the following adverse effects to a healthcare provider: gum overgrowth (gingival hyperplasia) or skin rash, tremors, weight gain, diarrhea, irregular menses, dizziness, nausea, or oversedation.
9. Hydantoins and related medications interact with many other drugs; do not add any other prescription, over-the-counter (OTC) drugs, or herbal supplements until a healthcare provider is consulted. Do not consume alcohol while taking these medications.

Regarding Succinimides

10. Report the following adverse effects to a healthcare provider: hiccups or epigastric pain with ethosuximide (Zarontin), drowsiness, or increased bleeding time.

SAFETY ALERT

Interpreting Physician Orders

It is extremely important for nurses to know their patients' needs and to clarify with the physician any medication order that is difficult to interpret or is questionable. For example, an error could be made if an order to discontinue "SSRI," intended to mean "sliding scale regular insulin," is misinterpreted as an order to discontinue the "selective serotonin reuptake inhibitor."

Safety Alerts highlight potential medication errors and The Joint Commission Safety Guidelines.

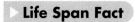

Life Span Fact

Onset of epilepsy is most common among the youngest and oldest age groups. About 50% of children have a generalized epilepsy syndrome compared with about 20% of adults. The incidence of epilepsy in older adults is greater than among the general population, perhaps because of the greater prevalence of mild strokes and cardiac arrest in this age group.

Life Span Facts provide important **pediatric and older adult considerations** for drug therapy, so students understand variations in nursing care and drug actions due to age.

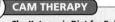

CAM THERAPY

The Ketogenic Diet for Epilepsy

The ketogenic diet may be used when seizures cannot be controlled through pharmaco-therapy or when there are unacceptable adverse effects to medications. Before antiepileptic drugs were developed, this diet was a primary treatment for epilepsy.

The ketogenic diet is a strict diet that is high in fat and low in carbohydrates and protein. It limits water intake and carefully controls caloric intake. Each meal has the same ketogenic ratio of 4 g of fat to 1 g of protein and carbohydrate. Extra fat is usually given in the form of cream.

Research suggests that the diet produces a high success rate for certain patients. The diet appears to be equally effective for every seizure type. The most frequently reported adverse effects include vomiting, fatigue, constipation, diarrhea, and hunger. Kidney stones, acidosis, and slower growth rates are possible risks. Those interested in trying the diet must consult with their healthcare provider; this is not a do-it-yourself diet and may be harmful if not monitored carefully by skilled professionals.

CAM (Complementary and Alternative Medicine) Therapy boxes present popular herbal or dietary supplements that may be considered along with conventional drugs.

Fast Facts Epilepsy

- Over two million Americans have epilepsy.
- One of every 100 teenagers has epilepsy.
- Of the U.S. population, 10% will have seizures within their lifetime.
- Most people with seizures are younger than 45 years of age.
- Epilepsy is not a mental illness and children with epilepsy have IQ scores equivalent to those of children without the disorder.
- Famous people who had epilepsy include Julius Caesar, Alexander the Great, Napoleon, Vincent van Gogh, Charles Dickens, Joan of Arc, and Socrates.
- Among adult alcoholics receiving treatment for withdrawal, over half will experience seizures within six hours upon arriving for treatment.

The **Fast Facts** feature puts the disease in a social and economic perspective.

END-OF-CHAPTER REVIEW RESOURCES

Student practical and vocational nurses from around the country told us that they start their chapter reading from the end of the chapter. So, to ensure students' success in the classroom, on the NCLEX-PN® exam, and in the workplace, we put dynamite review resources at the end of each chapter.

Core Concepts Summaries repeat the important points at the end of the chapter and provide a brief summary.

Review Questions serve as a post-test for the chapter and prepare students for the NCLEX-PN®. Tests include additional practice in calculating the correct dosage.

Case Study Questions help the student apply pharmacology and nursing care to a specific client scenario.

ACKNOWLEDGMENTS

We are grateful to all the educators who reviewed the manuscript of this text. Their insights, suggestions, and eye for detail helped us prepare a more relevant and useful book, one that focuses on the essential components of learning in the field of pharmacology. In particular, we would like to thank **Jeanine Brice**, RN, MSN, who reviewed and contributed to all nursing material including Nursing Process Focus Charts, Safety Alerts, Patients Need to Know, and all of the end-of-chapter questions. Your nursing experience, expertise, and dedication to the profession is evident in these materials.

Textbook Reviewers

Michaelann Allen, MA Ed, CMA
North Seattle Community College
Seattle, WA

Kevin Barnard, MS, CCEMT-P, NREMT-P, EMSI
Cuyahoga Community College
Cleveland, OH

Carole Berube, MA, MSN, BSN, RN
Bristol Community College
Fall River, MA

Ann Boeglin, MSN, RN
Vincennes University Jasper Campus
Jasper, IN

Charlene Chapman, BSN, RN
Pennsylvania Institute of Technology
Media, PA

Darlene Clark, MS, RN
Penn State University
University Park, PA

Kevin Dahlstedt, BA, MSN, RN
Western Nebraska Community College
Alliance, NE

David Flint, MEd, BSHS, EMT, WEMT, EMT-I
College of Technology
Idaho State University
Pocatello, ID

Michele Gerwick, PhD, RN
Indiana University of Pennsylvania
Indiana, PA

Bonita Gregg, MS Ed, RN
Community College of Allegheny County
West Mifflin, PA

Nancy Kennedy, MSN, RN
Ulster BOCES Career and Technical Center
Port Ewen, NY

Sharyn Ketcham, AAS, BS, MBA, MHSA, RMA
Phoenix College
Phoenix, AZ

Marlene Lazarus, DNP
Camden County College
Blackwood, NJ

Jo Ann Lindemann, MSN, RN
Dickinson State University
Dickinson, ND

Nelda New, PhD, APN, FNP-BC, ANP-BC, CNE
University of Central Arkansas
Conway, AR

Diana Rangaves, PharmD, RPh
Santa Rosa Junior College
Santa Rosa, CA

Tara Sadler, RN, BSN
South Arkansas Community College
El Dorado, AR

Lori Wahlberg, RN, MSN
Anoka Technical College
Anoka, MN

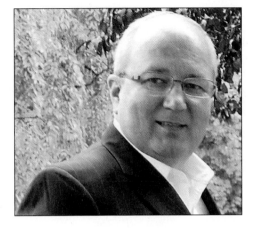

Leland Norman Holland, Jr., PhD (Norm), over 20 years ago, started out like many scientists, planning for a career in basic science research. Quickly he was drawn to the field of teaching in higher medical education, where he has spent most of his career since that time. Among the areas where he has been particularly effective are preparatory programs in nursing, medicine, dentistry, pharmacy, and allied health. Dr. Holland is both an affiliate and a supporter of nursing education nationwide. He brings to the profession a depth of knowledge in biology, chemistry, and medically related subjects such as microbiology, biological chemistry, and pharmacology. Dr. Holland's doctoral degree is in Medical Pharmacology. He is very much dedicated to the success of students and their preparation for work-life readiness. He continues to motivate students in the lifelong pursuit of learning.

I would like to acknowledge the willful encouragement of Farrell and Norma Jean Stalcup. I dedicate this book to my beloved wife, Karen, and my three wonderful children, Alexandria Noelle, my double-deuce daughter; Caleb Jaymes, my number one son; and Joshua Nathaniel, my number three "O"!
—LNH

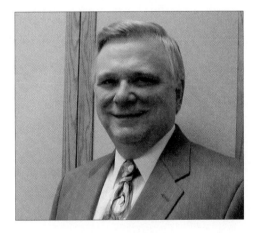

Michael Patrick Adams, PhD, RT(R), is an accomplished educator, author, and national speaker. The National Institute for Staff and Organizational Development in Austin, Texas, named Dr. Adams a Master Teacher. He has published two other textbooks with Pearson Publishing: *Pharmacology for Nurses: A Pathophysiologic Approach* and *Pharmacology: Connections to Nursing Practice.*

Dr. Adams obtained his master's degree in Pharmacology from Michigan State University and his Doctorate in Education at the University of South Florida. Dr. Adams was on the faculty of Lansing Community College and was Dean of Health Professions at Pasco-Hernando Community College for over 15 years. He is currently Professor of Anatomy and Physiology at Saint Petersburg College.

I dedicate this book to nursing educators, who contribute every day to making the world a better and more caring place.
—MPA

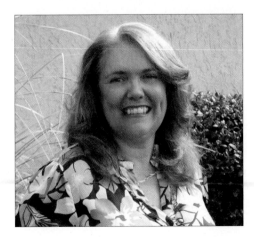

Jeanine L. Brice, RN, MSN, has been a nurse for over 26 years, initially graduating from the registered nursing program at Charles County Community College and continuing her nursing education, receiving a BS from the University of Maryland and an MSN from Bowie State University, specializing in nursing education and community health practice. Her clinical experience includes acute medical-surgical care, obstetrics, neonatology, and pediatric public health.

Ms. Brice has been involved in nursing/technical health education for over 23 years, formerly holding the positions of Professor of Nursing, Assistant Dean of Nursing Programs, and Coordinator of Technical Health Programs at Pasco-Hernando Community College. She currently is employed at St. Petersburg College tutoring nursing and allied health students.

I dedicate this book to my parents, William and Helen Davis, whom I had the privilege to care for during their final days . . . and to all those who will need the care of a nurse. May the information contained in this book help them receive competent and compassionate nursing care.
—JLB

CONTENTS

UNIT I
Basic Concepts in Pharmacology 1

CHAPTER 1 INTRODUCTION TO PHARMACOLOGY: DRUG REGULATION AND APPROVAL 2

Preclinical Investigation 7

Clinical Investigation 7

Submission of an NDA with Review 8

Postmarketing Studies 8

CHAPTER 2 DRUG CLASSES, SCHEDULES, AND CATEGORIES 12

CHAPTER 3 METHODS OF DRUG ADMINISTRATION 20

Tablets and Capsules 27

Sublingual and Buccal Drug Administration 27

Nasogastric and Gastrostomy Drug Administration 28

Transdermal Delivery System 29

Ophthalmic Administration 29

Otic Administration 31

Nasal Administration 31

Vaginal Administration 31

Rectal Administration 32

Intradermal and Subcutaneous Administration 33

Intramuscular Administration 36

Intravenous Administration 37

CHAPTER 4 WHAT HAPPENS AFTER A DRUG HAS BEEN ADMINISTERED 41

CHAPTER 5 THE NURSING PROCESS IN PHARMACOLOGY 51

CHAPTER 6 THE ROLE OF COMPLEMENTARY AND ALTERNATIVE THERAPIES IN PHARMACOLOGY 59

Herbal Products 61

Specialty Supplements 65

CHAPTER 7 SUBSTANCE ABUSE 69

Sedatives and Sedative-Hypnotics 74

Benzodiazepines 74

Opioids 75

Ethyl Alcohol 75

UNIT II
The Nervous System   85

CHAPTER 8   DRUGS AFFECTING FUNCTIONS OF THE AUTONOMIC
NERVOUS SYSTEM 86

DRUG PROTOTYPE *Bethanechol (Urecholine)* 93

NURSING PROCESS FOCUS Patients Receiving Direct- and Indirect-Acting
Cholinergic Drug Therapy 93

DRUG PROTOTYPE *Atropine (Atro-Pen)* 95

NURSING PROCESS FOCUS Patients Receiving Cholinergic Blocker
(Anticholinergic) Therapy 96

DRUG PROTOTYPE *Phenylephrine (Neo-Synephrine)* 98

NURSING PROCESS FOCUS Patients Receiving Adrenergic Drug Therapy 98

DRUG PROTOTYPE *Prazosin (Minipress)* 100

NURSING PROCESS FOCUS Patients Receiving Adrenergic Blocker Therapy 101

CHAPTER 9   DRUGS FOR ANXIETY AND INSOMNIA 105

Anxiety 106

Insomnia 109

DRUG PROTOTYPE *Escitalopram (Lexapro)* 113

NURSING PROCESS FOCUS Patients Receiving Antianxiety Therapy 115

DRUG PROTOTYPE *Lorazepam (Ativan)* 116

DRUG PROTOTYPE *Zolpidem (Ambien, Edluar, Others)* 118

CHAPTER 10   DRUGS FOR EMOTIONAL, MOOD, AND BEHAVIORAL
DISORDERS 122

Depression 123

Tricyclic Antidepressants 125

Selective Serotonin Reuptake Inhibitors 128

Atypical Antidepressants 129

DRUG PROTOTYPE *Imipramine (Tofranil)* 129

NURSING PROCESS FOCUS Patients Receiving Antidepressant Therapy 130

Monoamine Oxidase Inhibitors 132

DRUG PROTOTYPE *Sertraline (Zoloft)* 133

DRUG PROTOTYPE *Phenelzine (Nardil)* 133

Bipolar Disorder 133

Attention Deficit Hyperactivity Disorder 136

CNS Stimulants 137

Non-CNS Stimulants 137

DRUG PROTOTYPE *Methylphenidate (Ritalin)* 137

CHAPTER 11   DRUGS FOR PSYCHOSES 142

Schizophrenia 143

Conventional (First Generation) Antipsychotics 146

DRUG PROTOTYPE *Chlorpromazine* 147

Phenothiazines and Phenothiazine-Like Drugs 147

Nonphenothiazine Drugs 148

DRUG PROTOTYPE *Haloperidol (Haldol)* 149

NURSING PROCESS FOCUS Patients Receiving Phenothiazines and
Nonphenothiazine Therapy 149

Atypical (Second Generation) Antipsychotics 151

DRUG PROTOTYPE *Risperidone (Risperdal)* 152

NURSING PROCESS FOCUS Patients Receiving Atypical Antipsychotic
Therapy 153

Dopamine System Stabilizers (Third-Generation Antipsychotics) 154

CHAPTER 12 DRUGS FOR DEGENERATIVE DISEASES AND MUSCLES 157

Parkinson's Disease 159

Dopaminergic Drugs 160

DRUG PROTOTYPE *Levodopa, Carbidopa, and Entacapone (Stalevo)* 163

Cholinergic Blockers (Anticholinergics) 163

DRUG PROTOTYPE *Benztropine (Cogentin)* 164

Alzheimer's Disease 164

Acetylcholinesterase Inhibitors 165

Other Drugs That Slow Progression of AD 165

Drugs That Treat Behavioral Symptoms of AD 166

DRUG PROTOTYPE *Donepezil (Aricept)* 167

Multiple Sclerosis 167

Muscle Spasms 169

DRUG PROTOTYPE *Cyclobenzaprine (Amrix, Flexeril)* 171

Spasticity 171

NURSING PROCESS FOCUS Patients Receiving Drugs for Muscle Spasms
or Spasticity 172

DRUG PROTOTYPE *Dantrolene (Dantrium)* 175

CHAPTER 13 DRUGS FOR SEIZURES 180

Seizures 181

Partial Seizures 183

Generalized Seizures 183

Special Epileptic Syndromes 184

DRUG PROTOTYPE *Phenobarbital (Luminal)* 188

DRUG PROTOTYPE *Diazepam (Valium)* 188

DRUG PROTOTYPE *Phenytoin (Dilantin)* 190

DRUG PROTOTYPE *Valproic Acid (Depakene, Depakote)* 191

DRUG PROTOTYPE *Ethosuximide (Zarontin)* 192

NURSING PROCESS FOCUS Patients Receiving Antiseizure Drug Therapy 192

CHAPTER 14 DRUGS FOR PAIN MANAGEMENT 197

Acute or Chronic Pain 198

Opioid Analgesics for Severe Pain 203

Opioid Agonists 203

DRUG PROTOTYPE *Morphine (Astramorph PF, Duramorph, Others)* 203

Opioid Antagonists 205

DRUG PROTOTYPE *Naloxone (Narcan)* 205

Opioids with Mixed Agonist–Antagonist Effects 206

NURSING PROCESS FOCUS Patients Receiving Opioids 206

Nonopioid Analgesics for Moderate Pain 208

Nonsteroidal Anti-Inflammatory Drugs (NSAIDs) 208

DRUG PROTOTYPE *Aspirin (Acetylsalicylic Acid, ASA)* 208

Centrally Acting Drugs 210

Tension Headaches and Migraine 210

Triptans 211

Ergot Alkaloids 211

Other Antimigraine and Tension Headache Drugs 213

DRUG PROTOTYPE *Sumatriptan (Imitrex)* 213

CHAPTER 15 DRUGS FOR ANESTHESIA 217

Local Anesthesia 218

Esters 222

Amides 222

DRUG PROTOTYPE *Lidocaine (Xylocaine)* 222

NURSING PROCESS FOCUS Patients Receiving Local Anesthesia 223

General Anesthesia 224

DRUG PROTOTYPE *Nitrous Oxide* 225

DRUG PROTOTYPE *Isoflurane (Forane)* 225

Gases 226

Volatile Liquids 226

Intravenous Anesthetics 226

DRUG PROTOTYPE *Propofol (Diprivan)* 227

Adjuncts to Anesthesia 227

DRUG PROTOTYPE *Succinylcholine (Anectine)* 228

UNIT III
The Cardiovascular and Urinary Systems   233

CHAPTER 16 DRUGS FOR LIPID DISORDERS 234

DRUG PROTOTYPE *Atorvastatin (Lipitor)* 240

DRUG PROTOTYPE *Cholestyramine (Questran)* 240

NURSING PROCESS FOCUS Patients Receiving Drug Therapy with HMG-CoA Reductase Inhibitors (Statins) 241

DRUG PROTOTYPE *Gemfibrozil (Lopid)* 244

CHAPTER 17 DIURETICS AND DRUGS FOR ELECTROLYTE AND ACID–BASE DISORDERS 248

DRUG PROTOTYPE *Furosemide (Lasix)* 254

DRUG PROTOTYPE *Hydrochlorothiazide (Microzide)* 255

DRUG PROTOTYPE *Spironolactone (Aldactone)* 256

NURSING PROCESS FOCUS Patients Receiving Diuretic Therapy 257

Sodium Imbalances 259

Potassium Imbalances 259

DRUG PROTOTYPE Potassium Chloride (KCl) 260

DRUG PROTOTYPE Sodium Bicarbonate (NaHCO₃) 261

CHAPTER 18 DRUGS FOR HYPERTENSION 265

NURSING PROCESS FOCUS Patients Receiving ACE Inhibitor Therapy 276

DRUG PROTOTYPE Enalapril (Vasotec) 277

DRUG PROTOTYPE Nifedipine (Adalat CC, Procardia XL) 279

NURSING PROCESS FOCUS Patients Receiving Calcium Channel Blocker
Therapy 279

DRUG PROTOTYPE Doxazosin (Cardura) 282

DRUG PROTOTYPE Hydralazine (Apresoline) 283

CHAPTER 19 DRUGS FOR HEART FAILURE 287

DRUG PROTOTYPE Lisinopril (Prinivil, Zestril) 292

DRUG PROTOTYPE Digoxin (Lanoxin, Lanoxicaps) 295

DRUG PROTOTYPE Carvedilol (Coreg) 296

DRUG PROTOTYPE Milrinone (Primacor) 297

CHAPTER 20 DRUGS FOR ANGINA PECTORIS, MYOCARDIAL INFARCTION,
AND STROKE 301

Angina Pectoris 302

DRUG PROTOTYPE Nitroglycerin (Nitrostat, Nitro-Bid, Nitro-Dur, Others) 307

NURSING PROCESS FOCUS Patients Receiving Organic Nitrate Therapy 308

DRUG PROTOTYPE Atenolol (Tenormin) 309

DRUG PROTOTYPE Diltiazem (Cardizem, Cartia XT, Dilacor XR, Others) 309

Myocardial Infarction 310

DRUG PROTOTYPE Reteplase (Retavase) 312

Beta-Adrenergic Blockers 312

Antiplatelet and Anticoagulant Drugs 312

NURSING PROCESS FOCUS Patients Receiving Thrombolytic Therapy 313

Angiotensin-Converting Enzyme (ACE) Inhibitors 313

Pain Management 313

Stroke 314

CHAPTER 21 DRUGS FOR SHOCK AND ANAPHYLAXIS 319

Shock 320

Blood Products 322

Colloids 323

Crystalloids 323

DRUG PROTOTYPE Normal Serum Albumin (Albuminar, Plasbumin, Others) 323

NURSING PROCESS FOCUS Patients Receiving Intravenous Fluid Therapy 324

DRUG PROTOTYPE Norepinephrine (Levophed) 326

DRUG PROTOTYPE Dopamine (Dopastat, Intropin) 326

Anaphylaxis 326

DRUG PROTOTYPE *Epinephrine (Adrenalin)* 327

CHAPTER 22 DRUGS FOR DYSRHYTHMIAS 331

NURSING PROCESS FOCUS Patients Receiving Antidysrhythmic Drugs 336

DRUG PROTOTYPE *Procainamide* 339

DRUG PROTOTYPE *Propranolol (Inderal, InnoPran XL)* 340

DRUG PROTOTYPE *Amiodarone (Cordarone)* 341

DRUG PROTOTYPE *Verapamil (Calan, Isoptin SR, Others)* 342

CHAPTER 23 DRUGS FOR COAGULATION DISORDERS 346

Parenteral Anticoagulants 350

Oral Anticoagulants 352

DRUG PROTOTYPE *Heparin* 352

DRUG PROTOTYPE *Warfarin (Coumadin)* 353

NURSING PROCESS FOCUS Patients Receiving Anticoagulant and Antiplatelet Therapy 353

DRUG PROTOTYPE *Clopidogrel (Plavix)* 356

DRUG PROTOTYPE *Alteplase (Activase)* 357

DRUG PROTOTYPE *Aminocaproic Acid (Amicar)* 358

UNIT IV
The Immune System
361

CHAPTER 24 DRUGS FOR INFLAMMATION AND FEVER 362

Inflammation 363

DRUG PROTOTYPE *Naproxen (Naprosyn) and Naproxen Sodium (Aleve, Anaprox)* 366

NURSING PROCESS FOCUS Patients Receiving NSAID Therapy 367

DRUG PROTOTYPE *Prednisone* 369

Fever 369

DRUG PROTOTYPE *Acetaminophen (Tylenol)* 369

CHAPTER 25 DRUGS FOR IMMUNE SYSTEM MODULATION 373

Immunostimulants 376

DRUG PROTOTYPE *Hepatitis B Vaccine (Energix-B, Recombivax HB)* 378

DRUG PROTOTYPE *Interferon alfa-2b (Intron-A)* 380

DRUG PROTOTYPE *Cyclosporine (Gengraf, Neoral, Sandimmune)* 382

NURSING PROCESS FOCUS Patients Receiving Immunosuppressants 382

CHAPTER 26 DRUGS FOR BACTERIAL INFECTIONS 387

DRUG PROTOTYPE *Penicillin G Sodium/Potassium* 395

DRUG PROTOTYPE *Cefotaxime (Claforan)* 396

DRUG PROTOTYPE *Tetracycline (Sumycin, Others)* 397

DRUG PROTOTYPE *Erythromycin (E-Mycin, Erythrocin)* 398

DRUG PROTOTYPE *Gentamicin (Garamycin)* 400

DRUG PROTOTYPE *Ciprofloxacin (Cipro)* 401

DRUG PROTOTYPE *Trimethoprim–Sulfamethoxazole (Bactrim, Septra)* 402

DRUG PROTOTYPE *Vancomycin (Vancocin)* 403

NURSING PROCESS FOCUS Patients Receiving Antibacterial Therapy 404

Tuberculosis 406

DRUG PROTOTYPE *Isoniazid (INH, Nydrazid)* 406

NURSING PROCESS FOCUS Patients Receiving Antitubercular Drugs 407

CHAPTER 27 DRUGS FOR FUNGAL, VIRAL, AND PARASITIC DISEASES 412

Antifungal Drugs 413

DRUG PROTOTYPE *Amphotericin B (AmBisome, Fungizone, Others)* 416

DRUG PROTOTYPE *Nystatin (Mycostatin, Nystop, Others)* 416

NURSING PROCESS FOCUS Patients Receiving Superficial Antifungal Therapy 417

Antiviral Drugs 417

DRUG PROTOTYPE *Zidovudine (AZT, Retrovir)* 421

NURSING PROCESS FOCUS Patients Receiving Pharmacotherapy for HIV-AIDS 422

Treatment of Herpesvirus Infection 423

Treatment of Influenza Virus Infection 424

DRUG PROTOTYPE *Acyclovir (Zovirax)* 425

Treatment of Viral Hepatitis Infection 425

Antiparasitic Drugs 425

DRUG PROTOTYPE *Metronidazole (Flagyl)* 427

CHAPTER 28 DRUGS FOR NEOPLASIA 430

DRUG PROTOTYPE *Cyclophosphamide (Cytoxan)* 438

DRUG PROTOTYPE *Methotrexate (Rheumatrex, Trexall)* 440

DRUG PROTOTYPE *Doxorubicin (Adriamycin)* 441

DRUG PROTOTYPE *Vincristine (Oncovin)* 443

DRUG PROTOTYPE *Tamoxifen* 444

DRUG PROTOTYPE *Epoetin Alfa (Epogen, Procrit)* 446

NURSING PROCESS FOCUS Patients Receiving Antineoplastic Therapy 447

UNIT V
The Respiratory and Digestive Systems   453

CHAPTER 29 DRUGS FOR RESPIRATORY DISORDERS 454

Upper Respiratory Tract 455

Lower Respiratory Tract 455

Allergic Rhinitis 458

DRUG PROTOTYPE *Diphenhydramine (Benadryl, Others)* 460

NURSING PROCESS FOCUS Patients Receiving Antihistamine Therapy 461

DRUG PROTOTYPE *Fluticasone (Flonase, Veramyst)* 463

DRUG PROTOTYPE *Oxymetazoline (Afrin, Others)* 464

Asthma 465

NURSING PROCESS FOCUS Patients Receiving Bronchodilators 469

DRUG PROTOTYPE *Cromolyn (Intal)* 471

Chronic Obstructive Pulmonary Disease 471

CHAPTER 30 DRUGS FOR GASTROINTESTINAL DISORDERS 476

Peptic Ulcer Disease 479

DRUG PROTOTYPE *Omeprazole (Prilosec)* 483

DRUG PROTOTYPE *Ranitidine (Zantac)* 483

NURSING PROCESS FOCUS Patients Receiving Drug Therapy for Peptic
Ulcer Disease 484

Constipation 486

DRUG PROTOTYPE *Psyllium Mucilloid (Metamucil, Others)* 487

NURSING PROCESS FOCUS Patients Receiving Laxative Therapy 487

Diarrhea 488

DRUG PROTOTYPE *Diphenoxylate with Atropine (Lomotil)* 488

Nausea and Vomiting 489

DRUG PROTOTYPE *Ondansetron (Zofran, Zuplenz)* 490

Weight Loss 491

Pancreatic Enzymes 492

CHAPTER 31 VITAMINS, MINERALS, AND NUTRITIONAL SUPPLEMENTS 496

DRUG PROTOTYPE *Cyanocobalamin (Crystamine, Others)* 499

DRUG PROTOTYPE *Ferrous Sulfate (Feosol, Feostat, Others)* 501

NURSING PROCESS FOCUS Patients Receiving Iron Supplements 503

UNIT VI
The Endocrine and Reproductive Systems   **509**

CHAPTER 32 DRUGS FOR ENDOCRINE DISORDERS 510

Hypothalamic and Pituitary Disorders 514

DRUG PROTOTYPE *Desmopressin (DDAVP)* 514

Thyroid Disorders 516

DRUG PROTOTYPE *Levothyroxine (Levothroid, Synthroid, Others)* 518

DRUG PROTOTYPE *Propylthiouracil (PTU)* 519

NURSING PROCESS FOCUS Patients Receiving Thyroid Hormone Replacement 519

Adrenal Disorders 520

DRUG PROTOTYPE *Hydrocortisone (Cortef, Hydrocortone, Others)* 522

NURSING PROCESS FOCUS Patients Receiving Systemic Corticosteroid
Therapy 523

CHAPTER 33 DRUGS FOR DIABETES MELLITUS 528

Type 1 Diabetes Mellitus 529

DRUG PROTOTYPE *Regular Insulin (Humulin R, Novolin R)* 532

NURSING PROCESS FOCUS Patients Receiving Insulin Therapy 533

Type 2 Diabetes Mellitus 534

DRUG PROTOTYPE *Metformin (Fortamet, Glucophage, Glumetza, Others)* 537

NURSING PROCESS FOCUS Patients Receiving Pharmacotherapy for Type 2
Diabetes 538

CHAPTER 34 DRUGS FOR DISORDERS AND CONDITIONS
OF THE REPRODUCTIVE SYSTEM 542

Oral Contraceptives 546

DRUG PROTOTYPE *Estradiol with Norethindrone (Ortho-Novum, Others)* 547

NURSING PROCESS FOCUS Patients Receiving Oral Contraceptive Therapy 548

Menopause 549

Uterine Abnormalities 549

DRUG PROTOTYPE *Estrogen, conjugated (Cenestin, Enjuvia, Premarin)* 551

DRUG PROTOTYPE *Medroxyprogesterone (Depo-Provera,
Depo-SubQ-Provera, Provera)* 552

Labor and Breastfeeding 552

DRUG PROTOTYPE *Oxytocin (Pitocin)* 553

Hypogonadism 554

DRUG PROTOTYPE *Testosterone* 554

Erectile Dysfunction 555

DRUG PROTOTYPE *Sildenafil (Viagra)* 556

Benign Prostatic Hyperplasia 557

DRUG PROTOTYPE *Finasteride (Proscar)* 558

UNIT VII
The Skeletal System, Integumentary System, and Eyes and Ears 563

CHAPTER 35 DRUGS FOR BONE AND JOINT DISORDERS 564

Hypocalcemia 565

Osteomalacia and Rickets 566

DRUG PROTOTYPE *Calcium salts* 569

DRUG PROTOTYPE *Calcitriol (Calcijex, Rocaltrol)* 569

Osteoporosis 569

Selective Estrogen-Receptor Modulators 570

DRUG PROTOTYPE *Raloxifene (Evista)* 571

Calcitonin 572

Bisphosphonates 572

DRUG PROTOTYPE *Alendronate (Fosamax)* 572

NURSING PROCESS FOCUS Patients Receiving Pharmacotherapy for
Osteoporosis 572

Paget's Disease 573

Osteoarthritis 574

Rheumatoid Arthritis 575

DRUG PROTOTYPE *Hydroxychloroquine (Plaquenil)* 575

Gout 576

DRUG PROTOTYPE *Allopurinol (Lopurin, Zyloprim)* 578

CHAPTER 36 DRUGS FOR SKIN DISORDERS 582

Skin Parasites 586

DRUG PROTOTYPE *Permethrin (Acticin, Elimite, Nix)* 587

NURSING PROCESS FOCUS Patients Receiving Pharmacotherapy for Lice or Mite Infestation 588

Sunburn and Minor Skin Irritation 588

DRUG PROTOTYPE *Benzocaine (Americaine, Anbesol, Others)* 589

Acne And Rosacea 589

DRUG PROTOTYPE *Tretinoin (Avita, Retin-A, Others)* 591

Dermatitis and Eczema 591

Psoriasis 593

CHAPTER 37 DRUGS FOR EYE AND EAR DISORDERS 598

Glaucoma 600

DRUG PROTOTYPE *Latanoprost (Xalatan)* 601

Prostaglandins 602

Direct- and Indirect-Acting Cholinergics (Miotic Drugs) 602

Nonselective Sympathomimetics (Mydriatic Drugs) 602

Beta Adrenergic Blockers 603

Alpha$_2$-Adrenergic Drugs 603

Carbonic Anhydrase Inhibitors 603

DRUG PROTOTYPE *Timolol (Betimol, Timoptic, Others)* 604

Osmotic Diuretics 604

NURSING PROCESS FOCUS Patients Receiving Pharmacotherapy for Glaucoma 604

Eye Examinations and Minor Eye Conditions 605

Ear Conditions 606

APPENDIX A   References 611
APPENDIX B   Brief Answers to NCLEX-PN® and Case Study Questions 621
APPENDIX C   Calculating Dosages 624
INDEX 626
GUIDE TO SPECIAL FEATURES 657

***APPENDIX D** (Complete Answers and Rationales for NCLEX-PN® Review and Case Study Questions) and the **GLOSSARY** appear on the textbook's website.

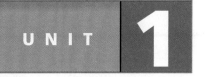
Basic Concepts in Pharmacology

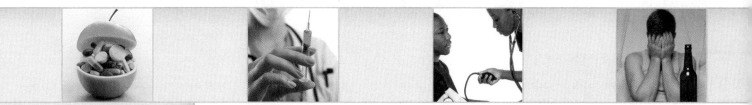

Unit Contents

Chapter 1   Introduction to Pharmacology: Drug Regulation and Approval / 2

Chapter 2   Drug Classes, Schedules, and Categories / 12

Chapter 3   Methods of Drug Administration / 20

Chapter 4   What Happens After a Drug Has Been Administered / 41

Chapter 5   The Nursing Process in Pharmacology / 51

Chapter 6   The Role of Complementary and Alternative Therapies in Pharmacology / 59

Chapter 7   Substance Abuse / 69

1 Introduction to Pharmacology: Drug Regulation and Approval

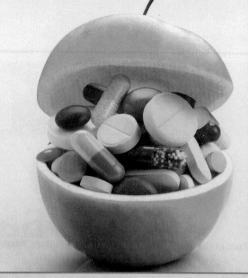

CORE CONCEPTS

1.1 Pharmacology is an expansive and challenging topic.

1.2 For healthcare providers, the fields of pharmacology and therapeutics are connected.

1.3 Agents may be classified as traditional drugs, biologics, and natural alternatives.

1.4 Drugs are available by prescription or over the counter (OTC).

1.5 Pharmaceutics is the science of pharmacy.

1.6 Drug regulations were created to protect the public from drug misuse.

1.7 U.S. drug standards have become increasingly complex.

1.8 There are four stages of approval for therapeutic and biologic drugs.

1.9 Governmental agencies face the dual challenge of increasing the speed of drug approval while still ensuring the safety of new drugs.

1.10 Healthcare providers must be prepared to deal with the threat of biological and chemical attack.

LEARNING OUTCOMES

After reading this chapter, the student should be able to:

1. Explain the interdisciplinary nature of pharmacology and give examples of subject area expertise needed to master the discipline.

2. Identify professions in which knowledge of pharmacology is important.

3. Explain how the disciplines of therapeutics and pharmacology are interconnected.

4. Distinguish between therapeutic drugs and agents such as foods, household products, and cosmetics.

5. Compare and contrast traditional drugs, biologics, and natural alternative therapies.

6. Identify the advantages and disadvantages of prescription and OTC drugs.

7. Distinguish between pharmaceutics and pharmacology.

8. Discuss the history of U.S. standards, acts, and organizations leading to the requirement that drug safety must be proven before marketing.

9. Discuss the role of the United States Food and Drug Administration (FDA) in determining the safety of drugs and whether they may be used for therapy.

10. Discuss the roles and responsibilities of branches within the FDA in overseeing traditional therapeutic drugs, biologics, and natural alternative therapies.

11. Identify four stages of approval for therapeutic and biologic drugs.

12. Discuss current challenges facing the FDA in approving new drugs for market.

13. Discuss the challenges facing healthcare providers in view of modern-day bioterrorist threats.

KEY TERMS

biologics (beye-oh-LOJ-iks) *4*

black box warnings *6*

clinical pharmacology *7*

complementary and alternative medicine (CAM) therapies *4*

formularies (FOR-mew-LEH-reez) *5*

natural alternative therapies *4*

off-label use *9*

pathophysiology (PATH-oh-fiz-ee-OL-oh-jee) *3*

pharmaceutics (far-mah-SOO-tiks) *5*

pharmacology (far-mah-KOL-oh-jee) *3*

pharmacopoeia (far-mah-KOH-pee-ah) *5*

pharmacotherapeutics (far-mah-koh-THER-ah-PEW-tiks) *3*

pharmacy (FAR-mah-see) *5*

therapeutics (ther-ah-PEW-tiks) *3*

More drugs are being administered to consumers than ever before. Because of the number of new drugs available for therapy, some experts are concerned that patients might be harmed if drugs are not thoroughly tested. The purpose of this chapter is to introduce the subject of pharmacology and to emphasize the role of the government in ensuring that drugs and natural alternatives are safe and effective for public use. It addresses the role that drug therapy has in fighting disease as governmental regulators, consumers, and healthcare professionals face new challenges in the years ahead. Drugs are the most powerful weapon we have against diseases and worldwide epidemics.

In addition, bioterrorist threats have led to widespread governmental changes in emergency preparedness planning. This chapter briefly introduces the role of pharmacology in the prevention and treatment of diseases or conditions that might develop due to global biological, chemical, or nuclear threats.

Pharmacology is an expansive and challenging topic.

CORE CONCEPT 1.1

The word **pharmacology** is derived from two Greek words: *pharmakon*, which means "medicine," and *logos*, which means "study." Thus, *pharmacology* is defined as "the study of medicine."

pharmaco = *medicine*
ology = *the study of*

Healthcare providers practice the discipline of pharmacology to study how drugs improve the health of the human body. If applied properly, drugs can dramatically improve patients' quality of life. If applied improperly, the consequences of drug action can be devastating.

The subject of pharmacology is an expansive topic ranging from a study of how drugs enter and travel throughout the body to the actual responses they produce. To learn the discipline well, students must master concepts from several interrelated areas, including anatomy, physiology, microbiology, chemistry, and **pathophysiology** (study of disease and functional changes that occur as a result of disease). The useful application of drugs depends on knowledge from at least these areas.

patho = *disease*
physio = *the nature of*
ology = *the study of*

Currently there are more than 10,000 brand and generic varieties of drugs available with many different names, interactions, adverse effects, and complicated mechanisms of action. Keeping up with the numbers of drugs is a huge challenge. Many drugs may be prescribed for more than one disease, and most produce multiple effects in the body. Further complicating the study of pharmacology is the fact that drugs may cause different responses depending on factors such as gender, age, health status, body mass, and genetics.

For healthcare providers, the fields of pharmacology and therapeutics are connected.

CORE CONCEPT 1.2

It is obvious that a thorough knowledge of pharmacology is important to those health professionals who prescribe drugs on a daily basis. This group includes physicians, physician's assistants, dentists, and advanced nurse practitioners. Depending on state law, members of other groups may also be permitted to prescribe medications. In this textbook, the group of professions that is allowed to prescribe drugs is referred to as *healthcare practitioners*.

A second group of professions includes nursing, allied health, and community service employees. These occupations have in common direct contact with patients or healthcare practitioners. Nurses and some other allied health workers are directly involved with drug administration as well as with issues related to drug education, management, and/or enforcement of drug laws. In this text, these professionals are referred to as *healthcare providers*.

Some healthcare providers, such as nurses, may administer drugs on a daily basis, whereas others may administer drugs occasionally. A strong knowledge of pharmacology is necessary to properly educate and advise patients regarding their healthcare needs. This knowledge is also essential to communicate effectively with healthcare practitioners, who rely heavily on nurses and allied health professionals to gather medical data from their patients and to follow up on results of therapy.

For healthcare providers studying pharmacology, it usually becomes apparent that the fields of pharmacology and therapeutics are connected. **Therapeutics** is the branch of medicine concerned with the treatment of disease and suffering. **Pharmacotherapeutics** is the use of medicine to treat disease.

CORE CONCEPT **1.3**	**Agents may be classified as traditional drugs, biologics, and natural alternatives.**

Drugs are chemicals that produce biologic responses within the body. From this perspective, drugs may be considered a part of the body's normal activities, from the essential gases that people breathe to the foods that they eat. Yet it is necessary to separate drugs from substances such as foods, household products, and cosmetics. Many agents, including antiperspirants, sunscreens, toothpastes, and shampoos, might alter the body's normal activities, but they are not considered to be medically therapeutic, as drugs taken for a medical disorder would be.

Therapeutic drugs are sometimes classified on the basis of how they are produced, either chemically or naturally. Most traditional drugs are chemically produced or synthesized in a laboratory. **Biologics** are agents naturally produced in animal cells, in microorganisms, or by the body itself. **Natural alternative therapies** are herbs, natural extracts, vitamins, minerals, or dietary supplements. Table 1.1 ◆ shows a summary of characteristics associated with traditional drug therapies, biologics, and natural alternative therapies. Although drugs may be described in many ways, this text limits its focus to agents used for therapy in a clinical or home setting. Traditional drugs and drug classes are discussed more thoroughly in Chapter 2. Natural alternatives are discussed more thoroughly in Chapter 6. In addition, most chapters include a feature called *Natural Alternatives* that highlights a specific herbal therapy or dietary supplement.

When studying the various approaches for therapy, the healthcare provider may encounter the category of treatment called **complementary and alternative medicine (CAM) therapies**. In addition to the herbs, vitamins, or supplements just described, CAM therapies include manipulative and body-based practices such as physical therapy, occupational therapy approaches, massage, biofeedback, hypnosis, and acupuncture. Although these and other approaches are successful in treating disease or a medical condition, traditional therapeutic drugs, biologics, and natural alternative therapies remain the primary focus of this textbook.

CORE CONCEPT **1.4**	**Drugs are available by prescription or over the counter (OTC).**

Legal drugs are obtained either with a prescription or by purchasing them over the counter. There are differences between the two methods of dispensing. To obtain prescription drugs, patients must get a physician's order authorizing them to receive the drugs. The advantages to this are numerous. Practitioners have an opportunity to examine their patients and determine a specific diagnosis. Practitioners can maximize therapy by ordering the proper drug for their patients' conditions and controlling the specific amount and frequency of the drug to be dispensed. Healthcare providers may give instructions on how to use the drug properly and what adverse effects to expect.

A drug's safety is related to its effectiveness. The difference between its usual effective dose and a dose that produces severe adverse effects is called its *margin of safety*. When drugs have been used over long periods and demonstrate wide margins of safety—that is, they are very safe and effective—regulators sometimes change them from being prescription drugs to being OTC drugs. Unlike prescription drugs, OTC drugs do not require an order from a healthcare practitioner.

Patients may treat themselves safely if they carefully follow instructions included with these OTC drugs. If patients do not follow these guidelines, OTC drugs can have serious adverse effects.

Patients prefer to take OTC medications for many reasons. OTC drugs can be obtained more easily than prescription drugs. They do not have to make an appointment with a physician, which saves time

TABLE 1.1	**Characteristics of Traditional Therapeutic Drugs, Biologics, and Natural Alternative Therapies**
Traditional Drug Therapies	■ Chemically produced in a laboratory ■ Routinely used by healthcare providers
Biologics	■ Naturally produced by the body itself, in animal cells, or in microorganisms ■ Include hormones and vaccines ■ Routinely used by healthcare providers
Natural Alternative Therapies	■ Naturally produced ■ Include herbs, extracts, vitamins, minerals, or dietary supplements ■ Sometimes used, depending on healthcare provider

and money. Without training, however, choosing the proper medication for a specific problem may be difficult. OTC drugs may react with foods, herbal products, and prescription or other OTC drugs. Patients may not be aware that some medications can impair their ability to function safely. Self-treatment is sometimes ineffective, and the potential for injury is much greater if the disease is allowed to progress without proper treatment.

Pharmaceutics is the science of pharmacy.

CORE CONCEPT 1.5

Pharmaceutics is the science of **pharmacy** (the preparation and dispensing of drugs) and is a very important part of pharmacotherapy. The general public often confuses pharmaceutics with pharmacology, or they recognize the root *pharm* and assume that *pharmacology* is the same as *pharmacy*. Correctly put, *pharmaceutics* is the science of pharmacy, and it involves dispensing a drug to a patient after he or she has been examined by a licensed healthcare practitioner. *Pharmacists* are the experts who catalogue signs, symptoms, adverse effects, and drug interactions. They often act as drug advisors to patients, making sure that they receive the proper medication and educating them about undesirable symptoms or interactions.

Concept Review   1.1

- Explain the meaning of this statement: "Pharmacotherapy involves the science of therapeutics and pharmaceutics."

Drug regulations were created to protect the public from drug misuse.

CORE CONCEPT 1.6

For many years, there were no standards or guidelines to protect the public from drug misuse. Patients could not be assured that available medicines were not a form of quackery. The archives of drug regulatory agencies are filled with examples of early medicines, such as rattlesnake oil for rheumatism. It became quite clear that drug regulations were needed to protect the public.

The first standards commonly used by pharmacists were early **formularies**, or lists of drugs and drug recipes. In 1820, the first comprehensive publication of drug standards, called the *U.S. Pharmacopoeia (USP)*, was established. (See the timeline in Figure 1.1 ■.) A **pharmacopoeia** is a medical reference summary indicating standards of drug purity and strength and directions for synthesis. In 1852, a national professional society of pharmacists—the American Pharmaceutical Association (APhA)—was founded. From 1852 until 1975, two major sources maintained drug standards in the United States: the USP and the APhA's *National Formulary (NF)*. All drug substances and products were covered in the USP; the NF focused on pharmaceutical ingredients. In 1975, the two organizations merged and created a single publication named the *U.S. Pharmacopoeia-National Formulary (USP-NF)*. Official updates for the *USP-NF* are published regularly. Today, the USP label can be found on some medication containers verifying the exact ingredients found within the container, as shown in Figure 1.2 ■. Although there is a lot of good information on the label of a drug container, newer labeling guidelines are being proposed in an effort to promote patient safety and to reduce drug misuse.

In the early 1900s, to protect the public, the government began to develop and enforce tougher drug legislation. In 1902, the Biologics Control Act was passed to standardize the quality of serums and other blood-related products. The Pure Food and Drug Act of 1906 gave the government power to control the labeling of medicines. In 1912, the Sherley Amendment prohibited the sale of drugs labeled with false therapeutic claims intended to cheat the consumer. In 1938, Congress passed the Food, Drug, and Cosmetic Act. This was the first law preventing the marketing of drugs that had not been thoroughly tested prior to marketing. According to the provisions of this law, drug companies were required to prove the safety and *efficacy* (i.e., effectiveness) of any drug before it could be sold within the United States.

U.S. drug standards have become increasingly complex.

CORE CONCEPT 1.7

Much has changed in the regulation of drugs since 1938. In 1988, the FDA was officially established as an agency of the U.S. Department of Health and Human Services. Today, the Center for Drug Evaluation and Research (CDER), a branch of the FDA, has powerful control over whether prescription drugs and OTC drugs may be used for therapy. The CDER states its mission as "facilitating the availability of safe effective drugs, keeping unsafe or ineffective drugs off the market, improving the health of Americans, and providing clear, easily understandable drug information for safe and effective use." Any pharmaceutical laboratory, whether private, public, or academic, must obtain FDA approval before marketing any drug. Another branch of the FDA, the Center for Biologics Evaluation and Research (CBER), regulates the use of biologics, including serums, vaccines, and products found in the bloodstream. In 1997, the FDA created *boxed warnings* to regulate drugs with "special problems." At the time no precedent had been established

FIGURE 1.1	
TIMELINE	**REGULATORY ACTS, STANDARDS, AND ORGANIZATIONS**
1820	A group of healthcare providers established the first comprehensive publication of drug standards called the **U.S. Pharmacopoeia (USP)**.
1852	A group of pharmacists founded a national professional society called the **American Pharmaceutical Association (APhA)**. The APhA then established the **National Formulary (NF)**, a standardized publication focusing on pharmaceutical ingredients. The *USP* continued to catalogue all drug-related substances and products.
1862	This was the beginning of the **Federal Bureau of Chemistry**, established under the administration of President Lincoln. Over the years and with added duties, it gradually became the Food and Drug Administration (FDA).
1902	Congress passed the **Biologics Control Act** to control the quality of serums and other blood-related products.
1906	**The Pure Food and Drug Act** gave the government power to control the labeling of medicines.
1912	**The Sherley Amendment** made medicines safer by prohibiting the sale of drugs labeled with false therapeutic claims.
1938	Congress passed the **Food, Drug, and Cosmetic Act**. It was the first law preventing the marketing of drugs not thoroughly tested. This law now provides for the requirement that drug companies must submit a New Drug Application (NDA) to the FDA prior to marketing a new drug.
1944	Congress passed the **Public Health Service Act**, covering many health issues, including biologic products and the control of communicable diseases.
1975	The *U.S. Pharmacopoeia* and *National Formulary* announced their union. The **USP-NF** became a single standardized publication.
1986	Congress passed the **Childhood Vaccine Act.** It authorized the FDA to acquire information about patients taking vaccines, to recall biologics, and to recommend civil penalties if guidelines regarding biologic use were not followed.
1988	The **FDA** was officially established as an agency of the **U.S. Department of Health and Human Services.**
1992	Congress passed the **Prescription Drug User Fee Act.** It required that nongeneric drug and biologic manufacturers pay fees to be used for improvements in the drug review process.
1994	Congress passed the **Dietary Supplement Health and Education Act** that requires clear labeling of dietary supplements. This act gives the FDA the power to remove supplements that cause a significant risk to the public.
1997	The **FDA Drug Modernization Act** reauthorized the Prescription Drug User Fee Act. This act represented the largest reform effort of the drug review process since 1938.
2002	The **Bioterrorism Act** implemented guidelines for registration of selected toxins that could pose a threat to human, animal, or plant safety and health.
2007	The **FDA Amendments Act** reviewed, expanded, and reaffirmed legislation to allow for additional comprehensive reviews of new drugs and medical products. This extended the reforms imposed from 1997. The **FDA's Critical Path Initiative** was a part of this reform.
2011	Provisions of the **Health Care Reform** law allowed the FDA to approve generic versions of biologic drugs. Additional drug rebates and benefits were provided to the American public. The **FDA Food Safety Modernization Act** represents the largest reform effort of food safety review since 1938.
2012	Renewal of the **Prescription Drug User Fee Act**.

Historical timeline of regulatory acts, standards, and organizations.

to monitor drugs with a potential for causing death or serious injury. **Black box warnings**, named after the black label appearing around drug safety information on package inserts, eventually became one of the primary alerts for identifying extreme adverse drug reactions discovered during and after review. The healthcare provider must be increasingly mindful about the level of precaution necessary to promote safety, including medication verification and special alerts. Because of their importance, black box warnings are included for all prototype drugs in this text.

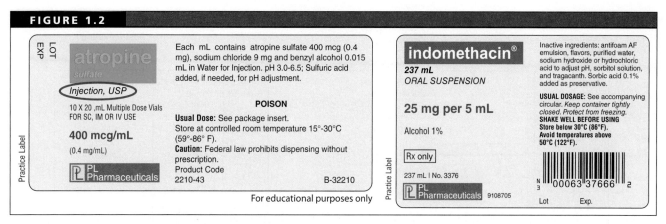

FIGURE 1.2

LOT
EXP

atropine
sulfate

Injection, USP

10 X 20 mL Multiple Dose Vials
FOR SC, IM OR IV USE

400 mcg/mL

(0.4 mg/mL)

PL
Pharmaceuticals

Practice Label

Each mL contains atropine sulfate 400 mcg (0.4 mg), sodium chloride 9 mg and benzyl alcohol 0.015 mL in Water for Injection. pH 3.0-6.5; Sulfuric acid added, if needed, for pH adjustment.

POISON

Usual Dose: See package insert.
Store at controlled room temperature 15°-30°C (59°-86° F).
Caution: Federal law prohibits dispensing without prescription.
Product Code
2210-43   B-32210

For educational purposes only

indomethacin®

237 mL
ORAL SUSPENSION

25 mg per 5 mL

Alcohol 1%

Rx only

237 mL I No. 3376

PL
Pharmaceuticals   9108705

Practice Label

Inactive ingredients: antifoam AF emulsion, flavors, purified water, sodium hydroxide or hydrochloric acid to adjust pH, sorbitol solution, and tragacanth. Sorbic acid 0.1% added as preservative.

USUAL DOSAGE: See accompanying circular. *Keep container tightly closed. Protect from freezing.*
SHAKE WELL BEFORE USING
Store below 30°C (86°F).
Avoid temperatures above 50°C (122°F).

N
3   00063 37666   2

Lot   Exp.

Some drug labels show the USP symbol; others do not.

The FDA also oversees administration of herbal products and dietary supplements, but the Center for Food Safety and Applied Nutrition (CFSAN) regulates use of these substances. Herbal products and dietary supplements are regulated by the Dietary Supplement Health and Education Act of 1994. This act does not provide the same degree of protection as the Food, Drug, and Cosmetic Act of 1938. For example, herbal and dietary supplements can be marketed without prior approval from the FDA; however, all package inserts and information are monitored once products have gone to market. The Dietary Supplement Health and Education Act is discussed in more detail in Chapter 6.

In 1998, the National Center for Complementary and Alternative Medicine (NCCAM) was established as the federal government's lead agency for scientific research and information about CAM therapies. Its mission has been to define "the usefulness and safety of complementary and alternative medicine interventions and their roles in improving health and health care." Among several areas of focus, this agency has supported research and serves as a resource for healthcare providers in establishing which alternative therapies are safe and effective.

> **Life Span Fact**

One historical achievement involving biologics is the 1986 Childhood Vaccine Act. This act authorized the FDA to acquire information about patients taking vaccines, to recall biologics, and to recommend civil penalties if guidelines regarding biologics were not followed.

There are four stages of approval for therapeutic and biologic drugs.

CORE CONCEPT 1.8

The amount of time spent in the review and approval process for both prescription and OTC drugs depends on several checkpoints in a well-developed and organized plan. Most therapeutic drugs and biologics are reviewed in four stages, which are summarized in Figure 1.3 ■. These stages are (1) preclinical investigation, (2) clinical investigation, (3) submission of a new drug application (NDA) with review, and (4) postmarketing studies.

Preclinical Investigation

Preclinical investigation involves basic science research. Scientists perform many tests on cells grown in the laboratory (a process called *culture*) or on animals to examine the effectiveness of a range of drug doses and to look for any adverse effects. Laboratory tests on cells and animals are important because they assist in predicting whether drugs will cause harm in humans. Because laboratory tests do not always reflect the way a human responds, preclinical investigation results are always inconclusive.

Clinical Investigation

Clinical investigation, the second stage of drug approval, takes place in three different phases, termed *clinical phase trials.* This is the longest part of the drug approval process and involves **clinical pharmacology**, an area of medicine devoted to the evaluation of drugs used for human benefit. During these phases, clinical pharmacologists, researchers, and healthcare providers examine data from volunteers and large groups of selected patients with certain diseases. Both scientists and healthcare providers establish drug doses and try to identify adverse effects. Clinical investigators address concerns such as whether the drug worsens other medical conditions, interacts unsafely with existing medications patients are taking, or affects one type of patient more than others.

Clinical Phase Trials. Clinical phase trials are essential because responses among patients vary. If a drug appears to be effective without causing serious adverse effects, approval for marketing may be accelerated, or the drug may be used for treatment immediately in special cases with careful monitoring. If the

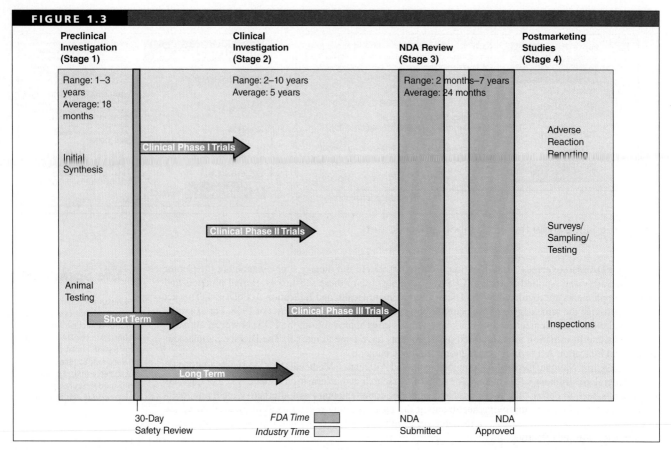

FIGURE 1.3

The approval of a new drug is a four-stage process: (1) preclinical investigation, (2) clinical investigation, (3) NDA submission and review, and (4) postmarketing studies. Within the second stage (clinical investigation), three phases of trials are conducted over two to ten years. Postmarketing studies, also called *postmarketing surveillance*, continue in large patient groups during the fourth stage of drug development.

drug shows promise but some minor problems are noted, the approval process is delayed until concerns are addressed. In any case, an NDA must be submitted before a drug is allowed to proceed to the next stage of the approval process.

Submission of an NDA with Review

A review of the NDA is the third stage of drug approval. During this stage, clinical phase III trials and animal testing may continue, depending on the results obtained from preclinical testing. If the NDA is approved, the process continues to the final stage. If the NDA is rejected, the process stops until concerns are addressed.

Postmarketing Studies

Postmarketing surveillance is the fourth stage of the drug approval process. It takes place after clinical trials and the NDA review process have been completed. Testing in humans is continued to check for any new harmful effects in larger and more diverse populations. Some adverse effects take longer to appear and are not identified until a drug is used by large numbers of patients.

Examples of this process have been approval of the COX-2 selective nonsteroidal anti-inflammatory drugs (NSAIDs), which were evaluated by the FDA during 2004 and 2005. Manufacturers of valdecoxib (Bextra), celecoxib (Celebrex), and rofecoxib (Vioxx) were originally asked to revise their labeling owing to emerging concerns that some NSAIDs exhibited extreme cardiovascular and gastrointestinal risks. In September 2004, manufacturers of rofecoxib voluntarily withdrew their product from the market due to safety concerns of heart attack and stroke. In April 2005, the FDA asked the manufacturers of valdecoxib to remove their product from the market due to similar concerns. Celecoxib has remained on the market, but the FDA announced that they would continue to analyze reports of COX-2 inhibitors to determine safety profiles and patient impact.

The FDA holds annual public meetings to hear comments from patients and professional and pharmaceutical organizations about the effectiveness and safety of new drug therapies. If the FDA discovers a serious problem, it will require that a drug be withdrawn from the market and its use discontinued.

Governmental agencies face the dual challenge of increasing the speed of drug approval while still ensuring the safety of new drugs.

CORE CONCEPT 1.9

The public once criticized the FDA and other regulatory agencies for being too slow in bringing new, potentially lifesaving drugs to the consumer. In the early 1990s, organized consumer groups and drug manufacturers pressured governmental officials to speed up the drug review process. Reasons for delays in the FDA drug approval process were outdated guidelines, poor communication, and agency understaffing.

In 1992, FDA officials, members of Congress, and representatives from pharmaceutical companies negotiated the Prescription Drug User Fee Act on a five-year trial basis. This act required drug and biologic manufacturers to pay substantial application fees at the time of an NDA to fund the approval process. This act requires that the FDA meet certain benchmarks, mostly related to speeding up the NDA process. With this extra income, the FDA hired more employees and restructured its organization to handle the greater number of drug applications more efficiently. Restructuring was a resounding success. From 1992 to 1996, the FDA approved double the number of drugs while cutting some review times by as much as half. In 1997, the FDA Modernization Act was passed, reauthorizing the Prescription Drug User Fee Act. It allowed drug companies to give healthcare providers information about *FDA-unapproved* uses of certain drugs. For example, sometimes drugs are approved to treat one condition, but not others; however, healthcare practitioners may discover that the drug is useful in treating a different problem. When such a benefit is found frequently, a drug company is allowed to share accurate information with other physicians about the drug's "unapproved" but effective use in treating another condition. When a drug is being prescribed for a condition for which it is not FDA-approved, it said to be an **off-label use**.

One concern now is that drugs are being developed at a faster rate than risks can be assessed. This is especially true for those drugs targeted to treat certain cancers. Officials have continued to call for patients, pharmacists, allied health workers, nurses, physicians, hospitals, and pharmaceutical companies to work together to minimize risks. Because of the higher numbers of drugs being approved for therapy, the potential for adverse drug–drug and drug–herbal interactions is greater than ever before.

Concept Review   1.2

■ Can you recall the major U.S. acts, standards, and organizations leading up to the present time? When was the FDA established? What current U.S. laws regulate how drugs are approved for marketing?

Healthcare providers must be prepared to deal with the threat of biological and chemical attack.

CORE CONCEPT 1.10

Prior to the September 11, 2001, terrorist attacks in the United States, concern about epidemic diseases mainly focused on the possible spread of traditional infectious diseases such as influenza, tuberculosis, cholera, and human immunodeficiency virus (HIV). Healthcare providers were also concerned about widespread food poisoning and sexually transmitted diseases other than HIV. Uncommon diseases such as anthrax produced fewer fatalities, so less attention was given to them.

Now, however, the healthcare community is more aware of the possibility of *bioterrorism*—the intentional use of infectious biological agents, chemical substances, or radiation to cause widespread harm or illness. Such federal agencies as the Centers for Disease Control and Prevention (CDC) and the U.S. Department of Defense have increased efforts to inform, educate, and prepare the public for disease outbreaks caused by bioterrorism. In 2002, the U.S. Department of Homeland Security was organized to provide additional security and defense for the United States in a terrorist attack. The department also prioritized the important issue of citizen preparedness, educating families how best to prepare for natural emergencies and disasters.

bio = *living organisms*
terrorism = *to induce fear*

Among the goals of a bioterrorist are to create widespread public panic and cause as many casualties as possible. The list of agents that can be used for this purpose is long. Some of these agents are easily obtainable and require little or no specialized knowledge to spread. The most worrisome threats are:

- Acutely infectious diseases such as anthrax, smallpox, plague, and hemorrhagic viruses
- Incapacitating chemicals such as nerve gas, cyanide, and chlorinated agents
- Nuclear and radiation emergencies

One can easily imagine what devastation would be caused if laboratories and healthcare professionals were not able to identify, isolate, and treat widespread diseases caused by bioterrorism. The following chapters contain important information related to bioterrorism. Chapter 26 reviews the topic of antibiotics for the treatment of anthrax. The treatment of chemical nerve warfare agents is discussed in Chapter 8. Chapter 32 includes a discussion of the treatment of radiation exposure.

CHAPTER REVIEW

CORE CONCEPTS SUMMARY

1.1 Pharmacology is an expansive and challenging topic.

Pharmacology, the study of medicine, is a subject devoted to proper drug treatment and health of the human body. It is an expansive topic utilizing concepts from human biology, pathophysiology, and chemistry.

1.2 For healthcare providers, the fields of pharmacology and therapeutics are connected.

Therapeutics is the science associated with the treatment of suffering and the prevention of disease. *Pharmacotherapeutics* is the useful application of drugs for the purpose of fighting disease. The study of pharmacology is important to health professionals from many different fields.

1.3 Agents may be classified as traditional drugs, biologics, and natural alternatives.

Drugs are chemical agents used to treat disease by producing biological responses within the body. Therapeutic drugs are classified as substances produced chemically or naturally. Biologics are natural agents produced by animal cells or microorganisms. Alternative therapies include natural herbs, plant extracts, or dietary supplements.

1.4 Drugs are available by prescription or over the counter (OTC).

There are two major methods of dispensing drugs. Prescription drugs require a physician's order; OTC drugs do not. There are advantages and disadvantages to both dispensing methods.

1.5 Pharmaceutics is the science of pharmacy.

Pharmaceutics involves the successful dispensation of drugs for therapeutic purposes. Dispensing medication safely is a major challenge for healthcare providers and patients.

1.6 Drug regulations were created to protect the public from drug misuse.

The first drug laws were acts created by Congress to protect patients from wrongful therapeutic claims. These and other standards form the basis of modern drug regulation agencies and organizations, such as the Food and Drug Administration and publications, such as the *U.S. Pharmacopoeia-National Formulary.*

1.7 U.S. drug standards have become increasingly complex.

The Food and Drug Administration (FDA), a branch of the U.S. Department of Health and Human Services, is the primary agency regulating drug safety. Three branches of the FDA control policies regarding drug therapies: the Center for Drug Evaluation and Research (CDER), the Center for Biologics Evaluation and Research (CBER), and the Center for Food Safety and Applied Nutrition (CFSAN). Black box warnings are a recent development enacted by the FDA. The National Center for Complementary and Alternative Medicine (NCCAM) is a newer agency established for scientific research and information about alternative therapies.

1.8 There are four stages of approval for therapeutic and biologic drugs.

Drug approval occurs in four stages: preclinical investigation, clinical investigation, submission of a new drug application (NDA) with review, and post-marketing studies. Clinical phase trials must be completed before drugs are approved for public use.

1.9 Governmental agencies face the dual challenge of increasing the speed of drug approval while still ensuring the safety of new drugs.

FDA officials, members of Congress, and pharmaceutical company representatives negotiated the Prescription Drug User Fee Act and FDA Modernization Act. These acts have sped up the approval process and require drug and biologic manufacturers to provide yearly product user fees. The concern now is that drugs are being approved at a rate faster than risks can be assessed.

1.10 Healthcare providers must be prepared to deal with the threat of biological and chemical attack.

Drugs are among the most powerful weapons to combat bioterrorism. Federal agencies have taken an active role in educating and preparing the public and the healthcare community about disease outbreaks caused by bioterrorism.

REVIEW QUESTIONS

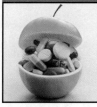

The following questions are written in NCLEX-PN® style. Answer these questions to assess your knowledge of the chapter material, and go back and review any material that is not clear to you.

1. Pathophysiology is defined as the study of:

1. How drugs enter and travel throughout the body and the responses they produce
2. How drugs improve the health of the human body
3. Drugs and how they elicit different responses
4. Diseases and functional changes occurring as a result of disease

2. Biologics are:

1. Produced in nature and include herbs, natural extracts, vitamins, and minerals
2. Chemically produced in a laboratory
3. Naturally produced in animal cells, microorganisms, or by the body itself
4. Not used routinely by physicians

3. Healthcare providers, such as Licensed Practical Nurses (LPN) and Licensed Vocational Nurses (LVN), are directly involved with drug administration and all of the following activities except:

1. Prescribing medications
2. Educating patients about their medications
3. Enforcing drug laws
4. Helping patients with medication management

4. What precautions should patients be aware of when taking OTC drugs? (Select all that apply.)

1. Self-treatment is sometimes ineffective.
2. OTC drugs may react with foods, herbal products, and prescription or other OTC drugs.
3. The potential for further injury or disease is not a consideration when taking OTC medications.
4. Instructions included with the medications should be read and followed as directed.

5. Dispensing of drugs to patients after they have been examined by a licensed healthcare provider is:

1. Pharmacology
2. Pharmaceutics
3. Therapeutics
4. Health care

6. The act that prevents the marketing of drugs that have not been thoroughly tested is the:

1. Pure Food and Drug Act (1906)
2. Food, Drug, and Cosmetic Act (1938)
3. Prescription Drug User Fee Act (1992)
4. FDA Modernization Act (1997)

7. The longest part of the drug approval process is typically:

1. Preclinical investigation
2. Clinical investigation
3. NDA submission and review
4. Postmarketing studies

8. The legislation responsible for cutting new drug application review times as much as 50% is the:

1. Pure Food and Drug Act
2. Sherley Amendment
3. Public Health Services Act
4. Prescription Drug User Fee Act

9. Black box warnings are:

1. Used to inform the consumer about general medication information
2. A list of ingredients within the medication
3. Located on the drug container label
4. The primary alert for notifying consumers of potential extreme adverse drug effects

10. Which of the following is considered a bioterrorist threat? (Select all that apply.)

1. Anthrax contamination
2. Incapacitating chemicals
3. Radiation exposure
4. Viruses that cause the common cold

NOTE: Answers to the Review Questions appear in Appendix B. The complete rationales and answers are located on the textbook's website.

Pearson Nursing Student Resources   Find additional review materials at **nursing.pearsonhighered.com.**

2 Drug Classes, Schedules, and Categories

CORE CONCEPTS

2.1 Drugs may be organized by their therapeutic and pharmacologic classifications.

2.2 Drugs have more than one name.

2.3 The differences between brand name drugs and their generic equivalents include price, formulations, and, most importantly, bioavailability.

2.4 Drugs with a potential for abuse are categorized into schedules.

2.5 In order to assess fetal risks, all prescription drugs are classified according to safety in pregnancy categories.

LEARNING OUTCOMES

After reading this chapter, the student should be able to:

1. Discuss the basis for placing drugs into therapeutic and pharmacologic classes.

2. Explain the prototype approach to drug classification.

3. Describe what is meant by a drug's mechanism of action.

4. Distinguish between a drug's chemical name, generic name, and trade name.

5. Explain why generic drug names are preferred to other drug names.

6. Discuss why drugs are sometimes placed on a restrictive list and why this is sometimes controversial.

7. Explain the meaning of the term *controlled substance*.

8. Explain the U.S. Controlled Substances Act of 1970 and the role of the U.S. Drug Enforcement Administration (DEA) in controlling drug abuse and misuse.

9. Identify the five drug schedules and provide examples of drugs at each level.

10. Identify the five pregnancy categories and explain what each category represents.

KEY TERMS

bioavailability (BEYE-oh-ah-VALE-ah-BILL-ih-TEE) 15
chemical name 14
combination drugs 15
controlled substance 16

generic name (je-NARE-ik) 14
mechanism of action 13
pharmacologic classification (FAR-mah-koh-LOJ-ik) 13
prototype drug (PRO-toh-type) 13

scheduled drugs 16
teratogen (tare-AT-oh-jen) 17
therapeutic classification (ther-ah-PEW-tik) 13
trade name 14

There are many ways that drugs can be classified, from a strict chemical group name to a trade name provided by the manufacturer. Because of the large number of drugs available, healthcare providers and consumers must have a system for identifying drugs and determining the limitations of their use. This chapter covers the methods by which drugs may be organized—by therapeutic or pharmacologic classification. This chapter also discusses drug schedules and pregnancy categories.

Drugs may be organized by their therapeutic and pharmacologic classifications.

CORE CONCEPT **2.1**

Medications may be classified in two major ways. Drugs may be organized by *therapeutic usefulness*. This is referred to as a **therapeutic classification**. Drugs may also be categorized by **mechanism of action** or *how they work pharmacologically*. This is referred to as a **pharmacologic classification**. Both methods are widely used in studying pharmacology, even though healthcare providers often do not make the distinction when the primary purpose of drug therapy is to improve the health of their patients.

Table 2.1 ◆ shows the method of therapeutic classification, using cardiac care as the example. The cardiovascular system is concerned with the proper functioning of the heart and blood vessels. Different types of drugs affect specific cardiovascular functions. Some drugs influence blood clotting, whereas others lower blood cholesterol or prevent the onset of stroke. Drugs may be used to lower blood pressure, treat heart failure, correct abnormal heart rhythm, alleviate chest pain, and treat or prevent circulatory shock. Drugs that affect cardiac disorders may be placed in numerous therapeutic classes. Drugs that influence blood clotting are called *anticoagulants*; those that lower blood cholesterol are called *antihyperlipidemics*, and those that lower blood pressure are called *antihypertensives*.

A therapeutic classification need not be complicated. For example, it is appropriate to classify a medication simply as "a drug used for stroke" or "a drug used for shock." The key to therapeutic classification is to state clearly what a particular drug does clinically. A few additional examples of therapeutic classification are antiemetics (to prevent vomiting or emesis), antacids (to reduce GI acid), anti-inflammatory drugs (to reduce inflammation), and antibiotics (to fight infective microorganisms).

Pharmacologic classification addresses *how* the medication produces its effects within the body. This method most directly applies to the foundational areas of science study including principles of cellular and molecular biology.

Table 2.2 ◆ shows various types of pharmacologic classifications using high blood pressure (hypertension) as an example. A *diuretic* is a class of drug used to treat hypertension by lowering plasma volume. Lowering plasma volume is the mechanism of action by which diuretics work. *Calcium channel blockers* treat hypertension by limiting the force of heart contractions. Other drugs, such as angiotensin-converting enzyme inhibitors, block components of the hormonal network called the *renin-angiotensin pathway*, thereby reducing hypertension. Notice that each example describes *how* hypertension may be controlled. Thus, the drug's pharmacologic classification is more specific than its therapeutic classification and requires application of human biochemical and physiological principles.

Before studying a particular drug's mechanism of action, it is recommended that students first become comfortable with the broad drug classes and then gradually move to more specific examples. Prototype drugs are an excellent place to start. A **prototype drug** is the well-understood drug model to which other medications in a pharmacologic class are compared. By learning the prototype drug, students may then predict the actions and adverse effects of other drugs in the same class. For example, by knowing the effects of penicillin V, students can apply this knowledge to the other drugs in the penicillin antibiotic class. *Students should be aware, however, that in many cases the original drug prototype is not the most widely used*

TABLE 2.1 Organizing Drugs by Therapeutic Classification	
Therapeutic Focus	
Cardiac care: Drugs affecting cardiovascular function	
Therapeutic Usefulness	**Therapeutic Classification***
influencing blood clotting	anticoagulant
lowering blood cholesterol	antihyperlipidemic
lowering blood pressure	antihypertensive
treating abnormal heartbeat	antidysrhythmic
treating chest pain (angina)	antianginal drug

Note: Although the names of some therapeutic categories may sound complicated, drug terminology will become more familiar as you begin to study drugs and drug classes. When studying this topic, always refer to a medical dictionary and reference drug guide.

TABLE 2.2 Organizing Drugs by Pharmacologic Classification

Focusing on Physiological Action

Therapy for high blood pressure may be achieved by:

Mechanism of Action	Pharmacologic Classification
lowering plasma volume	diuretic
blocking heart calcium channels	calcium channel blocker
blocking hormonal activity	angiotensin-converting enzyme inhibitor
blocking stress-related activity	adrenergic blocker (drug that inhibits actions of the sympathetic nervous system)
dilating peripheral blood vessels	vasodilator

drug in its class. As new drugs are developed, features such as antibiotic resistance, fewer side effects, or a more precise site of action might be factors that sway healthcare providers away from using the older drugs. Therefore, to master the subject of pharmacology, it is essential not only to be familiar with the drug prototypes but also to keep up with newer and more popular drugs. For all prototype drugs featured in this book, both therapeutic and pharmacologic classifications are provided to help students organize drug information.

Concept Review 2.1

■ What is the difference between a therapeutic classification and a pharmacologic classification? What is a *prototype drug,* and how is the prototype drug similar to and different from other drugs within the same pharmacologic or therapeutic class?

CORE CONCEPT 2.2 | Drugs have more than one name.

A major challenge when studying pharmacology is learning thousands of drug names. Adding to this difficulty is the fact that most drugs have multiple names. The three basic types of drug names are chemical, generic, and trade.

A **chemical name** is assigned using standard nomenclature established by the International Union of Pure and Applied Chemistry (IUPAC). A drug has only one chemical name, which is helpful in predicting its physical and chemical properties. Although chemical names convey a clear and concise meaning about the nature of a drug, they are often very complicated and difficult to pronounce and remember. For example, the chemical name of diazepam is 7-chloro-1, 3-ciphydro-1-methyl-5-phenyl-2H-1, 4-benzodiazepin-2-one. In only a few cases, usually when the name is brief and easily remembered, are chemical names commonly used. Examples of brief (and therefore useful) chemical names include lithium carbonate, calcium gluconate, and sodium chloride.

More practically, drugs are sometimes classified by *a portion* of their chemical structure, known as the chemical group name. Examples are antibiotic drugs, such as the fluoroquinolones and beta-lactam medications. Other common examples include the phenothiazines, thiazides, and benzodiazepines. Although names like these may seem complicated at first, familiarity with chemical group names will grow, and the nomenclature will become more manageable as students become more proficient and communicate with fellow healthcare providers.

The **generic name** of a drug is assigned by the U.S. Adopted Name Council. With few exceptions, generic names are less complicated and easier to remember than chemical names. Many organizations, including the FDA, the U.S. Pharmacopoeia, and the World Health Organization, routinely describe a medication by its generic name. Because there is only one generic name for each drug, healthcare providers routinely use this name, and pharmacology students generally must memorize it.

A drug's **trade name** is assigned by the company marketing the drug. The name is usually selected for marketability, and it is usually easy to remember. The trade name is also called the *proprietary, product,* or *brand* name. The term *proprietary* relates to ownership. In the United States, a drug developer is given exclusive rights to name and market a drug for 17 years after a new drug application (NDA) is submitted to the Food and Drug Administration (FDA). Because it takes several years before a drug can be approved, the amount of time spent in approval is subtracted from the 17 years. For example, if it takes seven years for a drug to be approved, competing companies will not be allowed to market a generic equivalent drug for another 10 years. The rationale for this is that the developing company must be allowed sufficient time to recoup the millions of dollars spent in research and the time needed to develop the new drug. After 17 years,

TABLE 2.3 Trade Name Products Containing Popular Generic Substances

Generic Substances	Trade Names
aspirin	Acuprin, Anacin, Aspergum, Bayer, Bufferin, Ecotrin, Empirin, Magnaprin, Miniprin, Ridiprin, Sloprin, Uni-Buff, Uni-Tren, Zorprin
diphenhydramine	Aler-Dryl, Allergia-C, Benadryl, Compoz Nighttime Sleep Aid, Diphedryl, Diphenadryl, Hydramine, Nytol, Pardryl, PediaCare Children's Allergy, Sominex, Unisom
ibuprofen	Advil, Dolgesic, Genpril, Haltran, IB Pro, Midol, Motrin, Nuprin, Rufen, Tab-Profen, Ultraprin

competing companies may sell a generic equivalent drug, using a different trade name, which the FDA must approve.

Trade names may be a challenge because of the dozens of product names containing similar ingredients. In addition, some **combination drugs** contain more than one active generic ingredient, making it difficult to match one generic name with one product name. As an example, refer to Table 2.3 ◆ and consider the drug diphenhydramine (generic name), also called Benadryl (one of many trade names). Diphenhydramine is an antihistamine. Low doses of diphenhydramine can be purchased over the counter; higher doses require a prescription. When looking for diphenhydramine, healthcare providers may find it listed under many trade names, such as Allerdryl and Compoz. Diphenhydramine may be provided alone or in combination with other active ingredients. Ibuprofen and aspirin are also examples of drugs with many different trade names. The rule of thumb is that a formulation's active ingredients are listed in the ingredients by their generic names. The generic name is usually written in lowercase, whereas the trade name is capitalized.

Concept Review 2.2

■ What are the differences between a chemical, a generic, and a trade name? Which name is most often used to describe the active ingredients within a drug product?

The differences between brand name drugs and their generic equivalents include price, formulations, and, most importantly, bioavailability.

CORE CONCEPT 2.3

Usually generic drugs are less expensive than brand name drugs. The reason is that a pharmaceutical company determines the price of a proprietary drug during its 17 years of exclusive rights to that new drug. Because there is no competition, the price can be kept quite high. The pharmaceutical company that developed a drug can sometimes use legal tactics to extend its exclusive rights to a drug, earning the company hundreds of millions of dollars per year in profits for a popular medicine. Once the exclusive rights end, competing companies market the generic drug for less money, and consumer savings may be considerable. In some states, pharmacists may routinely substitute a generic drug when the prescription calls for a brand name. In other states, the pharmacist must dispense drugs directly as written by the healthcare practitioner or obtain approval before providing a generic substitute.

The companies that market brand name drugs often aggressively oppose laws that might restrict the routine use of their products. They claim that significant differences exist between a trade name drug and its generic equivalent, and that switching to the generic drug may be harmful to the patient. Patient advocates, on the other hand, argue that generic substitutions should always be permitted because of the cost savings.

Are there real differences between a brand name drug and its generic equivalent? Despite the fact that the dosages may be identical, drug formulations are not always the same. The two drugs may have different *inert* ingredients or be processed differently. For example, in a tablet form, the active ingredients may be more tightly compressed in one of the preparations than in another, and this might affect how well the body can use the drug.

The key to comparing brand name drugs and their generic equivalents lies in measuring the *bioavailability* of the two preparations. **Bioavailability** is the physiologic ability of the drug to reach its target cells and produce its effect (Figure 2.1 ■). Anything that affects absorption of a drug or its distribution to the target cells will certainly affect drug action. Measuring how long a drug takes to exert its effect gives pharmacologists a crude measure of bioavailability. For example, if a patient is in circulatory shock and it takes a generic drug five minutes longer than the brand name drug to produce its effect, that difference would

bio = *in the living organism*
availability = *free to activate cellular targets*

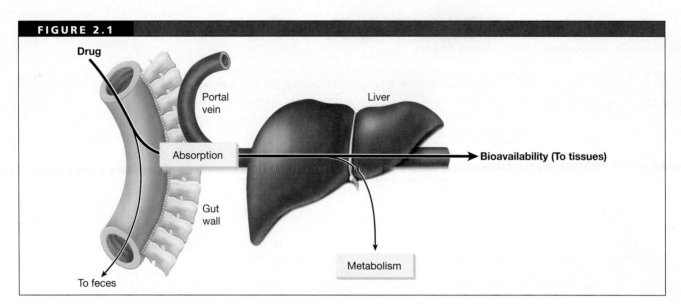

FIGURE 2.1

A drug's bioavailability will depend on the dosage form and how much will actually reach the target location.

be significant. However, if a generic medication for arthritis pain relief takes 45 minutes to act, compared with the brand name drug that takes 40 minutes, it probably does not matter which drug is prescribed.

In some cases, pharmacists must inform or notify patients of substitutions of generics for brand names. Pharmaceutical companies and some healthcare providers have supported disclosure of substitution, claiming that generic drugs—even those that have small differences in bioavailability and *bioequivalence* or same impact in the body—could adversely affect outcomes in patients with critical conditions or illnesses. Some states have compiled a *negative* formulary, a list of trade name drugs that pharmacists may *not* dispense as generic drugs. These drugs must only be dispensed exactly as written on the prescription, using the trade name drug the physician prescribed. However, laws frequently change: In many instances, the efforts of consumer advocacy groups have led to changes in or elimination of negative formulary lists.

bio = *in the living organism*
equivalence = *same impact*

Drugs with a potential for abuse are categorized into schedules.

Some drugs are frequently abused or have a high potential for becoming addictive. Technically, *addiction* refers to the overwhelming feeling that drives someone to use a drug repeatedly. *Dependence* is a related term, often defined as a physiologic or psychological need for a substance. *Physical dependence* refers to an altered physical condition caused by the nervous system adapting to repeated drug use. In this case, when the drug is no longer available, the individual experiences physical signs of discomfort known as *withdrawal*. In contrast, when an individual is *psychologically dependent*, there are few signs of physical discomfort when the drug is withdrawn; however, the individual feels an intense compelling desire to continue drug use. These concepts are discussed in detail in Chapter 7.

Drugs that cause dependency are restricted to use in situations of medical necessity, that is, if they are allowed at all. According to law, drugs that have a significant potential for abuse are placed into five categories called *schedules*. These **scheduled drugs** are classified according to their potential for abuse: Schedule I drugs have the highest potential for abuse, and Schedule V drugs have the lowest. Schedule I drugs have little or no therapeutic value or are intended for research purposes only. Drugs in the other four schedules may be dispensed only in cases when therapeutic value has been determined. Schedule V is the only category in which some drugs may be dispensed without a prescription because the quantities of the controlled drug are so low that the possibility of causing dependence is extremely remote. Table 2.4 ◆ shows the five drug schedules with examples. However, not all drugs with an abuse potential are regulated or placed into schedules. Tobacco, alcohol, and caffeine are significant examples.

In the United States, a **controlled substance** is a drug restricted by the Controlled Substances Act of 1970 and later revisions. The Controlled Substances Act is also called the Comprehensive Drug Abuse Prevention and Control Act. This act has several implications for the drugs in the controlled substances schedules. Hospitals and pharmacies must register with the Drug Enforcement Administration (DEA) and use their assigned registration numbers to purchase scheduled drugs. They must maintain complete records of all quantities purchased and sold. Drugs with higher abuse potential have more restrictions. For example, in the hospital a special drug order form must be used to obtain Schedule II drugs, and orders must be written and signed by the healthcare providers. Telephone orders to a pharmacy are not permitted. Refills for Schedule II drugs are not permitted; patients must visit their healthcare providers first. Those convicted of unlawful manufacturing, distributing, and dispensing of controlled substances face severe penalties.

TABLE 2.4   Drug Schedule and Examples

Drug Schedule	Abuse Potential	Physical Dependence	Psychological Dependence	Examples
I	Highest	High	High	heroin, lysergic acid diethylamide (LSD), peyote, methaqualone, and 3,4-methylenedioxymethamphetamine ("ecstasy")
II	High	High	High	hydromorphone, methadone, meperidine, oxycodone, and fentanyl; amphetamine, methamphetamine, methylphenidate, cocaine, amobarbital, glutethimide, and pentobarbital
III	Moderate	Moderate	High	combination products containing less than 15 mg of hydrocodone per dosage unit, products containing not more than 90 mg of codeine per dosage unit, buprenorphine products, benzphetamine, phendimetrazine, ketamine, and anabolic steroids
IV	Lower	Lower	Lower	alprazolam, clonazepam, clorazepate, diazepam, lorazepam, midazolam, temazepam, and triazolam
V	Lowest	Lowest	Lowest	cough preparations containing not more than 200 mg of codeine per 100 mL or per 100 g

The DEA authorizes healthcare providers to prescribe controlled substances. The federal legislation that gives the DEA the right to control drugs of abuse (and thus affects which drugs can be prescribed or not) is the Controlled Substances Act. See the Drug Enforcement Agency website.

In order to assess fetal risks, all prescription drugs are classified according to safety in pregnancy categories.

CORE CONCEPT 2.5

A major concern of expectant parents is whether a drug will harm their developing baby. Any substance that will harm a developing fetus or embryo is referred to as a **teratogen**. Pregnant patients should never take any prescribed, illegal, or OTC drug or any herbal or dietary supplement without the advice of their healthcare providers.

terato = *severe deformity*
gen = *something that produces*

To protect the fetus from the teratogenic effects of prescription drugs, the FDA has implemented a category system for classifying drugs based on how safe they are for the mother and the developing baby. According to this system, drugs are placed into one of five *pregnancy categories*, labeled as A, B, C, D, and X. These labels appear within package inserts and identify levels of risk to women and/or the fetus. The levels are based on degrees to which a drug has been proven to cause birth defects in laboratory animals or in human beings. These categories are summarized in Table 2.5 ◆.

Consumers sometimes question whether the testing of laboratory animals is an effective way to predict harm to a developing human fetus or embryo. Results from animal testing are not always transferable to the human body. In fact, results from animal experimentation often vary from species to species. For this reason, consumers should always be cautious, even when there is reasonable assurance that a drug is extremely safe.

TABLE 2.5   Categories of Safety in Pregnancy

Safety Category	Explanation	Examples
A Lowest Risk	Studies HAVE NOT shown a risk to women or to the fetus.	ferrous fumarate (Ferranol), levothyroxine (Synthroid), potassium chloride (KCl), potassium gluconate (Kaon Tablets), prenatal multivitamins, thyroglobulin (Proloid)
B	ANIMAL studies HAVE NOT shown a risk to the fetus or, if they have, studies in women have not confirmed this risk.	amoxicillin (Amoxil), fluoxetine (Prozac), insulin (Humulin R), loperamide (Imodium), penicillins, ranitidine (Zantac)
C	ANIMAL studies HAVE shown a risk to the fetus, but controlled studies have not been performed in women.	acyclovir (Zovirax), amitryptiline (Elavil), furosemide (Lasix), hydrochlorothiazide (HydroURIL), iron dextran (K FeRON), mineral oil (Fleet Mineral Oil), senna (Senokot)
D	Use of this drug category MAY cause harm to the fetus, but it may provide benefit to the mother in a life-threatening situation or when a safer therapy is not available.	ACE inhibitors, alcohol, cortisone acetate (Cortistan), nonsteroidal anti-inflammatory drugs in the third trimester, tetracyclines
X Highest Risk	Studies HAVE shown a significant risk to women and to the fetus.	castor oil (Purge), isotretinoin, methotrexate, most oral contraceptives, norethindrone (Norlutin), oxymetholone (Anadrol), progesterone (oral forms), statins, warfarin (Coumadin)

CHAPTER REVIEW

CORE CONCEPTS SUMMARY

2.1 Drugs may be organized by their therapeutic and pharmacologic classifications.

Two common ways to classify drugs are by therapeutic classification and pharmacologic classification. Therapeutic classes are based on a drug's clinical usefulness. Pharmacologic classes are based on a drug's mechanism of action. Prototype drugs are used to compare drugs within the same classification. Knowing about prototype drugs can help students understand other, similar drugs.

2.2 Drugs have more than one name.

Drugs may be described by a chemical, generic, or trade name. There are advantages and disadvantages to each naming method.

2.3 The differences between brand name drugs and their generic equivalents include price, formulations, and, most importantly, bioavailability.

In most states, generic drugs may be substituted for brand name products if the prescribing practitioner does not object. When generic drugs are substituted, differences in bioavailability may affect the safety and effectiveness of drug therapy.

2.4 Drugs with a potential for abuse are categorized into schedules.

Drugs that have the potential for abuse or dependency are placed into one of five schedules, Schedule I is the most restrictive category. Schedule V is the least restrictive category. The U.S. Drug Enforcement Administration (DEA) handles drug misuse.

2.5 In order to assess fetal risks, all prescription drugs are classified according to safety in pregnancy categories.

In the United States, all drugs are placed into one of five pregnancy categories: A, B, C, D, and X. Drugs in category A are the safest; those in category X are the most harmful.

REVIEW QUESTIONS

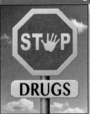

The following questions are written in NCLEX-PN® style. Answer these questions to assess your knowledge of the chapter material, and go back and review any material that is not clear to you.

1. Which of the following types of drug classification focuses on what a drug does clinically?

1. Therapeutic
2. Pharmacologic
3. Chemical
4. All of the above

2. *How* a medication produces its effects in the body is referred to as a drug's:

1. Therapeutic usefulness
2. Mechanism of action
3. Model for other drugs combating similar diseases
4. Clinical focus

3. In which of the following categories does a drug have only one name?

1. Chemical name
2. Generic name
3. Trade name
4. Both 1 and 2

4. Which of the following statements is correct?

1. Because chemical drug names are often complicated and difficult to remember or pronounce, the chemical structure of a drug is rarely considered in pharmacotherapy.
2. Matching one active ingredient with one trade name product is not a particularly challenging job for the healthcare provider.
3. When referring to a drug, the generic name is usually capitalized, whereas the trade name is written in lowercase.
4. The drug trade name is sometimes called the proprietary name, suggesting ownership.

5. When examining the question, "Are there real differences between brand name drugs and their generic equivalents?" the answer that emerges from reading this chapter is:

1. Drug formulations for brand name drugs are the same as their generic equivalents.
2. Brand name drugs are always more tightly compressed than generic drugs.
3. Generic drugs are always best because they generally cost less.
4. Brand name drugs are sometimes preferred because of differences in bioavailability compared to generic equivalents.

6. Which of the following are true statements about a negative formulary list of trade name drugs? (Select all that apply.)

1. It is a list of trade name drugs that cannot be substituted with generic drugs.
2. It is consistent throughout the United States.
3. The drugs on the list must be dispensed by the pharmacist using the drug's trade name as written on the prescription.
4. It was formed because of concern over the bioavailability of generic drugs and possible adverse effects on patient outcomes.

7. An altered physical condition caused by the nervous system adapting to repeated drug use is:

1. Addiction
2. Physical dependence
3. Psychological dependence
4. Withdrawal

8. The Controlled Substances Act of 1970 and later revisions enable the DEA to do which of the following?

1. Introduce drugs into the marketplace.
2. Restrict the use of drugs that have a significant potential for abuse.

3. Restrict the use of all drugs that have an abuse potential.
4. Allow patients to obtain Schedule II drug refills without visiting their healthcare provider first.

9. The drug schedule that allows therapeutic use of a drug with a prescription but contains drugs with relatively lower abuse and dependency potential than other scheduled drugs is:

1. Schedule II
2. Schedule III
3. Schedule IV
4. Schedule V

10. When preparing to administer medications to pregnant patients, nurses should know that their patients:

1. Are not at risk if they take drugs placed into pregnancy safety category X
2. Can take herbal or dietary supplements without fear of teratogenic effects to their developing baby
3. Are relatively safe if they take medications within pregnancy safety category B
4. Should never take drugs classified as pregnancy safety category D

NOTE: Answers to the Review Questions appear in Appendix B. The complete rationales and answers are located on the textbook's website.

Pearson Nursing Student Resources Find additional review materials at **nursing.pearsonhighered.com**.

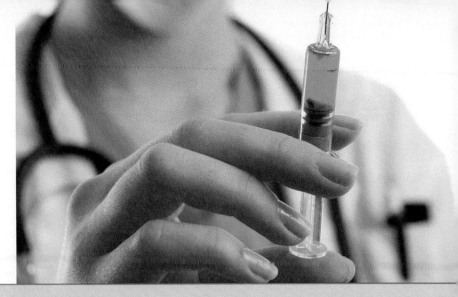

3 Methods of Drug Administration

CORE CONCEPTS

3.1 A major goal in pharmacotherapy is to limit the number and severity of adverse drug events.

3.2 The rights of drug administration form the basis of proper drug delivery.

3.3 Successful pharmacotherapy depends on patient compliance.

3.4 Healthcare providers use accepted abbreviations to communicate the directions and times for drug administration.

3.5 Three systems of measurement are used in pharmacology: metric, apothecary, and household.

3.6 Certain protocols and techniques are common to all methods of drug administration.

3.7 Enteral drugs are given orally or via nasogastric or gastrostomy tubes.

3.8 Topical drugs are applied locally to the skin and associated membranes.

3.9 Parenteral administration refers to dispensing medications by routes other than oral or topical.

LEARNING OUTCOMES

After reading this chapter, the student should be able to:

1. Discuss drug administration as a component of safe and effective health care.

2. Describe the roles and responsibilities of nurses, nursing assistants, therapists, and technicians regarding drug administration.

3. Explain how the six rights of drug administration affect patient safety.

4. Give specific examples of how the healthcare provider can increase patient compliance in taking medications.

5. Interpret abbreviations used in drug administration practices.

6. Compare and contrast the three systems of measurement used in pharmacology.

7. Explain the proper methods to administer enteral, topical, and parenteral drugs.

8. Compare and contrast the advantages and disadvantages of each route of drug administration.

KEY TERMS

adverse drug events *21*
adverse effects *21*
allergic reaction *22*
anaphylaxis (ANN-ah-fah-LAX-iss) *22*
apothecary system
　(ah-POTH-eh-kare-ee) *25*
astringent effect (ah-STRIN-jent) *31*
buccal route (BUCK-ahl) *27*

compliance (kom-PLY-ans) *22*
contraindications
　(CON-trah-EN-deh-KAY-shuns) *21*
enteral route (EN-tur-ul) *27*
enteric-coated (in-TARE-ik) *27*
household systems *25*
intradermal (ID) route
　(IN-trah-DERM-ul) *33*

intramuscular (IM) route
　(IN-trah-musk-u-lar) *36*
intravenous (IV) route
　(IN-trah-VEE-nus) *37*
metric system *24*
orally disintegrating tablets (ODTs) *27*
parenteral route (pah-REN-tur-ul) *32*
prn order *23*

routine orders *24*

single order *23*

six rights of drug
administration *22*

standing order *24*

STAT order *23*

subcutaneous (SC or SQ) route
(sub-kew-TAY-nee-us) *33*

sublingual (SL) route (sub-LIN-gwal) *27*

sustained-release *27*

three checks of drug
administration *22*

topical route (TOP-ik-ul) *28*

transdermal (trans-DER-mul) *29*

transmucosal (trans-mew-KOH-sul) *31*

Drug administration is an important part of providing comprehensive care to the patient. During drug administration, members of the healthcare team collaborate closely with pharmacists, physicians, their patients, and each other to ensure the safe delivery of prescribed medications. The purpose of this chapter is to introduce the roles and responsibilities of nurses and other healthcare providers, to define the practice of secure and effective distribution of medications, and to provide a basic overview of the major routes of drug administration.

A major goal in pharmacotherapy is to limit the number and severity of adverse drug events.

Whether administering drugs, supervising drug use, or providing assistance, the healthcare provider is expected to be familiar with the general principles of drug delivery. The large number of different drugs and the potential consequences of medication errors make this an enormous task.

The main responsibilities of the nurse include knowledge and understanding of the following:

- What drug is ordered
- Name (generic and trade) and drug classification
- Intended or proposed use
- Expected therapeutic effects on the body
- Situations under which drugs should not be used, or **contraindications**
- Special considerations (e.g., the effects of age, weight, body fat distribution, and individual pathophysiological states on pharmacotherapeutic response)
- Unwanted nontherapeutic effects, **adverse effects** (or *side effects*)
- Why the medication has been prescribed for this particular patient
- How the medication is supplied by the pharmacy
- How the medication should be administered, including dosage ranges
- What nursing process considerations related to the medication apply to this patient

contra = *opposing*
indications = *useful applications*

adverse = *negative*
effects = *drug responses*

Nursing assistants, therapists, and technicians work closely with nurses to provide care to the patients. Members of the health support staff who do not administer medications but who have an equally important role in providing care to the patients have a slightly different list of tasks than nurses. These tasks provide opportunities to monitor patients and make sure no unusual reactions or undesirable effects result from the medication. Tasks include:

- Monitoring blood pressure, pulse rate, and respiration rate
- Changing soiled or wet clothing, wraps, or bandages
- Dressing wounds, giving massages, and caring for the skin's surface
- Preparing food trays or helping to feed patients
- Observing patients and reporting significant symptoms, reactions, or changes in medical condition
- Reporting strange behaviors or habits in patients
- Helping transport patients
- Monitoring special equipment

Before any drug is administered, healthcare staff must obtain, process, and communicate important information to one another about the patient's medical history, physical assessment, disease processes, learning needs, and capabilities. They must consider growth and developmental factors and remember that many variables can influence how a patient responds to medications. Understanding these variables can increase the success of pharmacotherapy. A major goal of pharmacotherapy is to limit the number and severity of **adverse drug events**. Many adverse effects are preventable. By applying their experience and knowledge of pharmacotherapeutics to clinical practice, healthcare providers can avoid many serious adverse drug reactions. Some adverse events, however, are not preventable. It is vital that the healthcare team is prepared to recognize and respond to potentially damaging medication effects. Allergic and anaphylactic reactions are particularly serious effects that must be carefully monitored and prevented, when possible.

An **allergic reaction** is an acquired hyper-response of body defenses to a foreign substance (allergen). Signs of allergic reactions vary in severity and include skin rash with or without itching, edema, nausea, diarrhea, runny nose, or reddened eyes with tearing. On discovering that a patient is allergic to a product, it is the nurse's responsibility to first alert the charge nurse and patient's physician of the reaction in case it is necessary to give the patient medications to reverse the reaction. Next the nurse should document the allergy in the medical record and apply labels to the chart and medication administration record so that all healthcare personnel will be aware of the allergy. An agency-approved allergy bracelet should be placed on the patient. The pharmacist should also be told so that the medication can be checked for cross-sensitivity with other pharmacologic products. The pharmacotherapy of allergic reactions is covered in Chapter 25.

Anaphylaxis is a severe type of allergic reaction in which massive amounts of histamine and other chemical mediators of inflammation are released throughout the body. It can lead to life-threatening shock. Symptoms of anaphylaxis are severe shortness of breath, a sudden drop in blood pressure, and tachycardia. These symptoms require immediate attention. The pharmacotherapy of anaphylaxis is covered in Chapter 21.

CORE CONCEPT 3.2	**The rights of drug administration form the basis of proper drug delivery.**

The traditional **six rights of drug administration** form the operational basis for the safe delivery of medications and are recognized by such organizations as the Institute for Safe Medication Practices (ISMP). The six rights are simple and practical guidelines for nurses to use during drug preparation, delivery, and administration. The six rights are as follows:

- Right patient
- Right medication
- Right dose
- Right route of administration
- Right time of delivery
- Right documentation

Additional rights have been added over the years, depending on particular academic curricula or agency policies. Additions to the original six rights include the right to refuse medication, the right to receive drug education, and the right preparation.

The **three checks of drug administration** that nurses use with the six rights help to ensure patient safety and drug effectiveness. Traditionally these checks include the following:

- Checking the drug with the medication administration record (MAR) or medication information system when removing it from the medication drawer, refrigerator, or controlled substance locker
- Checking the drug when preparing it, pouring it, taking it out of the unit dose container, or connecting the IV tubing to the bag
- Checking the drug before administering it to the patient

Despite the use of these checks and rights to provide safe drug delivery, errors still occur, and some of them are fatal. Although the nurse is accountable for preparing and administering medications, many individuals—including physicians, pharmacists, and other healthcare providers—are also responsible for safe drug practices.

CORE CONCEPT 3.3	**Successful pharmacotherapy depends on patient compliance.**

Patient adherence or **compliance** is another major factor affecting the success of pharmacotherapy. Compliance means taking a medication in the way it was prescribed by the practitioner or, in the case of over-the-counter (OTC) drugs, following the instructions on the label. Patient noncompliance can include not taking the medication at all, taking it at the wrong time, or taking it in the wrong way.

Even when healthcare providers conscientiously use all the principles of effective drug administration, patients may not agree that the prescribed drug regimen is worthwhile. Before administering the drug, the nurse should use the nursing process to develop a personalized care plan that will allow the patient to be an active participant in his or her care. Support staff can help ensure that the care plan works. It is important to remember that a responsible, well-informed adult always has the legal option to refuse any medication. This right allows the patient to accept or reject the pharmacotherapy based on accurate information presented in a way the patient can understand.

Fast Facts Potentially Fatal Drug Reactions

Toxic Epidermal Necrolysis (TEN)

- Skin sloughing of 30% or more of the body (caused by skin cell breakdown)
- Severe and deadly allergic reaction caused by a drug
- Occurs when the liver fails to properly break down a drug, which then cannot be excreted normally
- Risk of death decreased if the drug is quickly withdrawn and supportive care is maintained

Stevens-Johnson Syndrome (SJS)

- Skin sloughing of 10% of the body
- Generalized blister-like lesions following within a few days
- Usually signaled initially by nonspecific upper respiratory infection (URI) with chills, fever, and malaise

In the plan of care, it is important to address information that the patient must know about the prescribed medications. This includes the name of the drug; why it was ordered; its expected actions; its possible side effects; and its potential interactions with other medications, foods, herbal supplements, or alcohol. Patients need to be reminded that they have an active role in ensuring the effectiveness and safety of their medications.

Many factors influence whether patients comply with pharmacotherapy. The drug may be too expensive or may not be approved by the patient's health insurance plan. Patients sometimes forget doses of medications, especially when they must be taken three or four times per day. Patients often stop using drugs that have annoying side effects or that affect lifestyle. Adverse effects such as headache, dizziness, nausea, diarrhea, or impotence often cause noncompliance. Patients sometimes self-adjust their doses. Some patients believe that if one tablet is good, two must be better. Others believe that they will become dependent on the medication if it is taken as prescribed, and so they take only half the required dose. Patients usually do not want to admit or report noncompliance to the nurse because they are embarrassed or fear being reprimanded. Because there are many reasons for noncompliance, the nurse must carefully question patients about their medications. When pharmacotherapy fails to produce the expected outcomes, noncompliance should be considered as a possible reason.

▶ **Life Span Fact**

Many older adults take at least three different drugs each day, with some taking as many as eight or more. This leads to poor compliance among older patients. Noncompliance can be even greater for elderly patients with dementia or Alzheimer's disease.

Healthcare providers use accepted abbreviations to communicate the directions and times for drug administration.

CORE CONCEPT 3.4

Table 3.1 ◆ lists common abbreviations that are used to give directions about drug administration. A **STAT order** refers to a medication that should be given immediately and only once. This order is often used with emergency medications that are needed for life-threatening situations. The physician normally notifies the nurse of any STAT order, so it can be obtained from the pharmacy and administered immediately.

A **single order** is for a drug that is to be given only once and at a specific time. An example is a preoperative order. A **prn order** is administered as required by the patient's condition. The nurse makes the judgment, based on patient assessment, as to when the medication should be administered. Orders

Fast Facts Grapefruit Juice and Drug Interactions

- Grapefruit juice may not be safe for people who take certain medications.
- Chemicals in grapefruit juice lower the activity of specific enzymes in the intestinal tract that normally break down medications. This allows a larger amount of medication to reach the bloodstream, resulting in increased drug activity.
- Drugs that may be affected by grapefruit juice include certain sedative-hypnotic drugs, antibiotics, drugs that lower blood cholesterol, some antihistamines, and antifungal agents.
- Grapefruit juice should be consumed at least two hours before or five hours after taking a medication that may interact with it.
- Some drinks that are flavored with fruit juice could contain grapefruit juice, even if grapefruit is not part of the name of the drink. Check the ingredients label.

TABLE 3.1 Drug Administration Abbreviations*

Abbreviation	Meaning	Abbreviation	Meaning
ac	before meals	prn	when needed/necessary
ad lib	as desired/as directed	q	every
AM	Morning	qh	every hour
ASAP	as soon as possible	qid	four times per day
bid	twice per day	q2h	every 2 hours (even)
cap	capsule	q4h	every 4 hours (even)
/d	per day	q6h	every 6 hours (even)
gtt	drop	q8h	every 8 hours (even)
h or hr	hour	q12h	every 12 hours
hs	hour of sleep/bedtime	Rx	take
no	number	SL	sublingual
pc	after meals; after eating	STAT	immediately; at once
PM	afternoon	tab	tablet
PO	by mouth	tid	three times per day

Many more abbreviations could be listed. The Joint Commission (formerly JCAHO) recommends that some previously used abbreviations be spelled out to avoid medication errors: Use "daily" (not qd); use "nightly" (not qhs); use "every other day" (not qod). For additional information, see The Joint Commission's official "Do Not Use List".

not written as single, STAT or prn are called **routine orders**. These are usually carried out within two hours of the time the order is written by the physician, but the exact timing is defined by each facility. A **standing order** is written in advance of a situation and should be carried out under specific circumstances. An example of a standing order is a set of postoperative prn prescriptions that are written for all patients who have undergone a specific surgical procedure. A common standing order for patients who have had a tonsillectomy is "Tylenol elixir 325 mg PO q6h prn sore throat." Because of the legal implications of putting all patients into a single treatment category, standing orders are no longer permitted in some facilities.

Agency policies dictate that drug orders be reviewed by the attending physician within specific time frames, usually at least every seven days. Prescriptions for narcotics and other scheduled drugs are often automatically stopped after 72 hours, unless specifically reordered by the physician. Automatic stop orders do not generally apply when the number of doses, or an exact period of time, is specified.

Some medications must be taken at specific times. If a drug causes stomach upset, it is usually administered with meals to prevent epigastric pain, nausea, or vomiting. Other medications should be administered between meals because food interferes with absorption. Some CNS drugs and antihypertensives are best administered at bedtime, because they may cause drowsiness. Others, such as sildenafil (Viagra), should be taken 30 to 60 minutes prior to intended sexual intercourse to achieve an erection. The nurse must pay careful attention when educating patients about when and how to take their medications to increase compliance and therapeutic success.

Once medications are administered, the nurse must correctly document that the medications have been given to the patient. Depending on the facility, documentation is done on the computer using a special program for medication administration or on a paper copy of the MAR. Either way, it is necessary that the drug name, dosage, time administered, and any assessments data be documented. For computer documentation, the identification of the nurse administering the medication is done when he or she logs on using an assigned password. On the paper copy of the MAR, the nurse must initial and sign his or her name. If a medication is refused or not given as ordered, this fact (along with the reasons) must be recorded on the appropriate form within the medical record.

Three systems of measurement are used in pharmacology: metric, apothecary, and household.

CORE CONCEPT 3.5

Dosages are labeled and dispensed according to their weight or volume. The most common system of drug measurement uses the **metric system**. The volume of a drug is expressed in terms of a liter (L) or a milliliter (mL). The abbreviation "cc" for cubic centimeter, a measurement of volume that is equivalent to 1 mL

TABLE 3.2   Metric, Apothecary, and Household Approximate Measurement Equivalents

Metric	Apothecary	Household
1 mL	15–16 minims	15–16 drops
4–5 mL (cc)	1 fluid dram	1 teaspoon or 60 drops
15 mL	4 fluid drams	1 tablespoon or 3–4 teaspoons
30 mL	8 fluid drams or 1 fluid ounce	2 tablespoons
240 mL	8 fluid ounces (1/2 pint)	1 glass or cup
500 mL	1 pint	2 glasses or 2 cups
1 L	32 fluid ounces or 1 quart	4 glasses or 4 cups or 1 quart
1 mg	1/60 grain	—
60–65 mg	1 grain	—
300–325 mg	5 grains	—
1 g	15–16 grains	—
1 kg	—	2.2 pounds

To convert grains to grams: Divide grains by 15 or 16.
To convert grams to grains: Multiply grams by 15 or 16.
To convert minims to milliliters: Divide minims by 15 or 16.

of fluid, is no longer recommended for use in medicine. The metric weight of a drug is stated in terms of kilograms (kg), grams (g), milligrams (mg), or micrograms (mcg). At one time, the abbreviation "µg" was used for micrograms, but this is no longer recommended. It is now recommended that "micrograms" and other small unusual measurements be spelled out.

The **apothecary system** and **household systems** are older systems of measurement. Although most physicians and pharmacies use the metric system, these older systems may still be seen. Until the metric system totally replaces the other systems, the healthcare provider must recognize dosages based on all three systems of measurement. Approximate equivalents among metric, apothecary, and household units of volume and weight are listed in Table 3.2 ◆.

Because Americans are familiar with the teaspoon, tablespoon, and cup, it is important for the nurse to be able to convert between the household and metric systems of measurement. In the hospital, a glass of fluid is measured in milliliters—an 8-ounce glass of water is recorded as 240 mL. If a patient being discharged is ordered to drink 2400 mL of fluid per day, the nurse may instruct the patient to drink ten 8-ounce glasses or 10 cups of fluid per day. Likewise, when a child is to be given a drug that is administered in elixir form, the nurse should explain that 5 mL of the drug is the same as one teaspoon. The nurse should encourage the use of accurate medical dosing devices at home, such as oral dosing syringes, oral droppers, cylindrical spoons, and medication cups. These are preferred over the traditional household measuring spoon because they are more accurate. Eating utensils that are commonly referred to as teaspoons or tablespoons often do not hold the volume that their names imply.

Certain protocols and techniques are common to all methods of drug administration.

CORE CONCEPT **3.6**

The three general routes of drug administration are enteral, topical, and parenteral, with subcategories among each general route. Each route has both advantages and disadvantages. Although some drugs are formulated to be given by several routes, others are made to be given by only one route. Pharmacokinetic considerations, such as how the route of administration affects drug absorption and distribution, are discussed in Chapter 4. Certain protocols and techniques are common to all methods of drug administration. The student should refer to the drug administration guidelines in the following list before reading about specific routes of administration in Table 3.3 ◆.

enteral = *ingestion*
topical = *surface*
parenteral = *equivalent to ingestion (as, for example, by intravenous route)*

- Review the medication order and check for drug allergies.
- Wash hands and put on gloves, if indicated.
- Use aseptic technique when preparing and administering medications.
- Identify the patient by asking the person to state his or her full name (or by asking the parent or guardian if the patient is confused), checking the patient's identification band, and comparing this information with the MAR.

- Ask the patient about known allergies, and check to see if he or she is wearing an allergy identification band.
- Ensure that the proper equipment and supplies, such as water and cups, are available at the bedside.
- Tell the patient what drug you are administering, the purpose of the drug, and how you will give it.
- Position the patient for the appropriate route of administration.
- If the drug is prepackaged as a unit dose, remove it from the packaging at the bedside.
- Unless specifically instructed to do so in the orders, do not leave drugs at the patient's bedside.
- Document the medication administration and any important patient responses on the MAR.

TABLE 3.3 Enteral Drug Administration	
Drug Form	**Administration Guidelines**
A. Tablet, capsule, or liquid	1. Assist the patient into a sitting position.
	2. Check to be sure that the patient is alert and can swallow.
	3. Place tablets or capsules into a medication cup.
	4. If the medication is liquid, shake the bottle to mix the agent, and measure the dose into the cup at eye level.
	5. Hand the patient the medication cup.
	6. Offer a glass of water to facilitate swallowing the medication. Milk or juice may be offered (if not contraindicated).
	7. Remain with the patient until all medication is swallowed.
B. Sublingual	1. Check that the patient is alert and can hold the medication under the tongue.
	2. Instruct the patient not to chew or swallow the tablet, or move it around with the tongue.
	3. Instruct the patient to allow the tablet to dissolve completely before swallowing saliva.
	4. Place the sublingual tablet under the patient's tongue.
	5. Remain with the patient to make sure that all of the medication has dissolved.
	6. Offer the patient a glass of water.
C. Buccal	1. Check that the patient is alert and can hold the medication between the gums and the cheek.
	2. Instruct the patient to allow the tablet to dissolve completely before swallowing saliva.
	3. Instruct the patient not to chew or swallow the tablet or move it around with the tongue.
	4. Place the buccal tablet between the gum line and the cheek.
	5. Remain with the patient to be sure that all of the medication has dissolved.
	6. Offer the patient a glass of water.
D. Nasogastric and gastrostomy	1. Administer liquid forms of the medication when possible to avoid clogging the tube.
	2. If the medication is solid, crush it into a fine powder and mix it thoroughly with at least 30 mL of warm water until dissolved. Undissolved medications may clog the tube.
	3. Turn off the feeding tube, if applicable.
	4. Verify tube placement. Verification can be done by testing the pH of stomach contents, by injecting 10–30 mL of air and listening with a stethoscope over the stomach area, or (the most reliable way) by x-ray.
	5. Attach a syringe (30 or 60 mL) with plunger. Aspirate the patient's stomach contents and measure the volume. This is termed the *gastric residual volume*. If it is greater than 100 mL (for an adult), check the facility's policy.
	6. Attach the syringe without plunger. Return the residual contents by allowing it to flow back into the tube via gravity. Flush the tube with about 10 mL (two teaspoons) of tap water. Amount of water may vary according to institutional policy or healthcare provider's order.
	7. Pour the medication into the syringe barrel, also allowing it to flow into the tube by gravity. Give each medication separately, flushing between each with water.
	8. Keep the head of the bed elevated at 45° angle for one hour to prevent aspiration.
	9. Reestablish continual feeding, as scheduled.

Enteral drugs are given orally or via nasogastric or gastrostomy tubes.

The **enteral route** includes drugs given orally and those administered through nasogastric (NG) or gastrostomy tubes. Oral drug administration (abbreviated PO, which refers to the Latin *per os*, meaning "by mouth") is the most common, most convenient, and usually the least costly of all routes. It is also considered the safest route because the skin's protective barrier is not broken. In cases of overdose, medications remaining in the stomach can be retrieved by causing vomiting. Oral preparations are available in tablet, capsule, caplet, and liquid forms. Medications administered by the enteral route take advantage of the large absorptive surfaces of the oral mucosa, stomach, or small intestine.

Tablets and Capsules

Tablets and capsules are the most common forms of drugs. Patients prefer tablets or capsules over other forms because they are easy to use. In some cases, tablets may be scored so they can easily be broken if the dose needs to be made smaller for a specific patient. **Orally disintegrating tablets (ODTs)** are a newer type of drug formulation that allows for quick dissolving and absorption of medications in the mouth or cheek. This approach is especially beneficial to patients who have difficulty swallowing (e.g., pediatric and geriatric patients) and for noncompliant patients (e.g., patients with psychiatric disorders).

The nurse should always check the manufacturer's instructions for administering the medication to be sure that crushing or opening is allowed. Some tablets and capsules should not be crushed or opened because their ingredients are inactivated by doing so. Other medications can severely irritate the stomach mucosa and cause nausea or vomiting. Occasionally, drugs should not be crushed because they irritate the oral mucosa, are extremely bitter, or contain dyes that stain the teeth. Most drug guides provide lists of drugs that may not be crushed. Guidelines for administering tablets or capsules are given in Table 3.3A.

The strongly acidic contents in the stomach can destroy some medications. To overcome this problem, tablets may have a hard, waxy coating that protects the medicine from acidity. These **enteric-coated** tablets are designed to dissolve in the alkaline environment of the small intestine. It is important that the nurse not crush enteric-coated tablets because the medication would then be directly exposed to the stomach environment.

Studies have clearly shown that patients are less compliant when they must take more than one dose of medicine per day, particularly if the number is three doses or more. With this in mind, pharmacologists have tried to design new drugs that need to be administered only once or twice daily. **Sustained-release** tablets or capsules are designed to dissolve very slowly. They release medication over a longer time, which increases the drug's duration of action (or length of time the medication works). Also called *extended-release (ER)*, *long-acting (LA)*, or *slow-release (SR) medications*, these forms allow convenient once or twice daily dosing. These sustained-release medications must not be crushed or opened.

Giving medications by the oral route has some disadvantages. The patient must be conscious and able to swallow properly. In addition, children and some adults do not like to swallow large tablets and capsules or take oral medications that are distasteful. Certain types of drugs, including proteins, are inactivated by digestive enzymes in the stomach and small intestine. Medications absorbed from the stomach and small intestine first travel to the liver, where they may be inactivated before they ever reach their target organs. This process, called *first-pass metabolism*, is discussed in Chapter 4. The significant variation in the motility of the GI tract among patients and in the tract's ability to absorb medications can create differences in bioavailability.

Sublingual and Buccal Drug Administration

For sublingual and buccal administration, the patient does not swallow the tablet but instead keeps it in the mouth until it dissolves. The mucosa of the oral cavity contains a rich blood supply that provides an excellent absorptive surface for certain drugs. Medications given by this route are not destroyed by digestive enzymes nor do they undergo first-pass metabolism in the liver.

For the **sublingual (SL) route**, the medication is placed under the tongue and allowed to dissolve slowly. The rich blood supply under the tongue results in a rapid onset of drug action. Sublingual dosage forms are most often formulated as rapidly disintegrating tablets or as soft gelatin capsules filled with liquid drug.

When multiple drugs have been ordered, the sublingual preparations should be administered after the oral medications have been swallowed. The patient should be instructed not to move the drug with the tongue, nor to eat or drink anything until the medication has completely dissolved. The sublingual mucosa is not suitable for extended-release formulations because it is a relatively small area and is constantly being bathed by saliva. Table 3.3B and Figure 3.1a ■ present important points about sublingual drug administration.

To administer by the **buccal route**, the tablet, capsule, lozenge, or troche is placed in the oral cavity between the gum and the cheek. The patient must be instructed not to touch the medication with the tongue, because it could get moved to the sublingual area where it would be more rapidly absorbed or to the back of the throat where it could be swallowed. Medications are absorbed more slowly from the buccal mucosa than from the sublingual area. The buccal route is preferred over the sublingual route for sustained-release delivery because of its greater mucosal surface area. Drugs formulated for buccal administration generally do not cause irritation and are small enough to not cause discomfort to the patient. Table 3.3C and Figure 3.1b ■ provide important guidelines for buccal drug administration.

▶ **Life Span Fact**

For children and elderly patients, as well as those who may have trouble swallowing, the nurse can sometimes crush tablets or open capsules and sprinkle the drug over food or mix it with juice to make it easier to swallow and to hide its taste.

FIGURE 3.1

(a) Sublingual (under the tongue) drug administration;
(b) buccal (between the gums and cheek) drug administration.

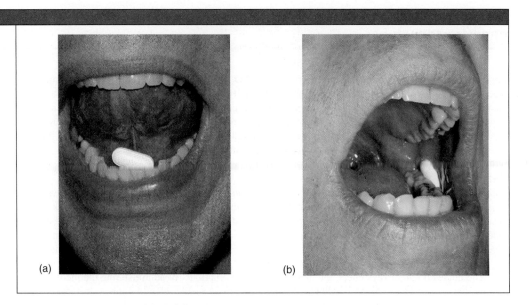

(a)   (b)

Nasogastric and Gastrostomy Drug Administration

Patients with a nasogastric (NG) tube or enteral feeding system such as a gastrostomy (G) tube may have their medications administered through these devices. The soft, flexible NG tube is inserted by way of the nasopharynx or oropharynx, with the tip lying in the stomach. A G tube is surgically placed directly into the patient's stomach. Generally, the NG tube is used for short-term treatment, whereas the G tube is inserted for patients who require long-term care. Drugs administered through these tubes are usually in liquid form. Although solid drugs can be crushed or dissolved, they tend to clog the tubes. Sustained-release drugs should not be crushed and administered through NG or G tubes. Drugs administered by this route are exposed to the same physiologic processes as those given orally. If a drug is ordered to be given through either tube, and the drug should not be crushed, the nurse will need to contact the healthcare practitioner for an appropriate replacement medication. Table 3.3D gives important guidelines for administering drugs through NG or G tubes.

CORE CONCEPT 3.8

Topical drugs are applied locally to the skin and associated membranes.

The **topical route** involves applying drugs locally to the skin or the membranous linings of the eye, ear, nose, respiratory tract, urinary tract, vagina, and rectum. These applications include the following:

- *Dermatologic preparations* These drugs are applied to the skin using formulations that include creams, lotions, gels, powders, and sprays. The skin is the most common topical route.

- *Instillations and irrigations* These drugs are applied into body cavities or orifices, including the eyes, ears, nose, urinary bladder, rectum, and vagina.

- *Inhalations* Inhalers, nebulizers, or positive-pressure breathing apparatuses are used to apply drugs to the respiratory tract. The most common indication for inhaled drugs is bronchoconstriction due to bronchitis or asthma. Many illegal, abused drugs are taken by this route because it provides a very rapid onset of drug action.

Drugs can be applied topically to produce a local or a systemic effect. Many drugs are applied topically to produce a local effect. For example, antibiotics may be applied to the skin to treat skin infections. Antineoplastic agents may be infused into the urinary bladder via catheter to treat tumors of the bladder mucosa. Corticosteroids are sprayed into the nostrils to reduce inflammation of the nasal mucosa due to allergic rhinitis. Local, topical delivery of these drugs produces fewer side effects than oral or parenteral delivery of the same drugs. When these drugs are given topically, they are absorbed very slowly, and only small amounts reach the general circulation.

Other drugs are given topically to ensure slow release and absorption of the drug in the general circulation. These agents are given for their systemic (system-wide) effects. For example, a nitroglycerin patch is not applied to the skin to treat a local skin condition, but to treat the systemic condition of coronary artery disease. Likewise, prochlorperazine (Compazine) suppositories are inserted rectally not to treat a disease of the rectum but to alleviate nausea. The distinction between topical drugs given for local effects and those given for systemic effects is an important one for the nurse to know. In the case of local drugs, absorption is undesirable and may cause side effects. For systemic drugs, absorption is necessary for the therapeutic action of the drug. With either type of topical agent, drugs should not be applied to abraded or denuded skin, unless the directions so indicate.

Transdermal Delivery System

Transdermal patches are an effective means of delivering certain medications. Examples include nitroglycerin for angina pectoris and scopolamine (Transderm-Scop) for motion sickness. Although transdermal patches contain a specific amount of drug, the rate of delivery and the actual dose received may vary. Patches are changed on a regular basis, using a site rotation routine, which should be documented in the MAR. Before applying a transdermal patch, the nurse should verify that the previous patch has been removed and disposed off appropriately. Drugs to be administered by this route avoid the first-pass effect in the liver and bypass digestive enzymes.Table 3.4A ◆ and Figure 3.2 ■ illustrate the major points of transdermal drug delivery.

Ophthalmic Administration

The ophthalmic route is used to treat local conditions of the eye and surrounding structures. Common indications include excessive dryness, infections, glaucoma, and dilation of the pupil during eye examinations. Ophthalmic drugs are available in the form of eye irrigations, drops, ointments, and medicated disks. Figure 3.3 ■ and Table 3.4B give guidelines for adult administration.

FIGURE 3.2

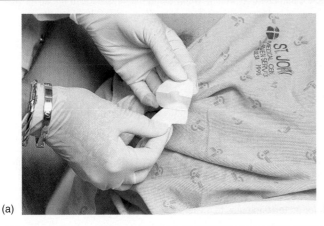 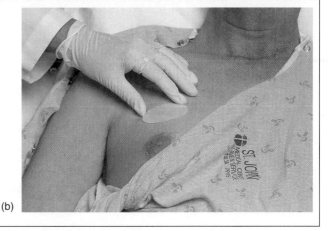

(a)   (b)

Transdermal patch administration: Put on gloves before handling the patch and read the manufacturer's directions. Label the patch with the date and time, and your initials. Remove any previous medication or patch, and cleanse the area. (a) Remove the protective coating from the patch and (b) apply the patch immediately to clean, dry, hairless skin.

FIGURE 3.3

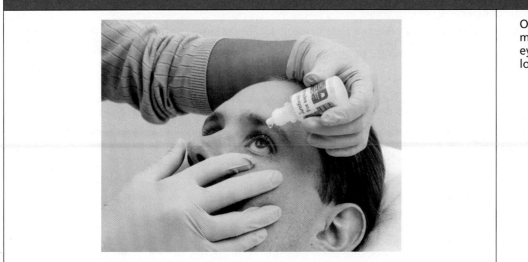

Ophthalmic drug administration: Instilling eye drops into the lower conjunctival sac.

TABLE 3.4	Topical Drug Administration
Drug Form	**Administration Guidelines**
A. Transdermal	**1.** Obtain the transdermal patch and read the manufacturer's guidelines. The application site and frequency of changing differ according to medication. **2.** Put on gloves before handling the patch to avoid absorbing any medication. **3.** Label the patch with the date, time, and your initials. **4.** Remove the previous medication or patch, and cleanse the area. **5.** If using a transdermal ointment, apply the ordered amount of medication in an even line directly on the premeasured paper that accompanies the medication tube. **6.** Press the patch or apply the medicated paper to clean, dry, and hairless skin. **7.** Rotate the sites to prevent skin irritation.
B. Ophthalmic	**1.** Instruct the patient to lie supine or sit with the head slightly tilted back. **2.** With your nondominant hand, pull the patient's lower lid down gently to expose the conjunctival sac, creating a pocket. **3.** Ask the patient to look upward. **4.** Hold the eyedropper 1/4 to 1/8 inch above the conjunctival sac. Do not hold the dropper over the patient's eye because this may stimulate the blink reflex. **5.** Instill the prescribed number of drops into the center of the pocket. Avoid touching the eye or conjunctival sac with the tip of the eyedropper. **6.** If applying ointment, follow steps 1–3, then apply a thin line of ointment evenly along the inner edge of the lower lid margin, from inner to outer canthus. **7.** Instruct the patient to gently close the eye. Apply gentle pressure with your finger to the nasolacrimal duct at the inner canthus for one to two minutes to avoid overflow drainage into the nose and throat. This minimizes the risk of absorption into the systemic circulation. **8.** With a tissue, remove the excess medication from around the patient's eye. **9.** Replace the dropper. Do not rinse the eyedropper.
C. Otic	**1.** Instruct the patient to lie on his or her side or to sit with the head tilted so that the affected ear is facing up. **2.** If necessary, use a clean washcloth to clean the pinna of the ear and the meatus to prevent any discharge from being washed into the ear canal during the instillation of the drops. **3.** Hold the dropper 1/4 inch above the ear canal, and instill the prescribed number of drops into the side of the ear canal, allowing the drops to flow downward. Avoid placing the drops directly on the tympanic membrane. **4.** Gently apply intermittent pressure to the tragus of the ear three or four times. **5.** Instruct the patient to remain on his or her side for up to 10 minutes to prevent loss of medication. **6.** If cotton ball is ordered, follow steps 1–2, then presoak with medication and insert it into the outermost part of ear canal. **7.** Wipe off any solution that may have dripped from the ear canal with a tissue.
D. Nasal drops	**1.** Ask the patient to blow his or her nose to clear the nasal passages. Have the patient lie supine. **2.** Draw up the correct volume of drug into the dropper. **3.** Instruct the patient to open and breathe through the mouth. **4.** Hold the tip of the dropper just above the patient's nostril, and without touching the nose with the dropper, direct the solution laterally toward the midline of the superior concha of the ethmoid bone—not at the base of the nasal cavity, where it will run down the throat and into the eustachian tube. **5.** Ask the patient to remain in this position for five minutes. **6.** Discard any remaining solution that is in the dropper.
E. Vaginal	**1.** Instruct the patient to assume a dorsal recumbent position with her knees bent and separated. **2.** Put on gloves; open the suppository and lubricate the rounded end of the suppository and the gloved forefinger of your dominant hand with a water-soluble lubricant. **3.** Expose the vaginal orifice by separating the labia with your nondominant hand. **4.** Insert the rounded end of the suppository about 8–10 cm along the posterior wall of the vagina, or as far as it will pass. **5.** If using a cream, jelly, or foam, gently insert the applicator 5 cm along the posterior vaginal wall and slowly push the plunger until empty. Remove the applicator and place on a paper towel. **6.** Ask the patient to lower her legs and remain lying in the dorsal recumbent position for five to ten minutes following insertion. Offer the patient a perineal pad.

TABLE 3.4 Topical Drug Administration (*continued*)	
Drug Form	**Administration Guidelines**
F. Rectal suppositories	**1.** Instruct the patient to lie on the left side (Sims' position). **2.** Put on gloves; open the suppository and lubricate the rounded end. **3.** Lubricate the gloved forefinger of your dominant hand with water-soluble lubricant. **4.** Inform the patient when the suppository is to be inserted; instruct the patient to take slow, deep breaths and deeply exhale during insertion to relax the anal sphincter. **5.** Gently insert the lubricated end of the suppository into the rectum, beyond the anal-rectal ridge to ensure retention. **6.** Instruct the patient to remain in the Sims' position or lie supine to prevent expulsion of the suppository. **7.** Instruct the patient to retain the suppository for at least 30 minutes to allow absorption, unless the suppository is administered to stimulate defecation.

Otic Administration

The otic route is used to treat local conditions of the ear, including infections and soft blockages of the auditory canal. Otic medications include eardrops and irrigations, which are usually ordered for cleaning. Figure 3.4 ■ and Table 3.4C present key points in administering otic medications.

Nasal Administration

The nasal route, a **transmucosal** method of drug delivery, is used for both local and systemic drug administration. The nasal mucosa provides an excellent absorptive surface for certain medications. Advantages of this route include ease of use and avoidance of the first-pass effect in the liver and the digestive enzymes. Nasal spray formulations of corticosteroids have revolutionized the treatment of allergic rhinitis because the medication is very safe when administered by this route.

Although the nasal mucosa provides an excellent surface for drug delivery, there is the potential for damage to the cilia within the nasal cavity, and mucosal irritation is common. In addition, unpredictable mucous secretion in some individuals may affect drug absorption from this site.

Drops or sprays are often used for their local **astringent effect**, which is to shrink swollen mucous membranes or to loosen secretions and facilitate drainage. This brings immediate relief from the nasal congestion caused by the common cold. The nose also provides the route to reach the nasal sinuses and the eustachian tube. Proper positioning of the patient prior to giving nose drops for sinus disorders depends on which sinuses are being treated. The same holds true for treatment of the eustachian tube. Table 3.4D and Figure 3.5 ■ illustrate important facts related to nasal drug administration.

Vaginal Administration

The vaginal route is used to deliver medications for treating local infections and to relieve vaginal pain and itching. Vaginal medications are inserted as suppositories, creams, jellies, or foams. It is important that the

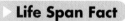

▶ **Life Span Fact**

Administration of otic drugs to infants and young children must be performed carefully to avoid injury to sensitive structures of the ear. Otic drops should be at room temperature before adding them to the ear. When giving otic drugs to young children, gently pull the pinna down and back. When giving otic drugs to older children and adults, gently pull the pinna down and forward.

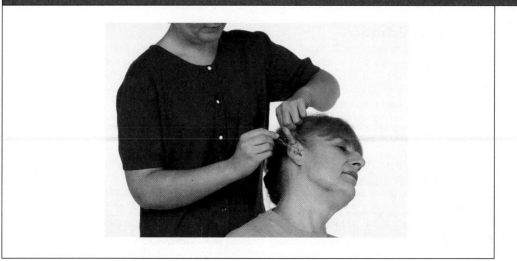

FIGURE 3.4

Otic drug administration: Instilling eardrops.
Source: Andy Crawford/Dorling Kindersley

FIGURE 3.5

Nasal drug
administration.

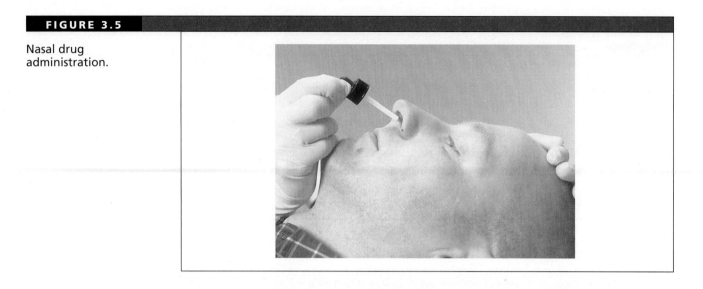

FIGURE 3.6

Vaginal drug adminis-
tration: (a) instilling a
vaginal suppository;
(b) using an applicator
to instill a vaginal cream.

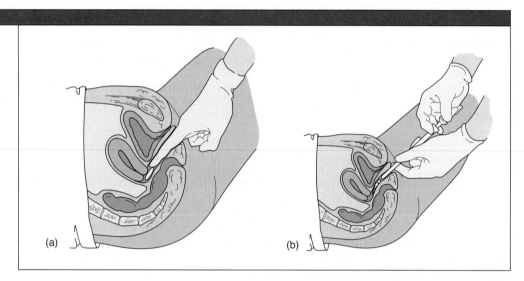

(a)   (b)

nurse explains the purpose of treatment and provides privacy for the patient. Before inserting vaginal drugs, the nurse should instruct the patient to empty her bladder. This lessens both discomfort during treatment and the possibility of irritating or injuring the vaginal lining. The patient should be offered a perineal pad following administration. Table 3.4E and Figure 3.6 ■ provide guidelines regarding vaginal drug administration.

Rectal Administration

The rectal route may be used for either local or systemic drug administration. It is a safe and effective means of delivering drugs to patients who are comatose or who are experiencing nausea and vomiting. Rectal drugs are normally in suppository form, although a few laxatives and diagnostic agents are given via enema. Although absorption is slower than by other routes, it is steady and reliable as long as the medication can be retained by the patient. Venous blood from the lower rectum is not transported by way of the liver. Therefore, the first-pass effect is avoided, as are the digestive enzymes of the upper GI tract. Table 3.4F gives details about rectal drug administration.

Parenteral administration refers to dispensing medications by routes other than oral or topical.

CORE CONCEPT 3.9

The **parenteral route** delivers drugs via a needle into the skin layers, subcutaneous tissue, muscles, or veins, with the needle inserted at different degrees, depending on the type of injection, as shown in Figure 3.7 ■. More advanced parenteral delivery includes administration into arteries, body cavities (such as intrathecal), and organs (such as intracardiac). Parenteral drug administration is much more invasive (meaning that the delivery method "invades" the barrier that the skin provides to protect the body) than topical or enteral administration. Because of the possibility of introducing pathogenic microbes directly into the blood or body tissues, aseptic techniques must be strictly used. The nurse is expected to identify and use appropriate materials for parenteral drug delivery, including specialized equipment and techniques involved in the preparation and administration of injectable products. The nurse must know the correct anatomical locations for parenteral administration and safety procedures regarding hazardous equipment disposal.

FIGURE 3.7

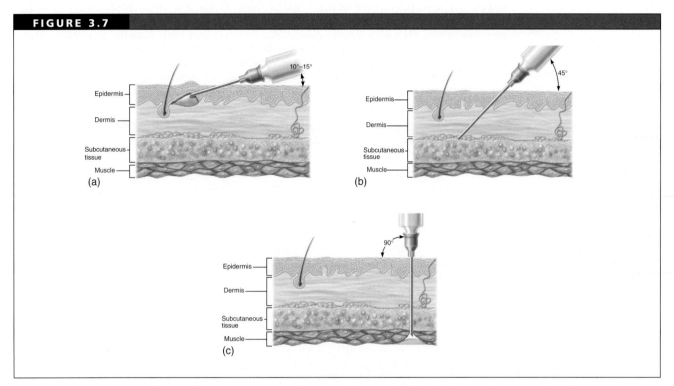

Parenteral drug administration: Gloves are worn at all times. (a) Intradermal administration is into the dermis at a 10–15° angle. See Figure 3.8. (b) Subcutaneous administration is into the subcutaneous tissue at a 45° angle. See Figure 3.9. (c) During intramuscular administration, a drug is injected into the muscle at a 90° angle. See Figure 3.10. Intravenous drug administration (not shown here) is given directly into the bloodstream.

Intradermal and Subcutaneous Administration

Injection into the skin delivers drugs to the blood vessels that supply the layers of the skin. Drugs may be injected either intradermally or subcutaneously. The major difference between these methods is the depth of injection, which is controlled by the angle of needle placement (see Figure 3.7). An advantage of both methods is that they offer a means of administering drugs to patients who are unable to take them orally. Drugs administered by these routes also avoid the first-pass effect in the liver and the digestive enzymes. Disadvantages are that only small volumes can be administered, and injections can cause pain and swelling at the injection site.

An **intradermal (ID) route** injection is administered into the dermis layer of the skin. Because the dermis contains more blood vessels than the deeper subcutaneous layer, drugs are more easily absorbed. This route is usually used for allergy and disease screening or for local anesthetic delivery prior to venous cannulation. Only very small volumes of drug, usually 0.1 to 0.2 mL, can be given by ID injections. The usual sites for ID injections are the nonhairy skin surfaces of the upper back, over the scapulae, the high upper chest, and the anterior forearm. Guidelines for intradermal injections are given in Table 3.5A ◆ and Figure 3.8 ■.

A **subcutaneous (SC or SQ) route** injection is delivered to the deepest layers of the skin. Insulin, heparin, vitamins, some vaccines, and other medications are given in this area because the sites are easy to reach and provide rapid absorption. Body sites that are ideal for subcutaneous injections include the following:

- Posterior upper arm (above the triceps muscle)
- Middle two thirds of the anterior thigh area

- Subscapular areas of the upper back
- Upper dorsogluteal and ventrogluteal areas
- Abdominal areas, above the iliac crest and below the diaphragm, 2 inches out from the umbilicus

Subcutaneous doses are small in volume, usually ranging from 0.5 to 1 mL, and are given at a 45° (normal weight patient) to 90° angle (obese patient). The needle size varies with the patient's quantity of body fat but is usually 1/2 to 5/8 inch. The needle length is usually one-half the size of a pinched skin fold that can be grasped between the thumb and forefinger. Insulin is administered using a special syringe that has "unit" markings made specifically for insulin. Tuberculin syringes (TB) are 1 mL syringes and are typically used when administering other medications less than 1 mL. Note that tuberculin syringes and insulin syringes are not interchangeable and should not be substituted for each other. It is important to rotate injection sites in an orderly and documented manner, to promote absorption, minimize tissue damage, and alleviate discomfort. For insulin, rotation should be within an anatomical area that promotes reliable absorption and maintains consistent blood glucose levels.

TABLE 3.5   Parenteral Drug Administration

Drug Form	Administration Guidelines
A. Intradermal route	1. Prepare the medication in a tuberculin or 1 mL syringe, using a 25–27 gauge, 3/8–5/8 inch needle. 2. Put on gloves and cleanse the injection site with an antiseptic swab, using a circular motion. Allow the site to air dry. 3. With the thumb and index finger of your nondominant hand, spread the patient's skin taut. 4. Insert the needle, with the bevel facing upward, at a 10°–15° angle. 5. Advance the needle until the entire bevel is under the skin; do not aspirate. 6. Slowly inject the medication to form a small wheal or bleb (small raised area). 7. Withdraw the needle quickly, and pat the site gently with a sterile 2 × 2 gauze pad. Do not massage the area. 8. Instruct the patient not to rub or scratch the area.
B. Subcutaneous route	1. Prepare the medication in a 1–3 mL syringe using a 23–25 gauge, 1/2–5/8 inch needle. For heparin, the recommended needle is 3/8 inch and 25–26 gauge. 2. Choose the site, avoiding bony areas, major nerves, and blood vessels. For heparin, check your facility's policy for the preferred injection sites. 3. Check the previous rotation sites and select a new area for injection. 4. Put on gloves and cleanse the injection site with an antiseptic swab using a circular motion. 5. Allow the site to air dry. 6. Pinch/lift the skin between the thumb and index finger of your nondominant hand. 7. Insert the needle at 45° or 90° angle, depending on the patient's body size and the length of the needle you are using: 90° angle for obese patients; 45° angle for average-weight patients. 8. Check facility policy on aspiration of subcutaneous injections. If policy allows, aspirate by gently pulling back on the plunger. If blood appears, withdraw the needle, discard the syringe, and prepare a new injection. *Do not aspirate heparin, low molecular weight heparin, or insulin.* 9. Inject the medication slowly. 10. Remove the needle quickly. Gently massage the site with an antiseptic swab. *Do not massage the site after injecting heparin or low molecular weight heparin because tissue damage may occur.*
C. Intramuscular route: ventrogluteal site	1. Prepare the medication using a 20–23 gauge, 1.5 inch needle. (Needle size may vary depending on the site and patient size.) 2. Put on gloves and cleanse the injection site with an antiseptic swab using a circular motion. Allow the site to air dry. 3. Locate the site by placing your hand with the heel on the greater trochanter and your thumb pointing toward the umbilicus. Point to the anterior iliac spine with your index finger, spreading your middle finger to point toward the iliac crest (forming a V). Injection of medication is given within the V-shaped area between the index and third finger. 4. Insert the needle with a smooth, dart-like movement at a 90° angle within the V-shaped area. 5. Aspirate and observe for blood. If blood appears, withdraw the needle, discard the syringe, and prepare a new injection. 6. Inject the medication slowly and with smooth, even pressure on the plunger. 7. Remove the needle quickly. 8. Apply pressure to the site with a dry, sterile 2 × 2 gauze and gently massage to promote absorption of the medication into the muscle.

TABLE 3.5 Parenteral Drug Administration (*continued*)

Drug Form	Administration Guidelines

D. Intravenous route	**1.** To add a drug to an IV fluid container:
	  a. Verify the order and compatibility of the drug with the IV fluid.
	  b. Prepare the medication in a 5–20 mL syringe using a 1–1.5 inch, 19–21 gauge needle.
	  c. Put on your gloves and assess the injection site for signs of inflammation or extravasation (oozing of tissue).
	  d. Locate the medication port on the IV fluid container and cleanse it with an antiseptic swab.
	  e. Carefully insert the needle or access device into the port and inject the medication.
	  f. Withdraw the needle and mix the solution by rotating the container end to end.
	  g. Hang the container and check the infusion rate.
	2. To administer an IV bolus (IV push) using an existing IV line or IV lock (reseal):
	  a. Verify the order and compatibility of the drug with the IV fluid.
	  b. Determine the correct rate of infusion.
	  c. Determine if IV fluids are infusing at the proper rate (IV line) and that the IV site is adequate.
	  d. Prepare the drug in a syringe with a 19–21 gauge needle.
	  e. Put on your gloves and assess the IV insertion site for signs of inflammation or extravasation (oozing of fluid within the tissue).
	  f. Select an injection port on the tubing that is closest to the insertion site (IV line).
	  g. Cleanse the tubing or lock port with an antiseptic swab and insert the needle into the port.
	  h. If administering medication through an existing IV line, occlude the tubing by pinching it just above the injection port.
	  i. Slowly inject the medication over the designated time (which is not usually faster than 1 mL/min, unless otherwise specified).
	  j. Withdraw the syringe. Release the tubing and ensure the proper IV infusion if using an existing IV line.
	  k. If using an IV lock, check your facility's policy for use of saline flush before and after injecting medications.

FIGURE 3.8

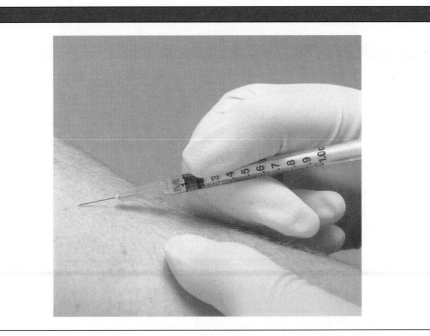

Intradermal drug administration: The needle is inserted, bevel up, at 10–15° angle.

When performing subcutaneous injections, it is usually not necessary to aspirate prior to the injection. It depends on what is being injected and the patient's anatomy. Aspiration might prevent inadvertent administration into a vein or artery in a thin person. Heparin and low molecular weight heparin, such as enoxaparin (Lovenox) should never be aspirated because of the drug's anticoagulant properties. Aspiration can cause bleeding, bruising and possible damage to the surrounding tissue. Massage after injection is also not recommended for the same reasons. Table 3.5B and Figure 3.9 ■ include important information regarding subcutaneous drug administration.

Intramuscular Administration

An **intramuscular (IM) route** injection delivers medication into specific muscles. Because muscle tissue has a rich blood supply, medication moves quickly into blood vessels to produce a more rapid onset of action than with oral, ID, or SC administration. The anatomical structure of muscle permits this tissue to receive a larger volume of medication than the subcutaneous region. An adult with well-developed muscles can safely tolerate up to 5 mL of medication in a large muscle, although only 2 to 3 mL is recommended. The deltoid and triceps muscles should receive a maximum of 1 mL.

A major consideration for the nurse regarding IM drug administration is the selection of an appropriate injection site. Injection sites must be located away from bones, large blood vessels, and nerves. Both the size and length of the needle are determined by body size and muscle mass, the type of drug to be administered, the amount of adipose (fat) tissue overlying the muscle, and the age of the patient. Information regarding IM injections is given in Table 3.5C and Figure 3.10 ■. The four common sites for IM injections are as follows:

- *Ventrogluteal site* This area provides the greatest thickness of gluteal muscles, contains no large blood vessels or nerves, is sealed off by bone, and contains less fat than the buttock area, thus eliminating the need to determine the depth of subcutaneous fat.
- *Deltoid site* Used in well-developed teens and adults for volumes of medication not to exceed 1 mL.
- *Dorsogluteal site* Used for adults and for children who have been walking for at least six months. The site is safe as long as the nurse appropriately locates the injection landmarks to avoid puncture or irritation of the sciatic nerve and blood vessels.
- *Vastus lateralis site* Usually thick and well developed in both adults and children, the middle third of the muscle is the site for IM injections.

> ▶ **Life Span Fact**
>
> The vastus lateralis is the site of choice for IM injections in pediatric patients.

FIGURE 3.9

Subcutaneous drug administration: Skin is pinched, and depending on amount of subcutaneous tissue, needle is inserted at a 45° or 90° angle.

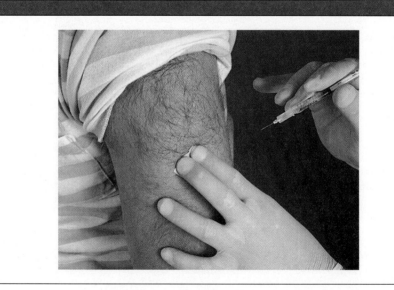

FIGURE 3.10

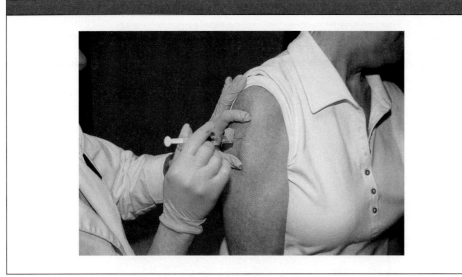

Intramuscular drug administration: Skin is spread taut between thumb and forefinger and the needle is inserted at a 90° angle.

Intravenous Administration

The **intravenous (IV) route** enables administration of medications and fluids directly into the bloodstream and allows their immediate availability for use by the body. The IV route is used when a very rapid onset of action is desired. Like other parenteral routes, IV medications bypass the enzymes of the digestive system and the first-pass effect of the liver. The three basic types of IV administration are as follows:

- *Large-volume infusion* This type of infusion is used for fluid maintenance, replacement, or supplementation. Compatible drugs may be mixed into a large-volume IV container with fluids such as normal saline or Ringer's lactate. Table 3.5D and Figure 3.11 ■ illustrate this technique.

- *Intermittent infusion* A small amount of IV solution is "piggy-backed" (added) to the primary large-volume infusion. This type of infusion, also illustrated in Figure 3.11, is used to give additional medications, such as antibiotics or analgesics over a short time.

- *IV bolus (push) administration* A concentrated single dose of medication is delivered directly to the circulation via syringe. Bolus injections may be given through an intermittent injection port or by direct IV push. Details on the bolus administration technique are given in Table 3.5D and Figure 3.12 ■.

Although the IV route provides the fastest onset of drug action, it is also the most dangerous. Once injected, the medication cannot be retrieved. If the drug solution or the needle is contaminated, pathogens have a direct route to the bloodstream and body tissues. Patients who are receiving IV injections must be closely monitored for adverse reactions. Some adverse reactions occur immediately after injection; others may take hours or days to appear. Antidotes for drugs that can cause potentially dangerous or fatal reactions must always be readily available. Several types of needleless IV systems are also available and have been shown to greatly reduce the chance of needlestick injuries among healthcare professionals.

SAFETY ALERT

Medication Administration Error–Mistaken Patient Identity

It is the responsibility of the nurse to check the patient's identification band, ask the patient to state name and date of birth, and verify that these pieces of information match those listed on the patient's medication administration record (MAR). Consider the evening nurse who entered Ms. Brown's room to administer medications. Ms. Brown was already in bed and asleep. The nurse gently shook her and said, "I have your 10 p.m. medication, Ms. Brown." Although the patient responded, she was not fully awake. She took the medication and quickly returned to sleep. Upon leaving, however, the nurse noticed the room number and realized that medication had just been given to Ms. Crown in the room next to Ms. Brown. This situation could have been avoided if the nurse had checked the ID band, asked the patient for identification information, and cross-checked the data against the MAR.

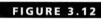

FIGURE 3.11

Administration of intravenous fluids: A large volume IV infusion bag with intermittent infusion bag "piggy-backed" into primary tubing.

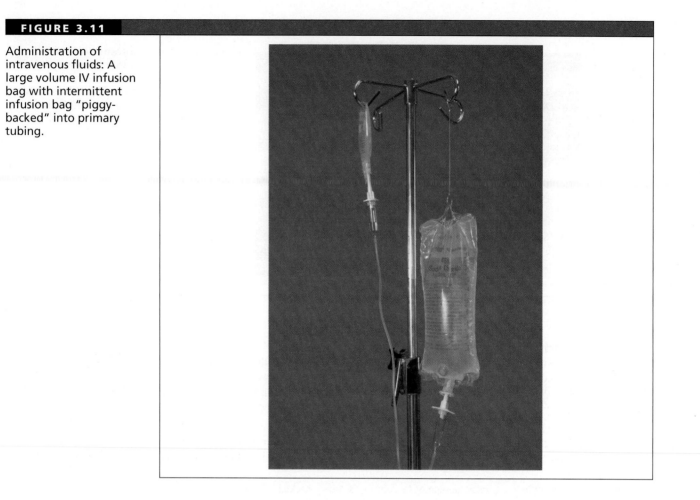

FIGURE 3.12

Injecting a medication by IV push.

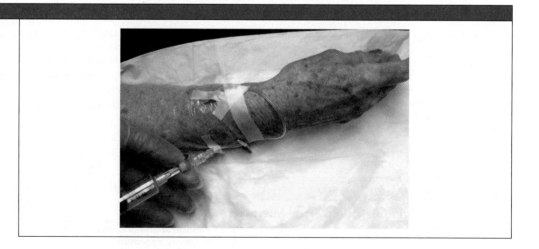

PATIENTS NEED TO KNOW

Patients need to know the following:

1. Always ask the healthcare provider or pharmacist which medications may be taken with food and water to reduce nausea and stomach irritation.
2. Do not crush, cut, or administer enteric-coated tablets with alkaline substances, such as antacids.
3. Establish a routine for taking medications by selecting a familiar time of the day, usually on the hour. Special organizers can be obtained to properly store medicines according to times, days, and dosages.
4. Follow the dosing times exactly. If a medication is missed, do not try to "catch up" on the next scheduled dose. If remembered soon after the scheduled time, it is appropriate to take the medicine. Otherwise, wait until the next scheduled dose. An exception would be if the next dose is not scheduled until the next day. For answers to specific questions, consult a healthcare provider.
5. Store medications in a safe, dry place. Discard them if they become old or outdated.
6. Use the measuring device provided by the drug manufacturer to take medications. Do not rely on kitchen utensils to judge the exact recommended dose.

CHAPTER REVIEW

CORE CONCEPTS SUMMARY

3.1 A major goal in pharmacotherapy is to limit the number and severity of adverse drug events.

Healthcare staff must be familiar with the general principles of drug delivery. The nurse must have a comprehensive knowledge of the actions and side effects of drugs before they are administered to limit the number and severity of adverse drugs events. Allergic and anaphylactic reactions are serious effects that must be carefully monitored and prevented, when possible.

3.2 The rights of drug administration form the basis of proper drug delivery.

The six rights and three checks are guidelines to safe drug administration, which involves a collaborative effort among nurses, physicians, and other healthcare professionals. The six rights are right patient, right medication, right dose, right route of administration, right time of delivery, and right documentation. The three checks are checking the MAR, checking the drug during preparation, and checking the drug before administering it to the patient.

3.3 Successful pharmacotherapy depends on patient compliance.

Pharmacologic compliance requires patients to understand and personally accept the value of the prescribed drug regimen. Understanding the reasons for noncompliance can help the healthcare team increase pharmacotherapeutic success.

3.4 Healthcare providers use accepted abbreviations to communicate the directions and times for drug administration.

There are established orders and time schedules by which medications are routinely administered. The single order (such as a preoperative order) is for a drug that is to be given only once and at a specific time. A prn order is administered as required by the patient's condition. Orders not written as single, STAT, or prn are called routine orders. A standing order is written in advance of a situation and is to be carried out under specific circumstances. Documenting drug administration and reporting side effects are important responsibilities of the nurse.

3.5 Three systems of measurement are used in pharmacology: metric, apothecary, and household.

Healthcare professionals must recognize dosages based on all three systems of measurement: the metric, apothecary, and household systems. The nurse must be able to convert between household and metric systems of measurement.

3.6 Certain protocols and techniques are common to all methods of drug administration.

The student should understand drug administration guidelines before proceeding to a study of specific drug administration routes. The three general routes of drug administration are enteral, topical, and parenteral.

3.7 Enteral drugs are given orally or via nasogastric or gastrostomy tubes.

Drugs administered via the enteral route are given orally or through nasogastric (NG) or gastrostomy (G) tubes. The enteral route is the most effective way to administer drugs.

3.8 Topical drugs are applied locally to the skin and associated membranes.

Topical drugs are applied locally to the skin or membranous linings of the eye, ear, nose, respiratory tract, urinary tract, vagina, and rectum.

3.9 Parenteral administration refers to dispensing medications by routes other than oral or topical.

Parenteral administration is the dispensing of medications via a needle, usually into the skin layers (ID), subcutaneous tissue (SC or SQ), muscles (IM), or veins (IV).

REVIEW QUESTIONS

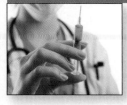

The following questions are written in NCLEX-PN® style. Answer these questions to assess your knowledge of the chapter material, and go back and review any material that is not clear to you.

1. A nurse enters the patient's room with medication along with a stethoscope, a fairly large-looking syringe, and container of water. In the course of administering the medication, the nurse will use all of these items. From your understanding of drug administration, which of the following routes will the nurse likely use?

1. Transdermal
2. Intravenous (parenteral)
3. Nasogastric (enteral)
4. Rectal

2. The nurse will not crush the extended-release medications ordered for his or her patient because:

1. They are very distasteful, and this reduces patient compliance.
2. Crushing alters the rate of absorption and medication delivery.
3. Multiple drug pieces cause obstructive symptoms.
4. Crushed oral medications have reduced bioavailability.

3. The reason why it is necessary to aspirate during an IM injection is to:

1. Avoid placement of the needle into a blood vessel.
2. Produce an air pocket for better drug distribution.
3. Avoid nerve puncture.
4. Remove air from the syringe.

4. Which of the following routes of drug administration has the fastest onset of action?

1. Transdermal
2. Intramuscular
3. Intravenous
4. Ophthalmic

5. After checking the doctor's orders, the nurse notes that the medication is to be given immediately. This type of order is a:

1. STAT order
2. Single order
3. prn order
4. Standing order

6. The nurse checks the label three times during the course of administering a medication: while getting the medication out of the container or drawer, before placing it into the medication cup, and before administering the medication or when placing the stock bottle back on the shelf. Of the "six rights of drug administration," this nurse is checking for the right:

1. Medication
2. Documentation
3. Patient
4. Time of delivery

7. When administering medications, the nurse's main responsibilities are to know and understand: (Select all that apply.)

1. The medication being ordered
2. The intended use of the medication
3. Any special considerations, such as the patient's age or pathophysiological state
4. Any possible side/adverse effects the medication may cause

8. Which information is not listed in the medication administration record (MAR)?

1. Date of medication administration
2. Route of drug administration
3. Dose of medication
4. Drug classification

9. The doctor ordered 5 mL of an oral decongestant twice a day for one of his or her pediatric patients. When teaching the mother of the patient about how much medication to give, the nurse tells her that 5 mL is equal to:

1. Two (2) teaspoons
2. One (1) tablespoon
3. 1/4 of a cup
4. One (1) teaspoon

10. The abbreviation "qod" was read in a patient's chart by a nursing student. The student knows that:

1. This abbreviation should not be used. Instead write out "every other day."
2. This abbreviation means "every hour."
3. The abbreviation should not be used. Instead, write out "nightly."
4. This abbreviation means "four times per day."

NOTE: Answers to the Review Questions appear in Appendix B. The complete rationales and answers are located on the textbook's website.

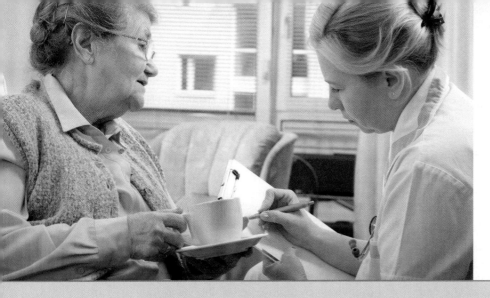

What Happens After a Drug Has Been Administered

CORE CONCEPTS

4.1 Pharmacokinetics focuses on what the body does to the drugs.

4.2 Absorption is the first step in drug transport.

4.3 Distribution refers to how drugs are transported throughout the body.

4.4 Metabolism is a process whereby drugs are made less or more active.

4.5 Excretion processes remove drugs from the body.

4.6 The rate of elimination and half-life characteristics influence drug responsiveness.

4.7 Pharmacodynamics focuses on what the drugs do to the body.

4.8 Drugs activate specific receptors to produce a response.

4.9 *Potency* and *efficacy* are terms often used to describe the success of drug therapy.

LEARNING OUTCOMES

After reading this chapter, the student should be able to:

1. Identify the four major processes of pharmacokinetics.

2. Discuss the factors affecting drug absorption.

3. Describe how plasma proteins affect drug distribution.

4. Explain the significance of the blood-brain barrier, blood-placental barrier, and blood-testicular barrier to drug therapy.

5. Explain the importance of the first-pass effect.

6. Describe how metabolic enzymes differ in younger and in older patients, and explain the significance of this difference to the success of drug therapy.

7. Explain how intermediate products of drug metabolism may produce more intense responses than the original drug.

8. Identify the major processes by which drugs are eliminated from the body.

9. Explain the importance of enterohepatic recirculation to drug therapy.

10. Explain how rate of elimination and plasma half-life ($t_{1/2}$) are related to the duration of drug action.

11. Discuss how successful pharmacotherapy depends on principles of pharmacodynamics.

12. Explain the significance of the receptor theory.

13. Describe how "blockers" of drug action work.

14. Compare and contrast the therapeutic terms *potency* and *efficacy*.

KEY TERMS

absorption (ab-SORP-shun) 43

agonists (AG-on-ists) 47

antagonists (an-TAG-oh-nists) 47

biotransformation (BEYE-oh-trans-for-MAY-shun) 43

distribution (dis-tree-BU-shun) 43

duration of drug action 46

efficacy (EFF-ik-ah-see) 47

enterohepatic recirculation (EN-ter-oh-HEE-pah-tik) 44

excretion (eks-KREE-shun) 44

first-pass effect 43

half-life ($t_{1/2}$) 45

metabolism (meh-TAHB-oh-liz-ehm) 43

minimum effective concentration 45

onset of drug action 45

peak plasma level 46

pharmacodynamics (FAR-mah-koh-deye-NAM-iks) 46

pharmacokinetics (FAR-mah-koh-kee-NET-iks) 42

potency (POH-ten-see) 47
prodrugs 43
receptor (ree-SEP-tor) 47

receptor theory 47
termination of drug
  action 46

therapeutic (THARE-ah-PEW-tick)
  range 45
toxic concentration 45

D rugs do not affect all patients the same way. Whether a drug achieves or falls short of achieving a therapeutic response is an important concern to patients and healthcare providers. Within a population, a dose of medication may produce a dramatic response in one patient while having no effect in another.

Many factors determine a drug's response. Patients sometimes take medications under conditions that interfere with drug activity. This interference is called a *drug interaction*. Food–drug interactions may occur when patients take their medication with food or beverages. Patients often take more than one medication at the same time. After drugs have been absorbed, the effectiveness of drug therapy may be altered by drug–drug interactions in the bloodstream.

To understand the impact that drug interactions have on drug safety and effectiveness, one must understand concepts from two important areas: pharmacokinetics and pharmacodynamics.

CORE CONCEPT 4.1

Pharmacokinetics focuses on what the body does to the drugs.

pharmaco = *drug related*
kinetics = *movement*

As the root words indicate, **pharmacokinetics** focuses on four processes: absorption, distribution, metabolism, and excretion, as shown in Figure 4.1 ■. A thorough knowledge of pharmacokinetics enables the healthcare provider to understand the therapeutic effects of a drug, as well as to predict potential adverse effects of drug therapy.

FIGURE 4.1

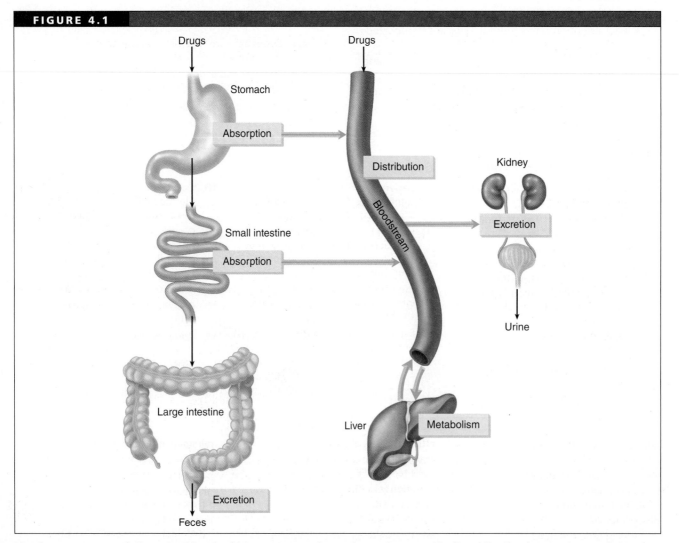

The four processes of pharmacokinetics (drug movement) are absorption, metabolism, distribution, and excretion.

Absorption is the first step in drug transport.

Absorption is the first step in how the body handles a drug. Absorption is a process involving the movement of a substance from its site of administration across one or more body membranes. A drug may be absorbed locally and produce a biologic effect at a remote site. Absorption may occur across the skin and associated mucous membranes, or drugs may move across membranes that line blood vessels. Ultimately, most drugs move across many membranes to reach their target cells. Many basic science textbooks cover the ways that foods and drugs are absorbed, including passive transport and energy-requiring transport processes. The presence of food in the digestive tract slows the absorption of drugs administered orally.

Distribution refers to how drugs are transported throughout the body.

Distribution is the process by which drugs are transported after they have been absorbed or administered directly into the bloodstream. Between the site of drug administration and the target tissue, many factors affect drug movement. One important example is the *binding* that occurs between drugs and other substances, such as plasma proteins, already present in the bloodstream. When a drug binds with a plasma protein such as albumin, the drug is held by the plasma protein in the bloodstream, where it is unable to reach its target cells. Often, a second drug will interfere with this binding by displacing the first drug from the plasma protein. In this case, the first drug's activity is intensified. The term *bioavailability* is often used to describe how much of a drug will be available after administration to produce a biological effect.

Even if a drug is not bound by plasma proteins, it still may not be able to reach all body tissues. Three important organs contain anatomic barriers that prevent some drugs from gaining access. These are the brain, the placenta, and the testes. Even though these organs have a larger blood supply compared to most other organs in the body, their cellular barriers only allow fat-soluble substances to cross. These special barriers are called the *blood-brain barrier*, *blood-placental barrier*, and *blood-testicular barrier*.

Some drugs are able to cross the blood-brain barrier without difficulty. These include antianxiety drugs, sedatives (sleep-inducing), and psychoactive (or mind-altering) drugs. Other medications, such as many antibiotics and anticancer medications, are absorbed easily in the intestinal tract but do not easily cross into the brain.

The blood-placental barrier serves an important protective function because it regulates which substances pass from the mother's bloodstream to the fetus. However, many potentially damaging agents such as cocaine and alcohol, and even some prescription or OTC medications, are not prevented from crossing this barrier. This is an extremely important issue. All food items and therapeutic drugs should be evaluated to assess their adverse effects on pregnant women and their unborn children, as discussed in Chapter 2. In males, the blood-testicular barrier prevents many drugs from reaching the testes, making it difficult to treat testicular disorders.

Metabolism is a process whereby drugs are made less or more active.

Metabolism is the next step in pharmacokinetics. It is often described as the total of all chemical reactions in the body. Metabolism occurs in almost every cell and organ—including the intestinal tract and kidneys—but the liver is the primary site. The individual chemical reactions of metabolism are called **biotransformation** reactions: They are the chemical conversion of drugs from one form to another that may result in increased or decreased activity. Metabolism is important to drug therapy because these chemical reactions deactivate most drugs. For this reason, patients with liver disease usually receive much lower doses than normal because their liver is unable to metabolize the drug to a safe, active form.

bio = *biologic*
transformation = *changing process*

Certain drugs called **prodrugs** require metabolism to make them active. In these cases, as the drug is broken down by chemical reactions of metabolism, the products formed by the breakdown produce a more intense response than does the original drug. An example of such a prodrug is sulfasalazine (Azulfidine), which is not active in its original form taken orally. Azulfidine is taken for the condition of ulcerative colitis. It is broken down by bacteria in the colon into two products that become active. Such cases of prodrugs are infrequent. Usually, metabolism is affected by the use of other drugs or the presence of other diseases.

pro = *before*
drug = *medication form*

An important mechanism that affects metabolism and drug action is the **first-pass effect**. Substances absorbed across the intestinal wall enter blood vessels known as the *hepatic portal circulation*, which carries blood directly to the liver (Figure 4.2 ■). Drugs administered orally are absorbed into the hepatic portal circulation and are taken directly to the liver for metabolism. The liver may then metabolize the drug to a less active form before it is distributed to the rest of the body and target organs. In some cases, this first-pass effect can inactivate more than 90% of an orally administered drug before it can reach the general circulation.

Many patients differ in how efficiently their metabolic enzymes work to metabolize drugs. Age, kidney and liver disease, genetics, and other factors can dramatically affect metabolism. Some patients metabolize drugs very slowly, others very quickly.

FIGURE 4.2

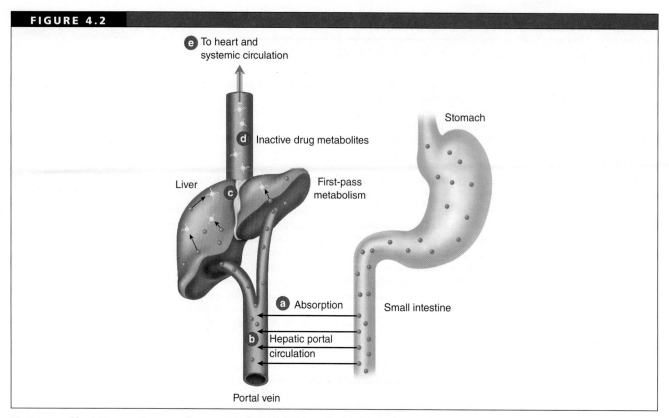

First-pass effect: Drugs given orally are absorbed (a) through the intestinal wall and enter the hepatic portal circulation (b). Absorbed drugs are taken directly to the liver (c) for metabolism (d) before reaching the heart and circulating throughout the rest of the body (e).

CORE CONCEPT 4.5	**Excretion processes remove drugs from the body.**

The last step of pharmacokinetics is **excretion**. Most substances that enter the body are removed by urination, exhalation, defecation, and/or sweating. Drugs are normally removed from the body by the kidneys, the respiratory tract, bile, or glandular activity.

The main organ of excretion is the kidney. The major role of the kidneys is to remove all nonnatural and harmful agents in the bloodstream while maintaining a balance of other natural substances. Most drugs are excreted by the kidneys. Therefore, kidney damage can significantly prolong drug action and is a common cause of adverse reactions. Drugs that affect the kidney and its filtration processes are presented in Chapter 17.

Drugs that are easily changed into gaseous form are especially suited for excretion by the respiratory system. The rate of respiratory excretion is dependent on the many factors that affect gas exchange, including diffusion, gas solubility, and blood flow. The greater the blood flow into lung capillaries, the greater the excretion. In contrast to other methods of excretion, the lungs excrete most drugs in their original unmetabolized form.

Some drugs are excreted through bile. However, most components of bile are circulated back to the liver by a process known as **enterohepatic recirculation**, as shown in Figure 4.3 ■. Recirculating drugs are then metabolized by the liver and excreted by the kidneys. The fraction of drug that is not recirculated continues on its way to the feces. Because of recirculation, elimination of drugs through bile may continue for several weeks after therapy has stopped, resulting in prolonged drug action.

Glands (other than the breast glands) that produce body fluids, such as saliva and sweat are less effective at excreting drugs. Most of the substances that are secreted in saliva and perspiration, such as urea or other waste products, are natural products. However, the breast glands can secrete any drug capable of crossing these membranes. Therefore, a breastfeeding mother should always check with her healthcare provider before taking any prescription drug, over-the-counter (OTC) drug, or natural alternative therapy.

▶ **Life Span Fact**

In general, metabolic enzyme activity is reduced in very young and in elderly patients. Therefore, pediatric and geriatric patients are usually more sensitive to medications than are other patients. Drug doses to the youngest and oldest age groups are often reduced to compensate for these differences.

Concept Review **4.1**

■ What does the term *pharmacokinetics* mean? Describe the four major parts of pharmacokinetics?

FIGURE 4.3

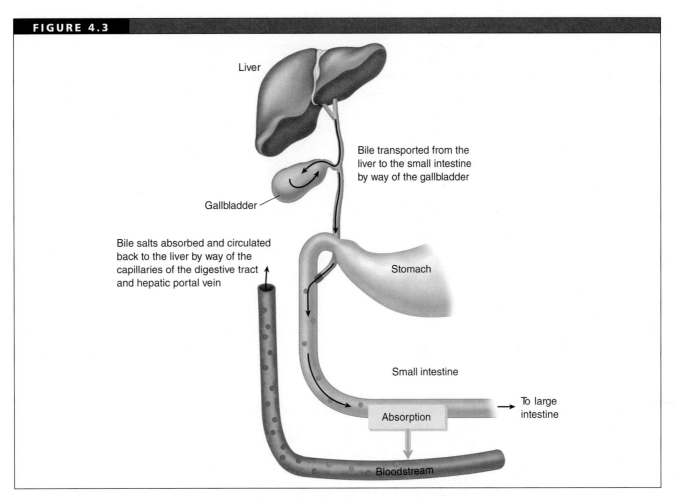

Liver

Bile transported from the
liver to the small intestine
by way of the gallbladder

Gallbladder

Bile salts absorbed and circulated
back to the liver by way of the
capillaries of the digestive tract
and hepatic portal vein

Stomach

Small intestine

To large
intestine

Absorption

Bloodstream

In the process of enterohepatic recirculation, bile is circulated back to the liver, where contained drugs are metabolized and then excreted by the kidneys. Elimination of drugs through the bile may result in prolonged drug action.

The rate of elimination and half-life characteristics influence drug responsiveness.

CORE CONCEPT 4.6

Elimination, which is another term for *excretion*, is often measured so that dosages of drugs can be determined more accurately. The term *rate of elimination* refers to the amount of drug removed per unit of time from the body by normal physiologic processes. The rate of elimination is helpful in determining how long a particular drug will remain in the bloodstream, and is thus an indicator of how long a drug will produce its effect.

The **half-life ($t_{1/2}$)** of a drug is a related measurement used to ensure that maximum therapeutic dosages are administered. Half-life is the length of time required for a drug's concentration in the plasma (i.e., in circulation) to decrease by one half. It is an indicator of how long a drug will produce its effect in the body. The larger the half-life value, the longer it takes for a drug to be eliminated. Some drugs have a half-life of just a few minutes, whereas others have a half-life of several hours or days. A drug with a half-life of 10 hours will take longer to be eliminated from the body than a drug with a half-life of five hours. Drugs with longer half-lives may be given less frequently—for example, once per day.

When a patient has a renal or hepatic disease, the plasma half-life of a drug increases. This reflects the important relationship of half-life to metabolism and excretion.

Several important pharmacokinetic principles can be illustrated by measuring the serum level of a drug following a single-dose administration. These pharmacokinetic values are shown graphically in Figure 4.4 ■. This figure demonstrates two plasma drug levels. First is the **minimum effective concentration**, the amount of drug required to produce a therapeutic effect. Second is the **toxic concentration**, the level of drug that will result in serious adverse effects. The plasma drug concentration *between* the minimum effective concentration and the toxic concentration is called the **therapeutic range** of the drug. The **onset of drug action** represents the amount of time it takes to produce a therapeutic effect after drug administration. Factors that affect drug onset may be many, depending on

FIGURE 4.4

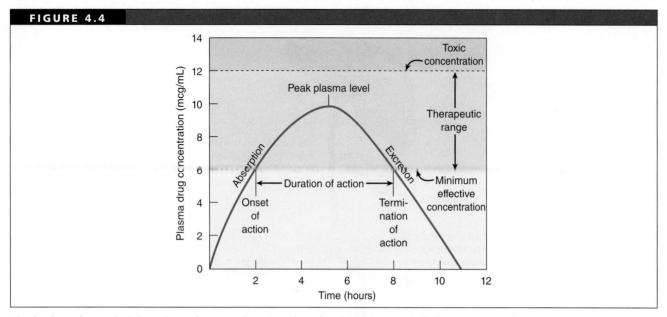

Single-dose drug administration: pharmacokinetic values for this drug are as follows: onset of action = two hours; duration of action = six hours; termination of action = eight hours after administration; peak plasma concentration = 10 mcg/mL; time to peak drug effect = five hours; $t_{1/2}$ = four hours.

numerous pharmacokinetic variables. As the drug is absorbed and then begins to circulate throughout the body, the level of medication reaches its peak. The **peak plasma level** occurs when the medication has reached its highest concentration in the bloodstream. Depending on accessibility of medications to their targets, peak drug levels are not necessarily associated with optimal therapeutic effects. Multiple doses of medication may be necessary to reach therapeutic drug levels. **Duration of drug action** is the amount of time it takes for a drug to maintain its desired effect. **Termination of drug action** is when the drug effect stops.

Concept Review 4.2

■ Why are rate of elimination and half-life ($t_{1/2}$) important to the healthcare provider?

CORE CONCEPT 4.7

Pharmacodynamics focuses on what the drugs do to the body.

As discussed already, many variables influence the effectiveness of drug therapy, such as rate of administration, frequency of drug dosing, and changing medical condition. Some of these factors are listed in Table 4.1 ◆.

Successful pharmacotherapy depends on these variables as well as how effectively the body responds to drugs at specific target locations. This leads to another important core area of pharmacology: the field of pharmacodynamics. The field of pharmacodynamics is complex and requires extensive knowledge of human physiology and biochemistry. **Pharmacodynamics** deals with the mechanisms of drug action, or how the drug exerts its effects. As the root words suggest, drugs have a powerful influence on body processes. The remaining part of this chapter is devoted to a few basic pharmacodynamic principles.

pharmaco = *drug related*
dynamics = *powerful change*

TABLE 4.1 Factors That Influence the Effectiveness of Drug Therapy	
Concentration (dose) of administered drug	Metabolic rate (lower in children and elderly patients)
Frequency of drug dosing	Genetics
Food–drug interactions	Excretion rate (rate of elimination)
Drug–drug interactions	Half-life ($t_{1/2}$) of administered drug
Absorption rate (refer to Core Concept 4.1)	Changing medical condition (liver or kidney disease)

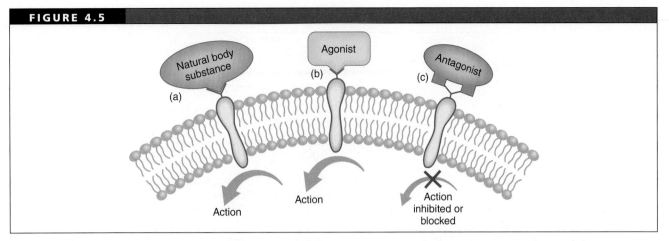

FIGURE 4.5

Cellular receptors: (a) A *neurotransmitter* or *hormone* binds to the receptor. A drug is a close "mimic" of the neurotransmitter or hormone and initiates a response by binding to the same receptor site. (b) An *agonist* is a drug that facilitates the pharmacologic response. (c) An *antagonist* is a drug that temporarily blocks or depresses the pharmacologic response.

Drugs activate specific receptors to produce a response.

CORE CONCEPT **4.8**

Successful pharmacotherapy is based on the principle that in order to treat a disorder, a drug must interact with specific receptors in its target tissue. The **receptor theory** is a classic theory referring to the cellular mechanism by which most drugs can change body processes. A **receptor** is any structural component of a cell to which a drug binds in a dose-related manner. Receptors can be located on the plasma membrane or in the cytoplasm or nucleus of the cell. The drug or natural body substance attaches to its receptor much like a thumb drive to a computer docking port (Figure 4.5 ■). Some drug actions are not linked to a receptor, but are connected directly with cell function, such as changing the membrane excitability or stability of a nerve or muscle cell.

recept = *receiving*
or = *entity*

The terms *agonist* and *antagonist* are often used to describe drug action at the receptor level. **Agonists** are drugs capable of binding with receptors and causing a cellular response; these are *facilitators* of cellular action. When they are present in the bloodstream, agonists cause the tissue to respond, resulting in a therapeutic action. **Antagonists** are drugs that inhibit or block the responses of agonists. Antagonists are called *blockers*.

ant = *against*
agonist = *activator*

therapeu = *healing treatment*
tic = *pertaining to*

Potency and *efficacy* are terms often used to describe the success of drug therapy.

CORE CONCEPT **4.9**

Potency refers to a drug's strength at a certain concentration or dose. As shown in Figure 4.6 ■, *dose-response curves* are used to compare potencies of different drugs. If drug A has a higher potency than drug B, it means that drug A will produce a more intense effect than drug B if both drugs are given at the same dose (Figure 4.6a). A higher potency also means that a much smaller dose of the medication will be needed to produce the same effect as another drug, as shown by the shift to the left of the dose-response curve for drug A in Figure 4.6a.

potency = *power quality*

Another core concept is **efficacy**. Efficacy refers to the ability of a drug to produce a more intense response as its concentration is increased. As an example, consider Figure 4.6b. If the doses of two similarly acting drugs (A and B) are increased, they will both produce a more intense effect, but drug B will have a maximum intensity that is lower than drug A. The drug reaching a lower maximum intensity compared to another drug is said to have a lower efficacy.

efficacy = *effectiveness*

In pharmacotherapeutics, it is generally more important to have a drug with higher efficacy than one with higher potency. For example, at recommended doses ibuprofen (200 mg) and aspirin (650 mg) are equally effective at relieving headache; thus, they have the *same efficacy*. The fact that ibuprofen relieves pain at a lower dose indicates that this agent is *more potent* than aspirin. If the patient is experiencing severe pain, however, neither aspirin nor ibuprofen has sufficient efficacy to bring relief. In this instance, morphine has a greater efficacy than aspirin or ibuprofen and can effectively treat this type of pain. In this example, the average dose is unimportant to the patient, but efficacy—the ability of the pain medication to bring essential relief—is crucial.

FIGURE 4.6

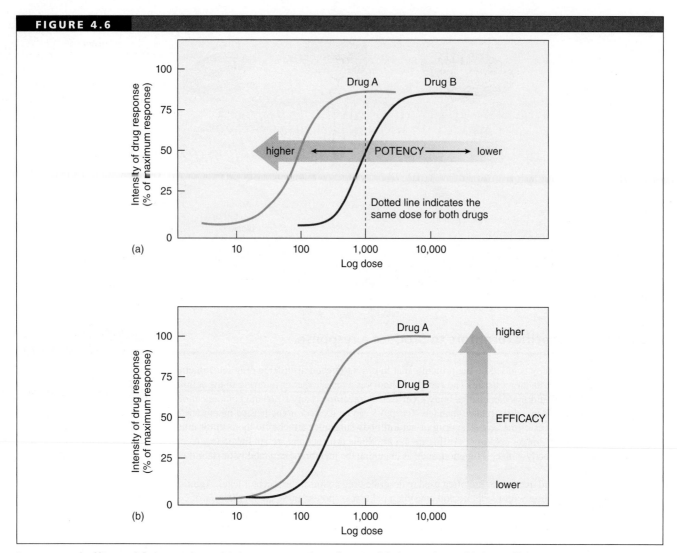

Potency and efficacy: (a) drug A has a higher potency than drug B; (b) drug A has a higher efficacy than drug B.

Concept Review 4.3

■ What does the term *pharmacodynamics* mean? Identify the importance of receptors, agonists, and antagonists in influencing drug action. What is the difference between a drug's potency and its efficacy?

CHAPTER REVIEW

CORE CONCEPTS SUMMARY

4.1 **Pharmacokinetics focuses on what the body does to the drugs.**

Pharmacokinetics is an area of pharmacology dealing with how drugs move throughout the body. There are four components of drug transport: absorption, distribution, metabolism, and excretion.

4.2 **Absorption is the first step in drug transport.**

Absorption is the first step in pharmacokinetics. It involves movement of a drug from its site of administration across body membranes. Drugs cross many membranes before reaching target organs. Drug absorption is affected by many factors.

4.3 Distribution refers to how drugs are transported throughout the body.

Distribution begins after absorption and continues until drug action. Drugs bound to plasma proteins may be isolated in the plasma and prevented from reaching their target cells. The blood-brain barrier, blood-placental barrier, and blood-testicular barrier all represent areas in the body where drug distribution may be limited.

4.4 Metabolism is a process whereby drugs are made less or more active.

Metabolic processes take place in the liver, and to a lesser extent, in organs such as the kidney and cells of the gastrointestinal tract. The first-pass effect is an important phenomenon. Many drugs absorbed across intestinal membranes are routed directly to the liver. Metabolic liver enzymes are usually less active in younger and in older patients; therefore, drug effects will most likely be greater in these age groups. Prodrugs are agents converted to a more active form when they are metabolically changed.

4.5 Excretion processes remove drugs from the body.

The kidneys, lungs, sweat glands, mammary glands, and gallbladder are the major structures involved in eliminating drugs from the body. The main organ involved with excretion is the kidney. Enterohepatic recirculation is a unique type of mechanism responsible for recirculating bile back into the bloodstream from the gastrointestinal tract.

4.6 The rate of elimination and half-life characteristics influence drug responsiveness.

The elimination rate of a drug is defined as the amount of drug removed from the body by normal physiologic processes per unit of time. Plasma half-life is the amount of time it takes for the body to remove half of the drug from the general circulation. These and other important factors affect the duration of drug action.

4.7 Pharmacodynamics focuses on what the drugs do to the body.

Pharmacodynamics is an area of pharmacology concerned with how drugs produce responses within the body. Successful drug therapy depends on the effectiveness of these responses.

4.8 Drugs activate specific receptors to produce a response.

Generally, the response of a drug begins when the agent encounters the receptor of its target cell. The receptor theory states that most responses in the body are caused by interactions of drugs with specific receptors. Receptors may be located on the plasma membrane, or they may be found in the cytoplasm or nucleus of the cell.

4.9 *Potency* and *efficacy* are terms often used to describe the success of drug therapy.

Potency relates to the concentration or amount of drug required to produce a maximum response. Efficacy refers to how great the maximal response of a drug will be.

REVIEW QUESTIONS

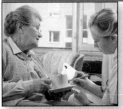 The following questions are written in NCLEX-PN® style. Answer these questions to assess your knowledge of the chapter material, and go back and review any material that is not clear to you.

1. Patients with liver disorders would most likely have problems with which pharmacokinetic phase?

1. Absorption
2. Distribution
3. Metabolism
4. Excretion

2. The patient asks the nurse why he or she must take his or her medication twice a day instead of just once. The nurse's best response would be:

1. "Taking it once a day is fine as long as it is taken at the same time every day."
2. "Taking the medication twice a day ensures that maximum concentrations are maintained within the body."
3. "You will need to speak to your physician about this."
4. "The first dose of the medication is blocked by deactivation and the second dose is metabolized by the body."

3. The nursing student learns that which of the following principles are true about how medications work? (Select all that apply.)

1. For a drug to be effective, it must be potent.
2. For drug efficacy to occur, a lower dose must be administered.
3. Antagonists bind to receptors and produce responses to block agonists.
4. The agonist-receptor interaction causes a cellular response, resulting in a therapeutic action.

4. The nurse is administering a drug that binds with a receptor to produce a therapeutic response. This type of drug is called a(n):

1. Antagonist
2. Facilitator
3. Agonist
4. Blocker

5. If a patient takes a medication on a full stomach, the nurse is aware that the medication will be:

1. Absorbed more rapidly
2. Absorbed more slowly
3. Neutralized by gastric enzymes
4. Activated by gastric enzymes

6. When planning care for a patient, the nurse takes into consideration which of the following factors that could directly influence the effectiveness of drugs that will be given? (Select all that apply.)

1. Drug–drug interactions
2. Food–drug interactions
3. Route of administration
4. Time of administration within the day

7. An antibiotic has been ordered for the patient with a brain abscess. The nurse understands that:

1. There are no antibiotics effective to treat brain abscesses because they cannot cross the blood-brain barrier.
2. Only fat-soluble substances will pass the blood-brain barrier so the antibiotic will need to be fat-soluble.
3. The half-life of the antibiotic will be decreased when crossing the blood-brain barrier.
4. The intestinal tract will prevent absorption from occurring.

8. When orally administered drugs are extensively metabolized by the liver, with only part of the drug dose reaching target organs, this is known as:

1. Half-life
2. Potency
3. First-pass effect
4. Rate of elimination

9. A patient asks the nurse how the body will "get rid of all the drugs" she is taking. The nurse responds by saying: (Select all that apply.)

1. "Drugs are normally removed from the body by the kidneys."
2. "Some drugs are removed from the body through some glands."
3. "Some drugs can be more effectively excreted through the sweat glands."
4. "Some drugs are changed into a gaseous form and are excreted by the lungs."

10. An elderly patient has reduced metabolic activity. The nurse may expect to see what change in the dosage of a drug given to this patient?

1. Increase the medication dosage.
2. Increase the number of times the patient has to take the medication.
3. Decrease the medication dosage.
4. Reduce the number of times the patient has to take the medication.

NOTE: Answers to the Review Questions appear in Appendix B. The complete rationales and answers are located on the textbook's website.

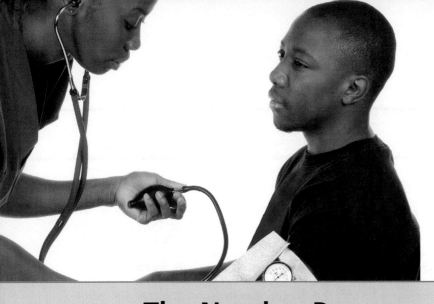

The Nursing Process in Pharmacology

5

CORE CONCEPTS

5.1 The first step of the nursing process is the assessment phase.

5.2 Nursing diagnoses are based on the data gathered in the assessment phase.

5.3 In the planning phase, the nurse creates an individualized plan of care for a patient based on the identified nursing diagnoses and etiologies.

5.4 The implementation phase puts the plan of care into action.

5.5 In the evaluation phase, the nurse obtains data to determine if the goal or outcome has been achieved.

LEARNING OUTCOMES

After reading this chapter, the student should be able to:

1. Describe the five steps of the nursing process.

2. Identify how the assessment phase of the nursing process can be used to gather data pertinent to medication administration.

3. Explain how nursing diagnoses can be used to improve medication administration.

4. Describe the steps in the planning phase of the nursing process.

5. Identify pharmacology applications included in the implementation phase of the nursing process.

6. Explain the importance of the evaluation phase in the nursing process as applied to pharmacotherapy.

KEY TERMS

assessment phase *52*

etiologies (e-tee-OL-o-gees) *53*

evaluation criteria *54*

evaluation phase *56*

goal *54*

implementation phase *55*

interventions *53*

nursing diagnosis *53*

nursing process *51*

outcome *54*

planning phase *53*

The **nursing process**, a systematic method of problem solving, forms the foundation of all nursing practice. The use of the nursing process is particularly essential during medication administration. By using the steps of the nursing process, the nurse can ensure that the interdisciplinary practice of pharmacology results in safe, effective, and individualized medication administration and outcomes for all patients under their care.

The nursing process is an ongoing activity involving five distinct phases: assessment, diagnosis, planning, implementation, and evaluation. The nursing process is cyclical and each phase is related to all the others; they are not separate entities but overlap. The licensed practical nurse (LPN) or licensed vocational nurse (LVN) contributes to each phase of the process under the direction of the registered nurse (RN). In this chapter, each phase is briefly reviewed, and each phase's use in pharmacology is emphasized. A summary of the phases is shown in Figure 5.1 ■.

| CORE CONCEPT 5.1 | **The first step of the nursing process is the assessment phase.** |

The **assessment phase** of the nursing process is the systematic collection, organization, validation, and documentation of patient data. The assessment phase serves two purposes. The first is to gather data that will enable the nurse to identify current patient health challenges and problems that the patient is at particular risk for developing. These data will eventually be used to identify appropriate nursing diagnoses and to develop a plan of care.

The second purpose of the assessment phase is to gather initial *baseline data* on the patient that will be compared to subsequent data during the evaluation phase of the nursing process. These comparisons will indicate to what extent the treatment goals have been achieved. When applying the nursing process to pharmacology, baseline data are necessary for the nurse to be able to evaluate therapeutic drug effects and adverse drug effects. For example, a common adverse effect of many antibiotics is the risk for allergic reaction, often identified by skin rash. To determine whether the rash is due to a medication, the nurse must first assess that a rash was not present prior to initiating drug therapy. As another example, if a patient is exhibiting elevated liver enzymes during hospitalization, the nurse will use baseline assessment data to determine whether the patient had this condition on admission, or whether it is a sign of a recent adverse drug reaction.

Data collected in the assessment phase come from many sources. These include the patient, caregivers, medical records, and other healthcare professionals. *Subjective* data include what the patient says or perceives, such as pain, anxiety, or nausea. Whenever possible, the subjective data are verified by *objective* data that are gathered through physical examination, medical history, laboratory tests, and other diagnostic sources.

Assessment must always include a comprehensive health history that includes the patient's use of prescription drugs, over-the-counter (OTC) agents, dietary supplements, and herbal products. The nurse should inquire about tobacco and alcohol use as well as past or current history of drug abuse because these may influence treatment outcomes. Any allergic or unusual reactions to drugs should be documented, including serious adverse drug reactions that may have occurred to close family members.

| FIGURE 5.1 |

The five overlapping phases of the nursing process. Each phase depends on the accuracy of the other phases. Each phase involves critical thinking.
Source: Berman, A., & Snyder, S. (2012). Kozier & Erb's fundamentals of nursing: Concepts, process, and practice (9th ed.). Upper Saddle River, NJ: Pearson Education.

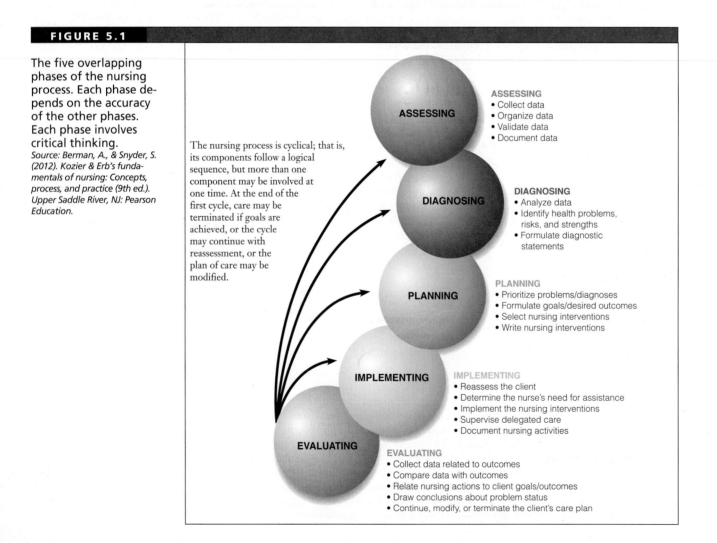

The nursing process is cyclical; that is, its components follow a logical sequence, but more than one component may be involved at one time. At the end of the first cycle, care may be terminated if goals are achieved, or the cycle may continue with reassessment, or the plan of care may be modified.

ASSESSING
- Collect data
- Organize data
- Validate data
- Document data

DIAGNOSING
- Analyze data
- Identify health problems, risks, and strengths
- Formulate diagnostic statements

PLANNING
- Prioritize problems/diagnoses
- Formulate goals/desired outcomes
- Select nursing interventions
- Write nursing interventions

IMPLEMENTING
- Reassess the client
- Determine the nurse's need for assistance
- Implement the nursing interventions
- Supervise delegated care
- Document nursing activities

EVALUATING
- Collect data related to outcomes
- Compare data with outcomes
- Relate nursing actions to client goals/outcomes
- Draw conclusions about problem status
- Continue, modify, or terminate the client's care plan

The initial health history gathered during the assessment phase is used to determine whether the patient has a contraindication that would present a risk for drug therapy. For example, the nurse may discover during assessment that the patient is pregnant and should not receive isotretinoin (Accutane) for her acne because it is a pregnancy category X drug. The nurse may discover that the patient has a history of allergy to penicillin, and therefore, should not be prescribed ampicillin due to the potential for cross-allergy. A thorough assessment is the best way to prevent adverse drug effects.

Concept Review	**5.1**

■ What types of assessments would be important for the nurse to perform on patients who will be required to self-administer their medications at home?

Nursing diagnoses are based on the data gathered in the assessment phase.

CORE CONCEPT 5.2

During the diagnosis phase of the nursing process, the nurse analyzes assessment data, identifies health problems, and formulates diagnostic statements. A **nursing diagnosis** is a clinical judgment of a patient's response to an actual or potential health problem, a problem that is within the nurse's scope of practice to address. It is the responsibility of the RN to identify the appropriate diagnosis and develop a plan of care. The LPN/LVN contributes to this phase by collecting data and collaborating with the RN.

dia = *through or complete*
gnosis = *knowledge*

Nursing diagnoses differ from medical diagnoses, which are determined by physicians. Whereas the medical diagnosis remains constant during a patient's hospital stay, nursing diagnoses are in constant flux as the patient responds to treatments. Nursing diagnoses address changes in the patient's condition—for example, alterations in mobility, nutritional intake, urinary elimination, knowledge, ability for self-care, and risk for injury. These nursing diagnoses are used to set goals and plan care.

Nursing diagnoses are often stated as a problem, or the risk for a problem, followed by a "related to" clause that identifies the **etiologies**, or those conditions that have caused or contributed to the problem. By altering one or more of these etiologies, nurses are able to effect improvements in the diagnosed problem. This is accomplished by planning and implementing **interventions**, which are actions that the nurse takes to achieve patient goals. The nurse chooses interventions that are patient focused and target the etiologies of the problem. The North American Nursing Diagnosis Association (NANDA) has developed standard wording, known as the nursing diagnosis, for identifying actual and potential patient health problems. For example, a nursing diagnosis may be, "*Activity Intolerance* related to acute knee pain." The nurse designs interventions to address the etiology (acute knee pain) that may include the administration of pain medications, heat, or ice packs.

etio = *cause*
ology = *study of*

Nursing diagnoses are prioritized by their level of importance and immediacy to the patient's clinical condition. For example, alterations in breathing would likely take precedence over the potential for skin breakdown. A primary nursing role is to enable patients to become active participants in their own care. Patients need to vocalize, to the extent possible, their priorities for care, which should be considered by the nurse when diagnoses are prioritized. By including patients when identifying needs, the nurse encourages them to take a more active role in working toward meeting the identified goals.

When applied to pharmacotherapy, the diagnosis phase of the nursing process addresses three main areas of concern:

■ Promoting therapeutic drug effects

■ Minimizing adverse drug effects and toxicity

■ Maximizing the ability of the patient for self-care, including the knowledge, skills, and resources necessary for safe and effective drug administration

The teaching of patients is one of the basic roles of nursing, and careful attention to drug teaching can promote therapeutic outcomes as well as minimize adverse effects. Examples of nursing diagnoses that intimately involve drug teaching include *Deficient Knowledge* related to a lack of information about new drug therapy and *Noncompliance* related to not taking the prescribed medication. The teaching of patients is discussed further in the planning phase. See Table 5.1 ◆ for selected nursing diagnoses for pharmacotherapy. For a complete list, the student should refer to a nursing fundamentals textbook.

In the planning phase, the nurse creates an individualized plan of care for a patient based on the identified nursing diagnoses and etiologies.

CORE CONCEPT 5.3

After a nursing diagnosis has been established, the nurse begins to plan ways to assist the patient to establish an optimum level of wellness. In the **planning phase** of the nursing process, the nurse prioritizes diagnoses, formulates desired goals, and selects nursing interventions.

TABLE 5.1 Common Nursing Diagnoses in Pharmacotherapy

Acute Confusion related to substance abuse

Risk for Confusion related to drug effects

Impaired Comfort related to drug effects

Deficient Fluid Volume related to drug effects

Excess Fluid Volume related to drug effects

Noncompliance related to lack of knowledge of drug therapy

Risk for Infection related to adverse drug effects

Risk for Injury related to adverse drug effects

Insomnia related to drug effects

Imbalanced Nutrition: Less than body requirements related to drug-induced nausea

Ineffective Health Maintenance related to drug therapy regimen

Activity Intolerance related to drug effects

Deficient Knowledge related to a lack of information about new drug therapy

*Other nursing diagnosis may be applicable depending on patient assessment and type of medication being used.

Source: NANDA International Nursing Diagnosis: Definitions and Classifications 2012–2014, Wiley-Blackwell (2011)

There are two main steps of the planning phase. The first step is to identify the desired **goal**, or **outcome**, to be achieved, and the specific **evaluation criteria** that will be used to determine if that goal has been met. The outcome may be a short-term or long-term goal, should include the time frame whenever possible, and must be realistic for the patient to achieve. The evaluation criteria should be specific and measurable. These criteria are often indicated by the abbreviation AEB (as evidenced by). The outcome should directly address the problem identified in the nursing diagnosis. For example, if the nursing diagnosis is *Risk for Dysfunctional Gastrointestinal Motility* related to opioid analgesic use, a goal might be: the absence of altered bowel elimination, AEB regular bowel evacuation, absence of difficulty passing stool, and absence of abdominal bloating or discomfort. Notice how this plan includes a clear goal as well as specific evaluation criteria.

The second step of the planning phase is to develop a list of interventions. The interventions are specific nursing actions designed to help move the patient toward the established goal.

When planning interventions the nurse should consider the specific health problem and etiologies, current practice guidelines, acceptability to the patient, and the nurse's own capabilities. In addition, the chosen nursing interventions should be safe and appropriate for the patient's age, health, and condition; congruent with the patient's values, beliefs, and culture; and appropriate to the other ordered therapies. The choice of nursing interventions will also depend on what is realistic and practical to the situation in terms of equipment availability, financial status of the patient, and available resources, including staff, agency, family, or community resources.

With respect to pharmacotherapy, the planning phase involves two main issues: drug administration and patient teaching. For the first issue, the nurse must plan how and when to administer the drug. For oral medications, does it need to be given with food or on an empty stomach? Is it more effective if administered at a certain time of day? Can it be crushed or split? For all medications, the nurse will plan interventions to enhance therapeutic outcomes and minimize or prevent adverse drug effects.

When planning patient drug teaching, the projected length of pharmacotherapy influences the amount and type of teaching provided by the nurse. Is the drug to be given for a short time during an acute care hospitalization, or is pharmacotherapy going to be long term and self-administered following discharge? If a drug is to be given short term, the patient should be told the name of the drug and its basic actions, why the patient is receiving it, and some of the drug's most common and major adverse effects, including any that should be promptly reported to the nurse or healthcare provider.

For drugs that will be taken after discharge, patient teaching should be comprehensive and be provided both orally and in writing. This teaching should include the drug name (both generic and trade), the drug class and its major effects, why the drug is being prescribed, the therapeutic effects and when they should occur, how and when to take the drug, the common and major adverse effects and which ones should be reported to the prescriber, the types of follow-up monitoring needed, potential drug interactions, the duration of drug therapy, the activities to avoid while taking the drug, and what to do if a dose is missed or forgotten. Table 5.2 ◆ gives tips for effective patient teaching that can be used for patients of all ages.

TABLE 5.2   Teaching Throughout the Life Span

Patient teaching is an essential component of the nursing process. To be effective, oral and written teaching must be age appropriate. The following are some tips for effective teaching.

CHILDREN

- Use family-centered approaches when providing drug teaching for children and adolescents.
- Engage young children and toddlers by using interactive strategies.
- Use simple, nonthreatening language.
- Provide a developmentally appropriate environment when teaching adolescents.
- Encourage problem solving to help adolescents make effective choices.

ADULTS

- Adult learners are independent; the nurse should facilitate learning.
- Adults learn best when the topic is of immediate value, and when new material is connected to previous experiences.
- Adults vary widely in their learning styles and preferences; teaching and learning is enhanced when patient learning styles are considered.
- Consider the literacy level of learners. It is recommended that written materials be on a fifth-grade reading level.
- Employ multiple methods of delivering information; a combination of verbal and written material is best.

OLDER ADULTS

- Plan several short learning sessions; repeat and review material covered; time needed for learning often increases with age.
- Relate new learning to the patient's real-life experiences.
- Provide printed material, videos, and/or pictures and diagrams that the patient can refer to at a later time.
- Modify teaching methods to sensory-perceptual deficits or cognitive decline. Ensure that the patient has the necessary aids (glasses, magnifying glass, hearing aid) to maximize the learning experience.
- Offer opportunities for practice of psychomotor skills related to administering medications.

The implementation phase puts the plan of care into action.

CORE CONCEPT 5.4

The **implementation phase** is when the nurse applies the knowledge, skills, and principles of nursing care to help move the patient toward the desired goal and optimal wellness. Implementation involves action on the part of the nurse or patient: administering a drug, providing patient teaching, and initiating actions identified by the nursing diagnoses and plan of care. The implementation phase should be designed to maximize therapeutic drug responses and prevent adverse reactions.

It must be remembered that implementation of the plan of care is subject to modification based on the patient's evolving condition. In implementing pharmacotherapy, an important decision that the nurse must make is whether it is appropriate to administer the drug at the planned time. To make this decision, the nurse needs to understand the drug's therapeutic and adverse effects well enough to know the circumstances under which it is appropriate, or not appropriate, to give the drug. After assessing a current vital sign, a laboratory result, a new health problem, or a physical assessment finding, it may be appropriate for the nurse to delay administration of an ordered drug until the prescriber can be contacted. For example, if the patient's current serum potassium level is below the normal range, and the nurse has an order to administer furosemide (Lasix), it would be an error for the nurse to administer the drug. Carrying out the order would cause serum potassium to fall, which could trigger cardiac dysrhythmias. Likewise, a patient who has a scheduled dose of morphine for pain relief but currently has a respiratory rate of less than eight should not receive the drug because it may cause respiratory failure.

As pharmacotherapy progresses, the nurse must be aware of circumstances that might require modification of the implementation phase. The patient may develop new symptoms that contraindicate the use of the drug being administered. For example, the patient may begin to show signs of a developing rash, changes in blood pressure, or alterations in mental status that call for discontinuation of the drug until the prescriber can be contacted. These examples help illustrate the cyclic nature of the

FIGURE 5.2

Teaching patients about drugs and their effects is an important step in the nursing process.

Source: Science Photo Library

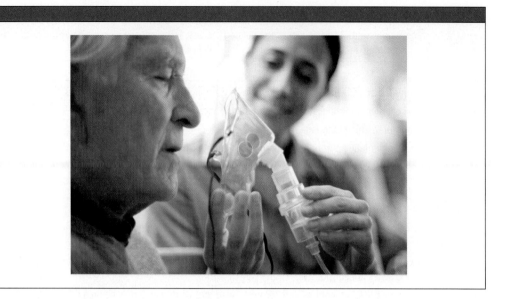

nursing process: the importance of continuous assessment and the revision of the planning and implementation phases.

Implementation also includes patient teaching (Figure 5.2 ■). Table 5.2 gives tips for effective patient teaching that can be used for patients of all ages. Patient drug teaching should start with what the patient already knows about a drug and build from there. The specific topics to include in this teaching are developed in the planning phase. When preparing to carry out the teaching, other factors that the nurse should consider are the patient's readiness to learn and whether or not it is an appropriate time for teaching. Patients who are in pain, sleepy, anxious, or distracted are less likely to understand instructions. Drug teaching should be tailored to the patient's developmental level, learning capacity, and preferred learning style. Patients may prefer that a family member or caregiver be present during the teaching. This is especially important for patients with limited English proficiency, pediatric patients, older adults with cognitive deficits, and patients with mental illnesses who may be incapable of safe self-administration. Patient teaching is sometimes a collaborative effort, requiring coordination with other medical disciplines as part of the sessions. Often a registered dietician, physical therapist, or diabetes educator collaborates in the patient teaching. When teaching, sufficient time must always be allotted to address any areas of concern for the patient.

Finally, documentation is an essential part of the implementation phase. This includes a thorough reporting of the interventions carried out, the drugs that were given (or withheld), the teaching that took place, and the patient's responses to the interventions.

In the evaluation phase, the nurse obtains data to determine if the goal or outcome has been achieved.

The **evaluation phase** compares the patient's current health status with the established outcome to determine if the plan of care is appropriate or if it needs revision. Essentially, the evaluation phase is used to determine if the goal or outcome has been met. If it has been met, the plan of care was appropriate. If the goal was partially met, the nurse may determine that the interventions may need to be continued for a longer time or otherwise modified to better resolve the health problem.

As it relates to pharmacotherapy, evaluation is used to determine whether the therapeutic effects of the drug have been achieved as well as whether adverse effects have been prevented or kept to acceptable levels. For example, if a drug is given for symptoms of pain, has the pain subsided? If an antibiotic is given for an infection, have the signs of that infection improved? If the evaluation data show no improvement in health status over the baseline data, the interventions will likely need to be revised, drug doses may need to be adjusted, more time may be needed to achieve a therapeutic drug response, or a different or additional drug may be needed. The data gathered during the evaluation phase becomes part of the assessment data and continues the cycle of nursing process as outcomes and interventions are revised. The evaluation data needs to be documented in the patient's record to ensure proper communication of the patient's response to the nursing interventions.

In an outpatient setting, lack of drug response determined during the evaluation phase may be caused by patient nonadherence to the drug regimen. During the assessment phase, the nurse must determine if the patient is taking the drug as prescribed. If nonadherence is discovered, the nurse must plan and implement strategies for increasing adherence, which includes identifying reasons for the nonadherence. Additional patient teaching is critical to obtain maximum patient adherence to the drug regimen: The nurse must help the patient to value pharmacotherapy as important to the improvement of the patient's health.

Concept Review 5.2

■ What strategies might the nurse implement to improve adherence to drug therapy for a geriatric patient?

> ### ▶ Life Span Fact
>
> When evaluating the success of drug therapy in older adults, the healthcare provider should understand that nonadherence may be due to physical or other limitations in. The inability to open childproof containers or to read the instructions on the label are possible causes of nonadherence. Older adults may be depending on caregivers to pick up or administer their medications on a regular basis. In many cases, simply forgetting to take a medication is a cause of lack of drug effect. The healthcare provider should assist older patients in overcoming these limitations so that pharmacotherapy can be optimized.

🍃 CAM THERAPY

Medication Errors and Dietary Supplements

Some herbal and dietary supplements have powerful effects on the body that can influence the outcomes of prescription drug therapy. In some cases, OTC supplements can enhance the effects of prescription drugs, whereas in other instances supplements may cancel the therapeutic effects of medications. For example, many patients with heart disease take garlic supplements in addition to warfarin (Coumadin) to prevent clots from forming. Because garlic and warfarin are both anticoagulants, taking them together could cause excessive bleeding. As another example, high doses of calcium supplements can cancel the beneficial antihypertensive effects of drugs, such as nifedipine (Procardia), a calcium channel blocker.

CHAPTER REVIEW

CORE CONCEPTS SUMMARY

5.1 **The first step of the nursing process is the assessment phase.**

Assessment is the careful, systematic collection of patient data. During this phase, the nurse gathers data that identify patient health challenges.

5.2 **Nursing diagnoses are based on the data gathered in the assessment phase.**

Nursing diagnoses are clinical judgments based on a patient's response to actual or potential patient problems; they include the etiologies of the health problem. These etiologies are factors that can be addressed by nursing interventions to address the health challenges of the patient.

5.3 **In the planning phase, the nurse creates an individualized plan of care for a patient based on the identified nursing diagnoses and etiologies.**

The first step of the planning phase is identification of a goal or outcome for the patient, including the evaluation criteria that will be used to determine whether or not the goal has been achieved. The second step is the formulation of nursing interventions to be used to help move the patient toward the established goal.

5.4 **The implementation phase puts the plan of care into action.**

When applied to pharmacology, the implementation phase involves administering the drug and providing patient drug teaching that maximizes therapeutic effects and minimizes side effects.

5.5 **In the evaluation phase, the nurse obtains data to determine if the goal or outcome has been achieved.**

By comparing the evaluation data to baseline data, the nurse is able to determine whether or not the established goal was met. Evaluation data are used to develop revised goals, plans, or interventions that will better resolve the health challenges of the patient.

REVIEW QUESTIONS

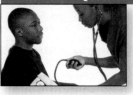

The following questions are written in NCLEX-PN® style. Answer these questions to assess your knowledge of the chapter material, and go back and review any material that is not clear to you.

1. The nurse reviews a patient record for drug allergies, current medications, and disease states that could affect drug responses. These actions are part of which phase of the nursing process?

1. Assessment
2. Planning
3. Implementation
4. Evaluation

2. The implementation phase of the nursing process involves which two main activities related to pharmacology?

1. Developing and performing nursing interventions
2. Providing and evaluating patient teaching
3. Administering drugs and providing patient education
4. Assessing and evaluating adverse drug effects

3. Which of the following would be most important for the nurse in the evaluation phase of the nursing process?

1. Patient satisfaction with drug therapy
2. Evidence of therapeutic drug effects
3. Development of minor adverse drug effects
4. The possibility of noncompliance with drug therapy

4. Which of the following is appropriate information to gather in the assessment phase of the nursing process? (Select all that apply.)

1. Drug allergies
2. Therapeutic response to the drug
3. History of renal or hepatic disease
4. Baseline physical assessment data

5. Ms. Smith is complaining of pain in her lower back. After asking Ms. Smith about her pain level, the nurse prepared the pain medication as ordered and is about to administer it to her. What phase of the nursing process is the nurse using?

1. Assessment
2. Planning
3. Implementation
4. Evaluation

6. The second phase of the nursing process involves analyzing data and identifying health problems, such as *Activity Intolerance* related to pain. This phase is known as:

1. Assessment
2. Implementation
3. Nursing diagnosis
4. Planning

7. The nursing process, as it relates to pharmacology, can best be described as a:

1. Way of determining whether a patient should use a cane or crutches when walking
2. Method of documentation that nurses use in their daily practice
3. Problem-solving method that encourages nurses to rely solely on their textbook knowledge of a patient's condition before determining a course of action
4. Systematic approach to problem solving that ensures the safe and effective administration of medication

8. The role of the LPN/LVN is to:

1. Work independently of the RN and other healthcare providers when establishing a plan of care for a patient.
2. Assist the physician in establishing a patient's plan of care.
3. Contribute to each phase of the process under the direction of the RN.
4. Rely completely on the RN to utilize the nursing process when caring for patients.

9. A male patient has just been diagnosed with diabetes mellitus. The interdisciplinary team, including the LPN/LVN, is in the process of developing a schedule of teaching sessions with him on subjects such as glucose monitoring, insulin injections and signs of hypoglycemia. What phase of the nursing process does this represent?

1. Assessment
2. Planning
3. Implementation
4. Evaluation

10. The nursing diagnosis statement is *Insomnia* related to anxiety as manifested by difficulty falling and staying asleep. The etiology of the problem is:

1. Insomnia
2. Anxiety
3. Difficulty falling asleep
4. Difficulty staying asleep

NOTE: Answers to the Review Questions appear in Appendix B. The complete rationales and answers are located on the textbook's website.

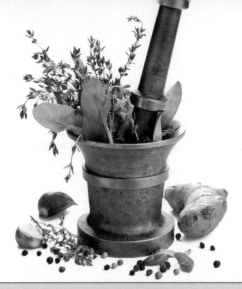

The Role of Complementary and Alternative Therapies in Pharmacology

CORE CONCEPTS

6.1 Complementary and alternative therapies are used by a large number of people to prevent and treat disease.

6.2 Natural products from plants have been used as medicines for thousands of years.

6.3 Herbal products are standardized with respect to a specific active ingredient.

6.4 Herbs can have significant pharmacologic actions and can interact with conventional drugs.

6.5 Specialty supplements are nonherbal products that are widely used to promote wellness.

6.6 Herbal products and specialty are not regulated in the same manner as prescription medications.

LEARNING OUTCOMES

After reading this chapter, the student should be able to:

1. Identify specific types of complementary and alternative therapies that are used by patients to promote wellness.

2. Discuss the reasons why herbal products and dietary supplements have steadily increased in popularity.

3. Identify the parts of an herb that may contain active ingredients and the types of formulations made from these parts.

4. Describe legislation that governs the use of herbal and dietary supplements.

5. Describe drug interactions and adverse effects that may be caused by herbal and dietary supplements.

6. Explain why it is important to standardize herbal products based on specific active ingredients.

7. Discuss the role of the healthcare provider in teaching patients about complementary and alternative therapies.

KEY TERMS

complementary and alternative medicine (CAM) *60*

dietary supplements *66*

Dietary Supplement and Nonprescription Drug Consumer Protection Act *67*

Dietary Supplement Health and Education Act (DSHEA) of 1994 *66*

herb *61*

specialty supplements *65*

omplementary and alternative therapies represent a multibillion dollar industry. Sales of dietary supplements alone exceed $26 billion annually, with over 200 million consumers using them. Consumers have turned to these treatments for a wide variety of reasons. Many people have the impression that natural substances have more healing power than synthetic medications. The ready availability of over-the-counter (OTC) herbal supplements and specialty supplements at a reasonable cost, combined with effective marketing strategies, has convinced many people to try them. This chapter examines the role of herbal and specialty supplements in the prevention and treatment of disease.

Complementary and alternative therapies are used by a large number of people to prevent and treat disease.

CORE CONCEPT 6.1

Complementary and alternative medicine (CAM) comprises an extremely diverse set of therapies and healing systems that are considered to be outside of mainstream health care. CAM systems have the following common characteristics:

- Focus on treating the individual
- Consider the health of the whole person
- Emphasize the integration of mind and body
- Promote disease prevention, self-care, and self-healing
- Recognize the role of spirituality in health and healing

Because of its popularity, the scientific community has focused considerable attention on determining the effectiveness or lack of effectiveness of CAM. Although some research into these alternative systems has been conducted, few CAM therapies have been subjected to rigorous clinical and scientific study. It is likely that some of these therapies will become mainstream treatments, whereas others will be found ineffective. The line between what is defined as an alternative therapy and what is considered mainstream is constantly changing. Increasing numbers of healthcare providers now recommend CAM therapies to their patients. Table 6.1 ◆ describes some of these therapies.

TABLE 6.1 Complementary and Alternative Therapies	
Healing Method	**Examples**
Biologic therapies	Herbal therapies
	Nutritional supplements
	Special diets
Alternate healthcare systems	Naturopathy
	Homeopathy
	Chiropractic
	Native American medicine (e.g., sweat lodges, medicine wheel)
	Chinese traditional medicine (e.g., acupuncture, Chinese herbs)
Manual healing	Massage
	Physical therapy
	Pressure-point therapies
Mind–body interventions	Yoga
	Meditation
	Hypnotherapy
	Guided imagery
	Biofeedback
	Movement-oriented therapies (e.g., music, dance)
Spiritual	Shamanism
	Faith and prayer

Fast Facts Alternative Therapies in America

One of the largest studies of Americans' use of complementary therapies conducted by the National Center for Complementary and Alternative Medicine (NCCAM) surveyed over 23,000 people (Barnes, Bloom, & Nahin, 2008). Findings of this study included the following:

- Thirty-eight percent of adults and about 12% of children are currently using CAM.

- Women and those with higher educational levels are most likely to use CAM.

- The most frequent conditions treated with CAM are back pain (17%), head or chest cold (10%), joint pain/arthritis (5%), neck pain (5%), and anxiety or depression (5%).

- People are more likely to use CAM when they are unable to afford conventional health care.

Healthcare providers have long known the value of CAM therapies in preventing and treating disease. For example, prayer, meditation, massage, and yoga have been used for centuries to treat both body and mind. From a therapeutic perspective, much of the value of CAM therapies is their ability to reduce the need for medications. If a patient can find anxiety relief through massage or biofeedback therapy, for example, the use of antianxiety drugs may be reduced or eliminated. Reduction of drug dose leads to fewer adverse effects and better compliance with drug therapy. This chapter focuses on two CAM therapies: herbs and specialty supplements.

Concept Review   6.1

- How does the healing philosophy of complementary and alternative medicine differ from that of conventional mainstream medicine?

HERBAL PRODUCTS

The number of people seeking herbal alternatives to conventional medical therapies has steadily increased over the past three decades. Many herbs are extensively used by patients as supplements to traditional pharmacotherapy.

Natural products from plants have been used as medicines for thousands of years.

CORE CONCEPT 6.2

Technically, an herb is a plant that lacks woody stems or bark. Over time, the term **herb** has come to refer to any plant product with a useful application, either as a food enhancer (such as a flavoring) or as a medicine.

The use of herbs in the treatment of disease has been recorded for thousands of years. One of the earliest recorded uses of plant products was a prescription for garlic in 3000 B.C. Eastern and Western medicine have recorded thousands of herbs and herb combinations claimed to have therapeutic value. Some of the most popular herbs and their primary uses are shown in Table 6.2 ◆.

The public's interest in herbal medicine began to decline when the pharmaceutical industry was born in the late 1800s. Drugs could be standardized and produced more cheaply than natural herbal products. In the early 1900s, regulatory agencies required that medicines be safe and effective. The focus of health care shifted to treating specific diseases, rather than promoting wellness and holistic care. Information about most herbal and alternative therapies was no longer taught in medical schools; these healing techniques were criticized as being unscientific relics of the past.

Beginning in the 1970s and continuing to the present day, herbal medicine has experienced a remarkable comeback. The majority of adult Americans are either currently taking herbal products on a regular basis or have taken them in the past. This increase in popularity has been due to a number of factors, including increased availability of herbal products, aggressive marketing by the herbal industry, increased attention to natural alternatives, and renewed interest in preventive medicine. The gradual aging of the population has led to more patients seeking therapeutic alternatives for chronic conditions such as pain, arthritis, prostate difficulties, and the need for hormone replacement. In addition, the high cost of prescription medicines has driven many people to seek less expensive alternatives.

TABLE 6.2 Popular Herbal Products

Common Name	Medicinal Part	Primary Use(s)
Aloe	Leaves	Treat skin ailments (topical) and constipation (oral)
Bilberry	Berries/leaf	Terminate diarrhea, improve and protect vision
Black cohosh	Roots	Relieve menopause symptoms
Cranberry	Berries/juice	Prevent urinary tract infection
Echinacea	Entire plant	Enhance immune system, reduce inflammation
Evening primrose	Oil extracted from seeds	Relieve pain and inflammation
Flaxseed	Seeds and oil	Reduce blood cholesterol, laxative
Garlic	Bulbs	Reduce blood cholesterol and blood pressure, as an anticoagulant
Ginger	Root	Relieve GI upset and motion sickness, as an anti-inflammatory
Ginkgo biloba	Leaves and seeds	Improve memory, reduce dizziness
Ginseng	Root	Relieve stress, enhance immune system, decrease fatigue
Horny goat weed	Leaves and roots	Enhance sexual function
Milk thistle	Seeds	As an antitoxin to protect against liver disease
Red yeast rice extract	Dried in capsules	Reduce blood cholesterol
Saw palmetto	Ripe fruit/berries	Relieve urinary problems related to prostate enlargement
Soy	Beans	Source of protein, vitamins, and minerals; relieve menopausal symptoms; prevent cardiovascular disease; as an anticancer agent
St. John's wort	Flowers, leaves, stems	Reduce depression, reduce anxiety, as an anti-inflammatory
Valerian	Roots	Relieve stress, promote sleep

▶ **Life Span Fact**

A wide range of dietary supplements, such as herbs and other specialty products, are being used to treat children. Unfortunately, the use of these therapies has not been well studied with children. Just as with conventional medicine, children may react differently than adults to herbal and other CAM therapies. The healthcare provider should assess for the use of supplements in all pediatric patients. It is important to ensure that caregivers know the importance of an accurate diagnosis from a licensed healthcare provider and that supplements or other CAM products should not replace or delay conventional medical care. In addition, caregivers should be taught to store all herbs/dietary supplements away from children, use only as directed, and report any side effects to the child's healthcare provider.

CORE CONCEPT 6.3

Herbal products are standardized with respect to a specific active ingredient.

The active ingredients in an herbal product may be present in only one specific part of the plant or in all parts. For example, the active chemicals in saw palmetto are in the berries. For ginger and black cohosh, the roots are used for their healing properties.

Most modern drugs contain only one active ingredient. This chemical is standardized and accurately measured so that the amount of drug received by the patient is precisely known. It is a common misconception that herbal products also contain one active ingredient, which can be extracted and delivered to patients in exact amounts, like drugs. Herbs, however, may contain dozens of active chemicals, many of which have not yet been isolated, studied, or even identified. It is possible that some of these substances work together synergistically and may not have the same activity if isolated. Furthermore, the strength of an herbal preparation often varies from batch to batch depending on where the herb was grown and how it was collected, prepared, and stored.

To achieve consistency in the strength or "dose" of an herbal product, scientists have attempted to standardize herbal products. Standardization allows the consumer to compare products and know the strength of the herb. Some of these standardizations are shown in Table 6.3 ◆. Until science can better characterize these substances, however, it is best to view the active ingredient of an herb as being the entire herb. An example of standardization—the ingredients of ginkgo biloba—is shown in Figure 6.1 ■.

The two basic formulations of herbal products are solid and liquid. Solid products include pills, tablets, and capsules made from dried herbs. Other solid products are salves and ointments that are administered topically. Liquid formulations are made by extracting the active chemicals from the plant and include teas, infusions, tinctures, and extracts. Some formulations of ginkgo biloba, one of the most popular herbals, are illustrated in Figure 6.2 ■.

TABLE 6.3   Standardization of Selected Herb Extracts

Herb	Standardization	Percent
Black cohosh	Triterpene glycosides	2.5
Echinacea	Echinacosides	4
Ginger	Pungent compounds (gingerols)	Greater than 10
Ginkgo leaf	Flavonglycosides	24–25
	Lactones	6
Ginseng root	Ginseosides	5–15
Milk thistle root	Silymarin	80
St. John's wort	Hypericins	0.3–0.5
	Hyperforin	3–5
Saw palmetto	Fatty acids and sterols	80–90

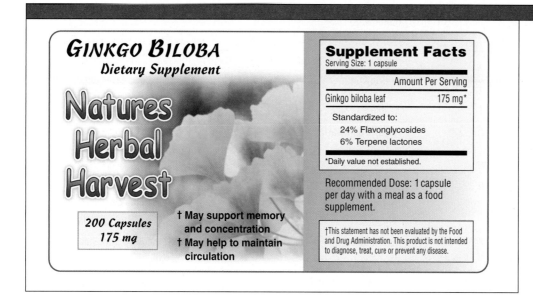

FIGURE 6.1

Ginkgo Biloba label. The label indicates the product is standardized to percent flavonglycosides and percent terpenes, active substances that are found in the ginkgo leaf. Also note the health claims on the label, which have not been evaluated by the FDA.

Herbs can have significant pharmacologic actions and can interact with conventional drugs.

CORE CONCEPT 6.4

A key concept to remember when dealing with alternative therapies is that natural does not always mean better or safe. There is no question that some herbs contain active chemicals as powerful as, and perhaps more effective than, currently approved medications. Thousands of years of experience, combined with current scientific research, have shown that some of these herbal remedies have therapeutic actions. Because a substance comes from a natural product, however, does not make it either safe or effective. For example, poison ivy is natural, but it certainly is not safe or therapeutic. Natural products may not offer an improvement over conventional therapy in treating certain disorders and, indeed, may be of no value whatsoever. Most importantly, a patient who substitutes an unproven alternative therapy for an established, effective medical treatment may delay healing, suffer harmful effects, and endanger his or her health.

Some herbal products contain ingredients that may interact with prescription drugs. For example, patients taking medications with potentially serious adverse effects, such as insulin, warfarin (Coumadin), or digoxin (Lanoxin), should be warned never to take any dietary supplement without first discussing their needs with their nurse practitioner or physician. Pregnant or lactating women should not take herbal products

FIGURE 6.2

Three different ginkgo formulations: tablets, tea bags, and liquid extract.

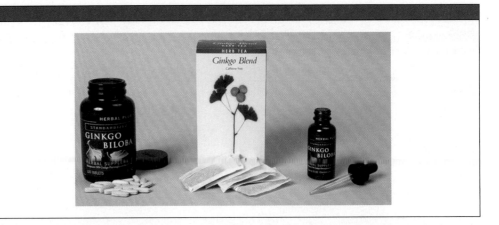

TABLE 6.4 Selected Herb–Drug Interactions

Common Name	Interacts With	Comments
Echinacea	Amiodarone, anabolic steroids, ketoconazole, methotrexate	Possible increased hepatotoxicity
Garlic	Aspirin and other NSAIDs, warfarin (Coumadin)	Increased bleeding risk
	Insulin, oral hypoglycemic agents	Additive hypoglycemic effects
Ginger	Aspirin and other NSAIDs, heparin, warfarin	Increased bleeding risk
Ginkgo biloba	Anticonvulsants	Possible decreased anticonvulsant effectiveness
	Aspirin and NSAIDs	Increased bleeding potential
	Heparin and warfarin (Coumadin)	Increased bleeding potential
	Tricyclic antidepressants	Possible decreased seizure threshold
Ginseng	CNS depressants	Increased sedation
	Digoxin (Lanoxin)	Increased toxicity
	Diuretics	Possible weakened diuretic effects
	Insulin and oral hypoglycemic agents	Increased hypoglycemic effects
	Warfarin	Decreased anticoagulant effects
St. John's wort	CNS depressants and opiates	Increased sedation
	Cyclosporine (Sandimmune)	Possible decreased cyclosporine levels
	Oral contraceptives	Decreased drug effectiveness
	Selective serotonin reuptake inhibitors (SSRIs), tricyclic antidepressants	Possible serotonin syndrome (headache, dizziness, sweating, agitation)
	Warfarin (Coumadin)	Decreased anticoagulant effects
Valerian	Barbiturates, benzodiazepines, and other CNS depressants	Increased sedation

without the approval of their healthcare provider. The health professional should also remember that the potential for any drug interaction increases in older adults, especially those with hepatic or renal impairment. Although the true extent of herb–drug interactions is largely unknown, some of the documented interactions are shown in Table 6.4 ◆.

Another warning that must be heeded with natural products is to beware of allergic reactions. Most herbal products contain a mixture of ingredients, and it is not unusual to find dozens of different chemicals in teas and infusions made from the flowers, leaves, or roots of a plant. Patients who have known allergies to certain foods or medicines should seek medical advice before taking an herbal product. It is always wise to take the smallest amount possible—less than the recommended dose—when starting herbal therapy to see if allergies or other adverse effects occur.

Healthcare providers have an obligation to seek the latest medical information on herbal products because there is a good possibility that their patients are using them to supplement traditional medicines. Patients should be advised to be skeptical of claims on the labels of dietary supplements and to seek their health information from reputable sources. Healthcare providers should never condemn patients' use of alternative therapies, but instead be supportive and seek to understand their goals for taking the supplements. The healthcare provider should teach patients the appropriate role of alternative therapies in the treatment of their disorders and discuss which treatments or combination of treatments will best meet their health goals.

SPECIALTY SUPPLEMENTS

Specialty supplements are *nonherbal* dietary supplements that can come from either plant or animal sources. Like herbal therapies, they are available OTC and are widely used by patients to enhance wellness.

Specialty supplements are nonherbal products that are widely used to promote wellness.

CORE CONCEPT 6.5

The actions of specialty supplements are more specific than those of herbal products, and they are generally targeted for one or a small number of conditions. Popular specialty supplements are listed in Table 6.5 ◆

In general, specialty supplements have a legitimate rationale for their use. For example, chondroitin and glucosamine are natural substances in the body necessary for cartilage growth and maintenance. Amino acids are natural building blocks of muscle protein. Fish oils contain omega fatty acids that have been shown to reduce the risk of heart disease in certain patients.

Unfortunately, the link between most specialty supplements and their benefits is unclear. In some cases, the body already has sufficient quantities of the substance; therefore, taking additional amounts may be of no benefit. In other cases, the supplement is marketed for conditions for which it has no proven effect (See Figure 6.3 ■). The good news is that these substances, when taken in amounts stated on the label, are generally not harmful. The bad news, however, is that they can give patients false hopes of an easy cure for a chronic condition such as heart disease or the pain of arthritis. As with herbal products, the healthcare provider should advise patients to be skeptical about the health claims regarding the use of these supplements.

Concept Review 6.2

■ Explain the differences between an herbal product and a specialty supplement.

Herbal products and specialty supplements are not regulated in the same manner as prescription medications.

CORE CONCEPT 6.6

Since the passage of the Food, Drug, and Cosmetic Act of 1935, Americans have come to expect that all prescription and OTC drugs have passed rigid standards of safety prior to being marketed. Furthermore, it

TABLE 6.5 Popular Specialty Supplements	
Name	**Common Uses**
Amino acids	Build protein, muscle strength, and endurance
Carnitine	Enhance energy and sports performance, heart health, memory, immune function, and male fertility
Coenzyme Q10	Treat heart disease, as an antioxidant
Dehydroepiandrosterone (DHEA)	Boost immune functions and memory
Fish oil	Reduce blood cholesterol, enhance brain function, increase visual acuity (due to presence of omega-3 fatty acids)
Glucosamine and chondroitin	Treat arthritis and other joint problems
Lactobacillus acidophilus	Maintain intestinal health
Melatonin	Restore normal sleep patterns
Methyl sulfonyl methane (MSM)	Reduce allergic reactions to pollen and foods, relieve pain and inflammation of arthritis and similar conditions
Selenium	Reduce the risk of certain types of cancer
Vitamin C	Prevent colds

FIGURE 6.3

L-carnitine is a popular dietary supplement. Notice the marketing targeted to improve (a) athletic performance and (b) weight loss, neither of which have been supported by the scientific literature.

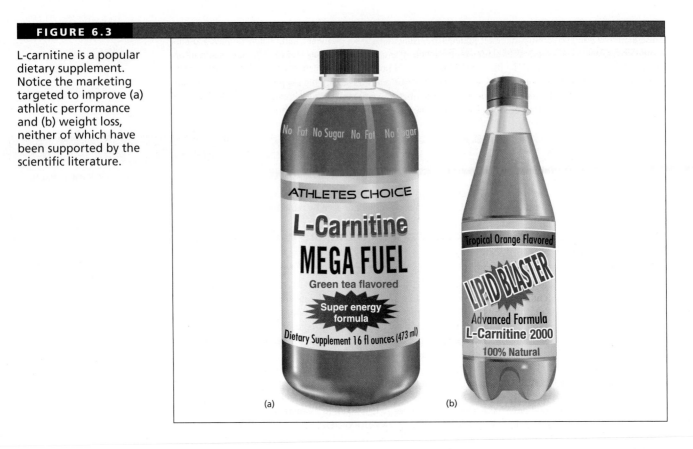

(a)   (b)

is assumed that the effectiveness of these drugs has been tested, and that they truly provide the therapeutic benefits claimed by the manufacturer. Indeed, most people would be outraged if they found out that the drug they purchased for pain relief or to cure an infectious disease was totally ineffective. Unfortunately, herbal products and specialty supplements are regulated by a far less restrictive law, the **Dietary Supplement Health and Education Act (DSHEA) of 1994**, than are drugs.

The DSHEA exempts dietary supplements from the Food, Drug, and Cosmetic Act, the legislation that regulates prescription drugs. **Dietary supplements** are defined as products intended to enhance or supplement the diet. They are not approved as drugs by the Food and Drug Administration (FDA). The DSHEA requires these products to be clearly labeled as dietary supplements. Figure 6.1 shows the label for ginkgo biloba clearly stating that the supplement is not approved by the FDA to treat any medical condition.

One strength of the legislation is that it gives the FDA the power to remove from the market any product that poses a "significant or unreasonable" risk to the public. The FDA used this legislative authority when the dietary supplement ephedra was removed from the market because of reported serious side effects in some patients. However, it took seven years from the time the FDA first warned consumers of the dangers of ephedra until it was removed from the market.

Unfortunately, the DSHEA has significant weaknesses that allow a lack of standardization in the dietary supplement industry and less protection of the consumer. These flaws include:

- Dietary supplements do not have to be tested by the manufacturer prior to marketing.
- The effectiveness of a dietary supplement does not have to be demonstrated by the manufacturer.
- The manufacturer does not have to prove the safety of the dietary supplement. It is the government's job to prove that the dietary supplement is *unsafe* and to take the necessary steps to remove it from the market.
- The label of a dietary supplement must clearly state that the product is not intended to diagnose, treat, cure, or prevent any disease. However, claims about a product's effect on body structure and function are allowed, including the following:
  - Helps promote healthy immune systems
  - Reduces anxiety and stress
  - Helps to maintain cardiovascular function
  - May reduce pain and inflammation
- The DSHEA does not regulate the *accuracy* of the label; the product may or may not contain the product listed in the amounts claimed.

Several steps have been taken to address the lack of purity and mislabeling of herbal and dietary supplements. In an attempt to protect consumers, Congress passed the **Dietary Supplement and Nonprescription Drug Consumer Protection Act**, which took effect in 2007. Companies marketing herbal and dietary supplements are now required to include contact information (address and phone number) on the product labels for consumers to use in reporting adverse events. Companies must notify the FDA of a "serious adverse event," which is defined as any adverse reaction resulting in death, a life-threatening experience, inpatient hospitalization, a persistent or significant disability, or a birth defect. Companies must notify the FDA of any serious adverse event reports within 15 days of receiving such reports.

Also in 2007, the FDA announced a final rule that requires the manufacturers of dietary supplements to evaluate the identity, purity, potency, and composition of their products. The labels must accurately reflect what is in the product, which must be free of contaminants such as pesticides, toxins, glass, or heavy metals.

Concept Review 6.3

■ How does the federal regulation of an herb by the DSHEA differ from the federal regulation of a prescription drug?

CHAPTER REVIEW

CORE CONCEPTS SUMMARY

6.1 Complementary and alternative therapies are used by a large number of people to prevent and treat disease.

Complementary and alternative medicine (CAM) is a set of therapies and healing systems used by many patients for disease prevention and self-healing. Complementary therapies offer nonpharmacologic alternatives to promote health and healing. They focus on the holistic treatment of each patient, integrate mind and body, and are often used in conjunction with conventional medical therapies.

6.2 Natural products from plants have been used as medicines for thousands of years.

Thousands of herbal therapies are recorded in Eastern and Western history. The popularity of alternative herbal remedies has steadily increased in recent years.

6.3 Herbal products are standardized with respect to a specific active ingredient.

Herbal products are marketed in a number of different formulations, some consisting of standardized extracts of specific chemicals, others containing whole herbs. Unlike drugs, herbs contain a large number of chemicals that may act in a coordinated manner to produce a therapeutic effect. The active ingredients may be in the flowers, leaves, stems, or roots of an herb.

6.4 Herbs can have significant pharmacologic actions and can interact with conventional drugs.

Just because a substance comes from a natural product does not make it safe or effective. Although herbal supplements may have therapeutic applications, they may not be the best product for treating the disease and may interact with prescription medicines.

6.5 Specialty supplements are nonherbal products that are widely used to promote wellness.

Specialty supplements include nonherbal therapies that are used to enhance a specific aspect of wellness. These products usually have a rational basis for therapy, although their benefits have not been conclusively proven.

6.6 Herbal products and specialty supplements are not regulated in the same manner as prescription medications.

The DSHEA loosely regulates herbal and dietary supplements. Dietary supplements and herbal products can be marketed without any proof that they are safe or effective. The Dietary Supplement and Nonprescription Drug Consumer Protection Act of 2007 required manufacturers to evaluate the purity, potency, and composition of their products. Labels must accurately reflect what is in the product, which must be free of contaminants.

REVIEW QUESTIONS

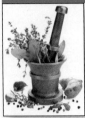

The following questions are written in NCLEX-PN® style. Answer these questions to assess your knowledge of the chapter material, and go back and review any material that is not clear to you.

1. The patient is to be started on warfarin (Coumadin) therapy. It is important for the nurse to check for the use of which herbs? (Select all that apply.)

1. Ginseng
2. Ginger
3. St. John's wort
4. Valerian

2. Patients often use herbal therapies for which of the following reasons?

1. To prevent overuse of prescription medications
2. To increase feelings of wellness and promote holistic treatment
3. Because herbal therapies are much more regulated than prescription drugs
4. Because herbal therapies are so much safer than man-made drugs

3. It is important that nurses ensure that their patients receive education regarding herbal products because:

1. Herbal products are approved under strict FDA regulations.
2. Labeling is not always reliable and herbal products should be used with caution.
3. There are so few side effects, and they can be purchased without a prescription.
4. The manufacturer has repeatedly demonstrated effectiveness.

4. An example of a specialty supplement is:

1. *Lactobacillus acidophilus*
2. Ginseng
3. Garlic
4. Ginkgo biloba

5. It is important for the nurse to collect information from the patient about the use of complementary and alternative medicine (CAM) because:

1. Patients must be warned that most CAM therapies are dangerous.
2. Additional treatment may not be needed.

3. CAM therapies could interact with prescription and OTC medications.
4. Most CAM therapies are totally ineffective.

6. The nurse understands that specialty supplements are used:

1. For a diverse range of disease conditions
2. For treatment of a targeted condition
3. When prescriptive medications are no longer effective
4. When the body no longer makes sufficient quantities of the substance

7. The Dietary Supplement Health and Education Act (DHSEA) is responsible for:

1. Strict herbal product testing
2. Ensuring that herbal products are labeled as "dietary supplements"
3. Sending the herbal product to the FDA for evaluation
4. Ensuring safety of the product

8. The patient is admitted with digoxin (Lanoxin) toxicity. The nurse checks for the use of which of the following herbal products?

1. St. John's wort
2. Valerian
3. Fish oil
4. Ginseng

9. The patient requests information on alternative treatments for her arthritis. The nurse provides the patient information on which of the following supplements?

1. Garlic and soy
2. Fish oil
3. Chondroitin and glucosamine
4. DHEA

10. Which of the following herbal products is commonly used to enhance the immune system?

1. Soy
2. Saw palmetto
3. Cranberry
4. Echinacea

NOTE: Answers to the Review Questions appear in Appendix B. The complete rationales and answers are located on the textbook's website.

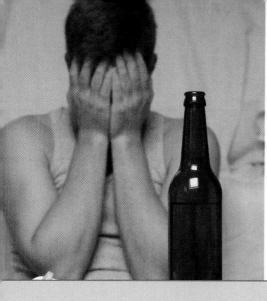

CHAPTER

7

Substance Abuse

CORE CONCEPTS

7.1 Abused substances belong to many different chemical classes.

7.2 Addiction depends on multiple, complex, and interacting variables.

7.3 Substance dependence is classified as physical dependence or psychological dependence.

7.4 Withdrawal results when an abused substance is no longer available.

7.5 Tolerance occurs when higher and higher doses of a drug are needed to achieve the initial response.

7.6 Central nervous system (CNS) depressants decrease the activity of the central nervous system.

7.7 Marijuana produces little physical dependence or tolerance.

7.8 Hallucinogens cause an altered state of thought and perception similar to that found in dreams.

7.9 CNS stimulants increase the activity of the central nervous system.

7.10 Nicotine is powerful and highly addictive.

7.11 Healthcare providers strive to remain free from impairment due to alcohol and drug addiction.

LEARNING OUTCOMES

After reading this chapter, the student should be able to:

1. Discuss the underlying causes of addiction.

2. Compare and contrast psychological and physical dependence.

3. Compare and contrast classic and conditioned withdrawal.

4. Explain the significance of drug tolerance to pharmacotherapy.

5. Explain the major characteristics of abuse, dependence, and tolerance resulting from alcohol, nicotine, marijuana, hallucinogens, CNS stimulants, sedatives, and opioids.

6. List the reasons why healthcare providers may have problems with alcohol or substance abuse.

7. Identify the signs of substance abuse exhibited by the healthcare provider.

KEY TERMS

addiction (ah-DIK-shun) 71

alcohol intoxication (AL-ku-hol in-tak-su-KA-shun) 75

analgesics (AN-ahl-GEE-siks) 70

attention deficit disorder (ADD) 78

attention deficit-hyperactivity disorder (ADHD) 78

club drugs 70

cross-tolerance (krause TOL-er-ans) 73

designer drugs (de-ZEYE-ner drugs) 70

narcolepsy (NAR-koh-lep-see) 78

opioids (OH-pee-oyds) 72

physical dependence (FI-zi-kul dee-PEN-dens) 72

psychedelics (seye-keh-DEL-iks) 76

psychological dependence (seye-koh-LOJ-i-kul dee-PEN-dens) 72

substance abuse 70

substance dependence 72

tetrahydrocannabinol (THC) (TEH-trah-HEYE-droh-cah-NAB-in-ol) 76

tolerance (TOL-er-ans) 73

withdrawal syndrome (with-DRAW-ul SIN-drom) 72

Substance abuse is the self-administration of a drug in a way that one's culture or society views as abnormal and not acceptable. Throughout history, individuals have consumed both natural and prescription drugs to increase physical or mental performance, cause a relaxed feeling, change a psychological state, or simply fit in with the crowd. Substance abuse has a tremendous economic, social, and public health impact on society.

CORE CONCEPT 7.1

Abused substances belong to many different chemical classes.

Substances from a wide variety of chemical classes are abused and can be taken by many different routes. Abused substances have in common an ability to affect the nervous system, particularly the brain. Some agents, such as opium, marijuana, cocaine, nicotine, caffeine, and alcohol, are obtained from natural sources. Others agents are synthetic or **designer drugs** that are created in illegal laboratories solely for making money in illegal drug trafficking. **Club drugs** are substances taken at dance clubs, all-night parties, and raves.

Although the public often connects substance abuse with illegal drugs, this is not necessarily the case: Alcohol and nicotine are the two most commonly abused drugs. Legal prescription medications such as oxycodone (OxyContin), methamphetamine, and alprazolam (Xanax) have become frequent drugs of abuse. Volatile inhalants, found in common household products such as aerosols and paint thinners, are often abused. Aerosols will make a user high with the practice of "huffing." Marijuana is the most frequently abused illegal drug nationwide. Other frequently abused substances include **analgesics** or *pain-reducing* drugs, sedatives, hallucinogens like lysergic acid diethylamide (LSD), and club drugs such as Ecstasy and flunitrazepam (Rohypnol), a powerful benzodiazepine depressant.

Several drugs once used therapeutically are now illegal because of their high potential for abuse. Cocaine was once widely used as a local anesthetic, but today all cocaine purchased and used in the private sector is illegal. LSD is now illegal, although in the 1940s and 1950s it was used in psychotherapy. Phencyclidine (PCP) was popular in the early 1960s as an anesthetic but was taken off the market in 1965 because patients reported hallucinations, delusions, and anxiety after recovering from anesthesia. Many of the amphetamines, once prescribed for bronchodilation, were stopped in the 1980s after psychotic episodes were reported. Some commonly abused substances are summarized in Table 7.1 ◆.

an = *without*

algesics = *causing pain*

sedatives = *causing sedation*

hallucinogens = *causing hallucinations*

Fast Facts Substance Abuse in the United States

- Over 28 million Americans have used illicit drugs at least once.
- Over 25% of high school students use an illegal drug monthly.
- An estimated 2.4 million Americans have used heroin during their lives.
- About one in five Americans has lived with an alcoholic while growing up. Children of alcoholic parents are four times more likely to become alcoholics than children of nonalcoholic parents.
- Alcohol is an important factor in 68% of manslaughters, 54% of murders, 48% of robberies, and 44% of burglaries.
- Among youth between the ages of 12 and 17, approximately 7.2 million have drunken alcohol at least once. Girls are as likely as boys to drink alcohol.
- Barbiturate overdose is a factor in almost one-third of all drug-related deaths.
- Thirty-six percent of 10th graders and 46% of 12th graders have reported using marijuana and hashish.
- Almost 8% of high school seniors have reported using cocaine.
- Two million Americans have used cocaine on a monthly basis; about 567,000 have used crack cocaine.
- Approximately 70% of the cocaine entering the United States comes from Colombia and passes through south Florida.
- Sixteen percent of 8th graders and 11% of 12th graders have reported using volatile inhalants.
- Thirty percent of all Americans are cigarette smokers, including 25% who are between the ages of 12 and 25.
- Forty-three percent of 10th graders and 54% of 12th graders have reported smoking cigarettes. Eight percent of 12th graders consume half a pack or more each day.
- Eight percent of 12th graders have reported using Ecstasy (MDMA).
- LSD is one of the most potent drugs known, with only 25–150 mcg constituting a dose. Almost 9% of 12th graders have reported using LSD.

TABLE 7.1 Commonly Abused Substances	Natural Substances	Medications
LEGAL SUBSTANCES WITHOUT PRESCRIPTION		
Ethyl alcohol	Drinking alcohol	OTC drugs
Aerosol inhalants	Solvents, varnishes	
Caffeine	Coffee	OTC drugs
Nicotine	Tobacco	Smoking cessation drugs
LEGAL SUBSTANCES WITH PRESCRIPTION		
Barbiturates		Sedatives; CNS depressants
Benzodiazepines		Sedatives; CNS depressants
Dextromethorphan (DMX)		OTC cough suppressants
Opioid Analgesics		Pain therapy
Ketamine		Anesthetic
Gamma hydroxybutyrate (GHB)		Anesthetic
Amphetamines, methamphetamines, and methylphenidate (Ritalin)		CNS stimulants
Anabolic steroids		Weight or muscle gain products
ILLEGAL SUBSTANCES OR DISCONTINUED IN TRADITIONAL THERAPIES		
Opioids	Opium	Heroin
Cannabinoids (THC)*	Marijuana	Glaucoma therapy
LSD	Rye/grain fungus	Psychiatric therapy
Psilocybin	Mushrooms	
Mescaline	Peyote	
Phencyclidine (PCP)*		Anesthetic
Cocaine	Coca plant	Local anesthetic
CLUB DRUGS WITH NO MEDICINAL USE—DESIGNER DRUGS		
MDA*		
MMDA* (Ecstasy)		
DOM* (STP)		

Chemical names are complicated and extensive; see Core Concepts 7.7 and 7.8 for more information.

Addiction depends on multiple, complex, and interacting variables.

Addiction, the progressive and chronic abuse of a substance, is an overwhelming feeling that drives someone to use a drug repeatedly despite serious health and social consequences. It is impossible to predict accurately whether a person will become an addict. Scientists have used psychological profiles and investigated genetic links in an attempt to predict a person's addictive tendency, but no firm connections have been found. Addiction depends on multiple, complex, and interacting variables. These variables fall into the following categories:

addict = *given over*

- *Agent or drug factors* Cost, availability, dose, method of administration (e.g., oral, IV, inhalation), speed of onset/duration of effect, and length of drug use

- *User factors* Genetic factors (e.g., metabolic enzymes, natural tolerance), tendency toward risk-taking behavior, prior experiences with drugs, disease that may require a scheduled drug

- *Environmental factors* Social/community *norms* (behavior accepted within a community), role models, peer influences, educational opportunities

Addiction may begin with a real need for pharmacotherapy. For example, narcotic analgesics may be prescribed for pain, or sedatives for a sleep disorder. A favorable experience of pain relief or being able to fall asleep may cause a patient to want to repeat these positive experiences.

It is a common misunderstanding, even among some health professionals, that the therapeutic use of scheduled drugs creates large numbers of patients with addiction. In fact, prescription drugs rarely cause addiction when used as prescribed. The risk of addiction for prescription medications is mostly a function of the dose and the length of therapy. For this reason, medications having a potential for abuse are usually prescribed at the lowest effective dose for the shortest time necessary to treat the medical problems (see Chapter 14 for more information on pain management). As mentioned in Chapters 1 and 2, numerous laws have been passed in an attempt to limit drug abuse and addiction.

CORE CONCEPT 7.3

Substance dependence is classified as physical dependence or psychological dependence.

Whether a substance is addictive relates to how easily an individual can stop taking it repeatedly. When a person has an overwhelming desire to take a drug and cannot stop, it is referred to as **substance dependence**. Substance dependence is classified into two categories: physical dependence and psychological dependence.

Physical dependence is an altered physical condition caused by the nervous system adapting to repeated substance use. Over time, the body's cells are tricked into believing that it is normal for the substance to continually be present. With physical dependence, uncomfortable symptoms, known as **withdrawal syndrome**, occur when the agent is stopped. **Opioids**, such as morphine and heroin, may produce physical dependence rather quickly with repeated doses, particularly when taken intravenously. Alcohol, sedatives, some stimulants, and nicotine are other examples of substances that may easily produce physical dependence with repeated use.

In contrast to physical dependence, **psychological dependence** causes no apparent signs of physical discomfort after the agent is stopped. The person, however, will have an intense craving and will display an overwhelming desire to continue using the substance even if there are obvious negative economic, physical, or social consequences. The intense craving may be associated with the individual's home environment or social contacts. Strong psychological cravings for a substance may continue for months or even years and is often responsible for *relapse* (return to the original drug-seeking behavior) during substance abuse therapy. Psychological dependence usually occurs only after relatively high doses of the substance have been used for a long time, such as with marijuana and antianxiety drugs. However, psychological dependence may develop quickly, perhaps after only one use, as with crack cocaine—a potent, inexpensive form of the drug.

re = *again*
lapse = *fall back*

CORE CONCEPT 7.4

Withdrawal results when an abused substance is no longer available.

Once an individual becomes physically dependent and the substance is stopped, withdrawal syndrome will occur. Symptoms of withdrawal syndrome may be severe for patients who are physically dependent on alcohol and sedatives. Helping a patient withdraw from these agents is best done in a substance abuse treatment facility. Examples of withdrawal syndromes related to different abused substances are listed in Table 7.2 ◆.

Prescription drugs may be used to reduce the severity of withdrawal symptoms. For example, alcohol withdrawal can be treated with a benzodiazepine such as diazepam (Valium), and opioid withdrawal might be treated with methadone. Other drugs used in the treatment of opioid dependence include buprenorphine (Subutex) and naloxone. These are discussed in Chapter 14. Symptoms of nicotine withdrawal may be relieved by nicotine replacement therapy (NRT) in the form of patches or chewing gum and the use of bupropion (Wellbutrin). No specific pharmacologic treatments are indicated for withdrawal from CNS stimulants, hallucinogens, marijuana, or inhalants.

With chronic substance abuse, patients will often associate their conditions and surroundings—including social contacts with other users—with use of the drug. Users tend to return to drug-seeking behavior when they interact with other substance abusers. Counselors often encourage patients to stop associating with past social contacts or having relationships with other substance abusers to lessen the possibility of relapse. With the assistance of self-help groups such as Alcoholics Anonymous, some patients are able to move to a drug-free lifestyle by making friends with new people who are drug free and alcohol free.

TABLE 7.2 Selected Drugs of Abuse, Withdrawal Symptoms, and Characteristics

Drug	Physiological and Psychological Effects	Signs of Toxicity
Alcohol	Tremors, fatigue, anxiety, abdominal cramping, hallucinations, confusion, seizures, delirium	Extreme somnolence, severe CNS depression, diminished reflexes, respiratory depression
Barbiturates	Insomnia, anxiety, weakness, abdominal cremps, tremor, anorexia, seizures, skin hypersensitivity reactions, hallucinations, delirium	Severe CNS depression, tremor, diaphoresis, vomiting, cyanosis, tachycardia, Cheyne–Stokes respirations
Benzodiazepines	Insomnia, restlessness, abdominal pain, nausea, sensitivity to light and sound, headache, fatigue, muscle twitches	Somnolence, confusion, diminished reflexes, coma
Cocaine and amphetamines	Mental depression, anxiety, extreme fatigue, hunger	Dysrhythmias, lethargy, skin pallor, psychosis
Hallucinogens	Rarely observed; dependent on specific drug	Panic reactions, confusion, blurred vision, increase in blood pressure, psychotic-like state
Marijuana	Irritability, restlessness, insomnia, tremor, chills, weight loss	Euphoria, paranoia, panic reactions, hallucinations, psychotic-like state
Nicotine	Irritability, anxiety, restlessness, headaches, increased appetite, insomnia, inability to concentrate, decrease in heart rate and blood pressure	Heart palpitations, tachyarrhythmias, confusion, depression, seizures
Opioids	Excessive sweating, restlessness, dilated pupils, agitation, goose bumps, tremor, violent yawning, increased heart rate and blood pressure, nausea/vomiting, abdominal cramps and pain, muscle spasms with kicking movements, weight loss	Respiratory depression, cyanosis, extreme somnolence, coma

Tolerance occurs when higher and higher doses of a drug are needed to achieve the initial response.

CORE CONCEPT 7.5

Tolerance is a biological condition that occurs when the body adapts to a substance after it is repeatedly administered. Over time, higher doses of the agent are needed to produce the initial effect. For example, at the start of pharmacotherapy, a patient may find that 2 mg of a sedative is effective for causing sleep. After taking the medication for several months, the patient notices that it takes 4 mg or perhaps 6 mg to fall asleep. Development of drug tolerance is common for substances that affect the nervous system. Tolerance should be thought of as a natural consequence of continued drug use and not be considered evidence of addiction or substance abuse.

Tolerance does not develop at the same rate for all actions of a drug. For example, patients usually develop tolerance to the nausea and vomiting produced by narcotic analgesics after only a few doses. Tolerance to the mood-altering effects of these drugs and to their ability to reduce pain develops more slowly but eventually may be complete. Tolerance never develops to these drugs' ability to constrict the pupils. Patients will often put up with annoying side effects of drugs, such as the sleepiness caused by antihistamines, if they know that tolerance to these effects will develop quickly.

Once tolerance develops to one substance, it often also occurs with use of closely related drugs. This reaction is known as **cross-tolerance**. For example, a heroin addict will be tolerant to the analgesic effects of other opioids such as morphine or meperidine. Patients who have developed tolerance to alcohol will show tolerance to other CNS depressants such as barbiturates, benzodiazepines, and some general anesthetics. This is important to know because doses of related medications may need to be adjusted so that the patient receives maximum therapeutic benefit.

The terms *immunity* and *resistance* are often confused with *tolerance*. These terms more correctly refer to the immune system and infections, and they should not be used to mean tolerance. For example, microorganisms become *resistant* to the effects of an antibiotic; they do not become *tolerant*. Patients become *tolerant* to the effects of pain relievers; they do not become *resistant*. Therefore, it is incorrect to say that patients are *immune* to drug therapy.

CAM THERAPY

Milk Thistle for Liver Damage

Milk thistle is a plant found growing in the Mediterranean region that has been used as an herbal medicine for centuries. The active ingredient in the milk thistle plant (*Silybum marianum*), silymarin, has been thought to protect the liver against injury. Some studies have indeed shown that silymarin is able to neutralize the effects of alcohol and actually stimulate liver regrowth. It acts as an antioxidant and free-radical scavenger. It is typically taken for liver cirrhosis, chronic hepatitis, and gallbladder disorders. The herb has few side effects other than mild diarrhea, bloating, and upset stomach.

Anti-inflammatory and anticarcinogenic properties of milk thistle have also been documented. Milk thistle has been claimed to reduce the growth of cancer cells, but this has not been confirmed by controlled research studies. The nurse should urge patients to report the use of this herb to their healthcare provider.

Concept Review   7.1

■ What is the difference between physical dependence and psychological dependence? How do patients know when they are physically dependent on a substance?

CORE CONCEPT 7.6

Central nervous system (CNS) depressants decrease the activity of the central nervous system.

depressant = *dispirited or lowered feeling*

CNS depressants form a group of drugs that cause patients to feel sedated or relaxed. Drugs in this group include barbiturates, nonbarbiturate sedative-hypnotics, benzodiazepines, alcohol, and opioids. Although the majority of these substances are legal, they are controlled because of their abuse potential.

Sedatives and Sedative-Hypnotics

tranquilizer = *causing a tranquil state*

Sedatives, sometimes referred to as *tranquilizers*, are prescribed mostly for sleep disorders and some forms of epilepsy. The two primary classes of sedatives are the barbiturates and the nonbarbiturate sedative-hypnotics. See Chapter 9 for discussion of their historic use in treating sleep disorders and Chapter 13 for their use in treating epilepsy. Their actions, indications, safety profiles, and addictive potential are generally the same. Physical dependence, psychological dependence, and tolerance develop when these agents are taken for long periods at high doses. Patients sometimes abuse these drugs by taking more doses than prescribed, sharing their medication with friends, or selling their medication. These drugs are frequently combined with other drugs of abuse such as CNS stimulants or alcohol. People with addiction often alternate between amphetamines, which keep them awake for several days, and barbiturates, which help them to relax and fall asleep. Methamphetamine, for example, is an amphetamine-like stimulant drug (Core Concept 7.9). It has the ability to keep someone awake and produce many of the signs that counter sleep such as an elevated breathing rate and heart rate, and increased blood pressure.

Many sedatives have a long duration of action. Effects may last an entire day, depending on the specific drug. Patients may appear dull or apathetic, with slurred speech and lack of motor coordination. High doses of these drugs suppress the respiratory centers in the brain, and the user may stop breathing or enter a coma. Death may result from overdose. Withdrawal symptoms from these drugs may also be life threatening.

eu = *healthy or well*
phoric = *bearing*

One drug of interest is gamma hydroxybutyric acid (GHB). GHB is approved by the Food and Drug Administration (FDA) as sodium oxybate (Xyrem) to treat patients with narcolepsy. Recreational users often abuse GHB by consuming this drug in high doses. Although used to produce a euphoric (pleasure) state, overdose of this drug can cause severe respiratory depression, seizures, and coma. Thus, its depressant effects warrant close attention in the nonbarbiturate sedative-hypnotic category.

Benzodiazepines

anxio = *anxiety/restlessness*
lytic = *destruction*

amnestic = *loss of memory*

Benzodiazepines are another group of CNS depressants that have a potential for abuse. They are one of the most widely prescribed classes of drugs and have largely replaced the barbiturates for certain disorders. Their primary indication is anxiety; thus, they are called *anxiolytic* drugs (see Chapter 9). They are also used for short-term treatment of seizures (see Chapter 13) and as muscle relaxants (see Chapter 12). Common benzodiazepines include alprazolam (Xanax), clonazepam (Klonopin), diazepam (Valium), temazepam (Restoril), triazolam (Halcion), and midazolam (Versed). Flunitrazepam (Rohypnol) is not approved by the FDA for any medical condition, but it is a club drug noted for its amnestic properties. Users will often feel carefree, without worry, and can even be subject to assault.

Although benzodiazepines are one of the most frequently prescribed drug classes, benzodiazepine abuse has various presentations. Those individuals who do abuse benzodiazepines may appear detached, sleepy, or disoriented. Death due to overdose is rare, even with high doses, unless benzodiazepines are used in combination with other CNS depressants. Abusers may combine these agents with alcohol, cocaine, or heroin to increase their drug experience. If combined with other agents, death due to overdose is very likely. Benzodiazepine withdrawal syndrome by itself is less severe than barbiturate withdrawal or alcohol withdrawal.

Opioids

Opioids are prescribed for severe pain, persistent cough, and diarrhea. The opioid class includes opium, morphine, and codeine, which are processed from natural substances found in the unripe seeds of the poppy plant, and synthetic drugs, such as hydromorphone (Dilaudid), oxycodone (OxyContin), fentanyl (Duragesic, Sublimaze), methadone (Dolophine), and heroin. The therapeutic effects of the opioids are discussed in detail in Chapter 14.

The effects of *oral* opioids begin within 30 minutes and may last over a day. *Parenteral* forms produce immediate effects, including the brief, intense rush of euphoria sought by heroin addicts. Individuals experience a range of CNS effects, from extreme pleasure to slowed body activities and extreme sedation. Signs include constricted pupils, an increase in the ability to withstand pain, and respiratory depression.

Addiction to opioids can occur rapidly, and withdrawal can produce intense symptoms. Although extremely unpleasant, withdrawal from opioids is not necessarily life threatening. Methadone is a narcotic sometimes used to treat opioid addiction. Although methadone has addictive properties of its own, it does not produce the same degree of euphoria as other opioids, and its effects are longer lasting. Heroin addicts may be switched to methadone to prevent unpleasant withdrawal symptoms. Because methadone is taken orally, the serious risks associated with intravenous drug use, such as hepatitis and AIDS, are eliminated. Patients sometimes remain on methadone maintenance for their lifetimes. Withdrawal from methadone is more prolonged than from heroin or morphine, but the symptoms are less intense.

Ethyl Alcohol

Ethyl alcohol, commonly known as alcohol, is one of the most widely abused drugs. Alcohol is a legal substance for adults and is available as beer, wine, and liquor. The economic, social, and health consequences of alcohol abuse are staggering. In contrast to the many negative consequences associated with long-term abuse of alcohol, drinking small quantities of alcohol on a daily basis has been found to reduce the risk of stroke and heart attack.

Alcohol is classified as a CNS depressant, because it slows the actions of the region of the brain responsible for alertness and wakefulness. Alcohol easily crosses the blood–brain barrier, and its effects can be noticed within 5 to 30 minutes. Effects of alcohol are directly related to the amount consumed within a certain time frame and include relaxation, sedation, memory impairment, loss of motor coordination, reduced judgment, and decreased inhibition. **Alcohol intoxication** occurs when muscle coordination is lost and mental function is affected. It results in a characteristic odor to the breath and increased blood flow in certain areas of the skin, causing a flushed face, pink cheeks, or red nose. Although these symptoms are easily recognized, the nurse must be aware that other substances and disorders may cause similar effects. For example, many antianxiety agents, sedatives, and antidepressants can cause drowsiness, memory difficulties, and loss of motor coordination. Certain mouthwashes, medicines, and other substances containing alcohol can give the breath an "alcoholic" smell.

The presence of food in the stomach will slow the absorption of alcohol, thus delaying the onset of drug action. *Metabolism*, or detoxification of alcohol by the liver, occurs at a slow, constant rate, which is not affected by the presence of food. The average rate is about 15 mL per hour—equal to one alcoholic beverage per hour. If consumed at a higher rate, alcohol will accumulate in the blood and produce greater effects on the brain. An overdose of alcohol produces vomiting, severe hypotension, respiratory failure, and coma. Death due to alcohol poisoning is common.

Chronic alcohol consumption produces both psychological and physiological dependence and results in a large number of adverse health effects. The organ most affected by chronic alcohol abuse is the liver. Alcoholism is a common cause of *cirrhosis*, a harmful and often fatal failure of the liver to perform its vital functions. Liver failure causes abnormalities in blood clotting and nutritional deficiencies and sensitizes the patient to the effects of all medications metabolized by the liver.

cirrh = *orange/yellow*
osis = *condition*

Alcohol withdrawal syndrome is severe and may be life threatening. The use of antiseizure medications for treating severe alcohol withdrawal symptoms is discussed in Chapter 13. Long-term treatment for alcohol abuse includes behavioral counseling and participation in self-help groups such as Alcoholics Anonymous. Disulfiram (Antabuse) may be given to discourage relapses. Disulfiram inhibits acetaldehyde dehydrogenase, the enzyme that metabolizes alcohol. If alcohol is consumed while taking disulfiram, the patient becomes violently ill within 5 to 10 minutes, with headache, shortness of breath, nausea/vomiting, and other unpleasant symptoms. Disulfiram is only effective in highly motivated patients, because the success of pharmacotherapy is entirely dependent on patient compliance. Alcohol sensitivity can continue for up to two weeks after disulfiram has been discontinued. As a pregnancy category X drug, disulfiram should never be taken during pregnancy.

In addition to disulfiram, acamprosate calcium (Campral, Forest) is an FDA-approved drug for maintaining alcohol abstinence in patients with alcohol dependence. Additional studies comparing the therapeutic benefit of disulfiram with acamprosate are needed. Adverse reactions to acamprosate include diarrhea, flatulence, and nausea. The drug is not recommended for patients who have impaired kidney functioning.

Concept Review 7.2

■ Compare the potential to cause coma or death of barbiturates and benzodiazepines.

CORE CONCEPT 7.7

Marijuana produces little physical dependence or tolerance.

Cannabinoids are substances obtained from the hemp plant *Cannabis sativa*, which grows in tropical climates. Cannabinoid agents are usually smoked and include marijuana, hashish, and hash oil. Although more than 61 cannabinoid chemicals have been identified, the ingredient responsible for most of the psychoactive properties is delta-9-**tetrahydrocannabinol (THC)**.

Marijuana (street names "grass," "pot," "weed," "reefer," or "dope") is a natural product obtained from *C. sativa*. It is the most commonly used illegal drug in the United States even though it has been legalized on a limited basis in some states. Use of marijuana slows motor activity, decreases coordination, and causes disconnected thoughts, paranoia, and euphoria. It increases thirst and craving for food, particularly chocolate and other candies. One hallmark symptom of marijuana use is red or bloodshot eyes, caused by dilation of blood vessels. THC also accumulates in the gonads.

para = *beside*
noia = *mind*

When inhaled, marijuana produces effects that occur within minutes and last up to 24 hours. Because marijuana smoke is inhaled more deeply and held within the lungs for a longer time than cigarette smoke, marijuana smoke introduces four times more tar into the lungs than tobacco smoke. Smoking marijuana on a daily basis may increase the risk of lung cancer and other respiratory disorders. Chronic use is associated with lack of motivation and loss of productivity.

Unlike many abused substances, marijuana produces little physical dependence or tolerance. Withdrawal symptoms are mild, if they are experienced at all. Metabolites of THC, however, remain in the body for months to years, allowing laboratory specialists to determine easily whether someone has used marijuana. For several days after use, THC can also be detected in the urine. Despite numerous attempts by scientists and clinicians to demonstrate therapeutic applications for marijuana, results have been controversial and the medical value of the drug remains to be proven.

Concept Review 7.3

■ Name three legal substances that are both used in traditional therapies and frequently abused. Are these substances natural or synthetic? Compare ethyl alcohol and marijuana in terms of common use.

CORE CONCEPT 7.8

Hallucinogens cause an altered state of thought and perception similar to that found in dreams.

Hallucinogens consist of an assorted class of chemicals that have in common the ability to produce an altered, dreamlike state of consciousness. Sometimes called **psychedelics**, the prototype substance for this class is LSD. All hallucinogens are Schedule I drugs and have no medical use.

For nearly all drugs of abuse, predictable symptoms occur in every user. Effects from hallucinogens, however, are highly variable and depend on the mood and expectations of the user and the surrounding environment in which the substance is used. Two patients taking the same agent will report completely different symptoms, and the same patient may report different symptoms with each use. Users who take LSD or *psilocybin* (Figure 7.1 ■) may experience symptoms such as laughter, visions, religious revelations, or deep personal insights. Common occurrences are hallucinations and afterimages (images that are projected onto people as they move). Users also report unusually bright lights and vivid colors. Some users hear voices; others report smells. Many experience a profound sense of truth and deep thoughts. Unpleasant experiences can be terrifying and may include anxiety, panic attacks, confusion, severe depression, or paranoia.

LSD (street names "acid," "the beast," "blotter acid," "California sunshine") is made from a fungus that grows on rye and other grains. LSD is almost always used in an oral form. It can be manufactured in capsules, tablets, or liquids. A common and inexpensive method for distributing LSD is to place drops of the drug on small pieces of paper that often contain images of cartoon characters or graphics related to the drug culture. After drying, the paper containing the LSD is swallowed to produce the drug's effects.

FIGURE 7.1

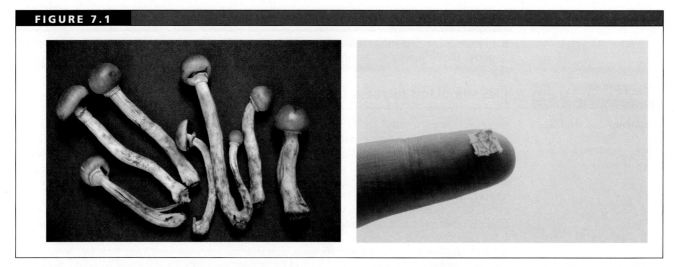

Comparison of psilocybin and LSD. Psilocybin is derived from a mushroom, shown in (a); an LSD "blot" is shown in (b).
Source: (left) Janine Wiedel Photolibrary/Alamy, (right) Joe Bird/Alamy

LSD is distributed throughout the body immediately after use. Effects are experienced within an hour and may last 6 to 12 hours. It affects the central and autonomic nervous systems, increasing blood pressure, elevating body temperature, dilating pupils, and increasing heart rate. Repeated use may cause memory loss and inability to reason. In extreme cases, patients may develop psychoses. One unusual adverse effect is flashbacks, in which the user experiences the effects of the drug again—sometimes weeks, months, or years after the drug was initially taken. Although users may experience tolerance, they have little or no dependence with hallucinogens.

Other hallucinogenic drugs that are abused include the following:

- *Mescaline* found in the peyote cactus of Mexico and Central America (Figure 7.2 ■)

- *MDMA (3,4-methylenedioxymethamphetamine, "XTC," or "Ecstasy")* an amphetamine originally created for research purposes but now extremely popular as a drug of abuse

- *DOM (2,5 dimethoxy-4-methylamphetamine, "STP")* a recreational drug often linked with rave parties

- *MDA (3,4-methylenedioxyamphetamine)* called the "love drug" because of a belief that it enhances sexual desires

- *PCP (chemical name phenylcyclohexylpiperadine; also called phencyclidine; street name "angel dust")* produces a trancelike state that may last for days and results in severe brain damage; used as an animal tranquilizer

- *Ketamine ("date rape" drug or "special K")* produces unconsciousness and amnesia; primary legal use is as an anesthetic

FIGURE 7.2

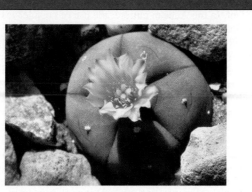

Mescaline is derived from the peyote plant (shown in photo).
Source: Konig/Jacana/Photo Researchers, Inc.

■ In examining and interviewing a patient, how could you determine whether he or she is under the influence of marijuana or hallucinogens?

CORE CONCEPT **7.9**

CNS stimulants increase the activity of the central nervous system.

stimulant = *arousing feelings*

narco = *numbness or stupor*

lepsy = *seizure*

Stimulants include a varied family of drugs with the ability to increase the activity of the CNS. Some are available by prescription for use in the treatment of **narcolepsy** (a sleep disorder in which people fall asleep unexpectedly), obesity, and **attention deficit disorder (ADD)** or **attention deficit hyperactivity disorder (ADHD)**. As drugs of abuse, CNS stimulants are taken to produce a sense of exhilaration, improve mental and physical performance, reduce appetite, prolong wakefulness, or simply "get high." Stimulants include amphetamines, cocaine, methylphenidate, and caffeine.

CNS stimulants have effects similar to the neurotransmitter norepinephrine, which is discussed in Chapter 8. Norepinephrine activates neurons in a part of the brain that affects awareness and wakefulness, called the *reticular formation* (see Chapter 9 for an in-depth discussion). High doses of amphetamines give the user a feeling of self-confidence, euphoria, alertness, and empowerment. Long-term use, however, often causes feelings of restlessness, anxiety, and fits of rage, especially when the user is coming down from a drug high.

Most CNS stimulants affect cardiovascular and respiratory activities, raising blood pressure and increasing respiration rate. Other symptoms include dilated pupils, sweating, and tremors. Overdoses of some stimulants lead to seizures and cardiac arrest.

Amphetamines and dextroamphetamines were once widely prescribed for depression, obesity, drowsiness, and congestion. In the 1960s, the healthcare profession realized that the risk for amphetamine dependence outweighed the drug's therapeutic usefulness. Because of the development of safer medications, the current therapeutic uses of these drugs are extremely limited. Most substance abusers get these agents from illegal laboratories, which can easily produce amphetamines and make tremendous profits.

Dextroamphetamine (Dexedrine) may be used to treat narcolepsy and for short-term weight loss when all other attempts to lose weight have been exhausted. Adderall (formulation of dextroamphetamine and amphetamine) is used to treat narcolepsy and ADHD.

Methamphetamine (street name "ice" or "crank") is often used as a recreational drug for those who like the "rush" that it provides. It is usually administered in powder or crystal form, but it also may be smoked. Methamphetamine is a Schedule II drug marketed under the trade name Desoxyn, although most abusers obtain it from illegal methamphetamine laboratories. A drug related to methamphetamine, called methcathinone (street name "cat"), is made illegally and snorted, taken orally, or injected intravenously. Methcathinone is a Schedule I agent.

Methylphenidate (Ritalin) is a CNS stimulant (Schedule II drug) that is widely prescribed for children diagnosed with ADD/ADHD (see Chapter 10). Ritalin has a calming effect on children who are inattentive or hyperactive. It stimulates the alertness center in the brain and allows the child to focus on tasks for longer periods. Lisdexamfetamine (Vyvanse) is another amphetamine-like substance used to treat ADHD. In adults and teens, Ritalin and Vyvanse usually produce the same effects as cocaine and amphetamines and are sometimes abused by adolescents and adults seeking euphoria. The tablets are crushed and used intranasally or dissolved in liquid and injected intravenously. Ritalin is also sometimes mixed with heroin (street name "speedball").

Cocaine is a natural substance obtained from the leaves of the coca plant, which grows in the Andes Mountain region of South America. The plant has been used by Andean cultures since 2500 B.C. Natives of this region chew the coca leaves or make teas of the dried leaves. Because it is taken orally, its absorption is slow, and the leaves contain only 1% cocaine, so users do not have the ill effects caused by chemically pure extracts from the plant. In the Andean culture, the use of coca leaves is not considered substance abuse because it is part of that society's culture.

Cocaine is a Schedule II drug that produces actions similar to those of the amphetamines, although its effects are usually more rapid and intense. It is the second most commonly abused illegal drug in the United States. Routes of administration include snorting, smoking, and injecting. In smaller doses, cocaine produces feelings of intense euphoria, a decrease in hunger, analgesia, delusions of physical strength, and increased sensory perception. Larger doses will magnify these effects and also cause rapid heartbeat, sweating, dilation of the pupils, and elevated body temperature. After euphoria diminishes, the user often feels irritable, depressed, and distrustful and usually has insomnia. Some users report the sensation that insects are crawling under their skin. Users who snort cocaine develop a chronic runny nose, a crusty redness around the nostrils, and deterioration of the nasal cartilage. Overdose can cause dysrhythmias, convulsions, stroke, or death due to respiratory arrest. The withdrawal syndrome for amphetamines and cocaine is much less intense than that from alcohol or barbiturates.

TABLE 7.3   Caffeine Content of Common Drugs, Foods, and Beverages

	Serving Size	Caffeine (mg)
OTC DRUGS		
NoDoz, maximum strength; Vivarin	1 tablet	200
Excedrin	2 tablets	130
NoDoz, regular strength	1 tablet	100
Anacin (also available in caffeine-free formulation)	2 tablets	64
COFFEES		
Coffee, brewed and instant	8 ounces	95–135
Coffee, decaffeinated	8 ounces	5
TEAS		
Tea, leaf or bag	8 ounces	50
Tea, green	8 ounces	30
Tea, instant	8 ounces	15
SOFT DRINKS		
Mountain Dew	12 ounces	55.5
Diet Coke	12 ounces	46.5
Coca-Cola Classic	12 ounces	34.5
Pepsi-Cola	12 ounces	37.5
CHOCOLATES AND CANDIES		
Hershey's Special Dark chocolate bar	1 bar (1.5 ounces)	31
Hershey Bar (milk chocolate)	1 bar (1.5 ounces)	10
Cocoa or hot chocolate	8 ounces	85

Caffeine is a natural substance found in the seeds, leaves, or fruits of more than 63 plant species throughout the world. Significant amounts of caffeine are consumed in chocolate, coffee, tea, and soft drinks (Table 7.3 ◆). Sometimes caffeine is added to over-the-counter (OTC) pain relievers to help relieve migraines and other conditions. Caffeine travels to almost all parts of the body after ingestion, and several hours are needed for the body to metabolize and eliminate the drug. Caffeine has a pronounced diuretic effect.

Caffeine is considered a CNS stimulant because it produces increased mental alertness, restlessness, nervousness, irritability, and insomnia. The physical effects of caffeine include bronchodilation, increased blood pressure, increased production of stomach acid, and changes in blood glucose levels. Repeated use of caffeine may result in physical dependence and tolerance.

Concept Review   7.5

■ Identify three groups of stimulants discussed in this section, and give examples for each group. Identify the major systems in the body affected by these stimulants.

Nicotine is powerful and highly addictive.

CORE CONCEPT 7.10

Nicotine is sometimes considered a CNS stimulant because of its ability to increase alertness. However, its actions and long-term consequences place it into a class by itself. Nicotine is unique among abused substances in that it is legal, strongly addictive, and highly carcinogenic. Furthermore, use of tobacco can cause harmful effects from secondhand smoke to those in the immediate area of the smoker. Patients often do not consider tobacco use to be substance abuse.

The most common method by which nicotine enters the body is through the inhalation of cigarette, pipe, or cigar smoke. Tobacco smoke contains more than 1,000 chemicals, many of which are carcinogens.

The primary addictive substance in cigarette smoke is nicotine. Effects of inhaled nicotine may last from 30 minutes to several hours.

Nicotine affects many body systems, including the nervous, cardiovascular, and endocrine systems. Nicotine stimulates the CNS directly, causing increased alertness and ability to focus, feelings of relaxation, and lightheadedness. The cardiovascular effects of nicotine include accelerated heart rate and increased blood pressure, caused by activation of nicotinic receptors located within the autonomic nervous system (see Chapter 8). These cardiovascular effects can be serious in patients taking oral contraceptives. The risk of a fatal heart attack is five times greater in smokers than in nonsmokers. Muscular tremors may occur with moderate doses of nicotine, and convulsions may result from very high doses. Nicotine affects the endocrine system by increasing the basal metabolic rate leading to weight loss. Nicotine also reduces appetite. Chronic use may lead to bronchitis, emphysema, and lung cancer.

Both psychological and physical dependence occur relatively quickly with nicotine. Once started on tobacco, patients tend to continue their drug use for many years, despite overwhelming medical evidence that their quality of life may be adversely affected and their life span shortened. Discontinuation results in agitation, weight gain, anxiety, headache, and an extreme craving for the drug. Although NRT (such as patches or gum), buproprion (Zyban, Wellbutrin), and varenicline tartrate (Chantix) assist patients in dealing with the unpleasant withdrawal symptoms, users often relapse because of stress, weight gain, and unpleasant symptoms.

Healthcare providers strive to remain free from impairment due to alcohol and drug addiction.

CORE CONCEPT 7.11

Healthcare providers play a key role in the identification, prevention, and treatment of substance abuse. Abusers are often reluctant to report their drug use, for fear of embarrassment or being arrested. Healthcare staff must be knowledgeable about the signs of substance abuse and withdrawal symptoms, and develop a keen sense of perception during interaction with their patients. A trusting healthcare provider–patient relationship is essential in helping patients deal with their dependence. By using therapeutic communication skills and by demonstrating a nonjudgmental, empathetic attitude, the healthcare team can build a trusting relationship with people that need medical assistance.

Impairment due to substance abuse is not only a behavioral or societal problem, but also a concern for the healthcare provider. Most nurses, for example, report that they have routinely encountered coworkers with perceived alcohol or substance abuse problems. Generally among nurses and other healthcare staff, alcohol is the most commonly abused legal substance; prescription drugs are abused secondly. Critical care nurses are especially likely to abuse stimulants and substances like marijuana or anxiolytic medications.

Reasons for these problems seem to be increasing tension due to the demands of the healthcare profession in general; social environments among medical professionals that promote self-reliance and independence; difficulty sleeping, in particular among workers with rotating shifts; and overall fatigue. Warning signs of substance abuse are overworking habits (e.g., arriving early and staying late for many days on end), high performance followed by deteriorating performance, isolation from other working staff, and frequent excuses (unexplained or complicated variables related to the worker's professional or social life).

Obvious signs may be frequent mood swings, irritability, or tearful outbursts followed by depression. Signs of substance abuse may be smell of alcohol on the breath covered up by mints or mouthwash, frequent absence from the unit to visit the restroom, or patients complaining of not receiving medications. Patients may complain about feeling pain despite having received seemingly adequate or repeated dosing of medication.

There are organizations that focus chiefly on addiction and the nursing profession as well as psychiatric disorders among nurses and other healthcare workers. The focus need not be just on disciplinary action but also on monitoring and support services. Agencies have adopted alternative disciplinary and peer assistance programs to make sure that both patients and healthcare providers receive proper assistance.

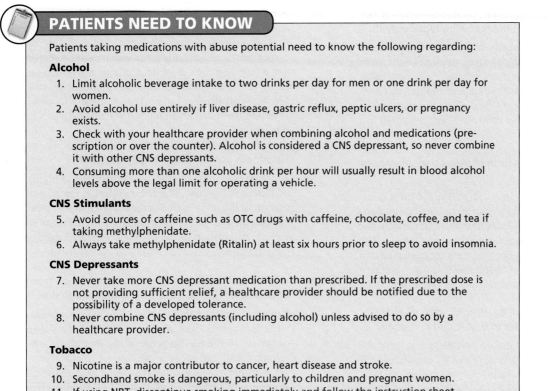

PATIENTS NEED TO KNOW

Patients taking medications with abuse potential need to know the following regarding:

Alcohol

1. Limit alcoholic beverage intake to two drinks per day for men or one drink per day for women.
2. Avoid alcohol use entirely if liver disease, gastric reflux, peptic ulcers, or pregnancy exists.
3. Check with your healthcare provider when combining alcohol and medications (prescription or over the counter). Alcohol is considered a CNS depressant, so never combine it with other CNS depressants.
4. Consuming more than one alcoholic drink per hour will usually result in blood alcohol levels above the legal limit for operating a vehicle.

CNS Stimulants

5. Avoid sources of caffeine such as OTC drugs with caffeine, chocolate, coffee, and tea if taking methylphenidate.
6. Always take methylphenidate (Ritalin) at least six hours prior to sleep to avoid insomnia.

CNS Depressants

7. Never take more CNS depressant medication than prescribed. If the prescribed dose is not providing sufficient relief, a healthcare provider should be notified due to the possibility of a developed tolerance.
8. Never combine CNS depressants (including alcohol) unless advised to do so by a healthcare provider.

Tobacco

9. Nicotine is a major contributor to cancer, heart disease and stroke.
10. Secondhand smoke is dangerous, particularly to children and pregnant women.
11. If using NRT, discontinue smoking immediately and follow the instruction sheet provided with the NRT of choice.

CHAPTER REVIEW

CORE CONCEPTS SUMMARY

7.1 Abused substances belong to many different chemical classes.

Some abused substances, such as alcohol and nicotine, are available without a prescription. Others, such as barbiturates, benzodiazepines, and most opioids, have legitimate medical uses. Still others, such as LSD and heroin, are illegal, having no current medical applications.

7.2 Addiction depends on multiple, complex, and interacting variables.

Addiction is an overwhelming feeling that causes someone to continue taking drugs. Although ideas about addiction have changed over the years, healthcare providers now recognize addiction as being related to drug, genetic, and environmental factors.

7.3 Substance dependence is classified as physical dependence or psychological dependence.

Dependence is an overwhelming need to take a drug on a continual basis. When physical dependence exists, the patient exhibits signs of withdrawal after the drug is discontinued. Psychological dependence is an intense craving for the drug.

7.4 Withdrawal results when an abused substance is no longer available.

When an abused drug is discontinued, patients may experience uncomfortable physical symptoms known as withdrawal syndrome. Symptoms vary depending on the specific drug of abuse and range from mild to life threatening.

7.5 Tolerance occurs when higher and higher doses of a drug are needed to achieve the initial response.

Tolerance occurs over time when patients adapt to continued drug use and require higher doses to produce the same effect. Cross-tolerance or tolerance resulting from prior exposure to a related drug also results in higher doses needed to produce the same effect.

7.6 Central nervous system (CNS) depressants decrease the activity of the central nervous system.

Substances that make patients feel relaxed and sleepy, and work by generally slowing neuronal activity in the brain, include sedatives, opioids, and ethyl alcohol. Examples of sedatives are barbiturates and benzodiazepines. Because of their abuse potential, many of these substances are controlled. Ethyl alcohol is a legal substance.

7.7 Marijuana produces little physical dependence or tolerance.

Despite legalization in some states, the most commonly abused illegal substance nationwide is marijuana. Marijuana produces less physical dependence than most other drugs and produces less tolerance. The medical value of this drug remains controversial and unproven. The risks of using this substance are lung cancer, respiratory problems, and lack of motivation.

7.8 Hallucinogens cause an altered state of thought and perception similar to that found in dreams.

Hallucinogens, also called psychedelics, have the ability to produce altered states of consciousness and dreams. They include LSD, mescaline, MDMA (Ecstasy), DOM (STP), MDA (love drug), and ketamine (an anesthetic).

7.9 CNS stimulants increase the activity of the central nervous system.

Amphetamines, methylphenidate, cocaine, and caffeine increase alertness by stimulating the central nervous system. Some substances are available by prescription and are used for narcolepsy, obesity, and attention deficit disorder. Caffeine is available in many consumer products, including chocolate, coffee, tea, soft drinks, and coffee ice cream. Cocaine is among the most commonly abused substances in America.

7.10 Nicotine is powerful and highly addictive.

Nicotine is a unique, legal, carcinogenic, and highly addictive substance. The most common method of entry into the body is by inhalation of cigarette, pipe, or cigar smoke. Important effects of inhaled nicotine include stimulation of the CNS and increased cardiovascular effects.

7.11 Healthcare providers strive to remain free from impairment due to alcohol and drug addiction.

Reasons why healthcare providers have problems with alcohol or drug abuse seem to be related to demands in the health profession, including self-reliant social and professional environments, rotating working shifts, and fatigue. Signs of impairment are frequent mood swings, irritability or depressive symptoms, smell of alcohol on the breath, frequent absences from the unit, and patients not receiving proper medications. Support groups and organizations assist with these related issues.

REVIEW QUESTIONS

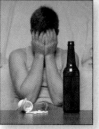

The following questions are written in NCLEX-PN® style. Answer these questions to assess your knowledge of the chapter material, and go back and review any material that is not clear to you.

1. The two most commonly abused drugs are:

1. Methylphenidate (Ritalin) and meperidine (Demerol)
2. Lysergic acid diethylamide (LSD) and phencyclidine (PCP)
3. Alcohol and nicotine
4. Opioids and inhalants

2. A patient has been admitted to the emergency room with a diagnosis of cocaine overdose. The nurse monitors the patient for:

1. Irritability, restlessness, and abdominal cramping
2. Dysrhythmias, convulsions, and stroke
3. Insomnia, hallucinations, and tremors
4. Delirium, extreme fatigue, hunger, and headaches

3. The patient requires a higher dose of the substance to produce the initial effect. The nurse recognizes this as:

1. Toxicity
2. Resistance
3. Immunity
4. Tolerance

4. The patient has developed an opioid addiction. The nurse anticipates that which of the following medications will be used for opioid withdrawal?

1. Methadone
2. Heroin
3. Diazepam (Valium)
4. Alprazolam (Xanax)

5. The nurse understands that which of the following substances produces little physical dependence or tolerance?

1. Heroin
2. Marijuana
3. Alcohol
4. Cocaine

6. The nurse recognizes that methylphenidate (Ritalin) is classified as a:

1. Schedule I drug
2. Schedule II drug
3. Schedule III drug
4. Schedule IV drug

7. The nurse checks the patient and finds the following: increased heart rate, dilated pupils, elevated body temperature, and sweating. The nurse suspects:

1. Marijuana use
2. Heroin use
3. Cocaine use
4. Amphetamine use

8. Which of the following would the nurse find when monitoring the patient for use of barbiturates?

1. Drowiness, lack of muscle coordination, decreased respirations
2. Euphoria and irritability

3. Increased pain threshold and hallucinations
4. Increased blood pressure and respirations

9. Physical dependence differs from psychological dependence in that with physical dependence:

1. There is an intense craving for the drug.
2. There is an overwhelming need to take the drug.
3. The patient exhibits signs of withdrawal after the drug is discontinued.
4. Higher doses are required to produce the initial effect of the drug.

10. The nurse educates the patient on disulfiram (Antabuse), explaining that:

1. Only small amounts of alcohol may be ingested while on this drug.
2. If alcohol is ingested, the patient may experience shortness of breath, nausea and vomiting, and headache.
3. It is safe for use in pregnancy.
4. It enhances alcohol metabolism within the body.

NOTE: Answers to the Review Questions appear in Appendix B. The complete rationales and answers are located on the textbook's website.

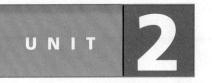

The Nervous System

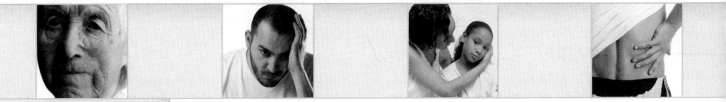

Unit Contents

Chapter 8 Drugs Affecting Functions of the Autonomic Nervous System / 86

Chapter 9 Drugs for Anxiety and Insomnia / 105

Chapter 10 Drugs for Emotional, Mood, and Behavioral Disorders / 122

Chapter 11 Drugs for Psychoses / 142

Chapter 12 Drugs for Degenerative Diseases and Muscles / 157

Chapter 13 Drugs for Seizures / 180

Chapter 14 Drugs for Pain Management / 197

Chapter 15 Drugs for Anesthesia / 217

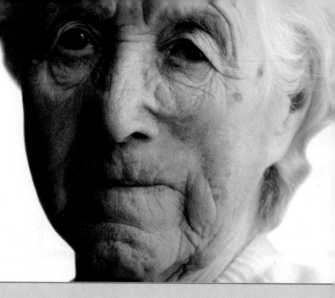

"I thought this was going to be a simple procedure. But after 4 days in bed, now I can't even urinate."

Mrs. Martha Wheaton

8

Drugs Affecting Functions of the Autonomic Nervous System

CORE CONCEPTS

8.1 The nervous system has two major divisions: central and peripheral.

8.2 The autonomic nervous system (a subdivision of the PNS) has sympathetic and parasympathetic branches.

8.3 Synapses are common sites of drug action.

8.4 Norepinephrine and acetylcholine are the two primary neurotransmitters in the autonomic nervous system.

8.5 Autonomic drugs are classified according to the receptors that they stimulate or block.

8.6 Cholinergic drugs have few therapeutic uses because of their numerous adverse effects.

8.7 Cholinergic blockers are mainly used to dry secretions and to treat asthma.

8.8 Adrenergic drugs are primarily used for their effects on the heart, bronchial tree, and nasal passages.

8.9 Adrenergic blockers are primarily used to treat hypertension and are the most widely prescribed class of autonomic drugs.

DRUG SNAPSHOT

The following drugs are discussed in this chapter:

DRUG CLASSES	DRUG PROTOTYPES
Cholinergic drugs	**Pr** bethanechol (Urecholine) **93**
Cholinergic blockers	**Pr** atropine (Atro-Pen) **95**
Adrenergic drugs	**Pr** phenylephrine (Neo-Synephrine) **98**
Adrenergic blockers	**Pr** prazosin (Minipress) **100**

LEARNING OUTCOMES

After reading this chapter, the student should be able to:

1. Identify the two primary divisions of the nervous system.

2. Identify the three primary functions of the nervous system.

3. Compare and contrast the actions of the sympathetic and parasympathetic nervous systems.

4. Describe the three parts of a synapse.

5. Identify the neurotransmitters important to the autonomic nervous system and the associated nerves.

6. Compare and contrast nicotinic and muscarinic receptors.

7. Compare and contrast the types of effects that occur when a drug stimulates alpha- and beta-receptors.

8. For each of the classes in the Drug Snapshot, identify representative drugs and explain their mechanisms of drug action, primary actions, and important adverse effects.

KEY TERMS

acetylcholine (Ach) (ah-SEET-ul-KOH-leen) 88

adrenergic (add-rah-NUR-jik) 90

adrenergic blockers 91

adrenergic drugs 91

alpha-receptor 90

anticholinergics 91

beta-receptor 90

cholinergic (kol-in-UR-jik) 90

cholinergic blockers 91

cholinergic drugs 91

epinephrine (EH-pin-NEF-rin) 90

ganglia (GANG-lee-ah) 90

muscarinic (MUS-kah-RIN-ik) 90

nicotinic (NIK-oh-TIN-ik) 90

norepinephrine (NE) (nor-EH-pin-NEF-rin) 88

parasympathetic nervous system (PAIR-ah-SIM-pah-THET-ik) 87

parasympathomimetics (PAIR-ah-SIM-path-oh-mah-MET-iks) 91

sympathetic nervous system (SIM-pah-THET-ik) 87

sympatholytics (SIM-path-oh-LIT-iks) 91

sympathomimetics (SIM-path-oh-mih-MET-iks) 91

Neuropharmacology represents one of the largest, most complicated, and least understood branches of pharmacology. Nervous system medications are used to treat a vast and diverse variety of conditions, including pain, anxiety, depression, schizophrenia, insomnia, and seizures. Through their effects on nerves, medications are also used to treat disorders common to the other organ systems. Examples include abnormalities in heart rate and rhythm, high blood pressure, pressure within the eyeball, asthma, and congestion.

Traditionally, the study of neuropharmacology begins with the autonomic nervous system. A firm grasp of autonomic pharmacology is necessary to understand and treat disorders of the affected organ systems. The remaining chapters in this unit are devoted to the specific treatment of nervous system conditions.

CORE CONCEPT 8.1   The nervous system has two major divisions: central and peripheral.

The nervous system is divided into the *central nervous system (CNS)* and the *peripheral nervous system (PNS)*. The CNS is made up of the brain and spinal cord. The PNS consists of all nervous tissue outside of the CNS. The basic functions of the nervous system are to:

- Recognize changes in the internal and external environments
- Process and integrate these environmental changes
- React to the environmental changes with a series of actions or responses

soma = *body*

auto = *self*
nom = *regulation*
ic = *relating to*

Figure 8.1 ■ shows the basic divisions of the PNS. Nerves in the PNS either recognize changes to the environment (*sensory* subdivision) or respond to these changes by moving muscles or secreting chemicals (*motor* subdivision). The *somatic nervous system* consists of nerves that provide voluntary control over skeletal muscle. Nerves of the *autonomic nervous system,* on the other hand, exert involuntary control over smooth muscle, cardiac muscle, and glands. Organs and tissues regulated by nerves from the autonomic nervous system include the heart, digestive tract, respiratory tract, reproductive tracts, arteries, salivary glands, and portions of the eye.

CORE CONCEPT 8.2   The autonomic nervous system (a subdivision of the PNS) has sympathetic and parasympathetic branches.

The autonomic nervous system has two branches called the **sympathetic nervous system** and the **parasympathetic nervous system**. Almost all organs and glands receive nerves from both branches of the autonomic nervous system.

The sympathetic nervous system is activated under conditions of stress and results in a set of reactions called the *fight-or-flight response.* The parasympathetic nervous system is activated under nonstressful conditions and results in reactions called the *rest-and-digest response.* Most of the reactions of the sympathetic branch are opposite to those of the parasympathetic branch. For example, activation of sympathetic nerves increases heart rate, whereas activation of parasympathetic nerves decreases heart rate. The major actions of the two branches are shown in Figure 8.2 ■. It is essential to learn these actions early in the study of pharmacology because knowledge of autonomic effects is used to predict the actions and adverse effects of many drugs.

FIGURE 8.1

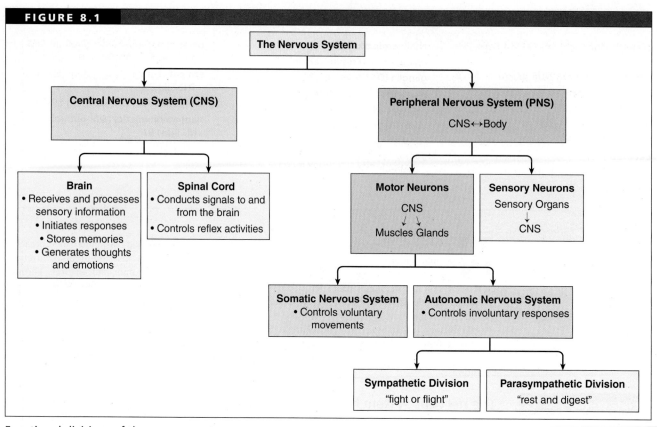

Functional divisions of the nervous system.

Concept Review 8.1

■ How would a person who is engaging in stressful or energetic activity benefit from the sympathetic effects of bronchodilation, slowed GI motility, and pupil dilation?

CORE CONCEPT 8.3

Synapses are common sites of drug action.

The basic functional unit of the nervous system is the nerve cell or *neuron*. For information to be transmitted throughout the nervous system, neurons must communicate with each other and with muscles and glands. A nerve impulse travels along a neuron to an area at the end of the neuron called a *synapse*. The synapse contains a space called the *synaptic cleft*, which must be crossed in order for impulses to reach the next neuron. The neuron generating the original impulse is called the *presynaptic neuron*. The nerve on the other side of the synapse, waiting to receive the impulse, is called the *postsynaptic neuron*. This basic structure is shown in Figure 8.3 ■.

pre = *before*
post = *after*
synaptic = *relating to the synapse*

Chemicals called *neurotransmitters* allow nerve impulses to cross the synaptic cleft. Neurotransmitters are released into the synaptic cleft when a nerve impulse reaches the end of a presynaptic neuron. The neurotransmitter travels across the synaptic cleft to reach receptors on the postsynaptic neuron, which then regenerates the impulse. Many different types of neurotransmitters are located throughout the nervous system, each related to distinct functions. *Many drugs are identical to or have the same general structure as neurotransmitters.* Drugs alter autonomic function by either blocking or enhancing the activity of these neurotransmitters.

CORE CONCEPT 8.4

Norepinephrine and acetylcholine are the two primary neurotransmitters in the autonomic nervous system.

The two primary neurotransmitters of the autonomic nervous system are **norepinephrine (NE)** and **acetylcholine (Ach)**. In the sympathetic nervous system, NE is released at the junction of the postsynaptic neuron and the organ or gland to be acted upon. For example, sympathetic nerves in the heart release NE onto cardiac muscle stimulating the heart to contract faster and with greater force. Sympathetic nerves also release NE onto the smooth muscle lining of the digestive tract, and its action is to slow contractions, or

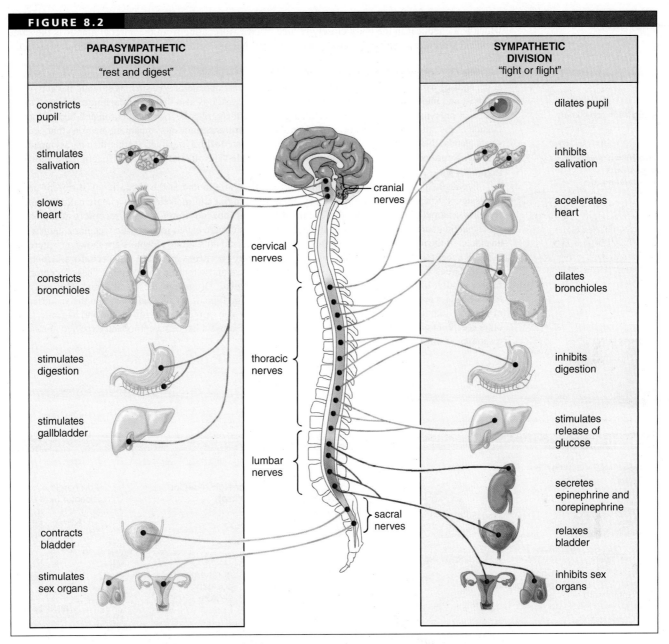

FIGURE 8.2

Effects of the sympathetic and parasympathetic nervous systems. *Source: Krogh, David. Biology: a guide to the natural world, 5th ed, 2011, Pearson Education. Reprinted and electronically reproduced by permission of Pearson Education, Inc., Upper Saddle River, NJ.*

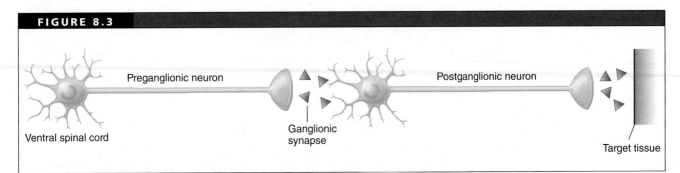

FIGURE 8.3

Basic structure of the autonomic pathway.

adren = *adrenal gland*
 (adrenaline)

ganglia = *nerve knots*

cholin = *acetylcholine*
erg = *work*
ic = *relating to*

adipose = *fat*

motility. Sympathetic nerves are sometimes called **adrenergic**. This term comes from the word adrenaline, which is a chemical in the body closely related to NE. Adrenaline from the adrenal glands is the same chemical structure as **epinephrine**. Epinephrine and NE are both released under conditions of extreme stress.

The physiology of Ach is more complicated because it is released in several locations. When released at the ends of parasympathetic neurons, it produces effects opposite of NE, such as slowing the activity of the heart and increasing the motility of the digestive tract. Ach is also the neurotransmitter released at the end of all presynaptic neurons at sites called **ganglia**, which are collections of neuron cell bodies located outside of the spinal cord. In addition, Ach is also a neurotransmitter of sympathetic neurons that activate sweat glands; this is a unique case in which Ach is associated with sympathetic rather than parasympathetic activity. Neurons that release Ach are called **cholinergic**. The sites of Ach and NE action are shown in Figure 8.4 ■.

Because Ach can stimulate receptors both at the ganglia and at the organ level, different names are assigned to these receptors. Ach receptors in the ganglia and in skeletal muscle are called **nicotinic** receptors, named after nicotine, the chemical found in tobacco products. Ach receptors at the end of postsynaptic neurons in the parasympathetic nervous system are called **muscarinic** receptors, named after an extract of the mushroom *Amanita muscaria*. Nicotinic and muscarinic receptors are shown in Figure 8.4.

NE receptors are of two basic subtypes: **alpha (α)-receptors** and **beta (β)-receptors**. *Alpha* and *beta* are Greek letters commonly used in naming chemical and scientific compounds. These receptors are further subdivided into beta$_1$, beta$_2$, beta$_3$, alpha$_1$, and alpha$_2$. Drugs may be selective and affect only one type of NE receptor, or they may affect all receptors. The type of response depends on the specific type of receptor that is activated. Drugs may also affect one type of receptor at low doses and begin to affect other receptors when the dose is increased. Table 8.1 ◆ shows a list of receptors and expected autonomic responses when receptors are activated.

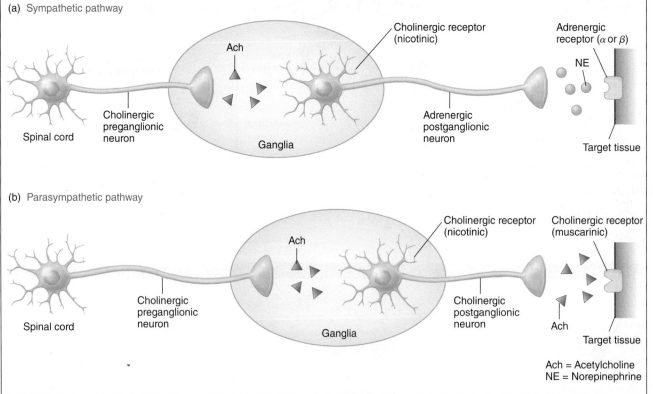

FIGURE 8.4

(a) Sympathetic pathway

(b) Parasympathetic pathway

Ach = Acetylcholine
NE = Norepinephrine

Norepinephrine (NE) receptors are adrenergic receptors (α and β) in the sympathetic pathway. Acetylcholine (Ach) receptors in the ganglia and skeletal muscles (not shown here) are called *nicotinic*. Ach receptors at the ends of postganglionic neurons in the parasympathetic pathway are called *muscarinic*.

TABLE 8.1   Types of Autonomic Receptors

Neurotransmitter	Receptor	Primary Locations	Responses
Acetylcholine (cholinergic)	Muscarinic	Parasympathetic target: organs other than the heart	Stimulation of smooth muscle contractions and gland secretions
		Heart	Decrease in heart rate and force of contraction
	Nicotinic	Cell bodies of postganglionic neurons (sympathetic and parasympathetic pathways)	Stimulation of smooth muscle contractions and gland secretions
Norepinephrine (adrenergic)	Alpha$_1$	All sympathetic target organs except the heart	Constriction of blood vessels, dilation of pupils
	Alpha$_2$	Presynaptic adrenergic neuron terminals	Inhibition of norepinephrine release
	Beta$_1$	Heart and kidneys	Increase in heart rate and force of contraction; release of renin
	Beta$_2$	All sympathetic target organs except the heart	Inhibition of smooth muscle contractions
	Beta$_3$	Adipose tissue	Breakdown of fat
		Bladder	Suppress emptying of bladder

Autonomic drugs are classified according to the receptors that they stimulate or block.

Because they can block or activate either the sympathetic or parasympathetic nervous system, autonomic drugs are classified based on one of four possible actions:

1. *Activation of the sympathetic nervous system.* These drugs are called **sympathomimetics** or **adrenergic drugs**. They produce the classic symptoms of the fight-or-flight response.

2. *Activation of the parasympathetic nervous system.* These drugs are called **cholinergic drugs** or **parasympathomimetics** and produce the classic symptoms of the rest-and-digest response.

3. *Inhibition of the sympathetic nervous system.* These drugs are called **adrenergic blockers** or **sympatholytics** and produce actions opposite to those of the sympathomimetics.

4. *Inhibition of the parasympathetic nervous system.* These drugs are called **anticholinergics** or **cholinergic blockers** and produce actions opposite to those of the parasympathomimetics.

sympatho = *sympathetic*
parasympatho = *parasympathetic*
mimetic = *to mimic*
lytic = *to undo*

Students beginning their study of pharmacology often have difficulty understanding the terminology and actions of autonomic drugs. It is only necessary to learn one group well because the others are logical extensions of the first. If the fight-or-flight symptoms of the adrenergic drugs are learned, the actions of the other three groups can be remembered as being either the same or opposite. For example, both the adrenergic drugs and the cholinergic blockers increase heart rate and dilate the pupils. The other two groups, the cholinergic drugs and the adrenergic blockers, have the opposite effects of slowing heart rate and constricting the pupils. Mastering the actions and terminology of autonomic drugs early in the study of pharmacology will reap rewards later in the course when these drugs are applied to various systems. See Table 8.2 ◆ for a quick review of the autonomic drug classes.

TABLE 8.2   Review of Autonomic Drug Classes

	Stimulation	Inhibition
Parasympathetic Nervous System	Cholinergic drugs (parasympathomimetics)	Cholinergic blockers (anticholinergics)
Sympathetic Nervous System	Adrenergic drugs (sympathomimetics)	Adrenergic blockers (sympatholytics)

CORE CONCEPT 8.6

Cholinergic drugs have few therapeutic uses because of their numerous adverse effects.

Remember the term *cholinergic* refers to neurons having Ach as the neurotransmitter. Cholinergic drugs or parasympathomimetics mimic actions of the parasympathetic nervous system. These drugs are associated with rest-and-digest responses. Because of their high potential for serious adverse effects, direct-acting cholinergic drugs are used only in a clinical setting. For instance, in ophthalmology, they are used to reduce intraocular pressure in patients with glaucoma (see Chapter 37). Others are used after anesthesia to stimulate the smooth muscles of the bowel or urinary tract. Potential adverse effects are increased salivation, sweating, abdominal cramps, and hypotension.

Indirect-acting cholinergic drugs, or drugs that inhibit the important enzyme acetylcholinesterase, have the same effects and adverse effects as direct-acting drugs including increased gland activity, sweating, increased muscle activity, and lowered heart rate. Acetylcholinesterase inhibitors facilitate the effects of the natural neurotransmitter Ach. Therefore, neostigmine (Prostigmin) and physostigmine (Antilirium) can induce actions in the body associated with rest and digestion. (Refer back to Figure 8.2.)

Several drugs in this class are used for their effects on Ach receptors *in skeletal muscle* rather than for their parasympathetic action. For example, myasthenia gravis is an autoimmune disorder characterized by destruction of cholinergic receptors found on the membranes of skeletal muscle tissue. Administration of pyridostigmine (Mestinon), neostigmine (Prostigmin), and other drugs (Table 8.3 ◆) will stimulate skeletal muscle contraction and diagnose or temporarily help to restore the severe muscle weakness found in this disease. Because several drugs useful in treating Alzheimer's disease are structurally similar to myasthenia drugs, the table includes drugs such as donepezil (Aricept), galantamine (Razadyne), rivastigmine (Exelon), and tacrine (Cognex). These drugs increase the amount of Ach binding to receptors located *within the brain* (see Chapter 12). Thus, cholinergic drugs may have effects in both the PNS *and* CNS.

Nerve agents (see Chapter 1) such as sarin and organophosphate insecticides are chemicals that inhibit acetylcholinesterase enzyme in the synaptic cleft throughout the entire nervous system. These agents can cause widespread and toxic parasympathomimetic effects. Symptoms are severe salivation, increased sweating, muscle twitching, involuntary urination and defecation, confusion, convulsions, and death. In an emergency, if nerve agents are released, Mark I injector kits containing the anticholinergic drug atropine or related medications are used to counteract toxic effects. Atropine blocks the attachment of Ach to receptor sites and prevents overstimulation caused by harmful nerve agents. In instances where too much anticholinergic activity occurs, as with atropine overdose or ingestion of poisonous substances, physostigmine (Antilirium) can be used as an antidote to counter overall adverse effects resulting from intense cholinergic blockade.

TABLE 8.3	Cholinergic Drugs (Parasympathomimetics)	
Type	**Drug**	**Primary Uses**
Direct acting	ⓟ bethanechol (Urecholine)	Stimulation of urination
	cevimeline HCl (Evoxac)	Treatment of dry mouth
	pilocarpine (Isopto Carpine, Ocusert, Salagen)	Glaucoma, treatment of dry mouth
Indirect acting (inhibitors of cholinesterase enzyme)	ambenonium (Mytelase)	Myasthenia gravis
	donepezil (Aricept) (see page 167 for the Drug Prototype box)	Alzheimer's disease
	edrophonium (Tensilon)	Diagnosis of myasthenia gravis
	galantamine (Razadyne)	Alzheimer's disease
	neostigmine (Prostigmin)	Myasthenia gravis
	physostigmine (Antilirium)	Cholinergic-blocking toxicity
	pyridostigmine (Mestinon, Regonol)	Myasthenia gravis
	rivastigmine (Exelon)	Alzheimer's disease
	tacrine (Cognex)	Alzheimer's disease

Drug Prototype: Ⓟ *Bethanechol (Urecholine)*

Therapeutic Class: Urinary retention (incomplete bladder emptying) treatment
Pharmacologic Class: Cholinergic receptor drug, parasympathomimetic

Actions and Uses: Bethanechol is a direct-acting parasympathomimetic that interacts with Ach receptors to cause actions typical of parasympathetic stimulation. It affects mostly the digestive and urinary tracts, where it stimulates smooth muscle contraction. These actions are particularly useful in stimulating the return of normal gastrointestinal (GI) and urinary tract function following general anesthesia.

Adverse Effects and Interactions: The adverse effects of bethanechol are parasympathetic actions: increased salivation,

sweating, abdominal cramping, and hypotension that can lead to fainting. It should not be given to patients with suspected urinary or intestinal obstruction or those with active asthma.

Do not use with ambenonium, neostigmine, and other cholinergic drugs; mecamylamine (blocker of Ach at the ganglia) may cause abdominal symptoms and hypotension. Procainamide, quinidine, atropine, and epinephrine reduce the effects of bethanechol.

NURSING PROCESS FOCUS   Patients Receiving Direct- and Indirect-Acting Cholinergic Drug Therapy

ASSESSMENT	POTENTIAL NURSING DIAGNOSES
Prior to administration: ■ Obtain a complete health history including cardiovascular, respiratory, GI, urinary, vision and neuromuscular conditions, allergies, and drug history for possible drug interactions. ■ Acquire the results of a complete physical examination including vital signs, height, weight, bowel sounds, ability to urinate, mental status, muscle strength, chewing ability, and signs such as ptosis and diplopia. ■ Evaluate laboratory blood findings: CBC, chemistry, renal and liver function studies.	■ *Urinary Incontinence* related to the adverse effects of direct-acting drugs ■ *Impaired Urinary Elimination* related to adverse effects of direct-acting drugs ■ *Impaired Physical Mobility* related to adverse effects of indirect-acting drugs ■ *Deficient Knowledge* related to a lack of information about drug therapy ■ *Risk for Injury* related to adverse effects of drug therapy ■ *Noncompliance* related to adverse effects of drug therapy

PLANNING: PATIENT GOALS AND EXPECTED OUTCOMES

The patient will:
■ Experience therapeutic effects: direct acting (an increase in bowel and bladder function and tone; regain normal pattern of elimination).
■ Experience therapeutic effects: indirect acting (a decrease in myasthenia gravis symptoms such as muscle weakness, ptosis, and diplopia).
■ Be free from or experience minimal adverse effects from drug therapy.
■ Verbalize an understanding of the drug's use, adverse effects, and required precautions.

IMPLEMENTATION

Interventions and (Rationales)	Patient Education/Discharge Planning
All Cholinergic drugs	
■ Monitor for therapeutic effects dependent on the reason drug is being given. (Improvement in mental status, urinary output and muscle strength indicates effectiveness of drug therapy.)	■ Encourage patient and caregivers to practice support measures to maximize therapeutic effects, e.g., adequate rest periods and assistance with ADLs.
■ Monitor for adverse effects and notify healthcare provider if pulse drops below 60 beats per minute or blood pressure is below approved parameters. (These drugs may decrease heart rate and BP, which may indicate cholinergic crisis that requires atropine.)	■ Instruct the patient to immediately report any of the following symptoms to their healthcare provider: nausea, vomiting, diarrhea, rash, jaundice, change in color of stool, feeling faint, tremors, or changes in behavior.
■ Monitor liver enzymes at the start of therapy and weekly for six weeks. (Drugs may cause liver toxicity.)	■ Instruct the patient to adhere to laboratory testing regimen for serum blood level tests of liver enzymes as directed.

continued . . .

NURSING PROCESS FOCUS *(continued)*

Interventions and (Rationales)	Patient Education/Discharge Planning
■ Administer medication correctly and evaluate the patient's knowledge of proper administration. (Proper administration helps to prevent complications.)	Instruct the patient to: ■ Take the drug as directed on regular schedule to maintain serum levels and control symptoms. ■ Not chew or crush sustained-release tablets. ■ Take oral cholinergic drugs on an empty stomach to lessen incidence of nausea and vomiting and to increase absorption.

Direct Acting

■ Monitor intake and output ratio. Palpate the abdomen for bladder distention. (Frequent monitoring will detect early signs of therapeutic or adverse effects. Drug onset of action is within 60 minutes, stimulating the smooth muscle of the bladder to contract and causing urination.)	■ Advise the patient to be near bathroom facilities after taking these drugs.
■ Provide for eye comfort such as adequately lighted areas and continue to monitor vision. (A cholinergic effect may cause blurred vision and difficulty seeing in low light.)	Advise the patient: ■ That blurred vision is a possible adverse effect and to take appropriate safety precautions. ■ Not to drive or engage in potentially hazardous activities until the drug's effects are known.
■ Help patients to rise from a lying to sitting or standing position until drug effects are determined. (Cholinergic drugs may cause orthostatic hypotension.)	■ Instruct the patient to avoid abrupt position changes and to avoid prolonged standing in one place.

Indirect Acting

■ Monitor neuromuscular status including muscle strength, ptosis, diplopia, and chewing. (Improvement demonstrates therapeutic effects.)	■ Instruct patients to report to their healthcare provider any difficulty with vision or swallowing.
■ Schedule the medication around mealtimes. Check drug reference material on administration with or without food. (Some drugs should be taken with food and others on an empty stomach.)	■ Instruct the patient about the appropriate time to take medications.
■ Schedule activities to avoid fatigue. (Excess fatigue can lead to cholinergic crisis.)	Instruct the patient to: ■ Plan activities according to muscle strength and fatigue. ■ Take frequent rest periods to avoid fatigue.
■ Monitor for muscle weakness after dose is given. (Depending on time of onset, it may indicate cholinergic crisis—overdose—OR myasthenic crisis—underdose.)	Instruct the patient to: ■ Report any severe muscle weakness that occurs 1 hour after administration of medication. ■ Report any muscle weakness that occurs three or more hours after medication administration because this is a major symptom of myasthenic crisis.

EVALUATION OF OUTCOME CRITERIA

Evaluate the effectiveness of drug therapy by confirming that patient goals and expected outcomes have been met (see "Planning"). *See Table 8.3 for a list of drugs to which these nursing actions apply.*

CORE CONCEPT 8.7

Cholinergic blockers are mainly used to dry secretions and to treat asthma.

Cholinergic blockers are drugs that have actions opposite those of the parasympathetic branch. They mimic the fight-or-flight response. Although the term *anticholinergic* is commonly used, a better term for this class of drugs would be *muscarinic blockers*, which more accurately describes blockade of the muscarinic receptor. Most therapeutic uses of the cholinergic blockers relate to their autonomic actions: dilation of pupils, increase in heart rate, drying of secretions, and dilation of the bronchi. Cholinergic blockers have been widely used in medicine for many disorders. A relatively high incidence of adverse effects and the development of safer, and sometimes more effective, medications has limited the current use of cholinergic blockers. For example, cholinergic blockers were once drugs of choice in treating peptic ulcers, but they have been replaced by proton-pump inhibitors and H_2-receptor blockers (see Chapter 30). Two important

TABLE 8.4   Cholinergic-Blocking Drugs (Anticholinergics)

Drug	Primary Uses
Pr atropine (Atro-Pen)	Poisoning with anticholinesterase agents; to increase heart rate, dilate pupils
benztropine (Cogentin) (see page 164 for the Drug Prototype box)	Parkinson's disease, neuroleptic side effects
cyclopentolate (Cyclogyl)	Dilation of pupils
dicyclomine (Bentyl, others)	Irritable bowel syndrome
fesoterodine (Toviaz)	Prevention of urgent, frequent, or uncontrolled urination
glycopyrrolate (Cuvposa, Robinul)	Production of a dry field prior to anesthesia, reduced salivation, peptic ulcers
ipratropium (Atrovent)	Asthma
methscopolamine (Pamine)	Motion sickness, ulcers
oxybutynin (Ditropan, Oxytrol)	Incontinence
propantheline (Pro-Banthine)	Irritable bowel syndrome, peptic ulcer
scopolamine (Hyoscine, Transderm-Scop)	Motion sickness, irritable bowel syndrome, adjunct to anesthesia
tiotropium (Spiriva)	Asthma
tolterodine (Detrol)	Overactive bladder with symptoms of urge urinary incontinence, urgency, and frequency
trihexyphenidyl	Parkinson's disease
tropicamide (Mydriacyl, Tropicacyl)	Mydriasis and cycloplegia for diagnostic procedures

incontinence = *not controlled (usually digestive or urinary)*

mydriasis = *prolonged pupil dilation*
cycloplegia = *ciliary eye muscle paralysis*

tachy = *rapid*
cardia = *heart beat*

adverse effects that limit their usefulness include tachycardia (fast heart rate) and the tendency to cause urinary retention in men with prostate disorders.

Some of the cholinergic blockers are used for their effects *in the CNS*, rather than their autonomic actions. Scopolamine (Hyoscine, Transderm-Scop) is used to produce sedation and prevent motion sickness (see Chapter 6); benztropine (Cogentin) and trihexyphenidyl (Artane) are prescribed to reduce the muscular tremor and rigidity associated with Parkinson's disease (see Chapter 12).

Some of the more common cholinergic blockers and their primary uses are listed in Table 8.4 ◆.

Drug Prototype: **Pr** *Atropine (Atro-Pen)*
Therapeutic Class: Antidote for anticholinestrase poisoning, antidysrhythmic, mydriatic (pupil dilating drug)
Pharmacologic Class: Anticholinergic, cholinergic receptor blocker

Actions and Uses: Atropine is a natural product found in the deadly nightshade plant, or *Atropa belladonna*. By blocking Ach (muscarinic) receptors, atropine causes symptoms of the fight-or-flight response, such as increased heart rate, bronchodilation, decreased motility in the GI tract, mydriasis (pupil dilation), and decreased secretions from glands. Throughout history, atropine has been used for a variety of purposes, although its use has declined because of the development of safer, more effective medications. Atropine is used to treat hypermotility diseases of the GI tract such as irritable bowel syndrome, to suppress secretions during surgical procedures, to increase the heart rate in patients with a slow heart beat bradycardia), to dilate the pupil during eye examinations, and to cause bronchodilation in patients with asthma. Atropine is an antidote for poisoning with nerve gas agents and organophosphate insecticides.

Adverse Effects and Interactions: The adverse effects of atropine limit its therapeutic usefulness. Adverse effects include dry mouth, constipation, urinary retention, and an increased heart rate. Atropine is usually contraindicated in patients with glaucoma because the drug may increase pressure within the eyeball.

Use of amantadine, antihistamines, tricyclic antidepressants, quinidine, disopyramide, and procainamide can increase the anticholinergic effects of atropine. Use with levodopa may decrease the effects of the latter. The antipsychotic effects of phenothiazines are generally decreased.

NURSING PROCESS FOCUS Patients Receiving Cholinergic Blocker (Anticholinergic) Therapy

ASSESSMENT	POTENTIAL NURSING DIAGNOSES
Prior to administration: ■ Obtain a complete health history including cardiovascular, respiratory, vision and neurological conditions, allergies, and drug history for possible drug interactions. ■ Evaluate laboratory blood findings: CBC, chemistry, renal and liver function studies. ■ Acquire the results of a complete physical examination including heart rate/rhythm, blood pressure, temperature, weight, bowel sounds, and elimination patterns.	■ *Deficient Knowledge* related to a lack of information about drug therapy ■ *Decreased Cardiac Output* related to adverse effects of drug therapy ■ *Risk for Imbalanced Body Temperature* related to inhibited sweat gland secretions ■ *Impaired Oral Mucous Membranes* related to decrease in exocrine secretions ■ *Constipation* related to adverse effect of drug therapy ■ *Urinary Retention* related to adverse effects of drug therapy ■ *Risk for Injury* related to neurological effects of medication

PLANNING: PATIENT GOALS AND EXPECTED OUTCOMES

The patient will:
■ Experience therapeutic effects (a decrease in symptoms for which the medication is prescribed).
■ Be free from or experience minimal adverse effects from drug therapy.
■ Verbalize an understanding of the drug's use, adverse effects, and required precautions.

IMPLEMENTATION

Interventions and (Rationales)	Patient Education/Discharge Planning
■ Closely monitor heart function and notify healthcare provider if BP or pulse exceeds established parameters or dysrhythmias develop. (Anticholinergic drugs stimulate heart rate, increasing the chance for dysrhythmias.)	■ Instruct the patient to monitor vital signs, ensuring proper use of home equipment.
■ Observe for adverse effects such as drowsiness, blurred vision, tachycardia, dry mouth, constipation, urinary hesitancy/retention, and decreased sweating. (Adverse effects are the result of the blockage of muscarinic receptors; can also be caused by an overdose of medication.)	Instruct the patient to: ■ Immediately report adverse effects such as palpitations shortness of breath or drowsiness to their healthcare provider. ■ Avoid driving and hazardous activities until effects of drugs are known.
■ Provide comfort measures. For dry mucous membranes, apply lubricant to moisten lips and oral mucosa, and assist in rinsing mouth. Use artificial tears for dry eyes, as needed. (Adverse effects of drug therapy can include dry mucous membranes and photosensitivity.)	Instruct the patient to: ■ Use oral rinses, sugarless gum or candy, and frequent oral hygiene to help relieve dry mouth. ■ Avoid alcohol-containing mouthwashes that can further dry oral tissue. ■ Wear sunglasses to decrease sensitivity to bright light.
■ Minimize exposure to heat or cold and strenuous exercise. (Cholinergic blockers can inhibit sweat gland secretions due to direct blockade of the muscarinic receptors on the sweat glands. Sweating is necessary for patients to cool down, so this inhibition of sweating can increase their risk for hyperthermia.)	■ Advise the patient to limit activity outside when the temperature is hot. Strenuous activity in a hot environment may cause heat stroke.
■ Monitor intake and output ratio. Palpate the abdomen for bladder distention. (Cholinergic blockers can cause urinary retention.)	■ Instruct the patient to notify the healthcare provider if difficulty in voiding occurs.
■ Monitor patients routinely for abdominal distention and auscultate for bowel sounds. (Cholinergic blockers may decrease tone and motility of the intestinal tract.)	■ Advise the patient to increase fluid intake and add bulk to the diet, if constipation becomes a problem.

EVALUATION OF OUTCOME CRITERIA

Evaluate the effectiveness of drug therapy by confirming that patient goals and expected outcomes have been met (see "Planning"). *See Table 8.4 for a list of drugs to which these nursing actions apply.*

Adrenergic drugs are primarily used for their effects on the heart, bronchial tree, and nasal passages.

Adrenergic drugs, or sympathomimetics, have actions similar to those produced by activation of the sympathetic nervous system (the fight-or-flight response). Again, remember that the term *adrenergic* refers to neurons having adrenaline-like substances in the nerve terminal. The adrenergic drugs produce many of the same symptoms as the cholinergic blockers. However, because the sympathetic nervous system activates alpha- and beta-receptors, the actions of the adrenergics are more specific and have wider therapeutic applications.

Although most effects of adrenergics are predictable based on their autonomic actions, their primary effects depend on which adrenergic receptors are stimulated. Drugs such as phenylephrine (Neo-Synephrine) stimulate alpha$_1$-receptors and are often used to dry nasal secretions. Because beta$_1$-receptors are predominant in the heart, beta$_1$-drugs such as dobutamine (Dobutrex) are used to stimulate the heart rate and increase its strength of contraction. Beta$_2$-drugs such as albuterol (Proventil) cause bronchodilation and are useful in the treatment of asthma.

Some adrenergic drugs are nonselective, stimulating more than one type of adrenergic receptor. For example, epinephrine stimulates all types of adrenergic receptors and is used for cardiac arrest and asthma. Pseudoephedrine (Sudafed and others) stimulates both alpha$_1$- and beta$_2$-receptors and is used orally as a nasal decongestant. Isoproterenol (Isuprel) stimulates both beta$_1$- and beta$_2$-receptors and is used to increase the rate, force, and conduction speed of the heart and, occasionally, to treat asthma. The nonselective drugs generally cause a wider variety of adverse effects all over the body.

Some of the more commonly used adrenergic drugs are shown in Table 8.5 ◆. Most drugs in this class are presented in other chapters of this book. For prototypes of drugs in this class, see epinephrine (Adrenalin) and norepinephrine (Levophed) in Chapter 22, oxymetazoline (Afrin, others) in Chapter 17, and salmeterol (Serevent) in Chapter 28.

nonselective = *not specifically directed*

hyper = *elevated*
tension = *blood pressure*

anaphylactic = *itchy rash, low blood pressure, swollen throat*

obstructive = *narrowed*
pulmonary = *lung passage*

dys = *abnormal*
rhythmias = *heart rhythms*

Concept Review 8.2

■ Why do the adrenergic drugs produce many of the same symptoms as the cholinergic blockers?

TABLE 8.5 Adrenergic Drugs (Sympathomimetics)

Drug	Primary Receptor Subtype	Primary Uses
albuterol (Proventil, Ventolin, VoSpire)	Beta$_2$	Asthma
clonidine (Catapres)	Alpha$_2$ in CNS	Hypertension
dobutamine (Dobutrex)	Beta$_1$	Cardiac stimulant
dopamine (Intropin) (see page 326 for the Drug Prototype box)	Alpha$_1$ and beta$_1$	Shock
epinephrine (Adrenalin, others) (see page 327 for the Drug Prototype box)	Alpha and beta	Cardiac arrest, asthma; anaphylactic and allergic reactions
formoterol (Foradil, Performist)	Beta$_2$	Asthma, chronic obstructive pulmonary disease (COPD)
isoproterenol (Isuprel)	Beta$_1$ and beta$_2$	Asthma, dysrhythmias, heart failure
metaproterenol	Beta$_2$	Asthma
methyldopa (Aldomet)	Alpha$_2$ in CNS	Hypertension
midodrine (ProAmatine)	Alpha	Hypertension
mirabegron (Myrbetriq)	Beta$_3$	Urinary incontinence
norepinephrine (Levophed) (see page 326 for the Drug Prototype box)	Alpha and beta$_1$	Shock
oxymetazoline (Afrin and others) (see page 464 for the Drug Prototype box)	Alpha	Nasal congestion
ⓟ phenylephrine (Neo-Synephrine)	Alpha	Maintain BP, nasal congestion
pseudoephedrine (Sudafed and others)	Alpha and beta	Nasal congestion
salmeterol (Serevent)	Beta$_2$	Asthma
terbutaline	Beta$_2$	Asthma

Drug Prototype: ℗ *Phenylephrine (Neo-Synephrine)*

Therapeutic Class: Nasal decongestant, mydriatic agent, antihypotensive

Pharmacologic Class: Adrenergic drug, alpha₁-adrenergic drug

Actions and Uses: Phenylephrine is a selective alpha-adrenergic drug that is available in several formulations, including intranasal, ophthalmic, IM, SC, and IV. All of its actions and indications result from sympathetic stimulation. When applied intranasally by spray or drops, it reduces nasal congestion by constricting small blood vessels in the nasal mucosa. Applied topically to the eye during ophthalmic examinations, phenylephrine can dilate the pupil without causing significant paralysis of the eye muscles (cycloplegia). The parenteral administration of phenylephrine can reverse acute hypotension caused by spinal anesthesia or vascular shock. Because it lacks beta-adrenergic activity, it produces relatively few cardiac adverse effects at therapeutic doses. Its longer duration of activity and lack of significant cardiac effects gives phenylephrine some advantages over epinephrine or norepinephrine in treating acute hypotension.

Adverse Effects and Interactions: When used topically or intranasally, adverse effects are uncommon. Prolonged intranasal use can cause burning of the mucosa and rebound congestion (see Chapter 37). Ophthalmic preparations can cause narrow-angle glaucoma because of their mydriatic effect. High doses can cause reflex bradycardia due to the elevation of blood pressure caused by stimulation of alpha₁-receptors. When given parenterally, the drug should be used with caution in patients with advanced coronary artery disease or hypertension. Anxiety, restlessness, and tremor may occur due to the drug's stimulatory effect on the CNS. Patients with hyperthyroidism may experience a severe increase in basal metabolic rate, resulting in increased blood pressure and tachycardia. Drug interactions may occur with monoamine oxidase (MAO) inhibitors, causing a hypertensive crisis. Increased effects may also occur with tricyclic antidepressants. This drug is incompatible with iron preparations (ferric salts).

> **BLACK BOX WARNING:**
> Severe reactions, including death, may occur with IV infusion even when appropriate dilution is used to avoid rapid diffusion. Therefore, restrict IV use for situations in which other routes are not feasible.

NURSING PROCESS FOCUS Patients Receiving Adrenergic Drug Therapy

ASSESSMENT	POTENTIAL NURSING DIAGNOSES
Prior to administration: ■ Obtain a complete health history including cardiovascular, respiratory, vision and liver conditions, allergies, and drug history for possible drug interactions ■ Obtain data regarding treatment of nasal congestion and current status of nasal mucosa for changes such as excoriation or bleeding ■ Acquire the results of a complete physical examination including vital signs, height, weight, cardiac and urinary output. ■ Evaluate laboratory blood findings: CBC, chemistry, renal and liver function studies.	■ *Deficient Knowledge* related to a lack of information about drug therapy ■ *Decreased Cardiac Output* related to bradycardia (disorder) ■ *Ineffective Cardiopulmonary Tissue Perfusion* related to bronchoconstriction (disorder) ■ *Risk for Injury* related to adverse effects of drug therapy ■ *Ineffective Breathing Pattern* related to nasal congestion ■ *Disturbed Sleep Pattern* related to adrenergic stimulation and drug-induced excitation

PLANNING: PATIENT GOALS AND EXPECTED OUTCOMES

The patient will:
■ Experience therapeutic effects (a decrease in symptoms for which the drug is being given).
■ Be free from or experience minimal adverse effects from drug therapy.
■ Verbalize an understanding of the drug's use, adverse effects, and required precautions.
■ Demonstrate proper nasal/ophthalmic medication instillation technique.

IMPLEMENTATION

Interventions and (Rationales)	Patient Education/Discharge Planning
■ Administer medication correctly and evaluate the patient's knowledge of proper administration. If drug is being administered IV, closely monitor IV insertion sites for extravasation and use an infusion pump to deliver medication. Use a tuberculin syringe when administering SC doses that are extremely small. For metered-dose inhalation, shake the container well, and wait at least two minutes between medications. Instill only the prescribed number of drops when using ophthalmic solutions.	Instruct the patient to: ■ Use the drug as prescribed and not "double up" on doses. ■ Take the medication early in the day to avoid insomnia. ■ Keep drug on hand for emergencies if using rescue inhalers or epinephrine kits; notify healthcare provider immediately after use.

continued . . .

NURSING PROCESS FOCUS   *(continued)*

Interventions and (Rationales)	Patient Education/Discharge Planning
■ Monitor the patient for adverse effects. (Adverse effects of adrenergic drugs may be serious and limit therapy.)	Instruct the patient to: ■ Immediately report shortness of breath, palpitations, dizziness, chest/arm pain or pressure, or other angina-like symptoms to the healthcare provider. ■ Consult the healthcare provider before attempting to use adrenergic drugs to treat nasal congestion or eye irritation. ■ Monitor blood pressure, pulse, and temperature to ensure proper use of home equipment.
■ Monitor breathing patterns and observe for shortness of breath and/or audible wheezing. Provide supportive nursing measures such as proper positioning for patients with dyspnea. (Monitoring provides information about effects of medication. Patients with respiratory problems should consult their healthcare provider to ensure the correct medication is being used for their condition.)	Instruct the patient: ■ To immediately report any difficulty breathing. ■ With a history of asthma to consult a healthcare provider before using over-the-counter (OTC) drugs to treat nasal stuffiness.
■ Observe the patient's responsiveness to light. (Some adrenergic drugs cause photosensitivity by affecting the pupillary light accommodation/response.)	■ Instruct patients using ophthalmic adrenergic drugs that transient stinging and blurred vision on instillation is normal. Headache and/or brow pain may also occur.
■ Provide eye comfort by reducing exposure to direct bright light in the environment; shield the eyes with a rolled washcloth or eye bandages for severe photosensitivity. (Adrenergic drugs can cause mydriasis and sensitivity to light.)	■ Instruct the patient to avoid driving and other activities requiring visual acuity until blurring subsides.
■ For patients receiving nasal adrenergic drugs, observe the nasal cavity. Monitor for rhinorrhea and epistaxis. (Vasoconstriction may cause transient stinging, excessive dryness, or bleeding.)	Instruct the patient to: ■ Observe the nasal cavity for signs of excoriation or bleeding before instilling nasal spray or drops; review procedure for safe instillation of nasal sprays or eyedrops. ■ Limit usage of OTC adrenergic drugs; inform the patient about rebound nasal congestion.

EVALUATION OF OUTCOME CRITERIA

Evaluate the effectiveness of drug therapy by confirming that patient goals and expected outcomes have been met (see "Planning"). *See Table 8.5 for a list of drugs to which these nursing actions apply.*

Adrenergic blockers are primarily used to treat hypertension and are the most widely prescribed class of autonomic drugs.

CORE CONCEPT 8.9

Adrenergic blockers inhibit the actions of the sympathetic nervous system. These drugs produce many of the same responses as the cholinergic drugs, but they are more widely used. Because the sympathetic nervous system has alpha- and beta-receptors, the actions of adrenergic blockers are specific and have wide therapeutic applications. In fact, they are the most widely prescribed class of autonomic drugs. Many of the adrenergic blockers are shown in Table 8.6 ◆.

Alpha-adrenergic blockers, or simply *alpha blockers*, are primarily used for their effects on vascular smooth muscle. By relaxing vascular smooth muscle in small arteries, alpha$_1$ blockers such as doxazosin (Cardura) cause vasodilation, which results in decreased blood pressure (hypotensive effect). Their primary use is in the treatment of hypertension, either alone or in combination with other drugs.

Some drugs in this class selectively block beta$_1$-receptors. Because beta$_1$-receptors are only present in the heart, the effects of drugs such as atenolol (Tenormin) are often called *cardioselective*. By slowing the heart rate, they lower blood pressure, which is their primary use.

Some beta blockers, such as propranolol (Inderal, InnoPran XL), are nonselective, blocking both beta$_1$- and beta$_2$-receptors. The nonselective beta blockers are used to treat hypertension, angina, and cardiac rhythm abnormalities. Their nonselective actions generally result in more adverse effects than the selective beta blockers. Prototypes of adrenergic blockers can be found for doxazosin (Cardura) in Chapter 18, carvedilol (Coreg) in Chapter 19, propranolol (Inderal, InnoPran XL) in Chapter 22, and atenolol (Tenormin) in Chapter 20.

vaso = *smooth muscle (blood vessel)*
dilation = *enlargement of diameter*

hypo = *lowered*
tensive = *blood pressure*

cardio = *the heart*
selective = *directed (toward)*

nonselective = *not specifically directed*

angina = *chest pain*

Concept Review 8.3

benign = *gentle*
prostatic = *prostate-related*
hyperplasia = *enlargement*

■ Both cholinergic drugs and adrenergic blockers produce similar actions. Why are adrenergic blockers used to treat hypertension, but cholinergic drugs are not used for this purpose?

TABLE 8.6 Adrenergic-Blocking Drugs (Sympatholytics)

Drug	Primary Receptor Subtype	Primary Uses
acebutolol (Sectral)	Beta$_1$	Hypertension, dysrhythmias, angina
alfuzosin (UroXatral)	Alpha$_1$	Benign prostatic hyperplasia (BPH)
atenolol (Tenormin) (see page 309 for the Drug Prototype box)	Beta$_1$	Hypertension, angina
carteolol (Cartrol)	Beta$_1$ and beta$_2$	Hypertension, glaucoma
carvedilol (Coreg) (see page 296 for the Drug Prototype box)	Alpha$_1$, beta$_1$, and beta$_2$	Hypertension, heart failure
doxazosin (Cardura) (see page 282 for the Drug Prototype Box)	Alpha$_1$	Hypertension
esmolol (Brevibloc)	Beta$_1$	Hypertension, dysrhythmias
metoprolol (Lopressor, Toprol)	Beta$_1$	Hypertension
nadolol (Corgard)	Beta$_1$ and beta$_2$	Hypertension
phentolamine (Regitine)	Alpha	Severe hypertension
℗ prazosin (Minipress)	Alpha$_1$	Hypertension
propranolol (Inderal, Innopran XL) (see page 340 for the Drug Prototype box)	Beta$_1$ and beta$_2$	Hypertension, dysrhythmias, heart failure
silodosin (Rapaflo)	Alpha$_1$	BPH
sotalol (Betapace)	Beta$_1$ and beta$_2$	Dysrhythmias
tamsulosin (Flomax)	Alpha$_1$	BPH
terazosin (Hytrin)	Alpha$_1$	Hypertension
timolol (Blocadren, Timoptic) (see page 604 for the Drug Prototype box)	Beta$_1$ and beta$_2$	Hypertension, angina, glaucoma

Drug Prototype: ℗ *Prazosin (Minipress)*

Therapeutic Class: Antihypertensive   **Pharmacologic Class: Sympatholytic, alpha$_1$-adrenergic blocker**

Actions and Uses: Prazosin is a selective alpha$_1$-adrenergic blocker that competes with NE at its receptors on vascular smooth muscle in arterioles and veins. Its major action is a rapid decrease in peripheral resistance that reduces blood pressure. It has little effect on cardiac output or heart rate, and it causes less reflex tachycardia than some other drugs in this class. Tolerance to its antihypertensive effect may occur. Its most common use is in combination with other drugs, such as beta blockers or diuretics, in the pharmacotherapy of hypertension. Prazosin has a short half-life and is often taken two or three times per day.

Adverse Effects and Interactions: Like other alpha blockers, prazosin has a tendency to cause orthostatic hypotension due to alpha$_1$-inhibition in vascular smooth muscle. In rare cases, this hypotension can be so severe as to cause unconsciousness about 30 minutes after the first dose. This is called the *first-dose phenomenon*. To avoid this situation, the first dose should be very low and given at bedtime. Dizziness, drowsiness, or lightheadedness may occur as a result of decreased blood flow to the brain due to the drug's hypotensive action. Reflex tachycardia may occur due to the rapid falls in blood pressure. The alpha blockade may also result in nasal congestion or inhibition of ejaculation.

Drug interactions include increased hypotensive effects with concurrent use of antihypertensives and diuretics.

NURSING PROCESS FOCUS Patients Receiving Adrenergic Blocker Therapy

ASSESSMENT	POTENTIAL NURSING DIAGNOSES
Prior to administration: ■ Obtain a complete health history including neurological, liver, GI and GU conditions; allergies; and drug history for possible drug interactions. ■ Acquire the results of a complete physical examination including vital signs, height, weight. For BPH (obtain urinary pattern and output). ■ Evaluate laboratory blood findings: CBC, chemistry, renal and liver function studies.	■ *Deficient Knowledge* related to a lack of information about drug therapy ■ *Risk for Injury* related to dizziness, syncope ■ *Impaired Urinary Elimination (frequency)* related to adverse effects of drug therapy ■ *Risk for Sexual Dysfunction* related to adverse effects of drug therapy

PLANNING: PATIENT GOALS AND EXPECTED OUTCOMES

The patient will:
■ Experience therapeutic effects (a decrease in blood pressure or ease of urination).
■ Be free from or experience minimal adverse effects from drug therapy.
■ Verbalize an understanding of the drug's use, adverse effects and required precautions.

IMPLEMENTATION

Interventions and (Rationales)	Patient Education/Discharge Planning
■ In patients with prostatic hypertrophy, monitor for urinary hesitancy/ feeling of incomplete bladder emptying, and interrupted urinary stream.	■ Instruct the patient to report increased difficulty with urination to a healthcare provider.
■ Monitor for syncope. (Alpha-adrenergic blockers produce first-dose syncope phenomenon and may cause loss of consciousness.)	Instruct the patient to: ■ Take this medication at bedtime, and to take the first dose *immediately* before getting into bed. ■ Avoid abrupt changes in position; warn the patient about first-dose phenomenon and reassure that this effect diminishes with continued therapy.
■ Take vital signs and notify healthcare provider if pulse or blood pressure drops below approved parameters. Monitor for dizziness, drowsiness, or lightheadedness. (These drugs can cause severe hypotension. Dizziness is a sign of decreased blood flow to the brain due to the drug's hypotensive action.)	Instruct the patient: ■ To monitor vital signs, especially blood pressure, ensuring proper use of home equipment. ■ Regarding the normotensive range of blood pressure; instruct the patient to consult the nurse regarding "reportable" blood pressure readings. ■ To rise from lying to sitting or standing slowly to avoid dizziness. ■ To report dizziness or syncope that persists beyond the first dose, as well as paresthesias and other neurologic changes.
■ Monitor level of consciousness and mood. (Adrenergic blockers can exacerbate existing mental depression.)	■ Instruct the patient to immediately report any feelings of depression. ■ Interview the patient regarding suicide potential; obtain a "no-self harm" verbal contract from the patient.
■ Observe for adverse effects that may include blurred vision, tinnitus, epistaxis, and edema.	Inform the patient: ■ That nasal congestion may be an adverse effect. ■ To report any adverse reactions to the healthcare provider. ■ About the potential danger of concomitant use of OTC nasal decongestants.
■ Monitor liver function. (These drugs increase the risk for liver toxicity.)	Instruct the patient: ■ To adhere to a regular schedule of laboratory testing for liver function as ordered by the healthcare provider. ■ To report signs and symptoms of liver toxicity: nausea, vomiting, diarrhea, rash, jaundice, abdominal pain, tenderness or distention, or change in color of stool. ■ About importance of ongoing medication compliance and follow-up.

EVALUATION OF OUTCOME CRITERIA

Evaluate the effectiveness of drug therapy by confirming that patient goals and expected outcomes have been met (see "Planning"). *See Table 8.6 for a list of drugs to which these nursing actions apply.*

PATIENTS NEED TO KNOW

Patients treated with autonomic medications need to know the following:

In General

1. Do not take any OTC cold, cough, or sinus drugs without seeking medical advice because these likely contain autonomic drugs.
2. Report any palpitations, shortness of breath, chest pain, or large changes in blood pressure immediately to a healthcare provider. Some of the most significant adverse effects of autonomic drugs relate to the cardiovascular system.
3. Notify a healthcare provider before taking autonomic drugs if the following conditions are present: thyroid disease, diabetes mellitus, dysrhythmias, or hypertension. Such medications have the potential to cause serious adverse effects in individuals with these conditions.
4. Move slowly when changing from a supine to an upright position to avoid dizziness and perhaps fainting. Many of the autonomic medications affect blood pressure.
5. Notify a healthcare provider if any significant change in bowel habits or abdominal cramping/constipation occurs after taking autonomic drugs.
6. Inform a healthcare provider before taking cholinergic blockers (anticholinergics) if urinating difficulty is present or if the diagnosis of benign prostatic hyperplasia (BPH) has been made.
7. Chew gum or suck on hard candies if dry mouth is experienced when taking autonomic drugs. Proper oral hygiene is important to avoid dental caries.

Regarding Adrenergic Blockers

8. Do not discontinue the use of beta blockers abruptly because doing so can result in chest pain or rebound hypertension.
9. Alpha blockers can sometimes cause impotence as an adverse effect. If there are difficulties with ejaculation, notify a healthcare provider so that other drug options can be explored.

CHAPTER REVIEW

CORE CONCEPTS SUMMARY

8.1 The nervous system has two major divisions: central and peripheral.

The central nervous system consists of the brain and spinal cord. The peripheral nervous system consists of a sensory portion and a motor portion. Outgoing motor signals are characterized as voluntary (somatic) or involuntary (autonomic).

8.2 The autonomic nervous system (a subdivision of the PNS) has sympathetic and parasympathetic branches.

Stimulation of sympathetic nerves causes symptoms of the fight-or-flight response. Stimulation of parasympathetic nerves induces the rest-and-digest response. With few exceptions, the actions of the two divisions oppose each other.

8.3 Synapses are common sites of drug action.

Synapses consist of a presynaptic nerve and a postsynaptic nerve with a space between them called the synaptic cleft. Neurotransmitters cross this synaptic cleft to regenerate the nerve impulse.

8.4 Norepinephrine and acetylcholine are the two primary neurotransmitters in the autonomic nervous system.

Norepinephrine is the neurotransmitter at the organ level in the sympathetic nervous system. Norepinephrine receptors may be alpha or beta subtypes. Acetylcholine is the neurotransmitter at the end of all presynaptic nerves (ganglia), at sweat glands, and in skeletal muscle. Acetylcholine receptors may be nicotinic or muscarinic.

8.5 Autonomic drugs are classified according to the receptors that they stimulate or block.

Adrenergic drugs stimulate sympathetic nerves, and cholinergic drugs primarily stimulate parasympathetic nerves. Adrenergic blockers inhibit the sympathetic division, whereas cholinergic blockers mostly inhibit the parasympathetic branch.

8.6 Cholinergic drugs have few therapeutic uses because of their numerous adverse effects.

Cholinergic drugs are used to treat glaucoma and to stimulate the urinary or digestive tracts following general anesthesia. Toxic nerve agents are cholinergic drugs, producing harmful effects in the body.

8.7 Cholinergic blockers are mainly used to dry secretions and to treat asthma.

The use of cholinergic blockers has declined due to their numerous adverse effects. They are used to dry secretions, dilate the bronchi, and dilate the pupils.

8.8 Adrenergic drugs are primarily used for their effects on the heart, bronchial tree, and nasal passages.

Adrenergic drugs may stimulate one or several subtypes of adrenergic receptors. Uses include increasing the heart rate, dilating the bronchi, and drying excess secretions caused by colds.

8.9 Adrenergic blockers are primarily used to treat hypertension and are the most widely prescribed class of autonomic drugs.

Adrenergic blockers are the most commonly prescribed autonomic medications. They may be selective for only one receptor subtype, such as the beta$_1$-blockers, or inhibit several subtypes. Hypertension is their primary indication.

REVIEW QUESTIONS

The following questions are written in NCLEX-PN® style. Answer these questions to assess your knowledge of the chapter material, and go back and review any material that is not clear to you.

1. While assisting the RN with the development of a plan of care for a patient with glaucoma, the LPN recognizes that which of the following drugs would be contraindicated for the patient?

1. Pilocarpine (Carpine)
2. Betaxolol HCl (Betoptic)
3. Timolol (Timoptic)
4. Atropine

2. The nurse is aware that the patient diagnosed with glaucoma would most likely be prescribed which of the following drugs?

1. Adrenergic drugs
2. Cholinergic drugs
3. Adrenergic blockers
4. Cholinergic blockers

3. The nurse informs the patient that rebound congestion can occur with long-term use of this adrenergic drug:

1. Albuterol (Proventil)
2. Neostigmine (Prostigmin)
3. Salmeterol (Serevent)
4. Phenylephrine (Neo-Synephrine)

4. The patient is diagnosed with urinary bladder urgency and incontinence. According to the physician's orders, the nurse administers which of the following cholinergic blockers for this condition?

1. Dicyclomine (Bentyl)
2. Ipratropium (Atrovent)
3. Oxybutynin (Ditropan)
4. Scopolamine (Transderm-Scop)

5. A patient is told that he is being given an alpha$_1$-adrenergic blocker. When he asks what this drug does, the nurse tells him that alpha-adrenergic blockers cause: (Select all that apply.)

1. Vasodilation
2. Decreased blood pressure
3. Increased blood pressure
4. Vasoconstriction

6. While obtaining a patient's medication history, the patient tells the nurse, "I'm on metoprolol (Lopressor)." The nurse knows that this drug is a(n):

1. Alpha blocker
2. Beta blocker
3. Cholinergic
4. Cholinergic blocker

7. Prior to administering atenolol (Tenormin), the nurse assesses:

1. Respirations and blood pressure
2. Respirations and heart rate
3. Heart rate and blood pressure
4. Temperature and blood pressure

8. The healthcare practitioner orders metaproterenol 20 mg, by mouth three times a day. The pharmacy sends metaproterenol sulfate syrup, 10 mg/5 mL. The nurse will administer _____ per day.

1. 20 mL
2. 60 mL
3. 30 mL
4. 40 mL

9. A patient has been prescribed phenylephrine to help relieve nasal congestion. The nurse informs her that prolonged use of this drug can cause:

1. Decreased heart rate
2. Decreased blood pressure
3. Drowsiness
4. Rebound congestion

10. The nurse suspects that the cholinergic blocker the patient is taking is causing which one of the following adverse effects?

1. Diaphoresis
2. Confusion
3. Dry mouth
4. Increased urination

CASE STUDY QUESTIONS

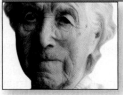

Remember Mrs. Wheaton, the patient introduced at the beginning of the chapter? Now read the remainder of the case study. Based on the information you have learned in this chapter, answer the questions that follow.

Mrs. Martha Wheaton, an 80-year-old woman, has been having problems with nonobstructive urinary retention following surgery, a retropubic urethral suspension. She required a Foley catheter for four days but was unable to void after removal of the catheter. The physician ordered bethanechol (Urecholine) for Mrs. Wheaton.

1. Mrs. Wheaton asks the nurse why the physician ordered bethanechol. The nurse explains that:

1. It causes the kidneys to produce more urine, which increases the pressure within the bladder, forcing her to urinate.
2. It inhibits smooth muscle contractions, causing the bladder to relax.
3. It stimulates smooth muscle contractions, causing the bladder to function normally.
4. It decreases the amount of urine produced in the kidneys so as not to put as much pressure on the bladder.

2. The nurse is reviewing information about bethanechol with Mrs. Wheaton. What information does the nurse provide? (Select all that apply.)

1. No adverse effects are significant to report when taking this medication.
2. The patient should avoid abrupt position changes.
3. Salivation and sweating may increase.
4. The patient should be near a bathroom after taking this medication.

A couple of months later, Mrs. Wheaton has been diagnosed with severe hypertension and is prescribed prazosin (Minipress).

3. The nurse informs Mrs. Wheaton that prazosin is a type of:

1. Cholinergic drug
2. Cholinergic blocker
3. Adrenergic drug
4. Adrenergic blocker

4. Mrs. Wheaton asks the nurse if there are any precautions she should know about. The nurse informs her that alpha-adrenergic blockers may cause: (Select all that apply.)

1. Dizziness when changing positions
2. Possible increased heart rate
3. Nasal congestion
4. Nausea

NOTE: Answers to the Review and Case Study Questions appear in Appendix B. The complete rationales and answers are located on the textbook's website.

Pearson Nursing Student Resources Find additional review materials at **nursing.pearsonhighered.com.**

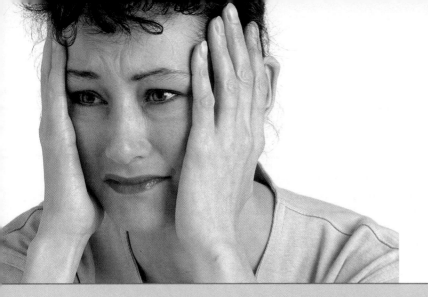

"I'm so nervous all the time; I can't even care for my children. All I can think of is that terrible accident."

Ms. Cynthia Reynolds

Drugs for Anxiety and Insomnia

CORE CONCEPTS

9.1 Anxiety disorders fall into categories of generalized anxiety, panic disorder, and anxiety due to fearful, recurrent, and traumatic life events.

9.2 Regions of the cerebral cortex, diencephalon, and brain stem are responsible for anxiety and wakefulness.

9.3 Anxiety is managed with both pharmacologic and nonpharmacologic strategies.

9.4 An inability to sleep is linked with anxiety.

9.5 Anxiety and insomnia are treated with many types of central nervous system (CNS) drugs.

9.6 When taken properly, antidepressants reduce symptoms of panic and anxiety.

9.7 Benzodiazepines are useful for the short-term treatment of anxiety and insomnia.

9.8 Barbiturates depress CNS function and cause drowsiness.

9.9 Additional drugs provide therapy for anxiety-related symptoms and sleep disorders.

DRUG SNAPSHOT

The following drugs are discussed in this chapter:

DRUG CLASSES	DRUG PROTOTYPES
Antidepressants	**Pr** escitalopram (Lexapro) *113*
Benzodiazepines	**Pr** lorazepam (Ativan) *116*
Barbiturates	
Nonbenzodiazepine, Nonbarbiturate CNS Drugs	**Pr** zolpidem (Ambien) *118*

LEARNING OUTCOMES

After reading this chapter, the student should be able to:

1. Identify the major categories of anxiety disorders.

2. Discuss factors contributing to anxiety and explain some nonpharmacologic therapies used to cope with this disorder.

3. Identify the four categories of CNS drugs used to treat anxiety and sleep disorders.

4. Explain the pharmacologic management of anxiety and insomnia.

5. Categorize drugs used for anxiety and insomnia based on their classification and mechanism of action.

6. For each of the classes listed in the Drug Snapshot, identify representative drugs and explain their mechanisms of drug action, primary actions, and important adverse effects.

KEY TERMS

antidepressants
   (AN-tee-dee-PRESS-ahnts) *110*

anxiety *106*

anxiolytics (ANG-zee-oh-LIT-iks) *109*

barbiturates (bar-bi-CHUR-ates) *116*

benzodiazepines (ben-zo-di-AZ-eh-
   peenz) *113*

black box warning *111*

CNS depressants (dee-PRESS-ahnts) *110*

generalized anxiety disorder (GAD) *106*

insomnia (in-SOM-nee-uh) *109*

limbic system (LIM-bik) *107*

obsessive–compulsive disorder (OCD) *106*

panic disorder *106*

phobias (FO-bee-ahs) *106*

posttraumatic stress disorder (PTSD) *106*

rebound insomnia *110*

reticular activating system (RAS) *107*

reticular formation (re-TIK-u-lurr) *107*

sedative-hypnotic (SED-ah-tiv
   hip-NOT-ik) *111*

sedatives (SED-ah-tivs) *111*

social anxiety disorder *106*

Patients experience nervousness and tension more often than any other symptoms. Seeking relief from these symptoms, patients often turn to a variety of pharmacologic and alternative therapies. Most healthcare providers agree that even though drugs do not cure the underlying problem, they can provide short-term help to calm patients who are experiencing acute anxiety or who have simple sleep disorders. This chapter discusses drugs that treat anxiety, cause sedation, or help patients sleep.

ANXIETY

According to the *International Classification of Diseases*, 10th edition (ICD-10), **anxiety** is a state of "apprehension, tension, or uneasiness that stems from the anticipation of danger, the source of which is largely unknown or unrecognized." Anxious individuals can often identify at least some factors that bring on their symptoms. Most people state that their feelings of anxiety are disproportionate to any factual dangers.

CORE CONCEPT 9.1

Anxiety disorders fall into categories of generalized anxiety, panic disorder, and anxiety due to fearful, recurrent, and traumatic life events.

The anxiety experienced by people faced with a stressful environment or situations is called *situational anxiety*. To a certain degree, situational anxiety is beneficial because it motivates people to accomplish tasks in a prompt manner—if for no other reason than to end the source of nervousness. Situational stress may be intense, but many people often learn to cope with this kind of stress without seeking conventional medical intervention.

Generalized anxiety disorder (GAD) is difficult-to-control, excessive anxiety that lasts six months or more. It occurs in response to a variety of life events or activities, and it interferes with normal, day-to-day functions. It is by far the most common type of stress disorder routinely observed by healthcare providers. Symptoms include restlessness, fatigue, muscle tension, nervousness, inability to focus or concentrate, an overwhelming sense of dread, and sleep disturbances. Autonomic signs of sympathetic nervous system activation involve sweating, blood pressure elevation, heart palpitations, varying degrees of respiratory change, and dry mouth. Parasympathetic responses may involve abdominal cramping, diarrhea, and urinary urgency. Additional motor symptoms experienced by the patient may include increased reflexes and numbness and tingling of the extremities. Females are slightly more likely to experience GAD, and its prevalence is highest in those ages 20 to 35.

A second category of anxiety, called **panic disorder**, is characterized by intense feelings of immediate apprehension, fearfulness, terror, or impending doom, accompanied by increased autonomic nervous system activity. Although panic attacks usually last less than 10 minutes, patients may describe them as seemingly endless. As many as 5% of the population will experience one or more panic attacks during their lifetimes, and women are affected about twice as often as men.

phobia = *fear*

Other categories of anxiety disorders include phobias, OCD, and PTSD. **Phobias** are fearful feelings attached to specific objects or situations. Attacks may occur when a person feels trapped, embarrassed, or unable to escape. Fear of crowds is termed **social anxiety disorder**, or *social phobia*. Performers may experience feelings of dread, nervousness, or apprehension termed *performance anxiety*. Some anxiety is normal when a person faces a crowd or performs for a crowd, but extreme fear is not normal. Phobias compel a patient to avoid the fearful stimulus entirely, to the point that his or her behavior is unnatural. **Obsessive–compulsive disorder (OCD)** involves recurrent, intrusive thoughts or repetitive behaviors that interfere with normal activities or relationships. Common examples include fear of exposure to germs and repetitive hand washing. **Posttraumatic stress disorder (PTSD)** is a type of extreme situational anxiety

Fast Facts Anxiety Disorders

- Millions of Americans experience anxiety every year.
- Other illnesses commonly coexist with anxiety, including depression, eating disorders, and substance abuse.
- The top five causes of anxiety affecting people between the ages of 18 and 54 are:
  - Phobias
    - About 9% of the U.S. population has some type of specific phobia.
    - Specific phobias usually begin in childhood and last for many years.
    - Over 15 million Americans have *social phobia*.
    - Over 1.8 million Americans have *agoraphobia*, an intense fear of crowds.
  - Posttraumatic stress disorder (PTSD)
  - More than 3% of the U.S. population has PTSD.
  - PTSD can develop at any age, although the average age of onset is 24 years old.
  - Generalized anxiety disorder (GAD)
    - About 3% of the U.S. population is diagnosed with GAD in a given year.
    - Generalized anxiety symptoms usually begin in an individual's early 30s.
  - Panic Disorder
    - About 3% of the U.S. population has panic disorder.
    - The average age of onset is 24 years old.
  - Obsessive–compulsive disorder (OCD)
    - One percent of the U.S. population has OCD.
    - Almost 51% of OCD cases is classified as severe.
    - The first symptoms of OCD usually begin in the late teenage years (average age 19 years old).
- For details, see the National Institutes of Mental Health website.

that develops in response to reexperiencing a previous life event. Traumatic life events such as war, physical or sexual abuse, natural disasters, or homicidal situations may lead to a sense of helplessness and reexperiencing of the traumatic event. The terrorist attacks on September 11, 2001, and Hurricanes Katrina and Sandy are examples of situations that triggered PTSD around the turn of the millennium through the century's first decade. Economic changes, global recession, and unemployment have been largely responsible for much persistent anxiety. People who experience lingering traumatic life events are at risk for developing signs and symptoms of PTSD.

Regions of the cerebral cortex, diencephalon, and brain stem are responsible for anxiety and wakefulness.

The emotional areas of the brain responsible for anxiety and restlessness are mostly the limbic system, hypothalamus, and the reticular activating system (Table 9.1 ◆). The **limbic system** is an area of the *cerebral cortex* responsible for emotional expression, learning, and memory. Signals routed through the limbic system connect with the hypothalamus, an area of the brain referred to as the *diencephalon*. Emotional states associated with this connection include anxiety, fear, anger, aggression, remorse, depression, euphoria, and changes in appetite and sexual drive.

The hypothalamus is an important center that triggers unconscious responses to extreme stress, such as increased blood pressure, elevated breathing rate, and dilated pupils. These are responses associated with the fight-or-flight response of the autonomic nervous system (see Chapter 8). The endocrine functions of the hypothalamus are discussed in Chapter 32.

The hypothalamus also connects with the **reticular formation**, a network of neurons found along the entire length of the *brainstem*. Stimulation of the reticular formation causes increased alertness and arousal; inhibition causes drowsiness and sleep.

The larger area in which the reticular formation is found is called the **reticular activating system** (**RAS**). The RAS controls sleeping and wakefulness and performs an alerting function for the cerebral cortex. It also helps a person focus attention on individual tasks by transmitting information to higher brain centers. The RAS is the neural mechanism thought to be responsible for emotions such as anxiety and fear. It is also the mechanism associated with restlessness and an interrupted sleeping pattern.

TABLE 9.1	Areas of the Brain Responsible for Anxiety and Restlessness	
Major Brain Region	**Specific Brain Region**	**Role in Anxiety Symptoms**
Cerebrum	Basal nuclei	Responsible for emotional expression, fear, dread, learning, and memory
	Limbic system	
Diencephalon	Thalamus	Triggers unconscious responses to extreme stress (fight-or-flight response)
	Hypothalamus	
	Epithalamus	
Brainstem	Midbrain	Responsible for overall level of heightened awareness
	Pons	
	Medulla oblongata	
	Reticular formation	
Cerebellum		

Cingulate gyrus (limbic lobe)

Reticular formation

Hypothalamus

Parahippocampal gyrus (limbic lobe)

Shaded areas and labels represent brain regions that have a specific role in anxiety symptoms.

CORE CONCEPT 9.3

Anxiety is managed with both pharmacologic and nonpharmacologic strategies.

Although stress itself may be incapacitating, it is often only a symptom of an underlying disorder. Uncovering and addressing the cause of the anxiety is more productive than merely treating the symptoms with medications. Patients should be encouraged to explore and develop nonpharmacologic coping strategies to deal with the underlying causes. Such strategies may include behavioral therapy, biofeedback techniques, meditation, and other complementary and alternative therapies. One model for anxiety management is shown in Figure 9.1 ■.

FIGURE **9.1**

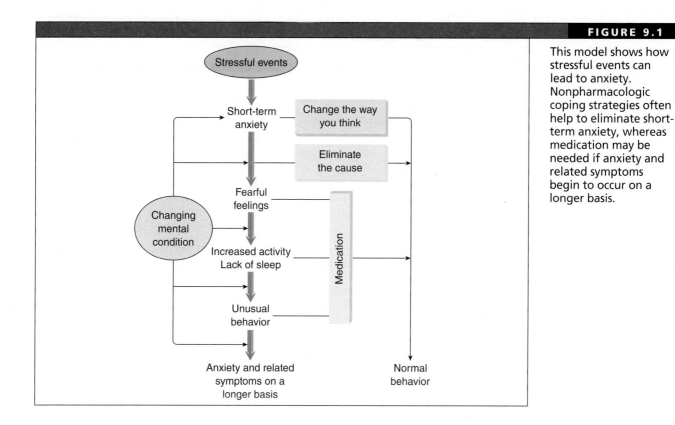

This model shows how stressful events can lead to anxiety. Nonpharmacologic coping strategies often help to eliminate short-term anxiety, whereas medication may be needed if anxiety and related symptoms begin to occur on a longer basis.

When anxiety becomes severe enough to significantly interfere with daily activities of life, pharmacotherapy is indicated. In most types of stress, **anxiolytics**, or drugs having the ability to relieve anxiety, are quite effective. These include medications in a number of therapeutic categories, involving drugs for depression (see Chapter 10) and seizures (see Chapter 13). Anxiolytics provide treatment for GAD, panic disorder, phobias, PTSD, and OCD.

anxio = *anxiety*
lytic = *to dissolve away; break*

Concept Review 9.1

■ What does the term *anxiolytic* mean? What disorders do anxiolytic drugs treat?

INSOMNIA

Insomnia is a condition characterized by a patient's inability to fall asleep or remain asleep. Pharmacotherapy may be needed if the sleeplessness interferes with normal daily activities.

in = *not (without)*
somnia = *sleep*

An inability to sleep is linked with anxiety.

Why is it that we need sleep? During an average lifetime, about 33% of our time is spent sleeping or trying to sleep. Insufficient sleep is associated with increased workplace and driving accidents. Although it is well established that sleep is essential for wellness, scientists are unsure of its function or how much is needed. Following are some theories:

■ Inactivity during sleep gives the body time to repair itself.

■ Sleep is a function that evolved as a protective mechanism. Throughout history, nighttime was the safest time of day, so deep rest (sleep) occurred during those hours.

■ Sleep deals with "electrical" charging and discharging of the brain. The brain needs time for processing and filing new information collected throughout the day. When this is done without interference from the environment, these vast amounts of data can later be retrieved through memory.

Fast Facts Insomnia

- One-third of the world's population has trouble sleeping during part of the year.
- Insomnia is more common in women than in men.
- Patients older than 65 years old sleep less than patients in any other age group.
- Only about 70% of people with insomnia ever report this problem to their healthcare provider.
- People buy over-the-counter (OTC) sleep medications and combination drugs with sleep additives more than any other drug category. Trade name products include Advil P.M., Excedrin P.M., Nytol, Equate Nighttime Sleep-Aid, Sominex, Compoz, Tylenol P.M., and Unicom.
- As a natural alternative for sleep, some people take melatonin, kava kava, or valerian.

The acts of sleeping and waking are synchronized with many different bodily functions. Body temperature, blood pressure, hormone levels, and respiration fluctuate cyclically throughout the 24-hour day. When this cycle is impaired, pharmacologic or other interventions may be needed to readjust it. Increased levels of the neurotransmitter serotonin help initiate the various processes of sleep.

Insomnia, or sleeplessness, is a disorder associated with anxiety. There are several major types of insomnia. *Short-term* or *behavioral insomnia* may be attributed to stress caused by a hectic lifestyle or the inability to resolve day-to-day conflicts within the home or workplace. Worries about work, marriage, children, and health are common reasons for short-term sleep loss. When stress interrupts normal sleeping patterns, patients cannot sleep because their minds are too active. *Long-term insomnia* may be caused by more intense emotional and mood-related illnesses such as depression, manic disorders, or chronic pain.

Foods or beverages containing stimulants such as caffeine may interrupt sleep. Patients may also find that using tobacco products makes them restless and edgy. Alcohol, although often enabling a person to fall asleep, may produce vivid dreams and frequent awakening that prevent restful sleep. Eating a large meal—especially one high in protein and fat—close to bedtime may interfere with sleep because metabolism increases to digest the food. Certain medications cause CNS stimulation, and these should not be taken immediately before bedtime. Stressful conditions—for example, too much light, an uncomfortable room temperature (especially one that is too warm), snoring, sleep apnea, and recurring nightmares—also interfere with sleep.

Nonpharmacologic means of relieving insomnia are usually tried before drug therapy, because long-term use of sleep medications will likely worsen insomnia and may cause physical or psychological dependence. Some patients experience a phenomenon called **rebound insomnia**. This effect occurs when a sedative drug is stopped abruptly or when it has been taken for a long time and drug dependence occurs. Alcohol abuse can also cause rebound insomnia.

> ### Life Span Fact
>
> Older adults are more likely to experience medication-related sleep problems. For the first night or two, drugs may seem to help the insomnia of an elderly patient, but as the medication accumulates in the system, it produces generalized brain dysfunction. The agitated patient may then be mistakenly overdosed with higher doses of medication.

Concept Review 9.2

- Why might a patient not be able to enjoy normal sleep? Why is long-term drug therapy for lack of sleep not a good idea?

CORE CONCEPT 9.5 Anxiety and insomnia are treated with many types of central nervous system (CNS) drugs.

CNS drugs are used to alter brain activity in patients with anxiety or sleep disorders. These medications are grouped into four major classes: (1) antidepressants, (2) benzodiazepines, (3) barbiturates, and (4) nonbarbiturate and nonbenzodiazepine CNS drugs.

Antidepressants have an ability to enhance mood by altering the levels of two important neurotransmitters in the brain—norepinephrine and serotonin. By restoring the balance of these neurotransmitters, antidepressants can reduce the symptoms associated with depression, panic, obsessive–compulsive behavior, and phobia. Antidepressants used to treat anxiety and insomnia include selective serotonin reuptake inhibitors (SSRIs), atypical antidepressants (such as serotonin–norepinephrine reuptake inhibitors (SNRIs)), tricyclic antidepressants (TCAs), and monoamine oxidase inhibitors (MAOIs). Use of the latter two types of drugs has declined in recent years. The mechanisms of action and important considerations of these drugs are covered in Chapter 10.

Another approach to relieving anxiety is the use of **CNS depressants** that slow neuronal activity in the brain. These drugs range from those that relax, to those that sedate, to those that cause sleep and

anti = *against*
depressant = *depressed neuronal function*

anesthesia. Coma and death are the end stages of CNS depression. Some drug classes can produce the full range of CNS depression from relaxation to full anesthesia, whereas others are less effective across this range. Medications that depress the CNS are sometimes called **sedatives** because of their ability to sedate or relax a patient. At higher doses, many of the same drugs can cause sleep and therefore are called *hypnotics*. The term **sedative-hypnotic** is often used to describe a drug with the ability to produce a calming effect at lower doses and sleep at higher doses. *Tranquilizer* is an older term used to describe a drug that produces a soothing or tranquil feeling.

CNS depressants used for anxiety and sleep disorders are categorized into two major classes: benzodiazepines and barbiturates. An additional category consists of miscellaneous drugs chemically unrelated to the other drug groups. These have additional therapeutic usefulness in the treatment of anxiety-related symptoms and insomnia:

sedative = *calming*
hypnotic = *sleep-inducing*

tranquilizer = *drug that soothes or makes you tranquil*

- Buspirone (BuSpar), a mild sedative

- Valproate (Depakote), an antiseizure medication

- Atenolol (Tenormin) and propranolol (Inderal, InnoPran XL), beta blockers to reduce stress

- Eszopiclone (Lunesta), zolpidem (Ambien), and zaleplon (Sonata), sleep disorder medications that directly activate benzodiazepine receptors in the brain

- Ramelteon (Rozerem), medication that activates melatonin receptors in the brain

- Diphenhydramine (Nytol and Sominex) and doxylamine (Unisom), OTC antihistamine sleep aids that cause drowsiness

As discussed in Chapter 7, long-term use of many CNS depressants can lead to physical or psychological dependence. The withdrawal syndrome for some CNS depressants can cause life-threatening neurologic reactions, including fever, psychosis, and seizures. Other withdrawal symptoms include increased heart rate and lowered blood pressure; loss of appetite; muscle cramps; impaired memory, concentration, and orientation; abnormal sounds in the ears and blurred vision; and insomnia, agitation, anxiety, and panic. Noticeable withdrawal symptoms typically last two to four weeks. Subtle ones can last months.

Concept Review 9.3

- Describe what each of the following terms means in relation to anxiety and alertness: *CNS depressants*, *sedatives*, *hypnotics*, *sedative-hypnotics*, and *tranquilizers*.

When taken properly, antidepressants reduce symptoms of panic and anxiety.

CORE CONCEPT 9.6

In the 1960s, antidepressants were mainly used for the treatment of depression or depression that occurred with anxiety. Today, antidepressants are used not only to treat major depressive disorder termed *clinical depression* (see Chapter 10) but also to treat symptoms of anxiety associated with panic disorder, OCD, social phobia, and PTSD. Because many of the features observed in patients with depressive disorder overlap with anxiety disorders, methods of intervention are often the same.

For most patients, panic symptoms come in two stages. The first stage is called *anticipatory anxiety*, when the patient begins to think about an upcoming challenge and starts to feel dread. The second stage is when physical symptoms such as shortness of breath, rapid heart rate, and muscle tension begin. Many of the stressful symptoms are associated with activation of the autonomic nervous system. The strategy in treating panic attacks is to help the patient face the fear and suppress symptoms during one or both of these stages. Drugs can lessen the negative thoughts associated with anticipating the panic, thereby reducing the stress. Drugs also decrease neuronal activity and suppress functions of the autonomic nervous system, helping the patient to remain calm. The patient can then use self-help skills to control behavior.

Antidepressants are often used to reduce persistent symptoms of panic and anxiety. These medications are summarized in Table 9.2 ◆. SSRIs and atypical antidepressants not only treat panic symptoms but also treat symptoms of PTSD, OCD, and phobias. Off-label uses are included. SSRIs and SNRIs produce fewer major adverse effects than the TCAs or MAOIs.

As with all CNS drugs, precautions must be taken to make sure that medications are effective. Because of adverse reactions, some patients might find antidepressant treatment unacceptable. In 2004, the Food and Drug Administration issued an advisory warning **(black box warning)** pointing out the potential warning signs of suicide in adults and children at the beginning of antidepressant therapy and when doses are changed. In the course of treatment, it is possible that several signs that are the focus of anxiety therapy—for example, irritability, panic attacks, agitation, insomnia, and hostility—may emerge. See Chapter 10

TABLE 9.2 Antidepressants for Anxiety Disorders

Drug	Route and Adult Dose	Clinical Uses
SELECTIVE SEROTONIN REUPTAKE INHIBITORS (SSRIs)		
citalopram (Celexa)	PO; start at 20 mg/day, may increase to 40 mg/day if needed	Depression
Pr escitalopram (Lexapro)	PO; 10 mg/day, may increase to 20 mg/day if needed after 1 week	Depression, GAD, social anxiety
fluoxetine (Prozac)	20 mg/day in a.m., may increase by 20 mg/day at weekly intervals (max: 80 mg/day); 20 mg/day in a.m.; when stable may switch to 90 mg sustained-release capsule every week (max: 90 mg/week)	Depression, social anxiety, OCD
fluvoxamine (Luvox)	PO; start with 50 mg/day, may increase slowly up to 300 mg/day given at bedtime or divided two times/day	Depression, social anxiety, OCD
paroxetine (Paxil)	PO; 20–60 mg/day	Depression, GAD, social anxiety, panic disorder, OCD, PTSD
sertraline (Zoloft) (see page 133 for the Drug Prototype box)	PO; begin with 50 mg/day, gradually increase every few weeks according to response (max: 200 mg)	Depression, social anxiety, panic disorder, OCD, PTSD
ATYPICAL ANTIDEPRESSANTS		
bupropion (Wellbutrin, Zyban)	PO; 75–100 mg tid (greater than 450 mg/day increases risk for adverse reactions)	Depression
duloxetine (Cymbalta)	PO; 40–60 mg/day in one or two divided doses	Depression, GAD, neuropathic pain, chronic fatigue syndrome, stress urinary continence, fibromyalgia
mirtazapine (Remeron)	PO; 15 mg/day in a single dose at bedtime; may increase every 1–2 weeks (max: 45 mg/day)	Depression
trazodone (Oleptro)	PO; 150 mg/day in divided doses, may increase by 50 mg/day every 3–4 days (max: 400–600 mg/day)	Depression, GAD
venlafaxine (Effexor)	Start with 37.5 mg sustained release every day and increase to 75–225 mg sustained release per day	Depression, social anxiety, GAD, neuropathic pain, migraines
TRICYCLIC ANTIDEPRESSANTS (TCAs)		
amitriptyline (Elavil)	PO; 75–100 mg/day, may gradually increase to 150–300 mg/day (use lower doses in outpatients)	Depression
clomipramine (Anafranil)	PO; 75–100 mg/day in divided doses	OCD, depression
desipramine (Norpramin)	PO; 75–100 mg/day at bedtime or in divided doses, may gradually increase to 150–300 mg/day (use lower doses in older adults)	Depression
doxepin (Silenor)	PO; 30–150 mg/day at bedtime or in divided doses, may gradually increase to 300 mg/day (use lower doses in older adults)	Depression
imipramine (Tofranil) (see page 129 for the Drug Prototype box)	PO; 75–100 mg/day in divided doses (max: 300 mg/day)	Depression, GAD
nortriptyline (Aventyl, Pamelor)	PO; 25 mg three times/day or four times/day, gradually increased to 100–150 mg/day	Depression
trimipramine (Surmontil)	PO; 75–100 mg/day (max: 300 mg/day) in divided doses	Depression
MONOAMINE OXIDASE INHIBITORS (MAOIs)		
phenelzine (Nardil) (see page 133 for the Drug Prototype box	PO; 15 mg three times/day, rapidly increase to at least 60 mg/day, may need up to 90 mg/day	Depression
tranylcypromine (Parnate)	PO; 30 mg/day in two divided doses (20 mg in a.m., 10 mg in p.m.), may increase by 10 mg/day at 3-week intervals (max: 60 mg/day)	Depression

Drug Prototype: ℞ Escitalopram (Lexapro)
Therapeutic Class: Antidepressant; anxiolytic
Pharmacologic Class: Selective serotonin reuptake inhibitor (SSRI)

Actions and Uses: Escitalopram is a selective serotonin reuptake inhibitor (SSRI). Selective inhibition of serotonin reuptake results in antidepressant activity without adverse autonomic effects such as increased heart rate or hypertension. This medication is indicated for generalized anxiety and depression. Off-label uses include the treatment of panic disorders.

Adverse Effects and Interactions: Serious reactions include dizziness, nausea, insomnia, somnolence, confusion, and seizures if taken in overdose. MAOIs should be avoided due to serotonin syndrome, marked by autonomic hyperactivity, hyperthermia, rigidity, diaphoresis, and neuroleptic malignant syndrome. Combination with MAOIs could result in hypertensive crisis, hyperthermia, and autonomic instability. Escitalopram will increase plasma levels of metoprolol and cimetidine. Concurrent use of alcohol and other CNS depressants may enhance CNS depressant effects; patients should avoid alcohol when taking this drug. Use caution with herbal supplements such as St. John's wort, which may cause serotonin syndrome and increase the effects of escitalopram.

BLACK BOX WARNING:
Antidepressants increase the risk of suicidal thinking and behavior in children, adolescents, and young adults with major depressive disorder and other psychiatric disorders.

for more detailed primary actions and adverse effects of these drugs. Following is a brief introduction to important considerations for each type of antidepressant:

- *SSRIs* These drugs are safer than the other classes of antidepressants and result in fewer occurrences of unfavorable sympathomimetic effects and anticholinergic effects (see Chapter 8). Because serotonin is thought to play a role in mood, these medications have received more attention in recent years. SSRIs can cause weight gain and sexual dysfunction. Excessive doses of these medications can cause confusion, anxiety, restlessness, hypertension, tremors, sweating, fever, blurred vision, constipation, and muscle incoordination. Serotonin syndrome is a potentially life-threatening drug reaction when taking too-high doses of SSRIs. Patients taking these drugs should avoid alcohol. SSRIs are often the preferred drugs for anxiety.

- *Atypical antidepressants* These are chemically unrelated to the other antidepressants. Their adverse effects are generally similar to those of SSRIs. SNRIs inhibit the reuptake of both serotonin and norepinephrine; therefore, these drugs are included here. Atypical antidepressants were the first effective alternatives to TCAs because of their more tolerable adverse effects. Common adverse effects are headache, insomnia, nervousness, dry mouth, dizziness, weight loss, sexual dysfunction, and chills.

- *TCAs* These are not recommended in patients with a history of heart attack, heart block, or abnormal heart rhythm. Patients often have annoying anticholinergic effects (see Chapter 8). Most TCAs are pregnancy category C or D. These drugs should not be used with alcohol or other CNS depressants. Patients with asthma, gastrointestinal disorders, alcoholism, schizophrenia, or bipolar disorder should use these drugs with extreme caution.

- *MAOIs* Patients should strictly avoid foods containing tyramine (a form of the amino acid tyrosine) and caffeine. MAOIs intensify the effects of insulin and other diabetes drugs. Common adverse effects include orthostatic hypotension, hypertension crisis, headache, and diarrhea. MAOIs are prescribed less often due to food interactions and serious adverse effects. Serotonin syndrome is a potentially life-threatening drug reaction when taking too-high doses of MAOIs.

Benzodiazepines are useful for the short-term treatment of anxiety and insomnia.

CORE CONCEPT 9.7

The **benzodiazepines** are one of the most widely prescribed drug classes. The root word *benzo* refers to an aromatic compound, one having a carbon ring structure attached to different atoms or to another carbon ring. Two nitrogen atoms incorporated into the ring structure are the reason for the *diazepine* portion of the name.

The benzodiazepines are used for panic disorder, generalized anxiety, phobias, and insomnia (Table 9.3 ◆). Since the introduction of the first benzodiazepines—chlordiazepoxide (Librium) and diazepam (Valium)—in the 1960s, the class has become one of the most widely prescribed in medicine. Although newer benzodiazepines are available, all have the same actions and adverse effects. They differ primarily in their onset and duration of action. Some, such as the induction drug midazolam (Versed), have a rapid onset

hyper = elevated
thermia = temperature

dia = across (through pores)
phoresis = to carry (implying sweat)

neuro = nerve
leptic = locked (seized up)

malignant = aggressive harm
syndrome = abnormal characteristic

benzo = aromatic or ring structure
di = two
azepine = nitrogen containing

TABLE 9.3 Benzodiazepines for Anxiety and Insomnia

Drug	Route and Adult Dose	Related Clinical Uses
ANXIETY		
alprazolam (Xanax)	For panic: PO; 1–2 mg three times/day For anxiety: PO; 0.25–0.5 mg three times/day	GAD, phobias, social anxiety, panic disorder
chlordiazepoxide (Librium)	Mild anxiety: PO; 5–10 mg three or four times/day Severe anxiety: PO; 20–25 mg three or four times/day	Phobias, alcohol withdrawal
clonazepam (Klonopin)	PO; 1–2 mg/day in divided doses (max: 4 mg/day)	Phobias, social anxiety, seizures, panic disorder
clorazepate (Tranxene)	PO; 15 mg/day at bedtime (max: 4 mg/day)	Alcohol withdrawal, seizures
diazepam (Valium) (see page 188 for the Drug Prototype box)	PO; 2–10 mg two times/day	Alcohol withdrawal, seizures, muscle spasms, induction of anesthesia
Pr lorazepam (Ativan)	For anxiety: PO; 2–6 mg/day in divided doses (max: 10 mg/day)	Panic disorder, phobias, alcohol withdrawal, seizures, induction of anesthesia
oxazepam (Serax)	PO; 10–30 mg three or four times/day	Phobias, alcohol withdrawal
INSOMNIA		
estazolam	PO; 1 mg at bedtime, may increase to 2 mg if necessary	Insomnia: 15–60 min onset and medium duration
flurazepam (Dalmane)	PO; 15–30 mg at bedtime	Insomnia: 30–60 min onset and long duration
quazepam (Doral)	PO; 7.5–15 mg at bedtime	Insomnia: 20–45 min onset and long duration
temazepam (Restoril)	PO; 7.5–30 mg at bedtime	Insomnia: 45–60 min onset and medium duration
triazolam (Halcion)	PO; 0.125–0.25 mg at bedtime (max: 0.5 mg/day)	Insomnia: 15–30 min onset and short duration

time of 15 to 30 minutes; others, such as oxazepam (Serax), take 2 to 3 hours to reach peak blood levels. In cases in which the benzodiazepines are used for insomnia therapy, this is important because *time of onset* translates to *time until sleep* for the patient. Duration of action translates to *time of anticipated sleep* or *drowsiness*. The benzodiazepines are categorized as Schedule IV drugs, although they produce considerably less physical dependence and result in less tolerance than the barbiturates.

These drugs intensify the effect of gamma-aminobutyric acid (GABA), which is a natural inhibitory neurotransmitter found throughout the brain. Most are metabolized in the liver to active metabolites and excreted primarily in urine. Death with routine use of benzodiazepines is unlikely, unless the benzodiazepines are taken in combination with other CNS depressants, or the patient suffers from sleep apnea.

Most benzodiazepines are given orally. Those that can be given parenterally, such as diazepam (Valium) and lorazepam (Ativan), should be monitored carefully because of their rapid onset of CNS effects and possible respiratory depression. Also, some benzodiazepines may be inappropriate for patients who have an existing diagnosis such as substance abuse.

Because of their greater safety, the benzodiazepines are primarily used for the short-term treatment of insomnia caused by anxiety. Benzodiazepines shorten the length of time it takes to fall asleep and reduce the frequency of interrupted sleep. Although most benzodiazepines increase total sleep time, some reduce Stage IV sleep, and some affect REM sleep. In general, the benzodiazepines used to treat short-term insomnia are different from those used to treat GAD (see Table 9.3).

Benzodiazepines have a number of other important indications. Diazepam (Valium) is featured as a prototype drug in Chapter 13 for its use in treating seizure disorders. Other uses include treatment of alcohol withdrawal symptoms (see Chapter 7), central muscle relaxation (see Chapter 12), and as induction drugs in general anesthesia (see Chapter 15).

NURSING PROCESS FOCUS Patients Receiving Antianxiety Therapy

ASSESSMENT	POTENTIAL NURSING DIAGNOSES
Prior to administration: ■ Obtain a complete health history including cardiovascular, neurological, and renal and liver conditions; allergies, drug history, likelihood of drug dependency, and possible drug interactions. ■ Identify factors that precipitate anxiety or insomnia and actions that have been previously tried to decrease symptoms. ■ Acquire baseline vital signs and neurological status including level of consciousness (LOC) and stress/coping patterns. ■ Evaluate laboratory blood findings: renal and liver function studies.	■ *Acute Confusion* related to adverse effects of drug therapy ■ *Deficient Knowledge* related to a lack of information about administration and adverse effects of drug therapy ■ *Ineffective Coping* related to anxiety and/or drug dependence ■ *Risk for Injury* related to sedative effect of drug ■ *Insomnia* related to anxiety or adverse effects of drug therapy

PLANNING: PATIENT GOALS AND EXPECTED OUTCOMES

The patient will:
■ Experience therapeutic effects (an increase in psychological comfort, normal sleep patterns).
■ Be free from or experience minimal adverse effects from drug therapy (absence of physical and behavioral manifestations of anxiety).
■ Verbalize an understanding of the drug's use, adverse effects, and required precautions.

IMPLEMENTATION

Interventions and (Rationales)	Patient Education/Discharge Planning
■ Monitor vital signs. Observe respiratory patterns, especially during sleep, for evidence of apnea or shallow breathing. (Benzodiazepines can reduce the respiratory drive in susceptible patients.)	Instruct the patient: ■ To consult a healthcare provider before taking this drug if snoring is a problem (snoring may indicate an obstruction in the upper respiratory tract, resulting in hypoxia). ■ Regarding methods to monitor vital signs at home, especially respirations.
■ Monitor neurologic status, especially level of consciousness. (Confusion or lack of response may indicate overmedication.)	■ Instruct the patient to report extreme lethargy, slurred speech, disorientation, or ataxia to the healthcare provider.
■ Ensure patient safety (i.e., nurses call light within reach). (Drug may cause excessive drowsiness.)	Instruct the patient to: ■ Not drive or perform hazardous activities until the effects of the drug are known. ■ Request assistance when getting out of bed and walking until the effect of the medication is known.
■ Monitor the patient's intake of stimulants, including caffeine (in beverages such as coffee, tea, cola, and other soft drinks and in OTC analgesics such as Excedrin), nicotine from tobacco products, and any drugs such as alcohol that produce drowsiness. (These products can reduce or enhance the drug's effectiveness.)	Instruct the patient to: ■ Avoid drinking or eating drinks or food with caffeine, especially before bedtime. ■ Avoid taking alcohol or OTC sleep-inducing antihistamines such as diphenhydramine. ■ Consult a healthcare provider before self-medicating with any OTC preparation.
■ Monitor effect and emotional status. (Drug may increase risk of mental depression, especially in patients with suicidal tendencies.)	Instruct the patient to: ■ Report significant mood changes, especially depression. ■ Avoid consuming alcohol or taking other CNS depressants while on benzodiazepines because these increase depressant effect.
■ Administer medication correctly and evaluate the patient's knowledge of proper administration. Avoid abrupt discontinuation of therapy. (Withdrawal symptoms, including rebound anxiety and sleeplessness, are possible with abrupt discontinuation after long-term use.)	Instruct the patient: ■ To take the drug exactly as prescribed. Discontinuation of medication must be done gradually. ■ To keep all follow-up appointments as directed by the healthcare provider to monitor response to medication. ■ About nonpharmacologic methods for reestablishing sleep regimen.

EVALUATION OF OUTCOME CRITERIA

Evaluate effectiveness of drug therapy by confirming that patient goals and expected outcomes have been met (see "Planning"). *See Tables 9.2 (SSRIs) and 9.3 for a list of drugs to which these nursing actions apply.*

Drug Prototype: ℞ *Lorazepam (Ativan)*

Therapeutic Class: Sedative-hypnotic, anxiolytic, anesthetic adjunct
Pharmacologic Class: Benzodiazepine, GABA receptor drug

Actions and Uses: Lorazepam is a benzodiazepine that acts by increasing the effects of GABA, an inhibitory neurotransmitter in the CNS. It is one of the most potent benzodiazepines. It has an extended half-life of 10 to 20 hours that allows for once or twice a day oral dosing. In addition to its use as an anxiolytic, lorazepam is used as a preanesthetic medication to provide sedation and for the management of status epilepticus.

Adverse Effects and Interactions: The most common adverse effects of lorazepam are drowsiness and sedation, which may decrease with time. When given in higher doses or by the intravenous (IV) route, more severe effects may be observed, such as amnesia, weakness, disorientation, ataxia, sleep disturbance, blood pressure changes, blurred vision, double vision, nausea, and vomiting.

Lorazepam interacts with multiple drugs; for example, concurrent use of CNS depressants, including alcohol, increases sedation effects and the risk of respiratory depression and death. Lorazepam may contribute to digoxin toxicity by increasing the serum digoxin level. Symptoms include visual changes, nausea, vomiting, dizziness, and confusion.

Lorazepam should be used with caution with herbal supplements. For example, sedation-producing herbs such as kava, valerian, chamomil, or hops may have an additive effect with medication. Stimulant herbs such as gotu-kola and ma huang may reduce the drug's effectiveness.

CORE CONCEPT 9.8 | ## Barbiturates depress CNS function and cause drowsiness.

barbiturate = *barbituric acid compound*

Barbiturates are drugs derived from barbituric acid. Until the discovery of the benzodiazepines, barbiturates were used extensively for anxiety and insomnia treatment (Table 9.4 ◆). Although barbiturates are still indicated for several conditions, they are rarely, if ever, prescribed for treating anxiety or insomnia because of their significant adverse effects and the availability of more effective medications. The risk of psychological and physical dependence is high—several are Schedule II drugs. The withdrawal syndrome from barbiturates is extremely severe and can be fatal. Overdose results in profound respiratory depression, hypotension, and shock. People have used barbiturates to commit suicide, and death due to overdose is not uncommon.

Barbiturates are capable of depressing CNS function at all levels. Like benzodiazepines, barbiturates act by binding to GABA receptor–chloride channel molecules, intensifying the effect of GABA throughout the brain. At low doses, they reduce anxiety and cause drowsiness. At moderate doses, they inhibit seizure activity (see Chapter 10) and promote sleep, probably by inhibiting brain impulses traveling through the limbic system and the RAS. At higher doses, some barbiturates can produce anesthesia (see Chapter 15).

TABLE 9.4 Barbiturates for Sedation and Insomnia

Drug	Route and Adult Dose
SHORT ACTING	
pentobarbital (Nembutal)	Sedative: PO; 20–30 mg two or three times/day
	Hypnotic: PO; 120–200 mg
secobarbital (Seconal)	Sedative: PO; 100–300 mg/day in three divided doses
	Hypnotic: PO; 100–200 mg
INTERMEDIATE ACTING	
amobarbital (Amytal)	Sedative: PO; 30–50 mg two or three times/day
	Hypnotic: PO; 65–200 mg (max: 500 mg)
butabarbital (Butisol)	Sedative: PO; 15–30 mg three or four times/day
	Hypnotic: PO; 50–100 mg at bedtime
LONG ACTING	
mephobarbital (Mebaral)	Sedative: PO; 32–100 mg three times/day
phenobarbital (Luminal) (see page 188 for the Drug Prototype box)	Sedative: PO; 30–120 mg/day

When taken for prolonged periods, barbiturates stimulate the microsomal enzymes in the liver that metabolize medications. Thus, barbiturates can stimulate their own metabolism as well as that of hundreds of other drugs that use these enzymes for their breakdown. With repeated use, tolerance develops to the sedative effects of these drugs, and cross-tolerance to other CNS depressants such as the opioids. Tolerance does not develop, however, to the respiratory depressant effects.

Concept Review 9.4

■ Identify the major drug classes used for sedation and insomnia. Why are CNS depressants especially dangerous if administered in high doses?

Additional drugs provide therapy for anxiety-related symptoms and sleep disorders.

The final group of CNS drugs used for anxiety and sleep disorders consists of miscellaneous drugs that are chemically unrelated to either benzodiazepines or barbiturates. These include the antiseizure medication valproate (Depakote) and the beta blockers atenolol (Tenormin) and propranolol (Inderal). Drugs used mainly for insomnia therapy include eszopiclone (Lunesta), zaleplon (Sonata), and zolpidem (Ambien). Buspirone (BuSpar) and zolpidem (Ambien) are commonly prescribed for their anxiolytic effects. Zolpidem (Ambien), ramelteon (Rozerem), and eszopiclone (Lunesta) are used primarily for their hypnotic effects. Dexmedetomidine (Precedex) is primarily used as an adjunctive medication during short surgical procedures (Table 9.5 ◆).

TABLE 9.5 Nonbenzodiazepine, Nonbarbiturate CNS Drugs for Anxiety and Insomnia

Drug	Route and Adult Dose	Clinical Uses
ANXIETY THERAPY		
Sedatives		
buspirone (BuSpar)	PO; 7.5–15 mg in divided doses, may increase by 5 mg/day every 2–3 days if needed (max: 60 mg/day)	GAD, OCD
dexmedetomidine (Precedex)	IV; loading dose 1 mcg/kg over 10 min; maintenance dose 0.2–0.7 mcg/kg/hr	Adjunctive medication during surgery, induction in anesthesia
Antiseizure Medication		
valproate/valproic acid (Depakene, Depakote)	For mania: PO; 250 mg three times/day (max: 60 mg/kg/day)	Panic disorder, seizures, smoking, bipolar disorder, prevention of migraines
Beta Blockers		
atenolol (Tenormin) (see page 309 for the Drug Prototype box)	PO; 25–100 mg once/day	Performance anxiety, social anxiety
propranolol (Inderal, InnoPran XL) (see page 340 for the Drug Prototype box)	For trembling: PO; 40 mg two times/day (max: up to 320 mg/day)	Performance anxiety, social anxiety

Drug	Route and Adult Dose	Onset and Duration
INSOMNIA THERAPY		
Nonbenzodiazepines		
eszopiclone (Lunesta)	PO; 1–2 mg at bedtime; depending on the age, clinical response, and tolerance of the patient	60 min onset and medium duration
zaleplon (Sonata)	PO; 10 mg at bedtime (max: 20 mg at bedtime)	15–30 min onset and short duration
℗ zolpidem (Ambien, Edular, others)	PO; 5–10 mg at bedtime	30 min onset and short (medium CR) duration
Melatonin Receptor Drug		
ramelteon (Rozerem)	PO; 8 mg at bedtime	30 min onset and short duration
Antihistamines		
diphenhydramine (Nytol and Sominex)	OTC medication	60–180 min onset and long duration
doxylamine (Unisom)	OTC medication	60–120 min onset and long duration

cognitive = *thinking, remembering, and reasoning*

motor = *producing motion or action*

The mechanism of action for buspirone (BuSpar) is unclear but appears to be related to D_2 dopamine receptors in the brain. The drug has profound effects on presynaptic dopamine receptors and a high attraction for serotonin receptors. Buspirone is less likely than benzodiazepines to affect cognitive and motor performance and rarely interacts with other CNS depressants. Common adverse effects include dizziness, headache, and drowsiness. Dependence and withdrawal problems are less of a concern with buspirone. Therapy may take several weeks to achieve optimal results.

The antiseizure medication valproate/valproic acid (Depakene, Depakote) is an important drug used to treat a variety of seizure types. Common uses include treatment for all partial and generalized seizures (see Chapter 13), the control of symptoms in patients with bipolar disorder (see Chapter 10), and to prevent migraine headaches (see Chapter 14). For these reasons, valproic acid is listed as one medication that might be helpful in reducing anxiety symptoms among patients predisposed to panic disorders, mood swings, or intense headaches. Adverse gastrointestinal effects such as nausea and vomiting are common. Rare life-threatening hepatotoxicity and pancreatitis are a concern.

Beta blockers were covered in Chapter 8 and are covered more thoroughly as they pertain to management of hypertension (see Chapter 18), angina (see Chapter 20), and cardiac dysrhythmias (see Chapter 22). Sweating, heart palpitations, and shaking are expected signs of situational, social, and performance anxiety. Low doses of beta blockers reduce symptoms connected with panic, tension, and excitement.

Zolpidem (Ambien) is a Schedule IV controlled substance limited to the short-term treatment of insomnia. It is highly specific to the GABA receptor and produces muscle relaxation (see Chapter 12) and antiseizure effects (see Chapter 13) only at doses much higher than hypnotic doses. As with other CNS depressants, zolpidem should be used cautiously in patients with respiratory impairment, in elderly persons, and in conjunction with other CNS depressants. Lower dosages may be necessary. In 2011, the FDA issued a statement saying that sleeping pills containing the drug zolpiden were dosed too high, especially for women, related to incidences of car crashes and accidents. Ambien has been shown to decrease sleep latency for up to 35 days in controlled clinical studies. Also, because of the rapid onset of this drug (within 30 minutes), zolpidem should be taken just prior to expected sleep. Adverse reactions are usually minimal (mild nausea, dizziness, diarrhea, daytime drowsiness). Rebound insomnia may occur when the drug is discontinued.

Drug Prototype: ℗ *Zolpidem (Ambien, Edluar, others)*
Therapeutic Class: Sedative-hypnotic
Pharmacologic Class: Nonbenzodiazepine, nonbarbiturate CNS depressant, GABA receptor drug

Actions and Uses: Although it is a nonbenzodiazepine, zolpidem acts in a similar fashion to facilitate GABA-mediated CNS depression in the brain. The only indication for zolpidem is short-term insomnia management (two to six weeks). It is available in immediate release, extended release, orally disintegrating tablet, and spray forms. Zolpidem is pregnancy category B (immediate release) or C (extended release).

Adverse Effects and Interactions: Adverse effects include daytime sedation, confusion, amnesia, dizziness, depression, nausea, and vomiting. The drug should be used with caution in depressed patients or those with a potential for suicide ideation.

Drug interactions with zolpidem include an increase in sedation when used concurrently with other CNS depressants, including alcohol. When taken with food, absorption is slowed significantly and the onset of action may be delayed.

🍃 CAM THERAPY

Valerian for Anxiety and Insomnia

Valerian (*Valeriana officinalis*) is a perennial plant that grows in Europe, Asia, and North America. Valerian has several substances in its roots that affect the CNS; the exact active chemical has yet to be identified. This herb has been used to treat nervousness, anxiety, and insomnia for thousands of years and is one of the most widely used herbal CNS depressants. The herb appears to have effects similar to benzodiazepines such as diazepam (Valium). The major side effects of valerian are extensions of its therapeutic effects: drowsiness and decreased alertness. Valerian should not be combined with alcohol or other drugs that cause sedation or drowsiness because excessive drowsiness may occur.

Although structurally unrelated to other drugs used to treat insomnia, eszopiclone (Lunesta) has properties similar to those of zolpidem (Ambien). Eszopiclone's longer elimination half-life, about twice as long as that of zolpidem, may give it an advantage in maintaining sleep and decreasing early-morning awakening. Eeszopiclone is more likely to cause daytime sedation.

Zaleplon (Sonata) may be useful for people who desire to fall asleep but need to awake early in the morning. It is sometimes used for travel purposes and has been advertised by pharmaceutical companies for this purpose.

Ramelteon is a melatonin receptor drug, which has been shown to speed the onset of sleep. It has a relatively short onset of action (30 minutes), and its duration is comparable to the noncontrolled release form of zolpidem. The FDA indications for remelteon or zolpidem are not limited to short-term use because they do not appear to produce dependence or tolerance to dose.

Drugs included in Table 9.5 without dosing information are diphenhydramine (Nytol and Sominex) and doxylamine (Unisom). These are OTC sleep aids. Antihistamines also produce drowsiness and are beneficial in calming patients. They offer the advantage of not causing dependence, although their use is often limited by anticholinergic adverse effects. Diphenhydramine is a common component of antihistamine combinations available OTC for allergic rhinitis and cough and for allergic reactions in general (see Chapter 25).

Concept Review   9.5

- What are the major drug classes used to treat GAD, panic disorder, and anxiety symptoms caused by fearful, recurrent, and traumatic life events?
- Name popular drugs used to treat symptoms of anxiety and insomnia.

PATIENTS NEED TO KNOW

Patients taking anxiolytics and CNS depressants need to know the following:

1. Stimulants such as coffee, tea, and chocolate should be avoided because they counteract anxiolytics and sedatives and increase the symptoms of anxiety.
2. Exercise, progressive muscle relaxation, and slow, deep breathing can assist with anxiety relief.
3. Alcohol, antihistamines, and other CNS depressants can increase the effects of anxiolytics. They should be avoided to decrease the risk of accidental depressant overdose and death.
4. Anxiolytics can cause drowsiness. Until effects of these drugs have been established, assistance with getting out of bed and driving may be needed and operation of machinery should be avoided.
5. Anxiolytics and sedatives should be stored in a secure place to avoid accidental ingestion by children and animals.
6. Avoid abrupt discontinuation of medication because withdrawal symptoms may occur after long-term use.
7. Report any significant changes in mood to the healthcare provider.
8. Do not take any OTC medications without first consulting the healthcare provider.
9. Smoking and nicotine dependence are increased in patients with anxiety disorders. Thus, it is believed that smoking and pharmacotherapy for anxiety-related disorders are counter effective. Quitting smoking can reduce anxiety.

SAFETY ALERT

Interpreting Physician Orders

It is extremely important for nurses to know their patients' needs and to clarify with the physician any medication order that is difficult to interpret or is questionable. For example, an error could be made if an order to discontinue "SSRI," intended to mean "sliding scale regular insulin," is misinterpreted as an order to discontinue the "selective serotonin reuptake inhibitor."

CHAPTER REVIEW

CORE CONCEPTS SUMMARY

9.1 Anxiety disorders fall into categories of generalized anxiety, panic disorder, and anxiety due to fearful, recurrent, and traumatic life events

There are at least five major types of anxiety disorders: generalized anxiety, panic disorder, phobias, obsessive–compulsive disorder, and posttraumatic stress disorder.

9.2 Regions of the cerebral cortex, diencephalon, and brain stem are responsible for anxiety and wakefulness.

The limbic system and the reticular activating system control anxiety and wakefulness. Neural signals passing between these two brain regions and the cerebral cortex are responsible for anxiety, fear, restlessness, and an interrupted sleep pattern.

9.3 Anxiety is managed with both pharmacologic and nonpharmacologic strategies.

Patients should be encouraged to explore and develop coping strategies for dealing with stress. In cases when anxiety becomes too severe, anxiolytics are an effective treatment.

9.4 An inability to sleep is linked with anxiety.

There are many reasons why a patient might experience sleeplessness. Stress is one factor in short-term insomnia. Others include caffeine, nicotine, room temperature, light, snoring, and sleep apnea. In long-term insomnia, psychological and physiological factors may be involved.

9.5 Anxiety and insomnia are treated with many types of central nervous system (CNS) drugs.

Antidepressants treat stress and related symptoms by altering levels of norepinephrine and serotonin in the brain. *Sedatives, sedative-hypnotics,* and *CNS depressants* are terms used to describe benzodiazepines,

barbiturates, and other drugs. These drugs suppress impulses traveling through the limbic and reticular activating systems, thereby reducing symptoms of stress, producing drowsiness, and promoting sleep.

9.6 When taken properly, antidepressants reduce symptoms of panic and anxiety.

Several classes of antidepressants treat panic and anxiety symptoms: tricyclic antidepressants (TCAs), monoamine oxidase inhibitors (MAOIs), selective serotonin reuptake inhibitors (SSRIs), and atypical antidepressants. The new SSRIs are preferred because they produce fewer sympathomimetic and anticholinergic effects.

9.7 Benzodiazepines are useful for the short-term treatment of anxiety and insomnia.

Benzodiazepines are commonly prescribed for insomnia. Several drugs are used; in general, they differ from the ones used to treat anxiety. Onset and duration of action help determine therapeutic application.

9.8 Barbiturates depress CNS function and cause drowsiness.

Barbiturates are rarely, if ever, prescribed for insomnia. The primary role of this class of drugs is sedation. They depress CNS function by binding to GABA receptors and causing drowsiness.

9.9 Additional drugs provide therapy for anxiety-related symptoms and sleep disorders.

Miscellaneous drugs provide relief from anxiety and anxiety-related symptoms. These include CNS depressants, antiseizure medications, and beta blockers. Additional drugs employed for insomnia therapy involve nonbenzodiazepines, melatonin receptor drugs, and antihistamines. Antihistamines are often found in OTC medications.

REVIEW QUESTIONS

The following questions are written in NCLEX-PN® style. Answer these questions to assess your knowledge of the chapter material, and go back and review any material that is not clear to you.

1. After eight months of use, the patient abruptly discontinues his zaleplon (Sonata). The patient is now complaining of anxiety and inability to sleep. The nurse suspects:

1. A panic disorder
2. Long-term insomnia
3. Behavioral insomnia
4. Rebound insomnia

2. Your patient was started on buspirone (BuSpar) for his anxiety disorder three days ago. The patient now calls the physician's office stating that it "just isn't working." The nurse's best response would be:

1. "BuSpar should give you immediate relief. I will notify the physician that this medication is not effective."
2. "It may take several weeks for BuSpar to be fully effective."
3. "You may need an increased dose of BuSpar for it to work."
4. "You will need additional medications to ease your anxiety."

3. The hospitalized patient is sleeping at the time the next sedative is ordered. The nurse should:

1. Wake the patient and administer the next dose of sedative.
2. Notify the physician.
3. Hold the dose and document the reason.
4. Hold this dose and administer it with the next dose.

4. The nurse informs the patient on zolpidem (Ambien) that it:

1. Will take a week for the medication to be effective
2. May be taken two to three hours before bedtime
3. Should be taken just prior to going to bed
4. Must be used long term to be effective

5. The patient has been taking barbiturates for the last few months for difficulty sleeping. The nurse's main concern for the patient who suddenly stops taking the barbiturate would be:

1. Respiratory depression
2. Severe withdrawal
3. Hypotension
4. Shock

6. Which of the following nursing interventions would be most appropriate for a patient who has just been administered a sedative?

1. Orient to surroundings.
2. Assess for respiratory dysfunction.
3. Shut off the lights and close the door.
4. Make sure the call light is within the patient's reach.

7. Anixety and insomnia are treated with: (Select all that apply.)

1. Benzodiazepines
2. Antidepressants
3. Antipsychotics
4. Barbiturates

8. It is important to ensure the patient knows to avoid _____, which can increase the effects of sedatives.

1. Nicotine
2. Alcohol
3. Chocolate
4. Tea

9. Which of the following is used in the treatment of generalized anxiety disorder (GAD)?

1. Alprazolam (Xanax)
2. Estazolam
3. Clonazepam (Klonopin)
4. Lorazepam (Ativan)

10. The nurse monitors the patient taking lorazepam (Ativan) for which of the following adverse effects?

1. Ataxia
2. Euphoria
3. Astigmatism
4. Tachypnea

CASE STUDY QUESTIONS

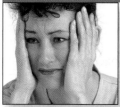

Remember Ms. Reynolds, the patient introduced at the beginning of the chapter? Now read the remainder of the case study. Based on the information you have learned in this chapter, answer the questions that follow.

Ms. Cynthia Reynolds is a 34-year-old interior designer who witnessed and was nearly involved in a fatal car accident on her way to a patient's house about 6 months ago. Since that time she has been having dreams about the accident, and during the day she often thinks about the events and the injured people she saw. She is fearful of driving and does all she can to avoid leaving her home-based office. When she hears a siren, she feels immediate anxiety and terror. After seeing a physician, Ms. Reynolds is diagnosed with Post Traumatic Stress Disorder (PTSD) and was given an SSRI to help relieve her anxiety.

1. There are a couple of SSRIs indicated for the signs and symptoms of PTSD. The nurse would expect Ms. Reynolds to take:

1. Celexa
2. Lexapro
3. Prozac
4. Paxil

2. While taking the SSRI, Ms. Reynolds is monitored for:

1. Diarrhea
2. Hypotension
3. Hallucinations
4. Weight gain

NOTE: Answers to the Review and Case Study Questions appear in Appendix B. The complete rationales and answers are located on the textbook's website.

Pearson Nursing Student Resources Find additional review materials at **nursing.pearsonhighered.com.**

"I hate my job. And my family is constantly nagging me about sleeping too much and eating too little. I don't know what's wrong with me."

Mrs. Rachel Coxilean

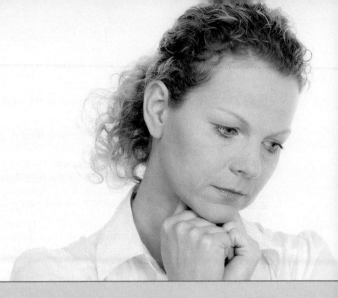

10 Drugs for Emotional, Mood, and Behavioral Disorders

CORE CONCEPTS

10.1 People suffer from depression for many reasons.

10.2 For best results, treatment of severe depression requires both medication and psychotherapy.

10.3 Antidepressants enhance mood by boosting the actions of neurotransmitters, including norepinephrine, dopamine, and serotonin.

10.4 Patients with bipolar disorder may experience emotions ranging from depression to extreme agitation.

10.5 Mood stabilization in patients with bipolar disorder is accomplished with lithium and other drugs.

10.6 Attention deficit hyperactivity disorder (ADHD) presents challenges for children and adults.

10.7 Central nervous system (CNS) stimulants have been the main course of treatment for ADHD.

DRUG SNAPSHOT

The following drugs are discussed in this chapter:

DRUG CLASSES	DRUG PROTOTYPES
Antidepressants	
Tricyclic antidepressants (TCAs)	**Pr** imipramine (Tofranil) *129*
Selective serotonin reuptake inhibitors (SSRIs)	**Pr** sertraline (Zoloft) *133*
Atypical antidepressants	
Monoamine oxidase inhibitors (MAOIs)	**Pr** phenelzine (Nardil) *133*

DRUG CLASSES	DRUG PROTOTYPES
Drugs for Bipolar Disorder	
Mood stabilizers	
Antiseizure drugs	
Atypical antipsychotic drugs	
Drugs for Attention Deficit–Hyperactivity Disorder (ADHD)	
CNS stimulants	**Pr** methylphenidate (Ritalin) *137*
Nonstimulant drugs for ADHD	

LEARNING OUTCOMES

After reading this chapter, the student should be able to:

1. Identify the general categories of mood disorders and their symptoms.

2. Explain the causes of major depressive disorder.

3. Discuss the pharmacologic management of patients with depression, bipolar disorder, and attention deficit–hyperactivity disorder (ADHD).

4. Identify symptoms of ADHD.

5. Categorize drugs used for mood, emotional, and behavioral disorders based on their classes and drug actions.

6. For each of the classes listed in the Drug Snapshot, identify representative drugs and explain their mechanisms of drug action, primary actions, and important adverse effects.

KEY TERMS

antidepressants (AN-tee-dee-PRESS-ahnts) *125*

antipsychotic drugs *135*

attention deficit disorder (ADD) *137*

attention deficit–hyperactivity disorder (ADHD) *136*

bipolar disorder (bi-PO-ler) *133*

clinical depression *123*

depression (dee-PRESS-shun) *123*

dysthymic disorder (dis-THIGH-mick) *124*

major depressive disorder *123*

monoamine oxidase inhibitors (MAOIs) (mon-oh-AHM-een OK-se-daze) *132*

mood stabilizers *134*

postpartum depression *124*

psychotic depression *124*

seasonal affective disorder (SAD) *124*

selective serotonin reuptake inhibitors (SSRIs) (sir-eh-TO-nin) *128*

serotonin–norepinephrine reuptake inhibitors (SNRIs) *129*

serotonin syndrome (SES) *129*

situational depression *124*

tricyclic antidepressants (TCAs) (treye-SICK-lick) *125*

Inappropriate or unusually intense emotions are among the leading causes of mental health disorders. Although mood changes are a normal part of life, when those changes become severe and impair functioning within the family, work environment, or interpersonal relationships, an individual may be diagnosed as having a mood disorder. The two major categories of mood disorders are depression and bipolar disorder. A third behavioral disorder, ADHD, is also included in this chapter.

DEPRESSION

Depression is an emotional disorder characterized by many symptoms, some of which are depressed mood, lack of energy, sleep disturbances, abnormal eating patterns, and feelings of despair, guilt, and misery (Table 10.1).

People suffer from depression for many reasons.

CORE CONCEPT 10.1

In some cases, depression may be situational or reactive, meaning that it results from challenging circumstances such as severe physical illness, loss of a job, death of a loved one, divorce, or financial difficulties coupled with inadequate psychosocial support. In other cases, the depression may be biological or physiological in origin, associated with dysfunction of neurologic processes associated with an imbalance of neurotransmitters. Family history of depression increases the risk of biological depression.

Among the most common forms of mental illness, **major depressive disorder** or **clinical depression** is estimated to affect 5% to 10% of adults in the United States. The American Psychiatric Association's *Diagnostic and Statistical Manual of Mental Disorders*, 5th edition (DSM-5), describes the following

---

TABLE 10.1 Situational and Biological Causes of Depression

Situational Causes of Depression

- Unpleasant life circumstances—grief from a lost loved one, divorce, loss of or dissatisfaction with a job, financial difficulty, excessive stress or responsibilities

- Negative thinking patterns—an environment that is likely to cause an individual to feel as if any attempts to escape or correct a situation are hopeless; poor self-image or lack of support from family or friends

- Substance abuse—substances that produce unpleasant adverse effects or withdrawal symptoms, such as opiates, alcohol, or other CNS depressants

- Medication intended for therapeutic use—unfavorable adverse effects from medication intended to treat a medical disorder (e.g., some antihypertensive drugs and oral contraceptives)

Biological Causes of Depression

- Genetic—history of depression in one's family

- Hormonal changes in the body—fluctuations of reproductive or metabolic hormones

- Neurobiological dysfunction—chemical disturbances in the brain; usually related to abnormal functioning or release of neurotransmitters (e.g., dopamine, norepinephrine, serotonin, or melatonin)

- Symptoms from a second disorder—almost any debilitating disorder, including head trauma, dementia, brain stroke or tumors, chronic pain, or thyroid dysfunction

criteria for diagnosis of a major depressive disorder: a depressed affect plus at least five of the following symptoms lasting for a minimum of two weeks:

- Difficulty sleeping or sleeping too much
- Extremely tired; without energy
- Abnormal eating patterns (eating too much or not enough)
- Vague physical symptoms (gastrointestinal [GI] pain, joint/muscle pain, or headaches)
- Inability to concentrate or make decisions
- Feelings of despair, guilt, and misery; lack of self-worth
- Obsessed with death (expressing a wish to die or to commit suicide)
- Avoiding psychosocial and interpersonal interactions
- Lack of interest in personal appearance or sex
- Delusions or hallucinations

The majority of depressed patients are not found in psychiatric hospitals but in mainstream society. For proper diagnosis and treatment to occur, recognition of depression is often a collaborative effort among healthcare providers. For example, it might be the pharmacist who recognizes that a customer is depressed when the customer buys natural or over-the-counter (OTC) remedies to control anxiety symptoms or to induce sleep.

Depression due to **situational depression** may be the result of circumstances in a person's life. **Dysthymic disorder** is a condition characterized by less severe depressive symptoms of an unknown origin that may prevent a person from feeling well or functioning normally. The process from recognizing depression to properly diagnosing and treating patients should be a collective attempt among healthcare providers. All staff members should be alert for signs and symptoms of depression in patients they treat.

Some women experience intense mood shifts associated with hormonal changes during the menstrual cycle, pregnancy, childbirth, and menopause. For example, up to 80% of women experience **postpartum depression** during the first several weeks after the birth of their baby. Many women face additional stresses such as responsibilities both at work and home, single parenthood, and caring for children and aging parents. If mood is severely depressed and persists long enough, many women will likely benefit from medical treatment.

Because of the possible consequences of perinatal mood disorders, some state agencies mandate that all new mothers receive information about mood shifts prior to their discharge after giving birth. Healthcare providers in obstetrician's offices, pediatric outpatient settings, and family medicine centers are encouraged to conduct routine screening for symptoms of perinatal mood disorders.

During the dark winter months, some patients experience a type of depression known as **seasonal affective disorder (SAD)**. This type of depression is associated with a reduced release of the brain neurohormone melatonin. Exposing patients on a regular basis to specific wavelengths of light may relieve SAD depression and prevent future episodes.

Psychotic depression is another condition characterized by the expression of mood shifts and unusual behaviors. Intense behaviors include hallucinations, combativeness, and disorganized speech patterns. For patients with psychosis and for patients with extreme mood swings, unusual behaviors are often treatable with antipsychotic drugs (see Chapter 11).

dys = *ill*
thymic = *mind*

meno = *monthly*
pause = *stop*

post = *after*
partum = *delivery*

peri = *around*
natal = *birth*

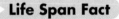 **Life Span Fact**

Depression is the most common mental health disorder of elderly patients, encompassing a variety of physical, emotional, cognitive, and social considerations.

CORE CONCEPT 10.2

For best results, treatment of severe depression requires both medication and psychotherapy.

The first step to treating depression is a complete health assessment. Drugs such as corticosteroids, levodopa, and oral contraceptives can cause symptoms of depression, and the healthcare provider should rule out this possibility. Medical and neurologic disorders, ranging from vitamin B deficiencies to thyroid gland disorders to early Alzheimer's disease, can mimic depression. Once physical causes for depression are ruled out, a psychological evaluation may be performed by a psychiatrist or psychologist to confirm the diagnosis.

During the health assessment, inquiries should be made about alcohol and drug use, and whether the patient has had thoughts about death or suicide. In addition, because depression is sometimes associated with heredity, the health history should include questions about whether other family members have had a depressive illness and, if treated, what therapies they received and which of them were effective.

After healthcare providers assess for symptoms of depression, it is necessary to determine the course of treatment. In general, severe depressive illness, particularly that which recurs, requires treatment with both medication and psychotherapy to achieve the best response. Counseling therapies help patients gain insight into and resolve their problems through verbal interaction with the therapist. Behavioral therapies help patients learn how to obtain more satisfaction and rewards through their own actions and how to unlearn the behavioral patterns that contribute to or result from their depression.

Two short-term psychotherapies that are helpful for some forms of depression are interpersonal and cognitive-behavioral therapies. *Interpersonal therapy* focuses on the patient's disturbed personal relationships that both cause and worsen the depression. *Cognitive-behavioral therapy* helps the patient change the negative styles of thought and behavior that are often associated with depression. *Psychodynamic therapies*, often postponed until the depressive symptoms are significantly improved, focus on resolving the patient's internal conflicts.

In patients with serious and life-threatening mood disorders that are unresponsive to pharmacotherapy, electroconvulsive therapy (ECT) has been the traditional treatment. Although ECT has been found to be safe, there may be serious complications related both to the anesthesia that is used and to the potential seizure activity caused by ECT. Studies suggest that repetitive transcranial magnetic stimulation (rTMS) may improve mood in major depressive disorder. In contrast to ECT, it has minimal effects on memory, does not require general anesthesia, and produces its effects without a generalized seizure.

trans = *across*
cranial = *head*

Even with the best professional care, the patient with depression may take a long time to recover. Individuals with major depression may have multiple bouts of the illness over the course of their lifetime. This can take its toll on the patient's family, friends, and other caregivers who may sometimes feel exhausted, frustrated, and even depressed themselves. They may experience episodes of anger toward the depressed loved one, only to subsequently suffer reactions of guilt about being angry. Such feelings can be distressing, and the caregiver may not know where to turn for help. It is often the healthcare provider who is best able to assist the family members of a person suffering from depression.

Antidepressants enhance mood by boosting the actions of neurotransmitters, including norepinephrine, dopamine, and serotonin.

CORE CONCEPT 10.3

Antidepressants are medications that combat depression by enhancing mood. Depression is thought to be associated with an imbalance of neurotransmitters in certain regions of the brain. Although medication does not completely restore these chemical imbalances, it does help to reduce depressive symptoms while the patient develops effective means of coping. Remember that antidepressants are often used off-label to treat a greater variety of symptoms, including anxiety and restlessness (see Chapter 9); so, many areas of the CNS are potentially targeted by this drug class. Antidepressants may also be used in pain management.

Antidepressants work by increasing the action of specific neurotransmitters in the brain, mainly norepinephrine, dopamine, and serotonin (chemical name, 5-hydroxytryptamine [5-HT]). There are two major ways in which most antidepressants work: (1) by blocking the enzymatic breakdown of norepinephrine and dopamine, and (2) by slowing the reuptake of serotonin and/or norepinephrine. The primary classes of antidepressant drugs, also shown in Table 10.2 ◆, are as follows:

- Tricyclic antidepressants (TCAs)
- Selective serotonin reuptake inhibitors (SSRIs)
- Atypical antidepressants
- Monoamine oxidase inhibitors (MAOIs)

Concept Review   10.1

- What are the major causes of depression? Identify symptoms of major depressive disorder. What is the name used to describe drugs that treat depression?

Tricyclic Antidepressants

Tricyclic antidepressants (TCAs) are drugs named for their three-ring chemical structure. They were the mainstay of depression pharmacotherapy from the early 1960s until the 1980s and are still used.

tri = *three*
cyclic = *rings*

TCAs act by inhibiting the reuptake of both norepinephrine and serotonin into presynaptic nerve terminals, as shown in Figure 10.1 ■. TCAs are used mainly for major depressive disorder and occasionally for situational depression. Clomipramine (Anafranil) is approved for treatment of obsessive–compulsive disorder, and other TCAs are sometimes used as off-label treatments for panic attacks (see Chapter 9). One use for TCAs, not related to psychopharmacology, is to treat childhood enuresis (bed-wetting). The mechanism for this is not completely understood. One idea is that since TCAs have anticholinergic effects, they decrease bladder tone and therefore allow more time for the bladder to fill.

pre = *before*
post = *after*
synaptic = *the synapse*

enuresis = *urination*

ortho = *standing up*
static = *still*
hypo = *reduced*
tension = *blood pressure*

Although TCAs treat depressive symptoms, they have some unpleasant and serious adverse effects. The most common adverse effect is orthostatic hypotension (feeling dizzy when changing to an upright or standing position), which occurs due to vasoconstriction of blood vessels. Sedation is a frequently reported complaint at the beginning of therapy, but patients usually become tolerant to this effect after several weeks of treatment. Most TCAs have a long half-life, which increases the risk of adverse effects for patients with delayed excretion. Anticholinergic effects, such as dry mouth, constipation, urinary retention, blurred vision, and tachycardia, are common (see Chapter 8). Significant drug interactions can occur with CNS depressants, sympathomimetics, anticholinergics, and MAOIs. Since the discovery of newer antidepressants, TCAs are less frequently used as first-line drugs in the treatment of anxiety mixed with depression.

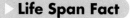 **Life Span Fact**

TCAs can cause heart block and other adverse cardiac effects. They must be used cautiously in older adults or those with cardiac disease.

TABLE 10.2 Antidepressants

Drug	Route and Adult Dose	Remarks
TRICYCLIC ANTIDEPRESSANTS (TCAs)		
amitriptyline (Elavil)	Adult: PO; 75–100 mg/day (may gradually increase to 150–300 mg/day); geriatric: PO; 10–25 mg at bedtime (may gradually increase to 25–150 mg/day)	For biological depression; inhibits gastric acid secretion by blocking histamine-2 receptors in the body
amoxapine (Asendin)	Adult: PO; begin with 100 mg/day, may increase on day 3 to 300 mg/day; geriatric: PO; 25 mg at bedtime, may increase every 3–7 days to 50–150 mg/day (max: 300 mg/day)	For situational and biological depression; not associated with cardiotoxicity; mild sedative
clomipramine (Anafranil)	PO; 75–300 mg/day in divided doses	For depression accompanying obsessive–compulsive disorder
desipramine (Norpramin)	PO; 75–100 mg/day, may increase to 150–300 mg/day	Active metabolite of imipramine
doxepin (Sinequan)	PO; 30–150 mg/day at bedtime, may gradually increase to 300 mg/day	For depression accompanying anxiety or alcohol dependence
ⓟ imipramine (Tofranil)	PO; 75–100 mg/day (max: 300 mg/day)	For biological depression or alcohol or cocaine dependence; may cause cardiac dysfunction and abnormal blood cell count; available IM; may control bed-wetting in children
maprotiline (Ludiomil)	Mild to moderate depression: PO; start at 75 mg/day and gradually increase every 2 weeks to 150 mg/day; severe depression: PO; start at 100–150 mg/day and gradually increase to 300 mg/day	For a broad range of depression from mild to severe
nortriptyline (Aventyl, Pamelor)	PO; 25 mg tid or qid; may increase to 100–150 mg/day	For biological depression; interactions similar to imipramine
protriptyline (Vivactil)	PO; 15–40 mg/day in three to four divided doses (max: 60 mg/day)	For symptoms of depression; few sedative qualities; causes increased heart rate
trimipramine (Surmontil)	PO; 75–100 mg/day (max: 300 mg/day)	For depression accompanied by a sleep disorder (has strong sedative effects)
SELECTIVE SEROTONIN REUPTAKE INHIBITORS (SSRIs)		
citalopram (Celexa)	PO; start at 20 mg/day (max: 40 mg/day)	Does not mimic the sympathetic response; has no acetylcholine blocking properties
escitalopram (Lexapro) (see page 113 for the Drug Prototype box)	PO; 10 mg daily, may increase to 20 mg after 1 week	May be used for generalized anxiety disorder
fluoxetine (Prozac)	PO; 20 mg/day in the a.m. (max: 80 mg/day)	May be used for obsessive–compulsive disorder and eating disorders
fluvoxamine (Luvox)	PO; start with 50 mg/day (max: 300 mg/day)	May be used for obsessive–compulsive disorder; no severe adverse cardiovascular effects; fewer acetylcholine blocking effects
paroxetine (Paxil, Pexeva)	Depression: PO; 10–50 mg/day (max: 80 mg/day); obsessive–compulsive disorder: PO; 20–60 mg/day; panic attacks: PO; 40 mg/day	May be used for obsessive–compulsive disorder and panic attacks
ⓟ sertraline (Zoloft)	Adult: PO; start with 50 mg/day, gradually increase every few weeks to a range of 50–200 mg; geriatric: start with 25 mg/day	Does not mimic sympathetic response; has no acetylcholine blocking properties
vilazodone (Viibryd)	Adult: PO; start with 10 mg/day for 7 days; follow with 20 mg once daily for an additional 7 days; increase to 40 mg once daily	For major depression; thought not to cause significant weight gain or decreased sexual desire
ATYPICAL ANTIDEPRESSANTS		
bupropion (Wellbutrin, Zyban)	PO; 75–100 mg tid (greater than 450 mg/day increases risk for adverse reactions)	For changing moods, schizoaffective disorders, and as an aid to quit smoking; increased risk for seizures; weaker blocker of serotonin and norepinephrine uptake
duloxetine (Cymbalta)	PO; 40–60 mg/day in one or two divided doses	For major depression, generalized anxiety disorder, neuropathic pain, chronic fatigue syndrome, stress urinary continence, and fibromyalgia

TABLE 10.2 Antidepressants *(continued)*

Drug	Route and Adult Dose	Remarks
mirtazapine (Remeron)	PO; 15 mg/day in a single dose at bedtime, may increase every 1–2 weeks (max: 45 mg/day)	Potent blocker of 5-HT$_2$ and 5-HT$_3$ receptor subtypes; blocks presynaptic alpha$_2$-receptors, enhancing norepinephrine release; use caution in patients with kidney or liver dysfunction
nefazodone	PO; 50–100 mg bid, may increase up to 300–600 mg/day	Minimal cardiovascular effects; fewer effects in blocking acetylcholine; less sedation; less sexual dysfunction compared to other antidepressants
trazodone (Oleptro)	PO; 150 mg/day, may increase by 50 mg/day every 3–4 days. (max: 400–600 mg/day for regular release and 375 mg/day for extended release)	Increases total sleep time; reduces night awakenings; has anxiolytic effects
venlafaxine (Effexor)	PO; start with 37.5 mg sustained release every day and increase to 75–225 mg sustained release per day	For major depression, situational depression, generalized anxiety disorder, neuropathic pain, and migraines
MONOAMINE OXIDASE INHIBITORS (MAOIs)		
isocarboxazid (Marplan)	PO; 10–30 mg/day (max: 30 mg/day)	May cause peripheral edema and high blood pressure; used in cases in which other approaches for treatment of depression are not successful
Pr phenelzine (Nardil)	PO; 15 mg tid (max: 90 mg/day)	May cause a hypertensive crisis or respiratory depression; use cautiously in patients with epilepsy or diabetes, or who are likely to abuse drugs and alcohol
selegiline (Emsam)	Transdermal patch; applied to dry, intact skin on the upper torso, upper thigh, or the outer surface of the upper arm once every 24 hours; the recommended starting dose and target dose is 6 mg/24 hours	Skin patch used to treat major depressive disorder. It is designed to deliver medication over a 24-hour period
tranylcypromine (Parnate)	PO; 30 mg/day (give 20 mg in a.m. and 10 mg in p.m.), may increase by 10 mg/day at 3-week intervals up to 60 mg/day	For severe depression in cases in which patients have not responded to other medications

FIGURE 10.1

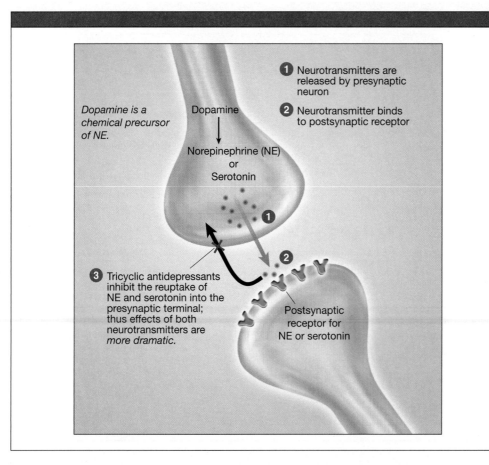

TCAs inhibit the reuptake of both norepinephrine and serotonin.

Selective Serotonin Reuptake Inhibitors

Selective serotonin reuptake inhibitors (SSRIs) are drugs that slow the reuptake of serotonin into presynaptic nerve terminals. They have become preferred drugs for the treatment of depression.

In the 1970s, it became increasingly clear that serotonin had a more substantial role in depression than once thought. Researchers knew that the TCAs altered the sensitivity of serotonin to certain receptors in the brain, but they did not know how this was connected with depression. Ongoing efforts to find antidepressants with fewer adverse effects led to the development of the SSRIs.

Serotonin (also called 5-HT) is a natural neurotransmitter in the CNS and is found in high concentrations in neurons of the hypothalamus, limbic system, medulla oblongata, and spinal cord. Serotonin is important to several body activities, including the cycling between nonrapid eye movement (NREM) and rapid eye movement (REM) sleep, pain perception, and emotional states (see Chapter 9). Lack of adequate serotonin in the CNS can lead to depression. Serotonin is metabolized to a less active substance by an enzyme located in presynaptic terminals called *monoamine oxidase (MAO)*. A second enzyme, *catecholamine O-methyl transferase (COMT)*, metabolizes serotonin in the synaptic cleft.

The TCAs inhibit the reuptake of both norepinephrine and serotonin into presynaptic nerve terminals. In contrast, the SSRIs are selective for just serotonin. Increased levels of serotonin in the synaptic cleft cause complex neurotransmitter changes in presynaptic and postsynaptic neurons in the brain. Presynaptic receptors become less sensitive, whereas postsynaptic receptors become more sensitive. This concept is illustrated in Figure 10.2 ■.

SSRIs have approximately the same efficacy at relieving depression as the MAO inhibitors and the tricyclics. The major advantage of the SSRIs, and the one that makes them first-line drugs, is their greater safety profile. Sympathomimetic effects (increased heart rate and hypertension) and anticholinergic effects (dry mouth, blurred vision, urinary retention, and constipation) are less common with this drug class. Sedation is also experienced less frequently and cardiotoxicity is not observed. All drugs in the SSRI class have equal efficacy and similar side effects. In general, SSRIs elicit a therapeutic response more quickly than TCAs.

One of the most common adverse effects of SSRIs relates to sexual dysfunction. Up to 70% of both men and women may experience decreased libido and lack of ability to reach orgasm. In men, delayed ejaculation and impotence may occur. For patients who are sexually active, these adverse effects may

mono = *one*
amine = *NH2 chemical formula*
oxidase = *water-forming enzyme (hydrogen reacts with oxygen)*

catecholamine = *sympathomimetic amine (dopamine, epinephrine, or norepinephrine)*

O-methyl transferase = *special CH₃ transferring enzyme (O = ortho position [chemical term])*

FIGURE 10.2

SSRIs selectively inhibit the reuptake of serotonin, causing complex changes in the presynaptic and postsynaptic neurons.

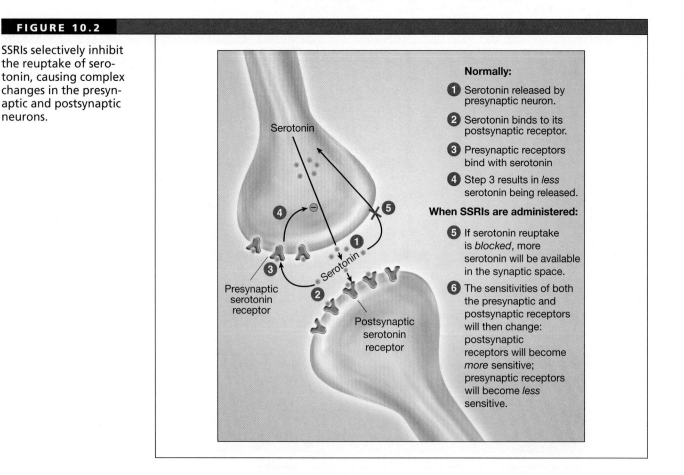

Normally:

1. Serotonin released by presynaptic neuron.
2. Serotonin binds to its postsynaptic receptor.
3. Presynaptic receptors bind with serotonin
4. Step 3 results in *less* serotonin being released.

When SSRIs are administered:

5. If serotonin reuptake is *blocked*, more serotonin will be available in the synaptic space.
6. The sensitivities of both the presynaptic and postsynaptic receptors will then change: postsynaptic receptors will become *more* sensitive; presynaptic receptors will become *less* sensitive.

Serotonin

Presynaptic serotonin receptor

Postsynaptic serotonin receptor

result in noncompliance with pharmacotherapy. Other common adverse effects of SSRIs include weight gain, nausea, headache, anxiety, and insomnia.

Serotonin syndrome (SES) is an adverse event that may occur when a patient is taking an SSRI and an additional medication that affects the metabolism, synthesis, or reuptake of serotonin. The result is that serotonin accumulates in the body. Symptoms can begin as early as two hours or as late as several weeks after taking the first dose. SES can be produced by the administration of an SSRI with an MAOI, a TCA, lithium, or a number of other medications. Symptoms of SES include mental status changes (confusion, anxiety, and restlessness), hypertension, tremors, sweating, fever, and lack of muscular coordination. Conservative treatment is to discontinue the SSRI and provide supportive care. In severe cases, mechanical ventilation and muscle relaxants may be necessary. If left untreated, death may occur.

Atypical Antidepressants

In terms of classification, the atypical antidepressants do not fit conveniently into the other antidepressant drug classes. Thus, "atypical" in this case really refers to the unique chemical structures represented in the group.

a = *not*
typical = *characteristic*

Duloxetine (Cymbalta) and venlafaxine (Effexor), sometimes considered to be in their own subgroup, are the **serotonin–norepinephrine reuptake inhibitors (SNRIs)**. They specifically inhibit the reabsorption of serotonin and norepinephrine and elevate mood by increasing the levels of these neurotransmitters in the CNS. In many cases, levels of dopamine are also affected with the SNRIs. In addition to being approved for the treatment of major depression, duloxetine (Cymbalta) is also approved for the treatment of generalized anxiety disorder and for neuropathic pain characteristic of fibromyalgia and diabetic neuropathy. Venlafaxine (Effexor), approved to treat depression and generalized anxiety disorder, is available in an intermediate-release form that requires two or three doses a day and an extended-release (XR) form that allows the patient to take the medication just once a day. Bupropion (Wellbutrin) not only inhibits the reuptake of serotonin but may also affect the activity of norepinephrine and dopamine. It should be used with caution in patients with seizure disorders because it lowers the seizure threshold. Bupropion is marketed as Zyban for use in cessation of smoking. Mirtazapine (Remeron) is used for depression and blocks presynaptic serotonin and norepinephrine receptors, thereby enhancing release of these neurotransmitters. Nefazodone is similar to Remeron. It was originally designed to treat depression, and causes minimal cardiovascular effects, fewer anticholinergic effects, less sedation, and less sexual dysfunction than the other antidepressants. Trazodone (Oleptro) is often used as a sleep aid, rather than as an antidepressant. The high levels of trazodone needed for the improvement of depression causes sedation in many patients.

Drug Prototype: Pr *Imipramine (Tofranil)*

Therapeutic Class: Antidepressant, treatment of nocturnal enuresis (bed-wetting) in children
Pharmacologic Class: Tricyclic antidepressant (TCA), serotonin and norepinephrine reuptake inhibitor (SNRI)

Actions and Uses: Imipramine blocks the reuptake of serotonin and norepinephrine into nerve terminals. It is mainly used for major depressive disorder, although it is occasionally used for the treatment of nocturnal enuresis in children. The nurse may find imipramine prescribed for a number of off-label uses, including intractable pain, anxiety disorders, and withdrawal syndromes from alcohol and cocaine.

Adverse Effects and Interactions: Adverse effects include sedation, drowsiness, blurred vision, dry mouth, and cardiovascular symptoms such as dysrhythmias, heart block, and extreme hypertension. Agents that mimic the action of norepinephrine or serotonin should be avoided because imipramine inhibits their metabolism and may produce toxicity. Some patients may experience photosensitivity. Concurrent use of other CNS depressants, including alcohol, may cause sedation. Cimetidine (Tagamet) may inhibit the metabolism of imipramine, leading to increased serum levels and possible toxicity. Clonidine may decrease its antihypertensive effects and increase risk for CNS depression. Use of oral contraceptives may increase or decrease imipramine levels. Disulfiram may lead to delirium and tachycardia.

Imipramine should be used with caution with herbal supplements, such as evening primrose oil or ginkgo biloba, which may lower the seizure threshold. St. John's wort used with imipramine may cause serotonin syndrome.

BLACK BOX WARNING:
Antidepressants can increase the risk of suicidal thinking and behavior, especially in children, adolescents, and young adults with major depressive disorder and other psychiatric disorders. This drug is not approved for use in pediatric patients.

Nursing Process Focus | Patients Receiving Antidepressant Therapy

ASSESSMENT	POTENTIAL NURSING DIAGNOSES
Prior to drug administration: ■ Obtain a complete health history including cardiovascular, thyroid, renal and liver conditions, allergies, drug history, likelihood of drug dependency, and possible drug interactions. ■ Evaluate laboratory blood findings: CBC, chemistry, clotting factors, glucose, renal and liver function studies. ■ Determine neurologic status, including history of mental previous disorders, seizure activity, level of consciousness (LOC), and identification of recent mood and behavior patterns. ■ Identify factors that may have precipitated the depressive episode and actions that have been previously tried to decrease symptoms.	■ *Ineffective Coping* related to inadequate level of confidence in ability to cope ■ *Risk for Injury* related to adverse effects of medications and depressive state ■ *Deficient Knowledge* related to a lack of information about drug therapy ■ *Noncompliance* related to length of time before medication reaches therapeutic levels and adverse effects of drug therapy ■ *Urinary Retention* related to adverse anticholinergic effects of drug

PLANNING: PATIENT GOALS AND EXPECTED OUTCOMES

The patient will:
■ Experience therapeutic effects (mood elevation and effectively engage in activities of daily living).
■ Be free from or experience minimal adverse effects from drug therapy.
■ Verbalize an understanding of the drug's use, adverse effects, and required precautions.

IMPLEMENTATION

Interventions and (Rationales)	Patient Teaching/Discharge Planning
■ Administer medication correctly and evaluate patient's knowledge of proper administration. (Proper administration helps to increase effectiveness of drugs and prevent severe adverse effects).	Instruct the patient to: ■ Take exactly as prescribed and use the same manufacturer's brand, if possible. ■ Take a missed dose as soon as it is noticed but do not take double or extra doses to catch up. ■ Take with food to decrease GI upset. ■ Not abruptly discontinue taking medication. ■ Practice reliable contraception and notify healthcare provider if pregnancy is planned or suspected.
■ Monitor vital signs, especially pulse and blood pressure. Notify healthcare provider if pulse or BP drop below approved parameters. (Tricyclic antidepressants may cause orthostatic hypotension.)	Instruct the patient to: ■ Report any change in sensorium, particularly impending syncope. ■ Avoid abrupt changes in position. ■ Monitor vital signs (especially blood pressure), ensuring proper use of home equipment. ■ Consult the healthcare provider regarding "reportable" blood pressure readings (e.g., lower than 80/50 mmHg).
■ Observe for serotonin syndrome in SSRI use: confusion, anxiety, restlessness, hypertension, tremors, diaphoresis, fever, lack of muscular coordination, and possibly death (usually occurs with concurrent use of St. John's wort or MAOIs). If suspected, discontinue the drug and initiate supportive care. Respond according to intensive care unit (ICU)/emergency department protocols.	Inform the patient: ■ That overdosage may result in serotonin syndrome, which can be life threatening. ■ To seek immediate medical attention for dizziness, headache, tremor, nausea/vomiting, anxiety, disorientation, lack of muscle coordination, sweating, and fever. ■ To seek medical attention if an increase in sweating is associated with nausea, vomiting, or chest pain.
■ Monitor cardiovascular status. Observe for hypertension and signs of impending stroke or MI and heart failure (CV symptoms may be a result of the sympathomimetic effects of MAOI and tricyclic antidepressants).	■ Instruct the patient to immediately report severe headache, dizziness, paresthesias, bradycardia, chest pain, tachycardia, nausea/vomiting, or diaphoresis.
■ Monitor neurologic status. Observe for somnolence and seizures. (Tricyclic antidepressants may cause somnolence related to CNS depression and may reduce the seizure threshold.)	Instruct the patient to: ■ Report any significant changes in neurologic status, such as seizures, extreme lethargy, slurred speech, disorientation, or ataxia to the healthcare provider, and to discontinue the drug. ■ Take the dose at bedtime to avoid daytime sedation.
■ Monitor mental and emotional status. Observe for suicidal ideation. (Therapeutic benefits may be delayed. Outpatients should have no more than a seven-day medication supply.) Also monitor for underlying or concomitant psychoses such as schizophrenia or bipolar disorders (may trigger manic states).	Instruct the patient: ■ To immediately report dysphoria or suicidal impulses ■ To commit to a "no-self harm" verbal contract ■ That it may take a couple of weeks before improvement is noticed, and about one month to achieve full therapeutic effect

continued . . .

NURSING PROCESS FOCUS   (continued)

▪ Monitor sleep–wake cycle. Observe for insomnia and/or daytime somnolence. (Sleep disturbances can be an effect of disease processes or use of certain antidepressants such as MAOIs.)	Instruct the patient to: ▪ Take the drug very early in the morning to promote normal timing of sleep onset. ▪ Avoid driving or potentially hazardous activities until the effects of the drug are known. ▪ Take at bedtime if daytime drowsiness persists. ▪ Take in the morning if insomnia persists.
▪ Monitor renal status and urinary output. (Medications may cause urinary retention due to muscle relaxation in the urinary tract. Imipramine is excreted through the kidneys. Fluoxetine is slowly metabolized and excreted, increasing the risk of organ damage.)	Instruct the patient to: ▪ Monitor fluid intake and output. ▪ Notify the healthcare provider of edema, dysuria (hesitancy, pain, diminished stream), changes in urine quantity or quality (e.g., cloudy, with sediment). ▪ Report fever or flank pain that may be indicative of a urinary tract infection related to urine retention.
▪ Use cautiously with elderly or young patients. (Diminished kidney and liver function related to aging can result in higher serum drug levels and may require lower doses. Children, due to an immature CNS, respond paradoxically to CNS-active drugs.)	Instruct the patient that: ▪ Elderly patients may be more prone to adverse effects such as hypertension and dysrhythmias. ▪ Children on imipramine for nocturnal enuresis may experience mood alterations.
▪ Monitor gastrointestinal status. Observe for abdominal distention. (Muscarinic blockade reduces tone and motility of intestinal smooth muscle and may cause paralytic ileus.)	Instruct the patient to: ▪ Exercise, drink adequate amounts of fluids, and add dietary fiber to promote stool passage. ▪ Consult the healthcare provider regarding a bulk laxative or stool softener if constipation becomes a problem.
▪ Continue to monitor laboratory studies, including CBC, clotting factors, and liver enzymes. Observe for signs and symptoms of liver toxicity. (Some antidressants may cause liver toxicity or cause gastrointestinal bleeding. Antidepressants need to be used cautiously with patients with a history of liver disease.)	Instruct the patient to: ▪ Report nausea, vomiting, diarrhea, rash, jaundice, epigastric or abdominal pain, tenderness, or change in color of stool to the healthcare provider. ▪ Adhere to laboratory testing regimen for blood tests and urinalysis as directed.
▪ Observe for signs of bleeding. (Imipramine may cause blood dyscrasias. Use with warfarin may increase bleeding time.)	▪ Instruct the patient to report excessive bruising, fatigue, pallor, shortness of breath, frank bleeding, and/or tarry stools to the healthcare provider. ▪ Conduct guaiac testing on stool for occult blood.
▪ Monitor for signs of dehydration. (Dehydration may cause lithium toxicity.)	▪ Inform the patient about the importance of staying well hydrated. ▪ Instruct the patient to report any nausea, emesis, diarrhea, weakness, lack of muscle coordination, confusion, lethargy, polyuria, or seizures (signs of lithium toxicity) to the healthcare provider.
▪ Monitor immune/metabolic status. Use with caution in patients with diabetes mellitus or hyperthyroidism. (If given in hyperthyroidism, this drug can cause agranulocytosis. Imipramine may either increase or decrease serum glucose. Fluoxetine may cause initial anorexia and weight loss, but prolonged therapy may result in weight gain of up to 20 pounds.)	Instruct the patient: ▪ With diabetes to monitor glucose level daily and to consult the nurse regarding reportable serum glucose levels. ▪ To monitor weight. Possible anorexia and weight loss will diminish with continued therapy.
▪ Observe for extrapyramidal and anticholinergic effects. In overdosage, 12 hours of anticholinergic activity is followed by CNS depression. Do not treat overdosage with quinidine, procainamide, atropine, or barbiturates. (Quinidine and procainamide can increase the possibility of dysrhythmia; atropine can lead to severe anticholinergic effects; and barbiturates can lead to excess sedation.)	Instruct the patient to: ▪ Immediately report any involuntary muscle movement of the face or upper body (e.g., tongue spasms), fever, anuria, lower abdominal pain, anxiety, hallucinations, psychomotor agitation, visual changes, dry mouth, and difficulty swallowing to the healthcare provider. ▪ Relieve dry mouth with (sugar-free) hard candies, by chewing gum, and by drinking fluids. ▪ Avoid alcohol-containing mouthwashes, which can further dry oral mucous membranes.
▪ Monitor visual acuity. Use with caution in narrow-angle glaucoma. (Imipramine may cause an increase in intraocular pressure. Anticholinergic effects may produce blurred vision.)	Instruct the patient to: ▪ Report any visual changes, headache, or eye pain to the healthcare provider. ▪ Inform an eye care professional of imipramine therapy.
▪ Ensure patient safety. (Dizziness caused by postural hypotension increases the risk of fall injuries.)	Instruct the patient to: ▪ Call for assistance before getting out of bed or attempting to ambulate alone. ▪ Avoid driving or performing hazardous activities until blood pressure is stabilized and effects of the drug are known.

EVALUATION OF OUTCOME CRITERIA

Evaluate the effectiveness of drug therapy by confirming that patient goals and expected outcomes have been met (see "Planning"). *See Table 10.2 for a list of drugs to which these nursing actions apply.*

Monoamine Oxidase Inhibitors

As discussed, the action of norepinephrine at adrenergic synapses is terminated through two means: (1) reuptake into the presynaptic nerve and (2) enzymatic destruction by the enzyme MAO. By decreasing the effectiveness of the enzyme MAO, **monoamine oxidase inhibitors (MAOIs)** limit the breakdown of norepinephrine, dopamine, and serotonin in the CNS. This creates higher levels of these neurotransmitters in the brain to facilitate neurotransmission and to alleviate the symptoms of depression (Figure 10.3 ■),

In the 1950s, the MAOIs were the first drugs approved to treat depression. They are just as effective as the TCAs and SSRIs in treating depression. However, because of drug–drug and food–drug interactions, hepatotoxicity, and the development of safer antidepressants, MAOIs are now reserved for patients who are not responsive to the other antidepressant classes.

Common adverse effects of the MAOIs include orthostatic hypotension, headache, insomnia, and diarrhea. A primary concern is that these agents interact with a large number of foods and other medications, sometimes with serious effects. A hypertensive crisis can occur when a MAOI is used together with other antidepressants or sympathomimetic drugs. Combining an MAOI with an SSRI can produce SES. If given with antihypertensives, the patient can experience excessive hypotension. MAOIs also increase the hypoglycemic effects of insulin and oral antidiabetic drugs. Extreme fever is known to occur in patients taking MAOIs with meperidine (Demerol), dextromethorphan (Pedia Care and others), and TCAs.

A hypertensive crisis can also result from an interaction between MAOIs and foods containing tyramine, a form of the amino acid tyrosine. In fact, tyrosine is a precursor to norepinephrine in the nervous system. In many respects, tyramine resembles norepinephrine. Tyramine is usually degraded by MAO in the intestines. If a patient is taking MAOIs, however, tyramine enters the bloodstream in high amounts and displaces norepinephrine in presynaptic nerve terminals. The result is a sudden increase in norepinephrine, causing acute hypertension. Symptoms usually occur within minutes of ingesting the food and include occipital headache, stiff neck, flushing, palpitations, profuse sweating, and nausea. Calcium channel blockers may be given as an antidote to reduce blood pressure. Examples of foods containing tyramine include smoked or pickled meats, most cheeses, yogurt, soy sauce, yeast, avocados, chocolate, pineapple and alcoholic beverages.

pre = before
menstrual = menstruation

FIGURE 10.3

MAOIs inhibit monoamine oxidase, an enzyme that stops the actions of neurotransmitters such as dopamine, norepinephrine, and serotonin.

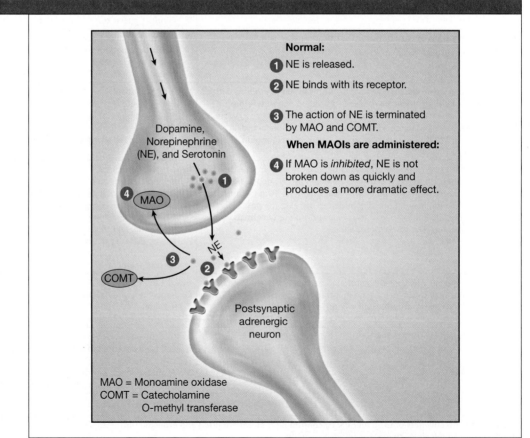

Normal:

1 NE is released.

2 NE binds with its receptor.

3 The action of NE is terminated by MAO and COMT.

When MAOIs are administered:

4 If MAO is *inhibited*, NE is not broken down as quickly and produces a more dramatic effect.

Dopamine, Norepinephrine (NE), and Serotonin

MAO

COMT

NE

Postsynaptic adrenergic neuron

MAO = Monoamine oxidase
COMT = Catecholamine
          O-methyl transferase

Drug Prototype: Pr *sertraline (Zoloft)*

Therapeutic Class: **Antidepressant**   Pharmacologic Class: **Selective serotonin reuptake inhibitor (SSRI)**

Actions and Uses: Sertraline is used for the treatment of depression, anxiety, obsessive–compulsive disorder, and panic. The antidepressant and anxiolytic properties of this drug can be attributed to its ability to inhibit the reuptake of serotonin in the brain. Other uses include premenstrual dysphoric disorder, posttraumatic stress disorder, and social anxiety disorder. Therapeutic actions include enhancement of mood and improvement of affect with maximum effects observed after several weeks.

Adverse Effects and Interactions: Adverse effects include agitation, insomnia, headache, dizziness, somnolence, and fatigue. Take extreme precautions in patients with cardiac disease, hepatic impairment, seizure disorders, suicidal ideation, mania, or hypomania. Concomitant use of sertraline and MAOIs or primozide is not advised. Antabuse should be avoided because of the alcohol content of the drug concentrate. Highly protein-bound medications such as digoxin and warfarin should be avoided due to risk of toxicity and increased blood concentrations leading to increased bleeding. MAOIs may cause neuroleptic malignant syndrome, extreme hypertension, and serotonin syndrome, characterized by headache, agitation, dizziness, fever, diarrhea, sweating, and shivering. Use cautiously with other centrally acting drugs to avoid adverse CNS effects. Patients should use caution if taking St. John's wort or L-tryptophan to avoid serotonin syndrome.

> **BLACK BOX WARNING:**
> Antidepressants can increase the risk of suicidal thinking and behavior, especially in children, adolescents, and young adults with major depressive disorder and other psychiatric disorders.

Concept Review 10.2

- Name the major classes of antidepressants. Name representative drugs within each class, and describe how each drug works pharmacologically.

Drug Prototype: Pr *Phenelzine (Nardil)*

Therapeutic Class: **Antidepressant**   Pharmacologic Class: **Monoamine oxidase inhibitor (MAOI)**

Actions and Uses: Phenelzine produces its effects by irreversible inhibition of MAO; therefore, it intensifies the effects of norepinephrine in adrenergic synapses. It is used to manage symptoms of depression not responsive to other types of pharmacotherapy, and it is occasionally used for panic disorder. Drug effects may continue for two to three weeks after therapy is discontinued.

Adverse Effects and Interactions: Common adverse effects are constipation, dry mouth, orthostatic hypotension, insomnia, nausea, and loss of appetite. It may increase heart rate and neural activity, leading to delirium, mania, anxiety, and convulsions. Severe hypertension may occur when ingesting foods containing tyramine. Seizures, respiratory depression, circulatory collapse, and coma may occur in cases of severe overdose. Many other drugs affect the action of phenelzine. Use with TCAs and SSRIs should be avoided, because the combination can cause temperature elevation and seizures. Opiates, including meperidine, should be avoided due to increased risk of respiratory failure or hypertensive crisis.

Phenelzine should be used with caution with herbal supplements such as ginseng, which could cause headache, tremors, mania, insomnia, irritability, and visual hallucinations. Concurrent use of ephedra could cause hypertensive crisis.

> **BLACK BOX WARNING:**
> Antidepressants can increase the risk of suicidal thinking and behavior, especially in children, adolescents, and young adults with major depressive disorder and other psychiatric disorders.

BIPOLAR DISORDER

Bipolar disorder is characterized by extreme and opposite moods. Patients may display signs of euphoria and depression or feelings of excitement and calm.

bi = *two*
polar = *extremes*

Patients with bipolar disorder may experience emotions ranging from depression to extreme agitation.

Once known as *manic depression*, bipolar disorder is characterized by extreme and opposite moods, such as euphoria and depression. Although the moods of patients may shift between extremes, usually patients will remain in one state for awhile, or they may remain in a normal state for prolonged times.

dys = *difficulty (as in illness)*
phoric = *bearing*

mania = *excessively intense or excited mood*

Depressed and slightly depressed or *dysphoric* signs and symptoms are the same as those described earlier in this chapter. Patients with bipolar disorder also display signs of *mania*, an emotional state characterized by high psychomotor activity and irritability. Symptoms of mania are shown in the following list; these are generally the opposite of depressive symptoms.

- Insomnia
- Activity for days without rest and without appearing tired
- Easy agitation and aggression
- Feelings of exaggerated confidence
- Making choices without regard for a long-term plan or consequences of action
- Attention seeking
- Unusual interest in sex
- Drug abuse, including alcohol, cocaine, or sleeping medications
- Denial that the behavior is a problem

Concept Review 10.3

- Identify the symptoms of mania. How do manic symptoms generally compare with depressive symptoms?

Mood stabilization in patients with bipolar disorder is accomplished with lithium and other drugs.

anti = *against*
psychotic = *psychosis, mental state*

seizure = *to take hold*

Drugs for bipolar disorder are called **mood stabilizers** because they have the ability to moderate extreme shifts in emotions between mania and depression. Currently, lithium, antiseizure drugs, and atypical antipsychotic drugs are the choices used for mood stabilization in patients with bipolar disorder. Table 10.3 ◆ lists selected drugs used to treat bipolar disorder.

For years, the traditional treatment of bipolar disorder has been lithium (Eskalith), which was used as monotherapy or in combination with other drugs. Lithium was approved in the United States in 1970. With lithium, serum levels must be checked every one to three days when beginning therapy, and every two to three months thereafter. To ensure therapeutic action, concentrations of lithium in the blood must remain within the range of 0.6 to 1.5 mEq/L. Close monitoring encourages compliance and helps to avoid toxicity. Lithium is taken as a salt, so it mixes in the bloodstream like sodium chloride.

CAM THERAPY

St. John's Wort for Depression

One of the most popular herbs in the United States, St. John's wort (*Hypericum perforatum*) grows throughout Asia, Europe, and North America. Its modern use is as an antidepressant. It gets its name from a legend that red spots once appeared on its leaves on the anniversary of the beheading of St. John the Baptist. The word wort is a British term for "plant."

Research suggests that substances found in St. John's wort selectively inhibit serotonin reuptake in certain brain neurons. A number of clinical studies suggest that St. John's wort is an effective treatment for mild to moderate depression, and that it may be just as effective as TCAs and SSRIs. Recent analyses also suggest that the herb may be effective for major depression and that it causes fewer adverse effects than traditional drugs. St. John's wort may interact with many medications, including oral contraceptives, warfarin, digoxin, and cyclosporine. It should not be taken concurrently with antidepressant medications.

St. John's wort is well tolerated, producing mild adverse effects such as gastrointestinal (GI) distress, fatigue, and allergic skin reactions. The herb contains compounds that photosensitize the skin; thus patients should be advised to apply sunscreen or to wear protective clothing when outdoors.

TABLE 10.3 Drugs for Bipolar Disorder: Mood Stabilizers

Drug	Route and Adult Dose	Remarks
lithium (Eskalith)	PO; initial 600 mg tid, maintenance 300 mg tid (max: 2.4 g/day)	For treatment of mania and depressive symptoms; must be used cautiously in epilepsy and in psychosis
ANTISEIZURE DRUGS		
carbamazepine (Tegretol)	PO; 200 mg bid, gradually increased to 800–1200 mg/day in three to four divided doses	For treatment of manic depressive and schizoaffective symptoms; used as antiseizure medication
lamotrigine (Lamictal)	PO; 50 mg/day for 2 weeks, then 50 mg bid for 2 weeks; may increase gradually up to 300–500 mg/day in two divided doses (max: 700 mg/day)	Used as antiseizure medication; fatal rash has been reported in children less than 16 years old
valproate/valproic acid (Depakene, Depakote) (see page 191 for the Drug Prototype box)	PO; 250 mg tid (max: 60 mg/kg/day)	For treatment of mania and prevention of migraine headache; used as antiseizure medication
ATYPICAL ANTIPSYCHOTIC DRUGS		
aripiprazole (Abilify)	PO; 10–15 mg/day (max: 30 mg/day)	For add-on treatment in adults with major depression; for mania or mixed episodes of bipolar disorder; for schizophrenia; for irritability associated with autistic disorder in pediatric patients
asenapine (Saphris)	Adult: 10 mg sublingually twice daily (monotherapy); 5 mg sublingually twice daily (adjunct to lithium or valproic acid therapy)	For the acute treatment of mania or mixed episodes associated with bipolar disorder in adults; taken alone or with a mood stabilizer (lithium or valproate)
olanzapine (Zyprexa)	Adult: PO; start with 5–10 mg/day; may increase by 2.5–5 mg every week (range 10–15 mg/day; max: 20 mg/day). Geriatric: PO; start with 5 mg/day	For schizophrenia and manic episodes of bipolar disorder
quetiapine (Seroquel)	PO; start with 25 mg bid; may increase to a target dose of 300–400 mg/day in divided doses	Approved as a once-daily monotherapy for the acute treatment of the depressive episodes associated with bipolar disorder
risperidone (Risperdal) (see page 152 for the Drug Prototype box)	PO; 1–6 mg bid; increase by 2 mg daily to an initial target dose of 6 mg/day	For symptoms of schizophrenia; for episodes of mania or mixed episodes of bipolar disorder; for behavior problems such as aggression, self-injury, and sudden mood changes in teenagers and children with autism
ziprasidone (Geodon)	PO; 20 mg bid (max: 80 mg bid)	For acute mania or mixed episodes associated with bipolar disorder; for maintenance treatment of bipolar disorder when added to lithium or valproate; for schizophrenia

Therefore, conditions in which sodium is lost (e.g., excessive sweating or increased urination which leads to dehydration) can cause the kidneys to reabsorb the lithium salts back into the blood, producing elevated serum levels of lithium known as lithium toxicity. Lithium overdose may be treated with hemodialysis and supportive care.

For the most complete control of bipolar disorder, it is not unusual for other drugs to be used in combination with lithium. During the depressed stage, a TCA or an atypical antidepressant such as bupropion (Wellbutrin) may be necessary. During manic phases, a benzodiazepine will moderate manic symptoms (see Chapter 9). In cases of extreme agitation, delusions, or hallucinations, antipsychotic drugs may be indicated (see Chapter 11). Continued patient compliance is essential to achieving successful pharmacotherapy because some patients do not perceive their condition as abnormal.

Today, antiseizure drugs (see Chapter 13) and atypical **antipsychotic drugs** (see Chapter 11) have emerged as probably the most effective agents for mood stabilization. For example, valproic acid (Depakene, Depakote), carbamazepine (Tegretol), and lamotrigine (Lamictal) are the antiseizure drugs most often used in the treatment of rapidly cycling and mixed states of bipolar disorder. Several atypical antipsychotics are very effective for the treatment of extreme mania. Important antipsychotic drugs for bipolar disorder are aripiprazole (Abilify), asenapine (Saphris), olanzapine (Zyprexa), quetiapine (Seroquel), risperidone (Risperdal), and ziprasidone (Geodon). Longer term stabilization of extreme and unusual behaviors with atypical antipsychotics is covered in Chapter 11. Lithium has remained effective for purely manic or purely depressive states.

Concept Review 10.4

■ Give the general name of drugs used to treat bipolar disorder. What has been the main drug used to treat bipolar disorder, and how does it work pharmacologically? What other drugs treat bipolar disorder?

ATTENTION DEFICIT HYPERACTIVITY DISORDER

A condition characterized by poor attention span, behavior control issues, and/or hyperactivity is called **attention deficit hyperactivity disorder (ADHD)**. Although the condition has most often been diagnosed in childhood, symptoms of ADHD may extend into adulthood, and an increasing number of adults are being evaluated for ADHD.

CORE CONCEPT 10.6

Attention deficit hyperactivity disorder presents challenges for children and adults.

ADHD is characterized by developmentally inappropriate behaviors involving difficulty in paying attention or focusing on tasks. ADHD may be diagnosed when a child's hyperactive behaviors significantly interfere with normal play, sleep, or learning activities. Hyperactive children usually have increased motor activity shown by a tendency to be fidgety and impulsive and to interrupt and talk excessively during their developmental years; therefore, they may not be able to interact with others appropriately at home or school. In boys, the activity levels are usually more overt. Girls show less aggression and impulsiveness but may show more anxiety, mood swings, social withdrawal, and cognitive and language delays. Girls also tend to be older at the time of diagnosis, so problems and setbacks related to the disorder exist for a longer time before treatment interventions are undertaken. Symptoms of ADHD are shown in the following list:

- Easy distractability
- Failure to receive or follow instructions properly
- Inability to focus on one task at a time and tendency to jump from one activity to another
- Difficulty remembering
- Frequent loss or misplacing of personal items
- Excessive talking and interrupting other children in a group
- Inability to sit still when asked repeatedly
- Impulsiveness
- Sleep disturbances

Most children with ADHD have associated challenges. Many find it difficult to concentrate on tasks assigned in school. Even if they are gifted, their grades may suffer because they have difficulty following a conventional routine; discipline may also be a problem. Teachers are often the first to suggest that a child should be examined for ADHD and receive medication when behaviors in the classroom escalate to the point of interfering with learning. A diagnosis is based on psychological and medical evaluations.

Fast Facts ADHD

- ADHD is the major reason why children are referred for mental health treatment.
- About 50% of children are also diagnosed with oppositional defiant or conduct disorder.
- Anxiety disorder is diagnosed in 25% of children.
- About one-third are also diagnosed with depression.
- Learning disabilities are present in about 20% of children.

The cause of ADHD is not clear. Evidence suggests that hyperactivity may be related to a deficit or dysfunction of dopamine, norepinephrine, and serotonin in the reticular activating system of the brain (see Chapter 9). ADHD was once thought to be caused by sugar, chocolate, high-carbohydrate foods and beverages, and certain food additives, but these have been disproved as causing or aggravating ADHD.

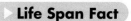

One-third to one-half of children diagnosed with ADHD also experience symptoms of attention dysfunction in their adult years. Symptoms of **attention deficit disorder (ADD)** in adults appear similar to those of mood disorders and include anxiety, mania, restlessness, and depression, which can also cause difficulties in interpersonal relationships. Attention dysfunction in adults is often linked with poor self-esteem, diminished social success, and introverted behaviors. Patients may have mood swings similar to bipolar disorder.

> **▶ Life Span Fact**
>
> ADHD affects as many as 5% of all children. Most children diagnosed with this condition are between the ages of three and seven years, and boys are four to eight times more likely to be diagnosed than girls.

Central nervous system (CNS) stimulants have been the main course of treatment for ADHD.

CORE CONCEPT 10.7

Traditional therapies for ADHD include CNS stimulants. Newer therapies have added non-CNS stimulants.

CNS Stimulants

These drugs stimulate specific areas of the CNS that heighten alertness and increase focus. In 2002, a non-CNS stimulant was first approved to treat ADHD. Agents for treating ADHD are listed in Table 10.4 ◆.

Stimulants reverse many of the symptoms and help patients to focus on tasks. The most widely prescribed drug for ADHD is methylphenidate (Ritalin). Other less prescribed CNS stimulants include d- and l-amphetamine racemic mixtures (Adderall), dextroamphetamine (Dexedrine), or methamphetamine (Desoxyn). More recently, extended release forms have been made available: dextroamphetamine mixture (Adderall XR), dexmethylphenidate (Focalin XR), and slow-releasing methylphenidate (Ritalin, LA/SR). Lisdexamfetamine (Vyvanse) is a psychostimulant prodrug of phenethylamine and amphetamine. It is a once-daily prescription medication thought to help increase attention and decrease impulsiveness and hyperactivity in patients with ADHD.

Patients taking CNS stimulants must be carefully monitored because the drugs may cause paradoxical hyperactivity. Adverse reactions include insomnia, nervousness, anorexia, and weight loss. Occasionally, a patient may suffer from dizziness, depression, irritability, nausea, or abdominal pain. These drugs are Schedule II controlled substances and pregnancy category C.

Non-CNS Stimulants

Non-CNS stimulants are now approved for treatment of ADHD. This is an advantage because they have no abuse potential. A fairly recent addition (2002) to the treatment of ADHD in children and adults is atomoxetine (Strattera). Although its exact mechanism is not known, it is classified as a norepinephrine reuptake inhibitor. Efficacy appears to be equivalent to methylphenidate (Ritalin). Patients on atomoxetine have demonstrated an improved ability to focus on tasks and reduced hyperactivity. Common adverse effects include headache, insomnia, upper abdominal pain, decreased appetite, and cough. Unlike methylphenidate,

Drug Prototype: ℞ *Methylphenidate (Ritalin)*

Therapeutic Class: Drug for attention deficit hyperactivity disorder, narcolepsy drug
Pharmacologic Class: Central nervous system stimulant, norepinephrine and dopamine releasing agent

Actions and Uses: Methylphenidate activates the reticular activating system, causing heightened alertness in various regions of the brain, particularly those centers associated with focus and attention. Activation is partially achieved by the release of neurotransmitters such as norepinephrine, dopamine, and serotonin. Impulsiveness, hyperactivity, and disruptive behavior are usually reduced within a few weeks. These changes promote improved psychosocial interactions and academic performance.

Adverse Effects and Interactions: In a patient with no ADHD, methylphenidate causes nervousness and insomnia. All patients are at risk for irregular heartbeat, high blood pressure, and liver toxicity. Methylphenidate is a Schedule II drug, indicating its potential to cause dependence when used for extended periods. Periodic drug-free "holidays" are recommended to reduce drug dependence and to assess the patient's condition.

Methylphenidate interacts with many drugs. For example, it may decrease the effectiveness of anticonvulsants, anticoagulants, and guanethidine. Use with clonidine may increase adverse effects. Antihypertensives or other CNS stimulants could increase the vasoconstrictive action of methylphenidate. MAOIs may produce hypertensive crisis.

> **BLACK BOX WARNING:**
> Methylphenidate is a Schedule II drug with high abuse potential. Administration for longer periods of time may lead to drug dependence. Misuse may cause sudden death or a serious cardiovascular adverse event.

TABLE 10.4 Drugs for Attention Deficit–Hyperactivity Disorder

Drug	Route and Adult Dose	Remarks
CNS STIMULANTS		
amphetamine (Adderall, Adderall-XR)	3–5 years old: PO; 2.5 mg one to two times/day, may increase by 2.5 mg at weekly intervals 6 years old: PO; 5 mg daily to bid, may increase by 5 mg at weekly intervals (max: 40 mg/day); Adult: 10 mg extended release, once daily (max: 30 mg/day)	May be used for daytime sleep disorder (narcolepsy); high potential for abuse
dexmethylphenidate (Focalin, Focalin-XR)	6 years old to adult: PO; 2.5 mg bid, may increase by 2.5–5 mg/week (max: 20 mg/day); 5 mg/day extended release may increase by 5 mg/week	Mild stimulant to the central nervous system; used to treat ADHD
dextroamphetamine (Dexedrine)	3–5 years old: PO; 2.5 mg daily to bid, may increase by 2.5 mg at weekly intervals; 6 years old: PO; 5 mg daily to bid, increase by 5 mg at weekly intervals (max: 40 mg/day)	Potent appetite suppressant; should only be used for short-term treatment of ADHD; safety in children less than 3 years old has not been established
lisdexamfetamine (Vyvanse)	6 years old to adult: PO: 20–70 mg once daily in a.m. (max: 70 mg/day); doses vary depending on age	Once-daily prescription medication for children, teens, and adults with ADHD; prodrug of dextroamphetamine
methamphetamine (Desoxyn)	6 years old: PO; 2.5–5 mg daily to bid, may increase by 5 mg at weekly intervals (max: 20–25 mg/day)	Abuse potential high in adults
ⓟ methylphenidate (Concerta, Daytrana, Metadate, Methylin, Ritalin, Quillivant XR)	6 years old: PO; 5–10 mg before breakfast and lunch, with gradual increase of 5–10 mg/week as needed (max: 60 mg/day) Adult: PO; 5–20 mg (prompt-release tablets) two to three times daily; may switch to extended release once the maintenance dose is determined; doses will vary depending on drug formulation	Most widely used drug for patients with ADHD; more dramatic effect on attention deficit than for hyperactivity; may be used for daytime sleep disorder (narcolepsy); once-daily extended release liquid form available
NONSTIMULANTS		
atomoxetine (Strattera)	Children less than 70 kg: PO; start with 0.5 mg/kg/day; may increase after 3 days to target dose of 1.2 mg/kg/day (max dose: 1.4 mg/kg/day or 100 mg) Adult: PO; start with 40 mg in a.m., may increase after 3 days to target dose of 80 mg/day given either once in the morning, divided morning, or late afternoon/early evening; may increase to max of 100 mg/day if needed	Inhibits reuptake of norepinephrine; safety and efficacy in children less than 6 years old has not been established
clonidine (Kapvay)	6 years old to 17 years old: PO; Start with 0.1 mg/day and gradually increase to desired response (max: 0.4 mg/day)	Sometimes prescribed when patients are extremely aggressive, active, or have difficulty sleeping; stimulates alpha$_2$-receptors in the brain; once-daily dosing provided; intermediate-releasing form and extended-release form available
guanfacine (Intuniv)	6 years old to 17 years old: PO; Start with 1 mg/day and gradually increase to desired response (max: 4 mg/day)	Treats high blood pressure; also used alone or together with other medicines to treat attention deficit hyperactivity disorder (ADHD)

it is not a scheduled drug; thus, parents who are hesitant to place their child on stimulants have a reasonable alternative.

Clonidine (Kapvay) is sometimes prescribed when patients are extremely aggressive or active or have difficulty falling asleep. Clonidine improves clinical symptoms of ADHD and is a centrally acting alpha$_2$-adrenergic drug. The extended release tablet offers the advantage of once-daily dosing. Blood pressure should be monitored during therapy due to hypotensive effects caused by clonidine.

Guanfacine (Intuniv) was approved in 2011, for use in combination therapy with stimulants. Because the drug is a known antihypertensive, blood pressure should always be monitored during therapy. Sedation is common especially at the initiation of drug therapy.

Concept Review   10.5

■ What are the symptoms experienced by patients with ADHD? Which drug is most often used in the treatment of these symptoms? What are the common symptoms experienced by adults with ADD?

PATIENTS NEED TO KNOW

Patients taking antidepressants need to know the following:

In General

1. Avoid driving or operating machinery until response to the medication is known. Its sedating effects can increase the risk for accidental injury.
2. Do not stop taking the medication without consulting your healthcare provider.
3. Antidepressants may take one to four weeks to become fully effective.

Regarding Tricyclics

4. Tricyclics may increase appetite, cause dizziness upon rapid change of position, and be sedating. Report dry mouth, constipation, urinary retention, increase in heart rate and palpitations, or blurred vision if they occur.
5. Avoid the use of alcohol; it increases sedative effects.

Regarding MAOIs

6. MAOIs may cause problems with sleep, agitation, dizziness when rapidly changing position, and dangerous interactions with other medications. Eating foods high in tyramine can cause a hypertensive crisis. Such foods include aged cheeses, wine, luncheon meats, and sausages.
7. Report any of the following adverse effects to your healthcare provider: increased heart rate or lightheadedness when changing positions.
8. Monitor weight; an increase or a decrease may occur.
9. A decrease in sexual interest or performance may occur. If this does, discuss a change in medication with your healthcare provider.

Regarding SSRIs

10. SSRIs may cause GI upset, dizziness, skin rash, and headache. Report these signs and symptoms to your healthcare provider.
11. Avoid foods containing large amounts of tryptophan, such as cottage cheese, poultry, peanuts, and sesame seeds.
12. Do not combine MAOIs and SSRIs. Do not take St. John's wort with any antidepressant. These combinations, such as confusion, mania, headache, respiratory problems, kidney failure, and possibly death, can cause serious adverse effects, termed SES.
13. If insomnia is a problem, take the medication in the morning.
14. If nausea is a problem, take the medication with food, unless otherwise instructed.

For Attention Deficit Hyperactivity Disorder (ADHD)

15. Many drugs used for the treatment of ADHD are controlled substances.
16. Dependence may occur due to the high abuse potential of CNS stimulants.
17. CNS stimulants often increase blood pressure. Nonstimulants may reduce blood pressure. Monitor blood pressure closely.
18. Take drugs at least six hours before bedtime to avoid insomnia.
19. Avoid giving drinks containing caffeine to children who are seizure prone and those with diabetes. (CNS stimulants lower the threshold in patients with seizure disorders and alter insulin needs in patients with diabetes.)
20. Monitor height and weight in children with prolonged therapy.
21. Take drugs after meals to reduce appetite-suppressive effects.
22. Do not take these medications for the purpose of combating fatigue.
23. Even though atomoxetine (Strattera) is a nonstimulant ADHD medication, it still has many of the adverse effects of the other ADHD medications.

CHAPTER REVIEW

CORE CONCEPTS SUMMARY

10.1 People suffer from depression for many reasons.

The two major categories of mood disorders are depression and bipolar disorder. Depression may involve both situational and biological causes. The recognition of depression is a collaborative effort among healthcare providers. A third emotional disorder is attention deficit–hyperactivity disorder.

10.2 For best results, treatment of severe depression requires both medication and psychotherapy.

After a health examination is performed to rule out physical causes of depression, a psychological evaluation may be performed. Patients diagnosed with a major depressive disorder have at least five symptoms of recognized depression. Treatment may include medication in addition to a number of other approaches, including counseling and behavioral therapy, short-term psychotherapies, interpersonal therapy, psychodynamic therapies, and in extreme cases, electroconvulsive therapy (ECT) and repetitive transcranial magnetic stimulation (rTMS). Most therapeutic approaches involve a long-term commitment from patients, healthcare providers, and family.

10.3 Antidepressants enhance mood by boosting the actions of neurotransmitters, including norepinephrine, dopamine, and serotonin.

Drugs for depression are called antidepressants. The major classes of antidepressants are tricyclic antidepressants (TCAs), selective serotonin reuptake inhibitors (SSRIs), atypical antidepressants, and monoamine oxidase inhibitors (MAOIs). All drug classes work mainly by increasing the amount of norepinephrine, serotonin, and possibly other neurotransmitters in the nerve synapse and thereby intensifying neurotransmitter action and enhancing mood.

10.4 Patients with bipolar disorder may experience emotions ranging from depression to extreme agitation.

Bipolar disorder is characterized by sometimes extreme and opposite moods, such as depression and euphoria. During the depressive stages, patients express signs of major depression. Patients may then change to signs of mania or high psychomotor activity and irritability.

10.5 Mood stabilization in patients with bipolar disorder is accomplished with lithium and other drugs.

Drugs for bipolar disorder are called mood stabilizers. Lithium (Eskalith) may be used alone or in combination with other drugs, including antidepressants and antianxiety agents. Antiseizure drugs and atypical antipsychotic drugs have emerged as more effective drug treatments for bipolar disorder. Drugs are selective for extreme mania, extreme depression, or cycling of mood that occurs between extreme emotional states.

10.6 Attention deficit hyperactivity disorder (ADHD) presents challenges for children and adults.

ADHD is a condition characterized by poor attention span, behavior control issues, and/or hyperactivity. ADHD is normally diagnosed in childhood, although one-third to one-half of children with symptoms of attention deficit experience them into adulthood. As adults, patients with ADD have symptoms similar to mood disorders.

10.7 Central nervous system (CNS) stimulants have been the main course of treatment for ADHD.

The traditional drugs used to treat attention deficit in children have been the CNS stimulants. Patients taking CNS stimulants must be carefully monitored to avoid adverse reactions. Recently, non-CNS stimulants, including the new drug atomoxetine (Strattera), have been used as a reasonable alternative to existing Schedule II controlled substances.

REVIEW QUESTIONS

The following questions are written in NCLEX-PN® style. Answer these questions to assess your knowledge of the chapter material, and go back and review any material that is not clear to you.

1. Patient education for the patient started on an SSRI would include:

1. The avoidance of tyramine-containing foods
2. The signs and symptoms of hypertension crisis
3. That tremors are a common adverse effect
4. That sexual dysfunction is one of the most common adverse effects

2. A patient is taking an MAOI for depression. In planning care for this patient, the nurse knows that a hypertensive crisis may be possible and plans on having what drug on hand as an antidote?

1. Meperidine (Demerol)
2. Dextromethorphan
3. Calcium channel blockers
4. Carbamazepine (Tegretol)

3. The nurse informs the patient to remain well hydrated while taking lithium because dehydration can lead to:

1. Lower serum lithium levels
2. Increased effectiveness
3. The need to increase the lithium dosage
4. Lithium toxicity

4. The patient on methylphenidate (Ritalin) should be monitored for:

1. Signs of weight loss
2. Hypotension
3. Renal toxicity
4. Extreme euphoria

5. Which of the following symptoms would indicate to the nurse that a patient may be at risk for lithium toxicity?

1. Increased urination and sweating
2. Dry mouth, vomiting, hypotension
3. Constipation, blurred vision, hypertension
4. Increased appetite, increased energy, memory loss

6. Imipramine (Tofranil) has been ordered in a patient experiencing depression. The nurse ensures the patient knows about which of the following?

1. The use of alcohol is permitted with this drug.
2. Avoid standing up too quickly.
3. Effectiveness occurs within a few hours of administration.
4. If a dose is missed, double up on the next dose.

7. The patient is taking phenelzine (Nardil). The nurse advises the patient to avoid eating:

1. Eggs
2. Aged cheeses
3. Onions
4. Apples

8. An older patient has a prescription for sertraline (Zoloft) 25 mg/day, PO, to be taken for 1 week and then increased to 50 mg/day the second week. The pharmacy gives the patient 50 mg tablets. How many tablets will the patient take per day during the first week?

1. One-quarter of the tablet
2. One tablet
3. Half tablet
4. One and one-half tablets

9. The nurse is providing education material to a patient just prescribed duloxetine (Cymbalta) for depression. The patient states that he has heard this medication is also used for: (Select all that apply.)

1. Phobias
2. Generalized anxiety
3. Neuropathic pain
4. Seizures

10. A patient asks how most antidepressants work. The nurse responds by saying that antidepressants improve mood by increasing levels of:

1. Epinephrine and norepinephrine
2. Reticular formation
3. Norepinephrine and serotonin
4. GABA and serotonin

CASE STUDY QUESTIONS

Remember Mrs. Coxilean, the patient introduced at the beginning of the chapter? Now read the remainder of the case study. Based on the information you have learned in this chapter, answer the questions that follow.

Mrs. Rachel Coxilean, a 32-year-old woman, visits her family doctor and explains that lately she has been experiencing frequent headaches, disinterest in eating and sex, and a hard time "keeping focused." For the past two years, she has been taking OTC medication to help her sleep. Two times within the past year, she missed work because of extreme fatigue. Mrs. Coxilean does not drink alcohol but admits, "The pressure is almost overwhelming sometimes." Mrs. Coxilean is diagnosed with major depressive disorder.

1. During the planning process, it is determined that the main reason why Mrs. Coxilean would not be treated with mood stabilizers is the lack of:

1. Complaints from the patient, suggesting attention deficit disorder
2. Toxicity concerns for this class of drug
3. Evidence that the patient feels her condition is normal
4. Extreme shifts between mania and depression

2. The physician is thinking of prescribing her phenelzine (Nardil). If Mrs. Coxilean were to take this medication, the nurse would most likely tell her:

1. "Avoid reducing your salt intake. It increases excretion of this medication."
2. "Avoid chocolate and some other foods when taking this medication."
3. "You can take herbal supplements without any risks."
4. "You can continue to take OTC medication for sleep, but monitor the frequency."

3. After considering Mrs. Coxilean's symptoms and noting that her lab values were normal, the nurse would expect that she would be started on which medication?

1. Doxepin (Sinequan)
2. Tranylcypromine (Parnate)
3. Sertraline (Zoloft)
4. Bupropion (Wellbutrin)

4. An SSRI was prescribed for Mrs. Coxilean. Which of the following effects might still remain a problem? (Select all that apply.)

1. Headaches
2. Loss of appetite
3. Poor sexual activity
4. Ability to focus

NOTE: Answers to the Review and Case Study Questions appear in Appendix B. The complete rationales and answers are located on the textbook's website.

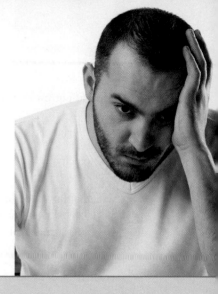

C
H
A
P
T
E
R

*"I don't need medication.
What I need is for you to tell
those FBI and CIA agents to
stop looking in my windows
every night."*

—Mr. Jeremy Wayne

11 Drugs for Psychoses

CORE CONCEPTS

11.1 Most psychoses have no identifiable cause and require long-term drug therapy.

11.2 Patients with schizophrenia experience many different symptoms that may change over time.

11.3 The experience and skills of the healthcare provider are critical to the pharmacologic management of psychoses.

11.4 Conventional antipsychotic drugs include the phenothiazines, phenothiazine-like drugs, and nonphenothiazines.

11.5 Atypical antipsychotic drugs and dopamine system stabilizers also address the needs of patients with psychoses.

DRUG SNAPSHOT

The following drugs are discussed in this chapter:

DRUG CLASSES	DRUG PROTOTYPES
Conventional Antipsychotics	
Phenothiazines	**Pr** chlorpromazine *147*
Nonphenothiazines	**Pr** haloperidol (Haldol) *149*
Atypical Antipsychotics	**Pr** risperidone (Risperdal) *152*
Dopamine System Stabilizers (Third-Generation Antipsychotics)	

LEARNING OUTCOMES

After reading this chapter, the student should be able to:

1. Identify the signs characteristic of psychosis.

2. Compare and contrast the positive and negative symptoms of schizophrenia.

3. Describe the theories for the cause of schizophrenia.

4. Explain the importance of patient drug compliance in the pharmacotherapy of schizophrenia.

5. Explain the symptoms associated with extrapyramidal adverse effects of antipsychotic drugs.

6. Explain the goals of pharmacotherapy and categorize

antipsychotic drugs based on their classification and drug action.

7. For each of the classes listed in the Drug Snapshot, identify representative drugs and explain their mechanisms of drug action, primary actions, and important adverse effects.

KEY TERMS

akathisia (ACK-ah-THEE-shea) *148*

extrapyramidal symptoms (EPS)
(peh-RAM-ed-el) *148*

negative symptoms *144*

neuroleptic malignant syndrome (NMS)
(noo-roh-LEP-tik) *147*

neuroleptics (noo-roh-LEP-ticks) *146*

parkinsonism *148*

positive symptoms *144*

schizoaffective disorder (SKIT-soh-
ah-FEK-tiv) *144*

schizophrenia (SKIT-soh-FREN-ee-uh) *143*

tardive dyskinesia (TAR-div dis-ki-NEE-
zee-uh) *148*

S evere mental illness can be incapacitating for the patient and intensely frustrating for family members dealing with the patient on a regular basis. Before the 1950s, patients with acute mental dysfunction were institutionalized, often for their entire lives. With the introduction of chlorpromazine in the 1950s and the development of subsequent drugs, antipsychotic drugs have revolutionized the treatment of mental illness. With proper medical management, patients with serious mental disorders can now lead normal or near-normal lives as functional members of society.

Most psychoses have no identifiable cause and require long-term drug therapy.

CORE CONCEPT **11.1**

Patients with psychoses often are unable to distinguish what is real from what is illusion. Because of this, patients may be viewed as medically and legally incompetent. The following signs are characteristic of psychosis:

- *Delusions* (strong beliefs in something that is false or not based on reality); for example, the patient may believe that someone is planting thoughts in his or her head.

- *Hallucinations* (seeing, hearing, or feeling something that is not there); for example, the patient may hear voices or see spiders crawling on walls that others around the patient do not hear or see.

- *Illusions* (distorted or misleading perceptions of something that is actually real); for example, the patient may see a shadow and believe it is really a person.

- *Disorganized behavior* For example, the patient may wear clothes in an entirely inappropriate manner and for no apparent reason, such as dressing up with layers of clothes including a hat, sunglasses, and several pairs of socks over the hands and feet.

- *Difficulty relating to others* For example, the patient may become withdrawn from other people in the room, showing signs of distress, maybe even turning combative if confronted or questioned. Behavior may range from total inactivity to extreme agitation.

- *Paranoia* For example, the patient may have an extreme suspicion that he or she is being followed, or that someone is trying to kill him or her.

Psychosis may be classified as *acute* or *chronic*. Acute psychotic episodes occur over hours or days, whereas chronic psychoses develop over months or years. Sometimes a cause may be attributed to the psychosis, such as brain damage, overdoses of certain medications, extreme depression, chronic alcoholism, or drug addiction. Genetic factors are known to play a role in some psychoses. Unfortunately, the vast majority of psychoses have no identifiable cause.

People with psychosis are usually unable to function in society without long-term drug therapy. Patients must see their healthcare provider periodically, and medication must be taken for life. Family members and social support groups are important sources of help for patients who cannot function without continuous drug therapy.

SCHIZOPHRENIA

Schizophrenia is a type of psychosis characterized by abnormal thoughts and thought processes, disordered communication, withdrawal from other people and the outside environment, and a high risk for suicide. Several subtypes of schizophrenic disorders are based on clinical presentation.

schizo = *split*
phrenia = *mind*

CORE CONCEPT 11.2

Patients with schizophrenia experience many different symptoms that may change over time.

Schizophrenia is the most common psychotic disorder, affecting 1% to 2% of the population. Symptoms generally begin to appear in early adulthood, with a peak incidence in men 15 to 24 years of age and in women 25 to 34 years of age. Patients experience a variety of symptoms that may change over time.

When observing patients with schizophrenia, healthcare workers should look for both positive and negative symptoms. **Positive symptoms** are those that *add on* to normal behavior. These include hallucinations, delusions, and disorganized thoughts or speech. **Negative symptoms** are those that *subtract from* normal behavior. These include lack of interest, motivation, responsiveness, or pleasure in daily activities. Proper diagnosis of positive and negative symptoms is important for selecting the most appropriate antipsychotic drug for treatment. The following symptoms may appear quickly or take several months or years to develop:

POSITIVE SYMPTOMS

- Hallucinations, delusions, or paranoia
- Strange behavior, such as talking in rambling statements or making up words
- Strange or irrational actions
- Changes from stupor to extreme hyperactivity

NEGATIVE SYMPTOMS

- Attitude of indifference toward or detachment from life activities
- Neglect of personal hygiene, job, and school
- Noticeable withdrawal from social activities and relationships
- Changes from extreme hyperactivity to stupor

Concept Review **11.1**

- What are the characteristic signs of schizophrenia? What distinguishes a positive symptom from a negative symptom?

Fast Facts Psychosis

- Symptoms of psychosis are often associated with other mental health problems, including substance abuse, depression, and dementia.
- More than 3 million Americans have schizophrenia.
- Patients with psychosis often develop symptoms between the ages of 13 and the early 20s.
- As many as 50% of homeless people in America have schizophrenia.
- The probability of developing schizophrenia is 1 in 100 for the general population, 1 in 10 if one parent has the disorder, and 1 in 4 if both parents are schizophrenic.
- There are a variety of services that help patients and the families of patients with schizophrenia:
  - Case management
  - Psychosocial rehabilitation programs
  - Self-help groups
  - Drop-in centers
  - Housing programs
  - Employment programs
  - "Talk" therapy and counseling
  - Crisis Services

schizo = *schizophrenia*
affective = *mood*

Schizoaffective disorder is a related condition in which the patient exhibits symptoms of both schizophrenia and mood disorder. For example, an acute schizoaffective reaction may include distorted perceptions, hallucinations, and delusions, followed by extreme depression. Over time, both positive and negative psychotic symptoms appear.

Many conditions can cause bizarre behavior, and these should be distinguished from schizophrenia. Chronic use of amphetamines or cocaine can create a paranoid syndrome. Certain complex partial seizures (see Chapter 13) can cause unusual symptoms that are sometimes mistaken for psychoses. Brain neoplasms, infections, or hemorrhage can also cause bizarre, psychotic-like symptoms.

FIGURE 11.1

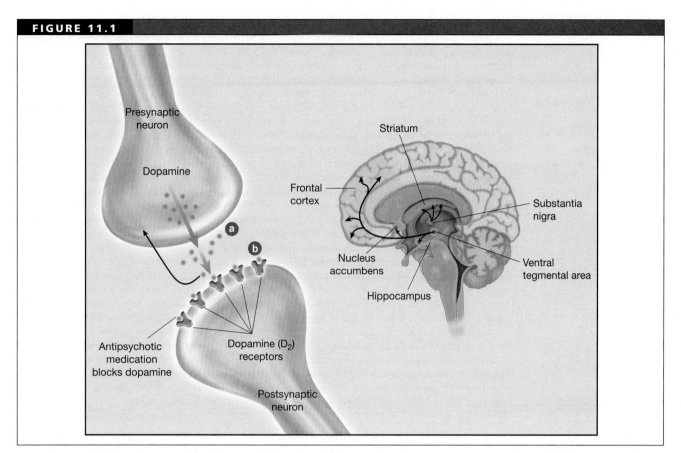

One theory of schizophrenia is that (a) too much dopamine is produced by neurons within the corpus striatum and other nuclei of the brain including locations in the frontal cortex and hippocampus. The extra dopamine overexcites the receptors. (b) Antipsychotic drugs act by attaching to D_2 receptors and preventing the extra dopamine from overstimulating the postsynaptic neurons.

The causes of schizophrenia have not been determined, although several theories have been proposed. There is a definite genetic component to schizophrenia, because many patients suffering from it have family members who have been afflicted with the same disorder. Another theory suggests that the disorder is caused by imbalances in neurotransmitters in specific brain areas. This theory suggests the possibility of overactive dopaminergic pathways found in the basal nuclei, an area of the brain that controls motor activity. The basal nuclei are responsible for starting and stopping synchronized motor activity, such as leg and arm motions during walking.

Synchronized motor activity seems to be associated with dopamine D_2-type receptors. The basal nuclei are particularly rich in D_2-type receptors, whereas the cerebrum contains very few. All antipsychotic drugs act by entering dopaminergic synapses and competing with dopamine. By blocking a majority of the D_2-type receptors, antipsychotic drugs reduce the symptoms of schizophrenia (Figure 11.1 ■).

Concept Review 11.2

■ What are the major types of psychoses, and how are they differentiated? How are the symptoms of schizophrenia reduced?

The experience and skills of the healthcare provider are critical to the pharmacologic management of psychoses.

CORE CONCEPT 11.3

The medical management of severe mental illness is extremely challenging. Many patients do not see their behavior as abnormal and have difficulty understanding the need for medication. If their medication produces undesirable adverse effects, such as severe muscle twitching or loss of sexual function, patient compliance diminishes and symptoms of their pretreatment illness quickly return. Agitation, distrust, and extreme frustration are common, because patients cannot comprehend why others are unable to think and see the same as they do.

The primary goal of pharmacotherapy for patients with schizophrenia is to reduce psychotic symptoms to a level that allows the patient to maintain satisfactory social relationships, as well as self-care and keeping a job. From a pharmacologic perspective, therapy has both a positive and a negative side. Although many symptoms of psychoses can be managed with current drugs, adverse effects are common and often severe. The antipsychotic drugs do not cure mental illness, and symptoms remain in remission only as long as the patient chooses to take the drug. The relapse rate for patients who discontinue their medication is 60% to 80%.

In terms of effectiveness, there is little difference among the various antipsychotic drugs; in other words, there is no single drug of choice for schizophrenia. Selection of a specific drug is based on clinician experience, the occurrence of adverse effects, and the needs of the patient. For example, patients with psychosis due to a degenerative disease may need an antipsychotic with minimal extrapyramidal adverse effects. (Extrapyramidal is named after the place in the brainstem where brain impulses exit the brain. These are motor impulses or nerve signals that may cause intense skeletal muscle contractions. Hence "extra" impulses or signals outside of the pyramids (named for the triangular-shaped bulges appearing along the brain stem) should be reduced for optimal pharmacotherapy in patients who are already susceptible to degenerative-related symptoms. Extrapyramidal symptoms are abbreviated "EPS.") Those who operate machinery need a drug that does not cause sedation. People, especially men who are sexually active, may want a drug without negative sexual effects. Erections are very difficult with antipsychotic medications. The experience and skills of the healthcare provider and mental health professionals are particularly valuable in achieving successful psychiatric pharmacotherapy. The patient's caregiver, when applicable, can be an essential partner in helping the healthcare team manage severe mental illness along with all of the challenges accompanying antipsychotic drug therapy.

The pharmacotherapy of psychosis has undergone two major "generations." Aripiprazole (Abilify) is the one example thought to reduce the risk of hyperglycemia and diabetes with longer-term use; therefore, this drug is sometimes grouped as a "third generation" antipsychotic. The first generation appeared in the early 1950s when the original drugs for treating severe mental illnesses were discovered. These drugs include *conventional* antipsychotics such as chlorpromazine. This essentially ended the era of placing all patients in insane asylums for their lifetimes. The second-generation or *atypical* antipsychotic drugs were discovered in the 1970s and 1980s and are more frequently prescribed because they produce significantly fewer adverse effects. Because of the common neurologic adverse effects, antipsychotic drugs are sometimes referred to as **neuroleptics**.

extra = *outside*
pyramidal = *brain stem pyramids*

neuro = *nervous*
leptic = *state of mind*

CONVENTIONAL (FIRST GENERATION) ANTIPSYCHOTICS

CORE CONCEPT 11.4

Conventional antipsychotic drugs include the phenothiazines, phenothiazine-like drugs, and nonphenothiazines.

Conventional or first-generation antipsychotic drugs were the first category of drugs to be developed. The conventional antipsychotics include the phenothiazines and phenothiazine-like drugs listed in Table 11.1 ◆. Within each category, drugs are named by their chemical structure. Both groups have similar actions and are considered first-generation antipsychotics.

TABLE 11.1 Conventional Antipsychotics: Phenothiazines

Drug	Route and Adult Dose	Remarks
℞ chlorpromazine	PO; 25–100 mg tid or qid (max: 1,000 mg/day) IM/IV; 25–50 mg (max: 600 mg every 4–6 hours)	Strong sedative properties; controls nausea and vomiting, dementia, and hiccups not treated by any other means; for agitated patients
fluphenazine	PO; 0.5–10 mg/day (max: 20 mg/day)	Also for dementia; available in IM or subcutaneous forms
perphenazine	PO; 4–16 mg bid to qid (max: 64 mg/day)	Also for dementia and nausea; available in IM and IV forms
prochlorperazine (Compazine)	PO; 0.5–10 mg/day (max: 20 mg/day)	Antiemetic drug used to treat nausea and vomiting
thioridazine (Mellaril)	PO; 50–100 mg tid (max: 800 mg/day)	Strong sedative properties; for moderate to severe depression and dementia
trifluoperazine	PO; 1–2 mg bid (max: 20 mg/day)	Also for dementia; use cautiously in patients with seizure disorders; available in IM form

Drug Prototype: ℗ᵣ *Chlorpromazine*

Therapeutic Class: Conventional antipsychotic, schizophrenia agent
Pharmacologic Class: Phenothiazine, D_2 dopamine receptor blocker

Actions and Uses: Chlorpromazine provides symptomatic relief of positive symptoms of schizophrenia and controls manic symptoms in patients with schizoaffective disorder. Many patients must take chlorpromazine for seven or eight weeks before they experience improvement. Extreme agitation may be treated with IM or IV injections, which begin to act within minutes. Chlorpromazine can also control severe nausea and vomiting.

Adverse Effects and Interactions: Strong blockade of $alpha_2$-adrenergic receptors and weak blockade of cholinergic receptors explain some of chlorpromazine's adverse effects. Common adverse effects are dizziness, drowsiness, and orthostatic hypotension.

EPS occur mostly in older adult patients, women, and pediatric patients who are dehydrated. **Neuroleptic malignant syndrome (NMS;** described in Table 11.2) may also occur. Patients taking chlorpromazine and exposed to warmer temperatures should be monitored more closely for symptoms of NMS.

Chlorpromazine interacts with several drugs. For example, use with sedative medications such as phenobarbital should be avoided. Taking chlorpromazine with tricyclic antidepressants can elevate blood pressure. Use of chlorpromazine with antiseizure medication can lower the seizure threshold.

Use with caution with herbal supplements, such as kava and St. John's wort, which may increase the risk and severity of dystonia.

> **BLACK BOX WARNING:**
> Older adult patients with dementia-related psychosis are at increased risk for death when taking conventional antipsychotics.

Phenothiazines and Phenothiazine-Like Drugs

The phenothiazines are most effective at treating the positive symptoms of schizophrenia, such as hallucinations and delusions, and have been the treatment of choice for psychoses for 50 years.

The first effective drug used to treat schizophrenia was the low-potency phenothiazine chlorpromazine, approved by the Food and Drug Administration (FDA) in 1954. Other phenothiazines are now available to treat mental illness. All block the excitement associated with the positive symptoms of schizophrenia, although they differ in their potency and adverse effect profiles. Hallucinations and delusions often begin to diminish within days. Other symptoms, however, may require as long as seven to eight weeks of pharmacotherapy to improve. Because of the high rate of recurrence of psychotic episodes, pharmacotherapy should be considered long term, usually for the life of the patient. Phenothiazines are thought to act by preventing both dopamine and serotonin from occupying critical neurologic receptor sites.

Although the phenothiazines once revolutionized treatment of severe mental illness, they exhibit numerous adverse effects that can limit pharmacotherapy. General adverse effects are listed in Table 11.2 ◆.

TABLE 11.2	Adverse Effects of the Conventional Antipsychotics
Effect	**Description**
Acute dystonia	Severe spasms, particularly the back muscles, tongue, and facial muscles; twitching movements
Akathisia	Constant pacing with repetitive, compulsive movements
Anticholinergic effects	Dry mouth, tachycardia, blurred vision
Hypotension	Particularly severe when moving quickly from a recumbent position to an upright position
Neuroleptic malignant syndrome	Symptoms include high fever, confusion, muscle rigidity, and elevated serum creatine kinase levels; NMS can be fatal
Parkinsonism	Tremor, muscle rigidity, stooped posture, and shuffling gait
Sedation	Usually diminishes with continued therapy
Sexual dysfunction	Impotence and diminished libido
Tardive dyskinesia	Bizarre tongue and face movements such as lip smacking and wormlike motions of the tongue; puffing of cheeks, uncontrolled chewing movements

Anticholinergic effects such as dry mouth, postural hypotension, and urinary retention are common. Ejaculation disorders occur in a high percentage of patients; delay in achieving orgasm (in both men and women) is a common cause for noncompliance. Menstrual disorders are common. Each phenothiazine has a slightly different spectrum of adverse effects.

Unlike many other drugs whose primary action is on the central nervous system (CNS) (e.g., amphetamines, barbiturates, anxiolytics, alcohol), antipsychotic drugs do not cause physical or psychological dependence. They also have a wide safety margin between a therapeutic dose and a lethal dose; deaths due to overdoses of antipsychotic drugs are uncommon.

Extrapyramidal symptoms (EPS) are a particularly serious set of adverse reactions to antipsychotic drugs. EPS include acute dystonia, akathisia, parkinsonism, and tardive dyskinesia. Acute *dystonias* (see Chapter 12) occur early in the course of pharmacotherapy and involve severe muscle spasms, particularly of the back, neck, tongue, and face. **Akathisia**, the most common EPS, is an inability to rest or relax. The patient paces, has trouble sitting or remaining still, and has difficulty sleeping. Symptoms of phenothiazine-induced **parkinsonism** include tremor, muscle rigidity, stooped posture, bradykinesia, and a shuffling gait. Parkinsonism results from abnormal neuronal activity in areas of the corpus striatum and substantia nigra. Long-term use of phenothiazines may lead to **tardive dyskinesia**, which is characterized by unusual tongue and face movements such as lip smacking and wormlike motions of the tongue. If extrapyramidal effects are reported early and the drug is withdrawn or the dosage is reduced, the adverse effects can be reversible. With higher doses given for prolonged periods, the EPS may become permanent.

With the conventional antipsychotics, it is not always possible to control the disabling symptoms of schizophrenia without producing some degree of extrapyramidal effects. In these patients, drug therapy may be warranted to treat EPS. Concurrent pharmacotherapy with an anticholinergic drug may prevent some of the extrapyramidal signs (see Chapter 12). For acute dystonia, benztropine (Cogentin) may be given parenterally. Levodopa medications are usually avoided, because of their ability to increase dopamine function and thus antagonize the action of the phenothiazines. Beta-adrenergic blockers and benzodiazepines are sometimes given to reduce signs of akathisia.

Nonphenothiazine Drugs

The nonphenothiazine antipsychotic class consists of drugs whose chemical structures are dissimilar to the phenothiazines (Table 11.3 ◆). Introduced shortly after the phenothiazines, the nonphenothiazines were initially expected to produce fewer adverse effects. Unfortunately, this appears not to be the case. The spectrum of adverse effects for the nonphenothiazines is identical to that for the phenothiazines, although the degree to which a particular effect occurs depends on the specific drug. In general, the nonphenothiazine drugs cause less sedation and fewer anticholinergic adverse effects than chlorpromazine but exhibit an equal or even greater incidence of extrapyramidal signs. Concurrent therapy with other CNS depressants must be carefully monitored because of the potential additive effects.

Drugs in the nonphenothiazine class have the same therapeutic effects and effectiveness as the phenothiazines. They are also believed to act by the same mechanism as the phenothiazines—that is, by blocking postsynaptic D_2 dopamine receptors. As a class, they offer no significant advantages over the phenothiazines in the treatment of schizophrenia.

brady = *slow*
kinesia = *movement*

corpus = *body*
striatum = *striped*

substantia = *substance*
nigra = *black*

tardive = *late*
dyskinesia = *abnormal movement*

non = *not having*
pheno = *chemical ring structure*
thiazine = *sulfur and nitrogen around four carbon atoms*

TABLE 11.3 Conventional Antipsychotics: Nonphenothiazines		
Drug	**Route and Adult Dose**	**Remarks**
(Pr) haloperidol (Haldol)	PO; 0.2–5 mg bid or tid	For severe psychosis, dementia, and Tourette's syndrome; available in IM form
loxapine (Loxitane)	PO; start with 20 mg/day and rapidly increase to 60–100 mg/day in divided doses (max: 250 mg/day)	Also for dementia
pimozide (Orap)	PO; 1–2 mg/day in divided doses; gradually increase every other day to 7–16 mg/day, whichever is less (max: 10 mg/day)	For Tourette's syndrome; use cautiously in patients with seizure disorders
thiothixene (Navane)	PO; 2 mg tid; may increase up to 15 mg/day (max: 60 mg/day)	Also for dementia; off-label use as an antidepressant

Drug Prototype: ⓅⓇ *Haloperidol (Haldol)*

Therapeutic Class: Conventional antipsychotic, schizophrenia agent
Pharmacologic Class: Nonphenothiazine, D₂ dopamine receptor blocker

Actions and Uses: Haloperidol is classified chemically as a butyrophenone. Its primary use is for the management of acute and chronic psychotic disorders. It may be used to treat patients with Tourette's syndrome and children with severe behavior problems such as unprovoked aggressiveness and explosive hyperexcitability. It is approximately 50 times more potent than chlorpromazine but has equal efficacy in relieving symptoms of schizophrenia. Haldol LA is a long-acting preparation that lasts for approximately three weeks following IM or SC administration. This is particularly beneficial for patients who are uncooperative or unable to take oral medications.

Adverse Effects and Interaction: Haloperidol produces less sedation and hypotension than chlorpromazine, but the incidence of EPS is high. Older adults are more likely to experience adverse effects and often are prescribed half the adult dose until the adverse effects of therapy can be determined. Although NMS is rare, it can occur.

Haloperidol interacts with many drugs. For example, the following drugs decrease the effects/absorption of haloperidol: aluminum- and magnesium-containing antacids, levodopa (also increases chances of levodopa toxicity), lithium (increases chance of severe neurologic toxicity), phenobarbital, phenytoin (also increases chances of phenytoin toxicity), rifampin, and beta blockers (may increase blood levels of haloperidol, thus leading to possible toxicity). Haloperidol inhibits the action of centrally acting antihypertensives.

Use with caution with herbal supplements such as kava, which may increase the effect of haloperidol.

> **BLACK BOX WARNING:**
> Older adult patients with dementia-related psychosis are at increased risk for death when taking conventional antipsychotics.

NURSING PROCESS FOCUS   Patients Receiving Phenothiazines and Nonphenothiazine Therapy

ASSESSMENT	POTENTIAL NURSING DIAGNOSES
Prior to administration: ■ Obtain a complete health history including cardiovascular, renal and liver conditions, allergies, drug history, and possible drug interactions. ■ Acquire baseline vital signs and ECG, laboratory blood levels (CBC, chemistry, drug screening, renal and liver function studies), and urine specimens for laboratory analysis. ■ Determine neurological status. (altered thought processes, level of consciousness (LOC), mental status, and identification of recent mood and behavior patterns). ■ Identify patient support system(s).	■ *Ineffective Therapeutic Regimen Management* related to noncompliance with medication regimen, presence of adverse effects, and need for long-term medication use ■ *Anxiety* related to symptoms of psychosis and adverse effects of drug therapy ■ *Risk for Injury* related to adverse effects of drug therapy and thought processes ■ *Noncompliance* related to length of time before medication reaches therapeutic levels and adverse effects of drug therapy ■ *Deficient Knowledge* related to a lack of information about disease process and drug therapy

PLANNING: PATIENT GOALS AND EXPECTED OUTCOMES

The patient will:
■ Experience therapeutic effects (reduction of psychotic symptoms).
■ Be free from or experience minimal adverse effects from drug therapy.
■ Verbalize an understanding of the drug's use, adverse effects, and required precautions.
■ Adhere to recommended treatment regimen.

IMPLEMENTATION

Interventions and (Rationales)	Patient Education/Discharge Planning
■ Administer medication correctly and evaluate the patient's knowledge of proper administration. (Ensuring proper administration helps to avoid unnecessary adverse effects and interactions with other medications while determining effectiveness.)	Instruct the patient: ■ Not to take any other medication or herbal therapies unless approved by the healthcare provider. ■ That it may take up to eight weeks for full therapeutic effects to be seen.
■ Monitor for therapeutic effects, e.g., decreased psychotic symptoms. (If the patient continues to exhibit symptoms of psychosis, he or she may not be taking the drug as ordered, may be taking an inadequate dose, or may not be affected by the drug; it may need to be discontinued and another antipsychotic begun.)	Instruct the patient to: ■ Notice increases or decreases of symptoms of psychosis, including hallucinations, abnormal sleep patterns, social withdrawal, delusions, or paranoia. ■ Contact the healthcare provider if no decrease of symptoms occurs over a six-week period.

continued . . .

NURSING PROCESS FOCUS   *(continued)*

Interventions and (Rationales)	Patient Education/Discharge Planning
■ Monitor for adverse effects of medications such as drowsiness, dizziness, lethargy, headaches, blurred vision, skin rash, diaphoresis, nausea/vomiting, anorexia, diarrhea, anuresis, depression, hypotension, or hypertension.	Instruct the patient: ■ Regarding the adverse effects specific to the type of antipsychotic medication being taken. ■ To report adverse effects to their healthcare provider.
■ Monitor for anticholinergic adverse effects such as orthostatic hypotension, constipation, anorexia, genitourinary problems, respiratory changes, and visual disturbances.	Instruct the patient to: ■ Avoid abrupt changes in position. ■ Not drive or perform hazardous activities until the effects of the drug are known. ■ Report vision changes. ■ Comply with required laboratory tests. ■ Increase dietary fiber, fluids, and exercise to prevent constipation. ■ Relieve symptoms of dry mouth with sugarless hard candy or gum and frequent drinks of water. ■ Notify the healthcare provider immediately if urinary retention occurs.
■ Monitor for extrapyramidal effects such as those associated with tardive dyskinesia, dystonia, akathisia, pseudoparkinsonism. (Presence of EPS may be sufficient reason for the patient to discontinue the antipsychotic. Monitor for NMS, which is life threatening and must be reported and treated immediately.)	Instruct the patient to: ■ Recognize that extrapyramidal effects such as the development of tremors, involuntary repetitive movements, decreased muscle tone, or increased restlessness may occur and not to stop taking medication until healthcare provider is seen. ■ Immediately seek treatment for elevated temperature, unstable blood pressure, profuse sweating, dyspnea, muscle rigidity, incontinence.
■ Monitor for weight gain, menstrual irregularities, impotence, and gynecomastia. (Some antipsychotic drugs may cause weight gain and have pituitary effects.)	■ Instruct the patient and caregivers to weigh the patient weekly and to report a weight gain of two pounds or more per week to the healthcare provider. ■ Instruct the patient to talk to healthcare provider about sexual concerns.
■ Monitor for alcohol/illegal drug use. (Patient may decide to use alcohol or illegal drugs as a means of coping with symptoms of psychosis, so he or she may stop taking the antipsychotic. Concurrent use will cause increased CNS depressant effect.)	■ Instruct the patient to refrain from alcohol and illegal drug use. Refer the patient to community support groups such as Alcoholics Anonymous (AA) or Narcotics Anonymous (NA) as appropriate.
■ Monitor caffeine use. (Use of caffeine-containing substances will negate effects of antipsychotics.)	Instruct the patient to: ■ Avoid caffeine. ■ Recognize common caffeine-containing products and assist in finding acceptable substitutes, such as decaffeinated coffee and tea, caffeine-free colas.
■ Continue to monitor vital signs, especially BP and heart rate. Monitor for cardiovascular changes, including hypotension, tachycardia, and electrocardiogram (ECG) changes. (Haloperidol has fewer cardiotoxic effects than other antipsychotics and may be preferred for patients with existing cardiovascular problems.)	■ Instruct the patient that dizziness and falls, especially on sudden position changes, may indicate cardiovascular changes. ■ Provide information on safety measures such as slowly rising from a sitting position.
■ Monitor for smoking. (Heavy smoking may decrease metabolism of haloperidol, leading to decreased effectiveness.)	■ Instruct the patient to stop or decrease smoking. Refer to smoking cessation programs, if indicated.
■ Monitor older adult patients closely. (Older adult patients may need lower doses and a more gradual dosage increase. Older adult women are at greater risk for developing tardive dyskinesia.)	Instruct the patient: ■ To look for unusual reactions such as confusion, depression, and hallucinations and for symptoms of tardive dyskinesia, and to report them immediately. ■ On ways to counteract anticholinergic effects of medication while taking into account any other existing medical problems.
■ Monitor laboratory results, including CBC, and drug levels.	■ Advise the patient of the necessity of having regular laboratory studies done.
■ Monitor for use of medication. (All antipsychotics must be taken as ordered for therapeutic results to occur.)	■ Instruct the patient that medication must be continued as ordered, even if no therapeutic benefits are felt, because it may take several months for full therapeutic benefits to take effect.
■ Monitor for seizures. (Drug may lower seizure threshold.)	■ Instruct the patient that seizures may occur and review appropriate safety precautions.

NURSING PROCESS FOCUS *(continued)*

Interventions and (Rationales)	Patient Education/Discharge Planning
■ Monitor the patient's environment. (Drug may cause the patient to perceive a brownish discoloration of objects or experience photophobia. Drug may also interfere with the ability to regulate body temperature.)	Instruct the patient to: ■ Wear dark glasses to avoid discomfort from photophobia. ■ Avoid temperature extremes. ■ Be aware that perception of brownish discoloration of objects may appear, but that it is not harmful.

EVALUATION OF OUTCOME CRITERIA

Evaluate the effectiveness of drug therapy by confirming that patient goals and expected outcomes have been met (see "Planning"). *See Tables 11.1 and 11.3 for lists of the drugs to which these nursing actions apply.*

ATYPICAL (SECOND GENERATION) ANTIPSYCHOTICS

Atypical antipsychotics treat both positive and negative symptoms of schizophrenia. They have become preferred drugs for treating psychoses.

Atypical antipsychotic drugs and dopamine system stabilizers also address the needs of patients with psychoses.

CORE CONCEPT 11.5

The approval of clozapine (Clozaril), the first atypical antipsychotic, marked the first major advance in the pharmacotherapy of psychoses since the discovery of chlorpromazine decades earlier. Clozapine and the other drugs in this class are called *second generation* or *atypical*, because they have a broader spectrum of action than the conventional antipsychotics, controlling both the positive and the negative symptoms of schizophrenia (Table 11.4 ◆). Furthermore, at therapeutic doses they exhibit their

TABLE 11.4   Atypical Antipsychotic Drugs

Drug	Route and Adult Dose	Remarks
aripiprazole (Abilify)	PO; 10–15 mg daily (max: 30 mg/day)	For schizophrenia; may cause loss of glycemic control in patients with diabetes. Often considered a "third generation" antipsychotic
asenapine (Saphris)	Sublingual; 5 mg twice daily (max: 10 mg twice daily)	For acute management of mania or mixed episodes associated with bipolar disorder in adults
clozapine (Clozaril)	PO; start at 25–50 mg/day and increase to a target dose of 50–450 mg/day in 3 days, may increase further (max: 900 mg/day)	For schizophrenia (adults older than 16 years); causes neutropenia and agranulocytosis
iloperidone (Fanapt)	PO; 12–24 mg/day administered twice daily	For schizophrenia (adults older than 16 years)
lurasidone (Latuda)	PO; 40 mg once daily (max: 80 mg/day)	For schizophrenia; once-a-day oral medication
olanzapine (Zyprexa)	PO adult: start with 5–10 mg/day, may increase by 2.5–5 mg every week (range 10–15 mg/day, max: 20 mg/day); geriatric: start with 5 mg/day	Blocks alpha receptors and acetylcholine
paliperidone (Invega)	PO; 6 mg/day (max: 12 mg/day)	For schizophrenia; for the treatment of schizoaffective disorder in adults and adolescents (12–17 years old)
quetiapine (Seroquel)	PO (regular release); start with 25 mg bid, may increase to a target dose of 300–400 mg/day in divided doses PO (extended release); 300 mg daily may increase to 400–800 mg daily (max: 800 mg/day)	Patients may experience hypotension when changing positions; use cautiously in older adults; also used for depression
ⓟ risperidone (Risperdal)	PO; 1–6 mg bid, increase by 2 mg daily to an initial target dose of 6 mg/day IM 25 mg once every 2 weeks (max: 50 mg)	Off-label use in behavioral disturbances (patients with intellectual and developmental disabilities)
ziprasidone (Geodon)	PO; 20 mg bid (max: 80 mg bid) IM 10–20 mg every 2–4 hours (max: 40 mg/ day)	Off-label use for Tourette's syndrome; patients may experience hypotension when changing positions

neutro = *neutrophil*
penia = *deficiency*

agranulo = *without granules*
cytosis = *greater than normal cells*

antipsychotic actions without producing the major EPS effects of the conventional drugs. Some atypical drugs, such as clozapine and risperidone, are especially useful for patients in whom other drugs have proved unsuccessful. Unfortunately, however, clozapine and other atypical antipsychotics can cause neutropenia (decreased neutrophil count) and agranulocytosis (*increased* WBCs without granules; *decreased* WBCs with granules).

Atypical antipsychotics are thought to act by blocking several receptor types in the brain. Like the phenothiazines, they block dopamine D_2 receptors. However, the atypicals also block serotonin and alpha$_2$-adrenergic receptors, which is thought to account for some of their properties. Because the atypical drugs are loosely bound to D_2 receptors, they produce fewer extrapyramidal adverse effects than the conventional antipsychotics.

Although there are fewer adverse effects with atypical antipsychotics, adverse effects are still significant, and patients must be carefully monitored. Most antipsychotics cause weight gain, and the atypical drugs are associated with obesity and its risk factors. Risperidone (Risperdal) and some of the other antipsychotic drugs increase prolactin levels, which can lead to menstrual disorders, decreased libido, and osteoporosis in women. In men, high prolactin levels can cause lack of libido and impotence. There is also concern that some atypical drugs alter glucose metabolism, which can lead to type II diabetes.

Concept Review 11.3

■ What is a neuroleptic drug? What are the two general classes of drugs used to treat psychoses? How does each drug category generally affect positive and/or negative symptoms of schizophrenia?

Drug Prototype: ℗ *Risperidone (Risperdal)*

Therapeutic Class: Atypical antipsychotic, schizophrenia agent, psychotic depression agent
Pharmacologic Class: Serotonin (5-HT) receptor antagonist, D$_2$ dopamine receptor antagonist (weaker affinity)

Actions and Uses: Therapeutic effects of risperidone include treatment and prevention of schizophrenia relapse and expression of bipolar mania symptoms. Risperidone also treats symptoms of irritability in children with autism. Expected results are a reduction of excitement, paranoia, or negative behaviors associated with psychosis. Effects result from blockade of dopamine type 2, serotonin type 2, and alpha$_2$-adrenergic receptors located within the CNS. For a full range of effectiveness, the drug is sometimes combined with lithium (Eskalith) or valproic acid (Depakene). Risperidone is a long-acting preparation, which, following IM administration, releases only a small amount. After a three-week lag, the rest of the drug releases and lasts for approximately four to six weeks. PO preparations release sooner and have a one- to two-week onset of action.

Adverse Effects and Interactions: If elderly patients with dementia-related psychoses are given risperidone, they are at an increased risk for heart failure, pneumonia, or sudden death. Patients with underlying cardiovascular disease may be especially prone to dysrhythmias and hypotension. Risperidone should be avoided in patients with a history of seizures, suicidal ideations, or kidney/liver disease. This medication may cause hyperglycemia and worsen glucose control in patients with diabetes. It is not known whether risperidone passes into breast milk or if it could harm a nursing baby. Due to its category C classification, safety in pregnancy has not been established.

Common adverse effects are extrapyramidal reactions (involuntary shaking of the head, neck, and arms), hyperactivity, fatigue, nausea, dizziness, visual disturbances, fever, and orthostatic hypotension. Risperidone may cause weight gain.

Patients taking risperidone should avoid CNS depressants such as alcohol, antihistamines, sedative-hypnotics, or opioid analgesics. These can increase some of the adverse effects of risperidone. Due to inhibition of liver enzymes, other drugs that increase the adverse effects of risperidone include the selective serotonin reuptake inhibitors (SSRIs) such as paroxetine, sertraline, and fluoxetine (Prozac), and antifungal drugs such as fluconazole, itraconazole, and ketoconazole. Risperidone may interfere with elimination by the kidneys of clozapine, also increasing the risk of adverse reactions.

Kava, valerian, or chamomile may increase risperidone's CNS depressive effects.

> **BLACK BOX WARNING:**
> Older adult patients with dementia-related psychosis are at increased risk for death when taking conventional antipsychotics.

NURSING PROCESS FOCUS Patients Receiving Atypical Antipsychotic Therapy

ASSESSMENT	POTENTIAL NURSING DIAGNOSES
Prior to administration: ■ Obtain a complete health history including cardiovascular, renal and liver conditions, allergies, drug history, and possible drug interactions. ■ Acquire baseline vital signs and ECG, laboratory blood levels (CBC, chemistry, drug screening, renal and liver function studies) and urine specimens for laboratory analysis. ■ Determine neurological status. (altered thought processes, hallucinations, level of consciousness [LOC], mental status, and identification of recent mood and behavior patterns). ■ Identify patient support system(s).	■ *Risk for Injury* related to adverse effects of drug therapy, and thought processes ■ *Ineffective Therapeutic Regimen Management* related to noncompliance with medication regimen, presence of adverse effects, and need for long-term medication use ■ *Anxiety* related to symptoms of psychosis ■ *Noncompliance* related to length of time before drug reaches therapeutic levels, desire to use alcohol or illegal drugs ■ *Deficient Knowledge* related to a lack of information about disease process and drug therapy

PLANNING: PATIENT GOALS AND EXPECTED OUTCOMES

The patient will:
■ Experience therapeutic effects (reduction of psychotic symptoms).
■ Be free from or experience minimal adverse effects from drug therapy.
■ Verbalize an understanding of the drug's use, adverse effects and required precautions.
■ Adhere to recommended treatment regimen.

IMPLEMENTATION

Interventions and (Rationales)	Patient Education/Discharge Planning
■ Administer medication correctly and evaluate the patient's knowledge of proper administration. (Ensuring proper administration helps to avoid unnecessary adverse effects and interactions with other medications while determining effectiveness.)	Instruct the patient: ■ Not to take any other medication or herbal therapies unless approved by the healthcare provider. ■ That it may take up to six weeks for full therapeutic effects to be seen.
■ Monitor RBC and WBC counts. (Agranulocytosis [WBCs below 3,500] can be a life-threatening adverse effect of these medications, which may also suppress bone marrow and lower infection-fighting ability.)	Instruct the patient to: ■ Keep appointments for laboratory testing. ■ Report any sore throat, signs of infection, fatigue without apparent cause, or bruising to the healthcare provider.
■ Observe for adverse effects. (These drugs may affect blood pressure, heart rate, and other autonomic functions.)	■ Instruct the patient to report any adverse effects such as drowsiness, dizziness, depression, anxiety, tachycardia, hypotension, nausea/vomiting, excessive salivation, changes in urinary frequency or urgency, incontinence, weight gain, muscle pain or weakness, rash, and fever to the healthcare provider.
■ Monitor for anticholinergic adverse effects. (These medications may cause mouth dryness, constipation, or urinary retention.)	Instruct the patient to: ■ Increase dietary fiber, fluids, and exercise to prevent constipation. ■ Relieve symptoms of dry mouth with sugar-free hard candy or chewing gum and frequent drinks of water. ■ Immediately notify the healthcare provider if urinary retention occurs. Possible catheter placement may be necessary.
■ Monitor for therapeutic effects, e.g., decrease of psychotic symptoms. (Decreased symptoms indicate an effective dose and type of medication.)	Instruct the patient to: ■ Notice increases or decreases of symptoms of psychosis, including hallucinations, abnormal sleep patterns, social withdrawal, delusions, or paranoia. ■ Contact the healthcare provider if symptoms do not decrease over a six-week period.
■ Monitor for alcohol or illegal drug use. (Used concurrently, these will cause increased CNS depression. The patient may decide to use alcohol or illegal drugs as a means of coping with symptoms of psychosis and may stop taking the drug.)	■ Instruct the patient to avoid alcohol or illegal drug use. Refer the patient to AA, NA, or other support group as appropriate.
■ Monitor caffeine use. (Use of caffeine-containing substances inhibits the effects of antipsychotics.)	Instruct the patient about: ■ Common caffeine-containing products. ■ Acceptable substitutes, including decaffeinated coffee and tea, and caffeine-free soda.
■ Monitor for smoking. (Heavy smoking may decrease blood levels of the drug.)	■ Instruct the patient to stop or decrease smoking. Refer to smoking cessation programs if indicated.
■ Monitor older adult patients closely. (Older patients may be more sensitive to anticholinergic adverse effects.)	■ Instruct older adult patients on ways to counteract anticholinergic effects of the medication while taking into account any other existing medical problems.

EVALUATION OF OUTCOME CRITERIA

Evaluate the effectiveness of drug therapy by confirming that patient goals and expected outcomes have been met (see "Planning"). *See Table 11.4 for a list of drugs to which these nursing actions apply.*

DOPAMINE SYSTEM STABILIZERS (THIRD-GENERATION ANTIPSYCHOTICS)

In 2002, due to side effects caused by conventional and atypical antipsychotic medications, a newer drug class was developed to better meet the needs of patients with psychoses. This class, sometimes considered a third-generation class of antipsychotics, consists of *dopamine system stabilizers (DSSs)* or dopamine partial agonists. Aripiprazole (Abilify) received FDA approval in 2002 for the treatment of schizophrenia and schizoaffective disorder. Because aripiprazole controls both the positive and the negative symptoms of schizophrenia, it is grouped in Table 17.4 with the atypical antipsychotic drugs.

Aripiprazole is generally well tolerated in patients with schizophrenia. In particular, its use seems to be associated with a lower incidence of EPS than haloperidol and fewer weight-gain issues than other atypical antipsychotics, for example, olanzapine. Anticholinergic adverse effects are virtually nonexistent. In fact, the incidence of adverse effects generally compared to the other atypical antipsychotic drugs is very low. Notable side effects, however, include headache, nausea/vomiting, fever, constipation, and anxiety. Healthcare providers are encouraged to balance the risks and benefits of medications when choosing an antipsychotic for an individual patient.

PATIENTS NEED TO KNOW

Patients being treated for psychoses of the nervous system need to know the following:

1. It is important to report the development of tremors, muscle spasms, involuntary repetitive movements, decreased muscle tone, or increased restlessness to the healthcare provider. These symptoms may indicate serious adverse effects that can be reversed if medication is changed soon after they start.
2. Consult a healthcare provider if dry mouth, rapid heart rate, constipation, or urinary retention occurs. An additional medication may be prescribed to relieve these signs and symptoms.
3. Avoid taking antacids with antipsychotics because they delay or decrease antipsychotic absorption.
4. Avoid alcohol or other sedatives while taking antipsychotics; it increases the depressant effects.
5. Extra protection from the sun is necessary; wear a hat and sunscreen.
6. Avoid driving or operating machinery until response to the medication is known. Its sedating effects can increase the risk for accidental injury.
7. Contact a healthcare provider for guidance if symptoms get worse or are not relieved by the medication. Do not stop the medication unless directed to do so.

CHAPTER REVIEW

CORE CONCEPTS SUMMARY

11.1 Most psychoses have no identifiable cause and require long-term drug therapy.

Psychosis is characterized by delusions, hallucinations, illusions, disorganized behavior, difficulty relating to others, and paranoia. Psychoses may be classified as acute or chronic. Sometimes a cause can be found for the psychosis, but the vast majority of cases have no identifiable cause. Most patients with psychoses are not able to function normally in society without long-term drug therapy.

11.2 Patients with schizophrenia experience many different symptoms that may change over time.

Schizophrenia is the most common psychiatric disorder; it is characterized by abnormal thoughts, disordered communication, withdrawal, and suicidal risk. Patients with schizophrenia exhibit positive (adding) or negative (subtracting) symptoms. Proper diagnosis of these symptoms is important for selecting the appropriate antipsychotic drug. The cause of schizophrenia has not been determined. Symptoms seem to be associated with neural *dopamine type 2 (D2) receptors* found in the basal nuclei. Schizoaffective disorders are characterized by symptoms of both schizophrenia and mood disorder.

11.3 **The experience and skills of the healthcare provider are critical to the pharmacologic management of psychoses.**

Management of severe mental illness is difficult. Many patients do not see themselves as abnormal and have difficulty understanding the need for medication. Although many symptoms of psychosis can be controlled with current drug therapy, adverse effects are common and often severe. Skills of the healthcare team are particularly valuable to achieving successful psychiatric drug treatment.

11.4 **Conventional antipsychotic drugs include the phenothiazines, phenothiazine-like drugs, and nonphenothiazines.**

Antipsychotic drugs are sometimes called *neuroleptics*. The two basic categories of drugs for psychosis are conventional antipsychotics and atypical antipsychotics. With conventional antipsychotics, it is not always possible to control *extrapyramidal symptoms (EPS)* which include muscle spasms (*dystonia*), inability to sit down (*akathisia*), and unusual tongue and facial movements (*tardive dyskinesia*). Phenothiazines, phenothiazine-like drugs, and nonphenothiazines treat positive signs of schizophrenia, but all have unpleasant adverse effects.

11.5 **Atypical antipsychotic drugs and dopamine system stabilizers also address the needs of patients with psychoses.**

Atypical antipsychotic drugs treat both positive and negative signs of schizophrenia and have become drugs of choice for treating psychoses. Like the phenothiazine drugs, atypical drugs block D$_2$ receptors. Although there are fewer adverse effects with atypical drugs, adverse effects are still significant, and patients must be carefully monitored. Dopamine system stabilizers (DSSs) represent the third-generation class of antipsychotics developed to better meet the needs of patients with psychoses.

REVIEW QUESTIONS

The following questions are written in NCLEX-PN® style. Answer these questions to assess your knowledge of the chapter material, and go back and review any material that is not clear to you.

1. While caring for a patient taking an antipsychotic drug, the nurse understands that:

1. Antipsychotic medications cure mental illnesses.
2. Some adverse effects of antipsychotic drugs can lead to noncompliance.
3. Antipsychotic medications are only administered when the patient is symptomatic.
4. Antipsychotic drugs improve symptoms within hours of administration.

2. Family members of a patient diagnosed with schizophrenia are being educated on the adverse effects of phenothiazines. Which of the following would the nurse include? (Select all that apply.)

1. The patient may experience a sedative effect that usually diminishes with continued therapy.
2. Severe muscle spasms may occur early in therapy.
3. Tardive dyskinesia can occur with long-term therapy.
4. Medications can be given to help prevent some adverse effects.

3. Which of the following symptoms does the nurse recognize as an anticholinergic effect of chlorpromazine?

1. Hallucinations, illusions, paranoia
2. Hypertension, polyuria, increased salivation
3. Dry mouth, tachycardia, blurred vision
4. High fever, confusion, muscle rigidity

4. The patient is on thioridazine (Mellaril) and has developed muscle spasms, difficulty sleeping, and a shuffling gait. The nurse recognizes this as:

1. Anticholinergic effects
2. Cholinergic effects
3. Extrapyramidal adverse effects
4. Serotonin syndrome

5. The patient states that he has not taken his antipsychotic drug for the past two weeks because it was causing sexual dysfunction. The nurse explains that it is important to continue taking his medication as prescribed because:

1. Hypertensive crisis may occur with abrupt withdrawal.
2. Muscle twitching may occur.
3. Noncompliance may bring on parkinsonism.
4. Symptoms of psychosis are likely to return.

6. The nurse understands that when evaluating the effects of certain antipsychotic medications, neuroleptic malignant syndrome (NMS) is most likely to occur with use of which of the following drug?

1. Chlorpromazine
2. Aripiprazole (Abilify)
3. Risperidone (Risperdal)
4. Clozapine (Clozaril)

7. The nurse understands that haloperidol (Haldol) may be ordered for which of the following reasons:

1. Seizures
2. Unprovoked aggressiveness
3. Severe mental depression
4. Alcoholism

8. The nurse monitors the patient taking which of the following drug groups because it can lead to type II diabetes?

1. Phenothiazines
2. Nonphenothiazines
3. Atypical antipsychotics
4. All antipsychotics

9. The nurse is speaking to a patient and his family about the use of herbal supplements. She warns them about possible interactions with prescribed medications, specifically combining herbal supplements with antipsychotic medication. When asked what herbal supplements are used to treat mental illness, the nurse suggests:

1. Echinacea
2. St. John's wort
3. Black cohosh
4. Saw palmetto

10. A patient is taking aripiprazole (Abilify). Which patient effects should the nurse observe to determine whether the drug is having a therapeutic effect?

1. Elevated mood and coping skills
2. Orthostatic hypotension and sedation
3. Decreased delusional thinking and hallucinations
4. Improved sleep and dietary habits

CASE STUDY QUESTIONS

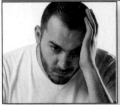

Remember Mr. Wayne, the patient introduced at the beginning of the chapter? Now read the remainder of the case study. Based on the information you have learned in this chapter, answer the questions that follow.

Mr. Jeremy Wayne, age 38, has been diagnosed with a psychosis characterized by the following symptoms: reports of seeing people who are not there, talking about government agents who are trying to kill him, and communicating with "double agents" about suspicious behavior. This patient has been in and out of the hospital for the past four weeks. Mr. Wayne's family reports difficulty in controlling him because he has not been taking his medication. Members in the community have seen Mr. Wayne pacing up and down the highway for several weeks. It becomes necessary to temporarily confine Mr. Wayne for medical treatment. He has had this disorder for 15 years and has a strong, supportive family (mother and father).

1. The symptoms described for Mr. Wayne are called _____ symptoms and respond best to treatment with which class of antipsychotic medication?

1. Positive; conventional or typical antipsychotics
2. Negative; conventional or typical antipsychotics
3. Positive; atypical antipsychotics
4. Negative; atypical antipsychotics

2. Mr. Wayne has been taking risperidone (Risperdal) for the past 10 years that he has been experiencing psychotic episodes. Mr. Wayne is placed back on his medication so the nurse monitors him closely for which of the following adverse effects: (Select all that apply.)

1. Hyperactivity
2. Spasms (shaking of head/neck)
3. Fatigue
4. Fever

3. According to the doctor's order, the nurse gives Mr. Wayne which of the following medications to help reduce the incidence of dystonia (spasms)?

1. Levodopa (Larodopa)
2. Benztropine (Cogentin)
3. Thioridazine (Mellaril)
4. Trifluoperazine

4. The physician orders the long-acting preparation of fluphenazine 15 mg SC. The pharmacy supplies fluphenazine 25 mg/mL. The nurse administers _____.

1. 0.4 mL
2. 1.4 mL
3. 0.6 mL
4. 1.6 mL

NOTE: Answers to the Review and Case Study Questions appear in Appendix B. The complete rationales and answers are located on the textbook's website.

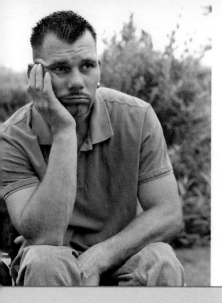

"It's hard to face the future, knowing what MS does to you."

Mr. Robert Wingate

Drugs for Degenerative Diseases and Muscles

CORE CONCEPTS

12.1 Medications are unable to cure most degenerative diseases of the CNS.

12.2 Parkinson's disease is progressive, with the occurrence of full symptoms taking many years.

12.3 Antiparkinson drugs act on the brain to restore the balance between dopamine and a_____line.

12.4 Patients with Alzheimer's d_____ a dramatic loss of ability _____ require acetylcholine as th_____

12.5 Alzheimer's _____ erase inhibit___

12.6 _____

12.7 _____

12.8 Muscle spasms are caused by injury, overmedication, hypocalcemia, and debilitating neurologic disorders.

12.9 Muscle spasms may be treated with nonpharmacologic or pharmacologic therapies.

12.10 Many muscle relaxants treat muscle spasms by inhibiting upper motor neuron activity, causing sedation, or altering simple reflexes.

12.11 Effective treatment for spasticity includes both physical therapy and medications.

12.12 Some drugs for spasticity provide relief by acting directly on muscle tissue, interfering with the release of calcium ions.

12.13 Neuromuscular blocking drugs block the effect of acetylcholine at the receptor.

DRUG S_____

The following _____

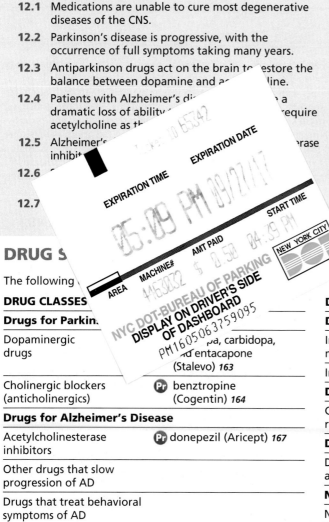

DRUG CLASSES	DRUG PROTOTYPES
Drugs for Parkin__	
Dopaminergic drugs	_pa, carbidopa, ___ entacapone (Stalevo) *163*
Cholinergic blockers (anticholinergics)	(Pr) benztropine (Cogentin) *164*
Drugs for Alzheimer's Disease	
Acetylcholinesterase inhibitors	(Pr) donepezil (Aricept) *167*
Other drugs that slow progression of AD	
Drugs that treat behavioral symptoms of AD	

DRUG CLASSES	DRUG PROTOTYPES
Drugs for Multiple Sclerosis	
Immune system modulating drugs	
Immunosuppressants	
Drugs for Muscle Spasms	
Centrally acting muscle relaxants	(Pr) cyclobenzaprine (Amrix, Flexeril) *171*
Drugs for Spasticity	
Direct-acting antispasmodics	(Pr) dantrolene (Dantrium) *175*
Neuromuscular Blocking Drugs	
Nondepolarizing blockers	
Depolarizing blockers	

LEARNING OUTCOMES

After reading this chapter, the student should be able to:

1. Identify the most common degenerative diseases of the CNS.

2. Describe symptoms of Parkinson's disease, Alzheimer's disease, multiple sclerosis, and spasticity.

3. Explain the neurochemical bases of central degenerative diseases and muscle spasms.

4. Explain the goals of pharmacotherapy and categorize drugs used in the treatment of degenerative diseases based on their class and drug action.

5. Describe the pharmacologic management of muscle spasms.

6. Discuss nonpharmacologic therapies used to treat muscle spasms and spasticity.

7. Discuss the pharmacology of neuromuscular blocking drugs.

8. Compare and contrast the roles of centrally acting skeletal muscle relaxants and direct-acting antispasmodics in treating muscle spasms and spasticity.

9. For each of the classes listed in the Drug Snapshot, identify representative drugs and explain their mechanisms of drug action, primary actions, and important adverse effects.

KEY TERMS

acetylcholinesterase (AchE) (AS-ee-til-KOH-lin-ES-ter-ays) 165

Alzheimer's disease (AD) (ALLZ-heye-mers) 164

dementia (dee-MEN-she-ah) 158

dystonia (diss-TONE-ee-ah) 172

multiple sclerosis (MS) (skle-ROH-sis) 167

neuromuscular blocking drugs (NEWR-oh-musc-you-lahr) 175

parkinsonism 159

spasticity (spas-TISS-ih-tee) 172

Central degenerative diseases and muscle disorders affect a patient's ability to perform daily activities and most often lead to immobility. Appropriate body movement depends on intact neural pathways and proper muscle functioning. Without medical intervention, neurologic disorders can result in major sensory, cognitive, and/or motor problems. Parkinson's disease, Alzheimer's disease (AD), and multiple sclerosis (MS) are three common debilitating and progressive neurologic disorders. Although medications are unable to stop or reverse the progressive nature of these diseases, therapy can often slow down the disorders and offer symptomatic relief. Common muscle disorders are muscle spasms and spasticity. This chapter focuses on the pharmacotherapy of neurodegenerative diseases and muscle disorders as well as treatments involving the neuromuscular junction.

CORE CONCEPT 12.1

Medications are unable to cure most degenerative diseases of the CNS.

Degenerative diseases of the central nervous system (CNS) include a variety of disorders with different causes and outcomes. Some, such as Huntington's disease, are quite rare, affect younger patients, and are caused by chromosomal defects. Others, such as AD, affect millions of people, mostly elderly patients, and have a devastating economic and social impact. Table 12.1 ◆ lists major degenerative diseases of the CNS.

TABLE 12.1 Degenerative Diseases of the Central Nervous System	
Disease	**Description**
Alzheimer's disease	Progressive loss of brain function characterized by memory loss, confusion, and **dementia** (a degenerative disorder characterized by progressive memory loss, confusion, and inability to think or communicate effectively)
Amyotrophic lateral sclerosis (ALS)	Progressive weakness and wasting of muscles caused by destruction of motor neurons
Huntington's chorea	Autosomal dominant genetic disorder resulting in progressive dementia and involuntary, spasmodic movements of limb and facial muscles
Multiple sclerosis (MS)	Demyelination of neurons in the central nervous system (CNS) resulting in progressive weakness, visual disturbances, mood alterations, and cognitive deficits
Parkinson's disease	Progressive loss of dopamine in the CNS causing tremor, muscle rigidity, and abnormal movement and posture

Fast Facts Neurodegenerative Diseases

Parkinson's Disease

- Over 1.5 million Americans have Parkinson's disease.
- Most patients with Parkinson's disease are above the age of 50.
- Greater than 50% of patients with Parkinson's disease who have difficulty with voluntary movement are less than 60 years of age.
- More men than women develop this disorder.

Dementia

- Of all patients with dementia, 60% to 70% have Alzheimer's disease.
- Over 4 million Americans have Alzheimer's disease.
- Alzheimer's disease mainly affects patients over the age of 65.

Multiple Sclerosis

- About 1.1 million people worldwide have MS.
- Onset of symptoms typically occurs between ages 15 and 40.
- Women are affected twice as often as men.
- MS occurs most often in Caucasian people of northern European origin.
- MS is about five times more prevalent in temperate climates than in tropical climates.

The cause of most neurologic degenerative diseases is unknown. Most progress from hardly noticeable signs and symptoms early in the disease to serious neurologic and cognitive deficits. In their early stages, disorders may be difficult to diagnose. With the exception of Parkinson's disease, pharmacotherapy provides only minimal benefit. Currently, medication is unable to cure any of the major neurodegenerative diseases.

PARKINSON'S DISEASE

Parkinson's disease is a degenerative disorder of the CNS caused by death of neurons that produce the brain neurotransmitter dopamine. It is the second most common degenerative disease of the nervous system, affecting many Americans. Pharmacotherapy is often successful in reducing some of the distressing symptoms of this disorder.

Parkinson's disease is progressive with the occurrence of full symptoms taking many years.

CORE CONCEPT 12.2

Parkinson's disease primarily affects patients older than 50 years of age; however, even teenagers can develop the disorder. Men are affected slightly more often than women. The disease is progressive. The appearance of full symptoms often takes many years. The symptoms of Parkinson's disease, described as **parkinsonism**, are summarized as follows:

- *Tremors* The hands and head develop a palsy-like motion or shakiness when at rest; *pill-rolling* is a common behavior in progressive states, in which patients rub the thumb and forefinger together as if a pill were between them.

- *Muscle rigidity* Stiffness may resemble symptoms of arthritis. Patients often have difficulty bending over or moving limbs. These symptoms may not be noticeable at first but become more obvious as the disease progresses.

- *Bradykinesia* This is the most noticeable of all symptoms. Patients may have difficulty chewing, swallowing, or speaking. Patients with Parkinson's disease have difficulties initiating movement and controlling fine muscle movements. Walking often becomes difficult, and patients shuffle their feet without taking normal strides.

brady = *slow*
kinesia = *movement*

- *Postural instability* Patients may be humped over slightly and may easily lose their balance. Stumbling results in frequent falls and injuries.

affective = *body emotion*
flattening = *without expression*

- *Affective flattening* Patients often have a "masked face" where there is little facial expression or blinking of the eyes.

Although Parkinson's disease is a progressive neurologic disorder primarily affecting muscle movement, other health problems often develop in these patients, including anxiety, depression, sleep disturbances, dementia, and disturbances of the autonomic nervous system (difficulty urinating and performing sexually). Several theories have been proposed to explain the development of parkinsonism. Because some patients with Parkinson's symptoms have a family history of this disorder, a genetic link is highly probable. Numerous environmental toxins, such as carbon monoxide, cyanide, manganese, chlorine, and pesticides, also have been suggested as a cause, but results of studies have not proven the cause–effect link. Viral infections, head trauma, and stroke have also been proposed as causes of parkinsonism.

substantia = *substance*
nigra = *black*

Symptoms of parkinsonism develop due to the degeneration and destruction of dopamine-producing neurons found within an area of the brain known as the *substantia nigra*. When not enough dopamine is released, this neurotransmitter cannot make contact with other critical areas of the brain.

corpus = *body*
striatum = *striped*

The most critical area for dopamine contact is the *corpus striatum*, an area responsible for controlling unconscious muscle movement. Patients with Parkinson's disease have difficulty initiating and controlling movements. Balance, posture, muscle tone, and involuntary muscle movements depend on the proper balance between dopamine (inhibitory) and acetylcholine (stimulatory). Under normal conditions, the inhibitory effects of dopamine and the excitatory effects of acetycholine balance one another to produce smooth coordinated muscle movement. If dopamine is absent, acetylcholine is able to overstimulate the corpus striatum. For this reason, drug therapy for parkinsonism focuses not only on restoring dopamine function but also on blocking the effect of acetylcholine within this sensitive area of the brain.

extra = *outside*
pyramidal = *medullary pyramidal tracts*
symptoms = *involuntary motor characteristics (e.g., EPS)*

Extrapyramidal symptoms (EPS) develop in response to the same neurochemical actions that cause Parkinson's disease. Recall that antipsychotic drugs act by blocking dopamine receptors. Treatment with some antipsychotic drugs may cause parkinsonism-like symptoms by interfering with the same neural pathway and functions affected by the lack of dopamine. Antiparkinson drugs are sometimes used to treat EPS caused by antipsychotic medications.

EPS may occur suddenly and become a medical emergency. With acute EPS, patients' muscles may spasm or lock up. Fever and confusion are other signs or symptoms of this reaction. If acute EPS occur in a healthcare facility, short-term medical treatment may be provided by administering diphenhydramine (Benadryl), which is an antihistamine that has acetylcholine-blocking properties. When symptoms are recognized outside a healthcare facility, the patient should be immediately taken to the emergency department. Untreated acute episodes of EPS can be fatal.

Concept Review **12.1**

- Parkinson's disease primarily affects which body functions? What are the five major symptoms of this disorder?

CORE CONCEPT 12.3

Antiparkinson drugs act on the brain to restore the balance between dopamine and acetylcholine.

The goal of pharmacotherapy for Parkinson's disease is to increase the ability of the patient to perform normal daily activities such as eating, walking, dressing, and bathing. Although pharmacotherapy does not cure this disorder, it can dramatically reduce symptoms in some patients.

anti = *against*
cholinergic = *acetylcholine action*

As mentioned, antiparkinson drugs are given to restore the balance of dopamine and acetylcholine within the corpus striatum of the brain. These drugs include dopaminergic drugs and anticholinergics (cholinergic blockers).

Dopaminergic Drugs

dopaminergic = *dopamine action*

Dopaminergic drugs, shown in Table 12.2 ◆, are used to increase dopamine action within critical areas of the corpus striatum. The basic ingredient in many of the preferred drugs for parkinsonism is levodopa, a dopaminergic substance that has been used more often than any other for this disorder. As shown in Figure 12.1 ■, levodopa is a precursor (a more basic chemical form) of dopamine. Supplying the nerve terminals directly with levodopa leads to increased synthesis of dopamine. Levodopa can cross the blood-brain barrier but dopamine cannot. Therefore, dopamine by itself is not used for therapy. The effectiveness of levodopa can be enhanced by combining it with carbidopa. This combination, marketed as Parcopa or Sinemet, makes more levodopa available to enter the CNS. Carbidopa (Lodosyn) alone can also increase the concentration of dopamine and levodopa in the brain.

Levodopa is chemically similar to some amino acids. Foods high in protein use the same pathways for the absorption into the bloodstream or brain, and therefore compete with levodopa (with or without

TABLE 12.2 Dopaminergic Drugs Used for Parkinsonism

Drug	Route and Adult Dose	Remarks
amantadine (Symmetrel)	PO; 100 mg daily or bid	Also for infection with influenza A virus; for relief of drug-induced EPS; may cause release of dopamine from nerve terminals
apomorphine	SC; 2 mg for the first dose; every few days, doses may be increased by 1 mg (max: 6 mg); if more than 1 week passes between doses, titration should be restarted at 2 mg	Activates dopamine receptors; may improve ability to walk, talk, and move
bromocriptine (Parlodel)	PO; 1.25–2.5 mg/day up to 100 mg/day in divided doses	Also for suppression of lactation, female infertility, and overproduction of growth hormone; activates the dopamine receptor directly
entacapone (Comtan)	PO; 200 mg given with levodopa–carbidopa up to 8 times/day	Blocks synaptic enzyme catecholamine O-methyl transferase (COMT) responsible for metabolizing dopamine
levodopa–carbidopa (Parcopa, Sinemet)	PO; 1 tablet containing 10 mg carbidopa/100 mg levodopa or 25 mg carbidopa/100 mg levodopa tid (max: 6 tablets/day)	Prevents metabolism of levodopa, enhancing dopamine action
Pr levodopa–carbidopa-entacapone (Stalevo)	PO; 1 tablet containing 10 mg carbidopa/100 mg levodopa or 25 mg carbidopa/100 mg levodopa tid (max: 6 tablets/day)	Chemical precursor to dopamine combined with a dopamine enhancer and a catecholamine O-methyl transferase (COMT) enzyme inhibitor
pramipexole (Mirapex)	PO; start with 0.125 mg tid for 1 week, double this dose for the next week, continue to increase by 0.25 mg/dose tid every week to a target dose of 1.5 mg tid	Activates dopamine receptors; also approved to treat restless legs syndrome
rasagiline (Azilect)	PO; 0.5–1 mg once daily	Blocks monoamine oxidase (MAO), the enzyme that degrades dopamine within brain nerve terminals
ropinirole (Requip)	PO; start with 0.25 mg tid, may increase by 0.25 mg/dose tid every week to a target dose of 1 mg tid	Activates dopamine receptors; approved to treat restless legs syndrome
rotigotine (Neupro)	Transdermal; start at 2 mg/24 hours for patients with early-stage Parkinson's disease; may be increased weekly by 2 mg/24 hours (max: 6 mg/24 hours); patients with advanced-stage Parkinson's disease may be initiated at 4 mg/24 hours (recommended: 8 mg/24 hours); for restless legs syndrome, start at 1 mg/24 hours (max: 3 mg/24 hours)	Approved to treat early-stage Parkinson's disease, advanced-stage Parkinson's disease and restless legs syndrome
selegiline (Eldepryl, Zelapar)	PO; 5 mg/dose bid; doses greater than 10 mg/day are potentially toxic	Blocks monoamine oxidase (MAO), the enzyme that degrades dopamine within brain nerve terminals; also for depression
tolcapone (Tasmar)	PO; 100 mg tid (max: 600 mg/day)	Blocks synaptic enzyme COMT responsible for metabolizing dopamine

carbidopa) for absorption. If levodopa is taken with foods high in protein, the effectiveness of the medication will be reduced. In addition, levodopa is absorbed in the small intestine, therefore any foods or conditions that delay gastric emptying will reduce drug availability.

Other approaches to enhancing dopamine are used in treating parkinsonism. Tolcapone (Tasmar), entacapone (Comtan), rasagiline (Azilect), and selegiline (Eldepryl, Zelapar) inhibit enzymes that normally destroy levodopa and dopamine. Rasagiline and selegiline are monoamine oxidase (MAO) inhibitors. Apomorphine (Apokyn), bromocriptine (Parlodel), pramipexole (Mirapex), and ropinirole (Requip) directly activate the dopamine receptor and are called *dopamine receptor drugs*. Amantadine (Symmetrel), an antiviral agent, causes the release of dopamine from nerve terminals. All these drugs are considered adjuncts to the pharmacotherapy of parkinsonism because they are not as effective as levodopa. In terms of

catecholamine = *neurotransmitter group synthesized from dopamine*

O-methyl-transferase = *degrading enzyme transferring a methyl (CH$_3$) group (e.g., COMT)*

monoamine oxidase (MAO) = *catecholamine degrading enzyme*

FIGURE 12.1

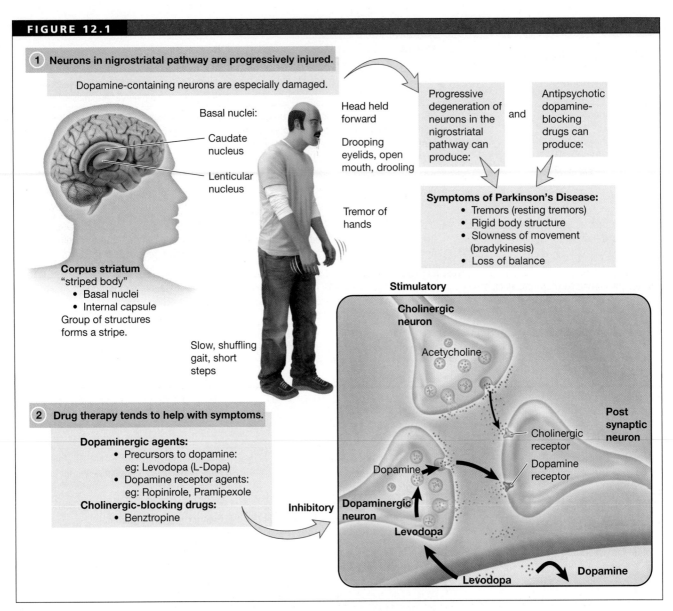

1 **Neurons in nigrostriatal pathway are progressively injured.**

Dopamine-containing neurons are especially damaged.

Basal nuclei:

— Caudate nucleus

— Lenticular nucleus

Corpus striatum
"striped body"
• Basal nuclei
• Internal capsule
Group of structures
forms a stripe.

Head held forward

Drooping eyelids, open mouth, drooling

Tremor of hands

Slow, shuffling gait, short steps

Progressive degeneration of neurons in the nigrostriatal pathway can produce:

and

Antipsychotic dopamine-blocking drugs can produce:

Symptoms of Parkinson's Disease:
• Tremors (resting tremors)
• Rigid body structure
• Slowness of movement (bradykinesis)
• Loss of balance

2 **Drug therapy tends to help with symptoms.**

Dopaminergic agents:
• Precursors to dopamine:
  eg: Levodopa (L-Dopa)
• Dopamine receptor agents:
  eg: Ropinirole, Pramipexole
Cholinergic-blocking drugs:
• Benztropine

Stimulatory

Cholinergic neuron

Acetycholine

Post synaptic neuron

Cholinergic receptor

Dopamine receptor

Dopamine

Dopaminergic neuron

Inhibitory

Levodopa

Levodopa

Dopamine

Dopamine cannot cross the blood–brain barrier. Levodopa, its precursor, can. Once levodopa crosses the blood–brain barrier and enters neurons, it is converted into dopamine, which normally inhibits firing of the next neuron. Natural acetylcholine in the brain stimulates the same postsynaptic neuron. Thus, to restore normal neuronal activity, drug therapy attempts to either (a) restore dopamine inhibitory action or (b) block acetylcholine (cholinergic) stimulatory activity.

activities of daily living (ADLs), most levodopa–carbidopa combination drugs are thought to control motor symptoms better. Pramipexole (Mirapex) and ropinirole (Requip) have proven to be safe and effective for initial sole therapy and also when combined with levodopa–carbidopa.

Additional drugs that reduce the requirements for levodopa–carbidopa include the catechol-O-methyl transferase (COMT) inhibitors. Entacapone (Comtan) and tolcapone (Tasmar) are COMT inhibitors. Like levodopa–carbidopa, these drugs increase concentrations of existing dopamine in nerve terminals and improve motor fluctuations related to the "wearing-off" effect. Entacapone combined with carbidopa and levodopa is marketed as Stalevo. Side effects of COMT inhibitors include mental confusion and hallucinations, nausea and vomiting, cramps, headache, diarrhea, and possible liver damage.

Rotigotine (Neupro) is a new dopamine receptor transdermal patch that can be applied once daily. In clinical trials (2012), it was shown to effectively treat early Parkinson's disease as monotherapy and was even shown to be effective in the treatment of advanced-stage Parkinson's disease and restless legs syndrome (RLS). The most common side effects of rotigotine for RLS are application site reactions, drowsiness, nausea, and headache.

Drug Prototype: ⓟ *Levodopa, Carbidopa, and Entacapone (Stalevo)*
Therapeutic Class: Antiparkinson drugs
Pharmacologic Class: Dopamine precursor, dopaminergic drugs

Actions and Uses: Stalevo restores the neurotransmitter dopamine in extrapyramidal areas of the brain, thus relieving some Parkinson's symptoms. To increase its effect, levodopa is combined with two other drugs, carbidopa and entacapone, which prevent its enzymatic breakdown. Several months may be needed to achieve maximum therapeutic effects.

Adverse Effects and Interactions: Side effects of Stalevo include uncontrolled and purposeless movements such as extending the fingers and shrugging the shoulders, involuntary movements, loss of appetite, nausea, and vomiting. Muscle twitching and spasmodic winking are early signs of toxicity. Orthostatic hypotension is common in some patients. The drug should be discontinued gradually, because abrupt withdrawal can produce acute parkinsonism. Foods high in protein and vitamin B6 will decrease the effectiveness of levodopa or levodopa–carbidopa.

Stalevo interacts with many drugs. For example, tricyclic antidepressants decrease effects of Stalevo, increase postural hypotension, and may increase sympathetic activity, with hypertension and sinus tachycardia. Stalevo cannot be used if an MAO inhibitor was taken within 14 to 28 days, because concurrent use may precipitate hypertensive crisis. Haloperidol taken concurrently may antagonize the therapeutic effects of Stalevo. Methyldopa may increase toxicity. Antihypertensives may cause increased hypotensive effects. Antiseizure medication may decrease the therapeutic effects of Stalevo. Antacids containing magnesium, calcium, or sodium bicarbonate may increase Stalevo absorption, which could lead to toxicity. Kava may worsen the Parkinson's symptoms.

Cholinergic Blockers (Anticholinergics)
A second approach to changing the balance between dopamine and acetylcholine in the brain is to give cholinergic blockers, or anticholinergics. By blocking the effect of acetylcholine, anticholinergics inhibit the overactivity of this neurotransmitter within the corpus striatum. These drugs are listed in Table 12.3 ◆.

Anticholinergics such as atropine were the first drugs used to treat parkinsonism. The large number of adverse effects has limited the use of these drugs. The anticholinergics now used for parkinsonism act within the CNS and produce fewer adverse effects. However, they continue to cause unpleasant autonomic symptoms such as dry mouth, blurred vision, tachycardia, urinary retention, and constipation (very troublesome). The centrally acting anticholinergics are not as effective as levodopa in relieving severe symptoms of parkinsonism. They are used early in the courses of the disease when symptoms are less severe, in patients who cannot tolerate levodopa, and in combination therapy with older antiparkinson drugs.

Concept Review   12.2

■ Antiparkinson drugs attempt to restore the balance of which two major CNS neurotransmitters?

TABLE 12.3 Anticholinergic Drugs Used for Parkinsonism

Drug	Route and Adult Dose	Remarks
ⓟ benztropine (Cogentin)	PO; 0.5–1 mg/day, gradually increase as needed (max: 6 mg/day)	Also used to relieve EPS from neuroleptic drugs; does not lighten tardive dyskinesia
biperiden (Akineton)	PO; 2 mg daily to qid	Blocks acetylcholine receptors; thus, actions associated with muscarinic blockade are observed (e.g., blurred vision, dry mouth); available in IM/IV forms.
diphenhydramine (Benadryl) (see page 460 for the Drug Prototype box)	PO; 25–50 mg tid or qid (max: 300 mg/day)	Also for allergic reactions, motion sickness, sedation, and coughing; blocks cholinergic function even though it is an antihistamine; available in IM/IV forms.
trihexyphenidyl (Artane)	PO; 1 mg for day 1; double this for day 2; then increase by 2 mg every 3–5 days up to 6–10 mg/day (max: 15 mg/day)	Also used to relieve EPS; off-label use for Huntington's chorea and spasmodic torticollis

Drug Prototype: (Pr) *Benztropine (Cogentin)*

Therapeutic Class: **Antiparkinson drug**

Pharmacologic Class: **Centrally acting cholinergic receptor blocker**

Actions and Uses: Benztropine acts by blocking excess cholinergic stimulation of neurons in the corpus striatum. It is used for relief of parkinsonism symptoms and for the treatment of EPS brought on by antipsychotic pharmacotherapy. This medication suppresses tremors but does not affect tardive dyskinesia.

Adverse Effects and Interactions: As expected from its autonomic action, benztropine can cause typical anticholinergic adverse effects such as sedation, dry mouth, constipation, and tachycardia.

Benztropine interacts with many drugs. For example, benztropine should not be taken with alcohol, tricyclic antidepressants, MAOIs, phenothiazines, procainamide, or quinidine because of combined sedative effects. Over-the-counter (OTC) cold medicines and alcohol should be avoided. Other drugs that enhance dopamine release or activation of the dopamine receptor may produce additive effects. Haloperidol will cause decreased effectiveness.

Antihistamines, phenothiazines, tricyclics, disopyramide, and quinidine may increase anticholinergic effects, and antidiarrheals may decrease absorption.

ALZHEIMER'S DISEASE

Alzheimer's disease (AD) affects memory, thinking, and behavior. It is one of the forms of dementia that gradually gets worse over time. As many as 50% of people are affected with this disease by the age of 85. The patient generally lives 5 to 10 years following diagnosis; AD is the fourth leading cause of death. Drugs help slow down the rate at which symptoms become worse.

Dementia is a degenerative disorder characterized by progressive memory loss, confusion, and inability to think or communicate effectively. Consciousness and perception are usually unaffected. Although the cause of most dementia is unknown, it is usually associated with cerebral atrophy or other structural changes within the brain.

Structural damage within the brain of patients with AD has been well documented. *Amyloid plaques* and *neurofibrillary tangles*, found at autopsy, are present in nearly all patients with AD. It is suspected that these structural changes are caused by chronic inflammatory or oxidative cellular damage to surrounding neurons. There is a loss in both the number and function of neurons in patients with AD.

CORE CONCEPT 12.4

Patients with Alzheimer's disease experience a dramatic loss of ability to perform tasks that require acetylcholine as the CNS neurotransmitter.

Patients with AD experience a dramatic loss of ability to perform tasks that require acetylcholine as the neurotransmitter. Because acetylcholine is a major neurotransmitter within the hippocampus (an area of the brain responsible for learning and memory) and other parts of the cerebral cortex, neuronal function within these brain areas is especially affected. Thus, an inability to remember and to recall information is among the early symptoms of AD. Symptoms of AD include the following:

- Impaired memory and judgment
- Confusion or disorientation
- Inability to recognize family or friends
- Aggressive behavior
- Depression
- Psychoses, including paranoia and delusions
- Anxiety

CORE CONCEPT 12.5

Alzheimer's disease is treated with acetylcholinesterase inhibitors.

acetylcholinesterase (AchE) = *Ach terminating enzyme*

inhibitor = *suppressing factor*

Drugs are used to slow memory loss and other progressive symptoms of dementia. Additional drugs may be given to treat associated symptoms such as depression, anxiety, or psychoses. The acetylcholinesterase inhibitors are the most widely used class of drugs for treating AD. Representative drugs used for treatment of AD are listed in Table 12.4 ◆.

TABLE 12.4	Drugs Used for Alzheimer's Disease	
Drug	**Route and Adult Dose**	**Remarks**
(Pr) donepezil (Aricept)	PO; 5–10 mg at bedtime	For mild to moderate dementia; may cause nausea, diarrhea, muscle cramps, and weight loss
galantamine (Razadyne, Reminyl)	PO; start with 4 mg bid at least 4 weeks; if tolerated, may increase by 4 mg bid every 4 weeks to target a dose of 12 mg bid (max: 8–16 mg bid)	For mild to moderate dementia; may cause weight loss, dizziness, nausea, vomiting, and hypotension when changing positions
memantine (Namenda)	PO; starting dose is 5 mg once daily; the dose usually is increased to 5 mg twice daily, then 5 mg and 10 mg as separate doses daily, and finally 10 mg twice daily	For moderate to severe dementia; NMDA receptor blocking drug; may cause a serious skin reaction, fatigue, dizziness, headache, confusion, vomiting, coughing, constipation, pain, and difficulty in breathing
rivastigmine (Exelon)	PO; start with 1.5 mg bid with food, may increase by 1.5 mg bid every 2 weeks if tolerated; target dose is 3–6 mg bid (max: 12 mg bid) Transdermal; 5 cm² patch (4.6mg/24 hours), 10 cm² patch (9.5mg/24 hours)	For mild to moderate dementia; may cause flu-like symptoms, dizziness, and weight loss
tacrine (Cognex)	PO; 10 mg qid, increase in 40 mg/day increments not sooner than every 6 weeks (max: 160 mg/day)	For mild to moderate dementia; off-label used for severe dementia in patients with HIV infection; may cause nausea, vomiting, and liver toxicity

Acetylcholinesterase Inhibitors

The Food and Drug Administration (FDA) has approved only a few drugs specifically for AD. The most effective of these medications acts by intensifying the effect of acetylcholine at the cholinergic receptor, as shown in Figure 12.2 ■ . Acetylcholine is naturally degraded in the synapse by the enzyme **acetylcholinesterase (AchE)**. When AchE is inhibited, acetylcholine levels increase and greatly impact the receptors. As described in Chapter 8, the AchE inhibitors *indirectly* stimulate the receptors for acetylcholine.

When treating AD, the goal of pharmacotherapy is to improve function in ADLs, behavior, and cognition. Although the AchE inhibitors improve functions in all three areas, their effectiveness is limited. These drugs do not cure AD—they only slow its progression. Therapy is begun as soon as the diagnosis of AD is established. These drugs are ineffective in treating the severe stages of this disorder, probably because so many neurons have been damaged. Increasing the levels of acetylcholine is only effective if there are functioning neurons present. Therefore, the AchE inhibitors are often discontinued as the disease progresses because their therapeutic benefit may not outweigh their expense or the risk of adverse effects. When discontinuing therapy, doses of the AchE inhibitors should be lowered gradually.

ADLs = *activities of daily living*

All AchE inhibitors used to treat AD are equally effective. Their adverse effects are those expected of drugs that enhance the parasympathetic nervous system (see Chapter 8). These include nausea, vomiting, and diarrhea. Of the drugs available for AD, tacrine (Cognex) is associated with liver toxicity. Rivastigmine (Exelon) is associated with weight loss, a potentially serious adverse effect in some older adults.

Other Drugs That Slow Progression of AD

Although AchE inhibitors are the mainstay of treatment for AD dementia, several other agents have been investigated for possible benefit in delaying the progression of this disease. Because at least some of the neuronal changes in AD are caused by oxidative cellular damage, antioxidants such as vitamin E have been examined. Other drugs purported to prevent or help slow the onset of AD progression have been NSAIDs and selegiline, an MAO inhibitor.

In 2003, memantine (Namenda) was approved by the FDA for combination treatment of moderate to severe AD. Its mechanism of action differs from that of the cholinesterase inhibitors. Unlike cholinesterase inhibitors that address the cholinergic defect in the brains of patients with AD, memantine reduces the abnormally high levels of glutamate. Glutamate exerts its neural effects through interaction with the N-methyl-D-aspartate (NMDA) receptor. When bound to the receptor, glutamate causes calcium to enter neurons, producing an excitatory effect. Too much glutamate in the brain may be responsible for brain cell death. Memantine, along with cholinesterase inhibitors such as donepezil, may have a protective function in reducing neuronal calcium overload.

Caprylidene (Axona) is a medical food approved for patients with AD. This food medication is metabolized into ketone bodies, which the brain can use for energy even when its ability to process glucose is impaired. Brain-imaging scans of older adults and those with AD have revealed an impaired ability to take up glucose, the brain's preferred source of energy. Thus, patients with AD may benefit from this type of therapy.

FIGURE 12.2

Alzheimer's medications work by intensifying the effect of acetylcholine at the receptor.

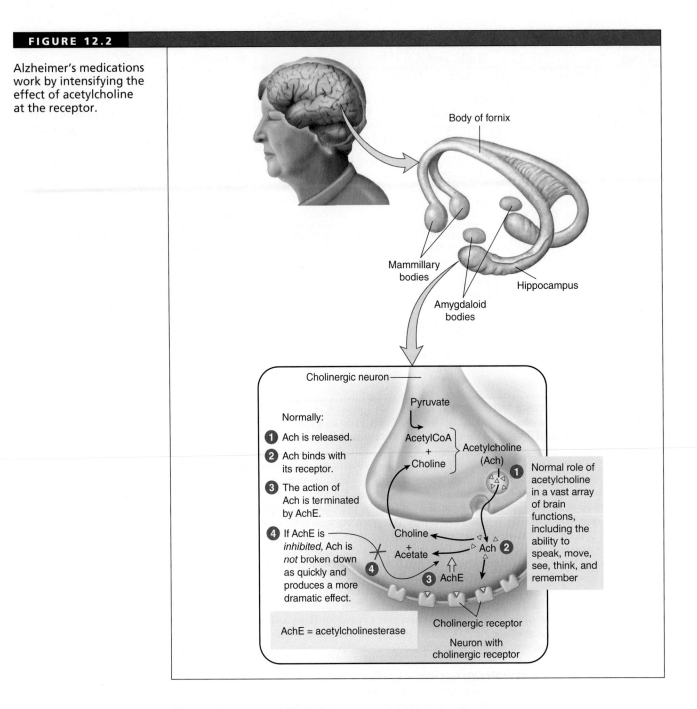

Drugs That Treat Behavioral Symptoms of AD

Agitation occurs in most patients with AD. This is often accompanied by delusional behavior, paranoia, hallucinations, or other psychotic symptoms. Atypical antipsychotic drugs such as risperidone (Risperdal) and olanzapine (Zyprexa) may be used to control these episodes. Conventional antipsychotics such as haloperidol (Haldol) are occasionally prescribed, although EPS often limit their use.

Although not as common as agitation, anxiety and depression may also occur in patients with AD. Anxiolytics such as buspirone (BuSpar) or some of the benzodiazepines are used to control excessive anxiety (see Chapter 9). Mood stabilizers such as sertraline (Zoloft), citalopram (Celexa), or fluoxetine (Prozac) may be given when major depression interferes with ADLs (see Chapter 10).

Concept Review   12.3

■ Alzheimer's disease is a dysfunction of which brain neurotransmitters? How do drugs for Alzheimer's disease restore neurotransmitter function and improve symptoms of dementia?

Drug Prototype: ℗ *Donepezil (Aricept)*

Therapeutic Class: Drug for Alzheimer's disease   **Pharmacologic Class: Acetylcholinerase inhibitor**

Actions and Uses: Donepezil is an AchE inhibitor that improves memory in cases of mild to moderate Alzheimer's dementia by enhancing the effects of acetylcholine in neurons in the cerebral cortex that have not yet been damaged. Patients should receive pharmacotherapy for at least six months prior to assessing the maximum benefits of drug therapy. Improvement in memory may be observed as early as one to four weeks following medication. The therapeutic effects of donepezil are often short-lived, and the degree of improvement is modest at best. An advantage of donepezil over other drugs in its class is that its long half-life permits it to be given once daily.

Adverse Effects and Interactions: Common adverse effects of donepezil are vomiting, diarrhea, and darkened urine. CNS adverse effects include insomnia, syncope, depression, headache, and irritability. Musculoskeletal adverse effects include muscle cramps, arthritis, and bone fractures. Generalized adverse effects include headache, fatigue, chest pain, increased libido, hot flashes, urinary incontinence, dehydration, and blurred vision. Unlike with tacrine, hepatotoxicity has not been observed. Patients with bradycardia, hypotension, asthma, hyperthyroidism, or active peptic ulcer disease should be monitored carefully. Anticholinergics will be less effective. Donepezil interacts with several other drugs. For example, bethanechol causes a synergistic effect. Phenobarbital, phenytoin, dexamethasone, and rifampin may speed elimination of donepezil. Quinidine or ketoconazole may inhibit metabolism of donepezil. Because donepezil acts by increasing cholinergic activity, two parasympathomimetics should not be administered at the same time.

CAM THERAPY

Ginkgo biloba for Dementia

The seeds and leaves of *Ginkgo biloba* have been used in traditional Chinese medicine for thousands of years. The tree is planted throughout the world, including the United States. In Western medicine, the focus has been on treating depression and memory loss. In Germany, an extract of *Ginkgo biloba* is approved for the treatment of dementia.

Ginkgo has been shown to improve mental functioning and stabilize AD. The mechanism of action seems to be related to increasing the blood supply to the brain by dilating blood vessels, decreasing the viscosity of the blood, and modifying the neurotransmitter system. The exact benefit of ginkgo remains unclear because some studies concluded that cognitive performance improved, whereas others have shown no improvement in the symptoms or progress of AD. Ginkgo is considered safe; however, it may increase the risk of bleeding in patients taking anticoagulants. A review of nine different trials of the effects of ginkgo on dementia concluded that the supplement was more effective than a placebo (Weinmann, Roll, Schwartzbach, Vauth & Willich, 2010)

MULTIPLE SCLEROSIS

Multiple sclerosis (MS) is a disorder characterized by damaged myelin located within the CNS. Antibodies produced by the patient slowly target and destroy myelin, axonal membranes, and supporting cells of the CNS, for example oligodendrocytes. As axons are destroyed, the ability of nerves to conduct electrical impulses is impaired. Inflammation accompanies damaged tissue, and multiple filamentous plaques called *scleroses* are formed.

oligo = *little*
dendro = *branched*
cytes = *cells*

scleroses = *thickened or hardened plaques*

Symptoms of multiple sclerosis result from demyelination of CNS nerve fibers.

During the early stages of MS, some damaged axons recover due to partial myelination and the development of alternative circuitry, but as antibodies continue to attack neural tissue, further damage and inflammation lead to neuronal death. Patients often have recurrent episodes of neurologic dysfunction, which progress at a fairly rapid rate.

The etiology of MS is unknown. Many clinicians and scientists suspect genetic or microbial factors due to reports that, in most cases, MS occurs in regions of colder climate. One theory proposes acquired

neurologic = *pertaining to the nervous system*

neuropathic = *nervous disease*

spasticity = *stiffness of muscle*

cognitive = *reasoning ability*

vertigo = *confusion and disorientation*

immunological resistance against pathogenic factors in warmer climates. Microscopic pathogens such as viruses have been suggested, though there is no strong evidence for this theory.

Signs and symptoms associated with axonal injury include fatigue, heat sensitivity, neuropathic pain, spasticity, impaired cognitive ability, disruption of balance and coordination, bowel and bladder symptoms, sexual dysfunction, dizziness, vertigo, visual impairment, and slurred speech. Although the disease is progressive, the precise course of MS is unpredictable, and each patient experiences a variety of symptoms depending on the extent and localization of demyelination.

Drugs for multiple sclerosis reduce immune attacks in the brain and treat unfavorable symptoms.

Like many neurodegenerative disorders, there are no drugs available that can cure MS or reverse the progressive nature of the disease. Existing drugs are only partially effective and some have serious adverse effects. Drugs are used in the treatment of MS to either modify the progression of the disease or to manage symptoms of the disease. Drugs for treating MS are shown in Table 12.5 ◆.

One approach to modify disease progression attempts to reduce inflammation and prevent attacks on the nervous system. Drugs also address impairment of movement due to demyelination of neurons. Goals are accomplished through the use of immune system modulating drugs, immunosuppressants, and drugs that block neuronal potassium channels.

The most treatable form of this disorder is *relapsing-remitting MS (RRMS)*. This condition involves unpredictable relapses (attacks) during which time new symptoms appear or existing symptoms become more severe. These symptoms can last for varying periods (days or months), followed by partial or total remission (recovery). In RRMS, the disease may be inactive for months or years. On average, people with RRMS have one or two attacks a year.

Immune system modulating drugs (also described later in the text as immunostimulants [see Chapter 25]) are used to treat the underlying causes of MS and to decrease the overall relapse rate. Interferon beta-1a (Avonex, Rebif) and interferon beta-1b (Betaseron, Extavia) are first-line therapies for slowing the neuronal damage caused by MS. Although generally well tolerated, the interferons have unfavorable adverse effects, including flu-like symptoms (e.g., headaches, fever, chills, muscle aches), anxiety, discomfort experienced at the injection site, and liver toxicity. Due to toxicity concerns and additive effects, caution should be exercised when taking these drugs in combination with chemotherapeutic agents or bone marrow-suppressing drugs.

Another first-line drug treatment, glatiramer (Copaxone) is an immunomodulating synthetic protein that resembles myelin basic protein, an essential part of the nerve's myelin coating. Because glatiramer resembles myelin, it is thought to curb the body's attack on the myelin covering and reduce the creation

TABLE 12.5 Drugs Used for Multiple Sclerosis

Drug	Comments	Administered
FOR IMMUNE ATTACKS AGAINST THE CNS		
dalfampridine (Ampyra)	Potassium channel blocker to treat walking impairment	PO
dimethyl fumarate (Tecfidera)	Myelin oxidative stress reducer	PO
fingolimod (Gilenya)	Immune system modulator	PO
glatiramer (Copaxone)	Immune system modulator; myelin protein protectant	SC
interferon beta-1a (Avonex, Rebif)	Immune system modulator	IM and SC
interferon beta-1b (Betaseron, Extavia)	Immune system modulator	SC
mitoxantrone (Novantrone)	Immunosuppressant drug	IV
natalizumab (Tysabri)	Immune system modulator	IV
teriflunomide (Aubagio)	Immune system modulator	PO

Drug	Comments	Symptoms Relieved
FOR THE RELIEF OF MS SYMPTOMS		
modafinil (Provigil)	Central adrenergic drug	Fatigue, memory loss, weakness
amantadine (Symmetrel)	Dopaminergic drug	Fatigue, memory loss, weakness
gabapentin (Neurontin)	Antiseizure drug	Anxiety, insomnia, neuropathic pain
methylprednisolone (Solu-Medrol)	Corticosteroid medication	Myelin swelling and inflammation

of new brain lesions. Glatiramer is available in prefilled syringes that can be kept at room temperature for several days. However, patients often complain of adverse effects and having to inject themselves. Adverse effects include redness, pain, swelling, itching, or a lump at the site of injection. Flushing, chest pain, weakness, infection, pain, nausea, joint pain, anxiety, and muscle stiffness are other common adverse effects.

Mitoxantrone (Novantrone) is an FDA-drug approved for patients with MS who have not responded to interferon or glatiramer therapy. Primarily a chemotherapeutic drug, mitoxantrone is substantially more toxic than the immune system modulating drugs. Toxicity is a concern due to irreversible cardiac injury and potential harm to a fetus. Notable adverse effects are reversible hair loss, gastrointestinal (GI) discomfort (nausea and vomiting), and allergic symptoms (itching, rash, hypotension). Some patients experience a blue-green tint to their urine, which is harmless.

Approved by the FDA in 2010, fingolimod (Gilenya) is an oral medication used for treating relapsing forms of MS. Its mechanism of action is unknown, although it may work by reducing the number of circulating lymphocytes, leading to reduced migration of leukocytes into the CNS. White blood cells cause inflammation and destruction of nerves in patients with MS. Fingolimod decreases the number of MS flare-ups and slows down the development of physical impairment caused by MS.

In 2010, dalfampridine (Ampyra) tablets were approved by the FDA as the first treatment to address walking impairment in patients with MS. It exerts an effect through its broad-spectrum potassium channel blockade and has been shown to increase nerve conduction and improve walking speed. The most bothersome adverse effect of dalfampridine is increased seizure activity. Because of this concern, this drug is contraindicated in patients with a prior history of seizures.

contraindicated = *not advisable*

Approved in 2012, teriflunomide (Aubagio) is one of the newest immunomodulator therapies for relapsing MS. Teriflunomide is the active metabolite of leflunomide (Arava), a drug previously approved to treat rheumatoid arthritis. Therapy with teriflunomide must be carefully monitored because the drug can cause severe liver damage, renal failure, and bone marrow suppression. It is contraindicated in pregnant patients due to possible teratogenic effects on the fetus.

teratogenic = *causing birth defects*

Miscellaneous drugs used for MS include modafinil (Provigil) and amantadine (Symmetrel) for treating fatigue, memory loss, and progressive weakness symptoms. Modafinil is an alpha$_1$-adrenergic drug thought to activate receptors that respond to the brain neurotransmitter norepinephrine. This agent increases alertness and energy and improves memory. Gabapentin (Neurontin) is an antiseizure drug used for treating mood disturbances, including depression and sensitivity to pain (see Chapter 13). Methylprednisolone (Solu-Medrol) and prednisone are steroidal anti-inflammatory agents that are administered for brief periods when the patient is experiencing acute MS symptoms caused by swelling and inflammation in the brain. Other medications not found the in the table may be used routinely to help treat fatigue and neurologic symptoms due to MS (i.e., pain and discomfort).

MUSCLE SPASMS

Muscle spasms are involuntary contractions of a muscle or groups of muscles. The muscles tighten, develop a fixed pattern of resistance, and lose functioning ability.

Muscle spasms are caused by injury, overmedication, hypocalcemia, and debilitating neurologic disorders.

CORE CONCEPT 12.8

Muscle spasms are a common condition usually associated with overuse of and local injury to the skeletal muscle. Other causes of muscle spasms include overmedication with antipsychotic drugs (see Chapter 11), epilepsy, hypocalcemia, pain, and debilitating neurologic disorders. Patients with muscle spasms may experience inflammation, edema, and pain at the affected muscle; loss of coordination; and reduced mobility. When a muscle goes into spasm, it freezes in a contracted state. A single, prolonged contraction is called a *tonic spasm*, whereas multiple, rapidly repeated contractions are called *clonic spasms*. Treatment of muscle spasms includes use of both nonpharmacologic and pharmacologic therapies.

hypo = *lowered*
calc = *calcium*
emia = *blood levels*

tonic = *single prolonged transient*
clonic = *multiple repetitive transient*
spasms = *involuntary contractions*

Muscle spasms may be treated with nonpharmacologic or pharmacologic therapies.

CORE CONCEPT 12.9

Identifying the etiology of muscle spasms requires a careful history and a physical exam. After a determination has been made, nonpharmacologic therapies are normally used in conjunction with medications. Nonpharmacologic measures may be immobilization of the affected muscle, application of heat or cold, hydrotherapy, ultrasound, supervised exercises, massage, or manipulation.

etiology = *cause or origin*

Fast Facts Muscle Spasms

- More than 12 million people worldwide have muscle spasms.

- Muscle spasms severe enough to warrant drug therapy are often found in patients who have had other debilitating disorders, such as neurodegenerative diseases, stroke, injury or cerebral palsy.

- Cerebral palsy is usually associated with events that occur before or during birth, but it may be caused by head trauma or infection during the first few months or years of life.

- Dystonia affects about 250,000 people in the United States; it is the third most common movement disorder after Parkinson's disease and essential tremor.

- Researchers have recognized multiple forms of inheritable dystonia and identified at least 10 genes or chromosomal locations responsible for the various manifestations.

Pharmacotherapy for muscle spasms may include combinations of analgesics, anti-inflammatory drugs, and centrally acting skeletal muscle relaxants. Most skeletal muscle relaxants relieve symptoms of muscular stiffness and rigidity that result from muscular injury. Drugs also help improve mobility. Therapeutic goals are to minimize pain and discomfort, increase range of motion, and improve the patient's ability to function independently.

Concept Review 12.4

- Give several reasons why muscle spasms develop. What is the main goal of therapy for muscle spasms?

CORE CONCEPT 12.10

Many muscle relaxants treat muscle spasms by inhibiting upper motor neuron activity, causing sedation, or altering simple reflexes.

Antispasmodic drugs relieve symptoms of muscular stiffness and rigidity. They improve mobility in cases in which patients have restricted movements.

Many antispasmodic drugs treat muscle spasms at the level of the CNS. The exact mechanisms of action are not fully known, but it is believed that these drugs affect the brain and/or spinal cord by inhibiting upper motor neuron activity, causing sedation, or altering simple reflexes.

Skeletal muscle relaxants are used to treat local spasms resulting from muscular injury and may be prescribed alone or in combination with other medications to reduce pain and increase range of motion. Commonly used centrally acting medications are baclofen (Lioresal), cyclobenzaprine (Amrix, Flexeril), tizanidine (Zanaflex), and benzodiazepines such as diazepam (Valium), clonazepam (Klonopin), and lorazepam (Ativan) (Table 12.6 ◆). All of the centrally acting drugs can cause sedation.

Baclofen (Lioresal) is structurally similar to the inhibitory neurotransmitter gamma amino butyric acid (GABA) and produces its effect by a mechanism that is not fully known. It inhibits neuronal activity within the brain and possibly the spinal cord. There is some uncertainty about whether the spinal effects of baclofen are associated with GABA. Baclofen may be used to reduce muscle spasms in patients with MS, cerebral palsy, or spinal cord injury. Common adverse effects of baclofen are drowsiness, dizziness, weakness, and fatigue. Baclofen is often the drug of first choice because of its wide safety margin.

Tizanidine (Zanaflex) is a centrally acting alpha$_2$-adrenergic agonist that inhibits motor neurons, mainly at the spinal cord level. It also affects some neural activity in the brain, patients receiving high doses report drowsiness. Though uncommon, one adverse effect of tizanidine is hallucinations. The drug's most frequent adverse effects are dry mouth, fatigue, dizziness, and sleepiness. Tizanidine is as effective as baclofen and is considered by some to be the drug of first choice.

As discussed in Chapter 13, benzodiazepines inhibit both sensory and motor neuron activities by enhancing the effects of GABA. Common adverse effects include drowsiness and ataxia (loss of coordination). Benzodiazepines are usually prescribed for muscle relaxation when baclofen and tizanidine fail to produce adequate relief.

tetany = *prolonged tightened muscles*

TABLE 12.6   Centrally Acting Antispasmodic Drugs

Drug	Route and Adult Dose	Remarks
baclofen (Lioresal)	PO; 5 mg tid (max: 80 mg/day)	May be administered orally or by an implantable pump, which infuses medication directly into the subarachnoid space
carisoprodol (Soma)	PO; 350 mg tid	CNS depressant; does not inhibit motor activity like other conventional muscle relaxers; muscle relaxation seems to be related to sedation
chlorzoxazone (Paraflex, Parafon Forte)	PO; 250–500 mg tid–qid (max: 3 g/day)	Depresses nerve transmission in the brain and spinal cord, possibly by sedation; not effective for cerebral palsy
clonazepam (Klonopin)	PO; 0.5 mg tid (max: 20 mg/day)	Benzodiazepine usually taken in combination with other drugs; used for the relief of skeletal muscle spasms; primarily for seizure disorders
Ⓟ cyclobenzaprine (Amrix, Flexeril)	PO; 10–20 mg bid–qid (max: 60 mg/day)	Short-term relief of muscle spasms associated with acute musculoskeletal conditions; not for cerebral palsy or central nervous system diseases
diazepam (Valium) (see page 188 for the Drug Prototype box)	PO; 4–10 mg bid–qid; IM/IV 2–10 mg, repeat if needed in 3–4 hours; IV pump; administer emulsion at 5 mg/min	Benzodiazepine used for the relief of skeletal muscle spasms associated with cerebral palsy, partial paralysis
lorazepam (Ativan) (see page 116 for the Drug Prototype box)	PO; 1–2 mg bid–tid (max: 10 mg/day)	Benzodiazepine used for extreme muscle tension
metaxalone (Skelaxin)	PO; 800 mg tid–qid for maximum of 10 days	For acute musculoskeletal conditions; causes its effect through sedation
methocarbamol (Robaxin)	PO; 1.5 g qid for 2–3 days, then reduce to 1 g qid	Adjunct to physical therapy for acute musculoskeletal disorders and tetany
orphenadrine (Banflex, Myolin, Norflex)	PO; 100 mg bid	IM/IV forms available
tizanidine (Zanaflex)	PO; 4–8 mg tid–qid (max: 36 mg/day)	To relax muscle tone associated with spasticity; effective at the spinal cord level

---

Drug Prototype: Ⓟ **Cyclobenzaprine (Amrix, Flexeril)**

Therapeutic Class: Skeletal muscle relaxant, centrally acting

Pharmacologic Class: Catecholamine reuptake inhibitor

Actions and Uses: Cyclobenzaprine relieves muscle spasms of local origin without interfering with general muscle function. This drug acts by depressing motor activity, primarily in the brainstem, with limited effects also occurring in the spinal cord. It increases circulating levels of norepinephrine, blocking presynaptic uptake. Its mechanism of action is similar to that of tricyclic antidepressants (see Chapter 10). It causes muscle relaxation in acute muscle spasticity, but it is not effective in cases of cerebral palsy or diseases of the brain and spinal cord. This medication is meant to provide therapy for only two to three weeks.

Adverse Effects and Interactions: Adverse reactions to cyclobenzaprine include drowsiness, blurred vision, dizziness, dry mouth, rash, and tachycardia. It should be used with caution in patients with myocardial infarction (MI), dysrhythmias, or severe cardiovascular disease. One reaction, although rare, is swelling of the tongue.

Alcohol, phenothiazines, and other CNS depressants may cause additive sedation. Cyclobenzaprine should not be used within two weeks of an MAOI because hyperpyretic crisis and convulsions may occur.

SPASTICITY

Spasticity is a condition in which muscle groups remain in a continuous state of contraction, usually as a result of damage to the CNS. The contracting muscles become stiff with increased muscle tone. Signs and symptoms may include mild to severe pain, exaggerated deep tendon reflexes, muscle spasms, scissoring (involuntary crossing of the legs), and fixed joints.

CORE CONCEPT 12.11

Effective treatment for spasticity includes both physical therapy and medications.

spasticity = *rigidly stiff muscles*

dys = *abnormal*
tonia = *tension*

Spasticity usually results from damage to the motor area of the cerebral cortex, which controls muscle movement. Etiologies most commonly associated with this condition include neurologic disorders such as cerebral palsy, severe head injury, spinal cord injury or lesions, and stroke. **Dystonia**, a chronic neurologic disorder, is characterized by involuntary muscle contraction that forces body parts into abnormal, occasionally painful movements or postures. It affects the muscle tone of the arms, legs, trunk, neck, eyelids, face, or vocal cords. Spasticity, whether short term or long term, can be distressing and greatly impacts an individual's quality of life. In addition to causing pain, it also impairs physical mobility, thereby influencing the person's ability to perform ADLs and diminishing his or her sense of independence.

NURSING PROCESS FOCUS Patients Receiving Drugs for Muscle Spasms or Spasticity

ASSESSMENT	POTENTIAL NURSING DIAGNOSES
Prior to administration: ■ Obtain a complete health history including cardiovascular, respiratory, and neuromuscular conditions, allergies, drug history and possible drug interactions. ■ Acquire baseline vital signs and ECG. ■ Evaluate laboratory blood levels: CBC, chemistry, drug screening, renal and liver function studies. ■ Determine neurologic status; especially LOC and neurological effects on the motor and respiratory function.	■ *Pain (acute/chronic)* related to muscle spasms ■ *Impaired Physical Mobility* related to acute/chronic pain ■ *Risk for Injury* related to adverse effects of drug therapy ■ *Deficient Knowledge* related to a lack of information about drug therapy or disease process

PLANNING: PATIENT GOALS AND EXPECTED OUTCOMES

The patient will:
■ Experience therapeutic effects (a decrease in pain, increase in range of motion and reduction of muscle spasms).
■ Be free from or experience minimal adverse effects from drug therapy.
■ Verbalize an understanding of the drug's use, adverse effects and required precautions.

IMPLEMENTATION

Interventions and (Rationales)	Patient Education/Discharge Planning
■ Monitor LOC and vital signs. (Some skeletal muscle relaxants alter the patient's LOC. Others within this class may alter blood pressure and heart rate.)	Instruct the patient to: ■ Avoid driving and other activities requiring mental alertness until the effects of the medication are known. ■ Report any significant change in sensorium, such as slurred speech, confusion, hallucinations, or extreme lethargy. ■ Report palpitations, chest pain, dyspnea, unusual fatigue, weakness, and visual disturbances. ■ Avoid using other CNS depressants such as alcohol that will intensify sedation.
■ Monitor pain and provide proper medication. Determine the location, duration, and precipitating factors of the patient's pain. (Drugs should diminish the patient's pain.)	Instruct the patient to: ■ Report the development of new sites of muscle pain. ■ Take medications as ordered.
■ Provide additional pain relief measures such as positional support, gentle massage, and moist heat or ice packs. (Drugs alone may not be sufficient in providing pain relief.)	Instruct the patient: ■ That complementary pain interventions such as positioning, gentle massage, and the application of heat or cold to the painful area may be helpful. ■ In relaxation techniques, deep breathing, and meditation methods to facilitate relaxation and reduce pain.
■ Monitor muscle tone, range of motion, and degree of muscle spasm. (Helps to determine the effectiveness of drug therapy and possible need for changes in drug therapy.)	Instruct the patient: ■ To perform gentle range of motion, only to the point of mild physical discomfort, throughout the day. ■ That medication may cause a decrease in muscle strength and dosage may need to be reduced.

Interventions and (Rationales)	Patient Education/Discharge Planning
■ Monitor for adverse effects such as drowsiness, weakness, fatigue, dry mouth, dizziness, faintness, rash, blurred vision, photosensitivity, rash, tachycardia, erratic blood pressure, photosensitivity, and urinary retention. (These adverse effects may occur with common antispasmodic drugs).	Instruct the patient: ■ To report any adverse effects to healthcare provider. ■ To take medication with food to decrease GI upset. ■ That frequent mouth rinses, sips of water, and sugarless candy or gum may help with dry mouth. ■ To report signs of urinary retention such as a feeling of urinary bladder fullness, distended abdomen, and discomfort. ■ To use sunscreen and protective clothing when outdoors.
■ Administer medication correctly and evaluate the patient's knowledge of proper administration. Do not abruptly stop providing medication and monitor for withdrawal symptoms. (Abrupt withdrawal of drugs such as baclofen may cause serious symptoms.)	■ Advise the patient not to abruptly discontinue medication. This action may result in withdrawal reactions such as visual hallucinations, paranoid ideation, and seizures.

EVALUATION OF OUTCOME CRITERIA

Evaluate the effectiveness of drug therapy by confirming that patient goals and expected outcomes have been met (see "Planning"). *See Tables 12.6 and 12.7 for lists of drugs to which these nursing actions apply.*

CAM THERAPY

Cayenne for Muscular Tension

Cayenne (*Capsicum annum*), also known as chili pepper, paprika, or red pepper, has been used as a remedy for muscle tension and associated pain. Applied in a cream base, it is commonly used to relieve muscle spasms in the shoulder and areas of the arm. Capsaicin, the active ingredient in cayenne, diminishes the chemical messengers that travel through the sensory nerves, thereby decreasing the sensation of pain. Its effect accumulates over time, so creams containing capsaicin need to be applied regularly to be effective. Although no known medical condition exists that would prevent the use of cayenne, it should never be applied over broken skin. External use of full-strength cayenne should be limited to no more than two days, because it may cause skin inflammation, blisters, and ulcers. It also needs to be kept away from eyes and mucous membranes to avoid burns. Hands must be washed thoroughly after usage. Commercial OTC creams containing capsaicin are available.

Effective treatment for spasticity includes both physical therapy and medications. Medications alone are not adequate to reduce the complications of spasticity, but regular and consistent physical therapy exercises have been shown to be effective in decreasing the severity of symptoms. Types of treatment include muscle stretching to help prevent contractures, muscle group strengthening exercises, and repetitive motion exercises for improvement of accuracy. In extreme cases, surgery for tendon release or to sever the nerve-muscle pathway has been used.

Some drugs for spasticity provide relief by acting directly on muscle tissue, interfering with the release of calcium ions.

CORE CONCEPT 12.12

Drugs that are effective in the treatment of spasticity include two centrally acting drugs, baclofen (Lioresal) and diazepam (Valium), and a direct-acting drug, dantrolene (Dantrium). The direct-acting drugs produce an antispasmodic effect at the level of the neuromuscular junction, as shown in Figure 12.3 ■.

Dantrolene relieves spasticity by interfering with the release of calcium ions in skeletal muscle. Other direct-acting drugs include incobotulinumtoxin A (Xeomin), onabotulinumtoxin A (Botox, Dysport), and rimabotulinumtoxin B (Myobloc). Although these botulinum toxins are generally known for their use in cosmetic procedures, in some instances they may offer temporary relief of dystonia symptoms.

Botulinum toxin is an unusual drug because in high doses it acts as a poison. *Clostridium botulinum* is the bacterium responsible for food poisoning or botulism. At lower doses, however, this drug is safe and effective as a muscle relaxant. It produces its effect by blocking the release of acetylcholine from cholinergic nerve terminals (see Chapter 8). Botulinum can cause extreme weakness, so its use may require the addition of other therapies to improve muscle strength. To prevent major problems with mobility or posture, botulinum toxin is often applied to small muscle groups. Sometimes this drug is administered together with centrally acting oral medications to further increase the functional use of a range of muscle groups.

FIGURE 12.3

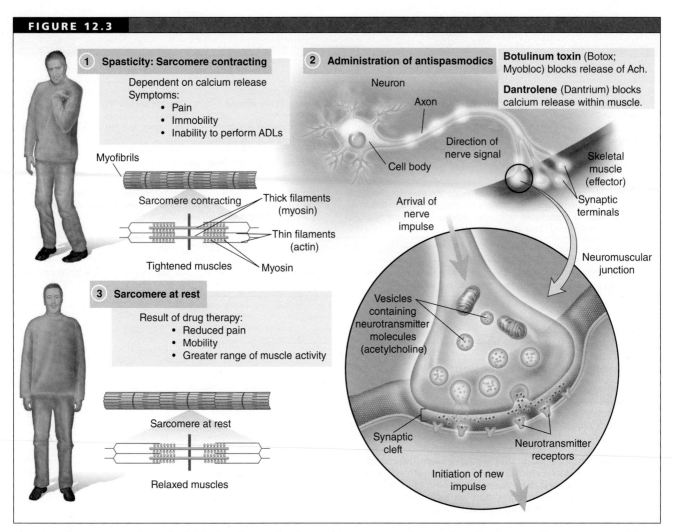

The use of antispasmodics, which block release of Ach or calcium, can result in reduced pain as well as greater mobility and range of motion.

blepharospasm =
involuntary blinking of the eyelids

Drawbacks to botulinum therapy are its delayed and limited effects. The treatment is mostly effective within six weeks of administration, and its effects last for only three to six months. Another drawback is the pain of injecting botulinum directly into the muscle. Local anesthetics are usually given to block this pain. Direct-acting antispasmotic drugs are summarized in Table 12.7 ◆.

TABLE 12.7   Direct-Acting Antispasmodic Drugs

Drug	Route and Adult Dose	Remarks
℗ dantrolene (Dantrium)	PO; 25 mg daily; increase to 25 mg bid–qid; may increase every 4–7 days up to 100 mg bid–tid	Hydantoin-like medication; also for the treatment of malignant hyperthermia; IV form available
incobotulinumtoxin A (Xeomin)	120 units injected per treatment session directly into target muscle	For treatment of cervical dystonia and involuntary blinking of the eyelids (*blepharospasm*)
onabotulinumtoxin A (Botox, Dysport)	25 units injected directly into target muscle (max: 30-day dose should not exceed 200 units)	Mainly used for cosmetic procedures, this drug has been used to treat excessive sweating and wrinkles; relaxes facial muscles around the eye and forehead
rimabotulinumtoxin B (Myobloc)	2,500–5,000 units/dose injected directly into target muscle; doses should be divided among muscle groups	May be used in cases of cervical dystonia

Drug Prototype: ⓟ *Dantrolene (Dantrium)*
Therapeutic Class: **Skeletal muscle relaxant, peripheral-acting**
Pharmacologic Class: **Skeletal muscle calcium release blocker**

Actions and Uses: Dantrolene is often used for spasticity, especially for spasms of the head and neck. It directly relaxes muscle spasms by interfering with the release of calcium ions from storage areas inside skeletal muscle cells. It does not affect cardiac or smooth muscle. Dantrolene is especially useful for muscle spasms when they occur after spinal cord injury or stroke and in cases of cerebral palsy, multiple sclerosis, and occasionally for the treatment of muscle pain after heavy exercise. It is also used for the treatment of malignant hyperthermia.

Adverse Effects and Interactions: Adverse effects include muscle weakness, drowsiness, dry mouth, dizziness, nausea, diarrhea, tachycardia, erratic blood pressure, photosensitivity, and urinary retention.

Dantrolene interacts with many other drugs. For example, it should not be taken with OTC cough preparations and antihistamines, alcohol, or other CNS depressants. Verapamil and other calcium channel blockers taken with dantrolene increase the risk of ventricular fibrillation and cardiovascular collapse. Patients with impaired cardiac or pulmonary function or hepatic disease should not take this drug.

BLACK BOX WARNING:
Dantrolene has a potential for hepatotoxicity. Liver dysfunction may be evidenced by blood chemical enzyme levels. The risk of hepatic injury is greater in females over 35 years of age and after 3 months of therapy. Therapy should be discontinued after 45 days if no observable benefit.

Quinine sulfate (Quinamm, Quiphile) has been used to treat nocturnal leg cramps, but in 2006 the FDA issued a warning that quinidine sulfate produces serious adverse effects such as cardiac dysrrhythmias, severe hypersensitivity reactions, and an abnormal platelet count. Labelling of the drug was modified to restrict the use of quinine sulfate for malaria only and not for leg cramps.

Neuromuscular blocking drugs block the effect of acetylcholine at the receptor.

CORE CONCEPT 12.13

Neuromuscular blocking drugs bind to nicotinic receptors located on the surface of skeletal muscle fibers. For pharmacotherapy drugs called *nicotinic blocking drugs* interfere with the binding of acetylcholine, thereby preventing voluntary muscle contraction. Nicotinic blocking drugs are *cholinergic* (see Chapter 8).

nicotin = *nicotine*
ic = *related to*

cholin = *acetycholine*
erg = *work (action)*
ic = *related to*

Neuromuscular blocking drugs are classified into two major categories: nondepolarizing blockers and depolarizing blockers. *Nondepolarizing blockers* compete with acetylcholine for the receptor. As long as drugs interfere with the binding of acetylcholine, muscles remain relaxed. By a related mechanism, *depolarizing blockers* bind to the acetylcholine receptor and produce a state of continuous depolarization. Remember that *depolarization* is the rapid cycling influx of sodium into neurons, propagating the electrical signal. This action first results in small fasciculations or a time of brief repeated muscle movements, followed by relaxation of muscle fibers. Relaxation is short-lived until charges across the muscle membrane are restored (repolarization). Importantly, patients treated with neuromuscular blockers are able to feel pain even though they cannot react to it. Thus, for surgical procedures, concomitant use of anesthetic agents is essential (see Chapter 15).

fascicu = *muscle fascicle (bundle)*
lation = *movement*

It is important to note that neuromuscular blocking drugs are different from *ganglionic blocking drugs* that target the autonomic nervous system. With ganglionic blocking drugs, acetylcholine does indeed bind to nicotinic receptors, but the resulting actions of these drugs are involuntary and do not involve skeletal muscle (see Chapter 8). Ganglionic blockers dampen parasympathetic tone and produce effects such as increased heart rate, dry mouth, urinary retention, and reduced GI activity. They also dampen sympathetic tone, resulting in reduced sweating and less norepinephrine being released from postsynaptic nerve terminals. As an example, mecamylamine (Inversine) is a ganglionic blocker primarily used to treat patients with essential hypertension (see Chapter 18).

ganglion = *cell bodies grouped outside CNS*

The classic example of a nondepolarizing blocker is tubocurarine. Tubocurarine and related blocking drugs are used to relax the muscles of patients being prepared for longer surgical procedures (Table 12.8 ◆). Although not preferred for mechanical ventilation or endotracheal intubation, small doses of these drugs may be used for intermediate surgical procedures. Concerns of tubocurarine-like treatment include over-relaxation of muscles. For example, normal breathing activity (involving the diaphragm, glottic, and intercostal muscles) and swallowing activity (involving the neck and certain esophageal muscles) require skeletal muscle contraction.

TABLE 12.8 Neuromuscular Blocking Drugs

Drug	Duration	Administration Route
NONDEPOLARIZING BLOCKERS		
atracurium (Tracrium)	Long duration	IV
cisatracurium (Nimbex)	Long duration	IV
mivacurium (Mivacron)	Shorter duration	IV
pipecuronium (Arduan)	Longest duration	IV
rocuronium (Zemuron)	Long duration	IV
tubocurarine	Longest duration; oldest of the nondepolarizing drugs	IV and IM
vecuronium (Norcuron)	Long duration	IV
DEPOLARIZING BLOCKERS		
succinylcholine (Anectine) (see page 228 for the Drug Prototype box)	Shortest duration	IV and IM

malignant = *harmful*
hyper = *elevated*
thermia = *fever*

post = *after*
operative = *surgery*

Depolarizing agents are used primarily to relax the muscles of patients receiving electroconvulsive therapy (ECT) (see Chapter 13) and for brief surgical procedures (see Chapter 15). Short surgical procedures involve mechanical ventilation and endotracheal intubation. Succinylcholine (Anectine) is the prototype example of a depolarizing blocker. Adverse effects include elevated blood levels of potassium, malignant hyperthermia, and postoperative muscle pain and persistent paralysis in some patients. As a specific antidote for persistent paralysis, patients are often given cholinesterase inhibitors.

PATIENTS NEED TO KNOW

Patients being treated for degenerative diseases and disorders of the neuromuscular system need to know the following:

Regarding Drugs for Parkinson's Disease or Dementia

1. Take levodopa–carbidopa at least 30–60 minutes before eating in order to allow the medication to be absorbed before food can interfere. Do not take with foods that contain protein, as these foods can decrease drug effectiveness.
2. Be extremely careful about getting up quickly from a seated position. Many dementia drugs cause dizziness, lightheadedness, blurred vision, and difficulty in concentrating.
3. Do not skip taking the medications, and do not take OTC preparations (especially medications for colds or pain) without checking with a healthcare provider.
4. Be aware that urine may become a little dark. This is a normal side effect of dopamine-like drugs.
5. Do not drink alcoholic beverages or take sedatives. Combined effects may be harmful.
6. Be familiar with adverse effects specific for the drugs being taken. Drugs used for Parkinson's may produce nausea, dry mouth, and diminished sweating in some cases. Drugs used for dementia may cause nausea, diarrhea, muscle cramps, weight loss, and change in urine color.

Regarding Drugs for Muscle Spasms and Spasticity

7. When receiving treatment for problems with mobility, it often takes several weeks for effectiveness to begin. Follow the advice of a healthcare provider in order to achieve full therapeutic effect.
8. Most antispasmodic drugs produce adverse effects such as drowsiness and dizziness. Therefore, avoid CNS depressants and alcohol.

Regarding Neuromuscular Blockers

9. Some patients react adversely to neuromuscular blockers. Inform the healthcare provider about any important family history, such as malignant hyperthermia, myasthenia gravis, cardiovascular disease, and any other unusual problems.
10. Be aware that unpleasant muscle pain may be associated with surgical procedures.

CHAPTER REVIEW

CORE CONCEPTS SUMMARY

12.1 Medications are unable to cure most degenerative diseases of the CNS.

Degenerative diseases of the CNS include Alzheimer's disease, multiple sclerosis, and Parkinson's disease. The cause of most neurologic degenerative disorders is unknown. With the exception of Parkinson's disease, drug therapy provides only minimal benefit.

12.2 Parkinson's disease is progressive, with the occurrence of full symptoms taking many years.

Parkinson's disease, or parkinsonism, is a degenerative disorder caused by death of neurons that produce the brain neurotransmitter dopamine. Dopamine-producing neurons in the substantia nigra supply nerve signals to the corpus striatum. When dopamine is depleted, symptoms of parkinsonism, including tremors, muscle rigidity, bradykinesia (slow movement), and postural instability, occur. These symptoms are the same EPS effects caused by prolonged antipsychotic drug treatment.

12.3 Antiparkinson drugs act on the brain to restore the balance between dopamine and acetylcholine.

Balance, posture, muscle tone, and involuntary muscle movement depend on the proper balance between the neurotransmitter dopamine (inhibitory) and acetylcholine (stimulatory) in the corpus striatum. Drug therapy for parkinsonism focuses on restoring dopamine function (dopaminergic drugs) and blocking the effect of acetylcholine overactivity (cholinergic blockers).

12.4 Patients with Alzheimer's disease experience a dramatic loss of ability to perform tasks that require acetylcholine as the CNS neurotransmitter.

Alzheimer's disease (AD) is a devastating, progressive, degenerative disease characterized by impaired memory, confusion or disorientation, inability to recognize family or friends, aggressive behavior, depression, psychoses, and anxiety. AD is responsible for 70% of all *dementia*. Although the cause of AD is unknown, structural brain damage and a dramatic loss of ability to perform tasks that require acetycholine as the neurotransmitter have been documented.

12.5 Alzheimer's disease is treated with acetylcholinesterase inhibitors.

Only a few drugs for AD have been approved. Most drugs act by intensifying the effect of acetylcholine at the cholinergic receptor. Acetylcholine is naturally degraded in the synapse by the enzyme acetylcholinesterase. When acetylcholinesterase is inhibited, acetylcholine levels increase and produce a greater effect on the receptor. This treatment improves function in activities of daily living, behavior, and cognition.

12.6 Symptoms of multiple sclerosis result from demyelination of CNS nerve fibers.

Multiple sclerosis is an autoimmune disorder of the CNS. Antibodies slowly destroy myelin in the brain and spinal cord, disrupting the ability of nerves to conduct electrical impulses. Over time, debilitating symptoms appear, including fatigue, heat sensitivity, pain, muscle cramps and spasms, impaired ability to think and reason, balance and coordination problems, and bowel and bladder symptoms.

12.7 Drugs for multiple sclerosis reduce immune attacks in the brain and treat unfavorable symptoms.

Two strategies for treating MS are reducing the immune response and relieving the symptoms. The most treatable form of MS is *relapsing-remitting MS (RRMS)*, in which unpredictable relapses occur. Drug treatments include immune system modulating drugs, immunosuppressants, and miscellaneous drugs used for treatment of MS symptoms such as inflammation, pain, fatigue, memory loss, and progressive weakness.

12.8 Muscle spasms are caused by injury, overmedication, hypocalcemia, and debilitating neurologic disorders.

Muscle spasms, or involuntary contractions of a muscle or group of muscles, occur for many reasons, including overmedication with antipsychotic drugs, epilepsy, hypocalcemia, pain, and incapacitating neurologic disorders. Two types of muscle spasms are tonic spasms and clonic spasms.

12.9 Muscle spasms may be treated with nonpharmacologic or pharmacologic therapies.

After a thorough medical exam, nonpharmacologic therapies such as immobilization, heat or cold, hydrotherapy, ultrasound, supervised exercises, massage, and manipulation may be used along with medications. Medications include analgesics, anti-inflammatory drugs, and centrally acting skeletal muscle relaxants.

12.10 Many muscle relaxants treat muscle spasms by inhibiting upper motor neuron activity, causing sedation, or altering simple reflexes.

Skeletal muscle relaxants treat local spasms resulting from muscular injury and may be prescribed alone or in combination with medications that reduce pain and increase range of motion. These include centrally acting drugs (affecting the brain and/or spinal cord) that have the potential to cause sedation and alter reflex activity.

12.11 Effective treatment for spasticity includes both physical therapy and medications.

Spasticity is a condition in which certain muscle groups remain in a state of contraction. Symptoms associated with spasticity include pain, exaggerated deep tendon reflexes, muscle spasms, scissoring, and fixed joints. Medications alone are not adequate in reducing the complications of spasticity.

12.12 Some drugs for spasticity provide relief by acting directly on muscle tissue, interfering with the release of calcium ions.

Direct-acting drugs produce an antispasmodic effect at the level of the neuromuscular junction. Drugs affect either calcium release from the muscle, or they interfere with the release of acetylcholine.

12.13 Neuromuscular blocking drugs block the effect of acetylcholine at the receptor.

Neuromuscular blocking drugs are classified as nondepolarizing blockers and depolarizing blockers. Both drugs bind to acetylcholine receptors, relaxing muscles by slightly different mechanisms and durations of action.

REVIEW QUESTIONS

The following questions are written in NCLEX-PN® style. Answer these questions to assess your knowledge of the chapter material, and go back and review any material that is not clear to you.

1. The patient taking levodopa is taught that he must wait at least one hour before or after eating foods high in:

1. Vitamin C
2. Carbohydrates
3. Folic acid
4. Protein

2. A patient in the early stages of Alzheimer's disease was started on donepezil (Aricept) a few weeks ago. She calls the nurse at the doctor's office and states that she has been experiencing what she believes to be adverse effects of the drug. Which of the following effects could the patient be experiencing? (Select all that apply.)

1. Sleepiness
2. Nausea
3. Diarrhea
4. Tinnitus

3. When administering levodopa to a patient with Parkinson's disease, the nurse understands that this drug:

1. Increases cholinergic stimulation within the brain
2. Restores acetylcholine and blocks dopamine within the brain
3. Restores dopamine function and blocks acetylcholine within the brain
4. Destroys dopamine receptors within the brain

4. The patient with Parkinson's disease is placed on haloperidol (Haldol) because of agitation and has started experiencing EPS. Which of the following drugs would the nurse anticipate being ordered?

1. Levodopa–carbidopa drugs
2. Risperidone (Risperdal)
3. Benztropine (Cogentin)
4. Cyclobenzaprine (Flexeril)

5. The patient with Alzheimer's disease has been started on rivastigmine (Exelon). The nurse will evaluate the patient for:

1. Liver toxicity
2. Weight loss
3. Renal failure
4. EPS

6. A patient had a surgical procedure in which succinylcholine (Anectine) was used to relax the muscles. The nurse taking care of this patient would monitor the patient for:

1. Hypothermia
2. Complaints of muscle pain
3. High sodium levels (hypernatremia)
4. Low levels of potassium (hypokalemia)

7. A patient is given a prescription for carisoprodol (Soma), 350 mg, po, three times a day. The pharmacy provides a bottle of 350 mg tablets. If the patient follows the directions, how many milligrams will the patient take in one day?

1. 900 mg
2. 1,115 mg
3. 1,050 mg
4. 1,015 mg

8. An interferon is prescribed for a patient with MS. The nurse includes which of the following points when educating the patient about drug therapy?

1. Report flu-like symptoms to the healthcare provider.
2. Expect urine to be orange.
3. Report the development of diarrhea.
4. The symptoms will get better over a period of a year.

9. A patient is being seen in the emergency room after an automobile accident. She complains that her lower back hurts. After an examination and x-ray, the patient is given a diagnosis of muscle strain, with associated spasms, and is placed on cyclobenzaprine (Flexeril) to help relax the muscles. In educating the patient about the cyclobenzaprine, the nurse informs her that: (Select all that apply.)

1. It can cause drowsiness.
2. If taken with alcohol, additional drowsiness may occur.
3. It is only intended for short-term use (2–3 weeks).
3. It can cause headaches.

10. A patient with a spinal cord injury is still suffering from muscle spasms. The physician has prescribed dantrolene to help control the spasms. The nurse informs the patient that he should report which of the following possible adverse effect(s) if they should occur:

1. Excessive salivation
2. Excessive urination
3. Muscle weakness
4. Insomnia

CASE STUDY QUESTIONS

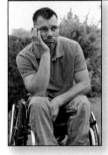

Remember Mr. Wingate, the patient introduced at the beginning of the chapter? Now read the remainder of the case study. Based on the information you have learned in this chapter, answer the questions that follow.

Mr. Robert Wingate, a 35-year-old man with MS, has persistent pain in his right hip and comes in for treatment. He explains that he has been taking enteric-coated aspirin for several weeks. He explains that he has been experiencing severe headaches. He has also been experiencing muscle twitches (multiple, rapidly repeating contractions) in his right hamstring. The muscle twitches have not been severe, but he is concerned that they may be related to his condition. Lately, he has been experiencing quite a bit of fatigue, and his vision is sometimes "blurry." Laboratory values show slight hypocalcemia. The patient explains that he hasn't had any trouble with his diet. No abnormalities in bone structure or peripheral inflammatory symptoms are observed on examination.

1. The nurse caring for Mr. Wingate just received a medication order to administer an immune system modulator. Which of the following medications might the nurse administer?

1. Amantadine (Symmetrel)
2. Interferon beta-1b (Betaseron)
3. Memantine (Namenda)
4. Gabapentin (Neurontin)

2. After being started on the immune system modulator, Mr. Wingate asks the nurse about this class of medications. The nurse responds by saying: (Select all that apply.)

1. "These drugs slow down the destruction of the neuron caused by MS."
2. "These drugs have very few adverse effects."
3. "There are no precautions when taking this type of drug with other drugs."
4. "Adverse effects can include fever, chills, and muscle aches."

3. In evaluating the effectiveness of Mr. Wingate's antispasmodic therapy, the nurse would expect that the medication would:

1. Improve Mr. Wingate's symptoms for the long term.
2. Improve Mr. Wingate's symptoms for the short term.
3. Make Mr. Wingate's symptoms worse.
4. Cause Mr. Wingate to be sedated.

4. If Mr. Wingate's condition and symptoms were to progress significantly, the nurse would expect to administer which of the following drugs?

1. Selegiline (Eldepryl, Zelapar)
2. Gabapentin (Neurontin)
3. Mitoxantrone (Novantrone)
4. Donepezil (ARICEPT)

NOTE: Answers to the Review and Case Study Questions appear in Appendix B. The complete rationales and answers are located on the textbook's website.

Pearson Nursing Student Resources
Find additional review materials at **nursing.pearsonhighered.com.**

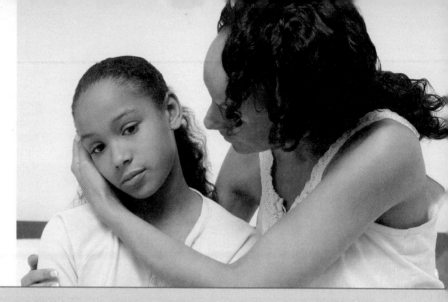

"I felt so helpless when I found out Destiny's problem was seizures. I'm glad there's a medication that will help her live a normal life."

Mrs. Kemi Anthonia

13 Drugs for Seizures

CORE CONCEPTS

13.1 Although some types of seizures involve convulsions, other seizures do not.

13.2 Many causes of seizure activity are known; a few are not.

13.3 Epileptic seizures are typically identified as partial, generalized, or special epileptic syndromes.

13.4 Effective seizure management involves strict adherence to safe drug therapy.

13.5 Antiseizure pharmacotherapy is directed at controlling the movement of electrolytes across neuronal membranes or affecting neurotransmitter balance.

13.6 By increasing the effects of gamma-aminobutyric acid or GABA in the brain, some drugs reduce a wide range of seizure types.

13.7 Hydantoin and related drugs are generally effective in treating partial seizures and tonic-clonic seizures.

13.8 Succinimides generally treat absence seizures.

DRUG SNAPSHOT

The following drugs are discussed in this chapter:

DRUG CLASSES	DRUG PROTOTYPES
Drugs That Potentiate GABA Action	
Barbiturates	(Pr) phenobarbital (Luminal) *188*
Benzodiazepines	(Pr) diazepam (Valium) *188*
Other GABA-Related Drugs	

DRUG CLASSES	DRUG PROTOTYPES
Hydantoin and Related Drugs	
Hydantoins	(Pr) phenytoin (Dilantin) *190*
Phenytoin-like drugs	(Pr) valproic acid (Depakene) *191*
Succinimides	(Pr) ethosuximide (Zarontin) *192*

LEARNING OUTCOMES

After reading this chapter, the student should be able to:

1. Compare and contrast the terms epilepsy, seizures, and convulsions.

2. Recognize possible causes of seizures.

3. Relate signs and symptoms to specific types of seizures.

4. Explain the importance of safety and patient drug compliance in the pharmacotherapy of epilepsy and seizures.

5. Describe the pharmacologic management of epilepsy and acute seizures.

6. Categorize drugs used in the treatment of seizures based on their classifications.

7. Explain the mechanisms of action by which barbiturates, benzodiazepines, and miscellaneous drugs control seizure activity.

8. For each of the classes listed in the Drug Snapshot, identify representative drugs and explain their mechanisms of drug action, primary actions, and important adverse effects.

KEY TERMS

action potential (poh-TEN-shial) *189*

convulsions (kon-VULL-shuns) *181*

eclampsia (ee-KLAMP-see-uh) *183*

epilepsy (EPP-ih-lepp-see) *181*

febrile seizures *182*

generalized seizures *183*

partial (focal) seizures *183*

pre-eclampsia (pree-ee-KLAMP-see-uh) *183*

seizure (SEE-zhurr) *181*

status epilepticus (ep-ih-LEP-tih-kus) *184*

A s the most common neurologic disorder, epilepsy affects more than 2 million Americans. By definition, **epilepsy** is any condition characterized by recurrent seizures. Symptoms of epilepsy depend on the type of seizure and may include signs such as blackout, fainting spells, sensory disturbances, jerking body movements, and temporary loss of memory. This chapter examines the drug therapies used to treat different kinds of seizures and epilepsy.

epilepsy = taking hold or to seize

SEIZURES

A **seizure** is a disturbance of electrical activity in the brain that may affect consciousness, motor activity, and sensation. Seizures are caused by abnormal or uncontrolled neuronal discharges. Uncontrolled charges start in one area of the brain and often move to other areas. As a valuable tool in measuring uncontrolled neuronal activity, the electroencephalogram (EEG) is useful in diagnosing seizure disorders. Figure 13.1 ■ compares normal and abnormal neuronal tracings.

Although some types of seizures involve convulsions, other seizures do not.

CORE CONCEPT 13.1

Seizures and *convulsions* are not interchangeable terms. **Convulsions** specifically refer to involuntary, violent spasms of large skeletal muscles of the face, neck, arms, and legs. Although some types of seizures involve convulsions, other seizures do not. Thus, it may be stated that all convulsions are seizures, but not all seizures are convulsions.

FIGURE 13.1

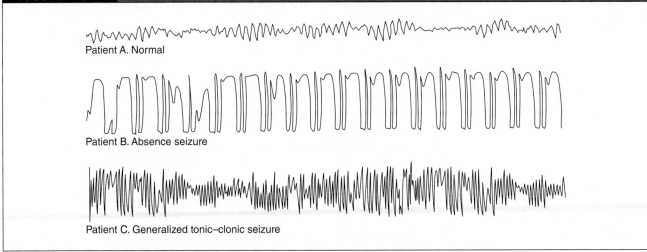

Patient A. Normal

Patient B. Absence seizure

Patient C. Generalized tonic–clonic seizure

Neurons produce tiny impulses when they communicate. These impulses may be detected by an electroencephalogram (EEG), a device that captures brain-wave activity. Brain waves have characteristic patterns termed *alpha*, *beta*, *delta*, and *theta*. Although interpretation of brain waves is a complex art, you can see from these examples that the EEG tracings of patients B and C are dramatically different from those of patient A, who has no seizures. Alpha waves are the predominant waveform observed in patients with normal brain activity.

Fast Facts Epilepsy

- Over two million Americans have epilepsy.
- One of every 100 teenagers has epilepsy.
- Of the U.S. population, 10% will have seizures within their lifetime.
- Most people with seizures are younger than 45 years of age.
- Epilepsy is not a mental illness and children with epilepsy have IQ scores equivalent to those of children without the disorder.
- Famous people who had epilepsy include Julius Caesar, Alexander the Great, Napoleon, Vincent van Gogh, Charles Dickens, Joan of Arc, and Socrates.
- Among adult alcoholics receiving treatment for withdrawal, over half will experience seizures within six hours upon arriving for treatment.

Drugs described in this chapter are generally referred to as *antiseizure drugs* rather than *anticonvulsants*. Recognizing also that antiseizure drugs are commonly called *antiepileptic drugs* (AEDs), the term *antiseizure* in this chapter applies to the treatment of all seizure-related symptoms, including signs of epilepsy.

CORE CONCEPT 13.2

Many causes of seizure activity are known; a few are not.

A seizure is considered symptomatic of an underlying disorder, rather than a disease in itself. Triggers include exposure to strobe or flickering lights or the occurrence of small fluid and electrolyte imbalances. Patients appear to have a lower tolerance to environmental triggers, and seizures often occur when patients are sleep deprived.

idio = *one's unknown arising*
pathic = *abnormal state*

There are many different causes of seizure activity. In some cases, the cause of seizure activity may be clear, but not in all situations. Seizures represent the most common serious neurologic problem affecting children, with an overall incidence approaching 2% for **febrile seizures** and 1% for idiopathic epilepsy. Certain medications for mood disorders, psychoses, and local anesthesia may cause seizures when given in high doses, possibly because of increased levels of stimulatory neurotransmitters or toxicity. Seizures may also occur from drug abuse, as with cocaine, or during withdrawal from alcohol or sedative–hypnotic drugs.

Seizures may present as an acute situation, or they may occur on a chronic basis. Seizures resulting from an acute complication are generally not recurrent after the situation has been resolved. On the other hand, if a brain abnormality exists following an acute complication, recurrent seizures are likely. The following are known causes of seizures:

- *Infectious diseases* Acute infections such as meningitis and encephalitis can cause inflammation in the brain.
- *Trauma* Physical trauma such as direct blows to the skull may increase intracranial pressure; chemical trauma such as the presence of toxic substances or the ingestion of poisons may cause brain injury.
- *Metabolic disorders* Changes in fluid and electrolytes such as hypoglycemia, hyponatremia, and water intoxication may cause seizures by altering electrical impulse transmission at the cellular level.
- *Vascular diseases* Changes in oxygenation such as those caused by respiratory hypoxia and carbon monoxide poisoning, and changes in perfusion such as those caused by hypotension, cerebral vascular accidents, shock, and cardiac dysrhythmias may be causes.
- *Pediatric disorders* Rapid increase in body temperature may result in a febrile seizure.
- *Neoplastic disease* Tumors, especially rapidly growing ones, may occupy space, increase intracranial pressure, and damage brain tissue by disrupting blood flow.

An important topic when discussing epilepsy and seizure treatment is birth control. Because several antiseizure drugs decrease the effectiveness of oral contraceptives, additional barrier methods of birth control should be practiced to avoid unintended pregnancy. Prior to pregnancy and considering the serious nature of epilepsy, patients should consult with their healthcare provider to determine the most appropriate plan of action for seizure control.

If patients become pregnant, extreme caution is necessary. Most antiseizure drugs are pregnancy category D. Some antiseizure drugs may cause folate deficiency, a condition correlated with fetal neural tube defects. Vitamin supplements may be necessary.

Pre-eclampsia and **eclampsia** are severe hypertensive disorders of pregnancy, characterized by seizures, coma, and perinatal mortality. Eclampsia is likely to occur from around the 20th week of gestation to at least one week following delivery of the baby. Roughly one-fourth of patients with eclampsia experience seizures within 72 hours postpartum.

post = *after*
partum = *delivery*

Seizures can have a significant impact on the quality of life. They may cause serious injury if they occur when a person is driving a vehicle or performing a dangerous activity. Without successful pharmacotherapy, epilepsy can severely limit participation in school, employment, or social activities and can affect self-esteem. Chronic depression may accompany poorly controlled seizures. Important considerations in health care include identifying patients at risk for seizures, documenting the pattern and type of seizure activity, and implementing safety precautions. In collaboration with the patient, the healthcare provider, pharmacist, and all healthcare staff are instrumental in achieving positive therapeutic outcomes. Through a combination of pharmacotherapy, patient–family support, and education, effective seizure control can be achieved in the majority of patients.

Epileptic seizures are typically identified as partial, generalized, or special epileptic syndromes.

CORE CONCEPT 13.3

Seizure symptoms vary depending on the areas of the brain affected by the abnormal electrical activity. These symptoms range from muscle twitching or slight tremor (shaking) of a limb to sudden, violent shaking and total loss of consciousness. Staring into space, altered vision, and difficult speech are other behaviors a person may exhibit during a seizure. It is important to determine the cause of recurrent seizures in order to plan for appropriate treatment options.

Methods of classifying epilepsy have changed over time. For example, the terms *grand mal* and *petit mal* epilepsy have been replaced by more descriptive and detailed categorization. Epilepsies are typically identified using the International Classification of Epileptic Seizures. Example nomenclatures are *partial* (less used term *focal*), *generalized*, and *special epileptic syndromes*. Types of partial or generalized seizures may be recognized based on symptoms observed during a seizure episode. Some symptoms are hard to notice and reflect the simple nature of neuronal misfiring in specific areas of the brain; others are more complex.

Partial Seizures

Partial (focal) seizures involve a limited portion of the brain. Abnormal electrical activity starts on one side and travels only a short distance before it stops. The area where the abnormal electrical activity starts is known as the abnormal *focus* (plural, *foci*).

Simple partial seizures have an onset from a small, limited focus. Patients may feel disoriented for a while, and they may hear and see things that are not there. Some patients smell and taste things that are not present, or have an upset stomach. Others may become emotional and experience a sense of joy, sorrow, or grief. The arms, legs, or face may twitch.

Complex partial seizures (formerly known as *psychomotor* or *temporal lobe seizures*) have sensory, motor, or autonomic symptoms with some degree of altered or impaired consciousness. Total loss of consciousness may not occur during a complex partial seizure, but a period of brief confusion and somnolence may follow the seizure. Such seizures are often preceded by an *aura*, sometimes described as an unpleasant odor or taste. Seizures may start with a blank stare, and patients may begin to chew or swallow repetitively. Some patients fumble with clothing; others try to take off their clothes. Most patients will not pay attention to verbal commands and will act as if they are having a psychotic episode. After a seizure, patients do not remember the seizure incident.

psycho = *mind*
motor = *motion or movement*

somno = *sleepiness*
lence = *filled with*

Generalized Seizures

As the name suggests, **generalized seizures** are not localized to one area but travel throughout the entire brain on both sides. The seizure is thought to originate bilaterally and symmetrically within the brain.

Absence seizures (formerly known as *petit mal seizures*) most often occur in children and last only for a few seconds. Because episodes are short-lived, they are difficult to detect. Absence epilepsy often goes unrecognized, or this disorder may be mistaken for daydreaming/signs of attention deficit disorder. Staring and temporary loss of responsiveness are the most common signs. There may be slight motor activity with eyelid fluttering or repetitive jerking motions.

bi = *two*
lateral = *sides*

sym = *same*
metrically = *measurement*

Atonic seizures are sometimes called *drop attacks*. Patients often stumble and fall for no apparent reason. Lasting for only a matter of seconds, episodes are very short.

a = *without*
tonic = *tension*

Tonic-clonic seizures (formerly known as *grand mal seizures*) are the most common type. This applies to all age groups. Seizures may be preceded by an aura (e.g., spiritual feeling, flash of light, special noise). Intense muscle contractions indicate the *tonic phase*. Due to air being forced out of the lungs, a hoarse cry may occur at the onset of the seizure. Patients may temporarily lose bladder or bowel control. Breathing may become shallow and even stop momentarily. The *clonic phase* is characterized by alternating contraction and relaxation of muscles. The seizure usually lasts one to two minutes, after which the patient becomes drowsy, disoriented, and sleeps deeply.

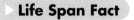

> **Life Span Fact**

Onset of epilepsy is most common among the youngest and oldest age groups. About 50% of children have a generalized epilepsy syndrome compared with about 20% of adults. The incidence of epilepsy in older adults is greater than among the general population, perhaps because of the greater prevalence of mild strokes and cardiac arrest in this age group.

> **Life Span Fact**

Preventing the onset of high fever is the best way to control febrile seizures in children.

Special Epileptic Syndromes

Special epileptic seizures include the febrile seizures of infancy, reflex epilepsies, and other forms of myoclonic epilepsies. Myoclonic epilepsies often go along with other neurologic abnormalities or progressively debilitating symptoms.

febrile = *fever*

Febrile seizures typically cause tonic-clonic motor activity lasting for one to two minutes, with rapid return of consciousness. These occur together with a rapid rise in body temperature and usually occur only once during any given illness. Febrile seizures are most likely to occur within the three-month to five-year-old age group.

myo = *muscle*
clonic = *repetitive jerking motions*

Myoclonic seizures are characterized by large, jerking body movements. Major muscle groups contract quickly, and patients appear unsteady and clumsy. They may fall from a sitting position or drop whatever they are holding. *Infantile spasms* are an example of a type of *generalized, myoclonic seizure* and are distinguished by short-lasting muscle spasms in the trunk and extremities. Such spasms are often not identified as seizures by parents or healthcare providers because the movements are much like the normal infantile startle reflex.

status = *state of*
epilepticus = *seizure activity*

hypo = *lowered*
glycemia = *blood sugar level*
thermia = *body temperature*

acid = *hydrogen ion accumulation (reduced pH; e.g., lactic acid)*
osis = *condition of*

Status epilepticus is a medical emergency caused by the repeated occurrence of seizures. This state could result with any type of seizure, but usually generalized tonic-clonic seizures are observed. When generalized tonic-clonic seizures are long and continuous, hypoxia may develop. Continuous muscle contractions also lead to hypoglycemia, acidosis, and hypothermia (due to increased metabolic needs, lactic acid production, and heat loss during muscle movement). Carbon dioxide retention also leads to acidosis. If not treated, status epilepticus can cause brain damage, and ultimately, death. Medical treatment involves the IV administration of antiseizure medications. During seizure activity, steps must be taken to make sure that the airway remains open.

Concept Review **13.1**

■ What is epilepsy? What is the difference between a seizure and a convulsion? Name and identify signs of the more common types of seizures.

CORE CONCEPT 13.4

Effective seizure management involves strict adherence to safe drug therapy.

The choice of drug for antiseizure pharmacotherapy depends on the patient's signs, previous medical history, and associated pathologies. Once a medication is selected, the patient is placed on a low initial dose. The amount is gradually increased until seizure control is achieved or until drug adverse effects prevent additional increases in dose. Serum drug levels may be obtained to assist the healthcare provider in determining the most effective drug concentration. If seizure activity continues, a different medication is added in small-dose increments while the dose of the first drug is slowly reduced. Because seizures are likely to occur if antiseizure drugs are abruptly withdrawn, the medication is usually discontinued over a period of 6 to 12 weeks.

Antiseizure drugs with indications are shown in Table 13.1 ◆. Some of the antiseizure drugs offer advantages over others. Owing to the limited induction of drug-metabolizing enzymes, the pharmacokinetic profiles of the more recently approved antiseizure drugs seem to be less complicated. In addition, the more recently approved antiseizure drugs are generally better tolerated.

One issue of antiseizure drug therapy relates to recent warnings issued by the Food and Drug Administration (FDA). In 2008, the FDA analyzed reports from clinical studies involving patients taking a variety of antiseizure medications. Epilepsy, bipolar disorder, psychoses, migraines, and neuropathic pain were among the disorders studied mainly because these were conditions emerging as disorders successfully treated with antiseizure-type medications. Currently all of these disorders are successfully treated with antiseizure medications as covered in Unit 2. Although antiseizure medications were originally designed to help people who have epilepsy, the nerve-calming qualities of these drugs have helped patients with migraines and nerve pain (neuralgia). Indeed, the usefulness of antiseizure drugs has extended beyond pain management and actually helped calm patients with behavioral and mood disturbances: attention-deficit hyperactivity disorder (ADHD), borderline personality disorder, and post-traumatic stress disorder (PTSD). Antiseizure drugs have even helped patients with schizophrenia. In a warning issued by the FDA, however, healthcare providers have been admonished to *balance carefully the clinical need for antiseizure drugs against the risk for suicidality among patients taking these drugs*. Patients and caregivers are encouraged to pay close attention to changes in mood and *not to make changes in antiseizure regimen* without consulting with their healthcare provider.

neur(o) = *nerve*
path = *disease*

Additional drawbacks include the fact that AED use may impact early child development. In 2013, a study of children whose mothers took AEDs while pregnant indicated an increased risk of early development issues. These children were not able to interact socially compared to children whose mothers did not take AEDs. Language and motor skills of the children were also impacted. Some children developed

TABLE 13.1   Selected Antiseizure Drugs with Indications

| Drug | Partial Seizures | Generalized Seizures | | Special |
		Absence	Tonic–Clonic	Myoclonic
DRUGS THAT POTENTIATE GABA				
diazepam (Valium)		✓	✓	✓
gabapentin (Neurontin)	✓			
lorazepam (Ativan)			✓	
phenobarbital (Luminal)	✓		✓	
pregabalin (Lyrica)	✓			
primidone (Mysoline)	✓		✓	
tiagabine (Gabitril)	✓			
topiramate (Topamax, Trokendi XR)	✓		✓	✓
HYDANTOIN AND RELATED DRUGS				
carbamazepine (Tegretol)	✓	✓		
lamotrigine (Lamictal)	✓	✓	✓	✓
levetiracetam (Keppra)	✓			
oxcarbazepine (Trileptal, Oxtellar XR)	✓		✓	
phenytoin (Dilantin)	✓		✓	
valproic acid (Depakene)	✓	✓	✓	✓
zonisamide (Zonegran)	✓	✓	✓	✓
SUCCINIMIDES				
ethosuximide (Zarontin)		✓		

autistic traits. This study compounds the fact that women who take oral contraceptives and antiseizure drugs together are at risk for pregnancy (see Chapter 34). This is a relatively well-known idea in health care. Thus, while many antiseizure drugs have advantages, they may also have disadvantages. A good fact to remember about all antiseizure drugs is that they can have serious clinical drawbacks if not taken safely.

Many of the antiseizure medications are used in adjunctive therapy. Some drugs have been investigated for their potential use in monotherapy. In most cases, effective seizure management can be obtained using only a single drug. For some patients, two antiseizure medications may be needed, although unwanted adverse effects may appear. Some antiseizure drug combinations may actually increase the incidence of seizures.

After several years of being seizure free, patients may question the need for their medication. In general, withdrawal of antiseizure drugs should be attempted only after at least three years of seizure-free activity and only under close direction from the healthcare provider. Doses of medications are reduced slowly, one at a time, over a period of several months. If seizures recur during the withdrawal process, pharmacotherapy is resumed, usually with the original stabilizing drug.

adjunctive = *joined or added*
mono = *only*
therapy = *treatment*

Concept Review   13.2

■ Give the names of antiseizure drugs used for the management of specific seizure types. Match the drugs with the types of seizures they best control. Which drugs are generally used for a broader range of seizures?

Antiseizure pharmacotherapy is directed at controlling the movement of electrolytes across neuronal membranes or affecting neurotransmitter balance.

CORE CONCEPT 13.5

In a resting state, neurons are normally surrounded by a higher concentration of sodium ions, calcium ions, and chloride ions. Potassium ion levels are higher inside the cell. An influx of sodium or calcium ions into the neuron *enhances* neuronal activity, whereas an influx of chloride ions *suppresses* neuronal activity.

The goal of antiseizure pharmacotherapy is to suppress neuronal activity just enough to prevent abnormal or repetitive firing. To this end, there are three general mechanisms by which antiseizure drugs work:

- Stimulating an influx of chloride ions, an effect associated with the neurotransmitter gamma-aminobutyric acid (GABA)
- Delaying an influx of sodium ions
- Delaying an influx of calcium ions

Some drugs act by more than one mechanism. This has prompted drug researchers to try to understand more clearly various drug mechanisms and to develop newer, better-controlled drugs. Recently a fourth mechanism has been studied: blocking of the primary excitatory neurotransmitter glutamate. Glutamate works in concert with the cell's Na^+-K^+ ATPase pump, which helps to restore ion balances across neuronal membranes after firing. Any drug that blocks glutamate activity prevents an influx of positive ions into the cell, so this is consistent with the last two mechanisms.

By increasing the effects of gamma-aminobutyric acid or GABA in the brain, some drugs reduce a wide range of seizure types.

CORE CONCEPT 13.6

Several important antiseizure drugs act by increasing the action of GABA, the primary inhibitory neurotransmitter in the brain. These drugs mimic the effects of GABA by stimulating an influx of chloride ions that interact with the GABA receptor–chloride channel molecule. A model of this receptor is shown in Figure 13.2 ■. When the receptor is stimulated, chloride ions move into the cell and suppress the firing of neurons.

A number of drugs, called GABA agonists, have been found to activate the GABA receptor. Drugs may bind directly to the GABA receptor through specific binding sites designated as $GABA_A$ or $GABA_B$. Most antiseizure drugs bind to the $GABA_A$ site. Drugs may enhance GABA release, or drugs may block the reuptake of GABA into nerve cells and other supporting cells in the central nervous system (CNS). Drugs have also been developed that inhibit GABA degrading enzymes.

Barbiturates, benzodiazepines, and several newer drugs reduce seizure activity by intensifying GABA action. These drugs are listed in Table 13.2 ◆. The predominant effect of GABA activation is CNS depression.

The antiseizure properties of phenobarbital were discovered in 1912, and this drug is still prescribed for seizures. As a class, barbiturates generally have a low margin for safety, a high potential for dependence, and may cause significant CNS depression. Phenobarbital, however, is able to suppress abnormal neuronal discharges without causing profound sedation. It is inexpensive, long acting, and produces a low incidence of adverse effects. When the drug is given orally, several weeks may be necessary to achieve optimum effects. Phenobarbital is a preferred drug used in the pharmacotherapy of neonatal seizures.

Other than phenobarbital, mephobarbital is occasionally used for epilepsy treatment. Mephobarbital (Mebaral) is converted to phenobarbital in the liver and offers no significant advantages over phenobarbital. Primidone (Mysoline) has a pharmacologic profile similar to phenobarbital and is among the drugs used to potentiate GABA action.

Like barbiturates, benzodiazepines and several other drugs intensify the effect of GABA in the brain. The benzodiazepines bind directly to the GABA receptor, suppressing abnormal neuronal firing.

FIGURE 13.2

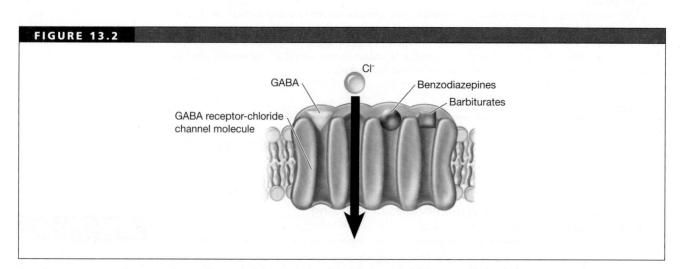

Model of the GABA receptor–chloride channel. The chloride selectivity filter allows the channel to open exclusively to chloride ions when GABA, benzodiazepines, or barbiturates bind to the cellular receptor (shown in green). Some antiseizure drugs are similar to the structure of GABA, or they may potentiate GABA indirectly. After the influx of chloride ions, the net result is inhibition of the neuron's action potential and suppression of the neuron's firing rate.

TABLE 13.2   Antiseizure Drugs That Activate GABA Receptors (GABA Agonists)

Drug	Route and Adult Dose	Remarks
BARBITURATES		
mephobarbital (Mebaral)	PO; 400–600 mg/day	Rarely used in the management of seizures; converted to phenobarbital by the liver.
(Pr) phenobarbital (Luminal)	For partial and generalized seizures: PO; 100–300 mg/day, IV/IM; 200–600 mg up to 20 mg/kg For status epilepticus: IV; 15–18 mg/kg in single or divided doses (max: 20 mg/kg)	For the management of tonic-clonic seizures, partial seizures, status epilepticus, and eclampsia; Schedule IV drug; may cause respiratory depression, agranulocytosis, laryngospasm, angioedema (swelling of the dermis).
primidone (Mysoline)	PO; 250 mg/day, increased by 250 mg/wk up to a maximum of 2 g in two to four divided doses	Similar treatment profile to phenobarbital.
BENZODIAZEPINES		
clonazepam (Klonopin)	PO; 1.5 mg/day in three divided doses, increased by 0.5–1 mg every three days until seizures are controlled	For absence seizures and minor motor seizures; also for panic disorder; Schedule IV drug; may cause drowsiness and impaired cognitive and motor performance.
clorazepate (Tranxene)	PO; 7.5 mg tid	For partial seizures; also for anxiety; Schedule IV drug.
(Pr) diazepam (Valium)	IV push, administer emulsion at 5 mg/min; IM/IV 5–10 mg (repeat as needed at 10–15 min intervals up to 30 mg; repeat again as needed every two to four hours)	Treatment for status epilepticus; also for anxiety-related symptoms and muscle spasms; see Drug Prototype box for adverse effects
lorazepam (Ativan) (see page 116 for the Prototype Drug box)	IV; 4 mg injected slowly at 2 mg/min; if inadequate response after 10 min, may repeat once	Most potent of the available benzodiazepines; for management of status epilepticus; also for nausea and vomiting, preoperative sedation, anxiety, and insomnia; Schedule IV drug.
OTHER GABA-RELATED DRUGS		
ezogabine (Potiga)	PO; start with 100 mg every eight hours; may increase dose at weekly intervals, not to exceed dosage increase of 150 mg/day/week. Optimize effective dosage between 200 mg three times daily (600 mg per day) to 400 mg three times daily (1,200 mg per day)	For use along with other medications to control partial onset seizures; often referred to as potassium channel openers due to their ability to suppress recurrent neuronal activity; may cause psychiatric and nervous system symptoms: confusion, memory impairment, blurred vision, balance disorder.
gabapentin (Neurontin)	For additional therapy: PO; start with 300 mg on day one, 300 mg bid on day two, 300 mg tid on day three, continue to increase over one week to a dose of 1,200 mg/day (400 mg tid); may increase to 1,800–2,400 mg/day	Chemical structure similar to GABA; speeds up the release of GABA from brain neurons; used for partial seizures or seizures that could become generalized; used in adults to treat nerve pain caused by herpes virus or shingles (herpes zoster), and to treat restless legs syndrome (RLS); may cause unsteadiness, weight gain, fatigue, dizziness.
pregabalin (Lyrica)	PO; start with 150 mg/day; may be increased up to 300 mg/day within 1 week, (max: 600 mg/day)	Chemical structure similar to GABA; used in the treatment of partial seizures; used for management of nerve pain associated with diabetes, nerve pain caused by herpes virus or shingles (herpes zoster), and fibromyalgia; similar adverse effects to gabapentin.
tiagabine (Gabitril)	PO; start with 4 mg/day, may increase by 4–8 mg/day every week up to 56 mg/day in two to four divided doses	Inhibits uptake of GABA into presynaptic neurons, prolonging GABA action; for the treatment of partial seizures; may cause confusion, stuttering; loss of sensation in the fingertips.
topiramate (Topamax, Trokendi XR)	PO (regular release); start with 50 mg/day, increase by 50 mg/week to effectiveness (max: 1,600 mg/day) PO (extended release); 200–400 mg once daily	Sugar-like chemical molecule; enhances the action of GABA; for partial seizures; useful in trigeminal neuralgia; may cause weight loss, numbness and tingling of the fingers and toes, behavioral issues including depression, agitation, hostility.
vigabatrin (Sabril)	PO; for infantile spasms, begin therapy at 50 mg/kg/day twice daily, increasing total daily dose per instructions to a maximum of 150 mg/kg/day; for adults with refractory complex partial seizures (CPS), initiate therapy at 500 mg twice daily, increasing total daily dose per instructions. The recommended dose is 1.5 grams twice daily	Increases GABA in the CNS; for the treatment of infantile spasms in babies one month to two years old and refractory complex partial seizures in adults; may cause fatigue, headache, irritability, gastrointestinal disturbances, inflamed throat, and irritated respiratory passages.

Benzodiazepines used in treating epilepsy include clonazepam (Klonopin), clorazepate (Tranxene), diazepam (Valium), and lorazepam (Ativan). Parenteral diazepam is used to terminate status epilepticus. Other short-term indications of benzodiazepines include absence seizures and myoclonic seizures. Because tolerance may begin to develop after only a few months of therapy, seizures may recur unless doses are periodically adjusted. Benzodiazepines and other GABA-related drugs are generally not used alone in seizure pharmacotherapy, but instead used in combination with other antiseizure medications.

Drug Prototype: ℗ *Phenobarbital (Luminal)*

Therapeutic Class: **Antiseizure drug, sedative-hypnotic**   Pharmacologic Class: **Barbiturate, GABA$_A$ receptor drug**

Actions and Uses: Phenobarbital is a long-acting barbiturate used for the management of a variety of seizures. It is also used for insomnia. Phenobarbital should not be used for pain relief, because it may increase a patient's sensitivity to pain.

Phenobarbital acts biochemically in the brain by enhancing the action of the neurotransmitter GABA, which is responsible for suppressing abnormal neuronal discharges that can cause epilepsy.

Adverse Effects and Interactions: Phenobarbital is a Schedule IV drug that may cause dependence. Common adverse effects include drowsiness, vitamin deficiencies (vitamin D, folate, B$_9$, and B$_{12}$), and laryngospasms. With overdose, phenobarbital may cause severe respiratory depression, CNS depression, coma, and death. Phenobarbital is a pregnancy category D drug.

Phenobarbital interacts with many other drugs. For example, it should not be taken with alcohol or other CNS depressants. These substances potentiate the action of barbiturates, increasing the risk of life-threatening respiratory depression or cardiac arrest. Phenobarbital increases the metabolism of many other drugs, reducing their effectiveness.

Drug Prototype: ℗ *Diazepam (Valium)*

Therapeutic Class: **Antiseizure drug, sedative-hypnotic, anxiolytic, anesthetic adjunct, skeletal muscle relaxant (centrally acting)**   Pharmacologic Class: **Benzodiazepine, GAB receptor drug**

Actions and Uses: Diazepam binds to GABA receptors located throughout the CNS. It produces its effects by suppressing neuronal activity in the limbic system and subsequent impulses that might be transmitted to the reticular activating system. Effects of this drug are suppression of abnormal neuronal foci that may cause seizures, calming without strong sedation, and skeletal muscle relaxation. When used orally, maximum therapeutic effects may take from one to two weeks. Tolerance may develop after about four weeks. When given IV, effects occur within minutes, and its anticonvulsant effects last for about 20 minutes.

Adverse Effects and Interactions: Diazepam should not be taken with alcohol or other CNS depressants because of combined sedation effects. Other drug interactions include cimetidine, oral contraceptives, valproic acid, and metoprolol, which potentiate diazepam's action, and levodopa and barbiturates, which decrease diazepam's action. Diazepam increases the levels of phenytoin in the bloodstream and may cause phenytoin toxicity. When given IV, hypotension, muscular weakness, tachycardia, and respiratory depression are common. Because of tolerance and dependency, use of diazepam is reserved for short-term seizure control or for status epilepticus.

Diazepam should be used with caution with herbal supplements, such as kava and chamomile, which may cause an increased effect.

CAM THERAPY

The Ketogenic Diet for Epilepsy

The ketogenic diet may be used when seizures cannot be controlled through pharmacotherapy or when there are unacceptable adverse effects to medications. Before antiepileptic drugs were developed, this diet was a primary treatment for epilepsy.

The ketogenic diet is a strict diet that is high in fat and low in carbohydrates and protein. It limits water intake and carefully controls caloric intake. Each meal has the same ketogenic ratio of 4 g of fat to 1 g of protein and carbohydrate. Extra fat is usually given in the form of cream.

Research suggests that the diet produces a high success rate for certain patients. The diet appears to be equally effective for every seizure type. The most frequently reported adverse effects include vomiting, fatigue, constipation, diarrhea, and hunger. Kidney stones, acidosis, and slower growth rates are possible risks. Those interested in trying the diet must consult with their healthcare provider; this is not a do-it-yourself diet and may be harmful if not monitored carefully by skilled professionals.

Since 2003, some of the GABA-related antiseizure drugs have been used for a variety of other conditions including depression, migraines, and for the management of neuropathic pain associated with diabetic peripheral neuropathy, postherpetic neuralgia, fibromyalgia, and spinal cord injury. In addition, some antiseizure drugs have been used for the management of anxiety and bipolar disorder symptoms. Two antiseizure drugs, gabapentin (Neurontin) and pregabalin (Lyrica) stand out as off-label approaches for the successful management of neuropathic pain and postherpetic neuralgia. Topiramate (Topamax, Trokendi XR) may be used in the treatment of trigeminal neuralgia.

neur = *nerve*
fibro = *fiber-related*
my = *muscle*
algia = *pain*

post = *after*
herpet = *herpes*
ic = *related*

Hydantoin and related drugs are generally effective in treating partial seizures and tonic-clonic seizures.

CORE CONCEPT 13.7

Hydantoins and related drugs dampen CNS activity by delaying an influx of sodium ions across neuronal membranes. Sodium movement is the major factor that determines whether a neuron will undergo an **action potential**. Sodium channels guide the movement of sodium ions into the cell. If sodium channels are temporarily inactivated, neuronal activity will be suppressed. If sodium channels are blocked, neuronal activity completely stops, as occurs with local anesthetic drugs (see Chapter 15). With hydantoin and related drugs, sodium channels are not blocked completely; they are just made to be less sensitive.

Several drugs in this group also affect the threshold of neuronal firing, or they may interfere with activation of the excitatory neurotransmitter glutamate. These approaches, although not directly connected with desensitization of sodium channels, result in the same effect (delayed depolarization of the neuron). Hydantoin and related drugs are listed in Table 13.3 ◆.

The oldest and most commonly prescribed antiseizure medication is phenytoin (Dilantin). Approved in the 1930s, phenytoin is a broad-spectrum hydantoin drug, useful in treatment of all kinds of epilepsy except absence seizures. It provides effective seizure suppression without the potential for abuse or extreme sedative effects. Patients vary significantly in their ability to metabolize phenytoin; therefore, dosages are highly individualized. Because of the very narrow range between therapeutic dose and toxic dose, patients must be carefully monitored. Hematologic toxicities have been associated with phenytoin drug use: thrombocytopenia, leukopenia, neutropenia, agranulocytosis, anemias, and other blood disorders have been reported. In addition, liver disease, renal dysfunction, and cardiac toxicity are severe potential hazards. Phenytoin and fosphenytoin (drug converted to phenytoin) are first-line drugs in the treatment of status epilepticus.

hematologic = *blood-related*

thrombocytopenia = *reduced platelets*

neutropenia = *reduced neutrophils*

agranulocytosis = *elevated agranulocytes (reduced granulocytes)*

anemias = *red blood cell deficiencies*

Some phenytoin-related drugs are used less frequently; others are more widely used. Most drugs share a mechanism similar to the hydantoins, including carbamazepine (Tegretol), oxcarbazepine (Trileptal, Oxtellar), and valproic acid (Depakene), which is also available as valproate and divalproex sodium. Because carbamazepine produces fewer adverse effects than phenytoin or phenobarbital, it is a preferred drug for treating tonic-clonic and partial seizures. Carbamazepine has been approved for the treatment of trigeminal neuralgia, a painful condition of the nerve responsible for facial sensation. Carbamazepine is also used off-label for a variety of indications, including ADHD, schizophrenia, borderline personality disorder, and PTSD. Oxcarbazepine is a derivative of carbamazepine, so its treatment profile is similar. Oxcarbazepine is slightly better tolerated, although serious skin and organ hypersensitivity reactions have been noted. Valproic acid is a preferred drug for absence seizures and is used in combination with other drugs for partial seizures. Valproic acid, carbamazepine, and lamotrigine are used in the treatment of bipolar disorder (see Chapter 10).

Newer approved antiseizure drugs show promise in treatment for a range of disorders, including absence seizures, partial seizures, myoclonic seizures, generalized tonic-clonic seizures, and mood

TABLE 13.3   Hydantoins and Related Drugs

Drug	Route and Adult Dose	Remarks
HYDANTOINS		
ethotoin (Peganone)	PO; initial dose 1 g/day or less in four to six divided doses with subsequent gradual dosage increases over a period of several days. Usual maintenance dosage is 2–3 g/day	For tonic-clonic and complex partial seizures; prevents the spread of seizure activity rather than to abolish the primary focus of seizure discharges; may cause swelling of the lips, tongue and throat, mood changes, chest pain, vision problems, fever.
fosphenytoin (Cerebyx)	IV; initial dose 15–20 mg PE/kg at 100–150 mg PE/min followed by 4–6 mg PE/kg/day (PE = phenytoin equivalents)	Converted to phenytoin in the body; for control of status epilepticus; short-term substitute for oral phenytoin.
Pp phenytoin (Dilantin)	PO; 15–18 mg/kg or 1 g initial dose, then 300 mg/day in one to three divided doses; may be gradually increased 100 mg/week	For tonic-clonic seizures, complex partial seizures, and seizures after head trauma; may cause unsteadiness and moderate cognitive problems, potential cosmetic issues (abnormal body/face hair and growth), skin blemishes, blood disorders, bone marrow suppression

(continued)

TABLE 13.3	Hydantoins and Related Drugs *(continued)*	
Drug	**Route and Adult Dose**	**Remarks**
PHENYTOIN-LIKE DRUGS		
carbamazepine (Tegretol)	PO; 200 mg bid, gradually increased to 800–1,200 mg/day in three to four divided doses	For tonic-clonic and complex partial seizures; useful in trigeminal neuralgia (condition characterized by intense pain along the angle of the jaw); also for bipolar disorder, ADHD, schizophrenia, borderline personality disorder, and PTSD; may cause rash (Stevens–Johnson syndrome), blood disorders, liver disease, reduced bone health.
felbamate (Felbatol)	Partial seizures: PO; start with 1,200 mg/day in three to four divided doses; may increase by 600 mg/day every 2 weeks (max: 3,600 mg/day) Lennox-Gastaut syndrome: PO; start at 15 mg/kg/day in three to four divided doses; may increase 15 mg/kg at weekly intervals to max of 45 mg/kg/day	For use in Lennox-Gastaut syndrome and partial seizures; may cause anemia and liver toxicity in some patients.
lamotrigine (Lamictal)	PO; 50 mg/day for 2 weeks, then 50 mg bid for 2 weeks; may increase gradually up to 300–500 mg/day in two divided doses (max: 700 mg/day)	For partial seizures, generalized tonic-clonic seizures, myoclonic seizures; also for bipolar disorder; may cause dizziness, fatigue, insomnia.
levetiracetam (Keppra)	PO; 500 mg twice daily (max: 3,000 mg total per day)	For use in partial seizures; may cause drowsiness, weakness, susceptibility to infections, nasal problems, nervousness.
oxcarbazepine (Trileptal, Oxtellar XR)	PO; initiation of monotherapy, 300 mg twice daily, increase 300 mg/day every third day up to 1,200 mg/day	Derivative of carbamazepine with similar treatment profile; may cause serious skin and organ hypersensitivity reactions in some patients.
rufinamide (Banzel)	PO; 400 to 800 mg per day, taken as two equal doses per day. The dose should be increased by 400 to 800 mg every two days until a maximum of 3,200 mg daily is reached	For the adjunctive treatment of seizures associated with Lennox-Gastaut syndrome in children four years and older and adults.
Pr valproic acid (Depakene, Depakote)**	PO/IV; 15 mg/kg/day in divided doses when total daily dose is greater than 250 mg; increase 5–10 mg every week until seizures are controlled (max: 60 mg/kg/day)	Broad-spectrum medication; for absence seizures, mixed generalized types of seizures; also for bipolar disorder; see Drug Prototype box for adverse effects.
zonisamide (Zonegran)	PO; 100–400 mg/day	Broad-spectrum medication; for partial seizures; it is a sulfonamide, which means that it may cause an allergic reaction in some patients.

**Other formulations of valproic acid include its salts, valproate, and divalproex sodium.

Drug Prototype: Pr *Phenytoin (Dilantin)*
Therapeutic Class: Antiseizure drug, antidysrhythmic   **Pharmacologic Class: Hydantoin, sodium influx suppressing drug**

Actions and Uses: Phenytoin acts by desensitizing sodium channels in the CNS responsible for neuronal responsivity. Desensitization prevents the spread of disruptive electrical charges in the brain that produce seizures. It is effective against most types of seizures except absence seizures. Phenytoin has antidysrhythmic activity similar to lidocaine (Class IB). An off-label use is for digoxin-induced dysrhythmias.

Adverse Effects and Interactions: Phenytoin may cause dysrhythmias such as bradycardia or ventricular fibrillation, severe hypotension, and hyperglycemia. Severe CNS reactions include headache, nystagmus, ataxia, confusion and slurred speech, paradoxical nervousness, twitching, and insomnia. Peripheral neuropathy may occur with long-term use. Phenytoin can cause multiple blood dyscrasias, including agranulocytosis and aplastic anemia. It may cause severe skin reactions, such as rashes, including exfoliative dermatitis, and Stevens–Johnson syndrome. Connective tissue reactions include lupus erythematosa, hypertrichosis, hirsutism, and gingival hypertrophy.

Phenytoin interacts with many other drugs, including oral anticoagulants, glucocorticoids, H_2 antagonists, antituberculin drugs, and food supplements such as folic acid, calcium, and vitamin D. It impairs the effectiveness of drugs such as digoxin, doxycycline, furosemide, estrogens and oral contraceptives, and theophylline. Phenytoin, when combined with tricyclic antidepressants, can trigger seizures.

Phenytoin should be used with caution with herbal supplements such as herbal laxatives (buckthorn, cascara sagrada, and senna), which may increase potassium loss.

Drug Prototype: ℗ᵣ *Valproic Acid (Depakene, Depakote)*

Therapeutic Class: Antiseizure drug, bipolar disorder drug, migraine prophylaxis **Pharmacologic Class:**
Valproate, sodium influx suppressing drug, calcium influx suppressing drug, GABA potentiating drug

Actions and Uses: The mechanism of action of valproic acid is the same as phenytoin, although effects on GABA and calcium channels may cause some additional actions. It is useful for a wide range of seizure types, including absence seizures and mixed types of seizures. Other uses include treatment of bipolar disorder and prevention of migraine headaches.

Valproic acid has several trade names and formulations, which sometimes causes confusion when studying this drug. These include the following.

- Valproic acid (Depakene) is the standard form of the drug given by the oral route.
- Valproate sodium is the sodium salt of valproic acid given orally or IV (Depacon).
- Divalproex sodium (Depakote ER) is a sustained release combination of valproic acid and its sodium salt. It is given orally and is available in an enteric-coated form.

Adverse Effects and Interactions: Adverse effects include sedation, drowsiness, gastrointestinal (GI) upset, and prolonged bleeding time. Other effects include visual disturbances, muscle weakness, tremor, psychomotor agitation, bone marrow suppression, weight gain, abdominal cramps, rash, alopecia, pruritus, photosensitivity, erythema multiforme, and fatal hepatotoxicity.

Valproic acid interacts with many drugs. For example, aspirin, cimetidine, chlorpromazine, erythromycin, and felbamate may increase valproic acid toxicity. Concomitant warfarin, aspirin, or alcohol use can cause severe bleeding. Alcohol, benzodiazepines, and other CNS depressants potentiate CNS depressant action. Lamotrigine, phenytoin, and rifampin lower valproic acid levels. Valproic acid increases serum phenobarbital and phenytoin levels. Use of clonazepam concurrently with valproic acid may induce absence seizures.

BLACK BOX WARNING:
May result in fatal hepatic failure, especially in children under the age of two years. Nonspecific symptoms often precede hepatic toxicity: weakness, facial edema, anorexia, and vomiting. Liver function tests should be performed prior to treatment and at specific intervals during the first six months of treatment. Valproic acid can produce life-threatening pancreatitis and teratogenic effects including spina bifida.

---

disorders. The most common adverse effects of the newer antiseizure drugs are drowsiness, dizziness, and blurred vision. Lamotrigine (Lamictal) has a broad spectrum of antiseizure activity and is FDA approved for long-term maintenance of bipolar disorder. This drug's duration of action is greatly affected by other drugs that inhibit or enhance hepatic metabolizing enzymes. Levetiracetam (Keppra) and zonisamide (Zonegram) are approved for adjunctive therapy of partial seizures in adults. Among the newer approved antiseizure drugs, levetiracetam has been generally less reactive than the other antiseizure medications. Conversely, zonisamide (a sulfonamide) has triggered hypersensitivity reactions in some patients. In addition, felbamate (Felbatol) has induced potentially harmful reactions, including liver toxicity and aplastic anemia.

In a severe form of epilepsy called *Lennox-Gastaut syndrome (LGS)*, valproic acid (Depakene, Depakote), lamotrigine (Lamictal), felbamate (Felbatol), topiramate (Topamax, Trokendi XR), and rufinamide (Banzel) are often used for treatment. LGS is characterized by tonic, atonic, atypical absence, and myoclonic symptoms. There is usually no single antiseizure medication that will control symptoms of this particular syndrome.

Succinimides generally treat absence seizures.

CORE CONCEPT **13.8**

Neurotransmitters, hormones, and some medications bind to neuronal membranes, stimulating the entry of calcium. Without calcium influx, neuronal transmission would not be possible. Succinimides delay entry of calcium into neurons by blocking calcium channels, increasing the electrical threshold of the neuron, and reducing the likelihood of an action potential. By raising the seizure threshold, succinimides keep neurons from firing too quickly, thus suppressing abnormal foci. The succinimides are generally effective only against absence seizures. These drugs are listed in Table 13.4 ◆.

Ethosuximide (Zarontin) is the most commonly prescribed drug in this class. It remains the preferred drug for absence seizures. It joins the other positive ion suppressing drugs that successfully treat absence seizures: valproic acid (Depakene, Depakote), lamotrigine (Lamictal), and zonisamide (Zonegran).

succin = *chemical related to succinic acid*
imide = *having an NH functional group*

Concept Review 13.3

- Name three general drug classes introduced by the Drug Snapshot feature at the beginning of this chapter. Identify the various stated chemical categories of antiseizure medications. Based on pharmacologic mechanisms, which of the drug examples do not conveniently fit into only one drug class? Which of the drugs control a wide range of seizure types? Which of the drugs have therapeutic applications other than seizure management?

TABLE 13.4	Succinimides	
Drug	**Route and Adult Dose**	**Remarks**
Pr ethosuximide (Zarontin)	PO; 250 mg bid, increased every 4–7 days (max: 1.5 g/day)	For absence seizures, myoclonic seizures, and akinetic epilepsy; may cause nausea, anorexia, abdominal pain, vomiting, gum overgrowth, blood disorders, behavioral changes, rash (Stevens–Johnson syndrome)
methsuximide (Celontin)	PO; 300 mg/day, may increase every 4–7 days (max: 1.2 g/day in divided doses)	For absence seizures; may be used in combination with other anticonvulsants in mixed types of seizure activity; may cause dizziness, drowsiness, blurred vision, increased risk for suicidal thoughts, fetal toxicity

Drug Prototype: Pr *Ethosuximide (Zarontin)*

Therapeutic Class: Antiseizure drug **Pharmacologic Class: Succinimide, low-threshold calcium channel blocking drug**

Actions and Uses: Ethosuximide is a drug of choice for absence (petit mal) seizures. It depresses the activity of neurons in the motor cortex by elevating the neuronal threshold. It is usually ineffective against psychomotor or tonic-clonic seizures; however, it may be given in combination with other medications that better treat these conditions. It is available in tablet and flavored syrup formulations.

Adverse Effects and Interactions: Ethosuximide may impair mental and physical abilities. Psychosis or extreme mood swings, including depression with suicidal intent, can occur. Behavioral changes are more prominent in patients with a history of psychiatric illness. CNS effects include dizziness, headache, lethargy, fatigue, ataxia, sleep pattern disturbances, attention difficulty, and hiccups. Bone marrow suppression and blood dyscrasias are possible, as is systemic lupus erythematosus.

Other reactions include gingival hypertrophy and tongue swelling. Common adverse effects are abdominal distress and weight loss.

Drug interactions include ethosuximide, which increases phenytoin serum levels. Valproic acid causes ethosuximide serum levels to fluctuate (increase or decrease). Serum drug levels should be done periodically to determine drug concentration.

Nursing Process Focus Patients Receiving Antiseizure Drug Therapy

ASSESSMENT	POTENTIAL NURSING DIAGNOSES
Prior to administration: ■ Obtain a complete health history including cardiovascular, renal and liver conditions, growth and developmental patterns, allergies, drug history, and possible drug interactions. ■ Evaluate laboratory blood findings: CBC, chemistry, renal and liver function studies, and drug screening. ■ Acquire the results of a complete physical examination including vital signs, ECG and neurological status (level of consciousness [LOC], mental status and identification of recent seizure activity).	■ *Risk for Injury* related to effects of seizure and adverse effects of drug therapy ■ *Noncompliance* related to length of time before medication reaches therapeutic levels and adverse effects of drug therapy ■ *Deficient Knowledge* related to a lack of information about disease process and drug therapy ■ *Ineffective Therapeutic Regimen Management* related to noncompliance with medication regimen, presence of adverse effects, and need for long-term medication use

PLANNING: PATIENT GOALS AND OUTCOMES

The patient will:
■ Experience therapeutic effects (absence of seizures or a reduction in the number or severity of seizures).
■ Be free from or experience minimal adverse effects from drug therapy.
■ Verbalize an understanding of the drug's use, adverse effects, and required precautions.

NURSING PROCESS FOCUS *(continued)*

IMPLEMENTATION

Interventions and (Rationales)	Patient Education/Discharge Planning
■ Monitor neurologic status, especially changes in level of consciousness and/or mental status. (Sedation may indicate overmedication or an adverse effect.)	Instruct the patient to: ■ Report any significant change in sensorium, such as slurred speech, confusion, hallucinations, or lethargy to the healthcare provider. ■ Report any changes in seizure quality or unexpected involuntary muscle movement such as twitching, tremor, or unusual eye movement to the healthcare provider. ■ Be aware of the risk for suicidality when not following proper medication regimen.
■ Protect the patient from injury during seizure events until the therapeutic effects of the drugs are achieved.	■ Instruct the patient to avoid driving and other hazardous activities until the effects of the drug are known.
■ Monitor effectiveness of drug therapy. (Observe for developmental and neurological changes; may indicate a need for dose adjustment.)	Instruct the patient to: ■ Keep a seizure diary to chronicle events during symptoms phase or during dose adjustment. ■ Take the medication exactly as ordered, including the same manufacturer's drug, each time the prescription is refilled. (Switching brands may result in alterations in seizure control.) ■ Take a missed dose as soon as remembered, but do not take double doses. (Doubling doses could result in toxic serum level.)
■ Monitor labs for drug levels: CBC renal and liver function studies. (Many antiseizure medications require blood testing to ensure therapeutic levels are achieved/maintained and are used to determine medication dosages. Some drugs can cause liver toxicity.)	■ Instruct the patient about the importance of keeping all laboratory appointments.
■ Monitor for adverse effects. Observe for hypersensitivity, nephrotoxicity, and hepatotoxicity.	■ Instruct the patient to report adverse effects (specific to the drug regimen) immediately to the healthcare provider.
■ Monitor oral health. Observe for signs of gingival hypertrophy, bleeding, or inflammation (phenytoin specific).	Instruct the patient to: ■ Use a soft toothbrush and oral rinses as prescribed by a dentist. ■ Avoid mouthwashes containing alcohol. ■ Report changes in oral health, such as excessive bleeding or inflammation of the gums. ■ Maintain a regular schedule of dental visits.
■ Monitor gastrointestinal status. (Valproic acid is a GI irritant and anticoagulant.) Conduct guaiac stool testing for occult blood. (Phenytoin's CNS depressant effects decrease GI motility, producing constipation.)	Instruct the patient to: ■ Take the drug with food to reduce GI upset. ■ Immediately report any severe or persistent heartburn, upper GI pain, nausea, or vomiting to the healthcare provider. ■ Increase exercise, fluid intake, and fiber intake to facilitate stool passage.
■ Monitor nutritional status. (Phenytoin's action on electrolytes may cause decreased absorption of folic acid, vitamin D, magnesium, and calcium. Deficiencies in these vitamins and minerals lead to anemia and osteoporosis. Valproic acid may cause an increase in appetite and weight.)	Instruct the patient: ■ In dietary or drug administration techniques specific to prescribed medications. ■ To report significant changes in appetite or weight gain.
■ Obtain information and monitor use of other medications. Antiseizure medications should not be used with CNS depressants or alcohol.	■ Instruct the patient to report use of any medication to the healthcare provider. ■ Inform the patient not to drink alcohol while taking these medications.
■ Administer medication correctly and evaluate the patient's knowledge of proper administration. Do not abruptly stop providing medication and monitor for presence of seizures. (Abrupt withdrawal of drugs can cause seizures to occur.)	■ Advise the patient not to discontinue medication abruptly. This action may result in status epilepticus.

EVALUATION OF OUTCOME CRITERIA

Evaluate effectiveness of drug therapy by confirming that patient goals and expected outcomes have been met (see "Planning"). *See Tables 13.2, 13.3, and 13.4 for a list of drugs to which these nursing actions apply.*

PATIENTS NEED TO KNOW

Patients taking antiseizure medications need to know the following:

In General

1. Never abruptly stop taking antiseizure medication; doing so can cause seizures to return.
2. Avoid alcohol and other CNS depressants because they can increase sedation.
3. Antiseizure medications may cause drowsiness; avoid driving and the use of machinery that could lead to injury.
4. It may require several dosage adjustments over many months to find the dosage that allows performance of normal daily activities while controlling seizures.
5. It is important to keep laboratory appointments because many antiseizure medications require blood testing to ensure that the drug is at a safe and effective level in the blood.
6. Consult a healthcare provider before trying to become pregnant; some antiseizure medications are not safe to use during pregnancy.
7. Report excess fatigue, drowsiness, agitation, confusion, or suicidal thoughts to a healthcare provider.

Regarding Hydantoins and Related Medications

8. Report the following adverse effects to a healthcare provider: gum overgrowth (gingival hyperplasia) or skin rash, tremors, weight gain, diarrhea, irregular menses, dizziness, nausea, or oversedation.
9. Hydantoins and related medications interact with many other drugs; do not add any other prescription, over-the-counter (OTC) drugs, or herbal supplements until a healthcare provider is consulted. Do not consume alcohol while taking these medications.

Regarding Succinimides

10. Report the following adverse effects to a healthcare provider: hiccups or epigastric pain with ethosuximide (Zarontin), drowsiness, or increased bleeding time.

CHAPTER REVIEW

CORE CONCEPTS SUMMARY

13.1 Although some types of seizures involve convulsions, other seizures do not.

Epilepsy is any disorder characterized by recurrent seizures. *Seizures* are abnormal and uncontrolled neuronal brain discharges. *Convulsions* are uncontrolled muscle contractions that accompany some major seizures. Drugs used to treat epilepsy are often referred to as *antiseizure drugs* or *antiepileptic drugs* (AEDs), rather than anticonvulsants.

13.2 Many causes of seizure activity are known; a few are not.

A seizure is considered a symptom of epilepsy rather than a disorder itself. In some cases, the exact cause of seizures is not known; however, there are many known causes. Seizures are the most common neurologic problem. Through a combination of pharmacotherapy, patient–family support, and education, effective seizure control can be achieved by most patients.

13.3 Epileptic seizures are typically identified as partial, generalized, or special epileptic syndromes.

Epilepsies are identified using the International Classification of Epileptic Seizures nomenclature, as partial (focal), generalized, or special epileptic syndromes. Partial seizures are further described as simple or complex seizures. Generalized seizures are described as absence seizures, atonic seizures, or tonic-clonic seizures. Special epileptic syndromes include febrile seizures, myoclonic seizures, and status epilepticus.

13.4 Effective seizure management involves strict adherence to safe drug therapy.

The choice of drug for epilepsy pharmacotherapy depends on the type of seizures the patient is experiencing, the patient's previous medical history, diagnostic studies, and the pathologic processes causing the seizures. In most cases, a single drug can effectively control seizures. In some patients, two antiseizure medications may be necessary. When discussing antiseizure medications, suicidality, developmental issues of children, birth control, and pregnancy are important topics for consideration.

13.5 Antiseizure pharmacotherapy is directed at controlling the movement of electrolytes across neuronal membranes or affecting neurotransmitter balance.

There are three general mechanisms by which antiseizure drugs work: stimulating an influx of chloride ions (an effect associated with the neurotransmitter GABA), delaying an influx of sodium, and delaying an influx of calcium. Antiseizure drugs are represented by these and possibly additional overlapping mechanisms: blocking of the excitatory neurotransmitter, glutamate, and delaying an efflux of potassium ions across neuronal membranes.

13.6 By increasing the effects of gamma-aminobutyric acid (GABA) in the brain, some drugs reduce a wide range of seizure types.

Some antiseizure drugs mimic the effects of GABA by stimulating an influx of chloride ions. Drugs may bind directly to the GABA receptor, enhance GABA release, block the reuptake of GABA into nerve cells and glia, or inhibit GABA degrading enzymes. Barbiturates, benzodiazepines, and several newer GABA-related drugs reduce seizure activity by potentiating GABA action.

13.7 Hydantoin and related drugs are generally effective in treating partial seizures and tonic-clonic seizures.

This class of drugs depresses CNS activity by desensitizing sodium channels and also by affecting the threshold of neuronal firing. Several widely used drugs, including phenytoin (Dilantin), carbamazepine (Tegretol), and valproic acid (Depakene), work by this mechanism. Some drugs act by more than one mechanism. Additional newer antiseizure drugs have been added to the regimen and may be used alone in therapy or as adjunctive drugs.

13.8 Succinimides generally treat absence seizures.

Succinimides delay entry of calcium into neurons by blocking calcium channels, increasing the electrical threshold, and reducing the likelihood that an action potential will be generated. Ethosuximide (Zarontin) is the most commonly prescribed drug in this class.

REVIEW QUESTIONS

The following questions are written in NCLEX-PN® style. Answer these questions to assess your knowledge of the chapter material, and go back and review any material that is not clear to you.

1. A young woman with a diagnosed seizure disorder asks the nurse about getting pregnant. In planning her response, the nurse knows that most antiseizure medications fall under which pregnancy category?

1. A
2. B
3. C
4. D

2. The patient on phenytoin (Dilantin) asks why he or she must have his or her labs checked. The nurse's best response would be:

1. "Dilantin can cause blood disorders."
2. "You will need to ask your doctor."
3. "We are checking to make sure you are getting enough but not too much medication."
4. "We must see if you are developing any adverse effects of the medication."

3. The patient on antiseizure medication wants to know how long he or she must take his or her medication before he or she is cured. The nurse's best response would be:

1. "You should be totally seizure free in one to three weeks."
2. "We may need to add additional medications before you are cured."

3. "It may take up to three years before you are cured."
4. "The goal of therapy is to control seizure activity."

4. A patient who has had repeated tonic-clonic seizures is admitted into the hospital. He has had a history of status epilepticus. In preparation for the possibility that status epilepticus may happen again, the nurse will have which drug available to terminate this serious type of seizure?

1. Diazepam (Valium)
2. Gabapentin (Neurontin)
3. Clorazepate (Tranxene)
4. Clonazepam (Klonopin)

5. The nurse is reviewing a patient's chart and reads that the patient experienced a generalized seizure involving alternating contractions and relaxation of the muscles. The nurse knows that this phase of the seizure is called the _____ phase.

1. Absence
2. Clonic
3. Febrile
4. Myoclonic

6. The nurse teaches the patient that one of the most common adverse effects of newer antiseizure drugs is:

1. GI upset
2. Spasms
3. Drowsiness
4. Dry mouth

7. A nurse is teaching a patient the importance of taking his or her antiseizure medication, phenobarbital (Luminal), every day at the same time. She informs the patient not to take more of this medication than prescribed because this antiseizure drug may cause: (Select all that apply.)

1. Severe respiratory depression
2. Coma
3. Confusion
4. Death

8. The nurse collects data on a patient taking ethosuximide (Zarontin) for which of the following possible adverse effects?

1. Urinary dysfunction
2. Gingival hyperplasia
3. Tremors
4. Depression

9. The nurse monitors for the occurrence of gingival hyperplasia for the patient who is taking which antiseizure medication?

1. Valproic acid (Depakene)
2. Carbamazepine (Tegretol)
3. Phenytoin (Dilantin)
4. Primidone (Mysoline)

10. The nurse checks a patient's phenytoin serum levels because, in addition to taking phenytoin, the patient is also taking:

1. Ethosuximide (Zarontin)
2. Phenobarbital (Luminal)
3. Carbamazepine (Tegretol)
4. Valproic acid (Depakene)

CASE STUDY QUESTIONS

Remember Mrs. Anthonia and her daughter, Destiny, who were introduced at the beginning of the chapter? Now read the remainder of the case study. Based on the information you have learned in this chapter, answer the questions that follow.

Mrs. Kemi Anthonia and her nine-year-old daughter, Destiny, recently visited the family physician. Mrs. Anthonia was concerned that Destiny's development might be stunted. Several complaints were noted: "Destiny sometimes acts very unusual, like she is not paying attention . . . on occasion she is unresponsive and bats her eyes . . . this sometimes lasts for a few seconds and everything appears normal again . . . lately she has been waking up a lot during the night." After a complete neurologic exam and set of laboratory tests, the family physician prescribed ethosuximide (Zarontin) for Destiny to be taken in gradually increased doses over seven days and then for a sustained period at the same dose. The physician then scheduled a return visit to the clinic in seven days.

1. The maintenance (sustained) dose of ethosuximide is usually based on 20 mg/kg/day in divided doses. Destiny weighs 66 pounds. How many kg does Destiny weigh? How many milligrams will she receive in a day? The nurse calculates the medication dosage and determines that Destiny weighs:

1. 33 kg and will receive 600 mg/day
2. 30 kg and will receive 660 mg/day
3. 30 kg and will receive 600 mg/day
4. 30 kg and will receive 630 mg/day

2. Mrs. Anthonia asks the nurse how ethosuximide (Zarontin) works to help her daughter's condition. The nurse replies that ethosuximide will:

1. Enhance the release of a neurotransmitter called GABA, which suppresses the firing of neurons.
2. Delay the amount of sodium going into the nerves, decreasing the ability of nerve impulses to travel.
3. Delay the entry of calcium into nerves keeping them from firing too quickly.
4. Activate the receptors that receive the neurotransmitter GABA.

3. The nurse lets Mrs. Anthonia know that Destiny will need to return to clinic to:

1. Be reexamined because Destiny's medication has a high potential for dependence
2. Be reexamined because Destiny's medication can cause anemia
3. Check serum drug levels to determine the most effective drug concentration
4. Check to be sure Destiny is OK because her medication has a low margin of safety

4. Which of the following medications, if prescribed for Destiny as a second medication, would cause ethosuximide (Zarontin) serum levels to fluctuate?

1. Phenobarbital (Luminal)
2. Diazepam (Valium)
3. Pregabalin (Lyrica)
4. Valproic acid (Depakene)

NOTE: Answers to the Review and Case Study Questions appear in Appendix B. The complete rationales and answers are located on the textbook's website.

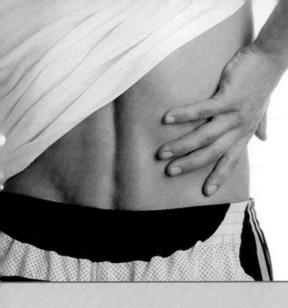

"I was playing tennis and it just popped. How many more months is this going to hurt?"

Mr. Damian Coidiuf

Drugs for Pain Management

CORE CONCEPTS

14.1 Pain assessment is the first step to pain management.

14.2 Pain transmission processes allow several major targets for pharmacologic intervention.

14.3 Nonpharmacologic techniques and adjuvant analgesics assist in providing adequate pain relief.

14.4 Opioid analgesic medications exert their effects by interacting with specific receptors.

14.5 Opioids have multiple therapeutic effects, including relief of severe pain.

14.6 Nonsteroidal anti-inflammatory drugs (NSAIDs) are the preferred nonopioid analgesics for inflammation and less severe pain.

14.7 Migraines can be effectively treated with a variety of drug classes.

DRUG SNAPSHOT

The following drugs are discussed in this chapter:

DRUG CLASSES	DRUG PROTOTYPES
Opioid Analgesics for Severe Pain	
Opioid agonists	**Pr** morphine (Astramorph PF, Duramorph, others) *203*
Opioid antagonists	**Pr** naloxone (Narcan) *205*
Opioids with mixed agonist–antagonist activity	
Nonopioid Analgesics for Moderate Pain	
Nonsteroidal anti-inflammatory drugs (NSAIDs)	
Aspirin and other salicylates	**Pr** aspirin (acetylsalicylic acid, ASA) *208*

DRUG CLASSES	DRUG PROTOTYPES
Ibuprofen and ibuprofen-like drugs	
Selective COX-2 inhibitors	
Centrally acting drugs	
Antimigraine and Tension Headache Drugs	
Triptans	**Pr** sumatriptan (Imitrex) *213*
Ergot alkaloids	
Other drugs	

LEARNING OUTCOMES

After reading this chapter, the student should be able to:

1. Relate the importance of pain assessment to effective pharmacotherapy.

2. Explain the neural mechanism for pain at the level of the spinal cord.

3. Explain how pain can be controlled by inhibiting the release of spinal neurotransmitters.

4. Describe the role of nonpharmacologic therapies and adjuvant analgesics in pain management.

5. Compare and contrast the types of opioid receptors and their importance to pharmacology.

6. Explain the role of opioid antagonists in the diagnosis and treatment of acute opioid toxicity.

7. Describe the long-term treatment of opioid dependence.

8. Compare the pharmacotherapeutic approaches of preventing migraines to those of aborting migraines.

9. Categorize drugs used in the treatment of pain based on their classifications and mechanisms of action.

10. For each of the classes listed in the Drug Snapshot, identify representative drugs and explain their mechanisms of drug action, primary actions, and important adverse effects.

KEY TERMS

Aδ fibers *199*

adjuvant analgesics (ADD-jeh-vent an-ul-JEE-ziks) *201*

analgesics (an-ul-JEE-ziks) *201*

auras (AUR-uhs) *211*

bradykinin (bray-dee-KYE-nin) *208*

C fibers *199*

cyclooxygenase (cox) (sye-klo-OK-sah-jen-ays) *208*

endogenous opioids (en-DAHJ-en-nuss O-pee-oyds) *200*

migraine (MYE-grayne) *211*

narcotic (nar-KOT-ik) *202*

nociceptor (no-si-SEPP-ter) *198*

opiates (OH-pee-ahts) *201*

opioid (OH-pee-oyd) *201*

patient-controlled analgesia (PCA) (patient-controlled an-ul-JEE-ziah *203*

prostaglandins (pros-tah-GLAN-dins) *208*

substance P *199*

tension headache *211*

P ain is a physiological and emotional experience characterized by unpleasant feelings, usually associated with a medical procedure, trauma, or disease. On a basic level, pain has always been described as a defense mechanism that helps the body avoid a potentially dangerous situation. Pain is a natural reaction prompting patients to seek medical help. Although the neural and chemical mechanisms for pain are well characterized, psychological and emotional processes modify pain; anxiety, fatigue, and depression can increase the perception of pain. Positive attitudes and support from caregivers can reduce the perception of pain. Patients are more likely to tolerate their pain if they know the source of the sensation and the course of medical treatment necessary to manage the pain.

ACUTE OR CHRONIC PAIN

The purpose of pain assessment is to guide the appropriate course of medical treatment. Pain can be characterized as acute or chronic. Acute pain is an intense pain occurring over a brief time, usually from time of injury until tissue repair. Chronic pain is longer lasting pain that may persist for weeks, months, or years. Pain lasting longer than six months can interfere with activities of daily living and can contribute to feelings of helplessness or hopelessness.

CORE CONCEPT 14.1

Pain assessment is the first step to pain management.

noci = *pain or injury*
ceptor = *receiver*

somatic = *referring to the body*

visceral = *deeper organ*

neur(o) = *nerve-related*
algia = *pain*
path(y) = *damage or disease state*
ic = *related to*

trigeminal = *fifth cranial nerve (tri = three branches; geminal = matching face)*

The psychological reaction to pain is a subjective experience. The same degree and type of pain may be described as excruciating and unbearable by one patient and not even be mentioned by another patient. Several numerical scales and survey instruments are available to help healthcare providers characterize the pain and measure the progress of drug therapy. Often the healthcare provider will simply ask, "How does your pain feel on a scale of zero to ten, ten being the most intense pain you have ever experienced?" Successful pain management depends on an accurate assessment of both the degree of pain and the source of pain experienced by the patient.

Besides being termed *acute* or *chronic*, pain can also be described by its source. Injury to *tissues* produces *nociceptor pain*. This type of pain may be further subdivided into *somatic pain*, which produces sharp, localized sensations in the body, or *visceral pain*, which produces generalized dull and internal throbbing or aching pain. The term **nociceptor** refers to activation of receptor nerve endings that receive and transmit pain signals to the central nervous system. *Neuropathic pain* is caused by direct injury to the nerves. Whereas *nociceptor* pain responds quite well to conventional pain relief medications, *neuropathic* pain responds less successfully. Common types of neuropathic pain are shown in Table 14.1 ◆.

TABLE 14.1 Common Types of Neuropathic Pain	
Examples	**Description**
Carpal tunnel syndrome	pain due to nerve compression in the wrist, thumb, and fingers
Central pain syndrome	general pain caused by damage of nerves in the CNS—that is, due to stroke or multiple sclerosis
Degenerative disk disease	back pain due to damage of nerves entering or exiting the spinal cord
Diabetic neuropathy	burning or stabbing pain in the hands and feet of patients suffering from diabetes
Intractable cancer pain	pain due to progressive or metastatic spread of cancer
Phantom limb pain	pain occurring in some patients after a limb is amputated
Postherpetic neuralgia	pain brought on by herpes and herpes–related viruses or the outbreak of shingles
Postsurgical pain	pain after a surgical procedure
Sciatica	leg pain due to compression or irritation of the sciatic nerve
Trigeminal neuralgia	shooting pain in the upper neck and jaw

Fast Facts Pain

- Pain is a common symptom.
- Approximately 16 million people experience chronic arthritic pain.
- At least 31 million adults report low back pain, with 19 million people experiencing this on a chronic basis.
- Currently, 50 million people are fully or partially disabled as a result of pain.
- Over 50% of adults experience muscle pain each year.
- Up to 40% of people with cancer report moderate to severe pain.
- About 28 million Americans suffer from headaches and migraines.
- Use of drug therapy and other measures controls 95% of migraines.
- After puberty, women have four to eight times more migraines than men.
- Before puberty, more boys have migraines than girls.
- Headaches and migraines appear mostly among people ages 20 to 40.
- Persons with a family history of headache or migraine have a greater chance of developing these disorders.

Concept Review 14.1

- What questions would you ask to identify a patient's type of pain? How would you distinguish between acute pain and chronic pain? Which is the more difficult type of pain to treat?

Pain transmission processes allow several major targets for pharmacologic intervention.

CORE CONCEPT 14.2

The process of pain transmission begins when nociceptors are stimulated. Nociceptors are free nerve endings located throughout the entire body. The nerve impulse signaling the pain is sent to the spinal cord along two types of sensory neurons, called Aδ and C fibers. **Aδ fibers** are sensory neurons that are *thinly wrapped in myelin*, a fatty substance that speeds up nerve transmission and signals sharp, well-defined pain. **C fibers** are *unmyelinated* fibers; thus, they carry nerve impulses more slowly and conduct dull, poorly localized pain.

Once pain impulses reach the spinal cord, neurotransmitters pass the message along to the next neuron. Here, a neurotransmitter called **substance P** is thought to be responsible for continuing the pain message, although other neurotransmitter candidates have been proposed. Spinal substance P is critical because it controls whether pain signals will continue to the brain. The activity of substance P may be affected by other neurotransmitters released from neurons in the central nervous system (CNS). One group

FIGURE 14.1

Neural pathways for pain.

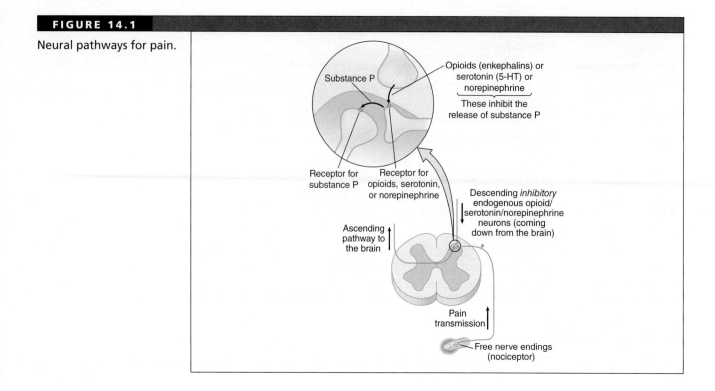

endo = *within*
genous = *coming from*

of these neurotransmitters, called **endogenous opioids**, includes endorphins, dynorphins, and enkephalins. Figure 14.1 ■ shows one point of contact where endogenous opioids modify sensory information at the level of the spinal cord. If pain impulses reach the brain, many possible actions may occur, ranging from immediate reaction to the stimulus, persistent aching and suffering, or thoughts of mental depression if the pain signal is repetitive and long-lasting.

Because pain signals begin at nociceptors located within peripheral body tissues and then proceed throughout the CNS, there are several targets where medications can work to stop pain transmission. In general, two major classes of drugs are employed to manage pain: opioid analgesics and nonopioid analgesics such as the nonsteroidal anti-inflammatory drugs (NSAIDs). Opioids act within the CNS, whereas NSAIDs act at the nociceptor level. There are multiple sites throughout the CNS where centrally acting drugs can produce their effects, and there are many peripheral targets as well, depending on the approach of drug therapy.

Concept Review 14.2

■ What is a nociceptor? Consider substance P and endogenous opioids, and describe the approaches of pain management.

Nonpharmacologic techniques and adjuvant analgesics assist in providing adequate pain relief.

somno = *drowsiness or sleepiness*
lence = *state of*

Although drugs are quite effective at relieving pain in most patients, they can have significant adverse effects. For example, at high doses, opioids can cause nausea, constipation, loss of appetite, and profound somnolence, and aspirin can cause gastrointestinal (GI) bleeding.

To help patients obtain adequate pain relief, nonpharmacologic techniques are often used as an essential form of adjunctive therapy. Rarely will nonpharmacologic techniques be used in place of pharmacotherapy, but when used together with medication, nonpharmacologic techniques allow medication doses to be lowered. Lowered doses typically mean fewer drug-related adverse effects. Some nonpharmacologic techniques employed for reducing pain include the following:

- Physical therapy
- Massage
- Biofeedback therapy

- Heat or cold packs
- Meditation or prayer
- Relaxation therapy
- Art or music therapy
- Imagery
- Chiropractic manipulation
- Hypnosis
- Therapeutic touch
- Transcutaneous electrical nerve stimulation (TENS)
- Energy therapies such as reiki and qi gong
- Acupuncture

Nonpharmacologic techniques have an advantage that they can help improve the patient's mood, reduce anxiety, and provide the patient with a sense of control. Depending on the technique, nonpharmacologic strategies often relax muscles, strengthen coping abilities, and generally improve the patient's quality of life. There are many determinants of successful therapy depending on the type of pain, its duration and severity. The success of therapy will also vary from patient to patient and will depend on many factors including the patient's age, attitude, tolerance, and level of compliance with overall therapy. The patient's coping skills, capabilities, and commitment will play a role in both pain management and recovery. Costs of health care, availability of support from family members, and support from members within the surrounding community are extremely important.

Patients with challenging or *intractable* (not easy to relieve) pain may require additional therapy. In this case, **adjuvant analgesics** or *co-analgesics* may be used. Antiseizure drugs (Chapter 13) and local anesthetics (Chapter 15) are examples of drug categories approved by the FDA for successful management of pain. Carbamazepine (Tegretol) is approved for treatment of pain due to trigeminal neuralgia. Valproic acid (Depakene or Depakote) is approved for the treatment of pain due to migraines. Gabapentin (Neurontin) is prescribed for the management of postherpetic neuralgia. Pregabalin (Lyrica) is approval for treatment of fibromyalgia, postherpetic neuralgia, and pain due to peripheral diabetic neuropathy. All of these drugs were originally developed to treat conditions other than pain, but now have found useful application for pain that is difficult to manage. Anesthetic nerve blocking drugs are another type of adjuvant analgesic used for the management of acute and chronic pain, and are administered in a variety of ways for different purposes. Lidoderm, for example, is a local anesthetic patch with 5% lidocaine used to reduce pain or discomfort caused by skin irritations such as sunburn, insect bites, plant resins, minor cuts, scratches, and burns. It is also used for post-surgical and post-shingles pain (Chapters 15 and 36). Corticosteroids reduce inflammation and can also control certain types of inflammatory pain (Chapter 24).

Many medications are appropriately used for pain management, even though the FDA has not specifically approved them for a particular use. Some well-established *off-label medications* for pain management are the tricyclic antidepressants (TCAs) (Chapter 10). Examples are amitriptyline (Elavil), nortriptyline (Aventyl, Pamelor) and imipramine (Tofranil), which have been used to suppress a variety of pain impulses characterized as chronic and neuropathic. Neuropathic pain impulses are even slowed by dysrhythmic drugs when TCAs are not effective. Thus, cardiovascular drugs have even found a place in pain management. Examples are mexiletine (Mexitil) and flecainide (Tambocor) (Chapter 22).

in = *opposite of*
tractable = *control*

Opioid analgesic medications exert their effects by interacting with specific receptors.

CORE CONCEPT 14.4

Analgesics are medications used to relieve pain. The two basic categories of analgesics are the opioids (narcotics) and the nonopioids. Terminology for the narcotic analgesics may be confusing. Several of these drugs are obtained from opium, a milky extract from the unripe seeds of the poppy plant, which contains more than 20 different chemicals having pharmacologic activity. Opium consists of 9% to 14% morphine and 0.8% to 2.5% codeine. These natural substances are called **opiates**. In a search for safer analgesics, chemists have created several dozen synthetic drugs with activity similar to that of the opiates. For example, morphine is a natural narcotic; meperidine is a synthetic narcotic. **Opioid** is a general term referring to any of these substances, natural or synthetic, and is often used interchangeably with the term *opiate*. An opioid analgesic is a natural or synthetic morphine-like substance responsible for reducing moderate to severe pain. Opioids are narcotic substances, meaning that they produce numbness or stupor-like symptoms.

an = *without*
algesia = *pain*

narc = *numbness or stupor*
otic = *like*

opi = *opium*
oid = *shape or form*

Narcotic is a general term often used to describe opioid drugs that produce analgesia and CNS depression. In common usage, a narcotic analgesic is the same as an opioid, and the terms are often used interchangeably. In the context of drug enforcement, however, the term *narcotic* describes a much broader range of abused illegal drugs such as hallucinogens, heroin, amphetamines, and marijuana. This is an important fact to remember when discussing use of opioids with members of law enforcement.

Opioids exert their actions by interacting with at least four major types of receptors: mu, kappa, delta, and an opioid-like receptor called nociceptin or orphanin FQ peptide. For pain management, the *mu receptors* and *kappa receptors* have been the ones traditionally targeted. Delta receptors also have a role in analgesia; they are connected with the emotional and affective components of the pain experience and thus, have become recent targets for drug development.

affective = *expressive*

Responses produced by activation of mu and kappa receptors are listed in Table 14.2 ◆. Some opioids, such as morphine, activate both mu and kappa receptors. Opioid blockers such as naloxone (Narcan) inhibit both the mu and kappa receptors. Other opioids, such as pentazocine (Talwin), exert mixed effects by activating the kappa receptors but blocking the mu receptors. This is the body's way of providing for a diverse set of body responses from one substance. Figure 14.2 ■ illustrates actions resulting from stimulation of mu and kappa receptors.

Concept Review   14.3

■ Distinguish between the following terms: *opioid*, *opiate*, and *narcotic*. Name four classes of opioid receptors, and identify those that are connected with analgesia.

TABLE 14.2 Responses Produced by Activation of Specific Opioid Receptors		
Response	**Mu Receptor**	**Kappa Receptor**
Analgesia	✓	✓
Decreased GI motility	✓	✓
Euphoria	✓	
Miosis (constricted pupils)		✓
Physical dependence	✓	
Respiratory depression	✓	
Sedation	✓	✓

FIGURE 14.2

Opioid receptors.

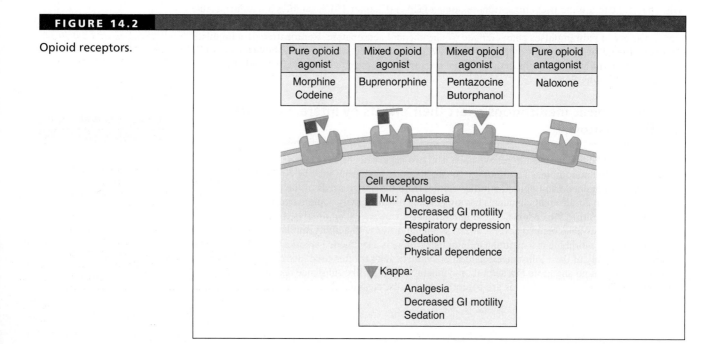

OPIOID ANALGESICS FOR SEVERE PAIN

Opioids have multiple therapeutic effects, including relief of severe pain.

Opioids are drugs for moderate to severe pain that cannot be controlled with other classes of analgesics. Narcotic opioids bind to opioid receptors and produce multiple responses throughout the body. As powerful CNS depressants, opioid narcotics can cause sedation, which may be a therapeutic effect or an adverse effect, depending on the patient's disease state. Some patients experience euphoria and intense relaxation, which are reasons why opiates are sometimes abused. There are many adverse effects, including respiratory depression, sedation, nausea, and vomiting. More than 20 different opioids are available as medications, and they can be classified by similarities in their chemical structures, by their mechanisms of action, or by their effectiveness. The most useful method is by effectiveness, which places opiates into categories of high or moderate narcotic activity (Table 14.3 ◆).

Opioid Agonists

Drugs that stimulate a particular opioid receptor are called *opioid agonists*. Morphine is the prototype opioid agonist used to treat severe pain. It is usually the standard by which the effectiveness of other opioids is compared.

All of the opioid agonists have the potential to cause physical and psychological dependence, as discussed in Chapter 7. Over the years, healthcare providers have been hesitant to administer the proper amount of opioid analgesic for fear of causing patient dependence or of producing serious adverse effects, such as sedation or respiratory depression. Because of this tendency, some patients have not received complete pain relief.

When used according to accepted medical practice, patients can, and indeed should, receive the pain relief they need without fear of addiction or adverse effects. One method available to accomplish this is **patient-controlled analgesia (PCA)**. In this instance, patients are allowed to self-medicate with opiate medication by pressing a button. Safe levels of pain medication are delivered with an infusion pump.

The fentanyl transdermal system (Duragesic patch) is another strong prescription medication used for the control of moderate to severe chronic pain. The patch enables longer-lasting relief from persistent pain. Fentanyl (Lazanda) nasal spray is available for quick delivery across nasal mucous membranes. Fentanyl is also administered as a lozenge (Oralet, Actiq), tablet (Fentora, Onsolis), or via sublingual (Abstral) administration. These slowly dissolve in the mouth, and drugs are absorbed via the mouth's mucous membranes.

Drug Prototype: ℗ *Morphine (Astramorph PF, Duramorph, Others)*

Therapeutic Class: Opioid analgesic
Pharmacologic Class: Opioid agonist receptor drug

Actions and Uses: Morphine binds with both mu and kappa receptor sites to produce strong analgesia. It causes euphoria, constriction of the pupils, and stimulation of cardiac muscle. It is used for relief of serious acute and chronic pain after non-narcotic analgesics have failed, as preanesthetic medication, to relieve shortness of breath associated with heart failure and pulmonary edema, and for acute chest pain connected with myocardial infarction (MI).

Adverse Effects and Interactions: Morphine may cause dysphoria (restlessness, depression, and anxiety), hallucinations, nausea, constipation, dizziness, and an itching sensation. Overdose may result in severe respiratory depression or cardiac arrest. Tolerance develops to the analgesic, sedative, and euphoric effects of the drug. Cross-tolerance also develops between morphine and other opioids such as heroin, methadone, and meperidine. Physical and psychological dependence develop when high doses are taken for prolonged periods. Morphine may intensify or mask the pain of gallbladder disease due to biliary tract spasms.

Morphine interacts with several drugs. For example, use with CNS depressants, such as alcohol, other opioids, general anesthetics, sedatives, and antidepressants such as monoamine oxidase inhibitors (MAOIs) and tricyclics, increases the action of opiates and thereby raises the risk of severe respiratory depression and death.

Use with caution with herbal supplements, such as yohimbe, which may increase the effect of morphine.

BLACK BOX WARNING:
When morphine is administered as an epidural drug, due to the risk of adverse effects, patients must be observed in a fully equipped and staffed environment for at least 24 hours. Morphine administered as extended-release tablets has an abuse liability similar to other opioid analgesics. Morphine is a Schedule II controlled substance and should be taken properly according to dispensing instructions (i.e., tablets/capsules should be taken whole and not broken, chewed, dissolved, or crushed). Alcohol should be avoided with morphine products (e.g., Avinza). Failure to follow these warnings could result in fatal respiratory depression.

TABLE 14.3 Opioids for Pain Management

Drug	Route and Adult Dose	Remarks
OPIOID AGONISTS WITH HIGH EFFECTIVENESS		
fentanyl (Actiq, Abstral Duragesic, Fentora, Lazanda, Onsolis, Oralet,)	IM; 0.05–0.1 mg Transdermal 25–100 mcg every 72 hours	Used with anesthesia for surgery and other procedures; also available by the buccal and nasal spray routes.
hydromorphone (Dilaudid, Exalgo)	PO; 1–4 mg every 4–6 hours prn	Also for cough; available in IM, IV, subcutaneous, and rectal forms.
levorphanol (Levo-Dromoran)	PO; 2–3 mg tid to qid prn	Also available in subcutaneous form.
meperidine (Demerol)	PO; 50–150 mg every 3–4 hours prn	For preoperative medication or obstetric analgesia; available in IM, IV, and subcutaneous forms.
methadone (Dolophine)	PO; 2.5–10 mg every 3–4 hours prn	For detoxification treatment of opioid dependency; available in IM and IV forms.
(Pr) morphine (Astramorph PF, Duramorph, others)	PO; 10–30 mg every 4 hours prn	Available in IM, IV, subcutaneous, intrathecal, epidural, and rectal forms.
oxymorphone (Opana)	Subcutaneous/IM; 1–1.5 mg every 4–6 hours prn; 5 mg every 4–6 hours prn	Also available in IV and rectal forms.
OPIOID AGONISTS WITH MODERATE EFFECTIVENESS		
codeine	PO; 15–60 mg qid	Also for cough; available in IM and subcutaneous forms; combination drug with aspirin is called Empirin; available also as combination drug with acetaminophen (Tylenol with codeine).
hydrocodone (Hycodan)	PO; 5–10 mg every 4–6 hours prn (max: 15 mg/dose)	Also for cough; combination drug with acetaminophen is called Vicodin.
oxycodone (OxyContin, Oxecta); oxycodone terephthalate (Percocet-5, Roxicet, others)	PO; 5–10 mg qid prn Controlled release; 10–20 mg every 12 hours	Combination drug with acetaminophen is called Percocet or Roxicet; with aspirin is called Percodan.
OPIOID ANTAGONISTS		
(Pr) naloxone (Narcan)	IV; 0.4–2 mg, may be repeated every 2–3 min up to 10 mg if necessary	For opioid overdose and postoperative opioid depression.
naltrexone (Trexan, ReVia, Vivatrol)	PO; 25 mg followed by another 25 mg in 1 hour if no withdrawal response (max: 800 mg/day)	For management of opiate or alcohol dependence; longer lasting effect than naloxone.
OPIOIDS WITH MIXED AGONIST–ANTAGONIST EFFECTS		
buprenorphine (Buprenex, Butrans, Suboxone)	IM/IV; 0.3 mg every 6 hours (max: 0.6 mg every 4 hours)	For moderate to severe pain; also available in subcutaneous, epidural, and rectal forms.
butorphanol (Stadol)	IM; 1–4 mg every 3–4 hours prn (max: 4 mg/dose)	For obstetrical analgesia during labor, cancer pain, renal colic, and burns; available in IV and intranasal forms.
nalbuphine (Nubain)	Subcutaneous/IM/IV; 10–20 mg every 3–6 hours prn (max: 160 mg/day)	For moderate to severe pain.
pentazocine (Talwin)	PO; 50–100 mg every 3–4 hours (max: 600 mg/day); subcutaneous/IM/IV; 30 mg every 3–4 hours (max: 360 mg/day)	For moderate to severe pain (much lower dose for women in labor).

Buccal fentanyl is indicated for the management of breakthrough cancer pain in adult patients who are already receiving and who might already be tolerant to traditional opioid therapy. These medications should not be used to treat pain other than chronic cancer pain or in the management of acute or postoperative pain, including headaches and migraines. Fentanyl may cause serious harm or death if used accidentally by a child or by an adult who does not have a higher level of tolerance to opioids. Respiratory depression and fatal overdose are risks. Alfentanil (Alfenta), remifentanil (Ultiva), and sufentanil (Sufenta) are used to provide continuous pain relief during and after surgery or for use during the induction and maintenance of general anesthesia; these are discussed further in Chapter 15.

In the pharmacologic management of pain, it is common practice to combine opioids and nonnarcotic analgesics into a single tablet or capsule (Core Concept 14.6). The two classes of analgesics work *synergistically* to relieve pain, and the dose of narcotic can be kept small to avoid dependence and opioid-related adverse effects. Examples of combination analgesics are as follows:

syn = *together*
erg = *work*
istically = *ability to*

- Vicodin (hydrocodone, 5 mg; acetaminophen, 500 mg)

- Percocet (oxycodone HCl, 5 mg; acetaminophen, 325 mg)

- Percodan (oxycodone HCl, 4.5 mg; oxycodone terephthalate, 0.38 mg; aspirin, 325 mg)

- Empirin with Codeine No. 2 (codeine phosphate, 15 mg; aspirin, 325 mg)

- Ascomp with Codeine or Fiorinal (codeine phosphate, 30 mg; aspirin, 325 mg; caffeine, 40 mg; butalbital, 50 mg)

- Fioricet with Codeine (codeine phosphate, 30 mg; acetaminophen, 325 mg; caffeine, 40 mg; butalbital, 50 mg)

- Tylenol with Codeine (single dose may contain from 15 to 60 mg of codeine phosphate and from 300 to 1,000 mg of acetaminophen)

Some opioids are used primarily for conditions other than pain relief. Codeine is often prescribed as a cough suppressant and is covered in Chapter 29. Opiates used in treating diarrhea are presented in Chapter 30.

Opioid Antagonists

Drugs that block an opioid receptor are called *opioid antagonists*. Opioid antagonists are substances that prevent the effects of opioid agonists. These drugs are considered *competitive antagonists* because they compete with opioid agonists for access to the opioid receptor site.

Opioid overdose can occur as a result of overly aggressive pain therapy or as a result of substance abuse. Any opioid may be abused for its psychoactive effects; however, morphine, meperidine, and heroin are sometimes preferred because of their potency. Although heroin is currently available as a legal analgesic in many countries, it is considered by the FDA to be too dangerous for therapeutic use and is a major drug of abuse. Once injected or inhaled, heroin rapidly crosses the blood–brain barrier to enter the brain, where it is metabolized to morphine. Thus, the effects and symptoms of heroin use are actually caused by the activation of mu and kappa receptors by morphine. The initial effect is an intense euphoria, called a *rush*, followed by several hours of deep relaxation.

Opioid antagonists are often used to reverse the symptoms of opioid toxicity or overdose. Symptoms of overdose include sedation or respiratory distress. Acute opioid intoxication is a medical emergency, with respiratory depression being the most serious problem. Infusion with the opioid antagonist naloxone (Narcan) may be used to reverse respiratory depression and other acute symptoms. Naltrexone mixed with morphine (Embeda) is used for moderate to severe pain control when a continuous, round-the-clock opioid analgesic is needed for an extended period. In cases in which the patient is unconscious or unclear as to which drug has been taken, opioid antagonists may be given to diagnose the overdose. If the opioid antagonist fails to quickly reverse the acute symptoms, the overdose may be attributed to a nonopioid substance.

Drug Prototype: ℞ *Naloxone (Narcan)*

Therapeutic Class: Drug for treatment of acute opioid overdose and misuse
Pharmacologic Class: Opioid receptor blocker

Actions and Uses: Naloxone is a pure opioid antagonist, blocking both mu and kappa receptors. It is used for complete or partial reversal of opioid effects in emergency situations when acute opioid overdose is suspected. Given intravenously, it begins to reverse opioid-initiated CNS and respiratory depression within minutes. It will immediately cause opioid withdrawal symptoms in patients physically dependent on opioids. It is also used to treat postoperative opioid depression (after-effect of the opioid therapy applied during surgery). It is occasionally given as adjunctive therapy to reverse hypotension caused by septic shock. Naloxone is pregnancy category B.

Adverse Effects and Interactions: Naloxone itself has minimal toxicity. However, in reversing the effects of opioids, the patient may experience rapid loss of analgesia, increased blood pressure, tremors, hyperventilation, nausea/vomiting, and drowsiness. It should not be used for respiratory depression caused by nonopioid medications.

Drug interactions include a reversal of the analgesic effects of narcotic agonists and agonist–antagonists.

BLACK BOX WARNING:
None; however, naltrexone, a similar opioid receptor antagonist, has the capacity to produce hepatic injury when taken in excessive doses or if taken by patients with hepatic injury or acute liver disease.

Opioids with Mixed Agonist–Antagonist Effects

Narcotic opioids that have mixed agonist–antagonist activity stimulate the opioid receptor; thus, they cause analgesia. However, withdrawal symptoms and adverse effects are not as intense due to partial activation of the receptor subtypes.

Although effective at relieving pain, the opioid agonists have a greater risk for dependence than almost any other class of medications. Tolerance develops relatively quickly to the euphoric effects of opioids, causing users to increase their doses and take the drugs more frequently. The higher and more frequent doses rapidly cause physical dependence in opioid abusers.

When physically dependent patients attempt to discontinue drug use, they experience extremely uncomfortable symptoms which generally cause them to continue taking the drugs. As long as the drugs are continued, they feel "normal" and continue to work and engage in social activities. If they abruptly discontinue the drugs, they experience withdrawal symptoms for about seven days before overcoming the physical dependence. Beyond this, the intense craving that characterizes psychological dependence may occur for many months, even years, following discontinuation of opioids. This often results in a return to drug-seeking behavior unless support groups are established.

One method of treating opioid dependence has been to switch the patient from IV and inhalation forms of illegal drugs to oral methadone (Dolophine). Although oral methadone is an opioid, it does not cause the euphoria of the injectable opioids. Methadone also does not cure the dependence, and the patient must continue taking the drug to avoid withdrawal symptoms. This therapy, called *methadone maintenance*, may continue for many months or years, until the patient decides to enter a total withdrawal treatment program. Methadone maintenance allows patients to return to productive work and social relationships without the physical, emotional, and criminal risks of illegal drug use.

A newer treatment option is to administer buprenorphine (Buprenex, Butrans, Suboxone), a mixed opioid agonist–antagonist, by the sublingual or transdermal route. Buprenorphine is used early in opioid abuse therapy to prevent opioid withdrawal symptoms. Suboxone, contains both buprenorphine and naloxone and is used later in the maintenance of opioid addiction.

Healthcare providers should always be aware that when administering mixed agonist–antagonists with opioid agonists, their pain-blocking properties are reduced. Thus, there may be a tendency to overprescribe mixed opioids, promoting drug misuse. This is true even though in most cases the potential for causing opioid addiction is lower with mixed agonist–antagonists drugs.

NURSING PROCESS FOCUS   Patients Receiving Opioids

ASSESSMENT	POTENTIAL NURSING DIAGNOSES
Prior to administration: ■ Obtain a complete health history including cardiovascular, respiratory, neurological, renal and liver conditions, allergies, drug history, likelihood of drug dependency, and possible drug interactions. ■ Evaluate complaints of pain (quality, intensity, location, duration). ■ Acquire the results of a complete phsycial examination including vital signs and ECG. ■ Evaluate laboratory blood findings: CBC, chemistry, renal and liver function studies, and drug screening. ■ Determine neurological status (level of consciousness [LOC], mental status and identification of recent mood and behavior patterns).	■ *Deficient Knowledge* related to a lack of information about drug therapy ■ *Acute or Chronic Pain* related to injury, disease process, surgical procedure or inadequate medication ■ *Ineffective Breathing Pattern* related to adverse effects of drug therapy ■ *Constipation* related to adverse effect of drug therapy ■ *Risk for Injury* related to adverse effect of drug therapy

PLANNING: PATIENT GOALS AND EXPECTED OUTCOMES

The patient will:
■ Experience therapeutic effects (report of pain relief or a reduction in pain intensity).
■ Be free from or experience minimal adverse effects from drug therapy.
■ Verbalize an understanding of the drug's use, adverse effects, and required precautions.

IMPLEMENTATION

Interventions and (Rationales)	Patient Education/Discharge Planning
■ Monitor the use of opioids. (Opioids are Schedule II controlled substances and can produce both physical and psychological dependence.)	■ Inform the patient and caregivers to take necessary steps to safeguard drug supply and to avoid sharing medications with others.
■ Administer medication correctly and evaluate the patient knowledge of proper administration. (Depending on the drug, they may be administered PO, subcutaneously, IM, IV, or epidural. Combining opioids with some medications or food items may be contraindicated.)	Instruct the patient: ■ That oral *capsules* may be opened and mixed with cool foods; extended-release *tablets*, however, may not be chewed, crushed, or broken. ■ That the oral solution for taking sublingually, may be more concentrated than the solution for swallowing. ■ To not use opioids concurrently with other medications (including herbal therapies) without consulting healthcare provider.

NURSING PROCESS FOCUS *(continued)*

Interventions and (Rationales)	Patient Education/Discharge Planning
◼ Monitor laboratory liver function studies. (Opioids are metabolized in the liver. Hepatic disease can increase blood levels of opioids to toxic levels.)	Instruct the patient to: ◼ Report to healthcare provider the following symptoms: nausea, vomiting, diarrhea, rash, jaundice, abdominal pain, tenderness, or distention, or change in color of stool. ◼ Adhere to laboratory testing regimen for liver function as ordered by the healthcare provider.
◼ Monitor vital signs, especially depth and rate of respirations/pulse oximetry. Withhold the drug if the patient's respiratory rate is below 12, and notify the healthcare provider. Keep resuscitative equipment and a narcotic antagonist such as naloxone (Narcan) accessible. (Opioid antagonists may reverse respiratory depression, decrease level of consciousness, and initiate other symptoms of narcotic overdose.)	Instruct the patient to: ◼ Monitor vital signs regularly, particularly respirations. ◼ Withhold medication for any difficulty in breathing or respirations below 12 breaths per minute; report symptoms immediately to the healthcare provider.
◼ Perform neuro checks regularly. Especially monitor for changes in LOC or seizure activity. (Decreased LOC and sluggish pupillary response may occur with high doses, and the drug may increase intracranial pressure.)	Instruct the patient to: ◼ Report headache or any significant change in sensorium, such as an aura or other visual effects that may indicate an impending seizure to the healthcare provider. ◼ Recognize seizures and methods to ensure personal safety during a seizure. ◼ Report any seizure activity immediately.
◼ If ordered prn, administer the medication upon patient's request or when nursing observations indicate expressions of pain by the patient.	Instruct the patient to: ◼ Alert the nurse immediately upon the return or increase of pain. ◼ Notify the healthcare provider regarding the drug's effectiveness.
◼ Monitor renal status and urinary output (may cause urinary retention, which may exacerbate existing symptoms of prostatic hypertrophy).	Instruct the patient to: ◼ Measure and monitor fluid intake and output. ◼ Report symptoms of dysuria (hesitancy, pain, diminished stream), changes in urine quality, or scanty urine output to the healthcare provider. ◼ Report fever or flank pain that may be indicative of a urinary tract infection.
◼ Monitor for other adverse effects such as restlessness, dizziness, anxiety, depression, hallucinations, nausea, and vomiting. (Hives or itching may indicate an allergic reaction due to the production of histamine. Depression, anxiety and hallucinations may indicate overdose.)	Instruct the patient to: ◼ Recognize adverse effects and symptoms of an allergic or anaphylactic reaction. ◼ Immediately report to healthcare provider any shortness of breath, tight feeling in the throat, itching, hives or other rash, feelings of dysphoria, nausea, or vomiting. ◼ Avoid the use of sleep-inducing over-the-counter (OTC) antihistamines without first consulting the healthcare provider.
◼ Monitor for constipation. (Drug slows peristalsis.)	Instruct the patient to: ◼ Maintain adequate fluid and fiber intake to facilitate stool passage. ◼ Use a stool softener or laxative as recommended by the healthcare provider.
◼ Ensure patient safety. Monitor ambulation until response to the drug is known. (Drug can cause sedation and dizziness.)	Instruct the patient to: ◼ Request assistance when getting out of bed. ◼ Avoid driving or performing hazardous activities until effect of the drug is known.
◼ Monitor frequency of requests and stated effectiveness of narcotic administered. (Opioids cause tolerance and dependence.)	Instruct the patient: ◼ Regarding cross-tolerance issues. ◼ To monitor medication supply to observe for hoarding, which may signal an impending suicide attempt. ◼ Who is suffering from a terminal illness about the issue of drug dependence as related to reduced life expectancy.

EVALUATION OF OUTCOME CRITERIA

Evaluate the effectiveness of drug therapy by confirming that patient goals and expected outcomes have been met (see "Planning"). *See Table 14.3 for a list of drugs to which these nursing actions apply.*

NONOPIOID ANALGESICS FOR MODERATE PAIN

Nonsteroidal anti-inflammatory drugs (NSAIDs) are the preferred nonopioid analgesics for inflammation and less severe pain.

The nonopioid analgesics involve NSAIDs and a few centrally acting drugs, including acetaminophen. The role of the NSAIDs in the treatment of inflammation and fever is discussed more thoroughly in Chapter 24. Therefore, there is only brief mention here. Table 14.4 ◆ highlights the more common nonopioid analgesics.

Nonsteroidal Anti-Inflammatory Drugs (NSAIDs)

NSAIDs are drugs for mild to moderate pain, especially for pain associated with inflammation. NSAIDs inhibit **cyclooxygenase**, an enzyme responsible for the formation of **prostaglandins**. When cyclooxygenase is inhibited, inflammation and pain are reduced. These drugs have many advantages over the opioids in that the NSAIDs have antipyretic, anti-inflammatory, and analgesic properties.

mediators = middle drugs

The NSAIDs act by inhibiting pain mediators at the nociceptor level. When tissue is damaged, local chemical mediators are released: histamine, potassium ion, hydrogen ion, bradykinin, and prostaglandins. **Bradykinin** is associated with sensory impulses of pain. Prostaglandins prompt pain through the formation of free radicals.

brady = slow
kinin = movement

Popular NSAIDs available OTC are aspirin and ibuprofen. Ibuprofen and related medications are available in many different formulations, including those designed for children. Most are safe and well tolerated by patients when used at low to moderate doses. Higher and more prolonged doses produce hepatotoxicity, which is a major concern with these classes of drugs (Chapter 24).

syn = together
thesis = put

After tissue damage, prostaglandins are formed with the help of two enzymes called *cyclooxygenase type 1 (COX-1)* and *cyclooxygenase typ. 2 (COX-2)*. Aspirin and ibuprofen-related drugs inhibit both COX-1 and COX-2. Thus, COX inhibition is the basis of NSAID therapy. Because the COX-2 enzyme is more specific for the synthesis of inflammatory prostaglandins, the selective COX-2 inhibitors provide a more focused peripheral pain relief. Celecoxib (Celebrex) is one of the COX-2 inhibitors still available in the United States; other COX-2 inhibitors have been discontinued. Figure 14.3 ■ illustrates the mechanism of pain transmission at the nociceptor level.

Drug Prototype: 🅿 Aspirin (Acetylsalicylic Acid, ASA)

Therapeutic Class: Nonopioid analgesic, nonsteroidal anti-inflammatory drug (NSAID), antipyretic; drug for myocardial infarction prophylaxis and transient ischemia

Pharmacologic Class: Salicylate, cyclooxygenase (COX) inhibitor, prostaglandin synthesis inhibitor, platelet aggregation inhibitor

Actions and Uses: Aspirin inhibits prostaglandin synthesis involved in the processes of pain and inflammation and produces mild to moderate relief of fever. It has limited effects on peripheral blood vessels, causing vasodilation and sweating. Aspirin has significant anticoagulant activity, and this property is responsible for its ability to reduce the risk of mortality following MI and to reduce the incidence of strokes. Aspirin has also been found to reduce the risk of colorectal cancer, although the mechanism by which it affords this protective effect is unknown.

Adverse Effects and Interactions: At high doses, such as those used to treat severe inflammatory disorders, aspirin may cause gastric discomfort and bleeding because of its antiplatelet effects. Hepatotoxicity, is also a concern, especially in patients with pre-existing liver disease. Enteric-coated tablets and buffered preparations are available for patients who experience GI adverse effects.

Because aspirin increases bleeding time, it should not be given to patients receiving anticoagulant therapy such as warfarin, heparin, and plicamycin. ASA may increase the action of oral hypoglycemic drugs. Effects of NSAIDs, uricosuric drugs such as probenecid, beta blockers, spironolactone, and sulfa drugs may be decreased when combined with ASA.

Use with phenobarbital, antacids, and glucocorticoids may decrease ASA effects. Insulin, methotrexate, phenytoin, sulfonamides, and penicillin may increase effects. When taken with alcohol, pyrazolone derivatives, steroids, or other NSAIDs, there is an increased risk for gastric ulcers.

Use with caution with herbal supplements, such as feverfew, which may increase the risk of bleeding.

TABLE 14.4 Nonopioid Analgesics		
Drug	**Route and Adult Dose**	**Remarks**
NSAIDS: ASPIRIN AND OTHER SALICYLATES		
(Pr) aspirin (acetylsalicylic acid, ASA)	PO; 350–650 mg every four hours (max: 4 g/day)	Also for fever, inflammation, and thromboembolic disorders, prevention of transient ischemic attacks and heart attacks; rectal form available
salsalate (Disalcid)	PO; 325–3,000 mg daily in divided doses (max: 4 g/day)	Also for fever, inflammation
NSAIDS: IBUPROFEN AND IBUPROFEN-LIKE DRUGS		
diclofenac (Cambia, Cataflam, Voltaren, Zipsor)	PO; 50 mg bid to qid (max: 200 mg/day)	Also for inflammation
diflunisal	PO; 1000 mg followed by 500 mg bid to tid	Also for inflammation
etodolac	PO; 200–400 mg tid to qid	Also for inflammation
fenoprofen (Nalfon)	PO; 200 mg tid to qid	Also for inflammation
flurbiprofen (Ansaid, Ocufen)	PO; 50–100 mg tid to qid (max: 300 mg/day)	Similar to ibuprofen
ibuprofen (Advil, Motrin, others)	PO; 400 mg tid to qid (max: 1,200 mg/day)	Also for fever and inflammation
indomethacin (Indocin)	PO; 25–50 mg bid or tid (max: 200 mg/day) or 75 mg sustained release one to two times/day	Also used for moderate to severe rheumatoid arthritis and acute gouty arthritis
ketoprofen (Actron, Orudis)	PO; 12.5–50 mg tid to qid	Also for inflammation
ketorolac (Toradol)	PO; 10 mg qid prn (max: 40 mg/day)	Also for allergic conjunctivitis, available in IM/IV forms
mefenamic acid (Ponstel)	PO; loading dose 500 mg, maintenance dose 250 mg every 6 hours prn	Used for short-term relief of mild to moderate pain, including menstrual cramps
meloxicam (Mobic)	PO; 7.5 mg daily (max: 15 mg/day)	Used for osteoarthritis
nabumetone (Relafen)	PO; 1,000 mg daily (max: 2,000 mg/day)	Inhibits COX-2 more than COX-1
naproxen (Naprosyn, Naprelan)	PO; 500 mg followed by 200–250 mg tid to qid (max: 1,000 mg/day)	Also for inflammation
naproxen sodium (Aleve, Anaprox, others)	PO; 250–500 mg bid (max: 1,000 mg/day naproxen)	Also for dysmenorrhea
oxaprozin (Daypro)	PO; 600–1200 mg daily (max: 1,800 mg/day)	Similar to naproxen; once-a-day dosage
piroxicam (Feldene)	PO; 10–20 mg daily to bid (max: 20 mg/day)	Has prolonged half-life
sulindac (Clinoril)	PO; 150–200 mg bid (max: 400 mg/day)	Also for inflammation
tolmetin (Tolectin)	PO; 400 mg tid (max: 2 g/day)	Also for inflammation
NSAIDS: SELECTIVE COX-2 INHIBITORS		
celecoxib (Celebrex)	PO; 100–200 mg bid or 200 mg/daily	Also for inflammation
CENTRALLY ACTING DRUGS		
acetaminophen (Tylenol) (see page 369 for the Drug Prototype Box)	PO; 325–650 mg every 4–6 hours	Also for fever; available in rectal form; centrally acting COX inhibitor
tramadol (Ultram)	PO; 50–100 mg every 4–6 hours prn (max: 400 mg/day), may start with 25 mg/day and increase by 25 mg every 3 days up to 200 mg/day	Causes less respiratory depression than morphine
ziconotide (Prialt)	Intrathecal; 0.1 mcg/hr via infusion, may increase by 0.1 mcg/hr every 2–3 days (max: 0.8 mcg/hr)	Also used for muscle spasticity

FIGURE 14.3

Mechanisms of pain at the nociceptor level.

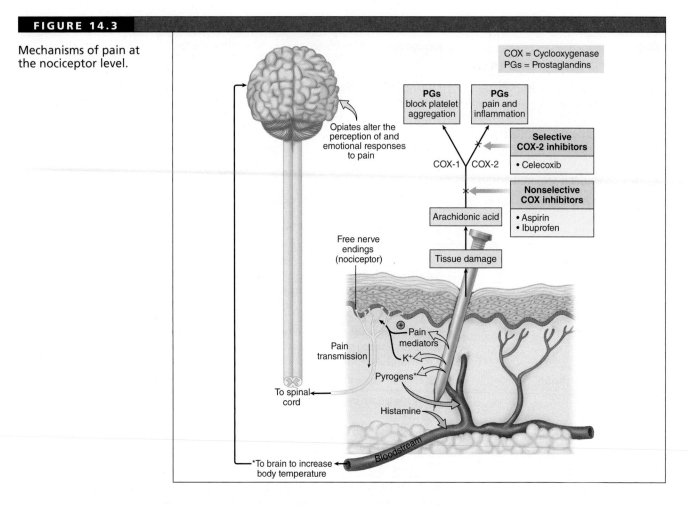

Centrally Acting Drugs

Centrally acting drugs are drugs that exert effects directly within the brain and spinal cord. Any analgesic drug, which has a *central effect* bypasses the nociceptor level. Acetaminophen is a centrally acting nonopioid analgesic. Acetaminophen reduces fever by direct action at the level of the hypothalamus and causes dilation of peripheral blood vessels, enabling sweating and dissipation of heat. It is the primary alternative to NSAIDs when patients cannot take aspirin or ibuprofen. Acetaminophen does not produce GI bleeding or ulcers and it does not exhibit cardiotoxicity. The safety profile of acetaminophen is excellent when administered in proper therapeutic doses; however, hepatotoxicity can occur with misuse and overdose. Aspirin and acetaminophen have similar efficacies in relieving pain and reducing fever. Acetaminophen is featured as a prototype drug for the treatment of fever in Chapter 24.

Tramadol (Ultram) and ziconotide (Prialt) are additional centrally acting analgesics. Of the two drugs, tramadol is the more widely prescribed. Tramadol has weak opioid activity, although it is not thought to relieve pain by this mechanism. Its main action is to inhibit reuptake of norepinephrine and serotonin in spinal neurons. Tramadol is well tolerated, but common adverse effects are vertigo, dizziness, headache, nausea, vomiting, constipation, and lethargy.

Concept Review 14.4

■ Think about cyclooxygenase inhibitors (NSAIDs) and prostaglandins, and then describe how pain might be regulated at the nociceptor.

TENSION HEADACHES AND MIGRAINE

Headache is one of the most common complaints of patients. Living with headaches can interfere with activities of daily living and can cause great distress. Pain and difficulty may result in work-related absences and neglect of home and family life. When headaches are persistent, or as migraines occur, drug therapy is needed.

Of the many types of headaches, the most common is the **tension headache**. It occurs when muscles of the head and neck tighten in response to stress. The tightness causes a steady and lingering pain. Although quite painful, tension headaches usually end when the stress is resolved. They are generally considered an annoyance rather than a medical emergency. Tension headaches are effectively treated with OTC analgesics such as aspirin, acetaminophen, or ibuprofen. More intense tension headache may be treated with additional classes of drugs.

The most painful type of headache is the **migraine**, which is characterized by throbbing or pulsating pain, sometimes preceded by an aura similar to those that warn of a seizure (see Chapter 13). The **auras** of migraines are sensory cues, such as seeing jagged lines or flashing lights, smelling, tasting, or hearing something strange. They let the patient know that a migraine attack is coming soon. Most patients with migraines also have nausea and vomiting. Triggers for migraines include nitrates and monosodium glutamate (MSG) found in many Asian foods, red wine, perfumes, food additives, caffeine, chocolate, and aspartame (a sugar substitute). By avoiding these substances, some patients can prevent the onset of a migraine attack.

Migraines can be effectively treated with a variety of drug classes.

CORE CONCEPT 14.7

There are two primary goals for the pharmacologic management of migraines. The first is to prevent migraines from occurring (*prophylaxis*), and the second is stop migraines in progress. For the most part, the drugs used to stop migraines are different than those used for prophylaxis; nevertheless, drug therapy is most effective if begun before a migraine has reached a severe level. It is not unusual for pharmacotherapy for mild migraines to begin with acetaminophen or NSAIDs. If OTC analgesics are unable to stop the migraine, then more specific drugs will be necessary.

pro = *before*
phylaxis = *guarding*

The two major drug classes used to terminate migraines are the triptans and the ergot alkaloids; both stimulate receptors to serotonin also called *5-hydroxytryptamine* (5-HT). A variety of other drugs classes are also used to treat migraines. Antimigraine drugs are listed in Table 14.5 ◆.

Triptans

Triptans were introduced in the 1990s for the treatment of migraine. As possible agonists to the 5-HT receptor, these drugs act to constrict blood vessels in the brain. They are effective in stopping migraines with or without auras. The first of the triptans marketed in the United States was sumatriptan (Imitrex). Since 1993, more triptans were developed. Although oral forms of the triptans are the most convenient, patients who experience unpleasant symptoms during a migraine, such as nausea and vomiting, may require an alternate dosage form. Intranasal formulation and prefilled syringes of triptans are available for patients who are able to self-administer.

Ergot Alkaloids

For patients who are unresponsive to triptans, the ergot alkaloids have been used to terminate migraines. The actions of the ergot alkaloids have been known for a long time. The first purified alkaloid, ergotamine (Ergostat), was isolated from the ergot fungus in 1920. Ergotamine is an inexpensive drug that is available in oral, sublingual, and suppository forms. Modification of the original molecule has produced another useful drug, dihydroergotamine (Migranal). Dihydroergotamine is given parenterally and as a nasal spray. Because the ergot alkaloids interact with adrenergic and dopaminergic receptors as well as serotonin receptors, they produce multiple actions and adverse effects such as tachycardia or bradycardia, nausea, vomiting, muscle pain and stiffness, peripheral constriction (leg weakness, numbness or tingling), lack of urination, and hypertension. Many ergot alkaloids are pregnancy category X drugs.

TABLE 14.5 Antimigraine Drugs

Drug	Route and Adult Dose	Remarks
TRIPTANS		
almotriptan (Axert)	PO; 6.25–12.5 mg, may repeat in 2 hours if necessary (max: two tablets/day)	May cause heart palpitations and rapid heartbeat
eletriptan (Relpax)	PO; 20–40 mg, may repeat in 2 hours if necessary (max: 80 mg/day)	May cause hypotension in older adult patients
frovatriptan (Frova)	PO; 2.5 mg, may repeat in 2 hours if necessary (max: 7.5 mg/day)	May cause chest pains and heart palpitations
naratriptan (Amerge)	PO; 1–2.5 mg, may repeat in 4 hours if necessary (max: 5 mg/day)	Serotonin stimulator; for migraine termination
rizatriptan (Maxalt)	PO; 5–10 mg, may repeat in 2 hours if necessary (max: 30 mg/day); 5 mg with concurrent propranolol (max: 15 mg/day)	May cause myocardial infarction
℗ sumatriptan (Imitrex)	PO; 25 mg for one dose (max: 100 mg)	Serotonin stimulator; subcutaneous and intranasal forms available; for termination of migraine
zolmitriptan (Zomig)	PO; 2.5–5 mg, may repeat in 2 hours if necessary (max: 10 mg/day)	Serotonin stimulator; for termination of migraine
ERGOT ALKALOIDS		
dihydroergotamine mesylate (D.H.E. 45, Migranal)	IM; 1 mg, may be repeated at 1-hour intervals to a total of 3 mg (max: 6 mg/week)	Also available as nasal spray; pregnancy category X; for migraine termination; may be used in combination with low-dose heparin to prevent postop deep vein thrombosis
ergotamine tartrate (Ergostat), ergotamine with caffeine (Cafergot, Ercaf, others)	PO; 1–2 mg followed by 1–2 mg every 30 minutes until headache stops (max: 6 mg/day or 10 mg/week)	Also available in sublingual, inhalant, or rectal forms; may cause physical dependence; pregnancy category X; for migraine termination
ANTISEIZURE DRUGS		
topiramate (Topamax)	PO; start with 50 mg/day, increase by 50 mg/week to effectiveness (max: 1,600 mg/day)	Sugar-like chemical molecule; enhances the action of GABA; also for partial seizures
valproic acid (Depakene, Depakote) (see page 191 for the Drug Prototype box)	PO; 250 mg bid (max: 100 mg/day)	Also for absence seizures and mixed generalized types of seizures and mania
BETA-ADRENERGIC BLOCKERS		
atenolol (Tenormin) (see page 309 for the Drug Prototype box)	PO; 25–50 mg daily (max: 100 mg/day)	Also used for hypertension and angina
metoprolol (Lopressor)	PO; 50–100 mg daily bid (max: 450 mg/day)	Also for angina and MI; sustained-release and IV forms available
propranolol (Inderal, InnoPran XL) (see page 340 for the Drug Prototype box)	PO; 80–240 mg/day in divided doses, may need 160–240 mg/day	Beta-adrenergic blocker for migraine prevention
timolol (Betimol, Timoptic) (see page 604 for the Drug Prototype box)	PO; 10 mg bid, may increase to 60 mg/day in two divided doses	Also for hypertension, angina, and glaucoma
CALCIUM CHANNEL BLOCKERS		
nifedipine (Adalat CC, Procardia XL) (see page 279 for the Drug Prototype box)	PO; 10–20 mg tid (max: 180 mg/day)	Selective for calcium channels in blood vessels; decreases peripheral vascular resistance and increases cardiac output; also for hypertension and angina; sustained-release form available
nimodipine (Nimotop)	PO; 60 mg every 4 hours for 21 days; start therapy within 96 hours of subarachnoid hemorrhage	Off-label use for migraines; primary use is for improvement of neurologic symptoms following a stroke
verapamil (Calan, Isoptin SR, others) (see page 342 for the Drug Prototype box)	PO; 40–80 mg tid	Off-label use for migraine prevention

TABLE 14.5	Antimigraine Drugs *(continued)*	
Drug	**Route and Adult Dose**	**Remarks**
TRICYCLIC ANTIDEPRESSANTS		
amitriptyline (Elavil)	PO; 75–100 mg/day	Off-label use for migraine prevention
imipramine (Tofranil) (see page 129 for the Drug Prototype box)	PO; 75–100 mg/day (max: 300 mg/day)	May cause cardiac dysfunction and abnormal blood cell count; also for alcohol or cocaine dependence; may control bedwetting in children; available IM
protriptyline (Vivactil)	PO; 15–40 mg/day in three to four divided doses (max: 60 mg/day)	For symptoms of depression; few sedative qualities; causes increased heart rate
MISCELLANEOUS DRUGS		
onabotulinumtoxin A (Botox)	IM; 155 units administered intramuscularly (IM) to muscles of the head and neck area	Direct-acting antispasmodic drug for muscle spasms and spasticity
methysergide (Sansert)	PO; 4–8 mg/day in divided doses	Similar to ergotamine; for migraine prevention
riboflavin (vitamin B_2)	PO; as a supplement: 5–10 mg/day; for deficiency: 5–30 mg/day in divided doses	Deficiency caused by chronic diarrhea, liver disease, alcoholism, or inadequate consumption of milk or animal products

Other Antimigraine and Tension Headache Drugs

Drugs for migraine prophylaxis include various classes of drugs that are discussed in other chapters of this textbook. These include antiseizure drugs (Chapter 13), beta-adrenergic blockers (Chapter 22), calcium channel blockers (Chapter 18), antidepressants (Chapter 10), and neuromuscular blockers (Chapter 12). Because all these drugs have the potential to produce side effects, prophylaxis is initiated only if the incidence of migraines is high and the patient is unresponsive to the drugs used to abort migraines. Of the various drugs, the beta blocker propranolol (Inderal) is one of the most commonly prescribed. Amitriptyline, an antidepressant, is often prescribed for patients who suffer from insomnia in addition to their migraines. In 2010, onabotulinumtoxinA (Botox) was approved for the treatment of chronic migraines in cases in which other medications were not successful. Botox inhibits neuromuscular transmission by blocking the release of acetylcholine from axon terminals innervating skeletal muscle. With this approach, IM injections are divided across specific muscles of the head and neck. When muscles are blocked, headaches due to intense muscle tension subside for a period of up to three months. More indications for Botox therapy are discussed in Chapter 12.

Drug Prototype: 🅟 *Sumatriptan (Imitrex)*

Therapeutic Class: Antimigraine drug

Pharmacologic Class: Triptan, 5-HT (serotonin) receptor drug, vasoconstrictor of intracranial arteries

Actions and Uses: Sumatriptan, a triptan, belongs to a relatively new group of antimigraine drugs known as the triptans. The triptans act by causing vasoconstriction of cranial arteries; this vasoconstriction is moderately selective and does not usually affect overall blood pressure. This medication is available in oral, intranasal, and subcutaneous forms. Subcutaneous administration ends migraine attacks in 10 to 20 minutes; the dose may be repeated 60 minutes after the first injection to a maximum of two doses per day. If taken orally, sumatriptan should be administered as soon as possible after the migraine is suspected or has begun.

Adverse Effects and Interactions: Some dizziness, drowsiness, or a warming sensation may be experienced after taking sumatriptan; however, these effects are not normally severe enough to warrant stopping therapy. Because of its vasoconstricting action, the drug can cause chest pressure and should be used cautiously, if at all, in patients with recent MI, or with a history of angina pectoris, hypertension, or diabetes.

Sumatriptan interacts with several drugs. For example, an increased effect may occur when taken with MAOIs and selective serotonin reuptake inhibitors (SSRIs). Further vasoconstriction can occur when taken with ergot alkaloids and other triptans.

PATIENTS NEED TO KNOW

Patients taking pain medication need to know the following facts and recommendations:

In General

1. Carefully describe pain to your healthcare provider so that the analgesic medication being taken is suited to the complaint.
2. Report any OTC medication taken for pain to your healthcare provider to minimize adverse effects and interactions.
3. Aspirin has many undesirable adverse effects mainly related to gastric upset and bleeding.
4. Follow instructions carefully and watch for drug interactions or contraindications.

Regarding Opiates

5. Avoid combining pain medications with alcohol and other CNS depressants (especially opioids).
6. Vital signs should be monitored with all opioid medications because of their CNS depressant effects.
7. Get up slowly from seated positions because certain pain medications cause lightheadedness.
8. Avoid operating machinery or driving a car if taking opiates because dizziness, blurred vision, and drowsiness can occur.
9. Do not abruptly stop taking opioids; this could result in withdrawal. Signs include chills, abdominal and muscle cramps, severe itching, sweating, restlessness, anxiety, yawning, and drug-seeking behavior.

CHAPTER REVIEW

CORE CONCEPTS SUMMARY

14.1 Pain assessment is the first step to pain management.

Pain is a subjective experience in which many patients describe discomfort differently. Pain may be classified as acute (from injury to recovery) or chronic (longer than six months). Pain may be classified as nociceptor pain and further divided into somatic or visceral pain and neuropathic pain.

14.2 Pain transmission processes allow several major targets for pharmacologic intervention.

Pain signals involve nerve impulses along two types of sensory neurons, Aδ and C fibers. Once impulses reach the spinal cord, substance P is thought to transmit pain at the spinal level. The release of substance P is controlled by ganglia that release neurotransmitters called *endogenous opioids*. If not blocked, the impulse travels to the brain, where pain information is sensed and a response to the sensation is initiated. Opioids act at the level of the central nervous system (CNS); nonsteroidal anti-inflammatory drugs (NSAIDs) act at the level of the peripheral nervous system (PNS).

14.3 Nonpharmacologic techniques and adjuvant analgesics assist in providing adequate pain relief.

Nonpharmacologic techniques may be used in place of drugs or as adjunctive to drug therapy. When used along with medication, nonpharmacologic techniques may allow lower doses to be given with possibly fewer drug-related adverse effects. Other adjunctive approaches include FDA approved antiseizure drugs, local anesthetics, and corticosteroids, which reduce inflammation and suppress pain in some cases. Off-label drug categories include TCAs, and drugs for dysrhythmia.

14.4 Opioid analgesic medications exert their effects by interacting with specific receptors.

Different types of receptors mediate analgesia (pain relief)—mu receptors and kappa receptors are the most commonly targeted. Both are opioid receptors that respond to natural or synthetic morphine-like substances. Natural substances extracted from unripe seeds of the poppy plant are called *opiates*. *Narcotic* is a general term referring to morphine-like drugs. In the context of drug enforcement, the term *narcotic* includes a much broader classification of abused illegal drugs.

14.5 Opioids have multiple therapeutic effects, including relief of severe pain.

Opioids produce many effects, including analgesia for intense pain, cough suppression, suppression of GI motility in diarrhea treatment, sedation, and euphoria. It is common practice to place opioids and nonnarcotic analgesics in a single tablet or capsule. Acute opioid intoxication is treated with the opioid antagonist naloxone. All of the narcotic analgesics have the potential to cause physical and psychological dependence. The opioids have a greater risk of dependency than most of the other classes of medications.

14.6 Nonsteroidal anti-inflammatory drugs (NSAIDs) are the preferred nonopioid analgesics for inflammation and less severe pain.

NSAIDs are nonopioid analgesics used to treat less severe pain associated with inflammation. NSAIDs have antifever and pain-reducing properties. These effects are achieved by inhibition of enzymes called cyclooxygenase type one (COX-1) and cyclooxygenase type two (COX-2). When cyclooxygenase (COX) is inhibited, prostaglandin synthesis is prevented. One medication is selective for the COX-2 receptor.

Another antifever drug is acetaminophen, a centrally acting drug that acts as a nonopioid analgesic.

14.7 Migraines can be effectively treated with a variety of drug classes.

Headaches in two categories—tension headaches and migraines—are the most common complaints of patients. The two primary goals of migraine therapy are migraine termination and migraine prevention. The two major classes of antimigraine drugs are ergot alkaloids and triptans. Drugs for migraine prophylaxis include beta-adrenergic blockers, calcium channel blockers, antidepressants, antiseizure drugs, and drugs for muscle tension.

REVIEW QUESTIONS

The following questions are written in NCLEX-PN® style. Answer these questions to assess your knowledge of the chapter material, and go back and review any material that is not clear to you.

1. The patient has osteoarthritis. Which of the following drugs would the nurse anticipate being ordered for both pain and inflammation?

1. Sumatriptan (Imitrex)
2. Acetaminophen (Tylenol)
3. Fentanyl (Sublimaze)
4. Meloxicam (Mobic)

2. The patient is starting on sumatriptan (Imitrex) for migraines. For which of the following should the nurse instruct the patient to notify his or her healthcare provider immediately?

1. Chest pressure
2. GI upset
3. Bleeding
4. Lethargy

3. A patient is receiving an NSAID, so the nurse monitors the patient for:

1. GI upset and bleeding
2. Urinary retention
3. Blurred vision
4. Anorexia

4. The patient is experiencing opioid dependency. The nurse would expect which drug to be used to treat this condition?

1. Oxycodone (OxyContin)
2. Tramadol (Ultram)
3. Hydromorphone (Dilaudid)
4. Methadone (Dolophine)

5. When planning care for a patient in pain, the nurse understands that pain signals begin at the _____ and proceed through the CNS.

1. Spinal cord
2. Viscera
3. Nociceptors
4. Substance P

6. Prior to administering pain medication, the nurse obtained which of the following information about the patient's pain? (Select all that apply.)

1. The patient's diagnosis
2. The location of the pain
3. When the patient last had a meal
4. The severity of the pain

7. The patient has been receiving morphine sulfate for pain control. An evaluation of the patient reveals a decreased level of consciousness and shallow respirations at a rate of 8 per minute. The nurse anticipates what opioid antagonist being ordered?

1. Butorphanol (Stadol)
2. Hydrocodone (Hycodan)
3. Naloxone (Narcan)
4. Oxycodone (OxyContin)

8. Since a patient is allergic to aspirin, the nurse administers what drug as an alternative for relief of mild pain?

1. Acetaminophen
2. Morphine
3. Etodolac
4. Fentanyl

9. The nurse monitors for which of the following adverse effects of ergotamine (Ergostate): (Select all that apply.)

1. Tachycardia
2. Nausea and vomiting
3. Peripheral dilation
4. Peripheral constriction

10. The healthcare provider orders ibuprofen 400 mg, po, three times a day. The pharmacy sends ibuprofen suspension 200 mg/5 mL. How many milliliters should the patient receive in each dose?

1. 2 mL
2. 15 mL
3. 5 mL
4. 10 mL

CASE STUDY QUESTIONS

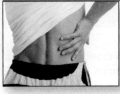

Remember Mr. Coidiuf, who was introduced at the beginning of the chapter? Now read the remainder of the case study. Based on the information you have learned in this chapter, answer the questions that follow.

Mr. Damian Coidiuf, age 32, sustained a back injury three years ago, which responded well to treatment with nonsteroidal anti-inflammatory medication. Over the last six months, Mr. Coidiuf has been seeing his healthcare provider again with complaints of "sharp painful sensations along his right hip." Despite careful attention, it appears that Mr. Coidiuf's pain is no longer responding to anti-inflammatory medication. His healthcare provider prescribes a narcotic analgesic (moderate effectiveness) with acetaminophen, hoping this treatment might provide relief. Following three physical therapy sessions, and the new medication, Mr. Coidiuf reports that he is "feeling better."

1. The nurse understands that when Mr. Coidiuf was given NSAIDs three years ago, the purpose was to: (Select all that apply.)

1. Reduce pain
2. Reduce inflammation
3. Acts within the CNS
4. Inhibit pain mediators at the nociceptors

2. According to the prescription, which of the following narcotic analgesics would the nurse expect to give to Mr. Coidiuf?

1. Percocet
2. Talwin
3. Dilaudid
4. Demerol

3. Mr. Coidiuf asks the nurse why the doctor put him on a narcotic that also contains acetaminophen. The nurse replies that: (Select all that apply.)

1. The two medications work well together to decrease pain.
2. A lower dose of the narcotic can be used when combined with acetaminophen.
3. Because narcotics can have serious adverse effects, using a low dose of a narcotic can help minimize these effects.
4. Combining the two medication helps to lower the cost.

4. While providing Mr. Coidiuf with information about the use of narcotics, the nurse informs him to report which of the following adverse effects to his healthcare provider?

1. Diarrhea
2. Hallucinations
3. Sedation
4. Insomnia

NOTE: Answers to the Review and Case Study Questions appear in Appendix B. The complete rationales and answers are located on the textbook's website.

Pearson Nursing Student Resources Find additional review materials at **nursing.pearsonhighered.com**.

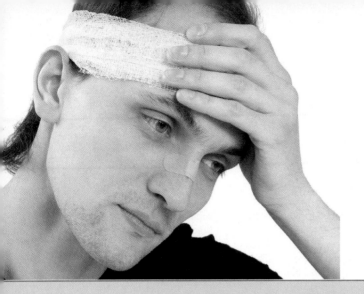

CHAPTER

15

Drugs for Anesthesia

CORE CONCEPTS

15.1 Local anesthesia causes a rapid loss of sensation to a limited part of the body.

15.2 Local anesthetics produce their therapeutic effect by blocking the entry of sodium ions into neurons.

15.3 Local anesthetics are classified by their chemical structures.

15.4 General anesthesia is a loss of sensation occurring throughout the entire body, accompanied by a loss of consciousness.

15.5 General anesthetics are usually administered by the inhalation or IV routes.

15.6 Intravenous anesthetics are important supplements to inhalant general anesthetics and include benzodiazepines, opioids, and miscellaneous IV drugs.

15.7 Nonanesthetic drugs are used as adjuncts to anesthesia before, during, and after surgery.

DRUG SNAPSHOT

The following drugs are discussed in this chapter:

DRUG CLASSES	DRUG PROTOTYPES	DRUG CLASSES	DRUG PROTOTYPES
Local Anesthetics		*Gases*	**Pr** nitrous oxide *225*
Esters		*Volatile liquids*	**Pr** isoflurane (Forane) *225*
Amides	**Pr** lidocaine (Xylocaine) *222*	Intravenous anesthetics	**Pr** propofol (Diprivan) *227*
Miscellaneous drugs		**Adjuncts to Anesthesia**	
General Anesthetics		Neuromuscular blockers	**Pr** succinylcholine (Anectine) *228*
Inhalation drugs			

LEARNING OUTCOMES

After reading this chapter, the student should be able to:

1. Compare and contrast the five major routes for administering local anesthetics.

2. Describe differences between the two major chemical classes of local anesthetics.

3. Explain why epinephrine and sodium hydroxide are sometimes included as part of the local anesthetic medicine.

4. Identify the actions of general anesthetics within the central nervous system (CNS).

5. Compare and contrast the two primary ways that general anesthesia may be induced.

6. Identify the four stages of general anesthesia.

7. Categorize drugs used for anesthesia based on their classifications and actions in the body.

8. For each of the classes listed in the Drug Snapshot, identify representative drugs and explain their mechanisms of drug action, primary actions, and important adverse effects.

KEY TERMS

amides (AM-ides) *220*

anesthesia (ANN-ess-THEE-zee-uh) *218*

esters (ES-turs) *220*

general anesthesia *218*

local anesthesia *218*

neuromuscular blockers *227*

an = *without*
esthesia = *sensation*

nesthesia is a medical procedure performed by administering drugs that cause a loss of sensation. **Local anesthesia** occurs when sensation is lost to a limited part of the body without loss of consciousness. **General anesthesia** requires different classes of drugs that cause loss of sensation to the entire body, usually resulting in a loss of consciousness. This chapter examines drugs used for both local and general anesthesia, including select drugs used before and after surgical procedures.

LOCAL ANESTHESIA

CORE CONCEPT 15.1

Local anesthesia causes a rapid loss of sensation to a limited part of the body.

Local anesthesia is loss of sensation to a relatively small part of the body without loss of consciousness to the patient. This technique may be necessary when a relatively brief dental or medical procedure is performed. Although local anesthesia often causes a loss of sensation to a small, limited area, it sometimes affects relatively large portions of the body, such as an entire limb. Because of this action, some local anesthetic treatments are more accurately called *surface anesthesia* or *regional anesthesia*, depending on how the drugs are administered and the results they produce.

The five major routes (Figure 15.1 ■) for applying local anesthetics are the following:

- Topical
- Infiltration
- Nerve block
- Spinal
- Epidural

The method used depends on the location and amount of anesthesia that is needed, as well as the specific procedure being performed. For example, some local anesthetics are applied topically before a needlestick or minor skin surgery. Others are used to block sensations to large areas such as limbs or the lower abdomen. The different methods of local and regional anesthesia are summarized in Table 15.1 ◆.

Fast Facts Anesthesia and Anesthetics

- The first medical applications of anesthetics involved ether (in 1842) and nitrous oxide (in 1846).
- Over 20 million people receive anestshetics each year in the United States.
- Most of the general public associate use of local anesthetic drugs with the practice of dentistry or topical skin medications.
- About half of the general anesthetics in medical practice are administered by a nurse anesthetist.
- Herbal products may interact with anesthetics—for example, St. John's wort may intensify or prolong the effects of some opioids and anesthetics.

Concept Review 15.1

- What is local anesthesia? Name the five general routes for local and regional anesthesia.

FIGURE 15.1

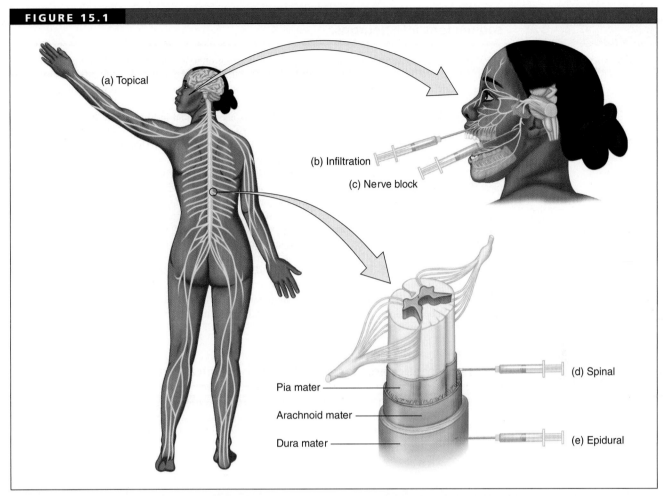

(a) Topical

(b) Infiltration

(c) Nerve block

Pia mater

Arachnoid mater

Dura mater

(d) Spinal

(e) Epidural

Routes for applying local anesthesia include (a) topical, (b) infiltration, (c) nerve block, (d) spinal, and (e) epidural.

TABLE 15.1 Methods of Local and Regional Anesthesia

Route	Formulation/Method	Description
Epidural anesthesia	Injection into the epidural space (the area between the vertebrae and the spinal cord).	Drug causes numbness, without paralysis, of the areas below the injection site. A small catheter is often placed into the epidural space to allow for multiple injections.
Infiltration (field block) anesthesia	Direct injection into tissue immediate to the surgical site.	Drug diffuses into tissue to block a specific group of nerves in a small area very close to the area to be operated on.
Nerve block anesthesia	Direct injection into tissue that may be distant from the operation site.	Drug affects the bundle of nerves serving the area to be operated on; used to block sensation in a limb or large area of the face.
Spinal anesthesia	Injection into the cerebrospinal spinal fluid (CSF).	Drug affects large, regional area such as the lower abdomen and legs.
Topical (surface) anesthesia	Creams, sprays, suppositories, drops, and lozenges.	Applied to mucous membranes, including the eyes, lips, gums, nasal membranes, and throat; very safe unless absorbed.

CORE CONCEPT 15.2

Local anesthetics produce their therapeutic effect by blocking the entry of sodium ions into neurons.

Local anesthetics are drugs that produce a rapid loss of sensation to a limited part of the body. The mechanism of action of local anesthetics is well known. Recall that the concentration of sodium is normally higher outside the neurons compared to the inside. A rapid influx of sodium ions into the cell is necessary for neurons to fire.

Local anesthetics act by blocking sodium channels, as illustrated in Figure 15.2 ■. The blocking of sodium channels is nonselective; therefore, both sensory and motor impulses are affected. Sensation and muscle activity in the treated area will be decreased temporarily. Because of their mechanism of action, local anesthetics are called *sodium channel blockers*.

During a medical or surgical procedure, it is essential for the anesthetic to last long enough to complete the procedure. Small amounts of epinephrine are sometimes added to the anesthetic solution in order to constrict blood vessels in the immediate area where the local anesthetic is applied. This keeps the drug active at the injected site and extends its duration of action. The addition of epinephrine to lidocaine (Xylocaine), for example, increases the anesthetic effect from about 20 minutes to 60 minutes. This is important for surgical and dental procedures that take longer than 20 minutes; otherwise, a second injection would be necessary.

Sometimes an alkaline substance, such as sodium hydroxide or sodium bicarbonate, is added to anesthetic solutions to increase the drug's effectiveness in areas with extensive local infection or abscesses. The reason for this is that bacteria tend to acidify an infected site, and local anesthetics are less effective in an acidic environment. Adding alkaline substances neutralizes the infected region and allows the anesthetic to work better.

CORE CONCEPT 15.3

Local anesthetics are classified by their chemical structures.

The two major classes of local anesthetics are **esters** and **amides** (Table 15.2 ◆). The terms *ester* and *amide* refer to types of chemical linkages found within the anesthetic molecules, as illustrated in Figure 15.3 ■. A small number of miscellaneous drugs are neither esters nor amides.

FIGURE 15.2

(a) In normal nerve conduction, sodium ions (Na+) enter the sodium channels along a neuron and allow the neuron to fire (set off an action potential) and conduct an impulse. (b) Local anesthetics (represented by the red x) block the sodium channels. Sodium ions are not able to enter the neuronal membrane through the sodium channels. Therefore, no action potential can be conducted along the nerve.

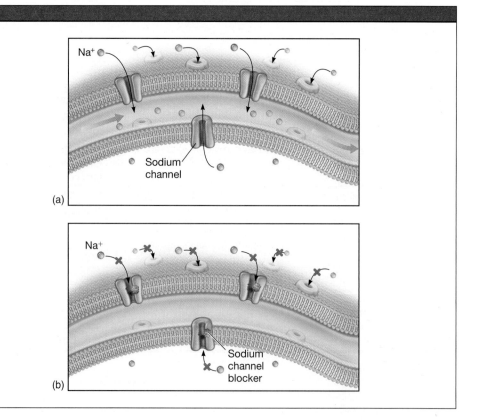

TABLE 15.2   Selected Local Anesthetics

Drug	Clinical Uses	Remarks
ESTERS		
benzocaine (Americaine, Anbesol, Solarcaine, others) (see page 589 for the Drug Prototype box)	Topical anesthesia	For sunburn, sore throat, earache, hemorrhoids, and other minor skins conditions
chloroprocaine (Nesacaine)	Infiltration, nerve block, and epidural anesthesia	Short duration
procaine (Novocain)	Infiltration, nerve block, epidural, and spinal anesthesia	Short duration
proparacaine (Alcaine, Ophthetic)	To numb the eye before surgery, certain tests, or procedures	Short duration
tetracaine (Pontocaine)	Topical and spinal anesthesia	Longer duration
AMIDES		
articaine (Septocaine, Zorcaine)	Infiltration and nerve block anesthesia	Longer duration
bupivicaine (Marcaine, Sensorcaine)	Infiltration and epidural anesthesia	Longer duration
dibucaine (Nupercainal)	Topical or spinal anesthesia	Longer duration
Pr lidocaine (Anestacon, Dilocaine, Xylocaine, others)	Topical anesthesia, infiltration, nerve block, epidural, and spinal anesthesia	May be combined as a mixture of lidocaine and prilocaine (EMLA cream) for topical application
mepivacaine (Carbocaine, Isocaine, Polocaine)	Infiltration, nerve block, and epidural anesthesia	Intermediate duration
prilocaine	Infiltration, nerve block, and epidural anesthesia	Intermediate duration
ropivacaine (Naropin)	Infiltration, nerve block, and epidural anesthesia	Longer duration
MISCELLANEOUS DRUGS		
dyclonine (Dyclone)	Topical anesthesia	For ear, nose, and throat procedures
ethyl chloride or chloroethane	Topical anesthesia	For minor medical procedures
pramoxine (Tronothane)	Topical anesthesia	For minor medical procedures

FIGURE 15.3

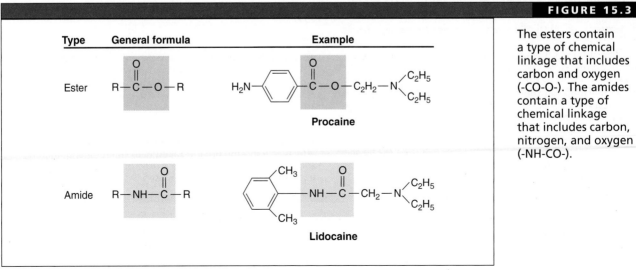

The esters contain a type of chemical linkage that includes carbon and oxygen (-CO-O-). The amides contain a type of chemical linkage that includes carbon, nitrogen, and oxygen (-NH-CO-).

Esters

Cocaine, the first local anesthetic widely used for medical procedures, was used as far back as the 1880s. Cocaine is a natural ester, found in the leaves of the plant *Erythroxylon coca*, native to the Andes Mountains of Peru. As late as the 1980s, cocaine was routinely used for eye surgery, nerve blocks, and spinal anesthesia. Although still available for local anesthesia, cocaine is a Schedule II drug and rarely used therapeutically in the United States. The abuse potential of cocaine is discussed in Chapter 7.

Another ester, procaine (Novocain), was the drug of choice for dental procedures from the mid-1900s to the 1960s. About that time, amide anesthetics were developed, and use of the ester anesthetics declined. One ester, benzocaine (Solarcaine and others), is used as a topical over-the-counter (OTC) drug for treating a large number of painful conditions, including sunburn, insect bites, hemorrhoids, sore throat, and minor wounds. Tetracaine is an ester that is often sprayed on the skin and mucous membranes to cause loss of feeling before and during surgery or for endoscopic procedures. For example, a topical anesthetic comprising benzocaine, butamben, and teratracaine (Cetacaine) is used in examinations of the esophagus or colon. Proparacaine (Alcaine, Ophthetic) is a drug used for short-term anesthesia in ocular procedures.

Amides

Amides have largely replaced the esters because they produce fewer adverse effects and generally have a longer duration of action. Lidocaine (Xylocaine) is the most widely used amide for short surgical procedures requiring local anesthesia. Ethyl chloride or cloroethane is a mild topical drug supplied as a liquid in a spray bottle. It is used for basic procedures such as removing splinters or small debris from the skin's surface.

Adverse effects to local anesthesia are uncommon. Allergy is rare. When it does occur, it is often due to sulfites, which are added as preservatives to prolong the shelf life of the anesthetic, or to methylparaben, which may be added to prevent bacterial growth in anesthetic solutions. Early signs of adverse effects of local anesthetics include symptoms of CNS stimulation such as restlessness or anxiety. Later, drowsiness and unresponsiveness may occur due to CNS depression. Cardiovascular effects, including hypotension and dysrhythmias, are possible. Patients with a history of cardiovascular disease are often given forms of local anesthetics that contain no epinephrine to reduce the possible effects of this sympathomimetic on the heart and blood pressure. CNS and cardiovascular adverse effects are rare unless the local anesthetic is absorbed rapidly or is accidentally injected directly into a blood vessel.

Concept Review   **15.2**

- How does a local anesthetic work? How does the anesthetic action of lidocaine with epinephrine differ from that of lidocaine without epinephrine?

Drug Prototype: ℗ *Lidocaine (Xylocaine)*
Therapeutic Class: Anesthetic (local/regional/topical), antidysrhythmic (class IB)
Pharmacologic Class: Sodium channel blocker; amide

Actions and Uses: Lidocaine is the most frequently used injectable local anesthetic. It is available in solutions ranging from 0.5% to 2% for infiltration, nerve block, spinal, or epidural anesthesia. A topical form is also available. When given for anesthesia, its onset of action is 5 to 15 minutes. Several hours may be needed for complete sensation to reappear. Lidocaine is also given IV, IM, or subcutaneously to treat dysrhythmias, as discussed in Chapter 22. Solutions of lidocaine containing preservatives or epinephrine are used for local anesthesia only and must never be given parenterally for dysrhythmias.

Adverse Effects and Interactions: When used for anesthesia, adverse effects are uncommon. An early symptom of toxicity is excitement, leading to irritability and confusion. Serious adverse effects include convulsions, respiratory depression, and cardiac arrest. Until the effect of the anesthetic diminishes, patients may injure themselves by biting or chewing areas of the mouth that have no sensation following a dental procedure.

Barbiturates may decrease activity of lidocaine. Increased effects of lidocaine occur if taken with cimetidine, quinidine, and beta blockers. If lidocaine is used on a regular basis, its effectiveness may diminish when used with other medications.

NURSING PROCESS FOCUS　Patients Receiving Local Anesthesia

ASSESSMENT	POTENTIAL NURSING DIAGNOSES
Prior to administration: ■ Obtain a complete health history including cardiovascular conditions, allergies (especially for amide-type drugs), drug history, and possible drug interactions. ■ Check for the presence of broken skin, infections, burns and wounds where medication is to be applied. ■ Determine character, duration, location, and intensity of pain where medication is to be applied.	■ *Deficient Knowledge* related to a lack of information about drug therapy ■ *Acute Pain* related to administration of drug ■ *Risk for Injury* related to lack of sensation to a part of the body caused by the anesthetic

PLANNING: PATIENT GOALS AND EXPECTED OUTCOMES

The patient will:
■ Experience therapeutic effects (no pain during surgical procedure).
■ Be free from or experience minimal adverse effects from drug therapy.

IMPLEMENTATION

Interventions and (Rationales)	Patient Education/Discharge Planning
■ Monitor for cardiovascular adverse effects. (These may occur if anesthetic is absorbed.)	■ Instruct the patient to report any unusual heart palpitations, lightheadedness, drowsiness, or confusion. If using medication on a regular basis, instruct the patient to see the healthcare provider regularly.
■ Check skin or mucous membranes for infection or inflammation. (Condition could be worsened by the drug.)	■ Instruct the patient to report any irritation or increase in discomfort in areas where medication was used to the healthcare provider.
■ Monitor for length of effectiveness. (Local anesthetics are effective for one to three hours.)	■ Instruct the patient to report any discomfort during the procedure.
■ Obtain information on and monitor the use of other medications.	■ Instruct the patient to report use of any medications to the healthcare provider.
■ Provide for patient safety. (There is a potential for injury related to the fact that the area being treated lacks sensation.)	■ Inform the patient about having no feeling in the anesthetized area and taking extra caution to avoid injury, including heat-related injury.
■ Monitor for gag reflex if used in the mouth or throat. (Xylocaine viscous may interfere with the swallowing reflex.)	Instruct the patient to: ■ Not eat within one hour of administration. ■ Not chew gum while any portion of the mouth or throat is anesthetized to prevent biting injuries.

EVALUATION OF OUTCOME CRITERIA

Evaluate the effectiveness of drug therapy by confirming that patient goals and expected outcomes have been met (see "Planning"). *See Table 15.2 for a list of drugs to which these nursing actions apply.*

CAM THERAPY

Oil of Cloves for Dental Pain

One natural remedy for tooth pain is oil of cloves, a natural substance whose use dates back thousands of years in Chinese medicine. Extracted from the clove plant Eugenia, eugenol is the active chemical that produces a numbing effect. It works especially well for dental caries (cavities). The herb is applied by soaking a piece of cotton and packing it around the gums close to the affected tooth. Dentists sometimes recommend it for temporary relief of a toothache. Clove oil has an antiseptic effect that has been reported to kill microorganisms.

Other uses of clove oil that lack reliable scientific evidence include treatment of premature ejaculation, low libido, and fever reduction. Clove oil is very safe, with rash and gastrointestinal (GI) upset being the most common adverse effects. Clove oil may increase the risk for bleeding and should be used cautiously in patients taking anticoagulants.

GENERAL ANESTHESIA

CORE CONCEPT 15.4

General anesthesia is a loss of sensation occurring throughout the entire body, accompanied by a loss of consciousness.

General anesthesia involves loss of sensation to the entire body. General anesthetics are used when it is necessary for patients to remain still and without pain for a period longer than could be achieved with local anesthetics. The goal of general anesthesia is to provide a rapid and complete loss of sensation. Signs of general anesthesia include total analgesia (no feeling of pain) and loss of consciousness, memory, and body movement. Although these signs are similar to those of sleeping, general anesthesia and sleep are not exactly the same. General anesthetics depress most nervous activity in the brain, whereas sleeping stops activity in only very specific areas. In fact, some brain activity actually increases during sleep, as described in Chapter 9.

General anesthesia is rarely achieved with a single drug. Instead, multiple medications are used to rapidly induce unconsciousness, cause muscle relaxation, and maintain deep anesthesia. This approach, called *balanced anesthesia*, allows the dose of inhalation anesthetic to be lower so that the procedure is safer for the patient.

General anesthesia is a progressive process that occurs in distinct steps, or stages. The most effective medications can quickly cause all four stages, whereas others are only able to cause stage 1 (light sedation). Most major surgery occurs in stage 3, where the patient is completely relaxed and sedated. Thus, stage 3 anesthesia is called *surgical anesthesia*. When seeking surgical anesthesia, the anesthesiologist will try to move quickly through stage 2 because this stage produces distressing symptoms. Often an IV drug will be given to calm the patient during this stage. The stages of general anesthesia are listed in Table 15.3 ◆.

There are two primary methods of causing general anesthesia. *Intravenous drugs* are usually administered first because they act within a few seconds. After the patient loses consciousness, *inhaled drugs* are used to maintain the anesthesia. During short surgical procedures or those requiring lower stages of anesthesia, the IV drugs may be used alone.

CORE CONCEPT 15.5

General anesthetics are usually administered by the inhalation or IV routes.

General anesthetics are drugs that rapidly produce unconsciousness and total analgesia. To supplement a general anesthetic, adjunctive drugs are given before, during, and after surgery. Inhaled general anesthetics, listed in Table 15.4 ◆, are gases or volatile liquids. These drugs produce their effects by preventing the flow of sodium into neurons in the CNS, thus delaying nerve impulses and producing a dramatic reduction in neural activity. The exact mechanism for how this occurs is not known, although it is likely that gamma-aminobutyric acid (GABA) receptors in the brain are activated. It is not the same mechanism as is known for local anesthetics. There is some inconclusive evidence suggesting that the mechanism may be related to that of some antiseizure drugs. There is no specific receptor that binds to general anesthetics, and they do not seem to affect neurotransmitter release.

TABLE 15.3	Stages of General Anesthesia
Stage 1	Loss of pain; the patient loses general sensation but may be awake. This stage proceeds until the patient loses consciousness.
Stage 2	Excitement and hyperactivity; the patient may be delirious and try to resist treatment. Heartbeat and breathing may become irregular, and blood pressure can increase. IV drugs are administered here to calm the patient.
Stage 3	Surgical anesthesia; skeletal muscles become paralyzed. Cardiovascular and breathing activities stabilize. Eye movements slow down and the patient becomes still.
Stage 4	Paralysis of the medulla region in the brain (responsible for controlling respiratory and cardiovascular activity). If breathing or the heart stops, death could result. This stage is usually avoided during general anesthesia.

TABLE 15.4   Inhaled General Anesthetics

Drug	Clinical Uses
GASES	
Pr nitrous oxide	Used alone in dentistry, obstetrics, and short medical procedures; used in combination with more potent inhaled anesthetics
VOLATILE LIQUIDS	
desflurane (Suprane)	Induction and maintenance of general anesthesia
enflurane (Ethrane)	Induction and maintenance of general anesthesia
Pr isoflurane (Forane)	Induction and maintenance of general anesthesia; most widely used inhalation anesthetic
sevoflurane (Ultane)	Induction and maintenance of general anesthesia

Drug Prototype: Pr *Nitrous Oxide*

Therapeutic Class: **General anesthetic**   Pharmacologic Class: **Inhalation gaseous drug**

Actions and Uses: The main action of nitrous oxide is analgesia caused by suppression of pain mechanisms in the CNS. This drug has a low potency and does not produce complete loss of consciousness or extreme relaxation of skeletal muscle. Because nitrous oxide does not cause surgical anesthesia (stage 3), it is commonly combined with other surgical anesthetic drugs. Nitrous oxide is ideal for dental procedures because the patient remains conscious and can follow instruction while experiencing full analgesia.

Adverse Effects and Interactions: When used in low to moderate doses, nitrous oxide produces few adverse effects. At higher doses, patients exhibit some adverse signs of stage 2 anesthesia, such as anxiety, excitement, and combativeness. Lowering the inhaled dose will quickly reverse these adverse effects. As nitrous oxide is exhaled the patient may temporarily have some difficulty breathing at the end of a procedure. Nausea and vomiting following the procedure are more common with nitrous oxide than with other inhalation anesthetics. Nitrous oxide has the potential to be abused by users (sometimes medical personnel) who enjoy the relaxed, sedated state that the drug produces.

Drug Prototype: Pr *Isoflurane (Forane)*

Therapeutic Class: **General anesthetic**   Pharmacologic Class: **Inhalation volatile liquid; GABA and glutamate receptor agonist**

Actions and Uses: Isoflurane produces a potent level of surgical anesthesia that is rapid in onset. It provides the patient with smooth induction with a low degree of metabolism by the body. This drug provides excellent muscle relaxation and may be used off-label as adjuvant therapy in the treatment of status asthmaticus. Isoflurane with oxygen or with an oxygen/nitrous oxide mixture may be used. Compared to other inhaled general anesthetics, cardiac output is well maintained.

Adverse Effects and Interactions: Mild nausea, vomiting, and tremor are common adverse effects. The drug produces a dose-dependent respiratory depression and a reduction in blood pressure. Malignant hyperthermia with elevated temperature has been reported. Patients with a known history of genetic predisposition to malignant hyperthermia should not use isoflurane. Caution should be used when treating patients with head trauma or brain neoplasms due to possible increases in intracranial pressure. Older adult patients are more susceptible to hypotension caused by the drug.

When isoflurane is used concurrently with nitrous oxide, coughing, breath holding, and laryngospasms may occur. If isoflurane is administered with systemic polymyxin and aminoglycosides, skeletal muscle weakness, respiratory depression, or apnea may occur. Additive effects may occur with isoflurane if administered with other skeletal muscle relaxants. Additive hypotension may result if used concurrently with antihypertensive medications such as beta blockers. Epinephrine, norepinephrine, dopamine, and other adrenergic agonists should be administered with caution due to the possibility of dysrhythmias. Other drugs may cause dysrhythmias including amiodarone, ibutilide, droperidol, and phenothiazines. Levodopa should be discontinued six to eight hours before isoflurane administration. St. John's wort should be discontinued two to three weeks prior to administration due to the possible risk of hypotension.

Gases

The only gas used routinely for anesthesia is nitrous oxide, commonly called *laughing gas*. Nitrous oxide is used for brief obstetrical and surgical procedures and dental procedures. It may also be used in conjunction with other general anesthetics, making it possible to decrease their doses with greater effectiveness.

Nitrous oxide should be used cautiously in patients with myasthenia gravis because it may cause respiratory depression and prolonged hypnotic effects. Patients with cardiovascular disease, especially those with increased intracranial pressure, should be monitored carefully because the hypnotic effects of the drug may be prolonged or potentiated.

Volatile Liquids

The volatile anesthetics are liquid at room temperature but are converted into a vapor and inhaled to produce their anesthetic effects. Volatile drugs include desflurane (Suprane), enflurane (Ethrane), isoflurane (Forane), and sevoflurane (Ultane). Some general anesthetics increase the sensitivity of the heart to drugs such as epinephrine, norepinephrine, dopamine, and serotonin. Most volatile liquids depress cardiovascular and respiratory function. Because isoflurane (Forane) has less effect on the heart and does not damage the liver, it has become the most widely used inhalation anesthetic. The volatile liquids are excreted almost entirely by the lungs through exhalation.

CORE CONCEPT 15.6

Intravenous anesthetics are important supplements to inhalant general anesthetics and include benzodiazepines, opioids, and miscellaneous IV drugs.

Intravenous Anesthetics

Intravenous anesthetics may be used alone, for short procedures, or in combination with inhalation anesthetics. IV general anesthetics, listed in Table 15.5 ◆ are important supplements to general anesthesia. Although occasionally used alone, they are more often administered with inhaled general anesthetics.

TABLE 15.5 Intravenous Anesthetics	
Drug	**Remarks**
BENZODIAZEPINES	
diazepam (Valium) (see page 188 for the Drug Prototype box)	For induction of anesthesia; prototype drug for the benzodiazepines
lorazepam (Ativan) (see page 116 for the Drug Prototype box)	For induction of anesthesia and to produce conscious sedation; for short medical procedures or surgery
midazolam (Versed)	For induction of anesthesia and to produce conscious sedation; for short diagnostic procedures
OPIOIDS	
alfentanil (Alfenta)	Rapid onset and short duration of action; for induction of anesthesia; used as a supplement to other anesthetic drugs
fentanyl (Sublimaze, others)	Short-acting analgesic used during the operative and perioperative period; used to supplement both general and regional anesthesia
remifentanil (Ultiva)	Approximately seven times more potent than fentanyl; onset and duration of action more rapid than fentanyl; for induction and maintenance of anesthesia
sufentanil (Sufenta)	Approximately seven times more potent than fentanyl; onset and duration of action more rapid than fentanyl; for induction and maintenance of anesthesia
MISCELLANEOUS IV DRUGS	
etomidate (Amidate)	For induction of anesthesia; for short medical procedures
fospropofol (Lusedra)	For induction and maintenance of general anesthesia; for short medical procedures
ketamine (Ketalar)	For sedation, amnesia, and analgesia; for short diagnostic, therapeutic, or surgical procedures; most often used in children
🅟🅟 propofol (Diprivan)	For induction and maintenance of general anesthesia; for short medical procedures

Drug Prototype: ℗ₚ Propofol (Diprivan)

Therapeutic Class: General anesthetic   **Pharmacologic Class: Intravenous induction drug; N-methy-D-aspartate (NMDA) receptor agonist**

Actions and Uses: Propofol is indicated for the induction and maintenance of general anesthesia. It has almost an immediate onset of action and is used effectively for conscious sedation. Emergence is rapid and few adverse effects occur during recovery. Propofol has an antiemetic effect that can prevent nausea and vomiting.

Adverse Effects and Interactions: Propofol is contraindicated in patients who have a known hypersensitivity reaction to the medication or its emulsion, which contains soybean and egg products. Diprivan injectable emulsion is not recommended for obstetrics, including cesarean section deliveries, or for use in nursing mothers. The drug should be used with caution in patients with cardiac or respiratory impairment.

The dose of propofol should be reduced in patients receiving preanesthetic medications such as benzodiazepines or opioids. Use with other CNS depressants can cause additive CNS and respiratory depression.

Concurrent administration of IV and inhaled anesthetics together allows the dose of the inhaled drug to be reduced, thus lessening the potential for serious adverse effects. Furthermore, when IV and inhaled anesthetics are combined, they provide greater analgesia and muscle relaxation than could be provided by the inhaled anesthetic alone. When IV anesthetics are administered alone, they are generally reserved for medical procedures that take less than 15 minutes.

anti = *against*
emetic = *vomiting*

Drugs employed as IV anesthetics include benzodiazepines, opioids, and miscellaneous drugs. Opioids offer the advantage of superior analgesia. Combining the opioid fentanyl (Sublimaze) with the antipsychotic drug droperidol (Inapsine) produces a state known as *neuroleptanalgesia*. In this state, patients are conscious but insensitive to pain and unaware of their surroundings. The premixed combination of these two drugs is marketed as Innovar. A similar conscious, *dissociated* (i.e., *unaware*) state is produced with the amnestic, ketamine (Ketalar).

amnestic = *loss of memory*

Concept Review   15.3

■ What is the role of IV anesthetics in surgical anesthesia? Why are these drugs not used alone for general anesthesia?

ADJUNCTS TO ANESTHESIA

Nonanesthetic drugs are used as adjuncts to anesthesia before, during, and after surgery.

CORE CONCEPT 15.7

A number of drugs are used either to complement the effects of general anesthetics or to treat anticipated adverse effects of the anesthesia. These drugs, shown in Table 15.6 ◆, are called *adjuncts* to anesthesia. They may be given prior to, during, or after surgery.

Preoperative drugs are given to relieve anxiety and to provide mild sedation. Opioids, such as morphine, may be given to reduce the amount of general anesthetic required or to reduce any pain that the patient will experience at the onset of surgery. Anticholinergics such as atropine may be administered to dry secretions and to suppress the bradycardia caused by some anesthetics. Sedative–hypnotic drugs help reduce fear, anxiety, or pain associated with the surgery.

pre = *before*
operative = *surgery*

sedative = *drowsy*
hypnotic = *sleep*

During surgery, the primary adjuncts are the **neuromuscular blockers** (see Chapter 12). Neuromuscular blockers cause paralysis without loss of consciousness, which means that without a general anesthetic, patients would be awake and without the ability to move. It is important to note that breathing muscles are skeletal muscle. This is why patients require intubation and mechanical ventilation. Administration of these drugs also allows a reduced amount of general anesthetic.

neuro = *nerve*
muscular = *muscle*

TABLE 15.6 Selected Adjuncts to Anesthesia

Drug	Remarks
ANTICHOLINERGIC	
atropine	Used in general anesthesia as a premedication, in emergency situations, or during surgery to increase heart rate and to reverse the effects of some cholinergic drugs
BENZODIAZEPINE	
midazolam (Versed)	Generally used before other intravenous agents for induction of anesthesia
CHOLINERGIC DRUG	
bethanechol (Urecholine) (see page 93 for the Drug Prototype box)	For relief of constipation and urinary retention caused by opioids; stimulates GI motility
DOPAMINE BLOCKER	
droperidol (Inapsine)	For nausea and vomiting caused by opioids; reduces anxiety and relaxes muscles
NEUROMUSCULAR BLOCKERS	
mivacurium (Mivacron)	Short duration; nondepolarizing type
Pr succinylcholine (Anectine)	Short duration; depolarizing type
tubocurarine	Long duration; nondepolarizing type
OPIOIDS	
alfentanil (Alfenta)	Short duration; for induction of anesthesia when endotracheal or mechanical ventilation is needed; provides analgesia
fentanyl (Sublimaze, others)	For analgesia during or after anesthesia; the combination of fentanyl and droperidol is called Innovar
morphine (see page 203 for the Drug Prototype box)	For analgesia during or after anesthesia
remifentanil (Ultiva)	For analgesia during or after anesthesia; shorter duration of action than fentanyl
sufentanil (Sufenta)	For primary anesthesia or to provide analgesia during or after anesthesia
PHENOTHIAZINE	
promethazine (Phenergan)	For nausea and vomiting associated with obstetric sedation and opioids

Drug Prototype: Pr *Succinylcholine (Anectine)*

Therapeutic Class: Skeletal muscle paralytic, neuromuscular blocker

Pharmacologic Class: Depolarizing blocker, acetylcholine receptor blocking drug

Actions and Uses: Like the natural neurotransmitter acetylcholine, succinylcholine acts on cholinergic receptor sites at neuromuscular junctions. At first, depolarization occurs, and skeletal muscles contract. After repeated contractions, however, the membrane is unable to repolarize as long as the drug stays on the receptor. Effects are first noted as muscle weakness and muscle spasms. Eventually paralysis occurs. Succinylcholine is rapidly broken down by the enzyme pseudocholinesterase; when the IV infusion is stopped, the duration of action is only a few minutes. Use of succinylcholine reduces the amount of general anesthetic needed for procedures.

Adverse Effects and Interactions: Succinylcholine can cause complete paralysis of the diaphragm and intercostal muscles; thus, mechanical ventilation is necessary during surgery. Bradycardia and respiratory depression are expected adverse effects. If doses are high, tachycardia, hypotension, and urinary retention may occur. Patients with certain genetic defects may experience rapid onset of extremely high fever with muscle rigidity—a serious condition known as malignant hyperthermia.

Additive skeletal muscle blockade will occur if succinylcholine is given concurrently with clindamycin, aminoglycosides, furosemide, lithium, quinidine, or lidocaine.

Increased effect of succinylcholine may occur if given with phenothiazines oxytocin, promazine; tacrine, or thiazide diuretics. Decreased effect of succinylcholine occurs if given with diazepam.

If this drug is given with nitrous oxide, an increased risk of bradycardia, dysrhythmias, sinus arrest, apnea, and malignant hyperthermia exists. If succinylcholine is given with cardiac glycosides, there is increased risk of cardiac dysrhythmias. If narcotics are given with succinylcholine, there is increased risk of bradycardia and sinus arrest.

BLACK BOX WARNING:
Succinylcholine should be administered in a facility with trained personnel to monitor, assist, and control respiration. Cardiac arrest has been reported resulting from hyperkalemia (elevated potassium blood level) rhabdomyolysis most frequently in infants or children with undiagnosed skeletal muscle myopathy, or Duchenne muscular dystrophy. In children, use of this drug is reserved for cases of emergency intubation (process of inserting an endotracheal tube for breathing) or when immediate securing of the airway is necessary.

Neuromuscular blocking agents are classified as *depolarizing blockers* and *nondepolarizing* blockers. The only depolarizing blocker is succinylcholine (Anectine), which works by binding to acetylcholine receptors at neuromuscular junctions to cause total skeletal muscle paralysis. Succinylcholine is used in surgery for ease of tracheal intubation. Mivacurium (Mivacron) is the shortest acting of the nondepolarizing blockers, whereas tubocurarine is a longer-acting neuromuscular blocker. The nondepolarizing blockers cause muscle paralysis by competing with acetylcholine for cholinergic receptors at neuromuscular junctions. Once attached to the receptor, the nonpolarizing blockers prevent muscle contraction.

junction = *connection*

Postoperative drugs include analgesics for pain and antiemetics, such as ondansetron (Zofran, Zuplenz) for the nausea and vomiting that sometimes occur during recovery from the anesthetic. Occasionally, following surgery, a parasympathomimetic, such as bethanechol (Urecholine) is administered to stimulate the urinary tract and the smooth muscle of the bowel (see Chapter 8).

post = *after*

PATIENTS NEED TO KNOW

Patients treated with local anesthetic medications need to know the following:
1. When using topical anesthetics for skin conditions, avoid touching the eyes.
2. Never apply topical medications to large patches of skin or to areas where there is an open lesion or cut unless instructed to do so by the healthcare provider.
3. Notify the dentist or healthcare providers of any previous adverse reactions to local anesthesia before being given additional anesthetic medications.
4. After receiving local anesthetic solutions for the mouth, do not consume food and drink until it is clear that the anesthetic has worn off.
5. While the area is still numb, do not chew or pick at an area where a dental procedure has been performed.
6. Be careful not to inhale anesthetic sprays used for topical application.
7. Get immediate assistance if drowsiness, confusion, or blurred vision has occurred after receiving a local anesthetic. Other signs/symptoms to look for include lightheadedness, an irregular heartbeat, or feeling faint.
8. Report all medications and conditions to the healthcare provider before receiving anesthetics.
9. For outpatient dental or medical procedures involving anesthesia, someone should be available to assist with activities such as transportation.
10. Follow postprocedure instructions carefully after anesthesia.
11. Have sufficient pain medication readily available so that postprocedure pain can be managed after the effects of the anesthesia are no longer felt.

CHAPTER REVIEW

CORE CONCEPTS SUMMARY

15.1   Local anesthesia causes a rapid loss of sensation to a limited part of the body.

Local anesthesia is loss of sensation to a relatively small part of the body without causing loss of consciousness. Sometimes local anesthesia is applied to an entire limb. In these cases, it is more accurately called *surface anesthesia* or *regional anesthesia*, depending on how the drugs are administered and the results they produce.

15.2   Local anesthetics produce their therapeutic effect by blocking the entry of sodium ions into neurons.

Blocking sodium entry into neurons prevents transmission of the electrical impulse along the nerve. Epinephrine is sometimes added to anesthetic solutions to increase the duration of action of the anesthetic. A base such as sodium hydroxide is added to make an infected tissue environment more alkaline.

15.3   Local anesthetics are classified by their chemical structures.

The two major classes of local anesthetics are esters and amides. Benzocaine (Solarcaine, others) is the most commonly used ester; lidocaine (Xylocaine) is the most widely prescribed amide.

15.4 General anesthesia is a loss of sensation occurring throughout the entire body, accompanied by a loss of consciousness.

General anesthesia proceeds in stages from light sedation to total loss of consciousness. The less potent anesthetics cause stage 1 anesthesia, whereas more potent drugs cause surgical anesthesia (stage 3).

15.5 General anesthetics are usually administered by the inhalation or IV routes.

Two primary methods for producing rapid unconsciousness and total analgesia are IV drugs and inhaled general anesthetics. Inhalation drugs include nitrous oxide, the only gaseous drug, and volatile liquids. Many drugs may be used alone or in combination with other drugs. The mechanism by which general anesthetics produce their effect is not completely known.

15.6 Intravenous anesthetics are important supplements to inhalant general anesthetics and include benzodiazepines, opioids, and miscellaneous IV drugs.

Intravenous drugs may be used along with inhaled anesthetics to lower the potential for serious adverse effects. Benzodiazepines, opioids, and other select IV drugs are generally reserved for quick medical procedures and treatments requiring superior analgesia.

15.7 Nonanesthetic drugs are used as adjuncts to anesthesia before, during, and after surgery.

A number of drugs are given prior to surgery to relieve anxiety, provide mild sedation, counteract pain, and dry secretions. Neuromuscular blockers, given during surgery, relax skeletal muscle and maintain a proper heart rate. Drugs after surgery include treatment for pain and vomiting and for stimulating the bowel and urinary tract.

REVIEW QUESTIONS

The following questions are written in NCLEX-PN® style. Answer these questions to assess your knowledge of the chapter material, and go back and review any material that is not clear to you.

1. The nurse informs the patient that which of the following herbal products may prolong or intensify the effects of anesthesia?

1. Kava kava
2. Oil of cloves
3. Anise
4. St. John's wort

2. While administering lidocaine, the nurse monitors for toxicity, which is manifested by: (Select all that apply.)

1. Excitement
2. Irritability
3. Tachypnea
4. Confusion

3. A patient in labor is advised that she can have epidural anesthesia to help relieve her pain. When she asks the nurse what will happen, the nurse tells her:

1. "An anesthetic drug will be injected directly into the area where the pain is occurring, affecting the nerves and blocking any sensations."
2. "A small tube (catheter) will be placed in the space between the vertebrae and the spinal cord and an anesthetic drug will be injected through the tube. The medication will cause numbness in the areas below the injection site, but you will still be able to move your legs."
3. "You will receive an injection of an anesthetic drug in your back, directly into the cerebrospinal spinal fluid, which will numb the lower half of your body."

4. "An anesthetic cream will be applied to the skin in the areas causing your pain. This cream will numb those areas."

4. Before administering propofol, the nurse checks a patient's record for allergies. After reviewing the records and talking to the patient, the nurse notifies the healthcare provider and the order is discontinued because the patient is allergic to:

1. Peanuts
2. Shellfish
3. Egg products
4. Milk

5. A patient is to receive nitrous oxide during surgery. The nurse understands that he or she will need to monitor the patient for which adverse effect?

1. Restlessness
2. Dysrhythmia
3. Hypertension
4. Mania

6. The patient being prepared for surgery asks the nurse why he or she is receiving morphine and atropine prior to surgery. The nurse's best response is:

1. "You will need to speak with your healthcare provider."
2. "The morphine will help to provide some pain relief before surgery and the atropine will help to decrease secretions."
3. "The morphine and atropine will help your anesthetic work more effectively."
4. "These medications are routinely used before we send a patient to surgery."

7. In reviewing a patient's preoperative paperwork, the nurse notes that the patient has a history of cardiovascular disease and therefore should not receive epinephrine along with the anesthetics because it can cause:

1. Tachycardia and hypertension
2. Bradycardia and hypotension
3. Tachycardia and hypotension
4. Bradycardia and hypertension

8. The nurse explains to the patient that he or she will receive both isoflurane (Forane) and nitrous oxide:

1. To provide the additional anesthesia to put him or her in a sleeplike state
2. To increase effectiveness of anesthesia with lower dosages of each drug
3. Because isoflurane is not effective when used alone
4. Because nitrous oxide should not be used alone

9. The anesthesiologist orders atropine, 1 mg IM for a patient in the recovery room. Available is 0.8 mg/mL. How many milliliters will be given?

1. 1 mL
2. 1.15 mL
3. 1.2 mL
4. 1.25 mL

10. The patient is experiencing nausea in the recovery room. The nurse anticipates which medication being ordered?

1. Meperidine
2. Bethanechol
3. Ondansetron
4. Succinylcholine

CASE STUDY QUESTIONS

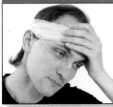

Remember Mr. Wayland, the patient introduced at the beginning of the chapter? Now read the remainder of the case study. Based on the information you have learned in this chapter, answer the questions that follow.

Mr. Jeffery Wayland, age 38, has a history of cardiovascular disease. He has collapsed and sustained an injury to his scalp. The wound is substantial, and Mr. Wayland is bleeding across his right forehead. The patient is rushed to the emergency department by his girlfriend. The girlfriend reports that Mr. Wayland is normally very fearful of doctors and nurses. It is unclear why Mr. Wayland collapsed. The doctor wants to inject the tissue surrounding the wound with 1% lidocaine with epinephrine for local anesthesia prior to suturing the laceration and asks the nurse to prepare the medication.

1. Because he is anxious, Mr. Wayland asks the nurse, "Is the doctor going to numb the area before he begins to put stitches in my head?" The nurse replies:

1. "Yes, the doctor will apply a topical (surface) anesthetic medication to numb the area."
2. "Yes, the doctor will inject an anesthetic medication directly around the area, or field, of the wound to help prevent pain."
3. "Yes, the doctor will inject an anesthetic medication that will block a bundle of nerve endings."
4. "Yes, the doctor will provide an anesthetic drug by injecting it into your epidural space."

2. The nurse understands that the addition of epinephrine to the lidocaine is to:

1. Prevent infection
2. Prevent an allergic reaction
3. Increase the duration of the anesthetic
4. Decrease pain after the procedure

3. Soon after administering the lidocaine, the nurse monitors Mr. Wayland for:

1. Constriction of airways
2. Anxiety
3. Tachycardia
4. Unresponsiveness

4. As the nurse, would it be advisable to give Mr. Wayland a barbiturate to help him calm down due to his fear of doctors and nurses in this case?

1. No, a barbiturate might increase toxicity symptoms if Mr. Wayland is allergic to lidocaine.
2. Yes, a barbiturate might increase the effectiveness of lidocaine in this situation and help the patient calm down.
3. No, a barbiturate might decrease the effectiveness of lidocaine in this situation and make the patient more irritable.
4. No, a barbiturate might decrease the effectiveness of lidocaine in this situation, although the medication would normally have a calming effect.

NOTE: Answers to the Review and Case Study Questions appear in Appendix B. The complete rationales and answers are located on the textbook's website.

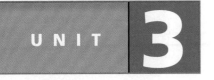
The Cardiovascular and Urinary Systems

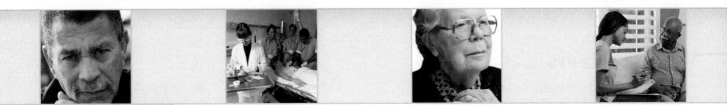

Unit Contents

Chapter 16   Drugs for Lipid Disorders / 234

Chapter 17   Diuretics and Drugs for Electrolyte and Acid–Base Disorders / 248

Chapter 18   Drugs for Hypertension / 265

Chapter 19   Drugs for Heart Failure / 287

Chapter 20   Drugs for Angina Pectoris, Myocardial Infarction, and Stroke / 301

Chapter 21   Drugs for Shock and Anaphylaxis / 319

Chapter 22   Drugs for Dysrhythmias / 331

Chapter 23   Drugs for Coagulation Disorders / 346

"I've lived too long to change my eating habits now. I've had bad blood tests for years and nothing has happened to me. Besides, I'm too busy to deal with one more problem in my life."

Mr. Edward Long

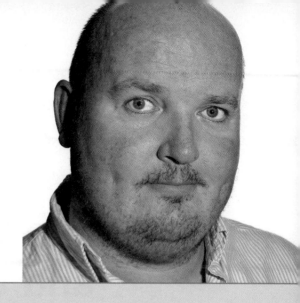

16 Drugs for Lipid Disorders

CORE CONCEPTS

16.1 Lipids serve essential roles in the body, but too much dietary fat can lead to disease.

16.2 Lipoproteins transport lipids through the blood for utilization by tissues, storage in adipose tissue, or excretion by the liver.

16.3 Elevated lipid levels can often be prevented or controlled through therapeutic lifestyle changes.

16.4 Statins are preferred drugs for reducing blood lipid levels.

16.5 Bile acid binding drugs can reduce LDL levels by increasing cholesterol excretion.

16.6 Niacin can reduce triglyceride and LDL-cholesterol levels.

16.7 Fibric acid drugs lower triglyceride levels, but have little effect on LDLs.

16.8 Other approaches to treating hyperlipidemia include ezetimibe, omega-3 fatty acids, and fixed-dose combination therapy.

DRUG SNAPSHOT

The following drugs are discussed in this chapter:

DRUG CLASSES	DRUG PROTOTYPES
HMG-CoA reductase inhibitors (statins)	Pr atorvastatin (Lipitor) *240*
Bile acid binding drugs	Pr cholestyramine (Questran) *240*
Fibric acid drugs (fibrates)	Pr gemfibrozil (Lopid) *244*

LEARNING OUTCOMES

After reading this chapter, the student should be able to:

1. Summarize the links among high blood cholesterol, low-density lipoprotein (LDL) levels, and cardiovascular disease.

2. Compare and contrast the different types of lipids.

3. Describe how lipids are transported through the body.

4. Compare and contrast the different types of lipoproteins.

5. Give examples of how blood lipid levels can be controlled through nonpharmacologic means.

6. Categorize antihyperlipidemic drugs based on their classifications and mechanisms of action.

7. For each of the classes in the Drug Snapshot, identify representative drugs and explain their mechanisms of drug action, primary actions, and important adverse effects.

KEY TERMS

atherosclerosis (ath-ur-oh-skler-OH-sis) *235*

bile acids (BEYE-ulz) *241*

dyslipidemia (dys-lip-i-DEEM-ee-uh) *235*

high-density lipoprotein (HDL) *236*

HMG-CoA reductase (ree-DUCK-tase) *238*

hypercholesterolemia (HEYE-purr-koh-LESS-tur-ol-EEM-ee-uh) *235*

hyperlipidemia (HEYE-purr-LIP-i-DEEM-ee-uh) *235*

hypertriglyceridemia (HEYE-purr-tri-gliss-ur-i-DEEM-ee-uh) *235*

lipoproteins (LIP-oh-PROH-teen) *236*

low-density lipoprotein (LDL) *236*

plaque (PLAK) *235*

therapeutic lifestyle changes *236*

triglycerides (tri-GLISS-ur-ide) *235*

very low-density lipoprotein (VLDL) *236*

Research has brought about a nutritional revolution as new knowledge about lipids and their relationship to obesity and cardiovascular disease has allowed people to make more intelligent lifestyle choices. Advances in the diagnosis of lipid disorders have helped to identify those patients at greatest risk for cardiovascular disease, and those most likely to benefit from pharmacologic intervention. Safe, effective drugs for lowering lipid levels are now available that decrease the risk of cardiovascular diseases. As a result of this knowledge and from advancements in pharmacology, the incidence of death due to cardiovascular disease has been declining, although it is still the leading cause of death in the United States.

Lipids serve essential roles in the body, but too much dietary fat can lead to disease.

CORE CONCEPT 16.1

Lipids, or fats, are organic compounds that are essential for good health. Lipid tissue provides cushioning and protection of organs and insulates the body to maintain core temperature. Phospholipid is the major component of all cell membranes in the body.

The most common lipids, the **triglycerides**, are the major storage form of fat in the body and the only type of lipid that serves as an important energy source. They account for 90% of the total lipids in the body.

Cholesterol is a lipid that is a major component of cell membranes and which serves as a building block for other lipid-based biochemicals such as vitamin D, bile salts, cortisol, estrogen, and testosterone. Its negative role in promoting **atherosclerosis** or plaque on the walls of arteries is well known. Fatty **plaque** deposits narrow arteries, thereby contributing to angina, myocardial infarction (MI), and stroke, as discussed in Chapter 20. Because the body needs only small amounts of cholesterol daily, it is not necessary to ingest excess amounts of cholesterol in the diet. Dietary cholesterol is obtained solely from animal food products; humans do not absorb the sterols produced by plants.

athero = *fatty*
sclera = *hard*
osis = *condition of*

Research is still uncovering the important roles of lipids in the diet. While it is clear that too much of certain types of dietary fat are associated with disease, some types actually promote wellness. For example, evidence is strong that intake of saturated fats and trans fats should be limited because they are associated with obesity, cardiovascular disease, and possibly cancer. However, omega-3 fatty acids, which are found in abundance in deep, cold-water fish such as salmon, tuna, and herring, may have health benefits. The richest plant source of omega-3 fatty acids is flaxseed, which has become a popular dietary supplement.

Several terms are used to describe lipid disorders. **Dyslipidemia** is a general term meaning an abnormal amount of lipid in the blood. **Hyperlipidemia** is a similar term that refers to high levels of lipids in the blood. Some patients have only one specific type of lipid that is elevated. Elevated blood cholesterol, or **hypercholesterolemia**, is the type of dyslipidemia that is most familiar to the general public. **Hypertriglyceridemia**, elevated triglycerides, is a less common disorder.

hyper = *above*
lipid = *fat*
emia = *blood*

Fast Facts High Blood Cholesterol

- Thirty million Americans (15% of U.S. adults) are believed to have both hypertension and high blood cholesterol levels.
- The incidence of high blood cholesterol increases until age 65.
- Moderate alcohol intake does not reduce LDL cholesterol, but it does increase high-density lipoprotein (HDL, or good) cholesterol.
- High blood cholesterol occurs more frequently in men than in premenopausal women, but after age 50, the disease is more common in women.
- To lower blood cholesterol, dietary intake of both cholesterol and saturated fats must be reduced.
- Familial hypercholesterolemia affects 1 in 500 people and is a genetic disease that predisposes people to high cholesterol levels.

CORE CONCEPT 16.2

Lipoproteins transport lipids through the blood for utilization by tissues, storage in adipose tissue, or excretion by the liver.

Knowledge of cholesterol metabolism is important to understanding cardiovascular disease and the pharmacotherapy of lipid disorders. In simplest terms, the greater the amount of cholesterol circulating in the blood, the greater the risk of cardiovascular disease. This is because the circulating cholesterol binds to vessel walls, increasing plaque buildup as years pass.

Because they are not soluble in the blood, cholesterol and other lipids are packaged as lipoprotein complexes by the liver. **Lipoproteins** contain an inner core of lipid surrounded by an outer shell of carrier protein, which makes them water soluble and able to be transported freely through the blood. The three most common lipoproteins are named based on their weight or density, which comes primarily from the amount of protein present in the complex. Figure 16.1 ■ illustrates the three basic lipoproteins and their composition. Each type of lipoprotein serves a different function in transporting lipids to their final destination.

Although cholesterol is packaged in all lipoproteins, **low-density lipoprotein (LDL)** has the greatest amount: Almost 50% of LDL consists of cholesterol. The liver makes LDL, which is then transported to tissues and organs, where it is used to build plasma membranes or to synthesize other steroids. Once in the tissues, cholesterol can also be stored for later use. Storage of cholesterol in the lining of blood vessels, however, contributes to plaque buildup and atherosclerosis. LDL is often called "bad" cholesterol because this lipoprotein contributes significantly to plaque deposits and coronary artery disease.

Under normal circumstances, the body makes all the cholesterol it needs to construct cell membranes and other vital functions. When cholesterol is ingested, the body simply makes less to compensate for the increased amounts in the diet. If a person includes too much cholesterol in the diet, however, this feedback loop fails and LDL-cholesterol builds, increasing the risk for health problems.

The body has a remarkable method for keeping blood cholesterol levels in check. A second type of lipoprotein, **high-density lipoprotein (HDL)**, picks up cholesterol in the blood and other tissues and returns it to the liver. Once in the liver, the cholesterol is used to make bile, which is essential for digestion of lipids. The cholesterol component of bile is then excreted in the feces, although some is reabsorbed back into the circulation. Excretion via bile is the only route the body uses to remove cholesterol. Thus HDL may be thought of as "cholesterol scavengers" that pick up cholesterol in blood and tissues and transport it for removal from the body. Because HDL transports cholesterol for destruction and removes it from the body, it is considered "good" cholesterol.

Of course, cholesterol is not the only type of lipid that can lead to cardiovascular disease. Triglycerides must also be monitored and maintained within normal levels. **Very low-density lipoprotein (VLDL)** is the primary carrier of triglycerides in the blood. VLDL is made in the liver and converted to LDL as it travels through the bloodstream as most of the triglycerides in VLDL are transported to adipose tissue for storage. The health consequences of high blood levels of VLDL are not as clear as for LDL levels. It has been demonstrated, however, that high levels of VLDL are associated with an increased risk of pancreatitis.

CORE CONCEPT 16.3

Elevated lipid levels can often be prevented or controlled through therapeutic lifestyle changes.

Most patients with dyslipidemias are asymptomatic and do not seek medical intervention until cardiovascular disease has progressed, resulting in hypertension or symptoms such as chest pain. For most patients, lipid disorders are the result of a combination of genetic and environmental (lifestyle) factors.

When a patient is found to have high LDL-cholesterol levels, a decision must be made regarding the initiation of drug therapy. Although the drugs used to control lipid levels are generally safe and effective, other risk factors are considered, such as age, family history of heart disease, hypertension, and cigarette smoking. The stage at which drug therapy is begun depends on the number and extent of these risk factors. The more risk factors present, the more aggressive is the therapy. Table 16.1 ◆ gives the desirable, borderline, and high laboratory values for each of the major lipids and lipoproteins.

Recommendations for the treatment of high blood cholesterol have been set by the National Cholesterol Education Program (NCEP) of the National Institutes of Health. These recommendations, which are revised periodically, are the gold standard for treating this disorder. In some patients, high blood cholesterol levels can be controlled by initiating **therapeutic lifestyle changes** without drug therapy. Many patients with borderline laboratory values can control their hyperlipidemia entirely through nonpharmacologic means. Even in patients with high risk for whom drug therapy is indicated, using these changes is important for reducing cholesterol levels. Following are the features of therapeutic lifestyle changes:

- Increase physical activity, which raises HDL levels and lowers triglycerides.
- Maintain weight within a normal range.
- Implement a medically supervised exercise plan.
- Reduce dietary saturated fat intake to 7% of total caloric intake.
- Reduce cholesterol intake to less than 200 mg/day.
- Increase intake of whole grains, vegetables, and fruits so that total dietary fiber is 10 to 25 g/day.
- Eliminate tobacco use.

FIGURE 16.1

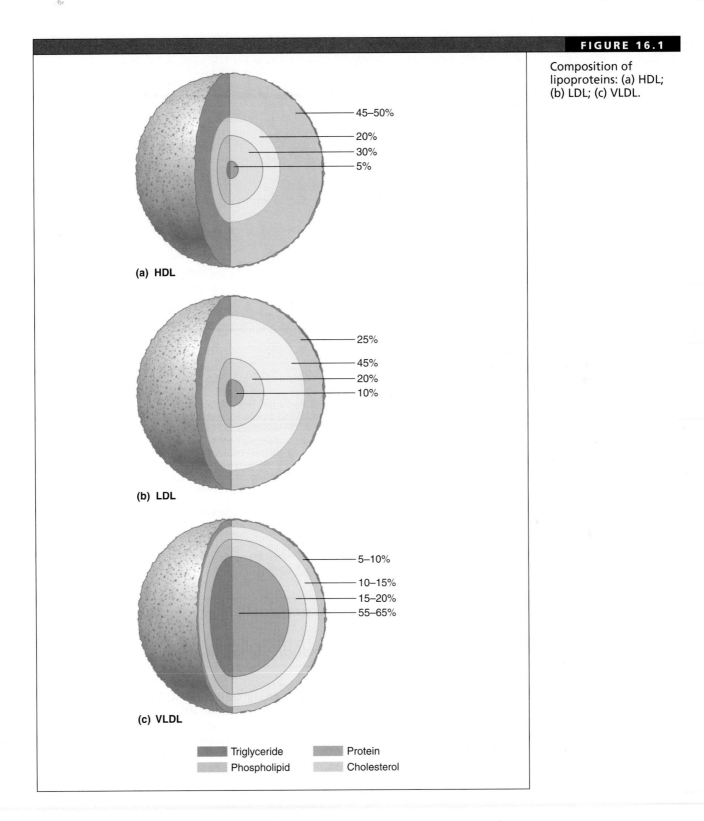

Composition of lipoproteins: (a) HDL; (b) LDL; (c) VLDL.

(a) HDL

45–50%
20%
30%
5%

(b) LDL

25%
45%
20%
10%

(c) VLDL

5–10%
10–15%
15–20%
55–65%

| Triglyceride | Protein |
| Phospholipid | Cholesterol |

In addition to the recommendations of the NCEP, other lifestyle changes likely contribute to keeping blood cholesterol levels within normal values and reducing the risk of heart disease. These factors include maintaining blood pressure within normal limits, reducing stress, and limiting the intake of high-sugar foods. Increased intake of omega-3 fatty acids has been shown to reduce the risk of cardiovascular disease. Because trans-fatty acids in the diet can raise blood cholesterol levels, patients should be advised to avoid foods that are fried or contain vegetable shortening or partially hydrogenated oils.

TABLE 16.1 Standard Laboratory Lipid Profiles		
Type of Lipid	**Laboratory Value (mg/dl)**	**Standard**
Total cholesterol	Less than 200	Desirable
	200–240	Borderline high risk
	Greater than 240	High risk
LDL cholesterol	Less than 100	Optimal
	100–129	Near or above optimal
	130–159	Moderate risk
	160–189	High risk
	Greater than 189	Very high risk
HDL cholesterol	Less than 35	High risk
	35–45	Moderate risk
	46–59	Low risk
	Greater than 60	Desirable
Triglycerides	Less than 149	Desirable
	150–199	Borderline high risk
	200–499	High risk
	Greater than 500	Very high risk

CAM THERAPY

Red Yeast Rice and Cholesterol

Red yeast rice is a supplement that is produced when rice is fermented with the yeast *Monascus purpureus*. The product is sometimes reduced to a powder and used as a coloring or flavoring. Red yeast rice has been used for centuries in Chinese medicine to treat various digestive and liver complaints, but more recently it has been used as a supplement to manage high blood cholesterol.

Red yeast rice clearly is effective at lowering blood cholesterol levels. This is likely because the product contains a chemical identical to the prescription drug lovastatin. In 2007, the Food and Drug Administration (FDA) decided that red yeast rice should be regulated as a prescription drug. Some supplement manufacturers remarketed the product after removing lovastatin from the red yeast rice. To avoid legal action, most red yeast labels do not mention a cholesterol-lowering effect. It is unclear whether the "lovastatin-removed" product has any ability to lower blood cholesterol. Patients should discuss this supplement with their healthcare provider before beginning therapy.

Concept Review 16.1

■ Why is the cholesterol in high-density lipoproteins considered to be "good" cholesterol?

CORE CONCEPT 16.4

Statins are preferred drugs for reducing blood lipid levels.

In the late 1970s, compounds were isolated from various species of fungi that were found to inhibit cholesterol production in human cells in the laboratory. This class of drugs, known as the *statins*, has since revolutionized the treatment of lipid disorders. Statins can produce a dramatic 20% to 40% reduction in LDL-cholesterol levels. In addition to decreasing LDL-cholesterol levels in the blood, statins can also lower triglyceride levels, lower VLDL levels, and raise "good" HDL-cholesterol levels. These effects have been shown to reduce the incidence of serious cardiovascular related events by 25% to 30%. Statins are now first-line drugs in the treatment of dyslipidemias and are among the most widely prescribed drugs in the United States.

Cholesterol is made in the liver by a series of more than 25 metabolic steps. Of the many enzymes involved in this complex pathway, **HMG-CoA reductase** (hydroxymethylglutaryl-CoenzymeA reductase) serves as the primary regulator of cholesterol biosynthesis. Under normal conditions, this enzyme is controlled through negative feedback: High levels of LDL cholesterol in the blood will shut down production of HMG-CoA reductase, thus turning off the cholesterol pathway. Figure 16.2 ■ illustrates some of the steps in cholesterol biosynthesis and the importance of HMG-CoA reductase.

The statins act by inhibiting HMG-CoA reductase. As the liver makes less cholesterol, the body responds by making more LDL receptors in order to scavenge more LDL from the blood, thus reducing blood levels of LDL. The drop in lipid levels is not permanent, however, patients need to remain on these drugs during the remainder of their lives or until their hyperlipidemia can be controlled through lifestyle changes. Statins have been shown to slow the progression of coronary artery disease and to reduce deaths from cardiovascular disease. Doses of the HMG-CoA reductase inhibitors are shown in Table 16.2 ◆.

FIGURE 16.2

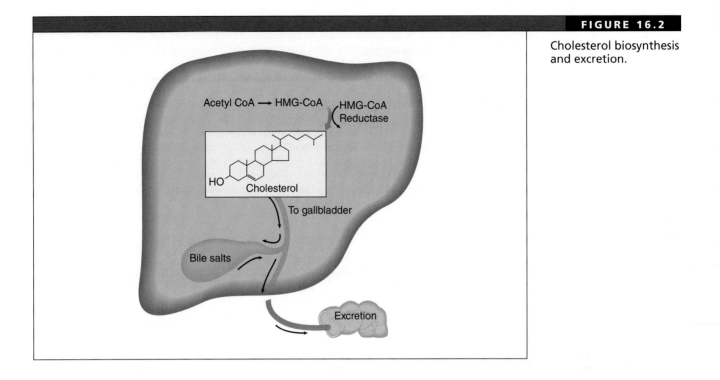

Cholesterol biosynthesis and excretion.

TABLE 16.2   Drugs for Dyslipidemias

Drug	Route and Adult Dose	Remarks
HMG-CoA REDUCTASE INHIBITORS		
Pr atorvastatin (Lipitor)	PO; 10–80 mg/day	May be taken with or without food at any time of the day
fluvastatin (Lescol)	PO; 20 mg/day (max: 80 mg/day)	May be taken with or without food in the evening
lovastatin (Altoprev, Mevacor)	PO; 20–40 mg 1–2 times/day	Should be taken with food in the evening
pitavastatin (Livalo)	PO; 1–4 mg/day (max: 4 mg/day)	May be taken with or without food at any time of the day
pravastatin (Pravachol)	PO; 10–40 mg/day	May be taken with or without food in the evening
rosuvastatin (Crestor)	PO; 5–40 mg/day	May be taken with or without food at any time of the day
simvastatin (Zocor)	PO; 5–40 mg/day	May be taken with or without food in the evening
BILE ACID BINDING DRUGS		
Pr cholestyramine (Questran)	PO; 4–8 g bid–qid	Take with large amounts of fluid; take other drugs one hour before or four hours after
colesevelam (Welchol)	PO; 1.9 g bid	Take with meals and with at least 8 oz of fluid
colestipol (Colestid)	PO; 5–20 g/day in divided doses	Taken with large amounts of fluid; take other drugs one hour before or four hours after
FIBRIC ACID DRUGS		
fenofibrate (Antara, Fibricor, Lofibra, Tricor, Trilipix)	PO; 43–200 mg/day, depending upon the specific product	Take with food. Assess periodically for symptoms of myopathy
Pr gemfibrozil (Lopid)	PO; 600 mg bid (max: 1500 mg/day)	Take 30 min before morning and evening meals
OTHER DRUGS FOR DYSLIPIDEMIAS		
ezetimibe (Zetia)	PO; 10 mg/day	Newer antihyperlipidemic; inhibits cholesterol absorption
icosapent (Vascepa)	PO; 4 g/day	Take with food
lomitapide (Juxtapid)	PO; 5–60 mg once daily	Newer drug for inherited hypercholesterolemia
mipomersan (Kynamro)	Subcutaneous; 200 mg once weekly	Newer drug for LDL and total cholesterol
niacin (Niacor, Niaspan, others)	PO; 1.5–3 g/day (max: 6 g/day)	Also used to treat niacin deficiency (10–20 mg/day). Take with food
omega-3-acid ethyl esters (Lovaza)	PO; 4 g/day	Take with food

Seven statins are currently available and all have very similar actions and adverse effects. All the statins are given orally. Some statins should be administered in the evening because cholesterol biosynthesis in the body is higher at night. Atorvastatin and rosuvastatin have longer half-lives and are effective regardless of the time of day they are taken.

The statins are generally safe drugs, having few serious adverse effects. Gastrointestinal (GI) disturbances such as indigestion, flatulence, cramping, and constipation are usually mild and disappear with continued use. Statins can cause muscle injury, resulting in symptoms such as weakness, soreness, and pain. Muscle-related side effects are dose related and tend to occur more often in elderly patients. Patients should be carefully monitored for these symptoms because muscle injury may progress to more serious conditions. In 2001, cerivastatin was removed from the market because of 31 fatalities due to severe rhabdomyolysis associated with the use of the drug. *Rhabdomyolysis* is a medical condition in which muscle tissue, including cardiac muscle, becomes extremely inflamed, resulting in breakdown of muscle. Patients reporting muscular soreness or weakness may have their statin dosage reduced, or they may be switched to a drug of a different class.

Drug Prototype: Pr *Atorvastatin (Lipitor)*
Therapeutic Class: Antihyperlipidemic drug   **Pharmacologic Class: HMG-CoA reductase inhibitor (statin)**

Actions and Uses: Atorvastatin slows the biosynthesis of cholesterol by blocking the rate-limiting enzyme, HMG-CoA reductase. The primary indication for atorvastatin is hypercholesterolemia. Although lovastatin (Mevacor) was the first HMG-CoA reductase inhibitor approved for use in the United States, atorvastatin has a long half-life and may be administered without regard to food or time of day. Maximum effects from atorvastatin are seen in 4–8 weeks. Effectiveness is measured by decreases in LDL, total cholesterol, and triglycerides, and an increase in HDL. Patients receiving this drug should be placed on a cholesterol-lowering diet, because this will enhance the drug's therapeutic effects. The primary goal in atorvastatin therapy is to reduce the risk of MI and stroke.

Adverse Effects and Interactions: Adverse effects of atorvastatin are rarely severe enough to cause discontinuation of therapy and include GI complaints such as intestinal cramping, diarrhea, and constipation. A small percentage of patients experience liver damage; thus, liver function is usually monitored periodically during therapy. The most serious adverse effect is rhabdomyolysis. Like other statins, atorvastatin is a pregnancy category X drug. Pregnancy testing should be conducted prior to treatment in women of childbearing years, and the patient should be advised to take precautions to prevent pregnancy during therapy.

Atorvastatin interacts with many other drugs. For example, it may increase digoxin levels by 20%, as well as increase levels of oral contraceptives. Erythromycin may increase atorvastatin levels by 40%.

Grapefruit juice inhibits the metabolism of statins, allowing them to reach toxic levels. Because HMG-CoA reductase inhibitors also decrease the synthesis of coenzyme Q10 (CoQ10), patients may benefit from CoQ10 supplements.

Drug Prototype: Pr *Cholestyramine (Questran)*
Therapeutic Class: Antihyperlipidemic drug   **Pharmacologic Class: Bile acid binding drug**

Actions and Uses: Cholestyramine is used to treat elevated levels of cholesterol and LDLs. The drug is formulated as a powder that is mixed with fluid before being taken once or twice daily. It is not absorbed or metabolized once it enters the intestine; thus, it does not produce systemic effects. It may take 30 days or longer to produce its maximum effect. Cholestyramine is sometimes combined with other cholesterol-lowering drugs, such as the statins or niacin to produce additive effects.

Adverse Effects and Interactions: Although cholestyramine rarely produces serious adverse effects, patients may experience constipation, bloating, gas, and nausea that may limit its use. Cholestyramine has the ability to bind to other drugs and interfere with their absorption. Examples include binding to vitamin K, thiazide diuretics, and penicillins. To prevent potential interactions, other medications should be taken one hour before or four hours after administration of cholestyramine. The drug is contraindicated in patients with biliary obstruction, biliary cirrhosis, or GI obstruction.

NURSING PROCESS FOCUS Patients Receiving Drug Therapy with HMG-CoA Reductase Inhibitors (Statins)

ASSESSMENT	POTENTIAL NURSING DIAGNOSES
Prior to administration: ■ Obtain a complete health history including cardiovascular, musculoskeletal, gastrointestinal, renal and liver conditions, diet, allergies, drug history, and possible drug interactions. ■ Evaluate laboratory blood findings: CBC, electrolytes, lipid panel, renal and liver function studies, glucose and pregnancy testing for women of childbearing age. ■ Acquire the results of a complete physical examination, including vital signs, height, and weight.	■ *Deficient Knowledge* related to a need for an altered lifestyle and lack of information about drug therapy ■ *Noncompliance* related to difficulty adhering to dietary and drug regimen ■ *Chronic Pain* related to drug-induced myopathy ■ *Ineffective Self-health Maintenance* related to insufficient knowledge of seriousness of disease and drug therapy regimen

PLANNING: PATIENT GOALS AND EXPECTED OUTCOMES

The patient will:
■ Experience therapeutic effects (lowered cholesterol and triglyceride levels).
■ Be free from or experience minimal adverse effects from drug therapy.
■ Verbalize an understanding of the drug's use, adverse effects, and required precautions.

IMPLEMENTATION

Interventions and (Rationales)	Patient Education/Discharge Planning
■ Monitor blood cholesterol and triglyceride levels at intervals during therapy. (Monitoring these levels will help to determine effectiveness of therapy.)	■ Advise the patient of the importance of keeping appointments for laboratory testing.
■ Monitor patient compliance with dietary regimen. (Maintenance of controlled saturated fat diet is essential to the effectiveness of medications.)	■ Ensure that patient/family understand that drug therapy is used in addition to diet therapy. Provide the patient with information needed to maintain a low-saturated fat, low-cholesterol diet.
■ Monitor the patient for alcohol abuse. (Excessive alcohol intake may result in liver damage and interfere with drug effectiveness.)	■ Instruct the patient to avoid or limit alcohol use.
■ Monitor the patient for adverse effects of drug therapy, e.g. GI effects, muscle soreness or joint pain unrelated to usual activity. (May indicate muscle inflammation related to medication.)	■ Instruct the patient to report symptoms of GI effects such as cramping and diarrhea; unexplained muscle tenderness and pain, tingling of extremities, or effects that hinder normal activities of daily living to the healthcare provider.
■ If complaints of increasing muscle soreness, monitor CPK level. (Elevated CPK may be indicative of myopathy.)	■ Instruct patient to see healthcare provider immediately if having increased muscle pain and weakness.
■ Obtain the patient's smoking history. (Smoking increases risk of cardiovascular disease and may decrease HDL levels.)	■ Encourage smoking cessation. Provide information about medications and smoking cessation programs.
■ Monitor patient's pregnancy status. (Statins are classified as pregnancy category X.)	■ Advise the patient of childbearing age of the dangers of using statins while pregnant; to report any prospects of pregnancy or possible side effects/symptoms.
■ Administer medication correctly and evaluate the patient's knowledge of proper administration. (Some medications interact with statins and grapefruit juice inhibits metabolism.)	Instruct the patient: ■ Not to take medication with grapefruit juice. ■ To notify healthcare practitioner when taking oral contraceptives, erythromycin and some cardiac medication such as digoxin, diltiazem, and verapamil.

EVALUATION OF OUTCOME CRITERIA

Evaluate the effectiveness of drug therapy by confirming that patient goals and expected outcomes have been met (see "Planning"). *See Table 16.2 for a list of drugs to which these nursing actions apply.*

Bile acid binding drugs can reduce LDL levels by increasing cholesterol excretion.

CORE CONCEPT **16.5**

Prior to the discovery of the statins, the primary means of lowering blood cholesterol was through use of bile acid binding drugs. **Bile acids**, contain a high concentration of cholesterol and are secreted by the liver to aid in the digestion of fats in the small intestine. Once bound in the intestine, the cholesterol in the bile acids is eliminated in the feces. Although they are no longer considered first-line drugs for dyslipidemias, they are sometimes combined with statins for patients who are unable to achieve sufficient response from the statins alone. Doses of these drugs are listed in Table 16.2. Bile acid binding drugs are also called bile acid resins and bile acid sequestrants. The prototype drug for this drug class is cholestyramine (Questran).

Although effective at producing a 20% decrease in LDL-cholesterol levels, the bile acid binding drugs tend to cause more frequent adverse effects than do the statins. Taken orally, bile acid binding drugs are not absorbed into the circulation; therefore, their adverse effects are limited to the GI tract. A high percentage of patients, however, experience constipation, bloating, nausea, or indigestion. Colesevelam (Welchol) is a newer drug in this class that is reported to have fewer adverse effects than the older drugs. Also of concern is that bile acid binding drugs can prevent the absorption of other medications and vitamins that may be taken at the same time. This can be avoided by teaching the patient to take these drugs one hour before, or four hours after, other medications.

| CORE CONCEPT 16.6 | **Niacin can reduce triglyceride and LDL-cholesterol levels.** |

Niacin, also called nicotinic acid, is a water-soluble B-complex vitamin whose primary action is to decrease VLDL levels. When VLDL is diminished, the patient also experiences a reduction in LDL-cholesterol and triglyceride levels. It also has the desirable effects of reducing triglycerides and increasing HDL levels. Thus, niacin is unique in that it can improve multiple types of dyslipidemias. As with other lipid-lowering drugs, maximum therapeutic effects may take a month or longer to achieve.

Its ability to lower lipid levels is unrelated to its role as a B-vitamin; very high doses are needed to achieve a lipid-lowering effect. For decreasing cholesterol, the usual dose is 2 to 3 g per day. When taken as a vitamin, the dose is only 25 mg per day.

Although effective at reducing LDL cholesterol by 20%, niacin produces more adverse effects than the statins. Flushing and hot flashes occur in almost every patient, although taking one aspirin tablet 30 minutes prior to niacin administration can reduce flushing in many patients. A variety of uncomfortable intestinal effects such as nausea, excess gas, and diarrhea are commonly reported. Although uncommon, more serious adverse effects such as liver toxicity and gout are possible. Because of these adverse effects, niacin is most often used in lower doses in combination with a statin or bile acid binding drug because the beneficial effects of these drugs are additive. Several fixed-dose combination drugs are available, including Advicor (niacin with lovastatin) and Simcor (niacin with simvastatin). Extended-release niacin, which is taken once daily, causes less flushing and GI adverse effects.

As a vitamin, niacin is available without a prescription. However, patients should be instructed not to attempt self-medication with this drug. One form of niacin, available over the counter as a vitamin supplement called *nicotinamide*, has no lipid-lowering effects. Patients should be informed that if niacin is used to lower cholesterol, it should be done under medical supervision.

| **Concept Review** | **16.2** |

■ How does the mechanism of the statins differ from that of niacin?

CAM THERAPY

Coenzyme Q10 for Heart Disease

Coenzyme Q10 (CoQ10) is a vitamin-like substance found in most animal cells. It is an essential component in the cell's mitochondria, which produce energy or adenosine triphosphate (ATP). Because the heart requires high levels of ATP, a sufficient level of CoQ10 is essential to that organ. Foods richest in this substance are pork, sardines, beef heart, salmon, broccoli, spinach, and nuts. Older adults appear to have an increased need for CoQ10.

Reports of the benefits of CoQ10 for treating heart disease began to emerge in the mid-1960s. Subsequent reports have claimed that CoQ10 may be beneficial in angina pectoris, dysrhythmias, periodontal disease, immune disorders, neurologic disease, obesity, diabetes mellitus, and certain cancers. Considerable research has been conducted on this antioxidant.

The statins decrease CoQ10 levels. Indeed, many of the adverse effects of statins may be due to the decrease in CoQ10 levels, including muscle weakness and rhabdomyolysis. Supplementation with CoQ10 may diminish myopathy symptoms. In addition, there is scientific evidence to suggest that CoQ10 causes a small decrease in blood pressure in patients with hypertension. Evidence to support the use of CoQ10 in treating patients with heart disease, neurologic disorders, or cancer is weak. As for most dietary supplements, controlled research studies are often lacking and give conflicting results.

Fibric acid drugs lower triglyceride levels, but have little effect on LDLs.

Once commonly prescribed to reduce lipid levels, the fibric acid drugs, or fibrates, have been largely re-placed by the statins for most indications. They are sometimes used in combination with the statins. In ad-dition they remain preferred drugs for treating extremely high triglyceride levels. Doses of the fibrates are listed in Table 16.2.

The first fibric acid drug, clofibrate (Atromid-S), was widely prescribed until studies demonstrated it did not reduce mortality from cardiovascular disease. Although clofibrate is no longer available in the United States, two other fibrates, fenofibrate (Antara, Lofibra Tricor, others), and gemfibrozil (Lopid), are sometimes prescribed for patients who have excessive triglyceride and VLDL levels. Fibrates are the most effective drugs for reducing VLDLs and blood triglyceride levels. Elevation of "good" HDL cholesterol is another effect of fibrate therapy. Unfortunately, these drugs have little effect on LDL-cholesterol levels.

Fibrates cause few serious adverse effects. Flushing, dizziness, fatigue, rashes, and GI complaints are the most common adverse effects. Like the statins, some patients experience muscle pain or weakness; therefore, patients receiving concurrent therapy with both statins and fibrates should be monitored carefully. The mechanisms of action of the fibrates and other drugs for dyslipidemias are shown in Figure 16.3 ■. Dosages of these drugs are listed in Table 16.2.

FIGURE 16.3

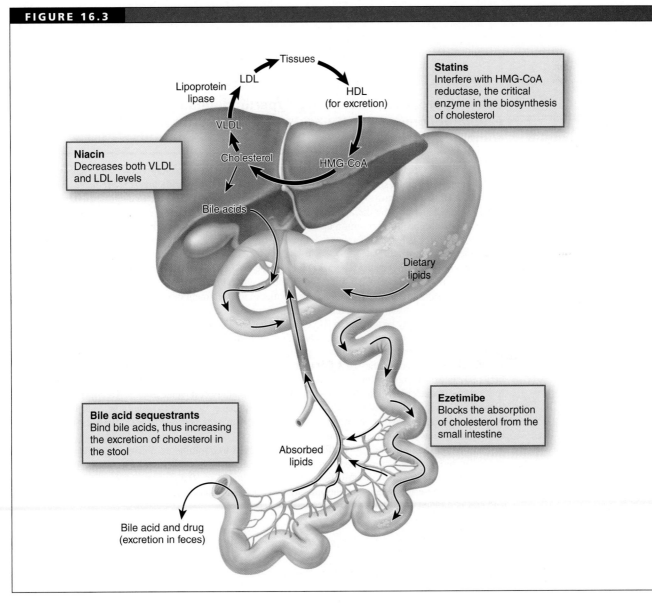

Mechanisms of action of lipid-lowering drugs.

Drug Prototype: ℗ *Gemfibrozil (Lopid)*

Therapeutic Class: Antihyperlipidemic drug   **Pharmacologic Class: Fibric acid drug**

Actions and Uses: Gemfibrozil can cause up to a 50% reduction in VLDL with a moderate increase in HDL. Because it is less effective than the statins, it is not a drug of first choice for reducing LDL-cholesterol levels. However, it is useful for patients with high triglyceride levels who have not responded favorably to diet modification and those at risk for pancreatitis.

Adverse Effects and Interactions: The most common adverse effects of gemfibrozil are related to the GI system: diarrhea, nausea, and abdominal cramping. The drug produces few serious adverse effects, but it may increase the likelihood of gallstones and occasionally affect liver function.

Using gemfibrozil with oral anticoagulants may increase the risk of bleeding. Concurrent use with statins should be avoided because this increases the risk of myopathy and rhabdomyolysis.

CORE CONCEPT 16.8

Other approaches to treating hyperlipidemia include ezetimibe, omega-3 fatty acids, and fixed-dose combination therapy.

A newer drug for treating high blood cholesterol levels is ezetimibe (Zetia). Ezetimibe blocks the absorption of cholesterol in the small intestine. LDL-cholesterol and triglyceride levels are reduced, with a slight increase in HDL cholesterol. When used as monotherapy, it can decrease blood cholesterol levels by about 20%. Adding a statin to the therapeutic regimen reduces LDL by an additional 15% to 20%. Adverse effects from ezetimibe are uncommon and include abdominal pain, back pain, diarrhea, and arthralgia. The dose for ezetimibe is listed in Table 16.2. In 2013, the FDA approved Liptruzet, a combination containing ezetimibe and atorvastatin.

Omega-3-acid ethyl esters (Lovaza) and icosapent (Vascepa) are two prescription forms of omega-3 fatty acids found in fish oil. Fish oil has long been a natural therapy for the treatment of high blood lipid levels. Both drugs are approved as an adjunct to diet in the treatment of severe hypertriglyceridemia. Most adverse effects are minor and include burping, fishy taste, and dyspepsia (indigestion). Those patients allergic to seafood may be allergic to fish oil. High doses of omega-3 fatty acids may prolong clotting time and should be used with caution in patients taking anticoagulants.

A recent trend in the treatment of hyperlipidemia is to combine drugs from two different classes in a single tablet. Vytorin combines 10 mg of ezetimibe with 10, 20, 40, or 80 mg of simvastatin. Advicor combines 20 mg of lovastatin with 500, 750, or 1000 mg of niacin. These fixed-dose combinations allow for lower doses of each individual drug, potentially resulting in fewer adverse effects. Taking a single tablet is easier for the patient to remember, which increases compliance. Because the combination drugs attack cholesterol levels using two distinct mechanisms of action, it may be possible to get a synergistic, or additive, effect of the drugs on blood cholesterol levels.

A second trend in treating cardiovascular disease is to combine an antihypertensive drug with an antihyperlipidemic medication. For example, Caduet combines the antihypertensive amlodipine with atorvastatin. Several fixed-dose combinations are available with 5 to 10 mg of amlodipine and 10 to 80 mg of atorvastatin. These combination agents are targeted for the millions of patients who have both hypertension and elevated blood cholesterol levels.

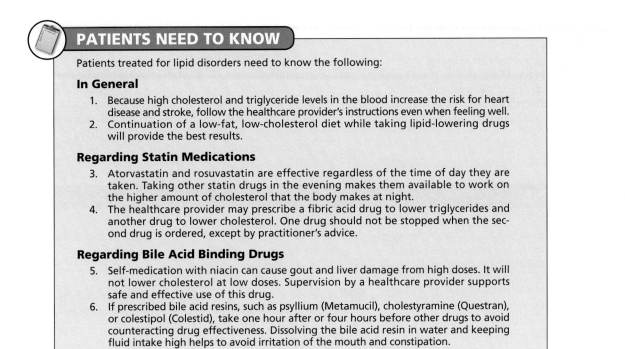

PATIENTS NEED TO KNOW

Patients treated for lipid disorders need to know the following:

In General

1. Because high cholesterol and triglyceride levels in the blood increase the risk for heart disease and stroke, follow the healthcare provider's instructions even when feeling well.
2. Continuation of a low-fat, low-cholesterol diet while taking lipid-lowering drugs will provide the best results.

Regarding Statin Medications

3. Atorvastatin and rosuvastatin are effective regardless of the time of day they are taken. Taking other statin drugs in the evening makes them available to work on the higher amount of cholesterol that the body makes at night.
4. The healthcare provider may prescribe a fibric acid drug to lower triglycerides and another drug to lower cholesterol. One drug should not be stopped when the second drug is ordered, except by practitioner's advice.

Regarding Bile Acid Binding Drugs

5. Self-medication with niacin can cause gout and liver damage from high doses. It will not lower cholesterol at low doses. Supervision by a healthcare provider supports safe and effective use of this drug.
6. If prescribed bile acid resins, such as psyllium (Metamucil), cholestyramine (Questran), or colestipol (Colestid), take one hour after or four hours before other drugs to avoid counteracting drug effectiveness. Dissolving the bile acid resin in water and keeping fluid intake high helps to avoid irritation of the mouth and constipation.

CHAPTER REVIEW

CORE CONCEPTS SUMMARY

16.1   Lipids serve essential roles in the body, but too much dietary fat can lead to disease

Lipids, or fats, have important roles in human physiology. Excessive dietary triglyceride or cholesterol can cause dyslipidemias, an abnormal amount of lipid in the blood. Dyslipidemias are major risk factors for cardiovascular disease.

16.2   Lipoproteins transport lipids through the blood for utilization by tissues, storage in adipose tissue, or excretion by the liver.

Lipids are packaged for travel through the blood in lipoprotein complexes. High VLDL and LDL are associated with an increased incidence of cardiovascular disease, whereas HDL provides a protective effect.

16.3   Elevated lipid levels can often be prevented or controlled through therapeutic lifestyle changes.

Before starting pharmacotherapy for hyperlipidemia, patients are usually advised to manage the condition through lifestyle changes, such as restriction of dietary saturated fats and cholesterol, increased exercise, and smoking cessation.

16.4   Statins are preferred drugs for reducing blood lipid levels.

Drugs in the statin class inhibit HMG-CoA reductase, a critical enzyme in the biosynthesis of cholesterol. They are safe and effective at lowering LDL cholesterol and are the most widely prescribed class of drugs for hyperlipidemias.

16.5   Bile acid binding drugs can reduce LDL levels by increasing cholesterol excretion.

The bile acid binding drugs are effective at lowering LDL cholesterol, although they produce more adverse effects than the statins. They should be taken separately from other medications because they can interfere with drug absorption.

16.6   Niacin can reduce triglyceride and LDL-cholesterol levels.

Niacin, or nicotinic acid, can be effective at lowering LDL cholesterol and triglycerides when given in large amounts. It is not usually a first-choice drug but is sometimes combined in smaller doses with other lipid-lowering drugs.

16.7 Fibric acid drugs lower triglyceride levels, but have little effect on LDLs.

Fibric acids such as gemfibrozil are effective at lowering triglycerides but less effective than the statins at lowering blood lipids. Their use is limited because of frequent adverse effects. However, they are sometimes combined with other drugs to produce an additive effect.

16.8 Other approaches to treating hyperlipidemia include ezetimibe, omega-3 fatty acids, and fixed-dose combination therapy.

Ezetimibe lowers LDL levels by blocking the absorption of cholesterol from the intestine. Omega-3 fatty acids are available by prescription to lower LDL cholesterol. Combination drugs such as Advicor and Vytorin attack high blood cholesterol levels using two different mechanisms.

REVIEW QUESTIONS

The following questions are written in NCLEX-PN® style. Answer these questions to assess your knowledge of the chapter material, and go back and review any material that is not clear to you.

1. This lipoprotein is responsible for transporting cholesterol from the blood to the liver.
1. LDL
2. VLDL
3. HDL
4. Triglycerides

2. The nurse understands that which of the following HMG-CoA reductase inhibitors should be taken with meals?
1. Atorvastatin (Lipitor)
2. Simvastatin (Zocor)
3. Lovastatin (Mevacor)
4. Rosuvastatin (Crestor)

3. The nurse is instructing a patient on how to take statin drugs. The patient is informed that statin drugs are most effective when taken:
1. In the morning
2. In the evening
3. With other medications
4. On an empty stomach

4. The healthcare practitioner orders lovastatin (Mevacor) 20 mg at bedtime. The supply is 10 mg tablets. How many tablets will the nurse give?
1. 1 tablet
2. 1½ tablets
3. 2 tablets
4. 2½ tablets

5. Which of the following patient complaint would the nurse consider to be an adverse reaction to a bile acid resin?
1. Constipation
2. Headache
3. Anxiety
4. Double vision

6. When administering colestipol (Colestid), the nurse:
1. Administers the drug with large amounts of fluid to prevent GI upset
2. Administers the drug 30 minutes prior to meals
3. Administers the drug at least one hour before or four hours after meals
4. Administers the drug at bedtime

7. A patient is interested in taking niacin to help reduce his or her cholesterol. When he or she asks the nurse about possible adverse effects, the nurse informs him or her that niacin can cause: (Select all that apply.)
1. Flushing
2. Excess gas
3. Constipation
4. Diarrhea

8. On assessment, the patient is found to have a total cholesterol level of 326 mg/dL and prehypertension. When assisting the RN in the development of a care plan, the LPN or LVN recognizes that the best treatment for this patient would be a low-fat diet and:
1. An exercise program only
2. Cholesterol-lowering medication
3. Over-the-counter supplements
4. An antihypertensive

9. After a review of a patient's chart, the nurse notices that the patient has developed gallstones and elevated liver enzymes. Which of the following cholesterol-lowering medications could cause this?
1. Cholestyramine (Questran)
2. Niacin (Nicotinic acid)
3. Gemfibrozil (Lopid)
4. Lovastatin (Mevacor)

10. A patient hears that taking fish oil is good for helping to bring down triglyceride levels. He asks the nurse about information concerning this form of treatment. The nurse would explain that: (Select all that apply.)
1. A minor adverse effect of this drug is dyspepsia.
2. Some people who are allergic to seafood may be allergic to fish oil.
3. Omega-3 fatty acids are the beneficial component found in fish oil.
4. No matter what the dose, omega-3-fatty acids may decrease the ability of the blood to clot.

CASE STUDY QUESTIONS

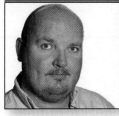

Remember Mr. Long, the patient introduced at the beginning of the chapter? Now read the remainder of the case study. Based on the information you have learned in this chapter, answer the questions that follow.

Mr. Edward Long is a 50-year-old office worker who has gained 50 pounds over the past five years. His blood pressure has consistently been high, but he has declined to take medication for the condition. His LDL-cholesterol level has been above 210 mg/dL on his last three office visits. He claims to have no chronic diseases and is at the office seeking assistance concerning his weight gain.

1. The physician ordered cholestyramine for Mr. Long. As the nurse, you inform Mr. Long that this drug acts by:

1. Inhibiting enzymes that make cholesterol.
2. Binding bile acids in the intestine, which increases cholesterol excretion.
3. Increasing the breakdown of cholesterol in the liver.
4. Making more bile acids, which bind cholesterol.

2. After two months of therapy, the physician switched the prescription to lovastatin (Mevacor). Mr. Long asks what makes this drug different from the other one he was on. You reply that this drug acts by:

1. Inhibiting enzymes that make cholesterol.
2. Binding bile acids in the intestine, which increase cholesterol excretion.
3. Increasing the breakdown of cholesterol in the liver.
4. Making more bile acids, which bind cholesterol.

3. After several weeks of lovastatin therapy, Mr. Long returns to the office for follow-up. What question should you ask to determine if he may be suffering from a very serious adverse effect of the statins?

1. "Do you have bloody diarrhea more than once a week?"
2. "Have you felt confused, lethargic, or drowsy since starting the drug?"
3. "Have you experienced excessive muscle weakness or pain?"
4. "Have you experienced acid indigestion or nausea?"

4. You are checking the results of Mr. Long's lab work. Which of the following therapeutic results would you expect to see now that he has been taking lovastatin?

1. Higher LDL level
2. Higher VLDL level
3. Lower HDL level
4. Higher HDL level

NOTE: Answers to the Review and Case Study Questions appear in Appendix B. The complete rationales and answers are located on the textbook's website.

Pearson Nursing Student Resources Find additional review materials at **nursing.pearsonhighered.com**.

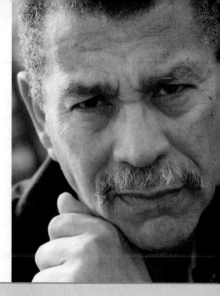

C
H
A
P
T
E
R

"I did everything the nurse told me to do. Why is my blood pressure so high when I've been taking all my medications?"

Mr. Joseph Grant

17 Diuretics and Drugs for Electrolyte and Acid–Base Disorders

CORE CONCEPTS

17.1 The kidneys regulate fluid volume, electrolytes, acids, and bases.

17.2 The composition of filtrate changes dramatically as a result of the processes of reabsorption and secretion.

17.3 Renal failure significantly impacts pharmacotherapy.

17.4 Diuretics are used to treat hypertension, heart failure, and fluid retention disorders.

17.5 The most effective diuretics are those that affect the loop of Henle.

17.6 The thiazides are the most widely prescribed class of diuretics.

17.7 Although less effective than the loop diuretics, potassium-sparing diuretics may help prevent hypokalemia.

17.8 Several less commonly prescribed diuretics have specific indications.

17.9 Electrolytes are charged substances that play important roles in maintaining homeostasis.

17.10 Acidic and basic drugs can be administered to correct pH imbalances.

DRUG SNAPSHOT

The following drugs are discussed in this chapter:

DRUG CLASSES	DRUG PROTOTYPES
Loop (high-ceiling) diuretics	Pr furosemide (Lasix) *254*
Thiazide diuretics	Pr hydrochlorothiazide (Microzide) *255*
Potassium-sparing diuretics	Pr spironolactone (Aldactone) *256*

DRUG CLASSES	DRUG PROTOTYPES
Miscellaneous diuretics	
Electrolytes	Pr potassium chloride (KCl) *260*
Acid–base agents	Pr sodium bicarbonate ($NaHCO_3$) *261*

LEARNING OUTCOMES

After reading this chapter, the student should be able to:

1. Explain the role of the kidneys in maintaining fluid, electrolyte, and acid–base balance.

2. Compare and contrast the loop, thiazide, and potassium-sparing diuretics.

3. Explain the pharmacotherapy of sodium and potassium imbalances.

4. Identify common causes of alkalosis and acidosis and the drugs used to treat these conditions.

5. Categorize drugs used in the treatment of urinary system electrolyte and acid–base disorders based on their classifications and mechanisms of action.

6. For each of the classes in the Drug Snapshot, identify representative drugs and explain their mechanisms of drug action, primary actions, and important adverse effects.

KEY TERMS

acidosis (ah-sid-OH-sis) *260*
aldosterone (al-DOH-stair-own) *256*
alkalosis (al-kah-LOH-sis) *260*
carbonic anhydrase (kar-BON-ik an-HY-drase) *256*
diuretic (dye-your-ET-ik) *252*
electrolytes (ee-LEK-troh-lites) *258*
end-stage renal disease (ESRD) *251*

erythropoietin (ee-rith-ro-po-EE-tin) *252*
filtrate (FIL-trate) *250*
hyperkalemia (heye-purr-kah-LEE-mee-ah) *256*
hypernatremia (heye-purr-nuh-TREE-mee-ah) *259*
hypokalemia (heye-poh-kah-LEE-mee-uh) *252*

hyponatremia (hy-po-nay-TREE-mee-uh) *259*
nephrons (NEF-ron) *249*
pH *260*
reabsorption *250*
renal failure *251*
secretion *251*

The volume and composition of fluids in the body must be maintained within narrow limits. Excess fluid volume can lead to hypertension or heart failure, whereas depletion may result in dehydration or shock. Body fluids must also contain specific amounts of essential ions or electrolytes and be maintained at specific pH values. The kidneys serve a remarkable role in keeping the volume and composition of body fluids within normal limits. This chapter examines diuretics and drugs used to reverse electrolyte and acid–base imbalances.

The kidneys regulate fluid volume, electrolytes, acids, and bases.

CORE CONCEPT 17.1

When most people think of the kidneys, they think of excretion. Although this is certainly one of their roles, the kidneys have many other essential functions. The kidneys are the primary organs for regulating fluid volume, electrolyte composition, and the acid–base balance of body fluids. They also secrete the enzyme renin, which helps to regulate blood pressure (see Chapter 18), and the hormone erythropoietin, which stimulates red blood cell production. In addition, the kidneys are responsible for the production of calcitriol, the active form of vitamin D, which helps maintain bone homeostasis (see Chapter 35). It is not surprising that overall wellness is strongly dependent on proper functioning of the kidneys.

The urinary system consists of two kidneys, two ureters, a urinary bladder, and a urethra. These structures are shown in Figure 17.1 ■. Each kidney contains more than 2 million **nephrons**, the functional units

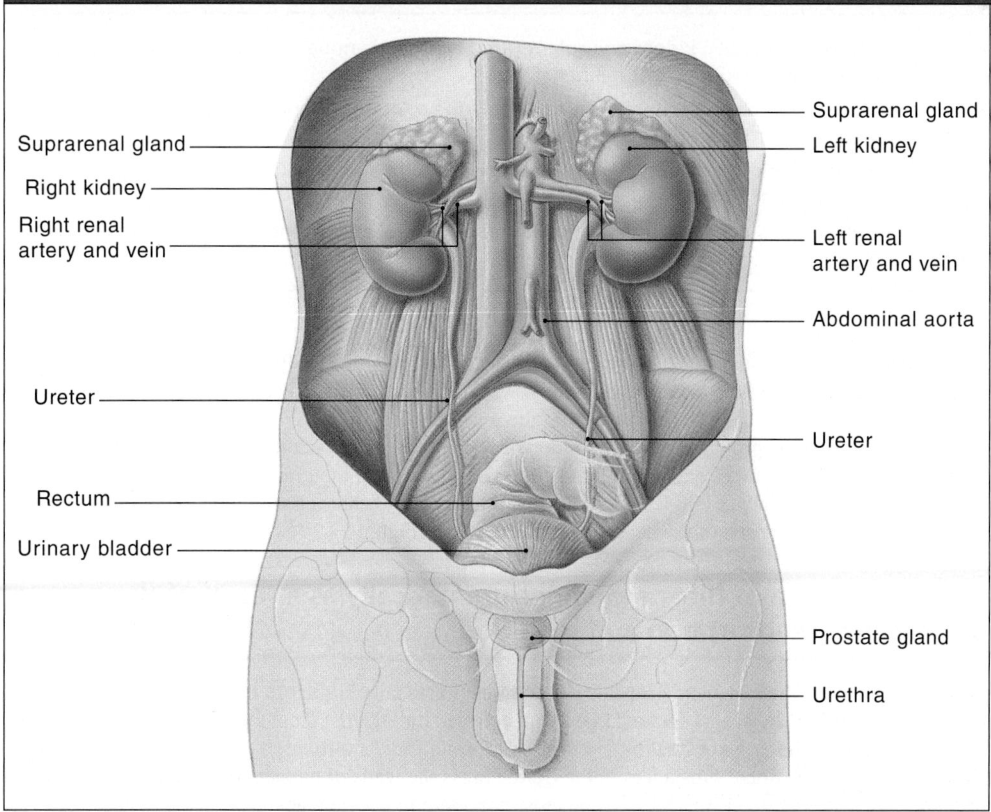

FIGURE 17.1

The urinary system.

Suprarenal gland
Right kidney
Right renal artery and vein
Ureter
Rectum
Urinary bladder

Suprarenal gland
Left kidney
Left renal artery and vein
Abdominal aorta
Ureter
Prostate gland
Urethra

FIGURE 17.2

The nephron.

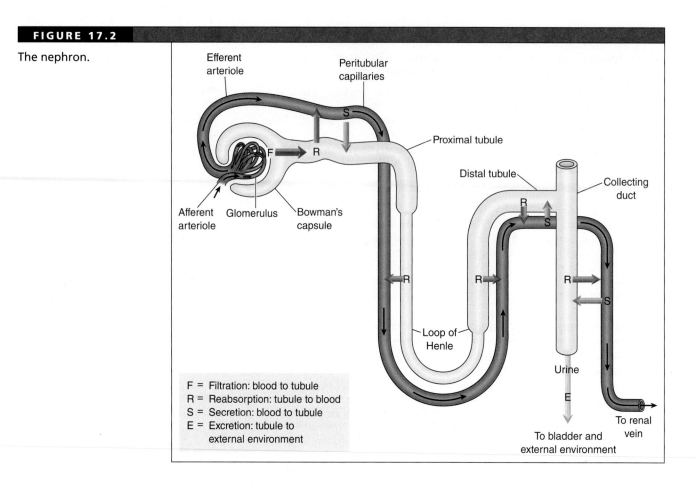

F = Filtration: blood to tubule
R = Reabsorption: tubule to blood
S = Secretion: blood to tubule
E = Excretion: tubule to
      external environment

Fast Facts Renal Disorders

- Although more than 16,000 kidney transplants are performed annually, more than 80,000 people are on a waiting list for kidney transplants.
- One out of every 750 people is born with a single kidney. A single kidney is larger and more vulnerable to injury from heavy contact sports.
- About 526,000 Americans suffer from chronic kidney failure, and 87,000 die annually from causes related to the disease.
- Type 2 diabetes is the leading cause of chronic kidney failure, accounting for 30–40% of all new cases each year.

of the kidney. As blood enters a nephron, it is filtered through a porous capillary known as the glomerulus. Once in the nephron, the fluid is called **filtrate**. Water and other small molecules readily pass through and enter the Bowman's capsule, the first section of the renal tubule. After leaving Bowman's capsule the filtrate travels through the proximal tubule, the loop of Henle, and, subsequently, the distal tubule. Nephrons empty their filtrate into tubes called common collecting ducts, and then into larger and larger collecting structures inside the kidney. Fluid leaving the collecting ducts and entering subsequent portions of the kidney is called urine. The parts of the nephron are illustrated in Figure 17.2 ■.

CORE CONCEPT 17.2

The composition of filtrate changes dramatically as a result of the processes of reabsorption and secretion.

When filtrate enters the Bowman's capsule, its composition is very similar to that of plasma. Plasma proteins such as albumin, however, are too large to have passed through the glomerulus and will not be present in the filtrate or in the urine of healthy patients. As filtrate travels through the nephron, its composition changes dramatically. Some substances in the filtrate cross the walls of the nephron to reenter the blood, a process known as **reabsorption**. Water is the most important molecule reabsorbed in the tubule. For every

180 liters (47 gallons) of water entering the filtrate each day, 178.5 liters (45.5 gallons) are reabsorbed, leaving only 1.5 liters to be excreted in the urine. Glucose, amino acids, and essential ions such as sodium, chloride, calcium, and bicarbonate are also reabsorbed.

Certain ions and molecules too large to pass through the glomerulus can still enter the urine by crossing from the blood to the filtrate through a process known as tubular **secretion**. Potassium, phosphate, hydrogen, and ammonium ions enter the filtrate through secretion. Examples of drugs secreted in the proximal tubule include penicillin G, ampicillin, nonsteroidal anti-inflammatory drugs (NSAIDs), furosemide, epinephrine, and trimethoprim.

Reabsorption and secretion are critical to the pharmacokinetics of many drugs. Some drugs are reabsorbed, whereas others are secreted into the filtrate. For example, approximately 90% of a dose of penicillin G enters the urine through secretion. When the kidney is damaged, reabsorption and secretion mechanisms are impaired and serum drug levels may be dramatically affected. The processes of reabsorption and secretion are depicted in Figure 17.2.

Concept Review   17.1

■ How does the composition of filtrate differ from that of blood?

Renal failure significantly impacts pharmacotherapy.

CORE CONCEPT 17.3

Renal failure is a decrease in the kidneys' ability to maintain electrolyte and fluid balance and to excrete waste products. If renal excretion is impaired, drugs will accumulate to high concentrations in the blood and tissues, resulting in toxicity. Because the kidneys excrete most drugs, the majority of medications will require a significant dosage reduction in patients with moderate to severe renal failure. *The importance of this cannot be overemphasized: Administering the "average" dose to a patient in severe renal failure can kill a patient.*

The healthcare provider has a critical role in preventing serious adverse drug effects in patients with renal impairment. Monitoring kidney function tests, such as urinalysis and serum creatinine helps to identify impending renal failure. Notifying the prescriber at the first indication of renal failure allows drug dosages to be lowered, thereby preventing toxicity. Because healthcare providers frequently encounter patients with renal failure, special note should be taken of nephrotoxic drugs when learning pharmacology. Once a diagnosis of renal impairment is established, all nephrotoxic medications should be either discontinued or used with extreme caution.

Renal failure is classified as acute or chronic, depending on its onset. Acute renal failure requires immediate treatment because accumulation of waste products, such as urea and creatinine can result in death if untreated. The cause of acute renal failure must be quickly identified and corrected. The most common cause of acute renal failure is lack of sufficient blood flow through the kidneys due to underlying conditions such as heart failure, dysrhythmias, hemorrhage, or dehydration.

Chronic renal failure occurs over a period of months or years. Over half of patients with chronic renal failure have a medical history of longstanding hypertension (HTN) or diabetes mellitus. Because of its long, gradual development and nonspecific symptoms, chronic renal failure may go undiagnosed for many years until the impairment becomes irreversible. When the kidneys are no longer able to function at a level necessary for day-to-day living, the patient has **end-stage renal disease (ESRD)** and dialysis and kidney transplantation become treatment alternatives.

CAM THERAPY

Cranberry for Urinary System Health

Nearly everyone is familiar with the bright red cranberries that are eaten during holiday times. Native Americans used the colorful, ripe berries to treat wounds and to cure anorexia and for other digestive complaints. In the 1900s, it was noted that the acidity of the urine increases after eating cranberries; thus began the belief that cranberry juice is a natural cure for urinary tract infections.

Cranberry juice or berries contain a significant amount of vitamin C and other antioxidants that can promote health. They contain a substance that can prevent bacteria from sticking on the walls of the bladder. Research suggests that cranberries can prevent symptomatic urinary tract infections in some patients, especially in women who have recurrent infections.

Cranberry is a safe supplement, although large amounts may cause GI upset and diarrhea. The juice should be 100% cranberry and not "cocktail" juice because that contains sugar, which enhances bacteria growth and may be contraindicated in patients with diabetes. Some individuals may prefer to take cranberry capsules, which are available at most pharmacies.

Pharmacotherapy of renal impairment includes administering diuretics, which can increase urine output. In addition, cardiovascular drugs are commonly administered to treat underlying HTN or heart failure. Dietary management, such as protein restriction and reduction of sodium, potassium, phosphorus, and magnesium intake, is often necessary to prevent worsening of renal impairment.

Many patients with chronic renal failure will also have a deficiency of **erythropoietin**, a hormone secreted by the kidney. Erythropoietin serves as a primary signal to increase red blood cell production in the bone marrow. A synthetic form of erythropoietin, epoetin alfa (Epogen, Procrit) is effective in treating several disorders caused by a deficiency in red blood cells. Epoetin is sometimes given to patients undergoing cancer chemotherapy to counteract the anemia caused by antineoplastic drugs (see Chapter 28). It is occasionally prescribed for patients prior to blood transfusions or surgery and to treat anemia in HIV-infected patients. Epoetin alfa is usually administered three times per week until an increase in the number of red blood cells is achieved.

CORE CONCEPT 17.4
Diuretics are used to treat hypertension, heart failure, and fluid retention disorders

dia = *thoroughly*
uretic = *to urinate*

A **diuretic** is a drug that increases urine output. The goal of most diuretic therapy is to reverse abnormal fluid retention by the body. Excretion of excess fluid in the body is particularly desirable in the following conditions:

- Hypertension
- Heart failure
- Kidney failure
- Pulmonary edema
- Liver failure or cirrhosis

The most common mechanism by which diuretics act is by blocking sodium ion (Na^+) reabsorption in the nephron, thus sending more Na^+ to the urine. Chloride ion (Cl^-) follows Na^+. Because water molecules travel with sodium, blocking the reabsorption of Na^+ will increase the volume of urination, or diuresis. Some drugs, such as furosemide (Lasix), act by preventing the reabsorption of Na^+ in the loop of Henle, and thus they are called loop diuretics. Because of the abundance of Na^+ in the loop of Henle, furosemide is capable of producing large increases in urine output. Other drugs, such as the thiazides, act on the distal tubule. Because most Na^+ has already been reabsorbed from the filtrate by the time it reaches this point in the nephron, the thiazides produce less diuresis than does furosemide. The sites at which the various diuretics act are shown in Figure 17.3 ■.

CORE CONCEPT 17.5
The most effective diuretics are those that affect the loop of Henle.

The most effective diuretics are the loop or high-ceiling diuretics. Drugs in this class act by blocking the reabsorption of Na^+ and Cl^- in the loop of Henle. When given by IV, they have the ability to cause large amounts of fluid to be excreted by the kidney in a very short time. Loop diuretics are used to reduce the fluid accumulation associated with heart failure, hepatic cirrhosis, or chronic renal failure. Furosemide (Lasix) and torsemide (Demadex) are also approved for HTN.

Furosemide is the most frequently prescribed loop diuretic. Unlike the thiazide diuretics, furosemide is able to increase urine output even when blood flow to the kidneys is diminished. Torsemide (Demadex) has a longer half-life than furosemide, which offers the advantage of once-a-day dosing. Bumetanide (Bumex) is 40 times more potent than furosemide but has a shorter duration of action.

de = *not/without*
hydration = *water*

hypo = *low or below normal*
kal = *potassium*
emia = *blood condition*

The rapid excretion of large amounts of water caused by loop diuretics may produce adverse effects such as dehydration and electrolyte imbalances. Signs of dehydration include thirst, dry mouth, weight loss, and headache. Hypotension, dizziness, and even fainting can result from the rapid fluid loss. When urine flow increases, potassium ion is lost from the body. Potassium depletion, or **hypokalemia**, may cause dysrhythmias, and thus potassium supplements may be indicated during loop diuretic therapy. Potassium loss is of particular concern to patients who are also taking digoxin (Lanoxin). Although rare, impairment of hearing or balance (ototoxicity) is possible. Because of the potential for serious adverse effects, the loop diuretics are normally reserved for patients with moderate to severe fluid retention, or

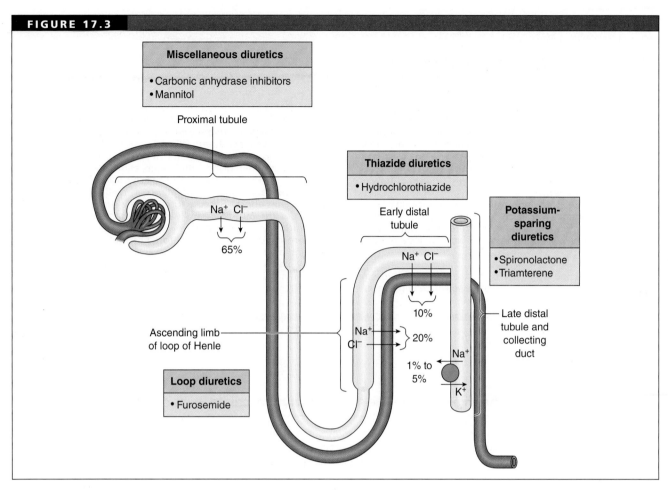

FIGURE 17.3

Sites of action of diuretics.

when other diuretics have failed to achieve therapeutic goals. Information on the loop diuretics is given in Table 17.1 ◆.

Concept Review 17.2

■ Why are drugs that block Na⁺ reabsorption at the loop of Henle more effective than those that act on the distal tubule?

TABLE 17.1 Loop Diuretics		
Drug	**Route and Adult Dose**	**Remarks**
bumetanide (Bumex)	PO; 0.5–2 mg daily (max: 10 mg/day)	IV form available; this drug is 40 times more potent than furosemide
ethacrynic acid (Edecrin)	PO; 50–100 mg once or twice per day (max: 400 mg/day)	IV form available; exhibits the most ototoxicity of the drugs in this class
Pr furosemide (Lasix)	PO; 20–80 mg daily (max: 600 mg/day) IV/IM; 20–40 mg in one or more divided doses (max: 600 mg/day)	IV and IM forms available
torsemide (Demadex)	PO; 4–20 mg daily (max: 200 mg/day)	IV form available; exhibits the lowest risk of ototoxicity of the drugs in this class

Drug Prototype ⓟ *Furosemide (Lasix)*

Therapeutic Class: Drug for heart failure (HF), edema, and HTN   **Pharmacologic Class: Diuretic (loop type)**

Actions and Uses: Furosemide is used for conditions in which the patient is retaining fluid. In the treatment of acute HF furosemide has the ability to remove large amounts of edema fluid from the patient in a short time. Patients often receive quick relief from their distressing symptoms. Compared to other diuretics, furosemide is particularly beneficial when cardiac output and renal flow are severely diminished.

Furosemide acts by preventing the reabsorption of sodium and chloride in the loop of Henle. By blocking sodium chloride (NaCl) reabsorption, furosemide interferes with water reabsorption. When water reabsorption is blocked, increased urination results.

Adverse Effects and Interactions: Adverse effects of furosemide, like those of most diuretics, include electrolyte imbalances, the most important of which is hypokalemia. Because hypokalemia may cause dysrhythmias in patients taking digoxin, combination therapy with furosemide and digoxin must be carefully monitored. When furosemide is given with corticosteroids and amphotericin B, it can increase the risk for hypokalemia. When given with lithium, elimination of lithium is decreased, causing higher risk of toxicity. When given with sulfonylureas and insulin, furosemide may diminish their hypoglycemic effects. Because furosemide is such a potent drug, fluid loss must be carefully monitored to prevent possible dehydration and hypotension.

Furosemide should be monitored carefully in patients receiving aminoglycoside antibiotics because additive ototoxicity may result. Patients allergic to sulfur or sulfonamide antibiotics should not receive furosemide because of potential allergic response.

CORE CONCEPT 17.6   ## The thiazides are the most widely prescribed class of diuretics.

The thiazides comprise the largest, most frequently prescribed class of diuretics. These drugs act on the distal tubule to block sodium reabsorption and increase water excretion. Their primary use is for the treatment of mild to moderate HTN. They are less effective at producing diuresis than the loop diuretics, and they are ineffective in patients with severe renal disease. All the thiazide diuretics are available by the oral route and have equivalent efficacy and safety profiles. Three drugs—chlorthalidone (Hygroton), indapamide (Lozol), and metolazone (Zaroxolyn)—are not true thiazides, although they are included with this drug class because they have similar mechanisms of action and adverse effects. The thiazide and thiazide-like diuretics are listed in Table 17.2 ◆.

The frequency of adverse effects with the thiazides is lower than that of the loop diuretics. As is true with other diuretics, dehydration is possible because of excessive or rapid fluid loss, and patients may experience dizziness due to hypotension when moving from a supine to an upright position. Electrolyte levels are monitored periodically to prevent hypokalemia. To avoid adverse effects from the drug, patients

TABLE 17.2 Thiazide and Thiazide-Like Diuretics		
Drug	**Route and Adult Dose**	**Remarks**
bendroflumethiazide and nadolol (Corzide)	PO; 1 tablet/day (40–80 mg nadolol/5 mg bendroflumethiazide)	Intermediate acting
chlorothiazide (Diuril)	PO; 250–500 mg one or two times/day	IV form available; short acting
chlorthalidone (Hygroton)	PO; 50–100 mg/day	Thiazide-like; long acting
ⓟ hydrochlorothiazide (Microzide)	PO; 25–100 mg/day	Short acting
indapamide (Lozol)	PO; 1.25–2.5 mg once daily	Thiazide-like; long acting
methyclothiazide (Aquatensen, Enduron)	PO; 2.5–10 mg/day	Long acting
metolazone (Zaroxolyn)	PO; 2.5–10 mg once daily	Thiazide-like; intermediate acting

Drug Prototype: Ⓟ *Hydrochlorothiazide (Microzide)*

Therapeutic Class: Drug for hypertension and edema   Pharmacologic Class: Thiazide diuretic

Actions and Uses: Hydrochlorothiazide is the most widely prescribed diuretic, belonging to a class of drugs known as the thiazides. Hydrochlorothiazide is approved to treat ascites, edema, HF, and HTN. Like many diuretics, it produces few serious adverse effects and is effective at producing a 10–20 mmHg reduction in blood pressure. Patients with severe HTN require the addition of a second drug from a different class to control the disease.

Hydrochlorothiazide acts on the kidney tubule to decrease the reabsorption of Na^+. When hydrochlorothiazide blocks this reabsorption, more Na^+ and water are sent into the urine, thus reducing blood volume and decreasing blood pressure. The volume of urine produced is directly proportional to the amount of Na^+ reabsorption blocked by the diuretic.

Adverse Effects and Interactions: The most common adverse effects of hydrochlorothiazide include possible electrolyte imbalances, especially loss of excessive K^+ and Na^+. Because potassium deficiency may cause cardiac conduction abnormalities, patients are usually asked to increase their intake of dietary potassium as a precaution.

Hydrochlorothiazide increases the action of antihypertensives and skeletal muscle relaxants. It may reduce the effectiveness of anticoagulants, antigout drugs, and antidiabetic drugs, including insulin.

Central nervous system (CNS) depressants such as alcohol, barbiturates, and opioids may increase the orthostatic hypotension caused by hydrochlorothiazide. Steroids or amphotericin B increase K^+ loss when given in conjunction with hydrochlorothiazide, leading to hypokalemia.

Hydrochlorothiazide increases the risk of serum toxicity of the following drugs: digoxin, lithium, allopurinol, anesthetics, and antineoplastics. It also alters vitamin D metabolism and calcium conservation; use of calcium supplements may cause hypercalcemia. It should be used with caution with ginkgo biloba, which may cause an increase in blood pressure.

taking thiazides should be advised to drink plenty of water and beverages containing electrolytes and to eat a balanced diet. Diabetic patients should be aware that thiazide diuretics sometimes raise blood glucose levels.

Hydrochlorothiazide is often combined with drugs from other classes for the pharmacotherapy of hypertension. The combination of hydrochlorothiazide with another antihypertensive allows for lower doses of each individual drug, thus decreasing the incidence of side effects. In addition, a combination drug can sometimes cause a greater reduction in blood pressure than using a single drug. Examples of combination drugs include the following:

Apresazide: hydrochlorothiazide with hydralazine (a direct vasodilator)

Benicar HCT: hydrochlorothiazide with olmesartan (an angiotensin II receptor blocker)

Lopressor HCT: with metoprolol (a beta adrenergic blocker)

Zestoretic: hydrochlorothiazide with lisinopril (an angiotensin-converting enzyme inhibitor)

Although less effective than the loop diuretics, potassium-sparing diuretics may help prevent hypokalemia.

CORE CONCEPT 17.7

Potassium depletion is a potentially serious adverse effect of the thiazide and loop diuretics. The therapeutic advantage of the potassium-sparing diuretics is that they are able to increase diuresis without adversely affecting blood potassium levels. These diuretics are shown in Table 17.3 ◆.

Normally, Na^+ and K^+ are exchanged in the distal tubule; Na^+ is reabsorbed into the bloodstream and K^+ is secreted into the tubule. Potassium-sparing diuretics block this exchange, causing sodium to stay in the tubule and ultimately leave through the urine. When Na^+ is blocked, the body retains more K^+. Because most of the Na^+ has already been removed by the time the filtrate reaches the distal tubule, potassium-sparing diuretics produce only a mild diuresis. Their primary use is in combination with thiazide or loop diuretics to minimize potassium loss.

TABLE 17.3 Potassium-Sparing Diuretics

Drug	Route and Adult Dose	Remarks
amiloride (Midamor)	PO; 5 mg/day (max: 20 mg/day)	Moduretic is a fixed-dose combination of amiloride and hydrochlorothiazide.
ⓟ spironolactone (Aldactone)	PO; 25–100 mg one or two times/day	Used in combination with other antihypertensives to increase diuresis; monitor serum potassium level carefully
eplerenone (Inspra)	PO; 25–50 mg once daily	Newer drug in class; actions very similar to spironolactone
triamterene (Dyrenium)	PO; 50–100 mg bid	Dyazide is a fixed-dose combination of triamterene and hydrochlorothiazide.

Spironolactone and eplerenone (Inspra) are potassium-sparing diuretics that act by blocking the actions of the hormone aldosterone; thus they are commonly called aldosterone antagonists. Secreted by the adrenal cortex, the normal function of **aldosterone** is to promote the retention of sodium ion. Although it produces only a mild diuresis, spironolactone has been found to significantly reduce mortality in patients with heart failure.

Unlike the loop and thiazide diuretics, patients taking potassium-sparing diuretics should not take potassium supplements and should not add potassium-rich foods to their diet. Intake of excess potassium when taking these medications may lead to **hyperkalemia**.

Drug Prototype: ⓟ *Spironolactone (Aldactone)*

Therapeutic Class: Antihypertensive, drug for reducing edema
Pharmacologic Class: Potassium-sparing diuretic, aldosterone antagonist

Actions and Uses: Spironolactone, the most frequently prescribed potassium-sparing diuretic, is primarily used to treat mild HTN, often in combination with other antihypertensives. It may also be used to reduce edema associated with kidney or liver disease, and it is effective in slowing the progression of heart failure.

Spironolactone blocks sodium reabsorption in the distal tubule by inhibiting aldosterone. Aldosterone is a hormone secreted by the adrenal cortex that is responsible for increasing the renal reabsorption of Na^+ in exchange for K^+, thus causing water retention. When blocked by spironolactone, sodium and water excretion is increased, and the body retains more potassium.

Adverse Effects and Interactions: Spironolactone does such an efficient job of retaining potassium that hyperkalemia may develop. The risk of hyperkalemia is increased if the patient takes potassium supplements or is also taking angiotensin-converting enzyme (ACE) inhibitors. Signs and symptoms of hyperkalemia include muscle weakness, fatigue, and bradycardia. When potassium levels are monitored carefully and maintained within normal values, adverse effects from spironolactone are uncommon. Spironolactone is contraindicated during pregnancy and lactation.

When spironolactone is combined with ammonium chloride, acidosis may occur. Aspirin and other salicylates may decrease the diuretic effect of the medication. Use of spironolactone with digoxin may decrease the effects of digoxin.

CORE CONCEPT 17.8

Several less commonly prescribed diuretics have specific indications.

intra = *within*
ocular = *eye*

A few miscellaneous diuretics have very limited and specific indications. Two of these drugs inhibit **carbonic anhydrase**, an enzyme involved with acid–base balance. Acetazolamide (Diamox) is a carbonic anhydrase inhibitor used to decrease intraocular pressure in patients with glaucoma (see Chapter 37). Unrelated to its diuretic effect, acetazolamide is also used to treat acute mountain sickness in patients at very high altitudes. The carbonic anhydrase inhibitors are not commonly used as diuretics, because they produce a very weak diuresis and have a higher incidence of adverse effects than other diuretics.

TABLE 17.4 Miscellaneous Diuretics		
Drug	**Route and Adult Dose**	**Remarks**
acetazolamide (Diamox)	PO; 250–375 mg/day in a.m.	Carbonic anhydrase inhibitor; IV form available
glycerin (Colace, Osmoglyn)	PO; 1–1.8 g/kg, 1–2 hours before ocular surgery	Osmotic type; also used to treat constipation and acute glaucoma
mannitol (Osmitrol)	IV; 100 g infused over 2–6 hours	Osmotic type
methazolamide (Neptazane)	PO; 50–100 mg bid or tid	Carbonic anhydrase inhibitor
urea (Ureaphil)	IV; 1–1.5 g/kg over 1–2.5 hours	Osmotic type

The osmotic diuretics also have very specific applications. Mannitol (Osmitrol) is used to maintain urine flow in patients with acute renal failure during prolonged surgery. Mannitol is also used to reduce swelling in the brain (increased intracranial pressure) and lower intraocular pressure in certain types of glaucoma. It is a very potent diuretic that is only given by the IV route. Osmotic diuretics are rarely drugs of first choice due to their potential toxicity. Table 17.4 ◆ lists some of the miscellaneous diuretics.

NURSING PROCESS FOCUS   Patients Receiving Diuretic Therapy

ASSESSMENT	POTENTIAL NURSING DIAGNOSES
Prior to administration: ■ Obtain a complete health history including cardiovascular disease, renal and liver conditions, diabetes, pregnancy, allergies, diet, and data on recent surgeries or trauma. ■ Acquire the results of a complete physical examination, including vital signs, height, and weight. ■ Obtain the patient's medication history, including cardiac medications, nicotine and alcohol consumption, and use of over-the counter/herbal supplements or alternative therapies. Determine possible drug allergies and/or interactions. ■ Evaluate laboratory blood findings: CBC, electrolytes, renal and liver function studies.	■ *Fluid Volume* related to effects of medical condition ■ *Deficient Fluid Volume* related to effects of drug therapy ■ *Urinary Elimination* related to diuretic use ■ *Risk for Electrolyte Imbalance* related to diuretic use ■ *Deficient Knowledge* related to a lack of information about drug therapy ■ *Noncompliance* related to adverse effects of medications

PLANNING: PATIENT GOALS AND EXPECTED OUTCOMES

The patient will:
■ Experience therapeutic effects (normal fluid balance and maintenance of normal electrolyte levels).
■ Be free from or experience minimal adverse effects from drug therapy.
■ Verbalize an understanding of the drug's use, adverse effects and required precautions.

IMPLEMENTATION

Interventions and (Rationales)	Patient Education/Discharge Planning
■ Monitor for fluid overload by measuring intake, output, and daily weights. (Intake, output, and daily body weight can be indications of the effectiveness of diuretic therapy.)	Instruct the patient to: ■ Immediately report any severe shortness of breath, frothy sputum, profound fatigue, edema in extremities, potential signs of heart failure, or pulmonary edema. ■ Accurately measure fluid intake, fluid output, and body weight, and report decrease in output or weight gain of 2 lb or more within two days. ■ Avoid excessive heat, which contributes to fluid loss through perspiration. ■ Consume adequate amounts of plain water.
■ Monitor laboratory findings, especially potassium and sodium. (Diuretics can cause electrolyte imbalances.)	■ Advise the patient of the importance of keeping appointments for laboratory testing. ■ Instruct the patient to inform laboratory personnel of diuretic therapy when providing blood or urine samples.

continued . . .

NURSING PROCESS FOCUS *(continued)*

Interventions and (Rationales)	Patient Education/Discharge Planning
■ Monitor vital signs, especially blood pressure. (Diuretics reduce blood volume, resulting in lowered blood pressure.)	Instruct the patient to: ■ Monitor blood pressure as specified by the healthcare provider and ensure proper use of home equipment. ■ Stop medication if severe hypotension exists, as specified by the healthcare provider (e.g., "hold for levels below 88/50 mmHg").
■ Observe for changes in level of consciousness, dizziness, fatigue, and postural hypotension. (Reduction in blood volume due to diuretic therapy may produce changes in level of consciousness or syncope.)	Instruct the patient to: ■ Immediately report any change in consciousness, especially feeling faint. ■ Change positions slowly. ■ Obtain blood pressure readings in sitting, standing, and lying positions.
■ Monitor nutritional status, especially intake of foods with sodium and potassium. (These electrolytes can become depleted with thiazide or loop diuretics. Potassium sparing diuretics may cause sodium loss but potassium increase.)	Instruct patients: ■ Receiving *loop or thiazide diuretics* to eat foods high in potassium. ■ Receiving *potassium-sparing diuretics* to avoid foods high in potassium. ■ To consult with healthcare provider before using vitamin/mineral supplements or electrolyte-fortified sports drinks. Combining potassium supplements with a high potassium diet may lead to hyperkalemia.
■ Observe for signs of hypersensitivity reaction. (Allergic responses may be life threatening.)	Instruct the patient or caregiver to report: ■ Difficulty breathing, throat tightness, hives or rash, or bleeding. ■ Flu-like symptoms such as shortness of breath, fever, sore throat, malaise, joint pain, profound fatigue.
■ Monitor hearing and vision. (Loop diuretics are ototoxic. Thiazide diuretics increase serum digoxin levels, which produce visual changes.)	■ Instruct the patient to report any changes in hearing or vision such as ringing or buzzing in the ears, becoming "hard of hearing," or experiencing dimness of sight, seeing halos, or having "yellow vision."
■ Monitor reactivity to light exposure. (Some diuretics cause photosensitivity.)	Instruct the patient to: ■ Limit exposure to the sun. ■ Wear dark glasses and light-colored loose-fitting clothes when outdoors.
■ Administer medication correctly and evaluate the patient's knowledge of proper administration. (Some medications interact with other medications.)	Instruct the patient: ■ About the appropriate dosing and administration of the specific diuretic being taken. ■ To take diuretic in the morning instead of at night to avoid interruption of sleep.

EVALUATION OF OUTCOME CRITERIA

Evaluate the effectiveness of drug therapy by confirming that patient goals and expected outcomes have been met (see "Planning"). *See Tables 17.1 through 17.4 for lists of drugs to which these nursing actions apply.*

CORE CONCEPT 17.9

Electrolytes are charged substances that play important roles in maintaining homeostasis.

electro = *conducts electricity*
lyte = *solution*

Minerals are inorganic substances needed in very small amounts by the body (see Chapter 31). When placed in water, some of these minerals become ions and possess a positive or negative charge. Small, inorganic molecules possessing a positive or negative charge are called **electrolytes**. Electrolytes are essential to many body functions, including nerve conduction, muscle contraction, and bone growth and remodeling. Too little or too much of an electrolyte may result in serious disease and must be quickly corrected.

Levels of electrolytes in body fluids are maintained within very narrow ranges, primarily by the kidney and gastrointestinal (GI) tract. As electrolytes are lost due to normal excretory functions, they must be replaced by adequate fluid intake; otherwise, electrolyte imbalances can result. Although imbalances can occur in any ion, sodium, potassium, and calcium are of greatest importance. Calcium homeostasis is presented in vitamins, minerals, and nutritional supplements because it is associated with the pharmacotherapy of bone disorders. Sodium and potassium are discussed in the following paragraphs. The major electrolyte imbalances and their treatments are described in Table 17.5 ◆.

An electrolyte imbalance is a sign of an underlying medical condition that needs attention. The most common cause is renal impairment. In some cases, drug therapy itself can cause the electrolyte imbalance. For example, aggressive therapy with loop diuretics such as furosemide (Lasix) can rapidly deplete the

TABLE 17.5 Electrolyte Imbalances

Ion	Condition	Abnormal Serum Value (mEq/L)	Supportive Treatment*
Calcium	Hypercalcemia	Greater than 11	Hypotonic fluid or calcitonin
	Hypocalcemia	Less than 4	Calcium supplements or vitamin D
Chloride	Hyperchloremia	Greater than 112	Hypotonic fluid
	Hypochloremia	Less than 95	Hypertonic salt solution
Magnesium	Hypermagnesemia	Greater than 4	Hypotonic fluid
	Hypomagnesemia	Less than 0.8	Magnesium supplements
Phosphate	Hyperphosphatemia	Greater than 6	Dietary phosphate restriction
	Hypophosphatemia	Less than 1	Phosphate supplements
Potassium	Hyperkalemia	Greater than 5	Hypotonic fluid, buffers, or dietary potassium restriction
	Hypokalemia	Less than 3.5	Potassium supplements
Sodium	Hypernatremia	Greater than 145	Hypotonic fluid or dietary sodium restriction
	Hyponatremia	Less than 135	Hypertonic salt solution or sodium supplement

For all electrolyte imbalances, the primary therapeutic goal is to identify and correct the cause of the imbalance.

body of Na^+ and K^+. Treatment includes correcting the electrolyte imbalance as well as treating the underlying medical condition. Treatments for electrolyte imbalances range from simple changes in dietary intake for mild imbalances to rapid electrolyte infusions in severe cases.

Sodium Imbalances

Because Na^+ is the major electrolyte in extracellular fluid, imbalances of this ion can have serious consequences. Sodium excess, or **hypernatremia**, is most commonly caused by kidney disease; Na^+ accumulates in the blood due to decreased excretion. Another cause of hypernatremia is high net water losses, such as occur from inadequate water intake, watery diarrhea, fever, or burns. A high serum Na^+ level can cause cellular dehydration with symptoms such as thirst, fatigue, weakness, muscle twitching, convulsions, and a decreased level of consciousness. For minor hypernatremia, a salt-restricted diet may be effective in returning serum Na^+ to normal levels. In patients with acute hypernatremia, however, IV fluids such as 5% dextrose in water or diuretics may be administered to quickly remove sodium from the body.

Sodium deficiency, or **hyponatremia**, may occur when Na^+ is lost because of serious skin burns, vomiting, diarrhea, kidney disease, and with conditions associated with excessive sweating or prolonged fever. Symptoms of hyponatremia include nausea, vomiting, anorexia, abdominal cramping, confusion, lethargy, convulsions, coma, and muscle twitching or tremors. Hyponatremia is usually treated with solutions of sodium chloride or with IV fluids containing salt, such as normal saline or lactated Ringer's solution. Tolvaptan (Samsca) is a newer drug administered to raise sodium levels in hospitalized patients with serious hyponatremia.

hyper = *high or above normal*
natri = *sodium*
emia = *blood condition*

Potassium Imbalances

Potassium levels must be carefully balanced between adequate dietary intake and renal excretion. Levels of K^+ in the blood must be maintained within narrow limits because too little or too much of this electrolyte is associated with fatal cardiac dysrhythmias and serious neuromuscular disorders.

Hyperkalemia may be caused by high consumption of potassium-rich foods or dietary supplements, particularly when patients are taking potassium-sparing diuretics such as spironolactone. Excess potassium may also accumulate when renal excretion is diminished due to kidney pathology. The most serious consequences of hyperkalemia are cardiac dysrhythmias.

In mild cases of hyperkalemia, K^+ levels may be returned to normal by restricting major dietary sources of potassium such as bananas, dried fruits, peanut butter, broccoli, and green leafy vegetables. If the patient is taking a potassium-sparing diuretic, the dose is lowered or an alternate drug is considered. In acute cases, administration of furosemide (Lasix) can increase potassium excretion within minutes. Serum potassium levels may also be lowered by administering sodium polystyrene sulfate (Kayexalate), a resin that removes K^+ by exchanging it for Na^+ in the large intestine. This drug is given concurrently with a laxative to promote rapid evacuation of the potassium. Sodium polystyrene sulfate is available in oral and enema formulations. An additional method of treating hyperkalemia is to administer glucose and insulin, which causes potassium to leave the extracellular fluid and enter cells.

Drug Prototype: Ⓟ *Potassium Chloride (KCl)*

Therapeutic Class: Potassium supplement **Pharmacologic Class: Electrolyte**

Actions and Uses: Potassium is one of the most important electrolytes in body fluids, and levels must be maintained within a narrow range of values between 3.5 and 5.5 mEq/L. Too much or too little K$^+$ may lead to serious consequences and must be immediately corrected. Neurons and muscle fibers are most sensitive to potassium loss. Muscle weakness, dysrhythmias, and cardiac arrest are possible consequences. KCl is also used to treat mild forms of alkalosis.

KCl is the drug of choice for treating or preventing hypokalemia. Therapy with loop or thiazide diuretics is the most common cause of excessive potassium loss. Patients taking thiazide or loop diuretics are usually instructed to take oral potassium supplements to prevent hypokalemia. Oral forms include tablets, powders, and liquids, usually heavily flavored because of the unpleasant taste of the drug. Intravenous forms may be given in critical care situations.

Adverse Effects and Interactions: KCl irritates the GI mucosa; therefore, nausea and vomiting are common. The drug may be taken with meals or antacids to lessen the gastric distress. Taking too much KCl can cause hyperkalemia, especially when it is combined with a diet that contains potassium-rich foods.

Potassium supplements interact with potassium-sparing diuretics and ACE inhibitors to increase the risk of hyperkalemia. If patients are taking these drugs, the healthcare provider should warn them not to take OTC potassium supplements.

Hypokalemia is a relatively common adverse effect resulting from high doses of loop diuretics such as furosemide. Strenuous muscular activity and severe vomiting or diarrhea can also result in significant potassium loss. Mild hypokalemia is treated by increasing the dietary intake of potassium-rich foods. More severe deficiencies require oral or parenteral potassium supplements. Potassium chloride (KCl) is available in IV and a wide variety of oral formulations to increase blood potassium levels.

CORE CONCEPT 17.10

Acidic and basic drugs can be administered to correct pH imbalances.

One of the most important homeostatic functions of the blood is to neutralize strong acids and bases. Much of the food we eat is either more acidic or more alkaline than body fluids. Furthermore, during the breakdown of food, the body generates significant amounts of acid. If body fluids become too acidic or too alkaline, enzymes will not function efficiently and cells may be injured.

The degree of acidity or alkalinity of a solution is measured by its **pH**. A pH of 7 is defined as neutral, above 7 as basic or alkaline, and below 7 as acidic. To maintain homeostasis, the pH of plasma and most body fluids must be kept within the very narrow range of 7.35 to 7.45. At pH values above 7.45, **alkalosis** develops, and symptoms of CNS stimulation occur that include nervousness and convulsions. **Acidosis** occurs below a pH of 7.35, and symptoms of CNS depression may result in coma. In either alkalosis or acidosis, death may result if large changes in pH are not corrected immediately.

Acidosis and alkalosis are not diseases; they are symptoms of underlying disorders. Primary treatment of acid–base disorders is always targeted to correct the underlying cause. Drugs are administered to support the patient's vital functions while the disease is being treated. Common causes of alkalosis and acidosis are listed in Table 17.6 ◆.

Treatment of alkalosis is directed toward addressing the underlying condition that is causing the excess bases to be retained. In mild cases, alkalosis may be corrected by administering sodium chloride concurrently with KCl. This combination increases the renal excretion of bicarbonate ion (a base), which indirectly increases the acidity of the blood. For acute patients, acidifying agents may be used. Hydrochloric acid and ammonium chloride are two drugs that can quickly lower the pH in patients with severe alkalosis.

In patients with acidosis, the goal is to quickly reverse the level of acids in the blood. A preferred treatment for acute acidosis is to administer infusions of sodium bicarbonate. Bicarbonate ion acts as a base to quickly neutralize acids in the blood and other body fluids. The patient must be carefully monitored during infusions because this drug can "over-correct" the acidosis, causing blood pH to turn alkaline. The correction of acid–base imbalances is illustrated in Figure 17.4 ■.

alkal = *basic*
osis = *condition*

TABLE 17.6 Causes of Acidosis and Alkalosis

Acidosis	Alkalosis
RESPIRATORY ORIGINS OF ACIDOSIS	**RESPIRATORY ORIGIN OF ALKALOSIS**
■ Hypoventilation or shallow breathing ■ Airway constriction ■ Damage to respiratory center in medulla	■ Hyperventilation due to asthma, anxiety, or high altitude
METABOLIC ORIGINS OF ACIDOSIS	**METABOLIC ORIGINS OF ALKALOSIS**
■ Severe diarrhea ■ Kidney failure ■ Diabetes mellitus ■ Excess alcohol ingestion ■ Starvation	■ Constipation for prolonged periods ■ Ingestion of excess sodium bicarbonate ■ Diuretics that cause potassium depletion ■ Severe vomiting

FIGURE 17.4

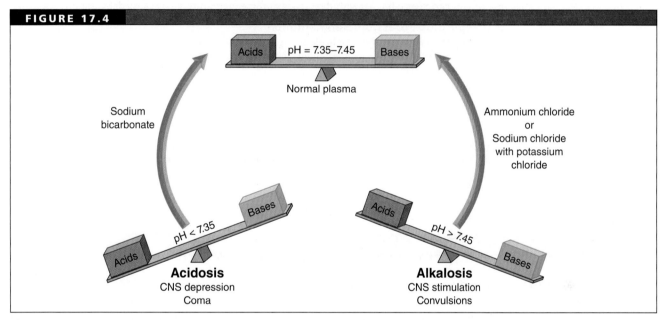

Correction of acid–base imbalances.

Drug Prototype: Ⓟⓡ *Sodium Bicarbonate (NaHCO₃)*

Therapeutic Class: Agent to treat acidosis or bicarbonate deficiency   **Pharmacologic Class: Electrolyte**

Actions and Uses: Acidosis is a more common event than alkalosis, occurring during shock or cardiac arrest, or with diabetes mellitus. Sodium bicarbonate is the drug of choice for correcting acidosis: The bicarbonate ion (HCO_3^-) directly raises the pH of body fluids. Sodium bicarbonate may be given orally if acidosis is mild, or IV in cases of acute disease. Although sodium bicarbonate neutralizes gastric acid, it is rarely used to treat peptic ulcers because of its tendency to cause gas and gastric distention.

Sodium bicarbonate may also be used to make the urine more basic. An alkaline urine will speed the excretion of acidic drugs, such as barbiturates and aspirin.

Adverse Effects and Interactions: Most of the adverse effects of sodium bicarbonate therapy are the result of alkalosis caused by *too much* bicarbonate ion. Symptoms may include confusion, irritability, slow respiration rate, and vomiting. Simply discontinuing the sodium bicarbonate infusion often reverses these symptoms; however, potassium chloride or ammonium chloride may be administered to reverse the alkalosis.

Sodium bicarbonate may decrease the absorption of ketoconazole and may decrease elimination of dextroamphetamine, ephedrine, pseudoephedrine, and quinidine. Sodium bicarbonate may increase the elimination of lithium, salicylates, and tetracyclines. Chronic use of sodium bicarbonate with milk or calcium supplements may cause milk–alkali syndrome, a condition characterized by very high serum calcium levels and possible kidney failure.

PATIENTS NEED TO KNOW

Patients treated for urinary, acid–base, and fluid disorders need to know the following:

Regarding Diuretics

1. See the healthcare provider regularly and have serum electrolytes, complete blood count (CBC), and glucose levels monitored as instructed.
2. When taking diuretics, drink plenty of water if dry mouth or thirst develops, unless otherwise directed by a healthcare provider.
3. Take diuretics in the morning or at least two hours before bedtime to avoid night-time diuresis.
4. If diabetes is present, monitor blood sugar levels very closely when taking thiazide diuretics because these drugs may elevate blood glucose levels.
5. Do not take thiazide diuretics during pregnancy or when breast-feeding.
6. When taking loop or thiazide diuretics, increase dietary sources of potassium-rich foods such as dark leafy vegetables, nuts, citrus fruits, bananas, and potatoes. If taking a potassium-sparing diuretic, avoid these foods unless otherwise instructed by a healthcare provider.
7. Avoid caffeinated beverages when taking diuretics. The diuretic effect of the caffeine combined with the effects of these medications may cause dehydration.

Regarding Potassium Supplements

8. Because KCl tablets are irritating to the GI mucosa, they should be taken with food. Do not crush or suck the tablets. If nausea or heartburn occurs, take antacids along with the KCl.

CHAPTER REVIEW

CORE CONCEPTS SUMMARY

17.1 The kidneys regulate fluid volume, electrolytes, acids, and bases.

The kidneys are essential to the overall health of the patient, and to control fluid volume, electrolyte composition, and acid–base balance. The functional unit of the kidney is the nephron.

17.2 The composition of filtrate changes dramatically as a result of the processes of reabsorption and secretion.

Filtrate entering the proximal tubule resembles plasma without proteins. Through the processes of reabsorption and secretion, the filtrate composition changes, producing urine.

17.3 Renal failure significantly impacts pharmacotherapy.

Because the kidneys excrete most drugs, a large number of medications require a significant dosage reduction in patients with moderate to severe renal failure. Renal failure is classified as acute or chronic. Pharmacotherapy of renal failure attempts to cure the cause of the dysfunction. Diuretics may be used to maintain urine output. Epoetin alfa is a form of erythropoietin used to treat anemia in which there is a deficiency in red blood cell production.

17.4 Diuretics are used to treat hypertension, heart failure, and fluid retention disorders.

Diuretics are drugs that increase urine output, usually by blocking sodium reabsorption. Indications for diuretics include hypertension, heart failure, kidney failure, and liver disease.

17.5 The most effective diuretics are those that affect the loop of Henle.

The high-ceiling or loop diuretics such as furosemide act by blocking sodium reabsorption in the loop of Henle. They are the most effective diuretics but are more likely to cause dehydration and electrolyte loss.

17.6 The thiazides are the most widely prescribed class of diuretics.

The thiazide diuretics block sodium reabsorption in the distal tubule. Although less effective than the loop diuretics, the thiazides are more frequently prescribed because of their lower incidence of serious adverse effects.

17.7 Although less effective than the loop diuretics, potassium-sparing diuretics may help prevent hypokalemia.

Potassium-sparing diuretics act on the distal tubule, although they are less effective than the loop diuretics. Their primary advantage is that they do not cause potassium loss.

17.8 Several less commonly prescribed diuretics have specific indications.

Carbonic anhydrase inhibitors and osmotic diuretics are not commonly prescribed. They have specific applications, such as decreasing intraocular pressure and maintaining urine flow during renal failure.

17.9 Electrolytes are charged substances that play important roles in maintaining homeostasis.

Electrolyte imbalances can cause significant signs and symptoms. Hypokalemia is a serious potential adverse effect of drug therapy with certain diuretics. Oral or IV potassium chloride can reverse symptoms of hypokalemia. Although less common, hyperkalemia may be just as serious and may be reversed by administration of glucose or insulin.

17.10 Acidic and basic drugs can be administered to correct pH imbalances.

Sodium chloride with potassium chloride may be administered to reverse mild to moderate alkalosis. Hydrochloric acid or ammonium chloride may be administered for acute alkalosis. Sodium bicarbonate is used to reverse acidosis.

REVIEW QUESTIONS

The following questions are written in NCLEX-PN® style. Answer these questions to assess your knowledge of the chapter material, and go back and review any material that is not clear to you.

1. Which of the following is not a function of the kidneys?

1. Acid–base balance
2. Secretion of renin
3. Production of white blood cells
4. Production of calcitriol

2. While collecting data on a patient suspected of being dehydrated, the nurse is looking for:

1. Headache and increased urinary output
2. Weight gain and edema
3. Hypertension and decreased urinary output
4. Hypotension, headache, and dry mouth

3. A patient, newly diagnosed with hypertension, was just seen by his or her healthcare provider. The office nurse was asked to give him or her samples of the most commonly prescribed diuretic used for this condition. The nurse gives the patient which of the following diuretics?

1. Ethacrynic acid (Edecrin)
2. Chlorothiazide (Diuril)
3. Spironolactone (Aldactone)
4. Mannitol (Osmitrol)

4. A female patient, recently started on diuretic therapy, is taught by the nurse that she should:

1. Take medication at night.
2. Rise slowly from a sitting position.
3. Increase sodium intake.
4. Decrease fluid intake.

5. A patient is receiving intravenous sodium bicarbonate for treatment of metabolic acidosis. During this infusion, how will the nurse monitor for therapeutic effect?

1. Liver function tests
2. White blood cell count
3. Serum pH
4. Glucose levels

6. The nurse is monitoring a patient for which of the following common adverse effects of oral potassium chloride?

1. Drowsiness
2. Nausea and vomiting
3. Hypoglycemia
4. Muscle weakness

7. When instructing a patient about taking potassium-sparing diuretics, the nurse teaches the patient to:

1. Take potassium supplements.
2. Not take potassium supplements
3. Add potassium rich foods to his or her diet.
4. Have his or her magnesium levels monitored regularly

8. The patient is receiving IV normal saline because of hyponatremia. On assessment, the nurse determines that the hyponatremia may have been caused by: (Select all that apply.)

1. Constipation
2. Severe diarrhea and vomiting
3. Prolonged fever and sweating
4. Hemorrhage

9. When taking diuretics, the patient is instructed to decrease or avoid the intake of:

1. Dark green, leafy vegetables
2. Nuts
3. Fruits
4. Caffeine

10. The healthcare provider orders 1,000 mL of 0.9% NaCl to infuse IV over eight hours. In monitoring the IV, how many mL should the nurse expect to infuse in one hour?

1. 100 mL
2. 125 mL
3. 135 mL
4. 150 mL

CASE STUDY QUESTIONS

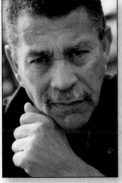

Remember Mr. Grant, the patient introduced at the beginning of the chapter? Now read the remainder of the case study. Based on the information you have learned in this chapter, answer the questions that follow.

Mr. Joseph Grant has been placed on hydrochlorothiazide (Microzide) for high blood pressure, and potassium chloride as a dietary supplement. His wife tells him to eat lots of bananas because she read that this was necessary when taking diuretics. After a few weeks, Mr. Grant becomes weak and feels as if his heart is skipping beats. His blood pressure remains high, despite the diuretic.

1. When providing education on his medications, which of the following should have been explained to Mr. Grant?

1. Never eat bananas when taking Microzide.
2. Eat lots of bananas when taking Microzide.
3. Limit potassium-rich foods when taking potassium supplements.
4. Never eat bananas and take Microzide at the same meal.

2. Given the previous information, the nurse believes it is quite possible that Mr. Grant's cardiac symptoms and weakness were caused by:

1. Hyperkalemia
2. Hypokalemia
3. Hypernatremia
4. Hyponatremia

3. The physician examines Mr. Grant and decides to administer a dose of sodium polystyrene sulfonate (Kayexalate). The nurse explains to Mr. Grant that the reason for administering this drug is to:

1. Increase fluid volume.
2. Decrease fluid volume.
3. Increase serum potassium levels.
4. Decrease serum potassium levels.

4. After Mr. Grant's condition stabilized, the physician decided to select furosemide (Lasix), a more effective diuretic to treat hypertension. Which of the following information should the nurse provide to Mr. Grant?

1. Never eat bananas when taking Lasix.
2. Eat lots of bananas when taking Lasix.
3. Limit potassium-rich foods when taking potassium supplements.
4. Never eat bananas and take Lasix at the same meal.

NOTE: Answers to the Review Questions appear in Appendix B. The complete rationales and answers are located on the textbook's website.

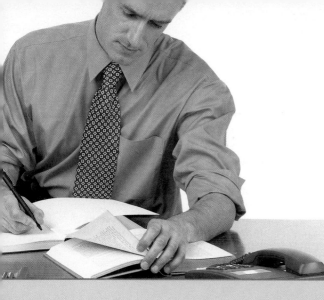

CHAPTER 18

Drugs for Hypertension

CORE CONCEPTS

18.1 Hypertension is characterized by the consistent elevation of arterial blood pressure.

18.2 Failure to treat hypertension can lead to stroke, heart failure, or myocardial infarction.

18.3 Blood pressure is caused by the pumping action of the heart.

18.4 The primary factors responsible for blood pressure are cardiac output, the resistance of the small arteries, and blood volume.

18.5 Many nervous and hormonal factors help to keep blood pressure within normal limits.

18.6 Positive lifestyle changes can reduce blood pressure and lessen the need for medications.

18.7 Selection of specific antihypertensive drugs depends on the severity of the disease.

18.8 Diuretics are often preferred drugs for treating mild to moderate hypertension.

18.9 Calcium channel blockers have emerged as important drugs in the treatment of hypertension.

18.10 Blocking the renin-angiotensin-aldosterone system leads to a decrease in blood pressure.

18.11 Adrenergic blockers are commonly used to treat hypertension.

18.12 Vasodilators lower blood pressure by relaxing arteriolar smooth muscle.

DRUG SNAPSHOT

The following drugs are discussed in this chapter:

DRUG CLASSES	DRUG PROTOTYPES
Diuretics	
Renin-angiotensin-aldosterone modifiers	Pr enalapril (Vasotec) *277*
Calcium channel blockers	Pr nifedipine (Adalat CC, Procardia XL) *279*

DRUG CLASSES	DRUG PROTOTYPES
Adrenergic blockers	Pr doxazosin (Cardura) *282*
Direct-acting vasodilators	Pr hydralazine (Apresoline) *283*

LEARNING OUTCOMES

After reading this chapter, the student should be able to:

1. Explain how hypertension is defined and classified.

2. Identify the long-term consequences of untreated hypertension.

3. Describe how the pumping action of the heart creates blood pressure.

4. Explain the effects of cardiac output, peripheral resistance, and blood volume on blood pressure.

5. Discuss nervous and hormonal factors that influence blood pressure.

6. Discuss the role of positive lifestyle changes in the management of hypertension.

7. Describe general principles that guide the selection of specific medications for hypertension.

8. For each of the classes listed in the Drug Snapshot, identify representative drugs and explain their mechanisms of drug action, primary actions, and important adverse effects.

KEY TERMS

aldosterone (al-DOH-stair-own) 274

angiotensin II (AN-geo-TEN-sin) 274

angiotensin-converting enzyme (ACE) (angeo-TEN-sin) 274

antidiuretic hormone (ADH) (ANT-eye-deye-your-ET-ik) 270

baroreceptors (BARE-oh-ree-sep-tours) 270

bradycardia (bray-dee-KAR-DEE-ah) 282

calcium channel blockers (CCBs) 278

cardiac output 269

diastolic pressure (DEYE-ah-stall-ik) 267

diuretics (deye-your-ET-ik) 269

electrolytes (ee-LEK-troh-lites) 273

false neurotransmitter (NYUR-oh-TRANS-mitt-ur) 282

hyperkalemia (heye-purr-kah-LEE-mee-ah) 274

hypertension (HTN) (heye-purr-TEN-shun) 266

hypokalemia (heye-poh-kah-LEE-mee-ah) 274

lumen (LOO-men) 269

orthostatic hypotension (or-tho-STAT-ik) 282

peripheral resistance (per-IF-ur-ul) 269

reflex tachycardia (ta-kee-CAR-dee-ah) 270

renin-angiotensin-aldosterone system (RAAS) (REN-in–an-geo-TEN-sin-al-DOS-ter-own) 274

systolic pressure (SIS-tol-ik) 267

vasomotor center (VAZO-mo-tor) 270

Cardiovascular disease, which includes all conditions affecting the heart and blood vessels, is the most common cause of death in the United States. Hypertension (HTN), or high blood pressure, is the most common of the cardiovascular diseases. Because healthcare providers encounter numerous patients with this disease, a firm grasp of the underlying principles of antihypertensive therapy is critical. By improving public awareness of HTN and teaching the importance of early intervention, the healthcare provider can contribute significantly to reducing cardiovascular mortality.

Hypertension is characterized by the consistent elevation of arterial blood pressure.

CORE CONCEPT 18.1

hyper = high
tension = pressure

Hypertension (HTN) is defined as the consistent elevation of arterial blood pressure. A patient is said to have chronic HTN if he or she presents with a sustained systolic blood pressure of greater than 140 mmHg or diastolic pressure of greater than 90 to 99 mmHg after multiple measurements are made over several clinic visits.

Many attempts have been made to further define HTN, with the goal of developing guidelines for treatment. The National High Blood Pressure Education Program Coordinating Committee of the National Heart, Lung, and Blood Institute of the National Institutes of Health has issued guidelines for treating HTN that have become well accepted in the medical community. The committee classified HTN into three categories—prehypertension, Stage 1, and Stage 2. The recommendations from Committee Report JNC-7 are summarized in Table 18.1 ◆. In addition to measurements of blood pressure, the classification of HTN also considers compelling conditions that have been shown to worsen the health outcomes for people with untreated HTN. These include heart failure, post-myocardial infarction, high risk for coronary artery disease, diabetes, chronic kidney disease, and previous stroke.

Blood pressure changes throughout the life span, gradually and continuously rising from childhood through adulthood. What is considered normal blood pressure at one age may be considered abnormal in someone older or younger. HTN has the greatest impact on older adults, affecting approximately 30% of those older than 50 years, 64% of men older than age 65, and 75% of women older than age 75.

TABLE 18.1 Classification and Management of Hypertension in Adults

Blood Pressure Classification	Systolic/Diastolic Blood Pressure (mmHg)	Initial Antihypertensive Therapy	
		Without Compelling Indication*	*With* Compelling Indication*
Normal	119/79 or lower	No antihypertensive indicated	No antihypertensive indicated
Prehypertension	120–139/80–89	—	—
Stage 1 Hypertension	140–159/90–99	Thiazide diuretic (for most patients)	Other antihypertensives, as needed
Stage 2 Hypertension	160 or higher/100 or higher	Two-drug combination antihypertensive (for most patients)	—

Compelling conditions include: heart failure, postmyocardial infarction, high risk for coronary artery disease, diabetes, chronic kidney disease, and recurrent stroke prevention.

Source: National High Blood Pressure Education Program National Heart, Lung, and Blood Institute. (2003). JNC-7 Express: The Seventh Report of the Joint National Committee on Prevention, Detection, Evaluation, and Treatment of High Blood Pressure.

Failure to treat hypertension can lead to stroke, heart failure, or myocardial infarction.

HTN is a complex disease that is caused by a combination of genetic and environmental factors. In 90% of the patients with HTN, no specific cause for the elevated blood pressure can be identified. This type of HTN is called *primary* or *essential*. Although the actual cause of primary HTN may not be known, many conditions or risk factors are associated with the disease. Advanced age and weight gain, particularly around the hips and thighs, tends to be associated with HTN. The disease is most prevalent in blacks and least prevalent in Mexican Americans. Men in all ethnic groups experience more HTN compared to women. The disease also has a hereditary component, with family members of patients with HTN having greater risk of acquiring the disease than nonfamily members. Other factors, such as tobacco use and high-fat diets, clearly contribute to the disease.

In 10% of patients, a specific cause of the HTN *can* be identified. This is called *secondary* hypertension. Certain diseases, such as Cushing's syndrome, hyperthyroidism, and chronic renal disease, cause elevated blood pressure. Certain drugs are also associated with HTN, including corticosteroids, oral contraceptives, and epoetin alfa (Epogen). The therapeutic goal for secondary HTN is to treat or remove the underlying condition that is causing the blood pressure elevation. In many cases, correcting this underlying condition will cure the associated HTN.

Because chronic HTN may produce no identifiable symptoms for as long as 10 to 20 years, many people are not aware of their condition. Convincing patients to control their diets, spend money on medication, and take drugs on a regular basis when they are feeling healthy is a difficult task for the healthcare provider. Failure to control HTN, however, can result in serious consequences. Prolonged high blood pressure can lead to accelerated narrowing of the arteries, resulting in strokes, kidney failure, and even cardiac arrest. One of the most serious consequences of chronic HTN is that the heart must work harder to pump blood to organs and tissues. This excessive workload can cause the heart to fail and the lungs to fill with fluid, a condition known as heart failure (HF). Drug therapy of HF is covered in Chapter 19.

The death rate from cardiovascular-related diseases has dropped significantly over the past 30 years because of the improved diagnosis and treatment of HTN, as well as the acceptance of healthier lifestyle habits. Early treatment is essential; the long-term cardiovascular damage caused by HTN is irreversible if the disease is allowed to progress unchecked.

Blood pressure is caused by the pumping action of the heart.

Although pressure can be measured in nearly any vessel in the body, the term *blood pressure* commonly refers to the pressure in the large arteries. Because the pumping action of the heart is the source of blood pressure, those arteries closest to the heart, such as the aorta, have the highest pressure. Pressure decreases gradually as the blood travels farther from the heart, until it falls close to zero in the largest veins. This is illustrated in Figure 18.1 ■.

When the ventricles of the heart contract and eject blood, the pressure created in the arteries is called **systolic pressure**. When the ventricles relax and the heart temporarily stops ejecting blood, pressure in the arteries will fall, and this results in **diastolic pressure**. Blood pressure is measured in units of millimeters of mercury, abbreviated as mmHg. (Hg is the chemical symbol for the element mercury.) The average normal systolic pressure in a healthy adult is considered to be less than 120 mmHg, whereas the average normal diastolic pressure is less than 80 mmHg. The systolic and diastolic pressures are usually measured and reported together, with the systolic given first. For example, average normal blood pressure is said to be less than 120/80 mmHg. Figure 18.2 ■ illustrates how the pumping action of the heart determines systolic and diastolic blood pressure.

Fast Facts Hypertension

- High blood pressure affects more than 70 million U.S. adults, or approximately one in three Americans.
- Among people with HTN, more than 28% do not realize they have the condition.
- African American men have the highest rate of HTN.
- Approximately 65% of Americans diagnosed with HTN do not have their condition under adequate control.
- HTN is the most common complication of pregnancy.
- Prehypertension (120–139/80–89 mmHg) affects over 20% of the adult population, almost 45 million people.
- Approximately 54,000 Americans die of HTN per year; it is a contributing factor in 300,000 additional deaths each year.

FIGURE 18.1

Blood pressure changes
throughout the
circulation.

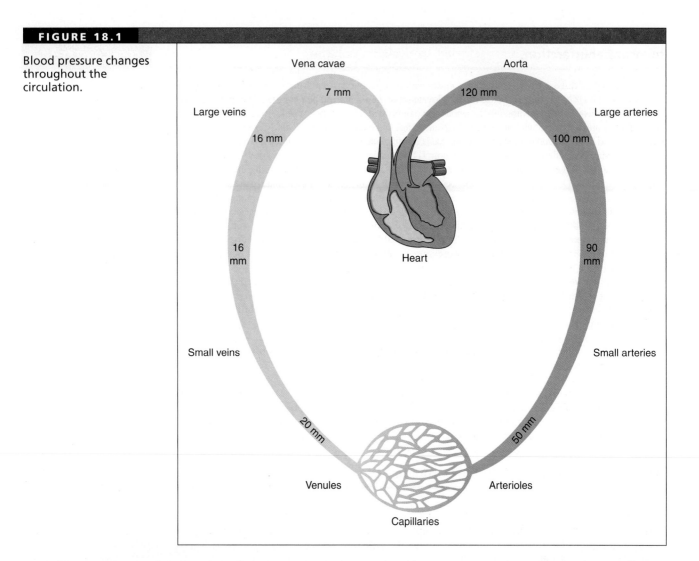

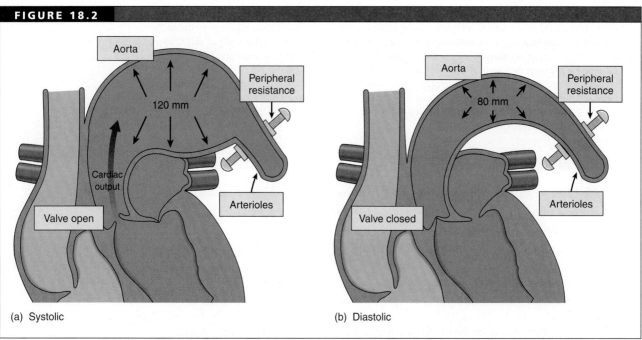

(a) Systolic pressure occurs when the heart ejects blood, creating high pressure in the arteries.
(b) Diastolic pressure occurs when the heart relaxes, resulting in less pressure in the arteries.

The primary factors responsible for blood pressure are cardiac output, the resistance of the small arteries, and blood volume.

In order to understand how drugs affect blood pressure, the student must have an excellent knowledge of cardiovascular physiology. Investing time to understand the details of how this system functions will reap great rewards later when studying the cardiovascular and respiratory drugs.

Although many factors can influence blood pressure, three factors are truly responsible for determining the pressure. The three primary factors—cardiac output, peripheral resistance, and blood volume—are shown in Figure 18.3 ■.

The volume of blood pumped per minute is called the **cardiac output**. Although resting cardiac output is approximately 5 liters per minute (L/min), strenuous exercise can increase this output to as much as 35 L/min. This is important to pharmacology because drugs that change the cardiac output have the potential to influence a patient's blood pressure. It is important to remember that the higher the cardiac output, the higher the blood pressure.

As blood flows at high speeds through the vascular system, it bumps and drags across the walls of the vessels. Although the vessel walls are extremely smooth, this friction reduces the velocity of the blood. This dragging or friction in the arteries is called **peripheral resistance**. Arteries have smooth muscle in their walls that, when constricted, will cause the inside diameter or **lumen** to become smaller, thus creating more resistance and higher pressure. This is how the body controls normal minute-by-minute changes in blood pressure. This is also important to pharmacology because a number of drugs affect vascular smooth muscle, causing vessels to constrict, thus raising blood pressure. Other drugs cause the smooth muscle to relax, thereby opening the lumen and lowering blood pressure. These drugs are among those used to treat HTN. The role of the autonomic nervous system in controlling peripheral resistance is presented in Chapter 8.

The third factor responsible for blood pressure is the total amount of blood in the vascular system, or *blood volume*. Although the average person maintains a relatively constant blood volume of approximately 5 L, this can change as a result of certain regulatory factors and with certain disease states. More blood in the vascular system will exert additional pressure on the walls of the arteries and raise blood pressure. For example, high sodium diets cause water to be retained by the body, thus increasing blood volume and raising blood pressure. On the other hand, drugs called **diuretics** can cause fluid loss through urination, thus decreasing blood volume and lowering blood pressure. Diuretics are discussed later in this chapter and were presented in Chapter 17.

Many nervous and hormonal factors help to keep blood pressure within normal limits.

It is critical that the body maintains a normal range of blood pressure and that it has the ability to safely and rapidly change pressure as it proceeds through daily activities, such as sleep and exercise. Too little blood pressure can cause dizziness and lack of urine formation, whereas too much pressure can cause vessels to rupture. A diagram explaining how the body maintains homeostasis during periods of blood pressure change is shown in Figure 18.4 ■

FIGURE 18.3

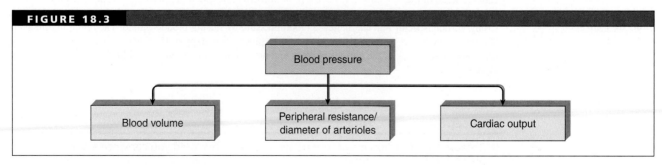

Primary factors affecting blood pressure.

FIGURE 18.4

Blood pressure is controlled by the actions of the cardio-vascular system and kidneys.

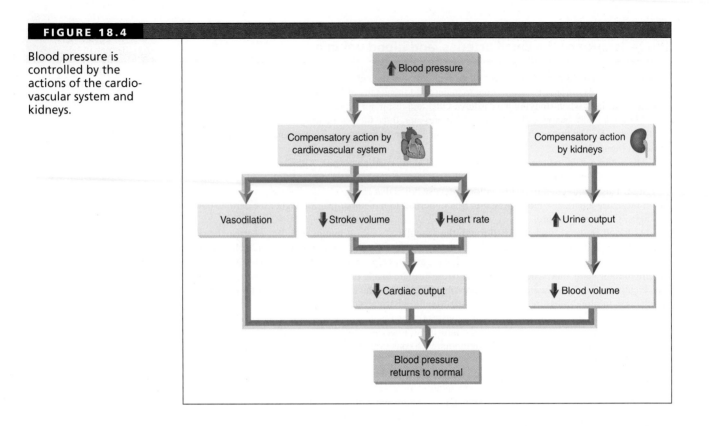

Blood pressure is regulated on a minute-to-minute basis by a cluster of neurons in the medulla oblongata called the **vasomotor center**. Nerves travel from the vasomotor center to the arteries, where the smooth muscle is directed to either constrict (raise blood pressure) or relax (lower blood pressure).

Receptors in the aorta and the carotid artery act as sensors to provide the vasomotor center with vital information on current conditions in the vascular system. Some of these neurons, called **baroreceptors**, have the ability to sense blood pressure within these large vessels. The baroreceptors are important to the pharmacotherapy of HTN. When a drug is given to lower blood pressure, the baroreceptors respond by trying to return pressure to its original (high) level. The baroreceptor response includes an immediate increase in heart rate, known as **reflex tachycardia**. In time, the body will recognize the lower blood pressure as normal, "reset" the baroreceptors, and reflex tachycardia will diminish. If reflex tachycardia does not decrease, a patient may be administered a beta-adrenergic blocker to prevent heart rate increase.

Emotions can also have a profound effect on blood pressure. Anger and stress can cause blood pressure to rise, whereas mental depression and lethargy may cause it to fall. Strong emotions, if present for a long time, may be important contributors to chronic HTN.

A number of hormones and other agents affect blood pressure on a daily basis. When given as medications, some of these agents may have a profound effect on blood pressure. For example, an injection of epinephrine or norepinephrine will immediately raise blood pressure. **Antidiuretic hormone (ADH)** is a strong vasoconstrictor that can increase blood pressure by raising blood volume. The renin-angiotensin-aldosterone system is particularly important in the pharmacotherapy of HTN and is discussed in core concept 18.9. A summary of the various nervous and hormonal factors influencing blood pressure is shown in Figure 18.5 ■.

baro = *pressure*
receptor = *sensor*

tachy = *rapid*
cardia = *heart*

anti = *against*
diuretic = *urination*

Concept Review 18.1

■ Because hypertension may cause no symptoms, how would you convince a patient to take his or her medication regularly?

FIGURE 18.5

Hormonal and nervous factors influencing blood pressure.

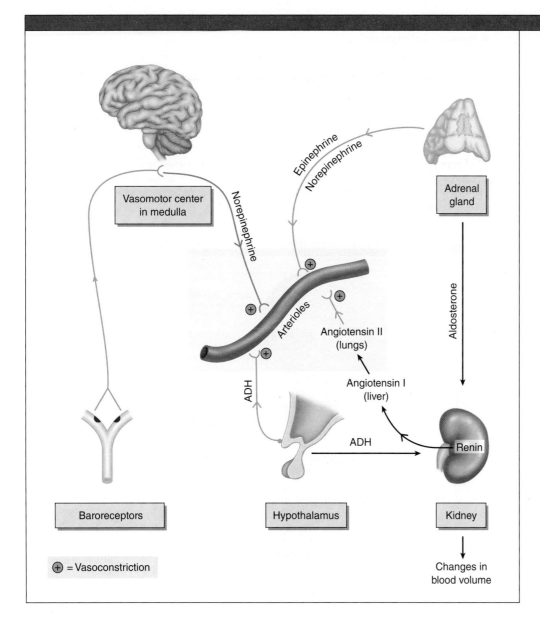

Positive lifestyle changes can reduce blood pressure and lessen the need for medications.

CORE CONCEPT 18.6

When a patient is first diagnosed with HTN, the healthcare provider obtains a comprehensive medical history to determine if the disease can be controlled without medications. Positive lifestyle changes should be recommended for all patients with prehypertension or HTN. Of great importance is maintaining optimum weight, because obesity is closely associated with blood lipid elevation and HTN. Combining a safe weight loss program with proper nutrition can delay the progression from prehypertension to HTN.

In many cases, implementing positive lifestyle changes may eliminate the need for pharmacotherapy altogether. Even if pharmacotherapy is required, it is important that the patients continue these lifestyle modifications so that dosages can be minimized. Because all blood pressure medications have potential adverse effects, it is important that patients attempt to control their disease through nonpharmacologic means to the greatest extent possible. Important nonpharmacologic methods for controlling HTN are as follows:

- Implement a medically supervised, safe weight-reduction plan, if 20% or more over normal body weight.
- Stop using tobacco.

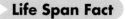

Life Span Fact

Control of blood pressure is particularly important in older adults. Age often causes blood vessels to be less elastic, thus impairing their ability to dilate or constrict with activities of daily living. Healthcare providers should emphasize to their older adult patients the importance of blood pressure monitoring and control.

- Restrict salt (sodium) intake and eat foods rich in potassium and magnesium.
- Limit alcohol consumption.
- Implement a medically supervised aerobic exercise plan.
- Reduce sources of stress and learn to implement coping strategies.

CORE CONCEPT 18.7

Selection of specific antihypertensive drugs depends on the severity of the disease.

The goal of antihypertensive therapy is to reduce blood pressure to normal levels so that the long-term consequences of HTN may be prevented. Keeping blood pressure within normal limits has been shown to reduce the risk of HTN-related diseases, such as stroke and heart failure. Several therapeutic strategies are used to achieve this goal, as summarized in Figure 18.6 ■.

FIGURE 18.6

Mechanism of action of antihypertensive drugs.

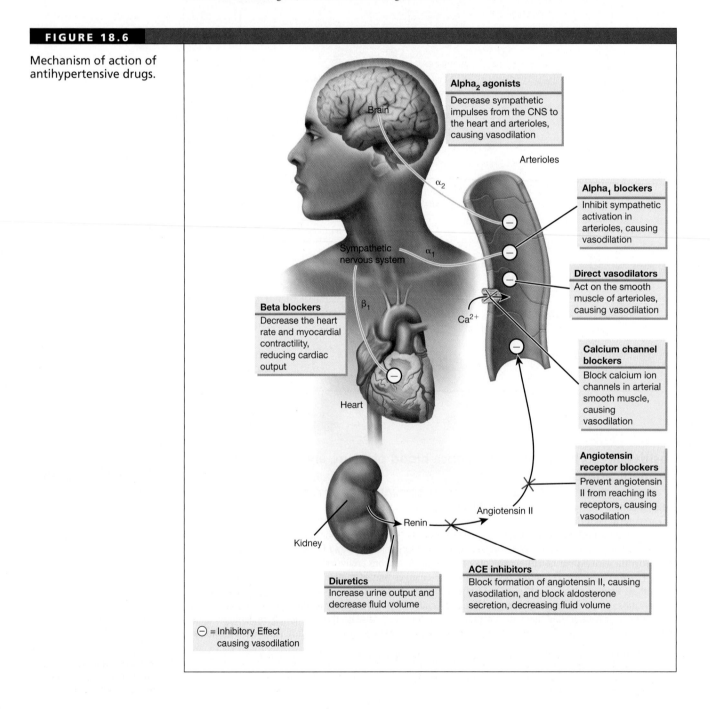

Alpha$_2$ agonists
Decrease sympathetic impulses from the CNS to the heart and arterioles, causing vasodilation

Alpha$_1$ blockers
Inhibit sympathetic activation in arterioles, causing vasodilation

Direct vasodilators
Act on the smooth muscle of arterioles, causing vasodilation

Calcium channel blockers
Block calcium ion channels in arterial smooth muscle, causing vasodilation

Angiotensin receptor blockers
Prevent angiotensin II from reaching its receptors, causing vasodilation

ACE inhibitors
Block formation of angiotensin II, causing vasodilation, and block aldosterone secretion, decreasing fluid volume

Beta blockers
Decrease the heart rate and myocardial contractility, reducing cardiac output

Diuretics
Increase urine output and decrease fluid volume

Brain
Arterioles
Sympathetic nervous system
Heart
Kidney
Renin
Angiotensin II
Ca^{2+}

⊖ = Inhibitory Effect causing vasodilation

The pharmacologic management of HTN is individualized to the patient's risk factors, comorbid medical conditions, and degree of blood pressure elevation. Patient responses to antihypertensive medications vary widely because of the many complex genetic and environmental factors affecting blood pressure. A large number of antihypertensive drugs are available, and choice of therapy is often based on the experience of the healthcare provider. Although antihypertensive treatment varies, there are several principles that guide pharmacotherapy.

Pharmacotherapy usually begins with low doses of a single antihypertensive medication. The patient is reevaluated after an appropriate time interval, when, if necessary, the prescriber may increase the dose of the initial drug or substitute another antihypertensive drug from a different drug class. The following are considered primary antihypertensive drug classes:

- Diuretics

- Renin-angiotensin-aldosterone inhibitors

- Calcium channel blockers (CCBs)

- Beta-adrenergic blockers

The *JNC-7* report recommends thiazide diuretics as the initial drugs for mild to moderate HTN. Patients with a compelling condition, however, may benefit from a second drug, either in combination with the diuretic or in place of the diuretic. The use of two drugs from different classes often produces an additive reduction in blood pressure. Another advantage of this approach is that it allows lower doses of each drug than would be needed if a single one were used. Lower doses usually produce fewer side effects, which improves patient adherence to therapy. However, adherence decreases when patients need to take more than one drug or when they need to take them more often. For convenience, drug manufacturers often combine two drugs into a single pill or capsule. The diuretic hydrochlorothiazide (Microzide) is the most common drug used in combination antihypertensive products. Examples of antihypertensive combination drugs include Diovan HCT (hydrochlorothiazide and valsartan), Zestoretic (hydrochlorothiazide and lisinopril), and Lotrel (benazepril and amlodipine).

Certain antihypertensive classes cause more frequent or serious adverse effects and are generally prescribed only when first-line medications do not produce a satisfactory response. The alternative antihypertensive drug classes include the following:

- Alpha$_1$-adrenergic blockers

- Alpha$_2$-adrenergic agonists (centrally-acting agents)

- Direct-acting vasodilators

In designing outcomes for patients with HTN, special attention should be placed on African Americans with this disorder. The incidence of HTN is significantly higher in African Americans than in other ethnic groups, and aggressive antihypertensive therapy may be necessary to manage the disorder. Some physicians recommend initiating therapy with two drugs to ensure adequate response. Based on clinical trials in African Americans, the Food and Drug Administration (FDA) recently approved BiDil, a fixed-dose combination of isosorbide dinitrate and hydralazine that appears to be particularly effective at lowering blood pressure in this population.

Diuretics are often preferred drugs for treating mild to moderate hypertension.

CORE CONCEPT 18.8

Diuretics act by increasing the amount of urine produced by the kidneys. They are widely used in the treatment of HTN, HF, and fluid balance disorders. Diuretics were presented in detail in Chapter 17, and prototype drug features for hydrochlorothiazide (Microzide), furosemide (Lasix), and spironolactone (Aldactone) are included in that chapter. This section focuses on the role of diuretics in treating hypertension. Table 18.2 ◆ lists diuretics commonly used to treat HTN.

Diuretics were the first widely prescribed class of drugs used to treat HTN in the 1950s. Despite many advances in drug therapy since then, diuretics are still considered drugs of first choice because they produce few adverse effects and are very effective at controlling mild to moderate HTN. For more advanced disease, they are prescribed in combination with antihypertensive medications from other classes.

Although many different diuretics are available for HTN, all produce a similar outcome: the reduction of blood volume through the urinary excretion of water and electrolytes. **Electrolytes** are ions such as sodium (Na^+), calcium (Ca^{2+}), chloride (Cl^-), and potassium (K^+). The mechanisms by which diuretics reduce blood volume differ among the various diuretics. Differences among the diuretic classes are presented in Chapter 17.

A common adverse effect of diuretic therapy is dehydration, the excessive loss of water from the body. Early signs of dehydration include thirst, dry mouth, dizziness, lethargy, and a fall in blood pressure.

de = *without or absence of*
hydra = *water*
tion = *condition*

TABLE 18.2 Diuretics for Hypertension

Drug	Route and Adult Dose	Remarks
amiloride (Midamor)	PO; 5–10 mg/day (max: 20 mg/day)	Potassium sparing type
bumetanide (Bumex)	PO; 0.25–2 mg once daily (max: 10 mg/day)	Loop diuretic type; decreases blood potassium levels; IV and IM forms available
chlorothiazide (Diuril)	PO/IV; 250 mg–1 g/day in one or two divided doses (max: 2 g/day)	Thiazide type; decreases blood potassium levels
chlorthalidone (Thalitone)	PO; 12.5–25 mg daily (max: 50 mg/day)	Thiazide type; decreases blood potassium levels
eplerenone (Inspra)	PO; 25–50 mg once daily (max: 100 mg/day)	A newer potassium-sparing diuretic
furosemide (Lasix) (see page 254 for the Drug Prototype box)	PO; 20–80 mg/day (max: 600 mg/day)	Loop diuretic type; decreases blood potassium levels; IV and IM forms available
hydrochlorothiazide (Microzide) (see page 255 for the Drug Prototype box)	PO; 25–100 mg in one to two divided doses (max: 200 mg/day)	Thiazide type; decreases blood potassium levels
indapamide (Lozol)	PO; 2.5–5 mg daily (max: 5 mg/day)	Similar to thiazide type; decreases blood potassium levels
spironolactone (Aldactone) (see page 256 for the Drug Prototype box)	PO; 25–100 mg 1–2 times/day (max: 400 mg/day)	Potassium-sparing type
torsemide (Demadex)	PO/IV; 10–20 mg/day (max: 200 mg/day)	Loop diuretic type; decreases blood potassium levels
triamterene (Dyrenium)	PO; 50–100 mg bid (max: 300 mg/day)	Potassium sparing type

> **Life Span Fact**

Older adults are especially at risk for dehydration and must be carefully monitored during the initial stages of diuretic therapy.

hyper = *high*
hypo = *low*
ka = *potassium*
emia = *blood*

Electrolyte imbalances of potassium, sodium, and magnesium ions are additional adverse effects of diuretic therapy. Loss of K⁺, **hypokalemia**, is of particular concern because it can lead to serious abnormalities in cardiac rhythm. When taking thiazide or loop diuretics, patients should be encouraged to include a potassium supplement or to eat foods rich in potassium content, such as bananas, oranges, tomatoes, milk, salmon, and beef.

Certain diuretics such as spironolactone (Aldactone) have fewer tendencies to cause K⁺ depletion, and, for this reason, are called *potassium-sparing diuretics*. Taking potassium supplements with potassium-sparing diuretics may lead to dangerously high K⁺ levels in the blood, or **hyperkalemia**, which can cause cardiac conduction abnormalities.

Concept Review 18.2

■ State the major reasons why patients should continue lifestyle changes even though their antihypertensive drugs appear to be effective.

CORE CONCEPT 18.9

Blocking the renin-angiotensin-aldosterone system leads to a decrease in blood pressure.

The **renin-angiotensin-aldosterone system (RAAS)** is one of the primary homeostatic mechanisms controlling blood pressure and fluid balance in the body. Drugs that modify the RAAS decrease blood pressure and increase urine output. They are widely used in the treatment of HTN, HF, and MI. Table 18.3 ◆ lists the RAAS modifiers commonly used to treat HTN.

angio = *vessels*
tensin = *pressure*

Renin is an enzyme secreted by specialized cells in the kidneys when blood pressure falls or when there is a decrease in Na⁺ flowing through the kidney tubules. In a series of enzymatic steps, **angiotensin II**, one of the most potent natural vasoconstrictors known, is formed. The enzyme responsible for the final step of this pathway is called **angiotensin-converting enzyme (ACE)**. The intense vasoconstriction of arterioles caused by angiotensin II raises blood pressure by increasing peripheral resistance.

A second, equally important effect of angiotensin II is stimulation of the secretion of **aldosterone**, a hormone from the adrenal gland that increases Na⁺ reabsorption in the kidney. The enhanced Na⁺ reabsorption causes the body to retain water, which raises blood volume and increases blood pressure. Drugs that inhibit the RAAS block the effects of angiotensin II, thus decreasing blood pressure through *two* mechanisms: dilating arteries and decreasing blood volume.

First detected in the venom of pit vipers in the 1960s, drugs that inhibit ACE have been approved for hypertension since the 1980s. Since then, the ACE inhibitors have become important drugs in the treatment of HTN. ACE inhibitors are preferred drugs for patients with both diabetes and HTN because they have

TABLE 18.3 ACE Inhibitors and Angiotensin-Receptor Blockers for Hypertension

Drug	Route and Adult dose	Remarks
ACE INHIBITORS		
benazepril (Lotensin)	PO; 10–40 mg in one to two divided doses (max: 40 mg/day)	May be used in combination with thiazide diuretics
captopril (Capoten)	PO; 6.25–25 mg tid (max: 450 mg/day)	Also for HF
Pr enalapril (Vasotec)	PO; 5–40 mg in 1–2 divided doses (max: 40 mg/day)	Also for HF; IV form available
fosinopril (Monopril)	PO; 5–40 mg daily (max: 80 mg/day)	Also for HF
lisinopril (Prinivil, Zestril) (see page 292 for the Drug Prototype box)	PO; 10 mg daily (max: 80 mg/day)	Also for HF
moexipril (Univasc)	PO; 7.5–30 mg daily (max: 30 mg/day)	Approved for HTN only
perindopril (Aceon)	PO; 4 mg once daily (max: 16 mg/day)	Also for HF, stable angina, and post MI therapy
quinapril (Accupril)	PO; 10–20 mg daily (max: 80 mg/day)	Also for HF
ramipril (Altace)	PO; 2.5–5 mg daily (max: 20 mg/day)	Also for HF, stroke prophylaxis and post-MI therapy
trandolapril (Mavik)	PO; 1–4 mg daily (max: 8 mg/day)	Also for post-MI therapy
ANGIOTENSIN-RECEPTOR BLOCKERS		
azilsartan (Edarbi)	PO; 40–80 mg once daily	Approved for HTN only. Newer drug in this class
candesartan (Atacand)	PO; start at 16 mg/day (max: 32 mg/day)	Also for HF
eprosartan (Teveten)	PO; 600 mg/day or 400 mg qid–bid (max: 800 mg/day)	Approved for HTN only
irbesartan (Avapro)	PO; 150–300 mg/day (max: 300 mg/day)	Approved for HTN only; Maximum effect may take 6–12 weeks
losartan (Cozaar)	PO; 25–50 mg in one to two divided doses (max: 100 mg/day)	Approved for HTN only
olmesartan (Benicar)	PO; 20–40 mg/day (max: 40 mg/day)	Approved for HTN only
telmisartan (Micardis)	PO; 40–80 mg/day (max: 80 mg/day)	Approved for HTN only
valsartan (Diovan)	PO; 80 mg/day (max: 320 mg/day)	Also for HF

been shown to reduce the progression of kidney failure that often occurs in patients with diabetes. Because of cardiovascular changes associated with diabetes, these patients often require therapy with at least two antihypertensive drugs. Adverse effects of ACE inhibitors are relatively minor and include persistent dry cough and hypotension following the first dose of the drug. Though rare, the most serious adverse effect of ACE inhibitors is the development of angioedema, an intense swelling around the lips, eyes, throat, and other body regions. In advanced cases, angioedema may lead to airway closure due to serious swelling in the neck. When angioedema does occur, it most often develops within hours or days after beginning ACE inhibitor therapy.

A second method of modifying the RAAS is blocking the action of angiotensin II *after* it is formed. This class of drugs is called the angiotensin-receptor blockers (ARBs). These drugs, which include irbesartan (Avapro), losartan (Cozaar), and valsartan (Diovan), block the receptors for angiotensin II in arteriolar smooth muscle and in the adrenal gland, thus causing blood pressure to fall. Their actions of arteriolar dilation and increased renal Na$^+$ excretion are quite similar to those of the ACE inhibitors. ARBs have relatively few adverse effects, such as headache, dizziness, and facial flushing, most of which are related to hypotension. Unlike the ACE inhibitors, they do not cause cough, and angioedema is rare. Drugs in this class are usually combined with drugs from other classes; for example, the drug Hyzaar combines losartan with the diuretic hydrochlorothiazide.

The newest method of modifying the RAAS is to inhibit the effects of renin itself. The direct renin inhibitors prevent the formation of angiotensin I and II. Aliskiren (Tekturna) was the first drug marketed in this class of antihypertensives. Pharmaceutical companies were quick to add aliskiren to other drugs to create fixed-dose combination drugs containing hydrochlorothiazide (Tekturna HCT), amlodipine (Tekamlo), and valsartan (Valturna). The most common adverse effects of aliskiren are diarrhea, cough, flu-like symptoms, and rash.

NURSING PROCESS FOCUS   Patients Receiving ACE Inhibitor Therapy

ASSESSMENT	POTENTIAL NURSING DIAGNOSES
Prior to administration: ■ Obtain a complete health history including cardiovascular conditions, neurological status, any incidence of angioedema, allergies, drug history, and possible drug interactions. ■ Acquire the results of a complete physical examination, including vital signs, height weight and ECG (compare to previous baseline values.) ■ Evaluate laboratory blood findings: CBC, electrolytes, lipid panel, and renal and liver function studies.	■ *Risk for Injury* related to orthostatic hypotension ■ *Deficient Knowledge* related to a lack of information about drug therapy ■ *Ineffective Tissue Perfusion* related to decreased blood volume ■ *Risk for Imbalanced Nutrition:* More than body requirements related to hyperkalemia ■ *Noncompliance* related to adverse effects of medications

PLANNING: PATIENT GOALS AND EXPECTED OUTCOMES

The patient will:
■ Experience therapeutic effects (a reduction in systolic/diastolic blood pressure and normal electrolyte levels).
■ Be free from or experience minimal adverse effects from drug therapy.
■ Verbalize an understanding of the drug's use, adverse effects, and required precautions.

IMPLEMENTATION

Interventions and (Rationales)	Patient Education/Discharge Planning
■ Monitor for first-dose phenomenon of profound hypotension. (First-dose phenomenon includes the relatively minor adverse effects of dry cough and hypotension.)	■ Warn the patient about the first-dose phenomenon; reassure that this effect diminishes with continued therapy.
■ Monitor vital signs, especially blood pressure. (ACE inhibitors can cause hypotension.)	Instruct the patient: ■ To monitor blood pressure as specified by the healthcare provider and ensure proper use of home equipment. ■ That changes in consciousness may occur due to rapid reduction in blood pressure and to immediately report feelings of faintness. ■ That the drug takes effect in approximately one hour and peaks in three to four hours. ■ To rest in the supine position beginning one hour after administration and for three hours after the first dose. ■ To always rise slowly, avoiding sudden posture changes.
■ Monitor for changes in level of consciousness, dizziness, drowsiness, or lightheadedness. (Signs of decreased blood flow to the brain are due to the drug's hypotensive action. Sudden fainting episodes are possible.)	Instruct the patient to: ■ Report dizziness or fainting that persists beyond the first dose as well as unusual sensations (e.g., numbness and tingling) or other changes in the face or limbs to the healthcare provider. ■ Contact the healthcare provider before the next scheduled dose of the drug if fainting occurs.
■ Ensure patient safety. (Postural hypotension may cause dizziness, affecting the ability to perform normal activities.)	Instruct the patient to: ■ Obtain help prior to getting out of bed or attempting to walk alone. ■ Avoid driving or other activities that require mental alertness or physical coordination until effects of the drug are known.
■ Observe for hypersensitivity reaction, particularly angioedema. (Angioedema may arise at any time during ACE inhibitor therapy, but it is generally expected shortly after initiation of therapy.)	Instruct the patient: ■ To immediately report any difficulty breathing, throat tightness, muscle cramps, hives or rash, or tremors to the healthcare provider. (These symptoms can occur as early as the first dose or much later as a delayed reaction.) ■ That angioedema can be life threatening and to call emergency medical services if severe dyspnea or hoarseness is accompanied by swelling of the face or mouth.
■ Monitor for persistent dry cough, a possible adverse effect of the drug. Monitor changes in cough pattern. (This may indicate another disease process.)	Instruct the patient to: ■ Expect persistent dry cough. ■ Report any change in the character or frequency of cough. (Any cough accompanied by shortness of breath, fever, or chest pain should be reported *immediately* to the healthcare provider because it may indicate MI.) ■ Sleep with the head elevated if cough becomes troublesome when in the supine position. ■ Use nonmedicated sugar-free lozenges or hard candies to relieve cough.

continued . . .

NURSING PROCESS FOCUS   (continued)

Interventions and (Rationales)	Patient Education/Discharge Planning
■ Monitor for dehydration or fluid overload. (Dehydration causes low circulating blood volume and will exacerbate hypotension. Severe dehydration may trigger syncope and collapse.)	Instruct the patient to: ■ Observe for signs of dehydration, such as oliguria, dry lips and mucous membranes, or poor skin turgor. ■ Report any bodily swelling that leaves sunken marks on the skin when pressed to the healthcare provider. ■ Measure and monitor fluid intake and output, and weigh daily. ■ Monitor increased need for fluids caused by vomiting, diarrhea, or excessive sweating. ■ Avoid excessive heat that contributes to sweating and fluid loss. ■ Consume adequate amounts of *plain* water.
■ Monitor for high potassium levels. (Hyperkalemia is a potentially life-threatening complication. Patients on ACE inhibitors should regularly have blood tests to measure potassium levels.)	Instruct the patient to: ■ Immediately report any signs of hyperkalemia to the healthcare provider: nausea, irregular heartbeat, profound fatigue/muscle weakness, and slow or faint pulse. ■ Avoid consuming electrolyte-fortified snacks, or sports drinks that may contain potassium. ■ Avoid using salt substitute (KCl) to flavor foods. ■ Consult the healthcare provider before taking any nutritional supplements containing potassium.
■ Monitor for liver and kidney function. (ACE inhibitors are metabolized by the liver and excreted by the kidneys.)	Instruct the patient to: ■ Report signs of liver toxicity such as nausea; vomiting; anorexia; diarrhea; rash; jaundice; abdominal pain, tenderness, or distension; or change in the color or character of stools to the healthcare provider. ■ Discontinue the drug immediately and contact the healthcare provider if jaundice occurs. ■ Adhere to laboratory testing regimen as ordered by the healthcare provider.
■ Administer medication correctly and evaluate the patient's knowledge level of proper administration. (Some medications interact with other medications.)	Instruct the patient: ■ That taking other antihypertensive drugs may increase risk for hypotension. ■ Not to take medication with grapefruit juice. ■ To consult a healthcare provider before taking potassium supplements or potassium-sparing diuretics. ■ That nonsteroidal anti-inflammatory drugs may reduce the actions of ACE inhibitors.

EVALUATION OF OUTCOME CRITERIA

Evaluate the effectiveness of drug therapy by confirming that patient goals and expected outcomes have been met (see "Planning"). *See Table 18.5 for a list of drugs to which these nursing actions apply.*

Drug Prototype: Pr *Enalapril (Vasotec)*

Therapeutic Class: **Drug for hypertension and heart failure**   Pharmacologic Class: **ACE inhibitor**

Actions and Uses: Enalapril is one of the most common ACE inhibitors prescribed for HTN. Unlike captopril, the first ACE inhibitor to be marketed, enalapril has a prolonged half-life, which permits administration once or twice daily. Enalapril acts by reducing angiotensin II and aldosterone levels to produce a significant reduction in blood pressure, with few adverse effects. Enalapril has effectiveness comparable to the thiazide diuretics and the beta-adrenergic blockers. It may be used by itself or in combination with other antihypertensives. Vaseretic is a fixed-dose combination of enalapril and hydrochlorothiazide.

Adverse Effects and Interactions: Unlike diuretics, ACE inhibitors such as enalapril have little effect on electrolyte balance, and unlike beta-adrenergic blockers, they cause few cardiac adverse effects. Like other antihypertensive drugs, enalapril may cause hypotension, especially when moving quickly from a supine to an upright position. This condition, known as postural or orthostatic hypotension, can cause lightheadedness and even

fainting. Care must be taken because a rapid fall in blood pressure may occur following the first dose. Most drugs in this class cause a persistent, dry cough. Other adverse effects include headache and dizziness.

Thiazide diuretics increase the risk of excessive potassium loss when used with enalapril. On the other hand, potassium-sparing diuretics increase the risk of hyperkalemia when used with ACE inhibitors.

Enalapril may induce lithium toxicity by reducing renal clearance of lithium. Nonsteroidal anti-inflammatory drugs (NSAIDs) may reduce the effectiveness of ACE inhibitors.

BLACK BOX WARNING:
Fetal injury and death may occur when ACE inhibitors or ARBs are taken during pregnancy. When pregnancy is detected, they should be discontinued as soon as possible.

CORE CONCEPT 18.10

Calcium channel blockers have emerged as important drugs in the treatment of hypertension.

Calcium channel blockers (CCBs) comprise a group of drugs that are used to treat a number of cardiovascular diseases, including angina pectoris, cardiac dysrhythmias, and HTN. When CCBs were first approved for the treatment of angina in the early 1980s, it was quickly noted that a "side effect" of the drugs was the lowering of blood pressure in patients with HTN. Although not usually prescribed as monotherapy for chronic HTN, CCBs are useful in treating patients who are unresponsive to other antihypertensive classes, such as elderly patients and blacks. Table 18.4 ◆ lists CCBs that are commonly used to treat HTN.

Contraction of a muscle is regulated by the amount of calcium ions inside the muscle cell. Muscular contraction occurs when Ca^{2+} enters the cell through channels in the plasma membrane. CCBs block these channels and prevent Ca^{2+} from entering the cell, thus inhibiting muscular contraction. At low doses, CCBs cause vasodilation in arterioles, thus decreasing blood pressure. Some CCBs, such as nifedipine (Adalat CC, Procardia XL), are selective for calcium channels in arterioles, whereas others, such as verapamil (Calan, Isoptin, others), affect channels in both arterioles and cardiac muscle. CCBs vary in their potency and in the frequency and types of adverse effects produced. The use of CCBs in the treatment of dysrhythmias and angina is discussed in Chapters 22 and 20, respectively.

Two CCBs, clevidipine (Cleviprex) and nicardipine (Cardene) are important drugs for treating patients with serious, life-threatening HTN. Clevidipine has an ultrashort half-life of one minute and is only available by the IV route for hypertensive emergencies.

The high safety profile of CCBs has contributed to their popularity in treating HTN. Common adverse effects related to their vasodilation action include headache, facial flushing, and dizziness. The CCBs that affect the heart should be used cautiously in patients with preexisting cardiac disease.

TABLE 18.4 Calcium Channel Blockers for Hypertension		
Drug	**Route And Adult Dose**	**Remarks**
amlodipine (Norvasc)	PO; 5–10 mg once daily (max: 10 mg/day)	Works primarily on peripheral circulation; reduces systolic, diastolic, and mean blood pressure; also for angina
diltiazem (Cardizem, Cartia XT, Dilacor XR, others) (see page 309 for the Drug Prototype box)	PO; 120–240 mg daily or 20–120 mg bid	Dilates coronary arteries; affects calcium channels in both heart and blood vessels; extended-release and IV forms are available; also for angina and dysrhythmias
felodipine (Plendil)	PO; 5–10 mg/day (max: 20 mg/day)	Selective for calcium channels in blood vessels; also for angina and HF
isradipine (DynaCirc)	PO; 1.25–10 mg bid (max: 20 mg/day)	Affects calcium channels in both heart and blood vessels; also for angina
nicardipine (Cardene)	PO; 20–40 mg tid (max: 120 mg/day) PO (Sustained release): 30–60 mg bid	Selective for calcium channels in blood vessels; also for angina; IV form is available
ⓟ nifedipine (Adalat CC, Procardia XL)	PO; 10–20 mg tid (max: 180 mg/day) PO (extended release); 30–60 mg once daily	Selective for calcium channels in blood vessels; decreases peripheral vascular resistance, and increases cardiac output; also for angina
nisoldipine (Nisocor)	PO; 10–20 mg bid (max: 60 mg/day)	Structurally similar to nifedipine; affects calcium channels in both the heart and blood vessels; also for angina and HF
verapamil (Calan, Isoptin SR, others) (see page 342 for the Drug Prototype box)	PO; 40–80 mg tid (max: 480 mg/day) PO (sustained release): 90–240 mg 1–2 times/day	Affects calcium channels in both heart and blood vessels; IV form available for specific dysrhythmias

Drug Prototype: ℗ *Nifedipine (Adalat CC, Procardia XL)*

Therapeutic Class: Drug for hypertension and angina   **Pharmacologic Class: Calcium channel blocker**

Actions and Uses: Nifedipine is a CCB prescribed for angina as well as for HTN. Nifedipine selectively blocks calcium channels in myocardial and vascular smooth muscle, including that in the coronary arteries. This results in reduced oxygen demands by the heart, an increase in cardiac output, and a fall in blood pressure. It is available as immediate-release capsules and as extended-release tablets (XL).

Adverse Effects and Interactions: Adverse effects of nifedipine are generally minor and related to vasodilation, such as headache, dizziness, and flushing. Fast-acting forms of nifedipine can cause significant reflex tachycardia. To avoid rebound hypotension, discontinuation of drug therapy should occur gradually.

Nifedipine may increase serum levels of digoxin, cimetidine, and ranitidine, and increase the effects of warfarin, resulting in increased partial thromboplastin time (PTT). It may also increase the effects of fentanyl anesthesia, resulting in severe hypotension and an increased need for fluids. Grapefruit juice may enhance the absorption of nifedipine.

Alcohol increases the vasodilating action of nifedipine and can lead to a severe drop in blood pressure. Nicotine causes vasoconstriction, countering the desired effect of nifedipine. Use with melatonin may increase blood pressure and heart rate.

NURSING PROCESS FOCUS   Patients Receiving Calcium Channel Blocker Therapy

ASSESSMENT	POTENTIAL NURSING DIAGNOSES
Prior to administration: ■ Obtain a complete health history including cardiovascular, respiratory, neurological, renal and liver conditions, allergies, drug history, and possible drug interactions. ■ Evaluate laboratory blood findings: CBC, electrolytes, lipid panel, and renal and liver function studies. ■ Acquire the results of a complete physical examination, including vital signs, height, weight, ECG, neurological status and signs of edema.	■ *Ineffective Self-health Maintenance* related to insufficient knowledge of seriousness of disease and drug therapy regimen ■ *Deficient Knowledge* related to a lack of information about drug therapy unfamiliarity with medication information ■ *Decreased Cardiac Output* related to effects of drug therapy ■ *Risk for Injury* related to possible orthostatic hypotension ■ *Noncompliance* related to adverse effects of medications

PLANNING: PATIENT GOALS AND EXPECTED OUTCOMES

The patient will:
■ Experience therapeutic effects (reduction in systolic/diastolic blood pressure).
■ Be free from or experience minimal adverse effects from drug therapy.
■ Verbalize an understanding of the drug's use, adverse effects, and required precautions.

IMPLEMENTATION

Interventions and (Rationales)	Patient Education/Discharge Planning
■ Monitor vital signs and ECG. Obtain blood pressure readings in sitting, standing, and supine positions to monitor fluctuations in blood pressure. (CCBs dilate the arteries, reducing blood pressure and possibly causing hypotension.)	Instruct the patient to: ■ Monitor vital signs as specified by the nurse, particularly the blood pressure, ensuring proper use of home equipment. ■ Withhold medication for severe hypotensive readings as specified by the nurse (e.g., "hold for levels below 88/50 mmHg"). ■ Immediately report palpitations or rapid heartbeat.
■ Observe for changes in level of consciousness, dizziness, fatigue, postural hypotension. (These adverse effects can be caused by vasodilation.) ■ Observe for paradoxical increase in chest pain, angina symptoms, or increase in heart rate. (These complaints may be related to severe hypotension.)	Instruct the patient to: ■ Report dizziness or lightheadedness to the healthcare provider. ■ Rise slowly from prolonged periods of sitting or lying down. ■ Inform patient to report chest pain or other angina-like symptoms immediately to the healthcare provider.
■ Monitor for signs of HF. (CCBs can decrease myocardial contractility, increasing the risk of HF.)	■ Instruct the patient to immediately report any severe shortness of breath, frothy sputum, profound fatigue, and swelling to the healthcare provider. These may be signs of HF or fluid accumulation in the lungs.

continued . . .

Interventions and (Rationales)	Patient Education/Discharge Planning
■ Monitor for fluid accumulation. Measure intake and output, and daily weights. (Edema is an adverse effect of some CCBs.)	Instruct the patient to: ■ Avoid excessive heat, which contributes to excessive sweating and fluid loss. ■ Measure and monitor fluid intake and output, and weigh daily. ■ Consume enough *plain* water to remain adequately, but not overly, hydrated.
■ Observe for hypersensitivity reaction. (Allergic responses may be life threatening.)	■ Instruct the patient to immediately report difficulty breathing, throat tightness, hives or rash, muscle cramps, or tremors to the healthcare provider.
■ Monitor liver and kidney function. (CCBs are metabolized in the liver and excreted by the kidneys.)	Instruct the patient to: ■ Report signs of liver toxicity to the healthcare provider: nausea, vomiting, anorexia, bleeding, severe upper abdominal pain, heartburn, jaundice, or a change in the color or character of stools. ■ Report signs of renal toxicity to the healthcare provider: fever, flank pain, changes in urine output, color, or character (cloudy, with sediment). ■ Adhere to laboratory testing regimens as ordered by the healthcare provider.
■ Observe for constipation. May need to increase dietary fiber or administer laxatives. (CCBs may cause constipation.)	Advise the patient to: ■ Maintain adequate fluid and fiber intake to facilitate stool passage. ■ Use a bulk laxative or stool softener, as recommended by the healthcare provider.
■ Ensure patient safety. Monitor ambulation until response to the drug is known. (Some CCBs may cause drowsiness.)	■ Instruct the patient to avoid driving or other activities that require mental alertness or physical coordination until the effects of the drug are known.
■ Administer medication correctly and evaluate the patient's knowledge level of proper administration. (Some medications interact with other medications.)	Instruct the patient: ■ That taking other antihypertensive drugs may increase risk for hypotension. ■ To avoid rebound hypotension, this drug should be discontinued gradually ■ Not to take nifedipine with grapefruit juice because it may enhance absorption. ■ That alcohol potentiates vasodilating action of nifedipine

EVALUATION OF OUTCOME CRITERIA

Evaluate the effectiveness of drug therapy by confirming that patient goals and expected outcomes have been met (see "Planning"). *See Table 18.4 for a list of drugs to which these nursing actions apply.*

CAM THERAPY

Grape Seed Extract for Hypertension

Grapes and grape seeds have been used to enhance wellness for thousands of years. Their primary use has been for cardiovascular conditions such as HTN, high blood cholesterol, atherosclerosis, and to generally improve circulation. Some claim that grape seed extract improves wound healing, prevents cancer, and lowers the risk for the long-term consequences of diabetes.

The grape seeds, usually obtained from winemaking, are crushed and placed into tablet, capsule, or liquid forms. Grape seed extract has antioxidant properties. In general, antioxidants improve wound healing and repair cellular injury. Preliminary evidence suggests that it may have some benefit in repairing blood vessel damage that could lead to atherosclerosis and HTN. Controlled, long-term studies on the effects of grape seed extract on HTN have not been conducted. It has few adverse effects, but caution should be used if taking anticoagulant drugs because increased bleeding may result. Overall, the benefits of grape seed extract are no different than those of a diet balanced with natural antioxidants and an occasional glass of red wine.

Adrenergic blockers are commonly used to treat hypertension.

Stimulation of the sympathetic division of the autonomic nervous system causes "fight-or-flight" responses such as faster heart rate, an increase in blood pressure, and bronchodilation. By blocking the sympathetic fight-or-flight responses, adrenergic drugs can cause the heart rate to slow, blood pressure to decline, and the bronchi to dilate. Adrenergic antagonists (or blockers) that are important in managing HTN are listed in Table 18.5 ◆.

Because of their beneficial effects on the heart and vessels, adrenergic blockers are used for a wide variety of cardiovascular disorders. These drugs can block the effects of the sympathetic division through a number of different mechanisms, although they all have in common the effect of lowering blood pressure. These mechanisms include the following:

- Blockade of alpha$_1$-receptors in the arterioles
- Blockade of beta$_1$-receptors in the heart
- Nonselective blockade of both beta$_1$- and beta$_2$-receptors
- Stimulation of alpha$_2$-adrenergic receptors in the brainstem (centrally acting)

TABLE 18.5   Adrenergic Blockers and Central-Acting Drugs for Hypertension

Drug	Route and Adult Dose	Remarks
acebutolol (Sectral)	PO; 400–800 mg/day (max: 1200 mg/day)	Selective beta$_1$-blocker; also for premature ventricular beats
atenolol (Tenormin) (see page 309 for the Drug Prototype box)	PO; 25–50 mg/day (max: 100 mg/day)	Selective beta$_1$-blocker; IV form available for MI; monitor apical pulse prior to administration
betaxolol (Kerlone)	PO; 10–40 mg/day (max: 40 mg/day)	Selective beta$_1$-blocker; approved for HTN only; discontinue drug gradually to avoid rebound HTN
bisoprolol (Zebeta)	PO; 2.5–5 mg daily (max: 20 mg/day)	Selective beta$_1$-blocker; also for angina; discontinue the drug gradually to avoid rebound HTN
carvedilol (Coreg) (see page 296 for the Drug Prototype box)	PO; 6.25 mg bid (max: 50 mg/day)	Blocks both alpha and beta receptors; also for HF
clonidine (Catapres)	PO; 0.1 mg bid–tid (max: 0.8 mg/day)	Central-acting alpha$_2$-adrenergic drug; transdermal patch available; epidural infusion form available for management of cancer pain
Pr doxazosin (Cardura)	PO; 1 mg at bedtime; may increase to 16 mg/day in one to two divided doses (max: 16 mg/day)	Selective alpha$_1$-blocker; also for benign prostatic hyperplasia (BPH)
methyldopa (Aldomet)	PO; 250 mg bid or tid (max: 3 g/day)	Central-acting alpha$_2$-adrenergic drug; IV form available; lowers standing and supine blood pressure
metoprolol (Lopressor, Toprol)	PO; 50–100 mg daily or bid (max: 450 mg/day)	Selective beta$_1$-blocker; sustained-release and IV forms available; also for angina and MI
nadolol (Corgard)	PO; 40 mg/day (max: 320 mg/day)	Nonselective beta blocker; also for angina
pindolol (Visken)	PO; 5 mg bid (max: 60 mg/day)	Nonselective beta$_1$- and beta$_2$-blocker; for HTN only
prazosin (Minipress) (see page 100 for the Drug Prototype box)	PO; 1 mg at bedtime; increase to 1 mg bid–tid (max: 20 mg/day)	Selective alpha$_1$-blocker used in combination with other antihypertensives; also for BPH, Raynaud's disease, and pheochromocytoma
propranolol (Inderal, InnoPran XL) (see page 340 for the Drug Prototype box)	PO; 40 mg bid but may be increased to 160–480 mg/day in divided doses (max: 480 mg/day)	Nonselective beta$_1$- and beta$_2$-blocker; also for angina, MI, dysrhythmias, and migraine prophylaxis; IV form available
Terazosin (Hytrin)	PO; 1 mg at bedtime; increase 1–5 mg/day (max: 20 mg/day)	Selective alpha$_1$-blocker; also for BPH
timolol (Betimol, Timoptic, others) (see page 604 for the Drug Prototype box)	PO; 10 mg bid (max: 60 mg/day)	Nonselective beta$_1$- and beta$_2$-blocker; also for MI and migraine prophylaxis and for glaucoma

Drug Prototype: Ⓟ *Doxazosin (Cardura)*

Therapeutic Class: Drug for hypertension and BPH   **Pharmacologic Class: Alpha₁-adrenergic blocker**

Actions and Uses: Doxazosin is an adrenergic blocker available only in oral form. Because it is selective for blocking alpha₁-receptors in vascular smooth muscle, it has few adverse effects on other autonomic organs and is sometimes preferred over nonselective beta blockers such as propranolol. Doxazosin dilates both arteries and veins and is capable of causing a rapid, profound fall in blood pressure. Although prazosin was the first alpha blocker available for hypertension, other alpha blockers such as doxazosin and terazosin (Hytrin) are more widely used because they can be taken once daily.

Doxazosin and several other alpha blockers also relax smooth muscle around the prostate gland. Patients who have difficulty urinating due to an enlarged prostate, a condition known as benign prostatic hyperplasia (BPH), sometimes receive these drugs to relieve symptoms of this disease, as discussed in Chapter 34.

Adverse Effects and Interactions: When starting doxazosin therapy, some patients experience orthostatic hypotension, although tolerance normally develops to this adverse effect after a few doses. Dizziness and headache are also common adverse effects, although they are rarely severe enough to cause discontinuation of therapy. Oral cimetidine may cause a mild increase (10%) in the half-life of doxazosin. Concurrent administration of doxazosin with phosphodiesterase–5 inhibitors, such as sildenafil (Viagra) can result in additive BP lowering effects and hypotension.

Some drugs, such as epinephrine, affect both beta- and alpha-adrenergic receptors and can cause serious adverse effects. Drugs that affect only one receptor subtype produce fewer adverse effects. Prazosin (Minipress), for example, is specific to alpha₁-receptors and thus has less effect on the heart, which contains beta₁-receptors. On the other hand, atenolol (Tenormin) and metoprolol (Lopressor, Toprol) are selective for beta₁-receptors and thus have little effect on the bronchi, which have beta₂-receptors. Of the adrenergic antagonists, only the beta-blockers are considered first-line drugs for the pharmacotherapy of HTN.

ortho = *straight*
static = *causing to stand*

brady = *slow*
cardia = *heart*

The adverse effects of adrenergic antagonists are predictable because they are extensions that would be expected from blocking the fight-or-flight response. The alpha₁-blockers tend to cause **orthostatic hypotension** in patients when they move quickly from a supine to an upright position. Dizziness, nausea, **bradycardia**, and dry mouth are also common. Less common, though sometimes a major cause for nonadherence, is their adverse effect on male sexual function (impotence). Because nonselective beta blockers slow the heart rate and cause bronchoconstriction, they should be used with caution in patients with asthma or HF.

Some adrenergic blockers affect the production of neurotransmitters in the *central* nervous system rather than affecting the *peripheral* nervous system. For example, methyldopa (Aldomet) is converted to a **false neurotransmitter** in the brainstem, thus causing a shortage of the "real" neurotransmitter and inhibition of the sympathetic nervous system. Clonidine (Catapres), an alpha₂ blocker, affects alpha-adrenergic receptors in the cardiovascular control centers in the brainstem. The central acting drugs have a tendency to produce sedation and are infrequently prescribed.

Concept Review 18.3

■ Why is it important for the patient to weigh himself or herself on a regular basis when taking antihypertensive drugs?

CORE CONCEPT 18.12

Vasodilators lower blood pressure by relaxing arteriolar smooth muscle.

Many of the antihypertensive drugs discussed thus far lower blood pressure through *indirect* means by affecting enzymes (ACE inhibitors), autonomic nerves (alpha and beta blockers), or fluid volume (diuretics). It would seem that a more efficient way to reduce blood pressure would be to cause a direct relaxation of arteriolar smooth muscle. Indeed, drugs that directly affect vascular smooth muscle are highly effective at lowering blood pressure, but they produce too many adverse effects to be drugs of first choice. The direct-acting vasodilators used for hypertension are listed in Table 18.6 ◆.

TABLE 18.6   Direct-Acting Vasodilators for Hypertension

Drug	Route and Adult Dose	Remarks
Pr hydralazine (Apresoline)	PO; 10–50 mg qid (max: 300 mg/day)	Diastolic response usually greater than systolic; IV and IM forms available.
minoxidil (Loniten)	PO; 5–40 mg/day (max: 100 mg/day)	Reserved for severe hypertension; topical form used to promote hair growth.
nitroprusside (Nitropress)	IV; 0.5–10 mcg/kg/min	For hypertensive crisis; produces both arteriolar and venous dilation; infusion not to exceed 10 min.

Direct vasodilators produce reflex tachycardia, a normal physiologic response to the sudden decrease in blood pressure caused by the drug. Reflex tachycardia forces the heart to work harder, and blood pressure increases, counteracting the effect of the antihypertensive drug. Patients with coronary artery disease could experience an acute angina attack. Fortunately, reflex tachycardia can be prevented by the concurrent administration of a beta blocker, such as propranolol.

A second potentially serious adverse effect of direct vasodilator therapy is sodium and water retention. As the kidney retains more sodium and water, blood volume increases, thus raising blood pressure and canceling the antihypertensive action of the vasodilator. A diuretic may be administered concurrently with a direct vasodilator to prevent fluid retention.

One direct-acting vasodilator, nitroprusside (Nitropress), is the traditional drug of choice for hypertensive emergency, a condition in which diastolic pressure is greater than 120 mmHg and there is evidence of organ damage, usually to the heart, kidney, or brain. This potentially life-threatening condition must be controlled quickly. Nitroprusside has the ability to lower blood pressure almost instantaneously on IV administration. Care must be taken not to decrease blood pressure too quickly because this can result in hypotension and severe restriction of blood flow to the cerebral, coronary, or renal capillaries.

Drug Prototype: **Pr** *Hydralazine (Apresoline)*
Therapeutic Class: **Drug for hypertension and heart failure**   Pharmacologic Class: **Direct-acting vasodilator**

Actions and Uses: Hydralazine was one of the first oral antihypertensive drugs marketed in the United States. Therapy is generally begun with low doses, which are gradually increased until the desired therapeutic response is obtained. After several months of therapy, tolerance to the drug develops and a dosage increase may be necessary. Although it produces an effective reduction in blood pressure, drugs in other antihypertensive classes have largely replaced hydralazine because of its many adverse effects. However, this may change due to the approval of BiDil, a fixed-dose combination of isosorbide dinitrate and hydralazine that appears to be effective at lowering blood pressure in African Americans.

Adverse Effects and Interactions: Headache, reflex tachycardia, palpitations, flushing, nausea, and diarrhea are common but may resolve as therapy progresses. Patients taking hydralazine often receive a beta blocker to counteract reflex tachycardia. The drug may produce a lupus-like syndrome with extended use. Sodium and fluid retention is another potentially serious adverse effect. The use of hydralazine is mostly limited to patients whose HTN cannot be controlled with safer medications.

Administering hydralazine with other antihypertensives or monoamine oxidase (MAO) inhibitors may cause severe hypotension. This includes all drug classes used as antihypertensives. NSAIDs may decrease the antihypertensive response of hydralazine.

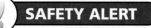

PATIENTS NEED TO KNOW

Patients treated for HTN need to know the following:
1. Take medications as prescribed.
2. Never discontinue the medication without approval from a healthcare provider.
3. To control HTN, incorporate lifestyle changes such as diet and exercise, even if blood pressure is brought into normal limits by the medication.
4. Check blood pressure on a regular basis and report significant variations to the healthcare provider.
5. Get out of bed slowly to avoid dizziness.
6. If taking loop or thiazide diuretics, potassium supplements or an increased intake of potassium-rich foods such as bananas, dried fruits, and orange juice may be necessary.
7. Take weight measurements regularly and report abnormal weight gains or losses.
8. Do not take any over-the-counter (OTC) medications for colds, flu, or allergies without first checking with a healthcare provider.

SAFETY ALERT

Drug-to-Food Interactions

Certain drug–food interactions can be very dangerous. For example, the combination of grapefruit juice and certain blood pressure-lowering drugs or some cholesterol-lowering drugs can cause toxic levels of the drug in the blood. It is advisable for patients to keep medications in their original, labeled containers so that instructions are readily available. The nurse should ensure that patients are fully informed about how to take their drugs by providing both oral and written instructions.

CHAPTER REVIEW

CORE CONCEPTS SUMMARY

18.1 Hypertension is characterized by the consistent elevation of arterial blood pressure.

A patient having a sustained blood pressure of 140/90 mmHg after multiple measurements made over several clinic visits is said to have hypertension (HTN). HTN is classified into three categories—prehypertension, Stage 1, and Stage 2.

18.2 Failure to treat hypertension can lead to stroke, heart failure, or myocardial infarction.

HTN is one of the most common diseases. Uncontrolled HTN can cause chronic and debilitating disorders such as stroke, heart attack, and heart failure.

18.3 Blood pressure is caused by the pumping action of the heart.

As the heart pumps, it creates pressure that is greatest in the arteries closest to the heart. The pressure created by the heart's contraction is called systolic pressure, and that present during the heart's relaxation is called diastolic pressure.

18.4 The primary factors responsible for blood pressure are cardiac output, the resistance of the small arteries, and blood volume.

As blood leaves the heart, its pressure depends on how much blood is present in the vessels (blood volume), how much is ejected per minute, and how much resistance it encounters from the small arteries (peripheral resistance). These are considered the primary factors controlling blood pressure.

18.5 Many nervous and hormonal factors help to keep blood pressure within normal limits.

Clusters of neurons in the medulla known as the vasomotor center regulate blood pressure. Feedback is provided to the vasomotor center by baroreceptors in the aorta and carotid arteries. Hormones such as epinephrine or ADH may have profound effects on blood pressure.

18.6 Positive lifestyle changes can reduce blood pressure and lessen the need for medications.

Because antihypertensive drugs may have uncomfortable adverse effects, lifestyle changes such as proper diet and exercise are often implemented prior to and during drug therapy to enable lower drug doses.

18.7 Selection of specific antihypertensive drugs depends on the severity of the disease.

Drug therapy of HTN often begins with low doses of a single drug. If ineffective, a second drug from a different class may be added to the regimen. Multidrug therapy is common.

18.8 Diuretics are often preferred drugs for treating mild to moderate hypertension.

Diuretics are often drugs of first choice for HTN because they have few adverse effects and can control minor to moderate HTN. Electrolytes should be carefully monitored in patients taking diuretics.

18.9 Blocking the renin-angiotensin-aldosterone system leads to a decrease in blood pressure.

Blocking angiotensin-converting enzyme (ACE) or the angiotensin II receptor can prevent the intense vasoconstriction caused by angiotensin. These drugs also decrease blood volume, which aids in producing their antihypertensive effect.

18.10 Calcium channel blockers have emerged as important drugs in the treatment of hypertension.

Calcium channel blockers (CCBs) block calcium ions from entering smooth muscle cells, causing arterioles to relax, thus reducing blood pressure. Some CCBs are also used to treat angina, heart failure, and dysrhythmias.

18.11 Adrenergic blockers are commonly used to treat hypertension.

Autonomic drugs that block alpha$_1$-receptors, block beta$_1$- and/or beta$_2$-receptors, or stimulate alpha$_2$-receptors in the brainstem (centrally acting) to lower blood pressure are available. Although acting by different mechanisms, these drugs all lower blood pressure.

18.12 Vasodilators lower blood pressure by relaxing arteriolar smooth muscle.

A few drugs lower blood pressure by directly relaxing arteriolar smooth muscle. Other than their use in treating hypertensive crisis, drugs in this class are not widely used because of their numerous adverse effects.

REVIEW QUESTIONS

The following questions are written in NCLEX-PN® style. Answer these questions to assess your knowledge of the chapter material, and go back and review any material that is not clear to you.

1. The nurse takes a patient's blood pressure at 142/92 mm Hg. In an adult patient, this level is considered:

1. Normal
2. Prehypertension
3. Hypertension, stage 1
4. Hypertension, stage 2

2. Just prior to starting antihypertensive therapy, the nurse obtains an ECG and the baseline heart rate of a patient. This was done because the effects of the medication he or she will be taking affects heart function and rate. What medication will the patient most likely be taking?

1. Cardizem
2. Micardis
3. Diuril
4. Nitropress

3. The patient is on two antihypertensive drugs. The nurse recognizes that the advantage of multidrug treatment is:

1. Blood pressure decreases faster.
2. Adverse effects are fewer.
3. There is less daily medication dosing.
4. Multidrug therapy treats the patient's other medical conditions.

4. The patient is taking furosemide (Lasix) 40 mg bid. The nurse monitors the patient's lab report for:

1. Hyperkalemia
2. Hypokalemia
3. Hypernatremia
4. Hypercalcemia

5. The patient has been taking losartan (Cozaar) for his hypertension. The physician has determined that the current medication regimen is not effective. Which of the following drugs may be added to the treatment plan?

1. Felodipine (Plendil)
2. Methyldopa (Aldomet)
3. Atenolol (Tenormin)
4. Hydrochlorothiazide (Microzide)

6. The patient has been started on antihypertensives. The nurse monitors the patient for:

1. Nausea and vomiting
2. Diarrhea
3. Dizziness
4. Tetany

7. A patient with hypertension has a medication order for diltiazem HCL 60 mg po twice a day. How many tablet(s) will the nurse administer in a day if the medication comes only as 120 mg per tablet:

1. Half tablet in the morning
2. Half tablet, once in the morning and one in the evening
3. One tablet in the morning
4. One tablet in the morning and one in the evening

8. The nurse is helping to develop a presentation on the different types of medications used for hypertension. The presentation will be conducted at a local church as part of their health ministry. One of the types of antihypertensive medications that will be included is the one that affects the renin-angiotensin-aldosterone system to increase urine. This medication is a(n):

1. Calcium channel blocker
2. Adrenergic blocker
3. ACE inhibitor
4. Direct-acting vasodilator

9. The patient has started on a direct-acting vasodilator. To make sure the patient understands how this medication works, the nurse includes what information in the teaching plan?

1. They block calcium from entering smooth muscle, causing arterioles to relax.
2. They block receptors in the brainstem to lower blood pressure.
3. They block the angiotensin-converting enzyme to prevent vessel constriction.
4. They relax smooth muscles in the blood vessels to decrease peripheral resistance.

10. The patient is on an ACE inhibitor. As a result of this therapy, the nurse checks for which of the following:

1. Hypokalemia
2. Hyperkalemia
3. Hypernatremia
4. Hyperglycemia

CASE STUDY QUESTIONS

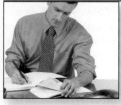 Remember Mr. Rodriguez, the patient introduced at the beginning of the chapter? Now read the remainder of the case study. Based on the information you have learned in this chapter, answer the questions that follow.

Mr. Paul Rodriguez was admitted to the emergency department unconscious with a nose bleed that wouldn't stop. His blood pressure was measured as 210/120 mmHg, and the doctor ordered that he be immediately placed on nitroprusside (Nitropress). He stayed in the hospital for two days and was discharged with a blood pressure of 135/88 mmHg. On discharge, Mr. Rodriguez was given a prescription for Hyzaar with instructions on how it works, monitoring, possible adverse effects, and precautions.

1. Why was nitroprusside, rather than Hyzaar, used in the emergency department?

1. Nitroprusside is safer.
2. Nitroprusside has a longer duration of action.
3. Nitroprusside has a faster onset of action.
4. Mr. Rodriguez is allergic to Hyzaar.

2. What two drug classes are contained in Hyzaar?

1. Thiazide diuretic and angiotensin-receptor blocker
2. Thiazide diuretic and potassium-sparing diuretic
3. ACE inhibitor and potassium-sparing diuretic
4. Alpha-adrenergic blocker and ACE inhibitor

3. What instructions did the nurse provide to Mr. Rodriguez about Hyzaar?

1. Always rise slowly and avoid sudden changes in posture.
2. Take a daily potassium supplement.
3. Eat plenty of calcium-rich foods such as yogurt.
4. Do not exercise regularly because exercise may interfere with blood pressure regulation.

4. After eight months on Hyzaar, the physician switched Mr. Rodriguez to nifedipine (Procardia). He then reported to the nurse that he stopped taking the Procardia because it made him dizzy, and he felt his heart was racing. The nurse explained that this common adverse effect was probably due to:

1. Electrolyte imbalance
2. Underdosing of nifedipine
3. Excessive vasodilation of arteries
4. Reflex tachycardia

NOTE: Answers to the Review and Case Study Questions appear in Appendix B. The complete rationales and answers are located on the textbook's website.

Pearson Nursing Student Resources   Find additional review materials at **nursing.pearsonhighered.com**.

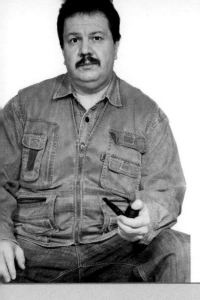

Drugs for Heart Failure

CORE CONCEPTS

19.1 Heart failure is closely associated with disorders such as chronic hypertension, coronary artery disease, and diabetes.

19.2 The central cause of heart failure is weakened heart muscle.

19.3 The three primary characteristics of heart function are force of contraction, heart rate, and speed of impulse conduction.

19.4 The specific therapy for heart failure depends on the severity of the disease.

19.5 Angiotensin-converting enzyme (ACE) inhibitors are the preferred drugs for heart failure.

19.6 Diuretics relieve symptoms of heart failure by reducing fluid overload and decreasing blood pressure.

19.7 Cardiac glycosides increase the force of myocardial contraction and were once the traditional drugs of choice for heart failure.

19.8 Beta-adrenergic blockers are used in combination with other drugs to slow the progression of heart failure.

19.9 Vasodilators reduce symptoms of heart failure by decreasing cardiac workload.

19.10 Phosphodiesterase inhibitors and other miscellaneous drugs are used for short-term therapy of advanced heart failure.

DRUG SNAPSHOT

The following drugs are discussed in this chapter:

DRUG CLASSES	DRUG PROTOTYPES
Angiotensin-converting enzyme (ACE) inhibitors	**Pr** lisinopril (Prinivil, Zestril) *292*
Diuretics	
Cardiac glycosides	**Pr** digoxin (Lanoxin, Lanoxicaps) *295*
Beta-adrenergic blockers	**Pr** carvedilol (Coreg) *296*

DRUG CLASSES	DRUG PROTOTYPES
Vasodilators	
Phosphodiesterase inhibitors and miscellaneous agents	**Pr** milrinone (Primacor) *297*

LEARNING OUTCOMES

After reading this chapter, the student should be able to:

1. Identify the major risk factors associated with the progression to heart failure.

2. Relate how the symptoms associated with heart failure may be caused by weakened heart muscle.

3. Identify drug classes that are used as first-line and second-line choices for the pharmacotherapy of heart failure.

4. Explain several means by which patients may manage their heart failure without drugs.

5. Categorize heart failure drugs based on their classifications and mechanisms of action.

6. For each of the classes listed in the Drug Snapshot, identify representative drugs and explain their mechanisms of drug action, primary actions, and important adverse effects.

KEY TERMS

afterload *289*
contractility (kon-trak-TILL-eh-tee) *289*
heart failure (HF) *288*
inotropic effect (in-oh-TRO-pik) *289*

natriuretic peptide (hBNP)
  (na-tree-ur-ET-ik) *297*
peripheral edema (purr-IF-ur-ul
  eh-DEE-mah) *289*

phosphodiesterase
  (fos-fo-die-ES-tur-ase) *297*
preload *289*

Heart failure (HF) is one of the most common and fatal of the cardiovascular diseases, and its incidence is expected to increase as the population ages. Despite the dramatic decline in death rates for most cardiovascular disease that has occurred over the past two decades, the death rate for HF has only recently begun to decrease. Although improved treatment of myocardial infarction (MI) and hypertension (HTN) has led to declines in mortality due to HF, approximately one in five patients dies within one year of diagnosis of HF, and 50% die within five years.

CORE CONCEPT 19.1

Heart failure is closely associated with disorders such as chronic hypertension, coronary artery disease, and diabetes.

Heart failure (HF) is the inability of the ventricles to pump enough blood to meet the body's metabolic demands. HF can be caused by any disorder that affects the heart's ability to receive or eject blood. Although weakening of cardiac muscle is a natural consequence of aging, the process can be accelerated by a number of diseases associated with HF that are shown in Table 19.1 ◆. There is no cure for HF; however, effective drug therapy can relieve many of the distressing symptoms of HF and may prolong patients' lives.

For many patients, HF is considered a *preventable* condition; controlling associated diseases will greatly reduce the risk of eventual HF. For example, controlling lipid levels and keeping blood pressure within normal limits will reduce the incidence of MI. Maintaining blood glucose within normal values can reduce the cardiovascular consequences of uncontrolled diabetes. Therefore, the therapy of HF is no longer just focused on end stages of the disorder. Pharmacotherapy is now targeted at prevention and slowing the progression of HF. This change in emphasis has led to significant improvements in survival and quality of life for patients with HF.

TABLE 19.1   Disorders Commonly Associated with Heart Failure

Disease	Description
Chronic hypertension	Sustained high systemic blood pressure
Coronary artery disease	Atherosclerosis of the coronary arteries
Diabetes	Lack of insulin or inability to tolerate carbohydrates
Mitral stenosis	Inability of the mitral valve to open fully
Myocardial infarction	Heart muscle death due to coronary artery obstruction

Fast Facts Heart Failure

- HF affects 10% of those over age 70.
- More than 58,000 people die of HF each year.
- African Americans have one-half to two times the incidence of HF as Whites.
- HF occurs slightly more frequently in men than in women.
- HF is twice as frequent in patients with hypertension and five times as frequent in persons who have experienced an MI.

The central cause of heart failure is weakened heart muscle.

Although a number of diseases can lead to HF, the end result is the same: The heart is unable to pump out the volume of blood required to meet the needs of the other organs. To understand how drugs act on the weakened heart muscle, it is essential to understand the underlying cardiac physiology.

The right side of the heart receives blood from the venous system and sends it to the lungs, where the blood receives oxygen and gives up its carbon dioxide. The blood returns to the left side of the heart, which sends it out to the rest of the body through the aorta. The amount of blood received by the right side should exactly equal that sent out by the left side. If this does not happen, HF may occur. The amount of blood pumped by each ventricle per minute is the cardiac output. The relationship between cardiac output and blood pressure is explained in Chapter 18.

Although many variables affect cardiac output, the two most important factors are preload and afterload. Just before the chambers of the heart contract (systole), they are filled to their maximum capacity with blood. The degree to which the cardiac muscle fibers are stretched just prior to contraction is **preload**. The more these fibers are stretched, the more forcefully they will contract. This is somewhat analogous to a rubber band: The more it is stretched, the more forcefully it will snap back. This strength of contraction of the heart is called **contractility**.

The second important factor affecting cardiac output is afterload. For the left ventricle to pump blood out of the heart, it must overcome a fairly substantial pressure in the aorta. The **afterload** is the amount of pressure in the aorta that must be overcome for blood to be ejected from the left ventricle. The greater afterload that occurs with chronic HTN creates a constant increased workload for the heart. This explains why patients with chronic HTN are more likely to experience HF. Lowering blood pressure results in less workload for the heart.

In HF, the myocardium becomes weakened, and the heart cannot eject all the blood it receives. This weakening may occur on the left side, the right side, or both sides of the heart. If it occurs on the left side, excess blood accumulates in the left ventricle. The wall of the left ventricle thickens and enlarges (*hypertrophy*) in an attempt to compensate for the increased workload. Because the left ventricle has limits to its ability to compensate, blood "backs up" into the lungs, resulting in the classic symptoms of cough and shortness of breath, particularly when the patient is lying down. Left HF is sometimes called *congestive* HF.

Although left-sided HF is more common, the right side of the heart can also become weak, either simultaneously with the left side or independently from the left side. In right HF, the blood "backs up" into the peripheral veins. This results in swelling of the feet and ankles, a condition known as **peripheral edema**, and engorgement of organs such as the liver. Figure 19.1 ■ illustrates the underlying pathophysiology of HF. Figure 19.2 ■ illustrates the signs and symptoms of the patient in HF.

The three primary characteristics of heart function are force of contraction, heart rate, and speed of impulse conduction.

Cardiac physiology is quite complex, particularly when the heart is challenged with a chronic disease such as HF. A simplified method for understanding cardiac function, and one that is quite useful for understanding drug therapy, is to visualize the heart as having three fundamental characteristics:

1. It contracts with a specific force or strength (contractility).
2. It beats at a certain rate (beats per minute).
3. It conducts electrical impulses at a particular speed.

The ability to change the force of contraction, or contractility, is of particular interest to the pharmacotherapy of HF. Because the fundamental cause of HF is a weak myocardium, causing the muscle to beat more forcefully seems to be an ideal solution. The ability to increase the strength of contraction is called a positive **inotropic effect** and is a fundamental characteristic of the class of drugs known as the cardiac glycosides.

ino = *fiber*
tropic = *to influence*

The ability of the heart to speed up or slow down is a second characteristic important to pharmacology. A faster heart works harder but not necessarily more efficiently. A slower heart has a longer time to rest between beats, thus decreasing the workload on the heart.

FIGURE 19.1

Pathophysiology of heart failure.

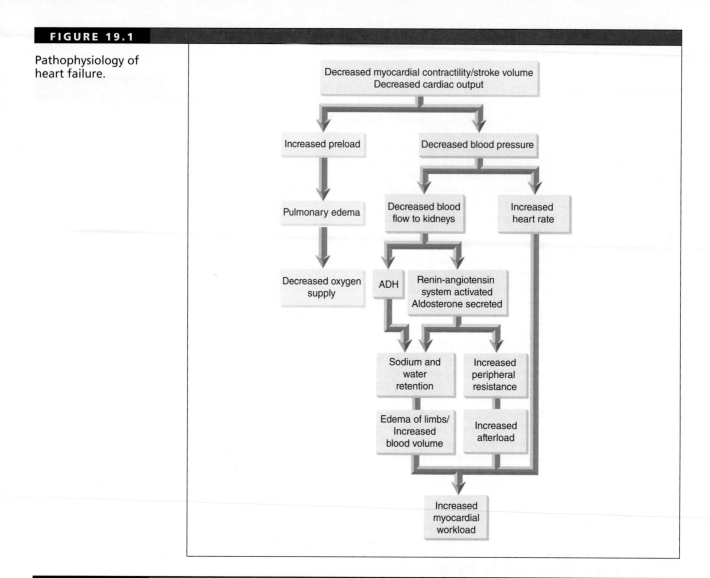

FIGURE 19.2

Signs and symptoms of the patient with heart failure.

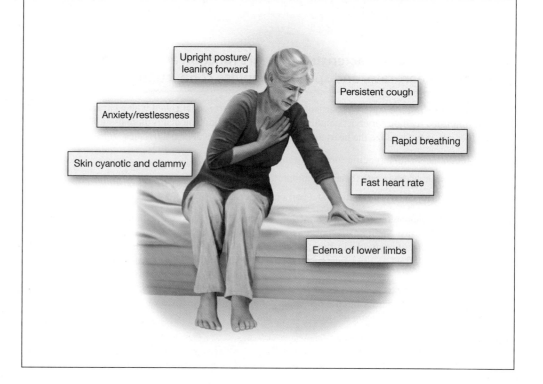

FIGURE 19.3

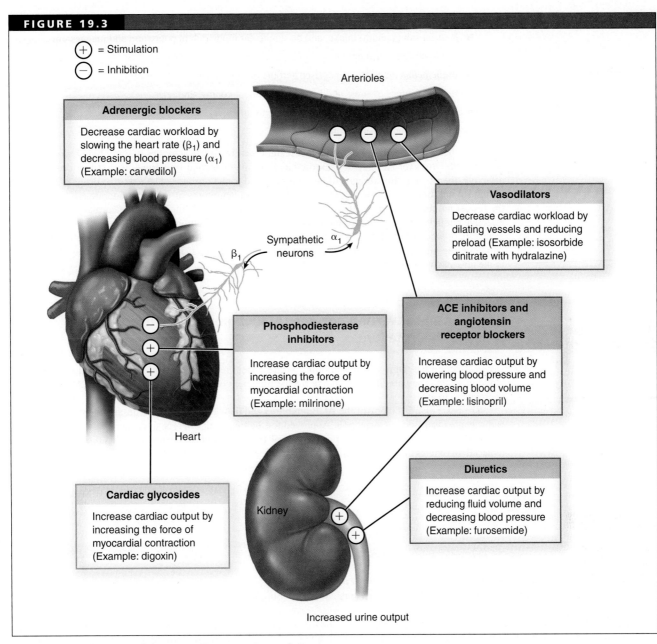

⊕ = Stimulation

⊖ = Inhibition

Arterioles

Adrenergic blockers

Decrease cardiac workload by slowing the heart rate (β_1) and decreasing blood pressure (α_1) (Example: carvedilol)

Vasodilators

Decrease cardiac workload by dilating vessels and reducing preload (Example: isosorbide dinitrate with hydralazine)

Sympathetic α_1
neurons

β_1

Phosphodiesterase inhibitors

Increase cardiac output by increasing the force of myocardial contraction (Example: milrinone)

ACE inhibitors and angiotensin receptor blockers

Increase cardiac output by lowering blood pressure and decreasing blood volume (Example: lisinopril)

Heart

Diuretics

Increase cardiac output by reducing fluid volume and decreasing blood pressure (Example: furosemide)

Cardiac glycosides

Increase cardiac output by increasing the force of myocardial contraction (Example: digoxin)

Kidney

Increased urine output

Mechanisms of action of drugs used to treat heart failure.

A third fundamental characteristic of cardiac physiology is the electrical conduction through the heart. Some cardiovascular drugs influence the speed of this conduction. Slowing the conduction speed through the heart will cause the heart to beat slower, thus lessening cardiac workload.

These primary characteristics of cardiac function can be modified through pharmacotherapy to assist the heart in meeting the body's metabolic demands. The mechanisms by which HF medications accomplish this are shown in Figure 19.3 ■.

The specific therapy for heart failure depends on the severity of the disease.

CORE CONCEPT 19.4

Although HF can be acute and require immediate treatment, it is often considered a progressive, chronic disorder. In its early stages, many of its symptoms can be improved through nonpharmacologic interventions. Through certain lifestyle changes, the patient can experience a higher quality of life either without drug therapy or with lower drug doses that have less risk for adverse effects. It should be noted that the following nonpharmacologic methods for controlling HF are the same strategies also used to manage hypertension.

- Stop using tobacco.
- Restrict salt (sodium) intake, and be sure to eat foods rich in potassium and magnesium.
- Limit alcohol consumption.
- Implement a medically supervised aerobic exercise plan.
- Reduce sources of stress and learn to implement coping strategies.
- Reduce weight to (or maintain it at) an optimum level.
- Limit caffeine consumption.

Once heart disease progresses such that it significantly affects activities of daily living, drug therapy is indicated. Drugs for HF may be classified as first-line or second-line drugs. If first-line drugs are not effective, then second-line drugs will be tried or added to the regimen. The first-line drugs are the ACE inhibitors and diuretics. These medications relieve most symptoms of mild to moderate HF and produce the fewest number of adverse effects. Sometimes considered first-line drugs, the cardiac glycosides are effective but have the potential for more serious adverse effects. Drugs of second choice are those used in acute HF, or when the ACE inhibitors and diuretics prove ineffective. Second-line drugs include the phosphodiesterase inhibitors, vasodilators, and beta-adrenergic blockers. The use of multiple drugs is common in the pharmacotherapy of HF.

CORE CONCEPT 19.5

Angiotensin-converting enzyme (ACE) inhibitors are the preferred drugs for heart failure.

Drugs affecting the renin-angiotensin-aldosterone system reduce the workload on the heart by lowering blood pressure. They are drugs of choice for the treatment of HF. Table 19.2 ◆ lists the ACE inhibitors approved to treat HF.

The basic pharmacology of the ACE inhibitors and their effects on the renin-angiotensin-aldosterone pathway are discussed in Chapter 18. Approved for the treatment of HTN since the 1980s, ACE inhibitors have since been shown to slow the progression of HF and to reduce deaths from this disease. They have replaced digoxin as the preferred drugs for the treatment of chronic HF.

Drug Prototype ⓟ *Lisinopril (Prinivil, Zestril)*
Therapeutic Class: Drug for HF, HTN, and MI prevention   **Pharmacologic Class: ACE inhibitor**

Actions and Uses: Lisinopril is one of the most frequently prescribed drugs for HTN and HF. An additional indication for this medication is to improve survival in patients when given within 24 hours of an acute MI.

Lisinopril lowers blood pressure by blocking ACE. Like other ACE inhibitors, doses of lisinopril may require two to three weeks of therapy for optimum effectiveness, and several months of therapy may be needed for a patient's cardiac function to return to normal. Because of their combined hypotensive action, concurrent therapy with lisinopril and diuretics should be carefully monitored.

Adverse Effects and Interactions: Lisinopril exhibits few serious adverse effects. The most common adverse effects are cough, headache, dizziness, orthostatic hypotension, and rash. Because high potassium levels may occur during therapy, use of potassium supplements or potassium-sparing diuretics should be avoided. Thus, electrolyte levels are usually monitored periodically. Angioedema is a rare, though potentially serious, adverse effect.

Lisinopril interacts with nonsteroidal anti-inflammatory drugs (NSAIDs) to cause decreased antihypertensive activity. Lisinopril may increase lithium levels and toxicity.

> **BLACK BOX WARNING:**
> Fetal injury and death may occur when ACE inhibitors are taken during pregnancy. When pregnancy is detected, they should be discontinued as soon as possible.

TABLE 19.2   First-Line Drugs for Heart Failure

Drug	Route and Adult Dose	Remarks
ACE INHIBITORS AND ANGIOTENSIN RECEPTOR BLOCKERS		
candesartan (Atacand)	PO; start at 4 mcg once daily, and slowly increase to a dose of 32 mg	Also for HTN
captopril (Capoten)	PO; 25–50 mg bid or tid (max: 450 mg/day)	Decreases central venous and pulmonary wedge pressure; also for HTN and post MI therapy
enalapril (Vasotec) (see page 277 for the Drug Prototype box)	PO; 2.5 mg qid–bid (max: 40 mg/day)	Increases cardiac output; IV form available; also for HTN
fosinopril (Monopril)	PO; 5–40 mg daily (max: 40 mg/day)	Also for HTN
(Pr) lisinopril (Prinivil, Zestril)	PO; 10 mg daily (max: 80 mg/day)	Therapy should not begin until two to three days after diuretics are stopped; also for HTN and post MI therapy.
quinapril (Accupril)	PO; 10–20 mg daily (max: 40 mg/day)	Observe for signs of hyperkalemia; also for HTN.
ramipril (Altace)	PO; 2.5–5 mg bid (max: 10 mg/day)	Also for HTN, stroke prophylaxis and post-MI therapy
valsartan (Diovan)	PO; Start with 40 mg bid and slowly increase 160 mg bid	Also for HTN
SELECTED DIURETICS		
bumetanide (Burinex, Bumex)	PO; 0.5–2 mg daily (max: 10 mg/day)	Affects loop of Henle; diuretic activity is 40 times greater and duration of action is shorter than furosemide; IM and IV forms available.
eplerenone (Inspra)	PO; 25–50 mg once daily (max: 100 mg/day)	Potassium-sparing diuretic; originally approved for HTN
furosemide (Lasix) (see page 254 for the Drug Prototype box)	PO; 20–80 mg in one or more divided doses (max: 600 mg/day)	Monitor for signs and symptoms of hypokalemia; also for HTN; IV and IM forms available; loop diuretic.
hydrochlorothiazide (Microzide) (see page 255 for the Drug Prototype box)	PO; 25–200 mg in one to three divided doses (max: 200 mg/day)	May bring on diabetes in patients with prediabetes; also for HTN; thiazide diuretic
spironolactone (Aldactone) (see page 256 for the Drug Prototype box)	PO; 5–200 mg in divided doses (max: 200 mg/day)	Used for refractory edema with HF; also for HTN; potassium-sparing diuretic
torsemide (Demadex)	PO; 10–20 mg/day (max: 200 mg/day)	Affects loop of Henle; also for HTN; IV form available

CAM THERAPY

Carnitine and Heart Disease

Carnitine is a natural substance structurally similar to amino acids. Its primary function in metabolism is to move fatty acids from the bloodstream into cells, where carnitine assists in the breakdown of lipids and the production of energy. The best food sources of carnitine are organ meat, fish, muscle meats, and milk products. Carnitine is available as a supplement in several forms, including L-carnitine, D-carnitine, and acetyl-carnitine. D-carnitine is associated with potential adverse effects and thus should be avoided.

Carnitine has been claimed to enhance energy and sports performance, heart health, memory, immune function, and male fertility. It is also being marketed as a "fat burner" for weight reduction.

Carnitine has been extensively studied. There is solid evidence to support supplementation in patients who are deficient in carnitine. Certain patients, such as vegetarians or those with heart disease, may need additional amounts. Carnitine supplementation has been shown to improve exercise tolerance in patients with angina. The use of carnitine may prevent the occurrence of dysrhythmias in the early stages of heart disease. Carnitine has also been shown to decrease triglyceride levels while increasing high-density lipoprotein (HDL) serum levels, thus helping to minimize one of the major risk factors associated with heart disease. Research has not shown carnitine supplementation to be of significant benefit in enhancing sports performance or weight loss.

dys = *difficult or bad*
rhythmia = *rhythm*

The ACE inhibitors produce their effects by blocking ACE, thus preventing the formation of angiotensin, an extremely potent vasoconstrictor. The primary actions of the ACE inhibitors are to lower blood pressure and reduce blood volume by enhancing the excretion of sodium and water. The resultant reduction of arterial blood pressure increases cardiac output. An additional effect of the ACE inhibitors is dilation of the veins returning blood to the heart. This action decreases preload and reduces pulmonary congestion and peripheral edema. The combined actions of ACE inhibitors substantially decrease the workload on the heart and allow it to work more efficiently. ACE inhibitors have been shown to reduce mortality following acute MI when therapy is started soon after the onset of symptoms (see Chapter 20).

A related group of drugs act by blocking the effects of angiotensin *after* it is formed. Angiotensin-receptor blockers (ARBs) are newer drugs that have similar effectiveness to the ACE inhibitors. Although the ARBs are usually prescribed for HTN, valsartan (Diovan) and candesartan (Atacand) are also approved for HF. Because research has not yet demonstrated a clear advantage of ARBs over other medications, their use in the treatment of HF is usually reserved for patients unable to tolerate the adverse effects of ACE inhibitors.

Diuretics relieve symptoms of heart failure by reducing fluid overload and decreasing blood pressure.

CORE CONCEPT 19.6

Diuretics are commonly used for the symptomatic treatment of HF. They produce few adverse effects and are effective at increasing urine flow, lowering blood volume, and reducing edema and congestion. When diuretics reduce fluid overload and lower blood pressure, the workload on the heart is reduced and cardiac output increases. They are widely used in the treatment of cardiovascular disease in patients with fluid overload. When used to treat HF, diuretics are usually prescribed in combination with ACE inhibitors and other HF medications in patients who have edema.

The most common adverse effects from diuretic therapy are electrolyte imbalances. Of greatest concern are the effects of diuretics on potassium levels, because too little or too much potassium can greatly affect a failing heart. This can be especially important in patients taking cardiac glycosides; patients with potassium or magnesium deficiencies are at greater risk for toxicity from digoxin. Potassium or magnesium supplements may be prescribed to prevent this adverse effect. Frequent laboratory testing may be necessary to monitor electrolyte levels in patients with HF.

The mechanism by which diuretics reduce blood volume, specifically where and how the nephron of the kidney is affected among the various drugs are discussed in Chapter 17. A Nursing Process Focus chart for diuretics, and prototype features for furosemide (Lasix), hydrochlorothiazide (Microzide) and spironolactone (Aldactone) are also included in Chapter 17.

Cardiac glycosides increase the force of myocardial contraction and were once the traditional drugs of choice for heart failure.

CORE CONCEPT 19.7

The value of the cardiac glycosides in treating heart disorders has been known for over 2,000 years. They have been used as arrow poisons by African tribes and as medicines by the ancient Egyptians and Romans.

Extracted from the common plants *Digitalis purpura* (purple foxglove) and *Digitalis lanata* (white foxglove), drugs from this class are sometimes called *digitalis glycosides*. Until the discovery of the ACE inhibitors, the cardiac glycosides were the mainstay of HF treatment. Digoxin (Lanoxin) is the only drug in this class available in the United States. The routes and dose for digoxin are listed in Table 19.3 ◆.

The primary action of digoxin is an increase in the force of myocardial contraction. This action, a positive inotropic effect, allows the weakened heart to eject more blood per beat, thus increasing cardiac output. The increased cardiac output helps the heart to meet the metabolic demands of the tissues.

A second important action of digoxin is its ability to slow electrical conduction through the heart. This results in fewer beats per minute. The reduced heart rate, combined with more forceful contractions, allows for much greater efficiency of the heart.

Unfortunately, digoxin has the potential to cause serious adverse effects at high doses and in certain patients. The margin of safety between a beneficial dose and a toxic dose is very small; thus, therapy should be closely monitored to prevent severe adverse effects. Serum digoxin levels above 1.8 mg/mL are considered toxic. Initial adverse effects are gastrointestinal (GI) related and include loss of appetite, vomiting, and diarrhea. Headache, drowsiness, confusion, and blurred vision may occur. Excessive slowing of the heart rate and other cardiac abnormalities can be fatal if not corrected.

The antidote for digoxin toxicity is administration of digoxin immune fab (Ovine). This drug binds digoxin, preventing it from reaching the tissues. Onset of action is rapid—less than one minute after the IV infusion is begun.

TABLE 19.3   **Second-Line Drugs for Heart Failure**

Drug	Route and Adult Dose	Remarks
CARDIAC GLYCOSIDE		
Pr digoxin (Lanoxin, Lanoxicaps)	PO; 0.125–0.5 mg/day (max: 0.5 mg/day)	Increases cardiac output; larger dose may be given to initiate therapy; IV form available; also used for dysrhythmias
BETA-ADRENERGIC BLOCKERS		
Pr carvedilol (Coreg)	PO; 3.125 mg bid for 2 weeks, then gradually increase dose (max: 25 mg bid)	Reduces cardiac workload; dose must be increased very slowly to prevent adverse effects; primary use is for HTN
metoprolol (Lopressor, Toprol XL)	PO; 25 mg/day for 2 weeks, then gradually increase dose; (max: 200 mg/day)	Also for HTN, angina, and post-MI therapy
DIRECT-ACTING VASODILATORS		
hydralazine with isosorbide dinitrate (BiDil)	PO; 1–2 tablets tid (each tablet contains 20 mg isosorbide dinitrate and 37.5 mg hydralazine) (max: 2 tablets/day)	Increases heart rate and cardiac output; decreases myocardial oxygen consumption; hydralazine also for HTN and isosorbide dinitrate for angina
nesiritide (Natrecor)	IV; 2 mcg/kg bolus followed by continuous infusion at 0.01 mcg/kg/min	Also called atrial natriuretic peptide; only for acute HF
PHOSPHODIESTERASE INHIBITORS		
inamrinone (Inocor)	IV; 0.75 mg/kg bolus given slowly over 2–3 min; then 5–10 mcg/kg/min (max: 10 mg/kg/day)	Larger dose is given to initiate therapy; peak effect reached in 10 min.
Pr milrinone (Primacor)	IV; 50 mcg/kg over 10 min; then 0.375–0.75 mcg/kg/min	Larger dose is given to initiate therapy; peak effect reached in 2 min.

Concept Review   **19.1**

- If cardiac glycosides are so effective at increasing myocardial contraction, why are they no longer first-line drugs for HF?

Drug Prototype: Pr *Digoxin (Lanoxin, Lanoxicaps)*

Therapeutic Class: Drug for heart failure   **Pharmacologic Class: Cardiac glycoside**

Actions and Uses: The primary benefit of digoxin is its ability to increase the strength of cardiac contraction (positive inotropic effect). Digoxin accomplishes this by inhibiting Na^+–K^+ ATPase, an enzyme in myocardial cells.

By increasing myocardial contractility, digoxin directly increases cardiac output, thus alleviating symptoms of HF and improving exercise tolerance. The increased cardiac output also results in increased urine production and a desirable reduction in blood volume, thus relieving the distressing symptoms of lung congestion and peripheral edema.

In addition to its positive inotropic effect, digoxin also has the ability to suppress the sinoatrial (SA) node (the pacemaker of the heart) and slow electrical conduction through the atrioventricular (AV) node. Because of these actions, digoxin is sometimes used to treat cardiac rhythm abnormalities known as dysrhythmias, which is discussed in Chapter 22. Pulse rate should be monitored daily, and values less than 60 beats per minute or greater than 100 beats per minute should be reported to the healthcare provider.

Adverse Effects and Interactions: The most dangerous adverse effect of digoxin is its ability to create dysrhythmias, particularly in patients who have hypokalemia. Because diuretics can cause hypokalemia and are also often used to treat HF, use of digoxin and diuretics together must be carefully monitored. Levels of potassium, magnesium, calcium, blood urea nitrogen (BUN), and creatinine should be monitored frequently (hypokalemia predisposes the patient to digoxin toxicity). Other adverse effects of digoxin therapy include nausea, vomiting, and anorexia and abnormalities of the nervous system such as blurred vision. Periodic serum levels are checked to determine if the digoxin level is within the therapeutic range, and the dosage may be adjusted based on the laboratory results. Digoxin also interacts with many other medications. Concurrent use with beta blockers may result in additive bradycardia. Because small changes in digoxin levels can produce serious adverse effects, the healthcare provider must constantly be alert for drug–drug interactions.

CORE CONCEPT 19.8
Beta-adrenergic blockers are used in combination with other drugs to slow the progression of heart failure.

Drugs that produce a positive inotropic effect, such as the cardiac glycosides and phosphodiesterase inhibitors, play important roles in treating the diminished contractility that is the hallmark of HF. It may seem somewhat unusual then to find medications that exhibit a *negative* inotropic effect prescribed for this disease. Yet such is the case with the beta-adrenergic blockers. Beta blockers have been shown to dramatically reduce the number of hospitalizations and deaths associated with HF.

Beta-adrenergic antagonists block the cardiac actions of the sympathetic nervous system, thus slowing the heart rate and reducing blood pressure. Workload on the heart is decreased. Carvedilol (Coreg) and metoprolol (Lopressor, Toprol XL) are the two beta blockers approved to treat HF. Patients with HF must be carefully monitored when taking beta blockers because these drugs have the potential to worsen HF. They are always used in combination with other agents, usually ACE inhibitors. The basic pharmacology of the beta blockers is presented in Chapter 8. Other indications, routes, and dosages of the beta-adrenergic blockers are discussed elsewhere in this text: hypertension in Chapter 18, dysrhythmias in Chapter 22, and angina/myocardial infarction in Chapter 20.

CORE CONCEPT 19.9
Vasodilators reduce symptoms of heart failure by decreasing cardiac workload.

The two direct-acting vasodilators, hydralazine (Apresoline) and isosorbide dinitrate (Isordil), act directly on vascular smooth muscle to relax blood vessels and lower blood pressure. Hydralazine acts on arterioles, whereas isosorbide dinitrate acts on veins. Because the two drugs act synergistically, isosorbide dinitrate is combined with hydralazine in the treatment of HF. BiDil is a fixed-dose combination of 20 mg of isosorbide dinitrate with 37.5 mg of hydralazine. Dosing for the drug is shown in Table 19.2.

Because of a high incidence of reflex tachycardia and orthostatic hypotension, vasodilators play a minor role in the drug therapy of HF. They are generally reserved for patients with more severe disease, or those who cannot tolerate ACE inhibitors. BiDil appears to be especially effective in treating HF in African American patients, who often exhibit resistance to standard therapies. Hydralazine is featured as a prototype drug for direct vasodilators in the treatment of HTN in Chapter 18. Isosorbide dinitrate belongs to a class of drugs called organic nitrates that are widely used in the treatment of angina pectoris (see Chapter 20).

Concept Review 19.2

■ Why are the ACE inhibitors preferred over both the nitrates and the diuretics in the treatment of HF?

Drug Prototype: ℗ *Carvedilol (Coreg)*
Therapeutic Class: Drug for heart failure and HTN **Pharmacologic Class: Beta-adrenergic blocker**

Actions and Uses: Carvedilol was the first beta-adrenergic blocker approved for the treatment of HF. It has been found to reduce symptoms, slow the progression of the disease, and increase exercise tolerance when combined with other HF drugs, such as ACE inhibitors. Unlike many drugs in this class, carvedilol blocks beta$_1$- and beta$_2$- as well as alpha$_1$-adrenergic receptors. The primary therapeutic effects relevant to HF are a reduction in heart rate and a drop in blood pressure. The lower blood pressure reduces the workload on the heart. The drug is also approved to treat HTN and for reducing cardiac complications following an MI.

Adverse Effects and Interactions: The most frequent adverse effects of carvedilol include back pain, bradycardia, dizziness, shortness of breath, fatigue, orthostatic hypotension, and weight gain. It should be used with caution in patients with asthma or cardiac dysrhythmias.

Carvedilol's effect in decreasing heart rate and contractility has the potential to worsen HF; therefore, dosage must be carefully monitored. Because of the potential for adverse cardiac effects, beta-adrenergic blockers such as carvedilol are usually given concurrently with other drugs in the treatment of HF.

Carvedilol interacts with many drugs. For example, levels of carvedilol are significantly increased when the drug is taken with rifampin. MAO inhibitors, clonidine, and reserpine can cause hypotension or bradycardia when given with carvedilol. When given with digoxin, carvedilol may increase digoxin levels. It may also enhance the hypoglycemic effects of insulin and oral hypoglycemic agents.

Drug Prototype: Pr *Milrinone (Primacor)*
Therapeutic Class: Drug for severe heart failure   Pharmacologic Class: **Phosphodiesterase inhibitor**

Actions and Uses: Of the two phosphodiesterase inhibitors available, milrinone is generally preferred because it has a shorter half-life and fewer adverse effects. It is given IV only and is primarily used for the short-term support of advanced HF. Peak effects occur in two minutes. Immediate effects of milrinone include an increased force of contraction and an increase in cardiac output.

Adverse Effects and Interactions: The most serious adverse effect of milrinone is ventricular dysrhythmia, which can occur in more than 1 of every 10 patients taking the drug. The patient's electrocardiogram (ECG) should be monitored continuously during the infusion of the drug. Less serious adverse effects include headache, nausea, and vomiting.

Use with disopyramide may cause excessive hypotension. Caution should be used when administering milrinone with digoxin, dobutamine, or other inotropic drugs because their positive inotropic effects on the heart may be additive.

Phosphodiesterase inhibitors and other miscellaneous drugs are used for short-term therapy of advanced heart failure.

CORE CONCEPT 19.10

Phosphodiesterase inhibitors are drugs with a very brief half-life that are occasionally used for the short-term control of acute HF. The doses of phosphodiesterase inhibitors are given in Table 19.3.

The two drugs in this class block the enzyme **phosphodiesterase** in cardiac and smooth muscle. Blocking phosphodiesterase has the effect of increasing the amount of calcium available for myocardial contraction. The inhibition results in two main actions that benefit patients with HF: an increased force of contraction (positive inotropic response) and vasodilation. Because of their toxicity, however, phosphodiesterase inhibitors are reserved for patients who have not responded to ACE inhibitors or cardiac glycosides, and they are generally used for two to three days only.

A third vasodilator used for HF is very different from hydralazine or isosorbide dinitrate. Nesiritide (Natrecor) is a small peptide hormone that is structurally identical to a hormone known as human beta-type **natriuretic peptide (hBNP)**, which is secreted by the heart when the heart begins to fail. Nesiritide reduces both preload and afterload, improving cardiac efficiency in patients with HF. Nesiritide has limited uses because of its ability to cause severe hypotension. The medication is given only by IV infusion, and patients require continuous monitoring. It is approved for patients with severe HF.

natri = *sodium*
uretic = *urinary excretion*

PATIENTS NEED TO KNOW

Patients treated for HF need to know the following:

In General
1. Take blood pressure regularly because many drugs for HF affect blood pressure. Report any persistent changes.
2. Take weight measurements regularly and report abnormal weight gains or losses.
3. Salt intake should be limited.

Regarding ACE Inhibitors
4. Avoid sudden position changes because these can cause lightheadedness.

Regarding Cardiac Glycosides
5. Check pulse rate before taking digoxin. If the rate is less than 60 beats per minute or the rate designated by a healthcare provider, the drug should not be taken.
6. Many drugs interact with digoxin to increase or decrease its effects on the heart. For this reason, it is important to consult with a healthcare provider before taking any other medication.
7. Report visual disturbances (seeing halos or a yellow-green tinge, blurring), nausea, headaches, or irregular heartbeat without delay because they are signs and symptoms of digoxin toxicity.

Regarding Diuretics
8. Limit salt intake as directed by the healthcare provider.
9. Drink at least six to eight glasses of water daily.
10. Report any of the following adverse effects: abdominal pain, jaundice, dark urine, flu-like symptoms.
11. To prevent dizziness, avoid sudden position changes.
12. An increased intake of potassium-rich foods such as bananas, dried fruits, and orange juice, or a potassium supplement may be necessary if certain diuretics are taken. Taking potassium supplements with food reduces stomach irritation.

CHAPTER REVIEW

CORE CONCEPTS SUMMARY

19.1 **Heart failure is closely associated with disorders such as chronic hypertension, coronary artery disease, and diabetes.**

Heart failure (HF) is not considered a distinct disease in itself. Instead, a number of diseases that affect the heart, such as chronic hypertension (HTN), coronary artery disease, and diabetes, lead to the collection of symptoms known as HF.

19.2 **The central cause of heart failure is weakened heart muscle.**

HF occurs when the heart cannot pump enough blood to meet the demands of the tissues. This usually occurs when the heart muscle cannot contract with sufficient force. HF may occur on the right side, left side, or both sides of the heart, producing symptoms such as shortness of breath, coughing, and peripheral edema.

19.3 **The three primary characteristics of heart function are force of contraction, heart rate, and speed of impulse conduction.**

The ability of the heart to effectively pump blood depends on the strength of contraction of the myocardial fibers. Heart rate and the speed of the impulse conduction across the myocardium also directly affect the ability of the heart to pump blood.

19.4 **The specific therapy for heart failure depends on the severity of the disease.**

Mild HF can be improved through lifestyle changes such as tobacco cessation and maintaining optimum weight. As HF progresses, pharmacotherapy with drugs of first choice, such as ACE inhibitors or diuretics, is indicated. More advanced disease may require therapy with cardiac glycosides, phosphodiesterase inhibitors, beta blockers, or vasodilators.

19.5 **Angiotensin-converting enzyme (ACE) inhibitors are the preferred drugs for heart failure.**

ACE inhibitors improve HF by reducing peripheral edema and increasing cardiac output. Because of their effectiveness and their relatively low potential for serious adverse effects, they have become preferred drugs in the treatment of HF.

19.6 **Diuretics relieve symptoms of heart failure by reducing fluid overload and decreasing blood pressure.**

Diuretics produce few serious adverse effects and are often used in combination with other HF drugs to reduce patients' symptoms. Potent diuretics such as furosemide are particularly valuable in treating acute HF.

19.7 **Cardiac glycosides increase the force of myocardial contraction and were once the traditional drugs of choice for heart failure.**

Cardiac glycosides, long the mainstay for pharmacotherapy of HF, increase myocardial contractility and are effective. The large number of drug–drug interactions and the potential for serious adverse effects such as dysrhythmias limit their use.

19.8 **Beta-adrenergic blockers are used in combination with other drugs to slow the progression of heart failure.**

Although beta blockers decrease myocardial contractility, they also lower heart rate and blood pressure, which is beneficial in reducing the symptoms of HF. When administered to treat patients with HF, they are nearly always used in combination with other drugs.

19.9 **Vasodilators reduce symptoms of heart failure by decreasing cardiac workload.**

Direct vasodilators are effective at relaxing blood vessels, thus reducing myocardial oxygen demand on the heart. BiDil is a combination of two vasodilators: isosorbide dinitrate and hydralazine. Their use is limited by their high incidence of adverse effects.

19.10 **Phosphodiesterase inhibitors and other miscellaneous drugs are used for short-term therapy of advanced heart failure.**

Phosphodiesterase inhibitors are a relatively new class of drugs used for the short-term treatment of HF. Although effective, they are given IV only and can produce potentially serious adverse effects. Nesiritide (Natrecor) is a small peptide hormone that is approved only for severe HF because of its potentially serious adverse effects.

REVIEW QUESTIONS

The following questions are written in NCLEX-PN® style. Answer these questions to assess your knowledge of the chapter material, and go back and review any material that is not clear to you.

1. The patient has developed a cough and shortness of breath when he or she lies down. After thoroughly collecting data on the patient, the nurse suspects:

1. Right HF
2. Left HF
3. Liver engorgement
4. Peripheral edema

2. The patient has been started on digoxin (Lanoxin) therapy. Which of the following should the nurse monitor carefully?

1. SGOT levels
2. Amylase levels
3. Sodium levels
4. Potassium levels

3. The nurse is teaching a patient about beta blockers. The patient states that he or she is already taking another kind of medication for his or her HF. The nurse tells him or her that this is not uncommon. What other drug is usually given with beta-blockers?

1. Cardiac glycosides
2. Diuretics
3. Phosphodiesterase inhibitors
4. ACE inhibitors

4. A patient who is taking hydralazine for HF is also experiencing angina. Which of the following drugs would be used in combination with hydralazine to help relieve this patient's symptoms?

1. Isosorbide dinitrate (Isordil)
2. Carvedilol (Coreg)
3. Chlorothiazide (Diuril)
4. Milrinone (Primacor)

5. The patient is admitted with HF. The physician orders IV milrinone (Primacor). The nurse observes for the most serious adverse effect of this drug, which is:

1. Headache
2. Dysrhythmias
3. Confusion
4. Drowsiness

6. The nurse is assisting in the development of a medication information pamphlet to be given to those patients taking ACE inhibitors. Which of the following should be included in the education provided to a patient on lisinopril (Prinivil)? (Select all that apply.)

1. "It may take several weeks for your blood pressure to return to normal."
2. "You must have your potassium monitored from time to time."
3. "This medication may change your vision from time to time."
4. "It interacts with NSAIDs to cause decreased antihypertensive activity."

7. In addition to decreasing cardiac contractility, the nurse informs the patient that beta blockers:

1. Lower heart rate and blood pressure.
2. Increase heart rate and afterload.
3. Produce systemic vasoconstriction.
4. Increase the force of myocardial contraction.

8. A patient is taking digoxin. Just in case the patient develops digoxin toxicity, which drug would the nurse expect to be ordered for this patient?

1. Digoxin immune fab
2. Milrinone (Primacor)
3. Inamrinone (Inocor)
4. Flecainide (Tambocor)

9. A patient is receiving digoxin and furosemide (Lasix). Which of the following electrolyte levels should the nurse most carefully monitor?

1. Potassium
2. Creatinine
3. Sodium
4. Calcium

10. The healthcare provider orders a patient to have 0.5 mg of digoxin. On hand, you have a bottle labeled digoxin 0.25 mg per tablet. How many tablet(s) will you give?

1. One tablet
2. One and one-half tablets
3. Two tablets
4. Half tablet

CASE STUDY QUESTIONS

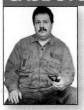

Remember Mr. Novi, the patient introduced at the beginning of the chapter? Now read the remainder of the case study. Based on the information you have learned in this chapter, answer the questions that follow.

Mr. Albert Novi, age 45, has smoked since age 12. He recently has had trouble breathing when mowing the lawn, and he coughs when he lies down to sleep at night. The physician has diagnosed Mr. Novi with early HF and is planning on *starting him on some medication to help his heart function more effectively, in addition to providing information on a smoking cessation program.*

1. Which of the following drugs would *most* likely be prescribed for Mr. Novi?

1. Isosorbide dinitrate (Isordil)
2. Enalapril (Vasotec)
3. Milrinone (Primacor)
4. Digoxin (Lanoxin)

2. Which of the following actions would be most desirable for a drug used to treat HF in Mr. Novi?

1. Increase the heart rate.
2. Increase cardiac output.
3. Increase arterial blood pressure.
4. Increase blood volume by retaining water.

3. After a year, Mr. Novi enters the emergency department with acute shortness of breath and severe congestion in both lungs. The nurse understands that the plan of care for a patient presenting in the emergency room with these symptoms will most likely include which medication?

1. Inamrinone (Inocor)
2. Captopril (Capoten)
3. Carvedilol (Coreg)
4. Spironolactone (Aldactone)

4. Mr. Novi has eventually been placed on digoxin and furosemide. Which of the following adverse effects of furosemide should nurse tell the patient about because it could lead to dysrhythmias and other cardiac disease while taking digoxin?

1. Hypotension
2. Bradycardia
3. Hypokalemia
4. Hyperkalemia

NOTE: Answers to the Review and Case Study Questions appear in Appendix B. The complete rationales and answers are located on the textbook's website.

Pearson Nursing Student Resources Find additional review materials at **nursing.pearsonhighered.com.**

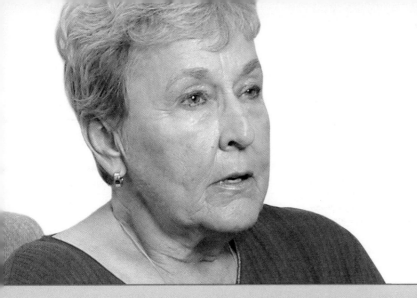

"Every time I mow the lawn it happens. The pain is so crushing, all I can do is cry in my yard."

Ms. Shirley Bush

Drugs for Angina Pectoris, Myocardial Infarction, and Stroke

CORE CONCEPTS

20.1 Coronary heart disease is caused by a restriction in blood flow to the myocardium.

20.2 Angina pectoris is characterized by severe chest pain caused by lack of sufficient oxygen flow to heart muscle.

20.3 Angina pain can often be controlled through positive lifestyle changes and surgical procedures.

20.4 The pharmacologic management of angina is achieved by reducing cardiac workload.

20.5 The organic nitrates relieve angina pain by dilating veins and the coronary arteries.

20.6 Beta-adrenergic blockers are sometimes preferred drugs for reducing the frequency of angina attacks.

20.7 Calcium channel blockers relieve angina pain by reducing the cardiac workload.

20.8 The early diagnosis and treatment of myocardial infarction (MI) increases chances of survival.

20.9 Thrombolytics dissolve clots blocking the coronary arteries.

20.10 Drugs are used to treat the symptoms and complications of acute MI.

20.11 Aggressive treatment of stroke can increase survival.

DRUG SNAPSHOT

The following drugs are discussed in this chapter:

DRUG CLASSES	DRUG PROTOTYPES
Organic nitrates	Pr nitroglycerin (Nitrostat, Nitro-Bid, Nitro-Dur, others) *307*
Beta-adrenergic blockers	Pr atenolol (Tenormin) *309*
Calcium channel blockers	Pr diltiazem (Cardizem, Cartia XT, Dilacor XR, others) *309*
Thrombolytics	Pr reteplase (Retavase) *312*

LEARNING OUTCOMES

After reading this chapter, the student should be able to:

1. Describe how the myocardium receives its oxygen and nutrient supply.

2. Explain the pathophysiology of angina pectoris.

3. Identify positive lifestyle changes that may be implemented to manage symptoms of angina.

4. Explain the pharmacologic treatment of MI.

5. Describe the pharmacologic treatment of stroke.

6. Categorize drugs used to treat angina, MI, and stroke based on their classification and mechanisms of action.

7. For each of the classes listed in the Drug Snapshot, identify representative drugs and explain their mechanisms of drug action, primary actions, and important adverse effects as they relate to the treatment of angina, MI, or stroke.

KEY TERMS

angina pectoris (an-JEYE-nuh
  PEK-tore-us) *302*
atherosclerosis (ath-ur-oh-skler-OH-sis) *302*
coronary arteries (KOR-un-air-ee
  AR-tur-ees) *302*
coronary artery bypass graft (CABG)
  surgery *304*
hemorrhagic stroke (hee-moh-RAJ-ik) *314*

myocardial infarction (MI) (meye-oh-KAR-
  dee-ul in-FARK-shun) *310*
myocardial ischemia (meye-oh-KAR-dee-
  ul ik-SKEE-mee-uh) *302*
percutaneous transluminal coronary
  angioplasty (PTCA) (per-cue-TAIN-ee-
  us trans-LOO-min-ul KOR-un-air-ee
  ANN-gee-oh-plas-tee) *304*

plaque (plak) *302*
stable angina *303*
stroke *314*
thrombotic stroke (throm-BOT-ik) *314*
unstable angina *303*
vasospastic (Prinzmetal's) angina *303*

cerebro = *head or brain*
vascular = *vessels*

All tissues in the body are dependent on a continuous supply of oxygen and vital nutrients to support life and health. The heart and brain are especially demanding. Should the blood supply to cardiac muscle become compromised, cardiovascular function may become impaired, resulting in angina pectoris, myocardial infarction (MI), and, possibly, death. Interruption of blood supply to the brain can cause fainting or stroke. This chapter focuses on the pharmacologic interventions related to angina pectoris, MI, and stroke (also called cerebrovascular accident or CVA).

CORE CONCEPT 20.1

Coronary heart disease is caused by a restriction in blood flow to the myocardium.

myo = *muscle*
cardium = *heart*

The heart is the hardest working organ in the body. Whereas the activity of most organs slows considerably during rest and sleep, the heart must continue pumping so that the tissues can receive the nutrients they need and dispose of the wastes they have accumulated. Because it is such a vital organ, the heart muscle (myocardium) must receive a continuous supply of oxygen and nutrients. Any disturbance in blood flow to the vital organs or to the myocardium itself—even for brief episodes—can result in life-threatening consequences.

Because the heart chambers fill with blood more than 60 times per minute, one would think that the myocardium would have an ample supply of oxygen and nutrients. The myocardium, however, receives essentially no nutrients from the blood traveling through the heart's chambers. Instead, heart muscle receives its nutrients from the first two arteries branching off the aorta, the right and left **coronary arteries**. As these arteries branch, they circle the heart, bringing cardiac muscle a continuous supply of oxygen and nutrients.

Coronary heart disease, also called coronary artery disease (CAD), is the term used to describe impaired blood flow in the coronary arteries. Moderate restriction of flow leads to angina pectoris. Severe impairment or complete loss of blood flow causes MI and a high risk of sudden death. CAD can also cause dysrhythmias and lead to heart failure.

ANGINA PECTORIS

Angina pectoris is acute chest pain caused by insufficient oxygen to a portion of the myocardium. Angina is characterized by chest pain on physical exertion or emotional stress. Although it produces many of the same symptoms as a heart attack, its pharmacologic treatment is quite different.

CORE CONCEPT 20.2

Angina pectoris is characterized by severe chest pain caused by lack of sufficient oxygen flow to heart muscle.

athero = *fatty*
sclera = *hard*
osis = *abnormal condition*

The most common cause of angina is **atherosclerosis**: a buildup of fatty, fibrous material called **plaque** in the walls of arteries. Although plaque may take as long as 40 to 50 years to accumulate to a level that would cause symptoms, plaque deposition actually begins very early in life. If plaque accumulates in a coronary artery, the myocardium downstream from the affected artery begins to receive less oxygen than it needs to perform its metabolic functions. This condition of having a reduced blood supply to cardiac muscle cells is called **myocardial ischemia**. Figure 20.1 ■ illustrates the progressive accumulation of plaque that is characteristic of atherosclerosis.

The classic presentation of angina pectoris is intense pain in the chest, often moving to the left side of the neck and lower jaw and down the left arm. Angina pain is usually preceded by physical exertion or emotional excitement—events associated with *increased myocardial oxygen demand*. The plaque-filled coronary artery is unable to supply the amount of nutrients needed by the stressed myocardium. With rest, angina pain usually diminishes in less than 15 minutes.

FIGURE 20.1

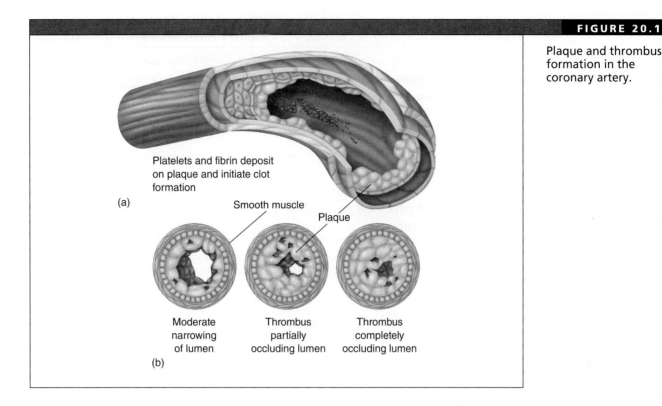

Plaque and thrombus formation in the coronary artery.

Platelets and fibrin deposit on plaque and initiate clot formation

(a)

Smooth muscle

Plaque

Moderate narrowing of lumen

Thrombus partially occluding lumen

Thrombus completely occluding lumen

(b)

There are several types of angina. Angina pectoris that is predictable in its frequency, intensity, and duration is called **stable angina**. If angina episodes become more frequent or severe and occur during periods of rest, the condition is called **unstable angina**. Unstable angina requires more aggressive medical intervention. It is sometimes considered a medical emergency because it is associated with an increased risk of MI. A third type of angina is known as **vasospastic or Prinzmetal's angina**. This type is caused by *spasms* of the coronary arteries, which may or may not contain plaque. Vasospastic angina pain occurs most often during periods of rest.

Angina pain may closely mimic that of an MI. It is necessary for the healthcare provider to distinguish quickly between the two diseases because the pharmacologic treatment of angina is much different than that of MI. Angina is rarely fatal. In contrast, MI has a high mortality rate if treatment is delayed, so drug therapy must begin immediately.

Chest pain is a common complaint of patients seeking care in physicians' offices and emergency departments. It is also one of the most frightening symptoms for patients, who often equate their pain to having MI with a real risk of sudden death. The pain experienced by the patient, however, is only a symptom of an underlying disorder. A number of diverse diseases can produce pain in the chest, and some of these are unrelated to the heart. A major goal of the healthcare provider is to quickly determine the cause of the pain so that the proper treatment can be administered. Table 20.1 ◆ lists some of the common diseases that can produce chest pain as a symptom.

TABLE 20.1   Examples of Disorders That May Produce Chest Pain

Name of Disease	Description
Coronary artery disease	Atherosclerosis of the coronary arteries
Diabetes	Lack of insulin or inability to tolerate carbohydrates
Gastric reflux	Backflow of stomach contents into the esophagus
Hypertension	High systemic blood pressure
Mitral stenosis	Inability of the mitral valve to fully open
Myocardial infarction	Cardiac muscle tissue death due to clots in coronary arteries
Peptic ulcer disease	Erosion of the mucosa of the stomach or small intestine

Fast Facts Angina Pectoris and Coronary Heart Disease

- Coronary heart disease causes one out of every five deaths in the United States.
- Almost 10 million Americans have angina pectoris; 500,000 new cases occur each year.
- Among ethnic groups, the incidence of angina is highest among African Americans, intermediate in Mexican Americans, and lowest in non-Hispanic Whites.
- Angina occurs more frequently in women than men; African American women have approximately twice the risk of African American men.

CORE CONCEPT 20.3

Angina pain can often be controlled through positive lifestyle changes and surgical procedures.

A combination of variables influences the development and progression of CAD, including dietary patterns and lifestyle choices. A number of dietary and lifestyle factors are associated with an increased incidence of angina. The healthcare provider should help the patient control the frequency of angina episodes by advising him or her to implement some or all of the following lifestyle changes:

- Limit alcohol consumption to small amounts.
- Eliminate foods high in cholesterol or saturated fats.
- Keep blood cholesterol and other lipid indicators within the normal ranges.
- Do not use tobacco.
- Keep blood pressure within the normal range.
- Exercise regularly and maintain optimum weight.
- Keep blood glucose levels within normal range.
- Limit salt (sodium) intake.
- Reduce stress levels as much as possible.

per = *through procedure*
cutaneous = *skin*

angio = *vessel*
plasty = *shaped or molded by a surgical procedure*

When the coronary arteries are significantly obstructed, the two most common interventions are **percutaneous transluminal coronary angioplasty (PTCA)** with stent insertion, and **coronary artery bypass graft (CABG) surgery**. PTCA is a procedure whereby the area of narrowing is dilated using either a balloon catheter or a laser. Because the artery may return to its narrowed state after the procedure, a stent is sometimes used in conjunction with balloon angioplasty. Angioplasty with stenting typically relieves 90% of the original blockage in the artery.

Concept Review 20.1

- How can a healthcare provider distinguish between stable angina and unstable angina?

CORE CONCEPT 20.4

The pharmacologic management of angina is achieved by reducing cardiac workload.

The treatment goals for a patient with angina are twofold: to *reduce the frequency* of angina episodes and to *terminate* acute angina pain in progress. Long-term goals include extending the patient's life span by preventing serious consequences of ischemic heart disease, such as dysrhythmias, heart failure, and MI. The primary means by which antiangina drugs act is by reducing the myocardial demand for oxygen. This reduced demand can be accomplished by at least four mechanisms:

- Slowing the heart rate
- Dilating veins so that heart receives less blood (reduced *preload*)
- Causing the heart to contract with less force (reduced *contractility*)
- Lowering blood pressure, thus offering the heart less resistance when ejecting blood from the ventricles (reduced *afterload*)

Three classes of drugs—organic nitrates, beta-adrenergic blockers, and calcium channel blockers—are used to treat angina. Rapid-acting organic nitrates are preferred drugs for *terminating* acute angina

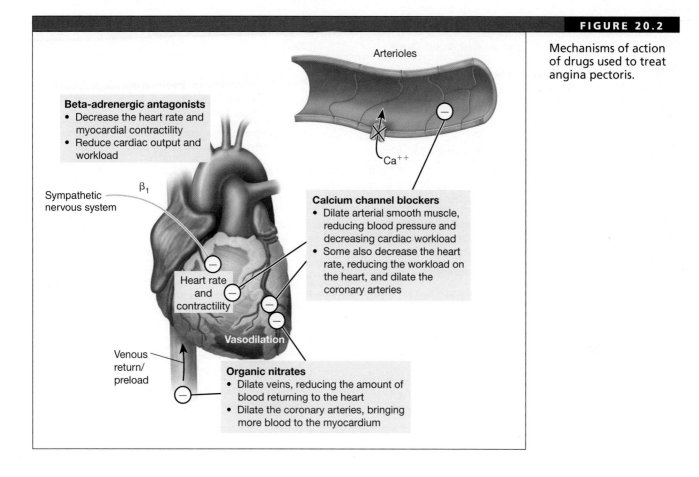

FIGURE 20.2

Mechanisms of action of drugs used to treat angina pectoris.

pain. Beta-adrenergic blockers are considered first-line drugs for *preventing* angina pain. Calcium channel blockers are used when beta blockers or long-acting organic nitrates are not tolerated well by a patient. It is important to understand that the antiangina medications relieve symptoms but do not cure the underlying disorder. A summary of the drugs used to prevent and treat CAD is shown in Figure 20.2 ■.

Patients with angina will also likely be taking several secondary medications. Daily low-dose aspirin reduces the risk of serious cardiovascular events. Statins may be prescribed to lower blood cholesterol levels and reduce the advancement of coronary atherosclerosis. Inclusion of omega-3 fatty acids is sometimes recommended in patients with stable CAD. Ranolazine (Ranexa) is a newer drug for angina that is approved for chronic angina that has not responded to other agents.

The organic nitrates relieve angina pain by dilating veins and the coronary arteries.

CORE CONCEPT 20.5

All drugs in this chemical class possess at least one nitrate (NO_2) group. The vasodilation effect of these agents is a result of the conversion of nitrate to its active form, nitric oxide (NO). Another nitrogen-containing drug, nitrous oxide (N_2O), is used in anesthesia (see the chapter on Chapter 13). Organic nitrates used to treat angina are listed in Table 20.2 ◆.

Since the discovery of their medicinal properties in 1857, the organic nitrates have been the mainstay for the treatment of angina. The primary therapeutic action of these agents is their ability to relax both arterial and venous smooth muscle. Dilation of veins reduces the amount of blood returning to the heart (preload), so the chambers contain a smaller volume. With less blood for the ventricles to pump, the workload on the heart is decreased, thereby lowering myocardial oxygen demand. The therapeutic outcome is that chest pain is terminated and episodes of angina become less frequent.

Organic nitrates also have the ability to dilate coronary arteries, and this was once thought to be their primary mechanism of action. It seems logical that dilating a partially occluded coronary vessel would allow more oxygen to reach ischemic myocardial tissue. Although this effect does indeed occur, it is not believed to be the primary mechanism of nitrate action in stable angina. This action, however, is important in treating the less common form of angina known as vasospastic angina. The organic nitrates can relax these spasms and stop the pain.

TABLE 20.2 Selected Drugs for Angina and Myocardial Infarction

Drug	Route and Adult Dose	Remarks
ORGANIC NITRATES		
isosorbide dinitrate (Dilatrate SR, Isordil)	PO; 2.5–30 mg qid (max: 480 mg/day)	For both acute attacks and long-term management; sublingual and chewable forms smaller dose is given to initiate therapy; extended-release form available
isosorbide mononitrate (Imdur, Ismo, Monoket)	PO (regular release); 20 mg bid; PO (sustained release); 30–60 mg once daily	For the prevention of angina; a smaller dose is given to initiate therapy; give in morning, if taking once daily
Pr nitroglycerin (Nitrostat, Nitro-Bid, Nitro-Dur, others)	Sublingual: 1 tablet (0.3–0.6 mg) or 1 spray (0.4–0.8 mg) every 3–5 minutes (max: three doses in 15 minutes)	Dilates both arteries and veins; sublingual, oral, translingual, IV, transmucosal, transdermal, and topical forms available; extended-release form available
BETA-ADRENERGIC BLOCKERS		
acebutolol (Sectral)	PO; 400–800 mg/day in 1–2 divided doses (max: 1,200 mg/day)	Cardioselective beta$_1$ blocker; decreases cardiac output; for hypertension, dysrhythmias, and stable angina
Pr atenolol (Tenormin)	PO; 25–50 mg daily (max: 100 mg/day)	Cardioselective beta$_1$ blocker; for angina, dysrhythmias, MI, and hypertension
metoprolol (Lopressor, Toprol XL)	For angina: PO; 100 mg bid (max: 400 mg/day) For MI: IV; 5 mg every two minutes for three doses followed by PO doses	Cardioselective beta$_1$ blocker; for angina, MI, and hypertension
nadolol (Corgard)	PO; 40 mg once daily (max: 320 mg/day)	Nonselective beta$_1$ and beta$_2$ blocker; for long-term prevention of angina and hypertension
propranolol (Inderal, InnoPran XL) (see page 340 for the Drug Profile box)	PO; 10–80 mg bid–tid (max: 320 mg/day)	Nonselective beta$_1$ and beta$_2$ blocker; IV form available; for angina, hypertension, dysrhythmias, MI, and migraine prophylaxis
timolol maleate (Betimol)	PO; 15–45 mg tid (max: 60 mg/day)	Nonselective beta$_1$ and beta$_2$ blocker; for hypertension, post MI and angina; topical form available for glaucoma
CALCIUM CHANNEL BLOCKERS		
amlodipine (Norvasc)	PO; 5–10 mg daily (max: 10 mg/day)	Also for hypertension; Lotrel contains amlodipine and the ACE inhibitor benazepril
bepridil (Vascor)	PO; 200 mg daily (max: 400 mg/day)	Also blocks sodium channels; usually reserved for patients unresponsive to safer antianginals
Pr diltiazem (Cardizem, Cartia XT, Dilacor XR, others)	PO (regular release); 30 mg tid-qid (max: 480 mg/day) PO (extended release); 20–240 mg bid (max: 540 mg/day)	Dilates coronary arteries and decreases coronary artery spasm; also for hypertension; IV form available for dysrhythmias
nicardipine (Cardene)	PO; 20–40 mg tid or 30–60 mg PO (sustained release); bid (max: 120 mg/day)	Also for hypertension; IV form available
nifedipine (Adalat CC, Procardia XL, others) (see page 279 for the Drug Profile box)	PO; 10–20 mg tid (max: 180 mg/day) PO (extended release); 30–90 mg once daily	Used in the treatment of vasospastic angina; also for hypertension
verapamil (Calan, Isoptin SR, others) (see page 342 for the Drug Profile box)	PO (regular release); 80 mg tid-qid (max: 480 mg/day) PO (sustained release); 180 mg once daily	Dilates coronary arteries and inhibits coronary artery spasm; also for hypertension; IV form available for dysrhythmias
MISCELLANEOUS DRUG		
ranolazine (Ranexa)	PO; 500–1,000 mg bid (max: 1,000 mg bid)	Acts by shifting myocardial metabolism from fatty acids to glucose, which decreases the oxygen demands of the heart

trans = *across or through*
dermis = *skin*

Organic nitrates are of two types: short acting and long acting. The short-acting agents, such as nitroglycerin, are taken sublingually to quickly stop an acute angina attack in progress. Long-acting nitrates, such as isosorbide dinitrate (Dilatrate SR, Isordil), are taken orally or delivered through a transdermal patch to decrease the frequency and severity of angina episodes. Long-acting nitrates are also useful in reducing the symptoms of heart failure (see Chapter 18).

Drug Prototype: ℗ *Nitroglycerin (Nitrostat, Nitro-Bid, Nitro-Dur, Others)*

Therapeutic Class: **Antiangina drug**   Pharmacologic Class: **Organic nitrate, vasodilator**

Actions and Uses: Nitroglycerin, the oldest and most widely used of the organic nitrates, can be delivered by a number of different routes, including sublingual, lingual spray, oral, IV, transmucosal, transdermal, topical, and extended-release forms. It is normally taken while an acute angina episode is in progress or just prior to physical activity. When given sublingually, it reaches peak plasma levels in only four minutes and thus can stop angina pain rapidly. Chest pain that does not respond quickly to sublingual nitroglycerin may indicate MI. The transdermal and oral sustained-release forms are for prophylaxis only, because they have a relatively slow onset of action.

Adverse Effects and Interactions: Adverse effects of nitroglycerin are usually cardiovascular and rarely life threatening. Because nitroglycerin can dilate vessels in the head, headache is common and may be persistent and severe. Occasionally, the venodilation created by nitroglycerin causes *reflex tachycardia*. A beta-adrenergic blocker may be prescribed to diminish this undesirable increase in heart rate. Many adverse effects of nitroglycerin diminish after a few doses.

Using with sildenafil (Viagra) may cause life-threatening hypotension and CV collapse. Nitrates should not be taken 24 hours before or after taking Viagra.

Although nitrates are safe drugs that have few serious adverse effects, some adverse effects may be troublesome to patients. Dilation of veins can reduce blood pressure and cause patients to become dizzy when moving to a standing position. This fall in blood pressure can result in reflex tachycardia, causing patients to feel as if their heart is having palpitations or skipping a beat. Dilation of cerebral vessels may cause headache, which can sometimes be severe. Flushing of the skin is common. Most of these effects are temporary and rarely cause discontinuation of drug therapy.

tachy = *rapid*
cardia = *heart*

Tolerance commonly occurs with the long-acting organic nitrates when they are taken for extended periods. The magnitude of the tolerance depends on the dosage and the frequency of drug administration. Patients are often instructed to remove the transdermal patch for 6–12 hours each day or withhold the nighttime dose of the oral organic nitrate to delay the development of tolerance.

Beta-adrenergic blockers are sometimes the preferred drugs for reducing the frequency of angina attacks.

CORE CONCEPT **20.6**

Beta-adrenergic blockers reduce the workload on the heart and are used for angina prophylaxis. Drugs for angina include cardioselective beta$_1$-blockers and mixed beta$_1$-beta$_2$-blockers. The beta-adrenergic blockers of importance in treating angina are listed in Table 20.2.

The pharmacology of the beta-adrenergic blockers, including a Nursing Process Focus, was presented in Chapter 8. Beta blockers are widely used in medicine, including for the treatment of hypertension (see Chapter 18), heart failure (see Chapter 19), and dysrhythmias (see Chapter 22). Because of their ability to reduce the workload on the heart by slowing heart rate and reducing contractility, several beta blockers are used to decrease the frequency and severity of angina attacks caused by exertion.

Beta-adrenergic blockers are well tolerated by most patients. In some patients, fatigue, lethargy, and depression occur. Because beta blockers slow the heart rate, they are contraindicated in patients with bradycardia and heart block. Heart rate should be closely monitored so that it does not fall below 60 beats per minute (bpm) at rest or 100 bpm during exercise. Patients with diabetes should be aware that blood glucose levels should be monitored more frequently and that insulin doses may need to be adjusted accordingly. Patients should be advised against abruptly stopping beta-blocker therapy because this may result in a sudden increase in workload on the heart and acute angina symptoms. Patients should also be advised to make position changes slowly when going from a recumbent to an upright position to prevent dizziness and possible fainting.

Calcium channel blockers relieve angina pain by reducing the cardiac workload.

CORE CONCEPT **20.7**

Several calcium channel blockers (CCBs) reduce myocardial oxygen demand by lowering blood pressure and slowing the heart rate. They are widely used in the treatment of cardiovascular diseases. The first approved use of CCBs was for the treatment of angina. CCBs' importance to the pharmacotherapy of angina is listed in Table 20.2.

NURSING PROCESS FOCUS Patients Receiving Organic Nitrate Therapy

ASSESSMENT	POTENTIAL NURSING DIAGNOSES
Prior to administration: ■ Obtain a complete health history including cardiovascular conditions, allergies, drug history, and possible drug interactions. ■ Acquire the results of a complete physical examination, including vital signs, height, weight, and ECG. ■ Evaluate laboratory blood findings: CBC, electrolytes, cardiac enzymes, lipid panel, and renal and liver function studies. ■ Attain information regarding cardiac related medications such as sildenafil (Viagra), vardenafil (Levitra), or tadalafil (Cialis) used within the past 24 hours.	■ *Risk for Ineffective Tissue Perfusion* related to hypotension from drug therapy ■ *Risk for Injury* (dizziness or fainting) related to hypotension from drug therapy ■ *Acute Pain* (headache) related to adverse effects of drug ■ *Deficient Knowledge* related to a lack of information about drug therapy ■ *Ineffective Self-health Maintenance* related to lack of knowledge about seriousnesss of disease and drug therapy regimen

PLANNING: PATIENT GOALS AND EXPECTED OUTCOMES

The patient will:
■ Experience therapeutic effects (relief or prevention of chest pain).
■ Be free from or experience minimal adverse effects from drug therapy.
■ Verbalize an understanding of the drug's use, adverse effects, and required precautions.

IMPLEMENTATION

Interventions and (Rationales)	Patient Education/Discharge Planning
■ In cases of chest pain, administer medication correctly and evaluate the patient's knowledge of proper administration. Ask the patient to describe and rate pain prior to and throughout drug administration for description/documentation of angina episode. (Location and quality of pain will determine need for medication; patients at risk for angina or MI will need to carry drug in case of emergencies for.)	In case of chest pain, instruct the patient to: ■ Place one tablet under the tongue every five minutes during an attack, up to three times/tablets, until pain is relieved. ■ Place SL tablet under the tongue or spray under the tongue; do not inhale spray. ■ Call emergency medical services (EMS) if chest pain is not relieved after two or three doses.
■ Obtain a 12-lead ECG to differentiate between angina and infarction. (Pharmacotherapy depends on which disorder is presenting.)	■ Explain to the patient the reason for and importance of conducting an ECG.
■ Monitor vital signs, especially blood pressure and pulse. Do not administer drug if the patient is hypotensive. (Drug will further reduce blood pressure.)	Instruct the patient to: ■ Monitor blood pressure as specified by the healthcare provider and ensure proper use of home equipment. ■ Sit or lie down before taking medication and to avoid abrupt changes in position. ■ Explain to the patient the reason for and importance of monitoring blood levels that indicate cardiac function.
■ Monitor laboratory findings, especially cardiac enzymes, CBC, blood urea nitrogen (BUN), creatinine, and liver function test. (Monitoring blood levels supplies valuable information on patient's status.)	■ Advise the patient of the importance of keeping appointments for laboratory testing.
■ Monitor alcohol use. (Use of alcohol with nitrates may cause extremely low blood pressure.)	■ Emphasize the importance of avoiding alcohol while taking nitroglycerin.
■ Monitor for headache in response to use of nitrates. (Nitrates cause vasodilation including vessels in the head, which may cause pain.)	Instruct the patient that: ■ Headache is a common adverse effect that usually decreases over time. ■ Over-the-counter (OTC) medicines usually relieve the headache. ■ He or she must notify the healthcare provider if headaches continue.
■ Monitor for use of erectile dysfunction drugs (e.g., sildenafil) concurrently with nitrates. (Life-threatening hypotension may result with concurrent use of these drugs.)	Instruct the patient to: ■ Not take erectile dysfunction drugs within 24 hours after taking nitrates. ■ Wait at least 24 hours after taking erectile dysfunction drugs to resume nitrate therapy.
■ For use of prophylactic nitrates, administer medication correctly and evaluate the patient's knowledge of proper administration. (Some patients may need the vasodilation effect of nitrates on a continuous basis.)	■ Instruct patient in the appropriate dosing and administration of the specific nitrate being taken. ■ Advise the patient to take medication prior to a stressful event or physical activity to prevent angina.

EVALUATION OF OUTCOME CRITERIA

Evaluate the effectiveness of drug therapy by confirming that patient goals and expected outcomes have been met (see Planning). *See Table 20.2 for a list of drugs to which these nursing actions apply.*

Drug Prototype: ℗ *Atenolol (Tenormin)*

Therapeutic Class: Drug for angina, hypertension, or MI   **Pharmacologic Class: Beta-adrenergic blocker**

Actions and Uses: Atenolol is one of the most frequently pre-scribed drugs in the United States due to its relative safety and effectiveness in treating a number of chronic disorders, includ-ing heart failure, hypertension, stable angina, and MI. Atenolol selectively blocks beta$_1$ receptors in the heart. Its effectiveness in angina is attributed to its ability to slow heart rate and reduce contractility (negative inotropic effect), both of which lower myocardial oxygen demand. Because of its seven- to nine-hour half-life, it may be taken once a day.

Adverse Effects and Interactions: As a cardioselective beta$_1$ blocker, atenolol has few adverse effects on the lungs and is useful for patients experiencing bronchospasm. Like other beta blockers, therapy generally begins with low doses, which are gradually increased until the therapeutic effect is achieved. The most frequent adverse effects of atenolol include fatigue, weak-ness, dizziness, and hypotension.

Using atenolol together with calcium channel block-ers may cause excessive cardiac suppression. Using atenolol together with digoxin may cause slowed atrioventricular conduction leading to heart block. Patients should avoid using this drug with nicotine or caffeine because their va-soconstriction action will diminish the beneficial effects of atenolol.

BLACK BOX WARNING:
Abrupt discontinuation of atenolol should be avoided in patients with ischemic heart disease because this can cause acute angina pain; doses should be reduced over a one- to two-week period.

Blockade of calcium ion channels has a number of effects on the heart, most of which are similar to those of beta-adrenergic blockers. Like beta blockers, actions of the CCBs are presented in several chapters in this text for the treatment of hypertension (see Chapter 18) and dysrhythmias (see Chapter 22). A Nurs-ing Process Focus for this drug class is included in Chapter 18.

CCBs cause arteriolar smooth muscle to relax, thus lowering peripheral resistance and reducing blood pressure. This decreases the myocardial oxygen demand, thus reducing the frequency of angina pain. Some CCBs are selective for arterioles. Others, such as verapamil and diltiazem, have an additional beneficial ef-fect of slowing the heart rate (negative chronotropic effect). An additional effect of the CCBs is their abil-ity to dilate the coronary arteries, bringing more oxygen to the myocardium. This is especially important in patients with vasospastic angina. Because they are able to relieve the acute spasms of vasospastic angina, CCBs are considered drugs of choice for this condition.

Most adverse effects of CCBs are related to vasodilation, such as headache, dizziness, and edema of the ankles and feet. CCBs should be used with caution in patients taking other cardiovascular medications that slow conduction through the atrioventricular (AV) node, particularly digoxin or beta-adrenergic block-ers. The combined effects of these drugs may cause partial or complete AV heart block, heart failure, or dysrhythmias.

Concept Review 20.2

■ How does decreasing the workload on the heart result in reduction in angina pain?

Drug Prototype: ℗ *Diltiazem (Cardizem, Cartia XT, Dilacor XR, Others)*

Therapeutic Class: Drug for angina and hypertension   **Pharmacologic Class: Calcium channel blocker**

Actions and Uses: Diltiazem inhibits the transport of calcium ions into myocardial cells and has the ability to relax both coronary and peripheral blood vessels. It is useful in the treatment of atrial dysrhythmias and hypertension as well as angina. When given as sustained-release capsules, it may be administered once daily.

Adverse Effects and Interactions: Adverse effects of diltiazem are generally not serious and are related to vasodilation such

as headache, dizziness, and edema of the ankles and feet. Al-though diltiazem produces few adverse effects on the heart or vessels, it should be used with caution in patients taking other cardiovascular medications, particularly digoxin or beta-adren-ergic blockers; the combined effects of these drugs may cause heart failure or dysrhythmias.

Diltiazem increases the levels of digoxin or quinidine if taken together. It should be used cautiously with ginger because this combination may interfere with blood clotting.

MYOCARDIAL INFARCTION

A **myocardial infarction (MI)** is the result of a sudden occlusion of a coronary artery. Immediate pharmacologic treatment may reduce patient mortality.

The early diagnosis and treatment of myocardial infarction (MI) increases chances of survival.

MIs are responsible for a substantial number of deaths each year. Some patients die before reaching a medical facility for treatment, and many others die within 48 hours after the initial MI. Clearly, MI is a serious and frightening disease and is responsible for a large percentage of sudden deaths.

The primary cause of MI is advanced CAD. Plaque buildup can severely narrow one or more branches of the coronary arteries. Pieces of plaque may break off and lodge in a small vessel that serves a portion of the myocardium. Deprived of its oxygen supply, the affected area of the myocardium becomes ischemic and cardiac muscle cells begin to die unless the blood supply is quickly restored. Figure 20.3 ■ illustrates this blockage and the resulting reperfusion process.

Goals for the pharmacologic treatment of acute MI include the following:

- Restore blood supply (perfusion) to the damaged myocardium as quickly as possible through the use of thrombolytics
- Reduce myocardial oxygen demand with organic nitrates, beta blockers, or CCBs to prevent another MI
- Control or prevent MI-associated dysrhythmias with beta blockers or other antidysrhythmics
- Reduce post-MI mortality with aspirin, beta blockers, and angiotensin-converting enzyme (ACE) inhibitors
- Manage severe chest pain and associated anxiety with analgesics
- Prevent enlargement of the clot with anticoagulants and antiplatelet drugs

Fast Facts Myocardial Infarction

- About 1.5 million Americans experience a new or recurrent MI each year.
- About one third of patients experiencing an MI will die; half the deaths occur prior to arrival at the hospital.
- About 60% of patients who died suddenly of MI had no previous symptoms of the disease.
- Mortality from MI is slightly higher in men than in women.
- More than 20% of men and 40% of women will die from an MI within 1 year of being diagnosed.

Thrombolytics dissolve clots blocking the coronary arteries.

Thrombolytics are medications that are administered to dissolve an existing blood clot. In the treatment of MI, the goal of thrombolytic therapy is to dissolve clots that are obstructing the coronary arteries and restore circulation to the myocardium as quickly as possible. Thrombolytics are most effective when administered from 20 minutes to 12 hours after the onset of MI symptoms. Quick restoration of cardiac circulation has been found to prevent permanent damage to the myocardium and reduce mortality from the disease. After the clot is successfully dissolved, anticoagulant or antiplatelet therapy is initiated to prevent the formation of additional thrombi.

Thrombolytics have a narrow margin of safety and the primary risk is excessive bleeding from interference in the clotting process. Older adults have an increased risk of serious bleeding and intracranial hemorrhage. Patients with recent trauma or surgery should not receive these drugs. Vital signs must be monitored continuously, and any signs of bleeding generally call for discontinuation of therapy. Because these medications are rapidly destroyed in the blood, stopping the infusion normally results in the rapid termination of any adverse effects.

FIGURE 20.3

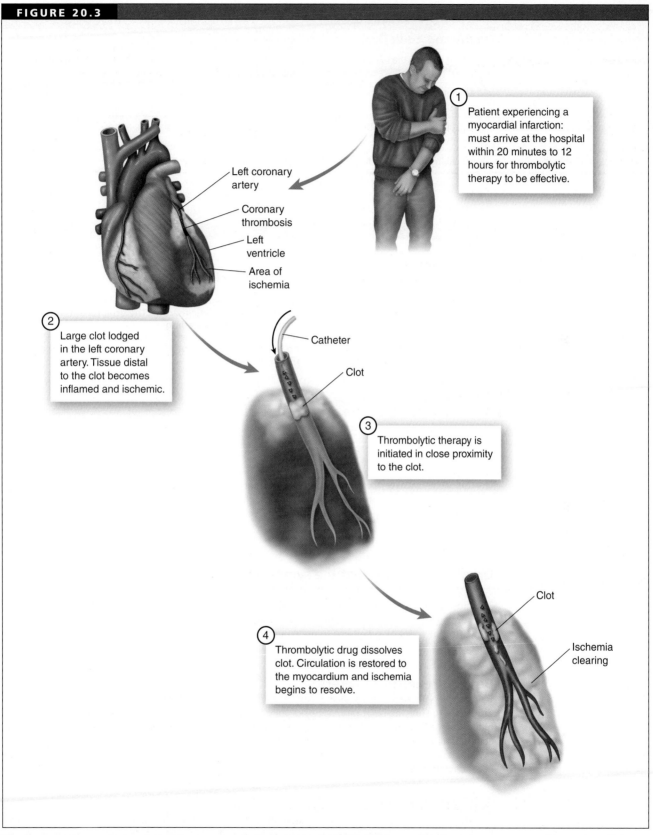

① Patient experiencing a myocardial infarction: must arrive at the hospital within 20 minutes to 12 hours for thrombolytic therapy to be effective.

Left coronary artery

Coronary thrombosis

Left ventricle

Area of ischemia

② Large clot lodged in the left coronary artery. Tissue distal to the clot becomes inflamed and ischemic.

Catheter

Clot

③ Thrombolytic therapy is initiated in close proximity to the clot.

④ Thrombolytic drug dissolves clot. Circulation is restored to the myocardium and ischemia begins to resolve.

Clot

Ischemia clearing

Blockade and reperfusion following myocardial infarction (MI): (1) blockage of left coronary artery with myocardial ischemia, (2) infusion of thrombolytics, (3) blood supply returning to myocardium, and (4) thrombus dissolving and ischemia clearing.

TABLE 20.3 Thrombolytics

Drug	Route and Adult Dose	Remarks
alteplase (Activase) (see page 357 for the Drug Profile box)	IV; 60 mg initially, then 20 mg/hr infused over next two hours	Naturally occurring tissue plasminogen activator; must be given within six hours of start of MI or three hours of thrombotic stroke
Pr reteplase (Retavase)	IV; 10 units over two minutes; repeat dose in 30 minutes	Given during an acute MI to decrease the risk of HF and death
streptokinase (Kabikinase)	IV; 250,000–1.5 million units over 60 minutes	For acute DVT, pulmonary embolism, and MI
tenecteplase (TNKase)	IV; 30–50 mg infused over five seconds	Newer thrombolytic with longer half-life

Drug Prototype: **Pr** *Reteplase (Retavase)*
Therapeutic Class: **Drug for dissolving clots** Pharmacologic Class: **Thrombolytic**

Actions and Uses: Like other drugs in this class, reteplase is most effective if given within 30 minutes but not later than 12 hours of the onset of MI symptoms. It usually acts within 20 minutes. A second bolus may be delivered after the first, if necessary. After the clot has been dissolved, therapy with heparin or another anticoagulant is started to prevent additional clots from forming.

Adverse Effects and Interactions: The major adverse effect of reteplase is hemorrhage. Healthcare providers must be vigilant in recognizing and reporting any abnormal bleeding that may occur during thrombolytic therapy. The drug is contraindicated in patients with active bleeding.

Drug interactions with anticoagulants and platelet aggregation inhibitors will produce an additive effect and increase the risk of bleeding.

Since the discovery of streptokinase, the first thrombolytic, there have been a number of generations of thrombolytics. The more recent drugs such as tenecteplase (TNKase) have a more rapid onset and a longer duration and may produce fewer adverse effects than older drugs in this class. Table 20.3 ◆ lists the major thrombolytics.

CORE CONCEPT 20.10

Drugs are used to treat the symptoms and complications of acute MI.

The most immediate needs of the patient with MI are to ensure that the heart continues functioning and that permanent damage from the infarction is minimized. Drugs from several classes are administered soon after the onset of symptoms to prevent reinfarction and, ultimately, to reduce mortality from the episode.

Beta-Adrenergic Blockers
Beta blockers are used for MI, as they are for angina, to reduce the cardiac workload. Beta blockers have the ability to slow the heart rate, decrease contractility, and reduce blood pressure. These three actions reduce the cardiac oxygen demand, which is beneficial for those who have experienced a recent MI. In addition, the ability of beta blockers to slow impulse conduction through the heart tends to suppress dysrhythmias, which can be serious and sometimes fatal complications can occur following MI. Their use has been found to reduce mortality following an MI if given within eight hours.

Antiplatelet and Anticoagulant Drugs
Aspirin has been found to dramatically reduce mortality, as much as 50%, in the weeks following an acute MI. Unless contraindicated, 160–324 mg of aspirin is given as soon as possible following a suspected MI. Clopidogrel (Plavix) is another effective antiplatelet agent that has been shown to reduce mortality associated with thrombi formation following an MI. Patients at high risk for thrombi formation may receive

NURSING PROCESS FOCUS   Patients Receiving Thrombolytic Therapy

ASSESSMENT	POTENTIAL NURSING DIAGNOSES
Prior to administration: ■ Obtain complete health history including cardiovascular, renal, and liver conditions; recent surgeries or trauma; allergies; drug history (especially cardiovascular and OTC); and possible drug interactions. ■ Acquire the results of a complete physical examination, including vital signs, height, and weight. ■ Evaluate laboratory blood findings: CBC, electrolytes, clotting factors (aPTT, PT, platelet count), and renal and liver function studies.	■ *Risk for Injury* (bleeding) related to adverse effects of thrombolytic therapy ■ *Ineffective Tissue Perfusion* related to increase in size of thrombus, altered blood flow ■ *Deficient Knowledge* related to a lack of information about drug therapy

PLANNING: PATIENT GOALS AND EXPECTED OUTCOMES

The patient will:
■ Experience therapeutic effects (dissolving of preexisting blood clot(s).
■ Be free from or experience minimal adverse effects from drug therapy.
■ Verbalize an understanding of the drug's use, adverse effects, and required precautions.

IMPLEMENTATION

Interventions and Rationales	Patient Education/Discharge Planning
■ Administer medication correctly; have IV lines initiated or Foley catheter inserted prior to beginning therapy. (This allows for monitoring the patient's condition.)	■ Instruct the patient about procedures and why they are necessary prior to beginning thrombolytic therapy.
■ Monitor vital signs every 15 minutes during the first hour of infusion, then every 30 minutes during the remainder of infusion. (A change in vital signs may indicate indication excessive bleeding, a major adverse effect of thrombolytic therapy.)	■ Advise the patient on the need for frequent monitoring of vital signs.
■ Patient should be moved as little as possible during the infusion. (This is done to prevent internal injury.)	■ Advise the patient that activity will be limited during infusion and that a pressure dressing may be needed to prevent any active bleeding.
■ If given for thrombotic stroke, monitor neurologic status frequently. (Changes in LOC can indicate excessive bleeding.)	■ Advise the patient about assessments and why they are necessary.
■ Have cardiac rhythm monitored while medication is infusing. (Dysrhythmias may occur with reperfusion of myocardium.)	■ Advise the patient that cardiac rhythm will be monitored during therapy.
■ Monitor laboratory findings (CBC, clotting factors and ABG) during and after therapy for indications of blood loss due to internal bleeding. (Patient has increased risk of bleeding for two to four days post infusion.)	■ Instruct the patient on increased risk for bleeding and on the need for activity restriction and frequent monitoring during this time.

EVALUATION OF OUTCOME CRITERIA

Evaluate the effectiveness of drug therapy by confirming that patient goals and expected outcomes have been met (see "Planning"). *See Table 23.4 for a list of drugs to which these nursing actions apply.*

anticoagulants such as heparin, low-molecular weight heparin, or warfarin (Coumadin) following an MI. Some patients may remain on anticoagulant therapy on a chronic basis after hospital discharge. The various coagulation modifiers are presented in Chapter 23.

Angiotensin-Converting Enzyme (ACE) Inhibitors

The ACE inhibitors captopril (Capoten) and lisinopril (Prinivil, Zestril) have also been found to reduce mortality following MI. These drugs are most effective when therapy is started within one or two days of the onset of symptoms. Oral therapy with the ACE inhibitors normally begins after thrombolytic therapy has been completed and the patient's condition has stabilized. The pharmacology of the ACE inhibitors is presented in Chapter 18.

Pain Management

Pain control is essential following acute MI to ensure the patient's comfort and reduce stress. Opioids such as morphine sulfate are sometimes given to ease the severe pain associated with acute MI and to sedate the anxious patient. Details on the pharmacology of the opioids were presented in Chapter 14.

Concept Review	20.3

- Why is it important to treat an MI within the first 24 hours after symptoms have begun? What classes of drugs are used for this purpose?

STROKE

A stroke is caused by a thrombus within or bleeding from a vessel serving the brain. Although drug therapy is limited, immediate treatment may reduce the degree of permanent disability resulting from a stroke.

CORE CONCEPT 20.11 | Aggressive treatment of stroke can increase survival.

Stroke is a major cause of permanent disability caused by blockage of blood to the brain or rupture of a blood vessel in the brain. The majority of strokes are caused by a thrombus in a vessel serving the brain (**thrombotic stroke**). Areas downstream from the clot lose their oxygen supply, and neural tissue will begin to die unless circulation is quickly restored. A smaller percentage of strokes, about 20%, are caused by rupture of a cerebral vessel and its associated bleeding into neural tissue (**hemorrhagic stroke**). Symptoms are the same for the two types of strokes. Specific symptoms will vary widely depending on the affected area of the brain and may include blindness, paralysis, speech problems, coma, and even dementia. Mortality from stroke is very high: As many as 40% of patients will die within the first year of a stroke.

Drug therapy of thrombotic stroke focuses on two main goals: prevention of strokes through the use of anticoagulants and antihypertensive agents, and restoration of blood supply to the affected portion of the brain as quickly as possible after an acute stroke through the use of thrombolytics.

Treatment for hemorrhage strokes depends on the cause and severity of the bleeding. Drugs used in the treatment of acute hemorrhagic stroke may include anticonvulsants to prevent seizure activity, antihypertensive agents to reduce BP, and osmotic diuretics to decrease intracranial pressure. Thrombolytic therapy is contraindicated in hemorrhagic strokes because its use would prolong bleeding into the intracranial space and cause further damage.

As discussed in Chapter 18, sustained, chronic hypertension is closely associated with stroke. Antihypertensive therapy with beta-adrenergic blockers, CCBs, diuretics, and ACE inhibitors can help manage blood pressure and reduce the probability of stroke.

In very low doses, aspirin reduces the incidence of stroke by discouraging the formation of thrombi by inhibiting platelet aggregation. Patients are often placed on low-dose aspirin therapy on a continual basis following their first stroke. Clopidogrel (Plavix) is an antiplatelet drug that may be used to provide antiplatelet activity in patients who cannot tolerate aspirin. Other anticoagulants such as warfarin may be given to prevent stroke in high-risk patients such as those with prosthetic heart valves.

The single most important breakthrough in the treatment of stroke was development of the thrombolytic agents. Prior to the discovery of these drugs, the treatment of thrombotic stroke was largely a passive, wait-and-see strategy. Now stroke is aggressively treated with thrombolytics as soon as the patient arrives at the hospital: These agents are most effective if administered within three hours of the attack. Use of aggressive thrombolytic therapy can completely restore brain function in a significant number of patients with stroke.

CAM THERAPY

Ginseng and Cardiovascular Disease

Ginseng is one of the oldest known herbal remedies. *Panax ginseng* is distributed throughout China, Korea, and Siberia, whereas *Panax quinquefolius* is native to Canada and the United States. American ginseng is not considered equivalent to Siberian ginseng.

Ginseng has been used for centuries to promote general wellness, boost immune function, and reduce fatigue. There are some claims that the herb lowers blood glucose and can help in the management of hypertension.

Ginseng is thought to have calcium channel blocking actions. The herb appears to improve blood flow to the heart in times of low oxygen supply, such as with myocardial ischemia. Some research has shown that ginseng lowers blood sugar levels in patients with type 2 diabetes. In addition, some studies have found ginseng to boost the immune system. The healthcare provider should caution patients who take ginseng, because herb–drug interactions are possible with CCBs, oral hypoglycemics, warfarin, and loop diuretics.

Fast Facts Stroke

- Stroke is the third leading cause of death, behind heart disease and cancer.
- The incidence of stroke increases with age, although 25% of all strokes occur in people younger than age 65:
  - 14% of those 65–74 years old have had a stroke
  - 25% of those 75–84 years old have had a stroke
  - 28% of those older than age 85 have had a stroke
- The highest incidence of stroke is in African American men—more than double that of white women.
- Stroke occurs more frequently in men than in women, although females account for about 60% of all deaths due to strokes.
- Over 160,000 Americans die of strokes each year.

PATIENTS NEED TO KNOW

Patients treated for chest pain need to know the following:

Regarding Drugs for Angina

1. Dissolve one nitroglycerin tablet under the tongue as soon as angina pain is felt. If pain is not relieved in five minutes, use another. Many practitioners recommend a third nitroglycerin tablet for pain not relieved five minutes after the second dose. If chest pain/pressure is not relieved by three doses of nitroglycerin, call EMS.
2. Rotate the application site of transdermal patches and do not apply a new patch until after the old patch has been removed.
3. Change positions slowly. Postural hypotension may cause dizziness and even fainting.
4. Monitor blood pressure regularly, and report any consistent changes to a healthcare provider.

Regarding Drugs for MI or Stroke

5. A variety of drugs are used in the treatment of MI and stroke. It is important to understand and comply with the drug therapy regimen prescribed by the healthcare provider.

CHAPTER REVIEW

CORE CONCEPTS SUMMARY

20.1 Coronary heart disease is caused by a restriction in blood flow to the myocardium.

The high metabolic rate of the heart requires that a continuous supply of oxygen be maintained in the coronary arteries. Restriction of flow can lead to angina pectoris or MI. Because both of these disorders can cause severe chest pain, the healthcare provider must quickly determine the cause of the pain, so that appropriate treatment may be administered.

20.2 Angina pectoris is characterized by severe chest pain caused by lack of sufficient oxygen flow to heart muscle.

The coronary arteries can become partially occluded with plaque, resulting in ischemia. Lack of sufficient oxygen to the myocardium upon emotional or physical exertion causes sharp chest pain, the characteristic symptom of angina.

20.3 Angina pain can often be controlled through positive lifestyle changes and surgical procedures.

A number of lifestyle changes can reduce the deposition of plaque in the coronary arteries and help prevent coronary heart disease. These include stopping tobacco use, limiting alcohol consumption, and getting adequate exercise. Surgical procedures may be necessary to control severe angina.

20.4 The pharmacologic management of angina is achieved by reducing cardiac workload.

Reducing the workload on the heart can relieve angina pain. This can be accomplished by slowing the heart rate, dilating the vessels, reducing the force of myocardial contraction, or reducing blood pressure.

20.5 The organic nitrates relieve angina pain by dilating veins and the coronary arteries.

Fast-acting organic nitrates can quickly terminate angina pain by causing venodilation, which reduces the workload on the heart. They also dilate the coronary arteries, bringing more oxygen to the myocardium. Long-acting nitrates can prevent acute angina episodes, but the patient may become tolerant to their protective effect.

20.6 Beta-adrenergic blockers are sometimes preferred drugs for reducing the frequency of angina attacks.

Beta blockers lower blood pressure, slow the heart rate, and reduce the force of contraction, thus reducing the workload on the myocardium. They are prescribed to reduce the frequency of acute angina episodes.

20.7 Calcium channel blockers (CCBs) relieve angina pain by reducing the cardiac workload.

CCBs are effective at lowering blood pressure, thus reducing the workload on the heart. They are prescribed to reduce the frequency of acute angina attacks.

20.8 The early diagnosis and treatment of myocardial infarction (MI) increases chances of survival.

MI is caused by a thrombus in a coronary artery and is responsible for a substantial number of sudden deaths. Fast, effective diagnosis and treatment can reduce mortality.

20.9 Thrombolytics dissolve clots blocking the coronary arteries.

When used within hours of the onset of an MI, thrombolytics can dissolve clots and restore circulation to the myocardium.

20.10 Drugs are used to treat the symptoms and complications of acute MI.

Beta blockers can slow the heart rate and reduce blood pressure and have been shown to reduce mortality when given soon after MI symptoms appear. Aspirin and ACE inhibitors have been shown to reduce mortality when given soon after the onset of MI. Narcotic analgesics are sometimes given to reduce the pain and anxiety associated with an MI.

20.11 Aggressive treatment of stroke can increase survival.

Stroke is now viewed as an emergency condition requiring immediate treatment to improve survival. Thrombolytics, when given quickly after the onset of thrombotic strokes, can restore some or all brain function. Some degree of stroke prevention can be achieved by using anticoagulants and by controlling blood pressure.

REVIEW QUESTIONS

The following questions are written in NCLEX-PN® style. Answer these questions to assess your knowledge of the chapter material, and go back and review any material that is not clear to you.

1. The patient is being discharged with nitroglycerin (Nitrostat) tablets. The nurse would teach the patient to:

1. "Swallow 3 tablets immediately for pain and call 911."
2. "Put one tablet under your tongue for chest pain."
3. "Call your physician when you have chest pain. The physician will tell you how many tablets to take."
4. "Place three tablets under your tongue and call 911."

2. The most common adverse effect of nitroglycerin that the nurse monitors the patient for is:

1. Headache
2. Hypertension
3. Diuresis
4. Bradycardia

3. The licensed practical/vocational nurse (LPN/LVN) is assisting the registered nurse in the development of a patient care plan. She recognizes that the patient is going to be receiving what class of medication that decreases heart rate, contractility, and blood pressure, and is used to increase survival rates in post-MI patients?

1. ACE inhibitors
2. Beta blockers
3. Vasodilators
4. Diuretics

4. The nurse assesses for the most common adverse effect of reteplase (Retavase), which is:

1. Dehydration
2. Bleeding
3. Confusion
4. Increased clotting times

5. The healthcare provider should be vigilant in observing for which of the following adverse effects during a reteplase infusion?

1. An increase in blood pressure
2. An increase in heart rate
3. Abnormal bleeding
4. Vomiting or diarrhea

6. The patient has a history of thrombotic stroke. Which of the following drug(s) might be used in her treatment? (Select all that apply.)

1. Aspirin
2. Warfarin (Coumadin)
3. Protamine sulfate
4. Ticlopidine (Ticlid)

7. The healthcare provider ordered an IV drip of D5W at 150 mL/hr. The tubing has a drip factor of 15 drops/mL. The nurse maintains the IV drip rate at how many drops per minute?

1. 25 drops/minute
2. 28 drops/minute
3. 35 drops/minute
4. 38 drops/minute

8. When treating angina, the nurse knows that the mechanism of action of a beta-adrenergic blocker is:

1. Slowed heart rate and decreased contractility of the heart
2. Relaxation of arterial and venous smooth muscle
3. Increased contractility and heart rate
4. Decreased peripheral resistance

9. The patient is instructed when taking calcium channel blockers that he should use extreme caution when taking which of the following medications?

1. Acetaminophen (Tylenol)
2. Ibuprofen (Motrin)
3. Digoxin (Lanoxin)
4. Ranitidine (Zantac)

10. The patient is complaining of a viselike pain in his chest and has been diagnosed with an MI. The nurse anticipates that he may be giving the patient which of the following medications? (Select all that apply.)

1. Aspirin
2. A beta blocker
3. Thrombolytics
4. An ACE inhibitor

CASE STUDY QUESTIONS

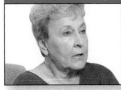

Remember Ms. Bush, the patient introduced at the beginning of the chapter? Now read the remainder of the case study. Based on the information you have learned in this chapter, answer the questions that follow.

Ms. Shirley Bush, a 65-year-old woman arrives in your office with a complaint of chest pain when she exercises. Subsequent tests show a 10% occlusion of two coronary arteries. Her blood pressure is 126/78 mmHg. The physician prescribes one aspirin per day, sublingual nitroglycerin, and metoprolol.

1. The nurse teaches Ms. Bush that the purpose of the nitroglycerin is to:

1. Prevent acute angina attacks.
2. End an angina attack in progress.
3. Prevent MI or stroke.
4. Relieve epigastric pain.

2. What instructions should the nurse provide to Ms. Bush about taking sublingual nitroglycerin?

1. Take before exercising.
2. Take on first indication of chest pain.
3. Take three or four times per day to prevent chest pain.
4. Take before bedtime and when rising.

3. Ms. Bush says, "What about the metoprolol?" The nurse tells her that she has been prescribed metoprolol to:

1. Prevent acute angina attacks.
2. End an angina attack in progress.
3. Prevent MI or stroke.
4. Lower blood pressure.

Ms. Bush discontinues her drugs without notifying her physician. Three months later, she arrives in the ED with a thrombotic stroke. Her blood pressure is 186/100 mmHg. The physician orders a reteplase infusion.

4. As the nurse starts the infusion, Ms. Bush asks, "What is this drug for?" The nurse tells her that the function of reteplase is to:

1. Dissolve existing blood clots.
2. Prevent possible formation of blood clots.
3. Stabilize blood pressure.
4. Reduce workload on the heart.

NOTE: Answers to the Review and Case Study Questions appear in Appendix B. The complete rationales and answers are located on the textbook's website.

Pearson Nursing Student Resources Find additional review materials at nursing.**nursing.pearsonhighered.com**.

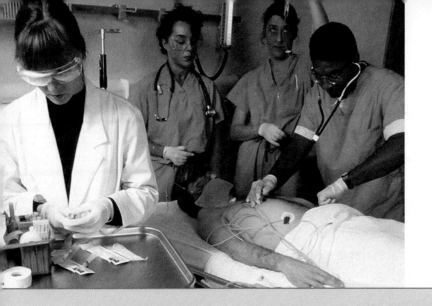

"*Where am I? What happened? I really hurt.*"

Mr. Joshua Hanks

Drugs for Shock and Anaphylaxis

21

CORE CONCEPTS

21.1 Shock is a syndrome characterized by the collapse of the circulatory system.

21.2 The initial treatment of shock includes basic life support and identification of the underlying cause.

21.3 Intravenous (IV) infusions are given to replace fluids lost during shock.

21.4 Vasoconstrictors are administered during shock to raise and maintain blood pressure.

21.5 Inotropic drugs are useful in reversing the decreased cardiac output that occurs during shock.

21.6 Anaphylaxis is a type of shock caused by a hyper-response of body defense mechanisms.

DRUG SNAPSHOT

The following drugs are discussed in this chapter:

DRUG CLASSES	DRUG PROTOTYPES
Fluid replacement drugs	**Pr** normal serum albumin (Albuminar, Plasbumin, others) *323*
Vasoconstrictors	**Pr** norepinephrine (Levophed) *326*
Inotropic drugs	**Pr** dopamine (Dopastat, Intropin) *326*
Drug for anaphylaxis	**Pr** epinephrine (Adrenalin) *327*

LEARNING OUTCOMES

After reading this chapter, the student should be able to:

1. Compare and contrast the different types of shock.

2. Relate the symptoms of shock to their physiologic causes.

3. Explain the initial treatment of a patient with shock.

4. Compare and contrast the use of blood products, colloids, and crystalloids in the pharmacotherapy of shock.

5. Identify the indications for the use of vasoconstrictors and inotropic drugs.

6. For each of the classes in the Drug Snapshot, identify representative drugs and explain their mechanisms of drug action, primary actions, and important adverse effects.

KEY TERMS

anaphylactic (ann-ah-fuh-LAK-tick) shock *320*
antigen (ANN-tuh-jen) *326*
cardiogenic shock (kar-dee-oh-JEN-ik) *320*

colloids (KO-loyds) *323*
crystalloids (KRIS-tuh-loyds) *323*
hypovolemic shock (high-poh-voh-LEEM-ik) *320*

inotropic drug (eye-noh-TROW-pik) *325*
neurogenic shock (nyoor-oh-JEN-ik) *320*
septic shock (SEP-tik) *320*
shock *320*

S hock is a condition in which vital organs are not receiving enough blood to function properly. Without an adequate supply of oxygen and other nutrients, cells cannot carry on normal metabolism. Shock is a medical emergency; failure to reverse the causes and symptoms of shock may lead to irreversible organ damage and death. This chapter examines how drugs are used to aid in the treatment of different types of shock.

SHOCK

CORE CONCEPT 21.1

Shock is a syndrome characterized by the collapse of the circulatory system.

There are several types of shock, each having different causes. A simple method for classifying shock is by naming the underlying pathologic process or organ system causing the disease. Table 21.1 ◆ describes the different types of shock and their primary causes. This chapter focuses on the pharmacologic therapy of three common types of shock: hypovolemic, cardiogenic, and anaphylactic.

Shock is a collection of signs and symptoms, many of which are nonspecific. Although symptoms vary among the different kinds of shock, there are some similarities. The patient may appear pale and claim to feel sick or weak without reporting any specific symptoms. Behavioral changes are often some of the earliest symptoms and may include restlessness, anxiety, confusion, depression, and lack of interest. Thirst is a common complaint. The skin may feel cold or clammy.

Assessing the patient's cardiovascular status may provide important clues for a diagnosis of shock. Blood pressure is usually low, with a diminished cardiac output. Heart rate may be rapid, with a weak pulse. Breathing is rapid and shallow. Figure 21.1 ■ illustrates some of the common symptoms of a patient in shock.

Diagnosis of shock is rarely based on such nonspecific symptoms. A careful medical history, however, will provide the healthcare provider with valuable clues as to what type of shock may be present. For example, obvious trauma or bleeding combined with the symptoms mentioned previously would suggest **hypovolemic shock**. If trauma to the brain or spinal cord is evident, **neurogenic shock** may be suspected. A history of heart disease would suggest **cardiogenic shock**, whereas a recent infection may indicate **septic shock**. A history of allergy with a sudden onset of symptoms following food or drug intake suggests **anaphylactic shock**.

The brain and heart are affected early in the progression of shock. Lack of blood to the brain may result in fainting, whereas disruption of blood supply to the myocardium can result in permanent damage to the heart. Immediate treatment is necessary to prevent failure of other organ systems, including respiratory collapse or renal failure.

hypo = *below*
vol = *volume*
emic = *pertaining to the blood*

neuro = *nervous system*
genic = *origin*

cardio = *heart*
genic = *origin*

CORE CONCEPT 21.2

The initial treatment of shock includes basic life support and identification of the underlying cause.

Acute shock is treated as a medical emergency, and the first goal is to provide basic life support. Rapid identification of the underlying cause is essential because the patient's condition may deteriorate rapidly without specific, emergency measures. Keeping the patient quiet and warm until specific therapy can be

TABLE 21.1 Classification of Shock		
Type of Shock	**Definition**	**Underlying Pathology**
Anaphylactic	Acute allergic reaction	Severe reaction to allergens such as penicillin, nuts, shellfish, or animal proteins
Cardiogenic	Failure of the heart to pump sufficient blood to tissues	Left heart failure, myocardial ischemia, MI, dysrhythmias, pulmonary embolism, and myocardial or pericardial infection
Hypovolemic	Loss of blood volume	Hemorrhage, burns, profuse sweating, excessive urination, vomiting, or diarrhea
Neurogenic	Vasodilation due to overstimulation of the parasympathetic nervous system or understimulation of the sympathetic nervous system	Trauma to the spinal cord or medulla, severe emotional stress or pain, drugs that depress the central nervous system
Septic	Multiple organ dysfunction as a result of pathogenic organisms in the blood	Widespread inflammatory response to bacterial, fungal, or parasitic infection

FIGURE 21.1

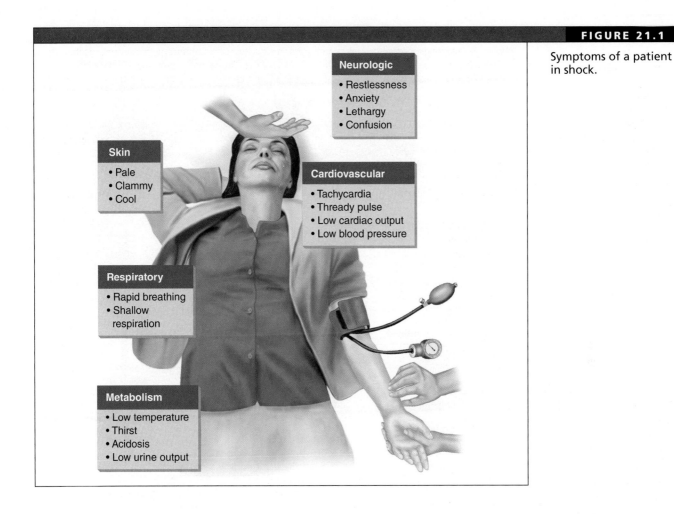

Symptoms of a patient in shock.

Neurologic
- Restlessness
- Anxiety
- Lethargy
- Confusion

Skin
- Pale
- Clammy
- Cool

Cardiovascular
- Tachycardia
- Thready pulse
- Low cardiac output
- Low blood pressure

Respiratory
- Rapid breathing
- Shallow respiration

Metabolism
- Low temperature
- Thirst
- Acidosis
- Low urine output

initiated is important. Maintaining the ABCs of life support—airway, breathing, and circulation—is critical. Once basic life support is established, the healthcare provider can begin more specific treatment of the underlying causes of the shock.

The remaining therapies for shock depend on the specific cause of the condition. The two primary pharmacotherapeutic goals are to restore normal fluid volume and composition and to maintain adequate blood pressure. Unless contraindicated, oxygen is administered. For anaphylaxis, an additional therapeutic goal is to prevent or stop the hypersensitive inflammatory response. Specific pharmacotherapies are illustrated in Figure 21.2 ■.

Concept Review   21.1

- What signs or symptoms might help a paramedic arriving on the scene of a motorcycle accident determine the cause of the patient's shock?

Fast Facts Shock

- Cardiogenic shock occurs in about 5–10% of the patients suffering from an acute myocardial infarction (MI).

- Cardiogenic shock is the leading cause of death in patients hospitalized with acute MI, with a mortality rate of up to 70–80%.

- The mortality rate for patients with sepsis who develop septic shock is 40–75%.

- The estimated death rate for anaphylaxis is 0.65–2% of all patients who experience the condition.

- Fewer than 100 fatal cases of anaphylaxis caused from insect stings occur annually in the United States.

FIGURE 21.2

Physiologic changes occurring during shock and their pharmacologic interventions.

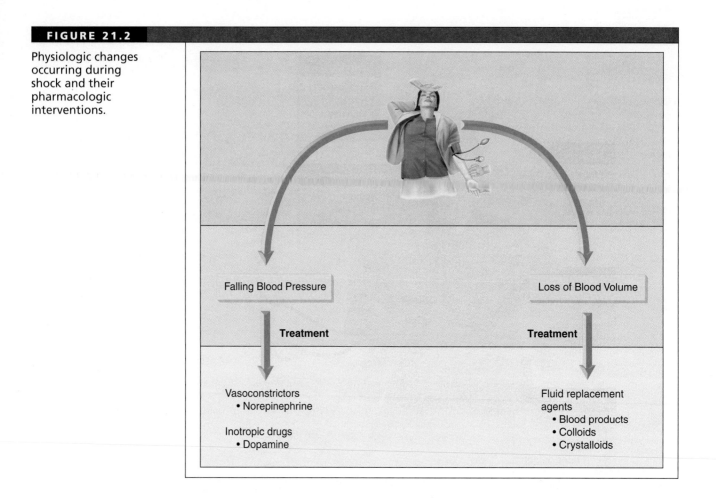

Falling Blood Pressure

Treatment

Vasoconstrictors
• Norepinephrine

Inotropic drugs
• Dopamine

Loss of Blood Volume

Treatment

Fluid replacement agents
• Blood products
• Colloids
• Crystalloids

CORE CONCEPT 21.3

Intravenous (IV) infusions are given to replace fluids lost during shock.

When a patient loses significant amounts of blood or other body fluids, immediate treatment with fluid replacement drugs is essential. Fluid loss can occur due to hemorrhage, extensive burns, severe dehydration, persistent vomiting or diarrhea, or aggressive diuretic therapy. Fluid loss can lead to dehydration and death if the fluid imbalance is not corrected. Fluid replacement drugs are sometimes referred to as *fluid expanders*.

The immediate goal in treating hypovolemic shock is to replace the lost fluid. In mild cases, this may be accomplished by drinking extra water or beverages containing electrolytes. In acute situations, therapy with IV infusions can immediately replace lost fluids. Regardless of how fluids are administered, careful attention must be paid to restoring normal levels of electrolytes as well as fluid volume.

Fluid replacement agents may be categorized as blood products, colloids, or crystalloids. Colloid and crystalloid infusions are often used when up to one-third of an adult's blood volume is lost. Examples of fluid replacement drugs are listed in Table 21.2 ◆.

Blood Products

Whole blood may be used for the treatment of acute, massive blood loss when there is the need to replace plasma volume and supply red blood cells. The supply of blood products, however, depends on human donors and requires careful cross-matching to ensure compatibility between the donor and the patient. Furthermore, the use of whole blood has the potential to transmit serious infections such as hepatitis or HIV. The administration of whole blood to expand fluid volume has been largely replaced with the use of specific blood components, along with colloids and crystalloids.

A single unit of whole blood can be separated into its specific constituents (red and white blood cells, platelets, plasma proteins, fresh frozen plasma, and globulins). This allows a single blood donation to be used to treat more than one patient.

TABLE 21.2 Fluid Replacement Drugs

Drug	Examples
Blood products	■ Whole blood ■ Plasma protein fraction ■ Fresh frozen plasma ■ Packed red blood cells
Colloids	■ Plasma protein fraction (Plasmanate, Plasma-Plex, Plasmatein, PPF, Protenate) ■ (Pr) Normal serum albumin (Albuminar, Plasbumin, others) ■ Dextran 40 (Gentran 40, Hyskon, Rheomacrodex) or dextran 70 (Macrodex) ■ Hetastarch (Hespan)
Crystalloids	■ Normal saline (0.9% sodium chloride), an isotonic solution ■ Lactated Ringer's, an isotonic solution ■ 0.45% normal saline (0.45% sodium chloride), a hypotonic solution ■ 5% dextrose in normal saline (D5W), a hypertonic solution ■ 5% dextrose in water (D5W), although the solution is isotonic, it becomes hypotonic once infused and metabolized

Colloids

Colloids are proteins or other large molecules that stay suspended in the blood for a long period and draw water molecules from the body's cells and tissues into the blood vessels. Colloids include normal human serum albumin, dextran, and hetastarch (Hespan). These drugs are administered to provide life-sustaining support following massive hemorrhage and to treat shock, burns, acute liver failure, and neonatal hemolytic disease.

Crystalloids

Crystalloids are IV solutions that contain electrolytes in amounts resembling those of natural plasma. Unlike colloids, crystalloid solutions can readily leave the blood and enter the cells or tissues. They are used to replace fluids that have been lost and to increase urine output. Crystalloid solutions are classified by their tonicity in relation to plasma. Tonicity refers to the concentration of dissolved molecules (solutes) within the solution. These solutions are classified as either *isotonic* (having the same concentration of solutes as plasma), *hypertonic* (having a greater concentration of solutes than plasma), or *hypotonic* (having a lesser concentration of solutes than plasma). The most common crystalloids used for the treatment of shock are isotonic solutions; they are primarily used to replace the loss of fluid volume.

Drug Prototype: (Pr) *Normal Serum Albumin (Albuminar, Plasbumin, Others)*
Therapeutic Class: **Fluid replacement drug**   **Pharmacologic Class:** **Blood product, colloid**

Actions and Uses: Normal serum albumin is a protein extracted from whole blood or plasma. Because of this, it may be classified as both a blood product and a colloid. Its functions are to maintain plasma osmotic pressure and to shuttle certain substances through the blood, including a substantial number of drug molecules. After extraction from blood or plasma, albumin is sterilized to remove possible contamination by the hepatitis viruses or HIV.

Administered IV, albumin is used to restore plasma volume during hypovolemic shock or to restore blood proteins in patients with hypoproteinemia. It has an immediate onset of action and is available in concentrations of 5% and 25%.

Adverse Effects and Interactions: Because albumin is a natural blood product, the patient may have antibodies to the donor's albumin, and allergic reactions are possible. Signs of allergy include fever, chills, rash, dyspnea, and possibly hypotension. Protein overload may occur if excessive albumin is infused.

No clinically significant drug interactions have been identified.

NURSING PROCESS FOCUS Patients Receiving Intravenous Fluid Therapy

ASSESSMENT	POTENTIAL NURSING DIAGNOSES
Prior to administration: ■ Obtain a complete health history including cardiovascular, respiratory, neurological, renal and skin conditions, allergies, drug history, and possible drug interactions. ■ Acquire the results of a complete physical examination, including vital signs, height, weight, presence of burns, lung sounds, LOC and urinary and cardiac output. ■ Evaluate laboratory blood findings: CBC, electrolytes, ABG, clotting factors, total protein/albumin, lipid panel, and renal and liver function studies.	■ *Deficient Fluid Volume* related to injury ■ *Ineffective Tissue Perfusion* related to decreased blood volume. ■ *Risk for Injury* related to loss of blood or adverse effect of drug therapy ■ *Risk for Electrolyte Imbalance* related to fluid loss ■ *Risk for Imbalanced Fluid Volume* related to drug therapy ■ *Deficient Knowledge* related to a lack of information about drug therapy

PLANNING: PATIENT GOALS AND EXPECTED OUTCOMES

The patient will:
■ Experience therapeutic effects (urinary output of at least 50 mL/hr and systolic blood pressure greater than 90 mm Hg).
■ Be free from or experience minimal adverse effects from drug therapy.
■ Verbalize an understanding of the drug's use, adverse effects, and required precautions.

IMPLEMENTATION

Interventions and (Rationales)	Patient Education/Discharge Planning
■ Administer intravenous fluids correctly, checking type of fluid and frequently monitoring flow rate and IV site. (Frequently monitoring the infusion of IV fluids will help prevent adverse effects.)	■ Inform patient about the need for IV fluids and the reason for frequent monitoring.
■ Monitor respiratory status: respirations, effort, O₂ saturation, and lung sounds. Report any signs of distress immediately to healthcare provider. (Effects of drugs and rapid infusion may result in fluid overload.)	Instruct the patient to: ■ Report any signs of respiratory distress such as shortness of breath to healthcare provider. ■ Report changes in sensorium such as lightheadedness, drowsiness, or dizziness to the healthcare provider.
■ Monitor cardiac function: BP, pulse, heart rate/rhythm, cardiac output, ECG, and laboratory blood tests. (Effects of drugs and rapid infusion may result in fluid overload and put stress on the circulatory system.) ■ Monitor renal function: Intake/output, urine color, BUN, creatinine, presence of edema, or dehydration. (Renal function changes with an increase or decrease in fluid volume. A decrease is usually seen with shock.)	■ Inform the patient about the rationale for monitoring cardiac function and to immediately report any palpitations, chest pain, or headache. ■ Instruct the patient about the rationale for monitoring fluid intake and output, laboratory tests, and possible need for a Foley catheter.
■ Weigh patient daily. (Daily weight is an accurate measure of fluid status.) ■ Monitor electrolytes. (Crystalloid drugs may cause hypernatremia and the resulting fluid retention.)	■ Teach the patient the rationale for monitoring weight to report any evidence of weight gain. ■ Instruct the patient to report any evidence of edema.
■ Observe the patient for signs of allergic reactions. (Administration of blood and blood products could cause allergic reactions.)	Instruct the patient: ■ To report itching, rash, chills, and difficulty breathing to the healthcare provider. ■ That frequent blood draws are necessary to monitor possible complications of drug administration.

EVALUATION OF OUTCOME CRITERIAM

Evaluate the effectiveness of drug therapy by confirming that patient goals and expected outcomes have been met (see Planning).

CORE CONCEPT 21.4

Vasoconstrictors are administered during shock to maintain blood pressure.

In the early stages of shock, the body compensates for the rapid fall in blood pressure by activating the sympathetic nervous system. This sympathetic activity causes vasoconstriction, which raises blood pressure and increases the heart rate and force of myocardial contractions. These compensatory measures help to maintain blood flow to vital organs such as the heart and brain and to decrease the flow to "less essential" organs such as the kidneys and liver.

The body's ability to compensate is limited, however, and profound hypotension may develop as shock progresses. In severe cases, vasoconstrictors, also called vasopressors, may be needed to help stabilize blood pressure. Because of the potential for serious adverse effects and potential organ damage due to the rapid and intense vasoconstriction, vasopressors are used only after fluid infusions have failed to raise blood pressure. Patients receiving these drugs must be monitored continuously during the infusion to avoid hypertension. Vasoconstrictor therapy is discontinued as soon as the patient's condition stabilizes. Discontinuation is always gradual, due to the possibility of rebound hypotension and undesirable cardiac effects.

Vasoconstrictors used to treat shock include dopamine (Dopastat, Intropin), norepinephrine (Levophed), phenylephrine (Neo-Synephrine), and epinephrine. Because dopamine also affects the strength of myocardial contraction, it is considered both a vasopressor and an inotropic drug (see Concept Section 21.5). Epinephrine is usually associated with the treatment of anaphylaxis (Section 21.6). The basic pharmacology of the sympathomimetic drugs is presented in Chapter 8. Table 21.3 ◆ gives the dosages for these drugs.

Inotropic drugs are useful in reversing the decreased cardiac output that occurs during shock.

As shock progresses, the heart begins to fail and cardiac output declines. This lowers the amount of blood reaching vital tissues and deepens the degree of shock. **Inotropic drugs**, also called *cardiotonic drugs*, have the potential to reverse the cardiac symptoms of shock by increasing the force of myocardial contraction. The role of the inotropic drug digoxin (Lanoxin) in treating patients with heart failure was presented in Chapter 19. Digoxin increases myocardial contractility and cardiac output, thus rapidly bringing tissues their needed oxygen. Chapter 19 should be reviewed because drugs prescribed for heart failure are sometimes used for the treatment of shock.

Dopamine is often a preferred drug for increasing the cardiac output in acute situations because it has both inotropic and vasoconstriction actions. Dobutamine (Dobutrex) is a beta$_1$-adrenergic agent that has value in the short-term treatment of certain types of shock because of its ability to cause the heart to beat more forcefully without significantly increasing heart rate. The resulting increase in cardiac output assists in maintaining blood flow to vital organs. Although very effective, dobutamine has a half-life of only 2 minutes, and therapy is limited to 72 hours.

TABLE 21.3   Vasoconstrictors and Inotropic Drugs for Shock

Drug	Rate and Adult Dose	Remarks
digoxin (Lanoxin, Lanoxicaps) (see page 295 for the Drug Prototype box)	IV; digitalizing dose 2.5–5 mcg every 6 hours for 24 hours; maintenance dose 0.125–0.5 mg/day	Doses are highly individualized for each patient; oral forms available; also for dysrhythmias and heart failure.
dobutamine (Dobutrex)	IV; infused at a rate of 2.5–40 mcg/kg/min for a max of 72 hours	Selective to beta$_1$-adrenergic receptors; for cardiac decompensation
🅟 dopamine (Dopastat, Intropin)	IV; 2–5 mcg/kg/min initial dose; may be increased to 20–50 mcg/kg/min	May activate dopaminergic, beta$_1$- or alpha$_1$-adrenergic receptors, depending on dose
🅟 epinephrine (Adrenalin)	Subcutaneous; 0.1–0.5 mL of 1:100 every 10–15 min; IV 0.1–0.25 mL of 1:1,000 every 10–15 min	Nonselective adrenergic drug; available by other routes for cardiac arrest and asthma and as an adjunct to local anesthesia
🅟 norepinephrine (Levophed)	IV; Initial 0.5–1 mcg/min, titrate to response; usual range 8–30 mcg/min	Activates alpha- and beta$_1$-adrenergic receptors; also for cardiac arrest
phenylephrine (Neo-Synephrine) (see page 98 for the Drug Prototype box)	IV; 0.1–0.18 mg/min until pressure stabilizes, then 0.04–0.06 mg/min for maintenance	Selective to alpha$_1$-receptors; used to maintain blood pressure during general anesthesia; also for certain dysrhythmias, nasal congestion, and glaucoma, and to dilate the pupil during eye exams; subcutaneous, IM, ophthalmic, and intranasal forms available

Drug Prototype (Pr) *Norepinephrine (Levophed)*

Therapeutic Class: **Drug for shock** Pharmacologic Class: **Sympathomimetic, vasoconstrictor**

Actions and Uses: Norepinephrine acts directly on alpha-adrenergic receptors in the smooth muscle of blood vessels to immediately raise blood pressure. Its stimulation of beta$_1$-receptors in the heart increases the force of contraction and increases cardiac output. It is given by the IV route and has a duration of only one to two minutes after the infusion is terminated.

Adverse Effects and Interactions: Norepinephrine is a powerful vasoconstrictor; thus, continuous monitoring of blood pressure is required to prevent the development of hypertension. When first administered, reflex bradycardia is sometimes experienced. It also has the ability to produce various types of dysrhythmias. Because of its potent effects on the cardiovascular system, it should be used with great caution in patients with heart disease.

Norepinephrine interacts with many drugs, including alpha and beta blockers, which may decrease the drug's effects on blood pressure. Conversely, ergot alkaloids and tricyclic antidepressants may increase vasopressor effects.

> **BLACK BOX WARNING:**
> Following extravasation, the affected area should be infiltrated immediately with 5–10 mg of phentolamine, an adrenergic blocker.

Drug Prototype (Pr) *Dopamine (Dopastat, Intropin)*

Therapeutic Class: **Drug for shock** Pharmacologic Class: **Nonselective adrenergic agonist, inotropic drug**

Actions and Uses: Dopamine is the immediate metabolic precursor to norepinephrine. Although classified as a sympathomimetic, the mechanism of dopamine's action is dependent on the dose. At low doses, dopamine selectively increases blood flow through the kidneys. This makes dopamine of particular value in treating hypovolemic and cardiogenic shock. At higher doses, dopamine stimulates beta$_1$-adrenergic receptors, causing the heart to beat with more force and increasing cardiac output. Another beneficial effect of dopamine when given in higher doses is its ability to stimulate alpha-adrenergic receptors, thus causing vasoconstriction and raising blood pressure.

Adverse Effects and Interactions: Because of its intense effects on the cardiovascular system, patients receiving dopamine are continuously monitored for signs of dysrhythmias and hypotension. Adverse effects are normally self-limiting because of the short half-life of the drug.

Dopamine interacts with many other drugs. For example, administering it with monoamine oxidase (MAO) inhibitors and ergot alkaloids increases alpha-adrenergic effects. Phenytoin may decrease dopamine action. Beta blockers may block the cardiac effects of dopamine. Alpha blockers decrease peripheral vasoconstriction. Halothane increases the risk of hypertension and ventricular dysrhythmias.

> **BLACK BOX WARNING:**
> Following extravasation, the affected area should be infiltrated immediately with 5 mg to 10 mg of phentolamine, an adrenergic blocker.

ANAPHYLAXIS

CORE CONCEPT 21.6

Anaphylaxis is a type of shock caused by a hyper-response of body defense mechanisms.

an = *without or against*
phylaxis = *protection*

Anaphylaxis is a condition in which the natural body defenses produce a hyper-response to an antigen. An **antigen** is anything that is recognized as foreign by the body. Certain foods, industrial chemicals, drugs, pollen, animal proteins, and even latex gloves can be antigens. A more detailed discussion of the immune system and the pharmacotherapy of immune disorders are included in Chapter 24.

Following the exposure to an antigen, the body normally responds with actions such as inflammation, antibody production, and activation of lymphocytes that rid the body of the foreign substance. During anaphylaxis, however, the body responds quickly—usually within minutes after exposure to the antigen—by releasing massive amounts of histamine and other inflammatory mediators. The patient may experience itching, hives, and a tightness in the throat or chest. Swelling occurs around the larynx, causing a hoarse voice and a nonproductive cough. As anaphylaxis progresses, the patient experiences a rapid fall in blood pressure and difficulty breathing due to bronchoconstriction. The fall in blood pressure causes *reflex tachycardia*, a rebound speeding up of the heart. Untreated anaphylactic shock may result in death. Figure 21.3 ■ illustrates the signs and symptoms of anaphylaxis.

FIGURE 21.3

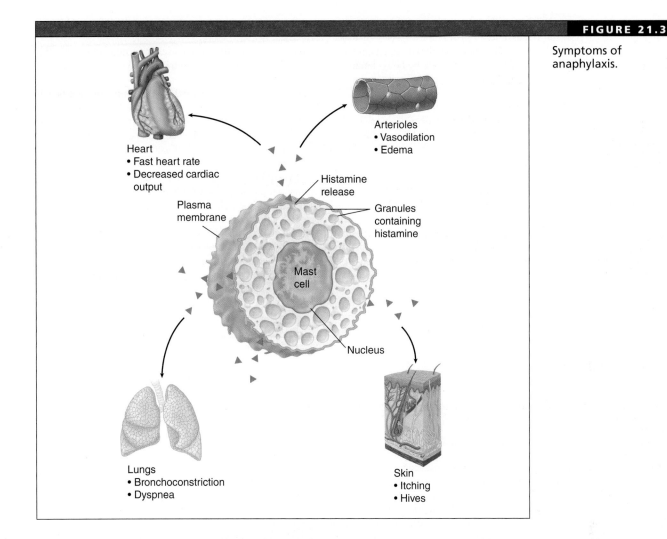

Symptoms of anaphylaxis.

Heart
• Fast heart rate
• Decreased cardiac output

Arterioles
• Vasodilation
• Edema

Histamine release

Plasma membrane

Granules containing histamine

Mast cell

Nucleus

Lungs
• Bronchoconstriction
• Dyspnea

Skin
• Itching
• Hives

It is always easier to *prevent* anaphylaxis than it is to *treat* it. Patients should be strongly advised to avoid substances that might trigger acute allergic reactions. This includes carefully reading all food and cosmetic labels to avoid exposure to known allergens. Individuals with known allergies to insect stings or food should carry a portable form of epinephrine, such as an EpiPen or Auvi-Q, a newer self-administration device that has built-in verbal instructions. The healthcare provider should always obtain a comprehensive drug allergy history before administering medications. Common allergens include the penicillin antibiotics and iodine-based contrast media used for radiologic exams. The patient should be observed in

Drug Prototype 💊 *Epinephrine (Adrenalin)*
Therapeutic Class: Drug for anaphylaxis and shock   Pharmacologic Class: Sympathomimetic, vasoconstrictor

Actions and Uses: Subcutaneous or IV epinephrine is a drug of choice for acute anaphylactic shock because it can reverse many of the distressing symptoms within minutes. Epinephrine is nonselective and activates both alpha- and beta-adrenergic receptors. Almost immediately after injection, blood pressure rises due to the stimulation of alpha$_1$-receptors. Activation of beta$_2$-receptors in the bronchi opens the airways to relieve shortness of breath. Cardiac output increases due to stimulation of beta$_1$-receptors in the heart. Epinephrine can also be administered topically, by inhalation, or by the intracardiac route.

Adverse Effects and Interactions: The most common adverse effects of epinephrine are nervousness, tremors, palpitations, dizziness, headache, and stinging/burning at the site of application. When administered parenterally, hypertension and dysrhythmias may occur rapidly; therefore, the patient is monitored continuously following IV or subcutaneous injections.

Epinephrine interacts with many drugs. For example, it may increase hypotension with phenothiazines and oxytocin. There may be additive toxicities with other sympathomimetics. MAO inhibitors, tricyclic antidepressants, and alpha- and beta-adrenergic drugs inhibit the actions of epinephrine.

the outpatient setting for 20 to 60 minutes after a drug injection because delayed anaphylactic reactions are possible.

The pharmacotherapy of anaphylaxis involves supporting the cardiovascular system and preventing further hyper-response by body defenses. Various medications are used to treat the symptoms of anaphylaxis, depending on the severity of the symptoms.

At the first suspicion of anaphylaxis, epinephrine is administered and IV fluid infusions are begun. Epinephrine is an initial drug for acute shock because it causes vasoconstriction and can rapidly relieve symptoms of bronchoconstriction. It may be necessary to use other vasoconstrictors (see Table 21.3) to overcome severe hypotension. Infusion of large amounts of fluids may be needed to overcome circulatory shock. These may include blood products, colloids, or crystalloids. Fluid infusions continue until systolic blood pressure reaches at least 90 mmHg and is stable.

A number of other drugs are useful in treating symptoms of anaphylaxis. Oxygen is usually administered immediately. Antihistamines such as diphenhydramine (Benadryl) may be administered intramuscularly or intravenously to prevent additional release of histamine. A bronchodilator such as albuterol (Ventolin, Proventil) is sometimes administered by inhalation to relieve the acute shortness of breath caused by histamine release. Corticosteroids such as hydrocortisone may be administered to dampen the acute inflammatory response that occurs during anaphylaxis. Corticosteroids may be administered for 24 hours or longer to prevent the possibility of delayed anaphylactic reactions. Additional effects of antihistamines are discussed in Chapter 24, bronchodilators in Chapter 29, and corticosteroids in Chapter 32, respectively.

Concept Review 21.2

■ How can inotropic drugs reduce the symptoms of shock without causing vasoconstriction?

PATIENTS NEED TO KNOW

Patients treated for shock need to know the following:

1. Seek emergency medical assistance immediately if signs or symptoms of shock are being experienced.
2. While waiting for medical assistance, keep warm by using blankets.
3. Have a caregiver, if present, monitor temperature, pulse, and blood pressure until emergency medical assistance arrives.
4. Do not move around. Lie down and elevate the feet.
5. Report any changes in mental status, such as depression, confusion, or anxiety, to the healthcare provider immediately.
6. If allergies to bee or wasp stings are known, carry medications such as an EpiPen for all outside activities. Inform others of any allergies, where medications are kept, and how to administer them.
7. Take medications for shock (such as epinephrine) exactly as prescribed.

CHAPTER REVIEW

CORE CONCEPTS SUMMARY

21.1 Shock is a syndrome characterized by the collapse of the circulatory system.

Basic types of shock include cardiogenic, hypovolemic, neurogenic, septic, and anaphylactic shock. Nonspecific symptoms of shock include hypotension, cold or clammy skin, reduced cardiac output, and behavioral changes such as confusion, apathy, or disorientation.

21.2 The initial treatment of shock includes basic life support and identification of the underlying cause.

Shock may be life threatening if allowed to proceed without medical intervention. Immediate therapy is targeted at restoring or maintaining vital processes such as respiratory function, blood pressure, and cardiac output. Immediate drug therapy includes vasoconstrictors, inotropic drugs, and IV fluid agents.

21.3 Intravenous (IV) infusions are given to replace fluids lost during shock.

Intravenous fluid agents include blood products, colloids, and crystalloids. These drugs help to maintain circulation and raise blood pressure.

21.4 Vasoconstrictors are administered during shock to maintain blood pressure.

An immediate concern for the patient in shock is a fall in blood pressure. A variety of adrenergic drugs, both selective and nonselective, are used to maintain blood pressure and cardiac function.

21.5 Inotropic drugs are useful in reversing the decreased cardiac output that occurs during shock.

Circulatory failure can occur during shock if the cardiac output falls below a critical level. A number of inotropic drugs are used to strengthen myocardial function and to improve cardiac output.

21.6 Anaphylaxis is a type of shock caused by a hyperresponse of body defense mechanisms.

When the body mounts a hyper-response to an antigen, anaphylactic shock may result. Epinephrine is a drug of choice for immediately reversing the cardiovascular symptoms. Intravenous fluid infusion agents, antihistamines, and corticosteroids also serve roles in treating this form of shock.

REVIEW QUESTIONS

The following questions are written in NCLEX-PN® style. Answer these questions to assess your knowledge of the chapter material, and go back and review any material that is not clear to you.

1. The patient with severe burns has just been admitted to hospital. The nurse will monitor for signs/symptoms of:

1. Cardiogenic shock
2. Hypovolemic shock
3. Septic shock
4. Anaphylactic shock

2. In the plan of care, the *most* important intervention for a patient experiencing shock is assessing:

1. Temperature
2. Heart rate
3. Respirations rate
4. Blood pressure

3. The nurse is preparing an IV solution for a patient in hypovolemic shock. Which IV solution would be most appropriate for this patient?

1. 0.45% NS
2. Normal serum albumin
3. 0.33% NS
4. D5W

4. The patient's family is asking questions about the medications used in the treatment for shock. The nurse explains that dopamine is one of the drugs being used and that it works: (Select all that apply.)

1. At low doses, to cause increased blood flow to the kidneys
2. At high doses, to increase cardiac output
3. To cause vasoconstriction and increases blood pressure
4. At high doses, to treat anaphylaxis

5. The patient is experiencing anaphylaxis. The nurse would administer which drug to increase blood pressure and treat bronchospasm related to anaphylaxis?

1. Epinephrine
2. Dobutamine (Dobutrex)

3. Digoxin (Lanoxin)
4. Dopamine

6. In reviewing a plan of care for a patient exhibiting the symptoms of anaphylaxis, which of the following medications would be avoided?

1. Antihistamines
2. Corticosteroids
3. Bronchodilators
4. Vasodilators

7. After administering an inotropic medication to a patient in shock, the nurse monitors the patient for signs of:

1. Decreased cardiac output
2. Increased cardiac output
3. Slowing of the heart rate
4. Increased afterload

8. When administering norepinephrine (Levophed), the nurse monitors the patient for:

1. Tachycardia
2. Hypotension
3. Hypertension
4. Liver failure

9. Dobutamine (Dobutrex) is used to treat shock because:

1. It increases myocardial contractility and heart rate.
2. It increases myocardial contractility without significantly increasing heart rate.
3. It decreases cardiac output.
4. It is a powerful vasoconstrictor.

10. The healthcare provider has ordered 1,000 mL of 0.9% sodium chloride to be administered intravenously over five hours. The drop factor on the tubing is 15 drops/mL. How many milliliters per hour will you administer and how many drops per minute?

1. 250 mL/hr and 50 drops/min
2. 200 mL/hr and 50 drops/min
3. 200 mL/hr and 45 drops/min
4. 250 mL/hr and 45 drops/min

CASE STUDY QUESTIONS

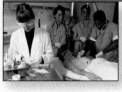

Remember Mr. Hanks from the beginning of the chapter? Now read the remainder of the case study. Based on the information you have learned in this chapter, answer the questions that follow.

Mr. Joshua Hanks arrives in the emergency department having lost a considerable amount of blood in an automobile accident. His blood pressure is 60/30 mmHg. His skin is clammy, and he is going in and out of consciousness. He is gasping for breath. The physician orders an infusion of 0.9% sodium chloride, IV dobutamine, IM hydrocortisone, and subcutaneous epinephrine.

1. The nurse notices that Mr. Hanks' breathing is labored and he appears anxious. The nurse administers which of the prescribed medications to help reduce Mr. Hanks' bronchospasm?

1. 0.9% sodium chloride
2. Dobutamine
3. Hydrocortisone
4. Epinephrine

2. Which drug was given to replace the fluids lost during Mr. Hanks' accident?

1. 0.9% sodium chloride
2. Dobutamine
3. Hydrocortisone
4. Epinephrine

3. Within two minutes, Mr. Hanks' blood pressure increases to 100/60 mmHg. The nurse understands that which drug most likely caused this effect?

1. 0.9% sodium chloride
2. Dobutamine
3. Hydrocortisone
4. Epinephrine

4. After four hours, Mr. Hanks has stabilized, but he still has some difficulty breathing. As ordered by the physician, which of the following drugs would the nurse most likely be administering to help Mr. Hanks with his breathing difficulties?

1. Diphenhydramine (Benadryl)
2. Hydrocortisone
3. Phenylephrine (Neo-Synephrine)
4. Albuterol (Ventolin)

NOTE: Answers to the Review and Case Study Questions appear in Appendix B. The complete rationales and answers are located on the textbook's website.

Pearson Nursing Student Resources Find additional review materials at **nursing.pearsonhighered.com**.

"I've never had anything happen like this. I was watching TV, and all of a sudden, my heart started racing."

Mrs. Margaret Duncan

Drugs for Dysrhythmias

CORE CONCEPTS

22.1 Some types of dysrhythmias produce no patient symptoms, whereas others may be life threatening.

22.2 Dysrhythmias are classified by the type of rhythm abnormality produced and its location.

22.3 The electrical conduction pathway in the myocardium keeps the heart beating in a synchronized manner.

22.4 Most antidysrhythmic drugs act by blocking ion channels in myocardial cells.

22.5 Antidysrhythmic drugs are classified by their mechanisms of action.

22.6 Sodium channel blockers slow the rate of impulse conduction through the heart.

22.7 Beta-adrenergic blockers reduce automaticity and slow conduction velocity in the heart.

22.8 Potassium channel blockers prolong the refractory period of the heart.

22.9 Calcium channel blockers are available to treat supraventricular dysrhythmias.

22.10 Digoxin and adenosine are used for specific dysrhythmias but do not act by blocking ion channels.

DRUG SNAPSHOT

The following drugs are discussed in this chapter:

DRUG CLASSES	DRUG PROTOTYPES	DRUG CLASSES	DRUG PROTOTYPES
Sodium channel blockers	(Pr) procainamide *339*	Calcium channel blockers	(Pr) verapamil (Calan, Isoptin SR, others) *342*
Beta-adrenergic blockers	(Pr) propranolol (Inderal, InnoPran XL) *340*	Miscellaneous drugs	
Potassium channel blockers	(Pr) amiodarone (Cordarone) *341*		

LEARNING OUTCOMES

After reading this chapter, the student should be able to:

1. Explain how rhythm abnormalities can affect cardiac function.

2. Illustrate the flow of electrical impulses through the normal heart.

3. Classify dysrhythmias based on their location and type of conduction abnormality.

4. Explain the importance of ion channels to cardiac function and the pharmacotherapy of dysrhythmias.

5. Identify the importance of nonpharmacologic therapies in the treatment of dysrhythmias.

6. Identify basic mechanisms by which antidysrhythmic drugs act.

7. Categorize antidysrhythmic drugs based on their classifications and mechanisms of action.

8. For each of the classes in the Drug Snapshot, identify representative drugs and explain their mechanisms of drug action, primary actions, and important adverse effects.

KEY TERMS

atrioventricular (AV) node (ay-tree-oh-
ven-TRIK-you-lur noad *333*

atrioventricular bundle (ay-tree-oh-ven-
TRIK-you-lur BUN-dul) *333*

automaticity (aw-toh-muh-TISS-uh-tee)
333

bundle branches (BUN-dul BRAN-chez)
333

calcium ion channels (KAL-see-um) *335*

depolarization (dee-po-lur-eye-ZAY-shun)
335

dysrhythmias (diss-RITH-mee-uh) *332*

ectopic foci/pacemakers (ek-TOP-ik FO-si)
335

electrocardiogram (ECG) (e-lek-tro-KAR-
dee-oh-gram) *333*

fibrillation (fi-bruh-LAY-shun) *332*

polarized (POLE-uh-rized) *335*

potassium ion channels (po-TASS-ee-um)
335

Purkinje fibers (purr-KEN-gee FI-burrs)
333

refractory period (ree-FRAK-tor-ee) *335*

sinoatrial (SA) node (si-no-AYE-tree-ul
noad) *333*

sinus rhythm (SI-nuss) *333*

sodium ion channels (SO-dee-um) *335*

---

dys = *difficult or bad*
rhythm = *rhythm*
ia = *condition*

Dysrhythmias are abnormalities of electrical conduction or rhythm in the heart. Sometimes called arrhythmias, they encompass a number of different disorders that range from harmless to life threatening. Diagnosis is often difficult because patients usually must be connected to an electrocardiogram (ECG) and be experiencing symptoms to determine the exact type of rhythm disorder. Proper diagnosis and optimum pharmacologic treatment can significantly reduce the frequency of serious dysrhythmias and their consequences.

CORE CONCEPT 22.1

Some types of dysrhythmias produce no patient symptoms, whereas others may be life threatening.

a = *no or not*
symptomat = *symptoms*
ic = *pertaining to*

Whereas some dysrhythmias produce no symptoms and have negligible effects on heart function, others are life threatening and require immediate treatment. Typical symptoms of a dysrhythmia include dizziness, weakness, decreased exercise tolerance, shortness of breath, and fainting. Many patients report palpitations or a sensation that their heart has skipped a beat. Persistent dysrhythmias are associated with increased risk of stroke and heart failure. Severe dysrhythmias may cause sudden death. Because asymptomatic patients may not seek medical attention, it is difficult to estimate the frequency of the disease, although it is likely that dysrhythmias are quite common in the population.

CORE CONCEPT 22.2

Dysrhythmias are classified by the type of rhythm abnormality produced and its location.

supra = *above*
ventricular = *cardiac ventricle*

There are many types of dysrhythmias, and they may be classified by a number of different methods. The simplest method is to name dysrhythmias according to the type of rhythm abnormality produced and their locations. A summary of the different types of dysrhythmias along with a brief description of each abnormality is given in Table 22.1 ◆. Dysrhythmias that originate in the atria are sometimes referred to as supraventricular. Those that originate in the ventricles are generally more serious because they are more likely to interfere with the normal function of the heart. Although obtaining a correct diagnosis of the type of dysrhythmia is sometimes difficult, it is essential for effective treatment. Atrial **fibrillation**, a complete disorganization of rhythm, is thought to be the most common type of dysrhythmia.

Fast Facts Dysrhythmias

- Dysrhythmias are responsible for more than 44,000 deaths each year.

- Atrial dysrhythmias occur more commonly in men than in women.

- The incidence of atrial dysrhythmias increases with age. They affect:
  - Less than 0.5% of those aged 25–35
  - About 1.5% of those up to age 60
  - About 9% of those over age 75

- About 15% of strokes occur in patients with atrial dysrhythmias.

- A large majority of sudden cardiac deaths are believed to be caused by ventricular dysrhythmias.

TABLE 22.1 Types of Dysrhythmias

Name of Dysrhythmia	Description
Atrial or ventricular flutter and/or fibrillation	Very rapid, uncoordinated beats; atrial may require treatment but is not usually fatal; ventricular flutter or fibrillation requires immediate treatment
Atrial or ventricular tachycardia	Rapid heartbeat greater than 100 beats per minute in adults; ventricular tachycardia is more serious than atrial tachycardia
Heart block	Area of nonconduction in the myocardium; may be partial or complete; classified as first, second, or third degree
Premature atrial or premature ventricular contractions (PVCs)	An extra beat often originating from a source other than the sinoatrial (SA) node; not normally serious unless it occurs in high frequency
Sinus bradycardia	Slow heartbeat, less than 60 beats per minute; may require a pacemaker

Dysrhythmias can occur in both healthy and diseased hearts. Although the actual cause of most dysrhythmias is elusive, dysrhythmias are often associated with certain conditions, primarily heart disease and myocardial infarction (MI). Following are some conditions associated with dysrhythmias:

- Hypertension (HTN)
- Cardiac valve disease, such as mitral stenosis
- Coronary artery disease
- Medications such as digoxin
- Low potassium levels in the blood
- Myocardial infarction
- Adverse effect from antidysrhythmic medication
- Stroke
- Diabetes mellitus
- Congestive heart failure

The electrical conduction pathway in the myocardium keeps the heart beating in a synchronized manner.

CORE CONCEPT 22.3

Although there are many different types of dysrhythmias, all have in common a defect in the formation or conduction of electrical impulses across the myocardium. These electrical impulses carry the signal for cardiac muscle cells to contract and must be coordinated precisely for the chambers to beat in a synchronized manner. For the heart to function properly, the atria must contract simultaneously, sending their blood into the ventricles. Following atrial contraction, the right and left ventricles then must contract simultaneously. Lack of synchronization of the atria and ventricles or of the right and left sides of the heart may have serious consequences. The normal conduction pathway in the heart is illustrated in Figure 22.1 ■.

Control of this synchronization begins in a small area of tissue in the wall of the right atrium called the **sinoatrial (SA) node**. The SA node or pacemaker of the heart has a property called **automaticity**, the ability of certain cells to spontaneously generate an electrical impulse known as an *action potential*, without instructions from the nervous system. The SA node generates a new action potential approximately 75 times every minute under resting conditions. This is referred to as the normal **sinus rhythm**.

On leaving the SA node, the action potential travels quickly across both atria to the **atrioventricular (AV) node**, a small area of specialized fibers that lies in the wall of the right atrium. The AV node also has the property of automaticity, although less than the SA node. If the SA node malfunctions, the AV node has the ability to spontaneously generate action potentials and continue the heart's contraction.

As the action potential leaves the AV node, it travels rapidly to the **atrioventricular bundle** or bundle of His, which is responsible for carrying the electrical signal from the atria to the ventricles. The impulse is then conducted down the right and left **bundle branches** (tissue that carries electrical signal impulse from the AV bundle to the Purkinje fibers). The **Purkinje fibers** carry the electrical impulse to all regions of the ventricles almost simultaneously.

The wave of electrical activity across the myocardium can be measured by an **electrocardiogram (ECG)**. The total time for the electrical impulse to travel across the heart is about 0.22 second. A normal ECG and its relationship to impulse conduction in the heart are shown in Figure 22.2 ■.

FIGURE 22.1

Normal conduction
pathway in the heart.

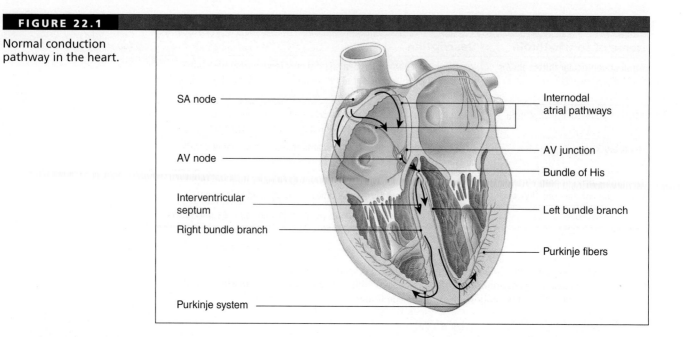

FIGURE 22.2

Normal ECG tracing.

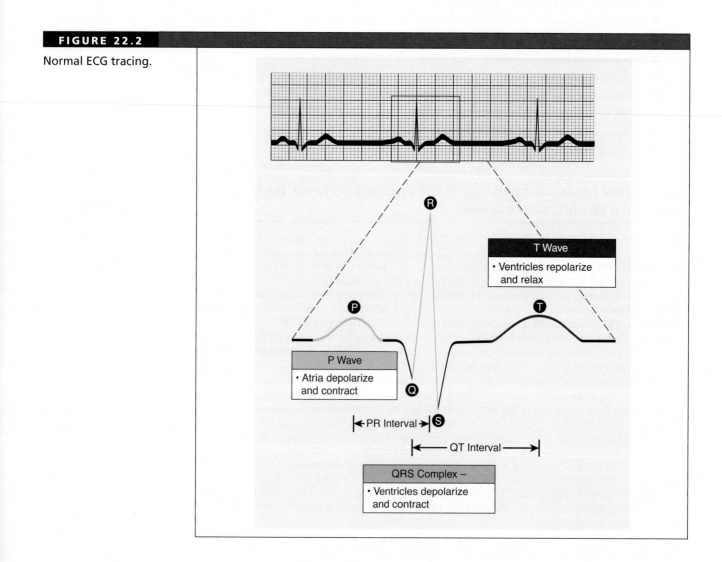

Although action potentials normally begin at the SA node and spread across the myocardium in a coordinated manner, other regions of the heart may begin to initiate beats. These areas, known as **ectopic foci** or **ectopic pacemakers**, may send impulses across the myocardium that compete with those from the normal conduction system. Although healthy hearts often experience an extra beat without incident, ectopic foci in diseased hearts have the potential to cause many of the types of dysrhythmias noted in Table 22.1.

It is important to understand that the underlying purpose of this conduction system is to keep the heart beating in a regular, synchronized manner so that cardiac output can be maintained. Some dysrhythmias occur sporadically, produce no symptoms, and cause little or no effect on cardiac output. These types of abnormalities may go unnoticed by the patient and rarely require treatment. Some dysrhythmias, however, seriously affect cardiac output, producing patient symptoms and resulting in potentially serious, if not mortal, consequences. It is these types of dysrhythmias that require pharmacotherapy.

ec = *outside*
top = *place*
ic =*pertaining to*

Concept Review   22.1

■ Trace the flow of electrical conduction across the heart. What would happen if the impulse never reached the AV node?

Most antidysrhythmic drugs act by blocking ion channels in myocardial cells.

CORE CONCEPT 22.4

Because most antidysrhythmic drugs act by interfering with the cardiac action potential, a firm grasp of this phenomenon is necessary for understanding drug mechanisms. Action potentials occur in both neurons and cardiac muscle cells due to differences in the concentration of certain ions found inside and outside the cell. Under resting conditions, sodium ions (Na^+) and calcium ions (Ca^{2+}) are found in higher concentrations *outside* the myocardial cells, whereas potassium ions (K^+) are found in higher concentrations *inside* these cells. These imbalances are, in part, responsible for the inside of a myocardial cell membrane being slightly negatively charged relative to the outside of the membrane. A cell having this negative membrane potential is said to be **polarized**.

An action potential begins when **sodium ion channels** located in the plasma membrane open and Na^+ rushes into the cell, producing a rapid **depolarization**, or loss of membrane potential. During this period, Ca^{2+} also enters the cell through **calcium ion channels**. It is this influx of Ca^{2+} that is responsible for the contraction of cardiac muscle. The cell returns to its polarized state by the removal of Na^+ from the cell via the sodium pump and movement of K^+ back into the cell through **potassium ion channels**. In cells located in the SA and AV nodes, it is the influx of Ca^{2+}, rather than Na^+, that generates the rapid depolarization of the membrane.

Although it may seem complicated to learn the different ions involved in an action potential, this knowledge is vital to understanding cardiac pharmacology. Blocking potassium, sodium, or calcium ion channels is the primary pharmacologic strategy used to prevent or terminate dysrhythmias. Figure 22.3 ■ illustrates the flow of ions during the action potential.

The pumping action of the heart requires alternating periods of contraction and relaxation. There is a brief period following depolarization when the cell cannot initiate another action potential. This time, known as the **refractory period**, ensures that the myocardial cell finishes contracting before a second action potential begins. Some antidysrhythmic drugs produce their effects by prolonging the refractory period.

Antidysrhythmic drugs are classified by their mechanisms of action.

CORE CONCEPT 22.5

The therapeutic goal of antidysrhythmic pharmacotherapy is to prevent or terminate dysrhythmias to reduce the risk for sudden death, stroke, or other complications resulting from the disease. All antidysrhythmic drugs have the potential to profoundly affect the heart's conduction system. Because they can cause serious adverse effects, antidysrhythmic drugs are normally reserved for patients experiencing symptoms of dysrhythmia or for those whose condition cannot be controlled by other means. Treating asymptomatic dysrhythmias with medications provides little or no benefit to the patient.

FIGURE 22.3

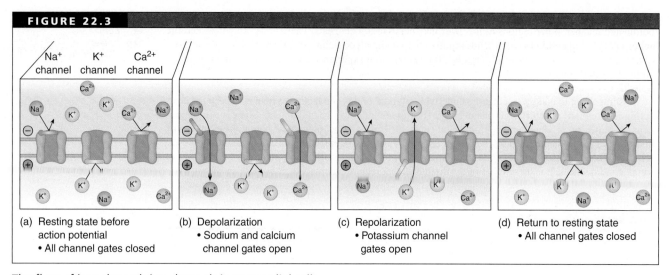

(a) Resting state before action potential
• All channel gates closed

(b) Depolarization
• Sodium and calcium channel gates open

(c) Repolarization
• Potassium channel gates open

(d) Return to resting state
• All channel gates closed

The flow of ions through ion channels in myocardial cells.

Antidysrhythmic drugs are grouped by the stage at which they affect the action potential. These drugs fall into four primary classes and a miscellaneous group that does not act by one of the first four mechanisms. Classes of antidysrhythmics include the following:

- Sodium channel blockers (Class I)
- Beta-adrenergic blockers (Class II)
- Potassium channel blockers (Class III)
- Calcium channel blockers (Class IV)
- Miscellaneous antidysrhythmic drugs

The use of antidysrhythmic drugs has significantly declined in the past 20 years. Research has determined that the use of antidysrhythmic medications for prophylaxis can actually *increase* mortality in some patients. This is because there is a narrow margin between a therapeutic effect and a toxic effect with drugs that affect cardiac rhythm. They have the ability not only to *correct* dysrhythmias but also to worsen or even *create* new dysrhythmias. The healthcare provider must carefully monitor patients taking antidysrhythmic drugs. Often, the patient is hospitalized during the initial stages of therapy so that the optimum dose can be accurately determined.

Another reason for the decline in antidysrhythmic drug use is the success of nonpharmacologic techniques. Research has demonstrated that catheter ablation and implantable cardioverter defibrillators (ICDs) are more successful in managing certain types of dysrhythmias than is the prophylactic use of medications. Catheter ablation is a treatment used to identify and destroy the myocardial cells responsible for the abnormal conduction. ICDs are devices that restore normal rhythm by either pacing the heart or giving it an electric shock when dysrhythmias occur.

NURSING PROCESS FOCUS   Patients Receiving Antidysrhythmic Drugs

ASSESSMENT	POTENTIAL NURSING DIAGNOSES
Prior to administration: ■ Obtain a complete health history including cardiovascular, neurological, renal and liver conditions, allergies, drug history, and possible drug interactions. ■ Evaluate laboratory blood findings: CBC, electrolytes, lipid panel, and renal and liver function studies. ■ Acquire the results of a complete physical examination, including vital signs, height, weight, ECG, LOC, and urinary output.	■ *Risk for Ineffective Tissue Perfusion* related to cardiac conduction abnormality ■ *Risk for Injury* related to adverse effects of drug therapy ■ *Deficient Knowledge* related to a lack of information about drug therapy ■ *Ineffective Self Health Maintenance* related to insufficient knowledge of seriousness of disease and drug therapy regimen

NURSING PROCESS FOCUS *(continued)*

PLANNING: PATIENT GOALS AND EXPECTED OUTCOMES

The patient will:
- Experience therapeutic effects (stabilization of heart rate, heart rhythm, sensorium, urinary output, and vital signs).
- Be free from or experience minimal adverse effects from drug therapy.
- Verbalize an understanding of the drug's use, adverse effects, and required precautions.

IMPLEMENTATION

Interventions and (Rationales)	Patient Education/Discharge Planning
Administer medication correctly and evaluate the patient's knowledge of proper administration. (Proper use of medication ensures that the patient will receive intended results and minimize adverse effects.)	Instruct the patient to: - Never discontinue the drug abruptly. - Take the drug exactly as prescribed, even if feeling well. - Take the pulse prior to taking the drug (may need to demonstrate technique). - Immediately notify the healthcare provider for further instructions if pulse is below the "reportable" pulse rate, usually 60 beats per minute. - Take blood pressure frequently if taking an antidysrhythmic medication that also lowers blood pressure.
Ensure cardiac rate and rhythm are monitored continuously if administering drug IV and regularly if administered orally. (IV route is used when rapid therapeutic effects are needed. Monitoring is needed to detect any potential serious dysrhythmias. Immediately report any changes in heart sounds or rhythm.)	- Explain the need for continuous ECG monitoring when administering the medication intravenously.
Monitor the IV site and administer all intravenous medications via an infusion pump. (Administering IV cardiac medications via an infusion pump helps to ensure safety and accuracy.)	- Instruct the patient to report any burning or stinging pain, swelling, warmth, redness, or tenderness at the IV insertion site.
Obtain information regarding possible causes of the dysrhythmia. (Electrolyte imbalances, hypoxia, pain, anxiety, caffeine ingestion, and tobacco use can contribute to dysrhythmias.)	Instruct the patient to: - Maintain a diet low in sodium and fat with sufficient potassium. - Report illness such as flu, vomiting, diarrhea, and dehydration to the healthcare provider to avoid adverse effects. - Avoid the use of caffeine and tobacco products.
Observe for adverse effects specific to the antidysrhythmic used. (These drugs affect heart function and can cause serious adverse effects. Continuing or worsening cardiac symptoms may indicate inadequate drug therapy.)	Instruct the patient to: - Report to healthcare provider any adverse effects specific to the prescribed antidysrhythmic, such as visual disturbances or skin rashes caused by potassium channel blockers. - Report any cardiac-related symptoms such as dizziness, hypotension, palpitations, chest pain, dyspnea, unusual fatigue and weakness.
Check for edema, noting location and character. Weigh patient daily and report a weight gain or loss of 1 kg or more in a 24-hour period. (Daily weight is an accurate measure of fluid status; weight gain or edema may indicate adverse drug effect or worsening cardiac disease.)	Have the patient: - Weigh and record their weight daily, ideally at the same time of day. - Report to healthcare provider a weight loss or gain of more than 1 kg (2 lb) in a 24-hour period.
Monitor ongoing laboratory results of electrolytes, especially potassium and magnesium; renal function and drug levels. (Hypokalemia or hypomagnesemia increases the risk of dysrhythmias. Inadequate or high drug levels may lead to increased dysrhythmias.)	Instruct the patient on the need to: - Return periodically for lab work. - Carry a wallet ID card or wear medical alert jewelry indicating antidysrhythmia medication.
Monitor lung sounds. Immediately report if patient is experiencing worsening dyspnea, crackles or pink, frothy pink-tinged sputum. (New or worsening dysrhythmias may cause lung congestion and possible heart failure.)	- Instruct the patient to immediately report to healthcare provider any severe shortness of breath, frothy sputum, profound fatigue, or swelling of extremities.

EVALUATION OF OUTCOME CRITERIA

Evaluate the effectiveness of drug therapy by confirming that patient goals and expected outcomes have been met (see "Planning"). *See Tables 22.2 through 22.5 for lists of drugs to which these nursing actions apply.*

CORE CONCEPT 22.6

Sodium channel blockers slow the rate of impulse conduction through the heart.

The first medical uses of the sodium channel blockers were recorded in the 18th century. Quinidine, the oldest antidysrhythmic drug, was originally obtained as a natural substance from the bark of the South American *Cinchona* tree. Although a prototype for many decades, quinidine (Quinidex, others) is rarely used today owing to the availability of safer antidysrhythmics. Sodium channel blockers used as antidysrhythmics are listed in Table 22.2 ◆.

Sodium channel blockers, the Class I drugs, are the largest group of antidysrhythmics. They are divided into three subgroups—IA, IB, and IC—based on subtle differences in their mechanisms of action. Because the action potential is dependent on the opening of sodium ion channels, a blockade of these channels will slow the spread of impulse conduction across the myocardium. This slowing of conduction will suppress ectopic pacemaker activity.

The chemical structures and actions of the sodium channel blockers are similar to those of the local anesthetics. In fact, the antidysrhythmic drug lidocaine is a prototype local anesthetic in Chapter 15. This anesthetic-like action slows impulse conduction across the heart. A few, such as quinidine and procainamide, are effective against many different types of dysrhythmias. The remaining Class I drugs are more specific and indicated only for life-threatening ventricular dysrhythmias.

All the sodium channel blockers have the potential to cause new dysrhythmias or worsen existing ones; thus, frequent ECGs should be obtained. The reduced heart rate caused by the drugs can result in hypotension, dizziness, and fainting. Some Class I drugs have significant anticholinergic adverse effects such as dry mouth, constipation, and urinary retention.

Concept Review 22.2

■ Why does slowing the speed of the electrical impulse across the myocardium sometimes correct a dysrhythmia?

TABLE 22.2 Sodium Channel Blockers (Class I)

Drug	Rate and Adult Dose	Remarks
disopyramide (Norpace)	PO (immediate release); 400–800 mg in divided doses PO (extended release); 300 mg bid	Class 1A; sustained-release form available; usually reserved for serious ventricular dysrhythmias
flecainide (Tambocor)	PO; 100 mg bid (max: 400 mg/day)	Class 1C; usually reserved for serious ventricular dysrhythmias
lidocaine (Xylocaine) (see page 222 for the Drug Prototype box)	IV; 1–4 mg/min infusion rate (max: 3 mg/kg per 5–10 min)	Class 1B; usually reserved for rapid control of ventricular dysrhythmias; IM, subcutaneous, and topical forms available; also widely used as a local anesthetic
mexiletine (Mexitil)	PO; 200–300 mg tid (max: 1,200 mg/day)	Class 1B; usually reserved for serious ventricular dysrhythmias
phenytoin (Dilantin) (see page 190 for the Drug Prototype box)	PO; 100–200 mg tid (max: 625 mg/day) IV; 50–100 mg every 10–15 min until dysrhythmia is terminated (max: 1 g/day)	Class 1B; off-label use for dysrhythmias induced by cardiac glycosides; oral form is used to treat convulsions
Pr procainamide	PO; 50 mg/kg/day in divided doses	Class 1A; IM, IV, and sustained-release forms available; for both atrial and ventricular dysrhythmias
propafenone (Rythmol)	PO (sustained release); 225 mg bid	Class 1C; usually reserved for serious ventricular dysrhythmias
quinidine sulfate	PO; 200–400 mg tid or qid (max: 3–4 g/day)	Class 1A; gluconate salt is also available in IM and IV forms; sustained-release forms available for the sulfate and gluconate salts

Drug Prototype: ℗ *Procainamide*

Therapeutic Class: Antidysrhythmic (Class 1A)   Pharmacologic Class: Sodium channel blocker

Actions and Uses: Procainamide is an older drug, approved in 1950, that is chemically related to the local anesthetic procaine. Procainamide blocks sodium ion channels in myocardial cells, thus slowing conduction of the action potential across the myocardium. This slight delay in conduction velocity prolongs the refractory period and can suppress dysrhythmias. Procainamide has the ability to correct many different types of dysrhythmias. The most common dosage form is the extended-release tablet; however, procainamide is also available in IV and IM formulations for emergency conditions.

Adverse Effects and Interactions: Procainamide has a narrow margin of safety, and dosage must be monitored carefully to avoid serious adverse effects. Nausea, vomiting, abdominal pain, and headache are common during therapy. The drug can cause fever accompanied by anorexia, weakness, and nausea/vomiting. High doses may produce central nervous system (CNS) effects such as confusion or psychosis.

Additive cardiac depressant effects may occur if procainamide is administered with other antidysrhythmics. Additive anticholinergic adverse effects will occur if procainamide is used concurrently with other medications that have anticholinergic effects.

> **BLACK BOX WARNING:**
> Chronic administration may result in a lupus-like syndrome in 30% to 50% of patients who are taking the drug for more than a year. Procainamide should be reserved for life-threatening dysrhythmias because it has the ability to produce new dysrhythmias or worsen existing ones.
>
> Complete blood counts should be monitored carefully and the drug discontinued at the first sign of potential blood abnormalities.

Beta-adrenergic blockers reduce automaticity and slow conduction velocity in the heart.

CORE CONCEPT 22.7

Beta-adrenergic blockers are used to treat a large number of cardiovascular diseases, including HTN, MI, heart failure, and dysrhythmias. Their ability to slow the heart rate and conduction velocity can suppress several types of dysrhythmias. Beta blockers of importance to dysrhythmias are listed in Table 22.3 ◆.

The basic pharmacology of beta-adrenergic blockers is explained in Chapter 8. Although the effects of beta blockers on the heart are complex, their basic actions are to slow the heart rate and decrease conduction velocity through the AV node. Myocardial automaticity is reduced, and many types of dysrhythmias are stabilized. The main value of beta blockers as antidysrhythmic drugs is to treat atrial dysrhythmias that are associated with heart failure.

Only a few beta blockers are approved for dysrhythmias because of the potential for adverse effects. Blockade of beta receptors in the heart may result in bradycardia, and hypotension may cause dizziness and possible fainting. Beta blockers that affect beta2-receptors will also affect the lungs, increasing the risk for bronchospasm. This is of particular concern in patients with asthma and in elderly patients with chronic obstructive pulmonary disease (COPD).

▶ **Life Span Fact**

Special attention should be given to older adults because anticholinergic adverse effects may worsen urinary hesitancy in patients with prostate enlargement.

TABLE 22.3	Beta-Adrenergic Blockers Used for Dysrhythmias (Class II)	
Drug	**Rate and Adult Dose**	**Remarks**
acebutolol (Sectral)	PO; 200–600 mg bid (max: 1,200 mg/day)	Cardioselective beta$_1$ blocker; usually reserved for ventricular dysrhythmias; also for HTN and angina
esmolol (Brevibloc)	IV; 50 mcg/kg/min maintenance dose (max: 200 mcg/kg/min)	Cardioselective beta$_1$ blocker; usually reserved for immediate control of severe atrial dysrhythmias; very short half-life of 9 minutes
℗ propranolol (Inderal, InnoPran XL)	PO; 10–30 mg tid or qid (max: 480 mg/day) IV; 0.5–3.1 mg every 4 hours	Sustained-release forms available; also for HTN, prevention of MI, angina, and migraines

Drug Prototype: (Pr) *Propranolol (Inderal, InnoPran XL)*

Therapeutic Class: **Antidysrhythmic (Class II)**   Pharmacologic Class: **Beta-adrenergic blocker**

Actions and Uses: Propranolol is a nonselective beta-adrenergic blocker, affecting both beta1-receptors in the heart and beta2-receptors in the lungs. Propranolol reduces heart rate, slows conduction velocity, and lowers blood pressure. Propranolol is most effective in treating tachycardia. It is approved to treat a wide variety of disorders, including HTN, angina, and migraine headaches, and to prevent MI.

Adverse Effects and Interactions: Frequent adverse effects of propranolol include hypotension and bradycardia. Because of its ability to slow the heart rate, patients with serious cardiac disorders such as heart failure must be carefully monitored. Adverse effects such as diminished sex drive and impotence may result in nonadherence.

Propranolol interacts with many other drugs, including phenothiazines, which have additive hypotensive effects. Propranolol should not be given within two weeks of a monoamine oxidase (MAO) inhibitor. Beta-adrenergic drugs such as albuterol block the actions of propranolol.

BLACK BOX WARNING:
Abrupt withdrawal is not advised in patients with angina or heart disease. Dosage should gradually be reduced over one to two weeks and the drug should be restarted if angina symptoms develop during this period.

Concept Review   22.3

■ Why are selective alpha-adrenergic blockers such as doxazosin (Cardura) of no value in treating dysrhythmias?

CORE CONCEPT 22.8   **Potassium channel blockers prolong the refractory period of the heart.**

Although a small class of drugs, the potassium channel blockers (Class III) have important applications to the treatment of dysrhythmias. Potassium channel blockers used as antidysrhythmics are listed in Table 22.4 ◆.

The drugs in Class III exert their actions by blocking potassium ion channels in myocardial cells. After the action potential has passed and the myocardial cell is in a depolarized state, repolarization depends on removal of potassium from the cell. The Class III drugs prolong the duration of the action potential by lengthening the refractory period (resting stage), which tends to stabilize dysrhythmias.

Potassium channel blockers are reserved for serious dysrhythmias because of potentially serious adverse effects. Like other antidysrhythmics, potassium channel blockers slow the heart rate, resulting in bradycardia and possible hypotension. These adverse effects occur in a significant number of patients. These medications can worsen dysrhythmias, especially following the first few doses. Older adults with preexisting heart failure must be carefully monitored because they are particularly at risk for adverse cardiac effects of potassium channel blockers.

TABLE 22.4   Potassium Channel Blockers (Class III)

Drug	Rate and Adult Dose	Remarks
(Pr) amiodarone (Cordarone, Pacerone)	PO; 400–600 mg/day (max: 1,600 mg/day as loading dose)	IV form available; usually reserved for serious ventricular dysrhythmias
dofetilide (Tikosyn)	PO; 125–500 mcg bid based on creatinine clearance	Usually for atrial dysrhythmias
dronedarone (Multaq)	PO; 400 mg bid	Newer drug; given to reduce the risk of cardiovascular hospitalization in patients with atrial dysrhythmias
ibutilide (Corvert)	IV; 1 mg (10 mL) infused over 10 minutes	Usually reserved for atrial flutter or fibrillation
sotalol (Betapace, Betapace AF, Sorine)	PO; 80 mg bid (max: 320 mg/day)	Usually reserved for serious ventricular dysrhythmias; also a nonselective beta-adrenergic blocker

DRUG PROTOTYPE: Pr *Amiodarone (Cordarone)*

Therapeutic Class: Antidysrhythmic (Class III)   Pharmacologic Class: Potassium channel blocker

Actions and Uses: Amiodarone is approved for the treatment of resistant ventricular tachycardia that may prove life threatening, and it is a preferred drug for treating atrial dysrhythmias in patients with heart failure. In addition to blocking potassium ion channels, some of amiodarone's actions on the heart relate to its blockade of sodium ion channels. Amiodarone is available as oral tablets and as an IV infusion. IV infusions are limited to short-term therapy, normally only two to four days. Its onset of action may take several weeks when the drug is given orally. Its effects, however, can last four to eight weeks after the drug is discontinued because it has an extended half-life that may exceed 100 days.

Adverse Effects and Interactions: Amiodarone may cause blurred vision, rashes, photosensitivity, nausea, vomiting, anorexia, fatigue, dizziness, and hypotension. Because this medication is concentrated by certain tissues and has a prolonged half-life, adverse effects may be slow to resolve. As with other antidysrhythmics, patients must be closely monitored to avoid serious toxicity.

Amiodarone interacts with many other drugs. For example, it increases digoxin levels in the blood and enhances the actions of anticoagulants. If used together with beta blockers, sinus bradycardia may increase, and sinus arrest and atrioventricular block may occur. Amiodarone increases phenytoin levels two- to threefold.

Use cautiously with herbal supplements such as echinacea, which may cause increased liver toxicity. Aloe may increase the effect of amiodarone.

BLACK BOX WARNING:
(oral form only): Amiodarone causes a pneumonia-like syndrome in the lungs. Because the pulmonary toxicity may be fatal, baseline and periodic assessment of lung function is essential. Amiodarone has prodysrhythmic action and may cause bradycardia, cardiogenic shock, or AV block. Mild liver injury is frequent with amiodarone.

Calcium channel blockers are available to treat supraventricular dysrhythmias.

CORE CONCEPT 22.9

Like the beta blockers, the calcium channel blockers (Class IV) are widely prescribed for various cardiovascular disorders. By slowing conduction velocity, they are able to stabilize certain dysrhythmias. Although about 10 calcium channel blockers (CCBs) are available to treat cardiovascular diseases, only a limited number have been approved for dysrhythmias. Doses for the CCBs used for treating dysrhythmias are listed in Table 22.5 ◆. The basic pharmacology of this drug class is presented in Chapter 18. Diltiazem is featured as a prototype drug in Chapter 20.

Blockade of calcium ion channels produces effects on the heart that are similar to those of beta-adrenergic blockers. Effects include reduced automaticity in the SA node and slowed impulse conduction

TABLE 22.5 Calcium Channel Blockers (Class IV) and Miscellaneous Drugs for Dysrhythmias		
Drug	**Rate and Adult Dose**	**Remarks**
diltiazem (Cardizem, Cartia XT, Dilacor XR, others) (see page 309 for the Drug Prototype box)	IV; 5–15 mg/hr continuous infusion for a maximum of 24 hours (max: 15 mg/hr)	Oral and sustained-release forms available for HTN and angina
Pr verapamil (Calan, Isoptin SR, others)	PO; 240–480 mg/day IV; 5–10 mg direct: may repeat in 15–30 minutes if needed	Sustained-release and IV forms available; also for HTN, angina, and migraines
MISCELLANEOUS DRUGS		
adenosine (Adenocard, Adenoscan)	IV; 6–12 mg given as a bolus injection every 1–2 minutes as needed (max: 12 mg/dose)	Usually reserved for atrial dysrhythmias; half-life is only 10 seconds
digoxin (Lanoxin) (see page 295 for the Drug Prototype box)	PO; 0.125–0.5 mg qid; dose is individualized for each patient	Usually reserved for atrial dysrhythmias; IV and IM forms available; also for heart failure

---

DRUG PROTOTYPE: ℗℗ *Verapamil (Calan, Isoptin SR, Others)*
Therapeutic Class: **Antidysrhythmic (Class IV)**   Pharmacologic Class: **Calcium channel blocker**

Actions and Uses: Verapamil was the first CCB approved by the Food and Drug Administration (FDA). The drug acts by inhibiting the flow of Ca2+ into myocardial cells and in vascular smooth muscle. In the heart, this action slows conduction velocity and stabilizes dysrhythmias. In the vessels, calcium ion channel inhibition lowers blood pressure. Verapamil also dilates the coronary arteries, an action that is important when the drug is used to treat angina (see Chapter 20).

Adverse Effects and Interactions: Adverse effects are generally minor and may include headache, constipation, and hypotension. Because verapamil can cause bradycardia, patients with heart failure should be carefully monitored. Like many other antidysrhythmics, it has the ability to elevate blood levels of digoxin. Because both digoxin and verapamil have the effect of slowing conduction through the AV node, their concurrent use must be carefully monitored.

Grapefruit juice may increase verapamil levels. The drug should be used cautiously with hawthorn, which may have additive hypotensive effects.

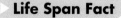

Life Span Fact

The healthcare provider should carefully monitor older adults with preexisting heart failure because these patients are particularly at risk from the cardiac effects of potassium channel blockers.

through the AV node. This prolongs the refractory period and stabilizes many types of dysrhythmias. CCBs are only effective against atrial dysrhythmias.

CCBs are well tolerated by most patients. As with other antidysrhythmics, patients should be carefully monitored for bradycardia and hypotension. Because their cardiac effects are almost identical to those of beta-adrenergic blockers, patients concurrently taking drugs from both classes are especially at risk for bradycardia and possible heart failure. Because older patients often have multiple cardiovascular disorders, such as HTN, heart failure, and dysrhythmias, it is not unusual to find elderly patients taking drugs from multiple classes.

Concept Review   22.4

■ Remembering the effects of digoxin on the heart from Chapter 19, explain why most antidysrhythmic drugs have the potential to cause serious adverse effects in patients taking cardiac glycosides.

CORE CONCEPT 22.10

Digoxin and adenosine are used for specific dysrhythmias but do not act by blocking ion channels.

Two other drugs, adenosine and digoxin, are used to treat specific dysrhythmias, but they do not act by the mechanisms described previously. These drugs are summarized in Table 22.5.

Adenosine (Adenocard, Adenoscan) is given as a one- to two-second bolus IV injection to terminate serious atrial tachycardia by slowing conduction through the AV node and decreasing automaticity of the SA node. Its primary indication is a specific dysrhythmia known as paroxysmal supraventricular tachycardia (PSVT), for which it is a preferred drug. Although dyspnea is common, adverse effects are generally brief, because of its 10-second half-life.

Although digoxin (Lanoxin) is primarily used to treat heart failure, it is also prescribed for certain types of atrial dysrhythmias because it decreases automaticity of the SA node and slows conduction through the AV node. Excessive levels of digoxin can produce serious dysrhythmias, and interactions with other medications are common; therefore, patients must be carefully monitored during therapy. The adverse effects of digoxin are described in Chapter 19.

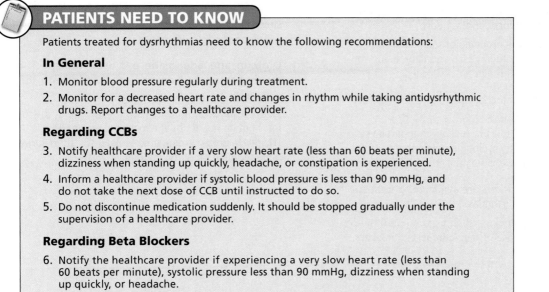

PATIENTS NEED TO KNOW

Patients treated for dysrhythmias need to know the following recommendations:

In General

1. Monitor blood pressure regularly during treatment.
2. Monitor for a decreased heart rate and changes in rhythm while taking antidysrhythmic drugs. Report changes to a healthcare provider.

Regarding CCBs

3. Notify healthcare provider if a very slow heart rate (less than 60 beats per minute), dizziness when standing up quickly, headache, or constipation is experienced.
4. Inform a healthcare provider if systolic blood pressure is less than 90 mmHg, and do not take the next dose of CCB until instructed to do so.
5. Do not discontinue medication suddenly. It should be stopped gradually under the supervision of a healthcare provider.

Regarding Beta Blockers

6. Notify the healthcare provider if experiencing a very slow heart rate (less than 60 beats per minute), systolic pressure less than 90 mmHg, dizziness when standing up quickly, or headache.
7. Notify dentists, surgeons, and eye doctors if taking propranolol (Inderal, InnoPran XL). This drug lowers intraocular pressure.
8. For those with diabetes, check blood glucose regularly while taking beta blockers. These medications can change how the body uses sugars and starches.

CHAPTER REVIEW

CORE CONCEPTS SUMMARY

22.1 Some types of dysrhythmias produce no patient symptoms, whereas others may be life threatening.

Some dysrhythmias produce no symptoms and are harmless, whereas others are life threatening. The frequency of dysrhythmias is difficult to ascertain, although they are thought to be quite common, particularly in the geriatric population.

22.2 Dysrhythmias are classified by the type of rhythm abnormality produced and its location.

Dysrhythmias are classified by their site of origin, either atrial or ventricular, and by the type of rhythm abnormality produced, such as tachycardia, flutter, or fibrillation. Dysrhythmias are associated with diseases such as HTN and heart failure.

22.3 The electrical conduction pathway in the myocardium keeps the heart beating in a synchronized manner.

The normal rhythm of the heart is established by the SA node, which ensures that the chambers beat in a synchronized manner. The central problem with dysrhythmias is their potential to affect the function of the heart, reduce cardiac output, and

cause certain consequences such as stroke or heart failure.

22.4 Most antidysrhythmic drugs act by blocking ion channels in myocardial cells.

Antidysrhythmic drugs affect the action potential in myocardial cells. They act by blocking sodium, potassium, or calcium channels in the cell membrane.

22.5 Antidysrhythmic drugs are classified by their mechanisms of action.

All antidysrhythmic drugs have the ability to cause rhythm abnormalities or worsen existing ones. Most antidysrhythmic medications are placed into one of five classes, based on their mechanisms of action. Class I drugs are further subdivided into IA, IB, and IC. Nonpharmacologic treatments such as cardioversion or catheter ablation are sometimes preferred over drug therapy.

22.6 Sodium channel blockers slow the rate of impulse conduction through the heart.

Sodium channel blockers stabilize dysrhythmias by slowing the spread of impulse conduction across the myocardium. Quinidine, a Class IA drug, is the oldest antidysrhythmic drug.

22.7 Beta-adrenergic blockers reduce automaticity and slow conduction velocity in the heart.

Beta blockers such as propranolol stabilize dysrhythmias by slowing the heart rate and decreasing the conduction velocity through the AV node.

22.8 Potassium channel blockers prolong the refractory period of the heart.

Potassium channel blockers such as amiodarone stabilize dysrhythmias by prolonging the duration of the action potential and extending the refractory period.

22.9 Calcium channel blockers are available to treat supraventricular dysrhythmias.

Calcium channel blockers such as verapamil have effects similar to those of beta-adrenergic blockers.

These include reduced automaticity in the SA node, slowed impulse conduction through the AV node, and a prolonged refractory period.

22.10 Digoxin and adenosine are used for specific dysrhythmias but do not act by blocking ion channels.

Digoxin and adenosine are used for specific dysrhythmias but do not act by the mechanisms of Class I, II, III, or IV drugs. Adenosine is used for short-term, rapid termination of dysrhythmias.

REVIEW QUESTIONS

The following questions are written in NCLEX-PN® style. Answer these questions to assess your knowledge of the chapter material, and go back and review any material that is not clear to you.

1. The nurse is monitoring the electrolytes and ECG of a patient with a cardiac dysthymia because he knows that which of the following electrolytes produces depolarization when it rushes into cardiac cells?

1. Potassium
2. Magnesium
3. Sodium
4. Chloride

2. A patient has been ordered a sodium channel blockers. In explaining to the patient how this class of drug works, the nurse says that sodium channel blockers:

1. Increase automaticity
2. Slow impulse conduction
3. Prolong the refractory period
4. Increase impulse conduction

3. The physician has ordered propranolol, 15 mg by mouth (po), three times a day. The pharmacy has propranolol in 30-mg tablets. How many tablets will the nurse give per dose and how many mg will the patient receive in a day?

1. One-half tablet per dose, 30 mg per day
2. One-half tablet per dose, 45 mg per day
3. One and one-half tablets per dose, 45 mg per day
4. One and one-half tablets per dose, 35 mg per day

4. When the patient is on amiodarone (Cordarone). What changes will the nurse expect to see to the patient's digoxin order?

1. Discontinued
2. Increased

3. Decreased
4. Doubled

5. The nurse is monitoring a patient taking an antidysrhythmic drug. What outcome would the nurse expect to see?

1. Decreased heart rate
2. Increased heart rate
3. Increased renal insufficiency
4. Increased hepatic insufficiency

6. The patient taking an antidysrhythmic is instructed by the nurse to notify the physician if:

1. Constipation occurs.
2. The heart rate is less than 60 beats per minute.
3. The heart rate is greater than 90 beats per minute.
4. Blood pressure does not decrease.

7. A group of patients is being taught about the common adverse effects of antidysrhythmic medications. Some of the adverse effects they are being taught about include: (Select all that apply.)

1. Dizziness
2. Hypotension
3. Weakness
4. Anorexia

8. Which of the following would be included in the teaching plan for a patient taking an antidysrhythmic medication?

1. "Take the drug only when you are feeling excessively tired."
2. "Take your pulse prior to taking your medication."
3. "Do not drink alcohol unless you have spoken with your physician."
4. "You will need to increase your sodium and potassium intake."

9. A patient is taking an antidysrhythmic medication and learns in a patient education session that sometimes this medication is also used to treat angina. What medication is the nurse discussing?

1. Digoxin (Lanoxin)
2. Verapamil (Calan)
3. Adenosine (Adenocard)
4. Quinidine sulfate

10. When administering this antidysrhythmic, the nurse also knows that this drug is used to treat hypertension and angina. What drug is the nurse administering?

1. Diltiazem (Cardizem)
2. Digoxin (Lanoxin)
3. Adenosine (Adenocard)
4. Quinidine sulfate

CASE STUDY QUESTIONS

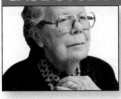

Remember Mrs. Duncan, the patient introduced at the beginning of the chapter? Now read the remainder of the case study. Based on the information you have learned in this chapter, answer the questions that follow.

Mrs. Margaret Duncan, age 72, who has a history of hypertension, has arrived in the emergency department with a life-threatening ventricular dysrhythmia. She is frightened and is wondering what is happening. The physician has ordered that an IV lidocaine infusion be started on Mrs. Duncan.

1. The nurse explains to Mrs. Duncan that lidocaine would be expected to terminate her dysrhythmia primarily by which of the following mechanisms?

1. Speeding up the heart rate
2. Lowering blood pressure
3. Increasing the strength of myocardial contractions
4. Slowing the speed of electrical conduction across the myocardium

2. When Mrs. Duncan is discharged from the hospital, she is placed on propranolol. The nurse informs the patient that this drug should:

1. Raise her blood pressure
2. Lower her blood pressure

3. Have no effect on her hypertension
4. First raise her blood pressure, then lower it

3. The physician lowers the dose of propranolol and adds amiodarone (Cordarone) to the drug regimen. Mrs. Duncan begins to experience dizziness, fainting spells, and fatigue. The nurse recognizes that this is most likely caused by which of the following?

1. Mrs. Duncan is not eating enough potassium-rich foods.
2. The drug combination is causing bradycardia or hypertension.
3. The drug combination is causing respiratory depression.
4. Mrs. Duncan's hypertension is out of control.

4. When taking these medications, Mrs. Duncan is instructed to:

1. Check her pulse rate frequently.
2. Keep a log of weight gain or loss.
3. Eat plenty of foods containing potassium.
4. Avoid taking aspirin, unless instructed to do so by the physician.

NOTE: Answers to the Review and Case Study Questions appear in Appendix B. The complete rationales and answers are located on the textbook's website.

Pearson Nursing Student Resources   Find additional review materials at: **nursing.pearsonhighered.com.**

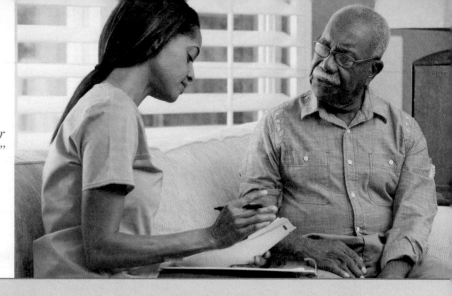

"Let me see if I understand this . . . I need to go to the lab and get stuck every other day for the next two weeks?"

Mr. Thomas Hawkins

23 Drugs for Coagulation Disorders

CORE CONCEPTS

23.1 Hemostasis is a complex process involving multiple steps and many clotting factors.

23.2 Removing a blood clot is essential to restoring normal circulation.

23.3 Drugs are used to modify the coagulation process.

23.4 Anticoagulants prevent the formation and enlargement of clots.

23.5 Antiplatelet drugs prolong bleeding time by interfering with platelet aggregation.

23.6 Thrombolytics are used to dissolve existing clots.

23.7 Hemostatics are used to promote the formation of clots.

DRUG SNAPSHOT

The following drugs are discussed in this chapter:

DRUG CLASSES	DRUG PROTOTYPES		DRUG CLASSES	DRUG PROTOTYPES
Anticoagulants	(Pr) heparin *352*		Thrombolytics	(Pr) alteplase (Activase) *357*
	(Pr) warfarin (Coumadin) *353*		Hemostatics	(Pr) aminocaproic acid (Amicar) *358*
Antiplatelet drugs	(Pr) clopidogrel (Plavix) *356*			

LEARNING OUTCOMES

After reading this chapter, the student should be able to:

1. Explain the importance of hemostasis.

2. Construct a diagram that illustrates the primary steps of hemostasis and fibrinolysis.

3. Describe the types of disorders for which coagulation modifier drugs are prescribed.

4. Identify the primary mechanisms by which coagulation modifier drugs act.

5. Categorize coagulation modifier drugs based on their classifications and mechanisms of action.

6. For each of the classes in the Drug Snapshot, identify representative drugs and explain their mechanisms of drug action, primary actions, and important adverse effects.

KEY TERMS

activated partial thromboplastin time (aPTT) (throm-bow-PLAS-tin) *352*
anticoagulant (ANT-eye-co-AG-you-lent) *350*

antiplatelet drugs (ant-eye-PLAY-tuh-let) *350*
clotting factors *347*
coagulation (co-ag-you-LAY-shun) *347*

coagulation cascade (cass-KADE) *347*
deep venous thrombosis (DVT) *349*
embolus (EM-boh-luss) *349*
fibrin (FEYE-brin) *347*

fibrinogen (feye-BRIN-oh-jen) *347*
fibrinolysis (feye-brin-OL-oh-sis) *349*
glycoprotein IIb/IIIa (GLEYE-koh-proh-
   teen) *356*
hemostasis (hee-moh-STAY-sis) *347*
hemostatics (hee-moh-STAT-iks) *350*
international normalized ratio (INR) *352*

low molecular weight heparins
   (LMWHs) *351*
plasmin (PLAZ-min) *349*
plasminogen (plaz-MIN-oh-jen) *349*
prothrombin (PRO-throm-bin) *347*
prothrombin time (PT) *352*
thrombin (THROM-bin) *347*

thromboembolic disorder (THROM-bow-
   EM-bow-lik) *349*
thrombolytics (throm-bow-LIT-iks) *350*
thrombus (THROM-bus) *349*
tissue plasminogen activator
   (tPA) *349*

E veryone is familiar with the bleeding associated with simple cuts and scrapes, and we take for granted that bleeding will stop in a few minutes. **Hemostasis**, or the stopping of blood flow, is an essential mechanism protecting the body from both external and internal injury. Without efficient hemostasis, bleeding from wounds would lead to shock and perhaps death. Too much clotting, however, can be just as deadly as too little. Thus, hemostasis must maintain a delicate balance between blood fluidity and coagulation.

hemo = *blood*
stasis = *stopping*

Many diseases and conditions affect hemostasis. Some common disorders that often require pharmacotherapy with coagulation modifiers are described in Table 23.1 ◆.

Hemostasis is a complex process involving multiple steps and many clotting factors.

CORE CONCEPT 23.1

Hemostasis is complex and involves a number of substances called **clotting factors**. The clotting factors are activated in a series of sequential steps, sometimes referred to as a *cascade*. Drugs can be used to modify several of these steps.

When an injury occurs, cells lining damaged blood vessels release chemicals that begin the process of hemostasis. The vessel immediately spasms, which limits blood flow to the injured area. Platelets become sticky, adhere to the injured area, and aggregate or clump to plug the damaged vessel. Blood flow is further slowed, resulting in **coagulation**, the formation of an insoluble clot. The basic steps of hemostasis are shown in Figure 23.1 ■.

The **coagulation cascade** is a complex series of steps that begins when the injured cells release a chemical called *prothrombin activator* or prothrombinase. Prothrombin activator converts the clotting factor **prothrombin** to an enzyme called **thrombin**. Thrombin then converts **fibrinogen**, a plasma protein, to long strands of **fibrin**. Thus two of the factors essential to clotting, thrombin and fibrin, are only formed *after* injury to the vessels. The fibrin strands form an insoluble web over the injured area to stop blood loss. Normal blood clotting occurs in about six minutes. The primary steps in the coagulation cascade are illustrated in Figure 23.2 ■.

pro = *before*
thrombin = *clot*

It is important to note that several clotting factors, including thromboplastin and fibrinogen, are proteins made by the liver that are constantly circulating through the blood in an *inactive* form. Vitamin K is required for the liver to make four of the clotting factors. Because the liver supplies many of the clotting factors, patients with serious hepatic impairment usually exhibit abnormal coagulation.

thrombo = *clot*
plastin = *to form*

TABLE 23.1 Disorders Commonly Treated with Coagulation Modifier Drugs	
Disorder/Condition	**Description**
Angina	Pain due to narrowing of the coronary vessels that interferes with blood flow to cardiac muscle
Deep venous thrombosis (DVT)	Clot within a vein in the legs
Indwelling devices	Mechanical heart valves, stents
Myocardial infarction	Death of cardiac muscle tissue due to blockage of a coronary artery
Postoperative hemorrhage	Bleeding following a surgical procedure
Pulmonary embolus	Clot within a pulmonary artery that blocks blood flow to the lungs
Stroke (cerebrovascular accident)	Clot within an artery that blocks blood flow to the brain
Valvular heart disease	Disease of heart valves or replacement of a heart valve

Basic steps in hemostasis.

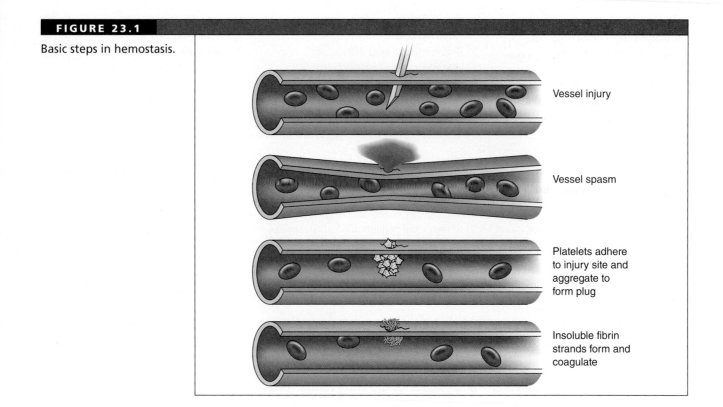

Vessel injury

Vessel spasm

Platelets adhere
to injury site and
aggregate to
form plug

Insoluble fibrin
strands form and
coagulate

Major steps in the
coagulation cascade.

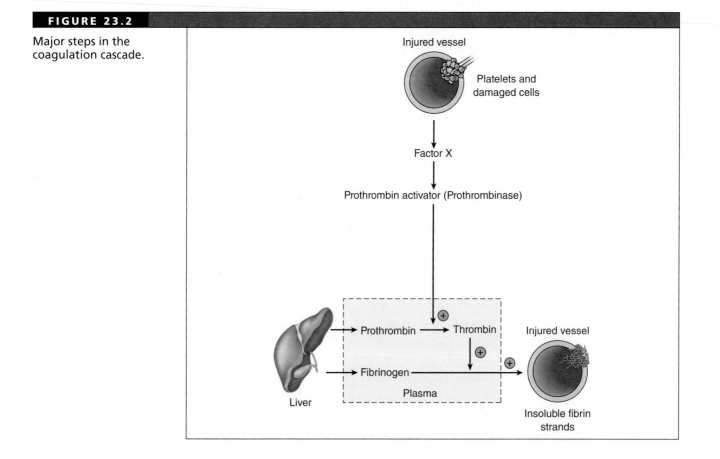

Injured vessel

Platelets and
damaged cells

Factor X

Prothrombin activator (Prothrombinase)

Liver

Prothrombin ⟶ Thrombin

Fibrinogen

Plasma

Injured vessel

Insoluble fibrin
strands

Fast Facts Clotting Disorders

- More than 60,000–100,000 patients die each year of pulmonary emboli. For 25% of these patients, sudden death will be the first sign of the condition.
- Von Willebrand's disease is the most common hereditary platelet disorder, affecting about 1.4 million Americans.
- Hemophilia A, or classic hemophilia, is a hereditary condition in which a person lacks clotting factor VIII; it accounts for 80% of all hemophilia cases.
- More than 20,000 people in the United States have hemophilia.

Removing a blood clot is essential to restoring normal circulation.

CORE CONCEPT 23.2

The goal of hemostasis has been achieved once a blood clot is formed, and the body is protected from excessive hemorrhage. Large clots, however, may prevent adequate blood flow to the affected area; circulation must eventually be restored so that the tissue can resume normal activities. The process of clot removal is called **fibrinolysis**.

fibrin = *fiber*
lysis = *break apart*

Fibrinolysis also involves several sequential steps. When the fibrin clot is formed, nearby blood vessel cells secrete **tissue plasminogen activator (tPA)**. tPA converts the inactive protein **plasminogen**, which is present in the fibrin clot, to its active form called **plasmin**. Plasmin then digests the fibrin strands to remove the clot. The body normally regulates fibrinolysis such that *unwanted* fibrin clots are removed, whereas fibrin present in wounds is left to maintain hemostasis. The steps of fibrinolysis are shown in Figure 23.3 ■.

Drugs are used to modify the coagulation process.

CORE CONCEPT 23.3

There are many types of disorders in which abnormal coagulation might occur. The term **thromboembolic disorder** is used to describe conditions in which the body forms undesirable clots. Thromboembolic disorders may occur in either veins or arteries and can place patients in extreme danger. Once a stationary clot, or **thrombus**, forms in a vessel, it often grows larger as more fibrin is added. Thrombi in the venous system usually form in the veins of the legs in patients due to sluggish blood flow, a condition called **deep venous thrombosis (DVT)**. Pieces of a thrombus may break off and travel in the bloodstream to lodge in other vessels. A traveling clot is called an **embolus**. When thrombi or emboli form, drug therapy is indicated.

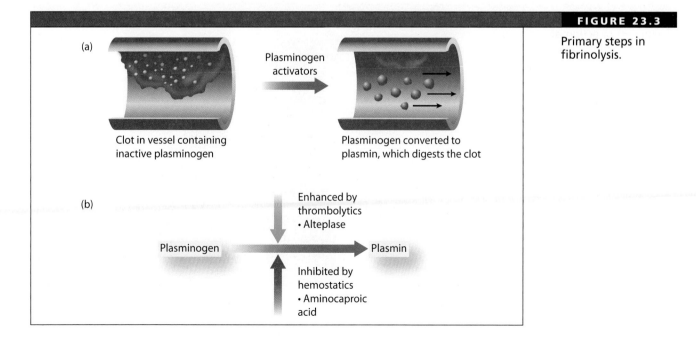

FIGURE 23.3

Primary steps in fibrinolysis.

(a) Clot in vessel containing inactive plasminogen → Plasminogen activators → Plasminogen converted to plasmin, which digests the clot

(b) Plasminogen → Plasmin

Enhanced by thrombolytics
• Alteplase

Inhibited by hemostatics
• Aminocaproic acid

anti = *against*
coagulation = *clotting*

Drugs can be used to modify hemostasis in a number of ways. **Anticoagulants** are drugs used to prevent excessive clotting, usually by interfering with some aspect of the coagulation cascade. The **anti-platelet drugs**, also frequently prescribed to modify hemostasis, act by diminishing the clotting action of platelets. Regardless of the mechanism, all anticoagulant and antiplatelet drugs will increase the time the body takes to form clots. These drugs are often referred to as *blood thinners*, which is an incorrect term, because they do not change the thickness of the blood.

Once an abnormal clot has formed, it may be critical to quickly remove it in order to restore normal function. This is particularly important for blood vessels serving the heart, lungs, and brain. A specific class of drugs, the **thrombolytics**, is used to dissolve such life-threatening clots.

thrombo = *clot*
lytic = *remove/destroy*

In some cases, the blood may not clot quickly enough—for example, following surgery. In this case, it is sometimes desirable to administer medications that make the blood clot more quickly in order to prevent excessive bleeding. These drugs, called **hemostatics**, inhibit the normal removal of fibrin, thus keeping the clot in place for a longer period. Hemostatics are used to speed clot formation, thereby limiting bleeding from a surgical site (see Figure 23.3).

Concept Review 23.1

■ Which clotting factors are always circulating in the blood? Which are formed only once coagulation is underway?

CORE CONCEPT 23.4

Anticoagulants prevent the formation and enlargement of clots.

Anticoagulants are drugs that inhibit certain clotting factors, thus lengthening clotting time and preventing thrombi from forming or growing larger. Because thromboembolic disease can be life threatening, therapy is often begun by administering anticoagulants intravenously or subcutaneously to achieve a rapid onset of action. As the disease stabilizes, the patient is switched to oral anticoagulants. Anticoagulants act by a number of different mechanisms, which are illustrated in Figure 23.4 ■. Table 23.2 ◆ lists the primary anticoagulants.

The most frequent, and potentially serious, adverse effect of anticoagulant and antiplatelet drugs is bleeding. The patient must be observed for signs of hemorrhage, such as bruising, bleeding gums, and blood in the urine or stools. Patients who have recently experienced a traumatic injury or recent surgery are especially at risk. Any symptoms of bleeding must be immediately reported to the healthcare provider. Specific blockers may be administered to reverse the anticoagulant effects: Protamine sulfate is used for heparin, and vitamin K is administered for warfarin.

Parenteral Anticoagulants

The traditional drug of choice for rapid anticoagulation is heparin. Heparin inactivates thrombin and several other clotting factors within minutes after it is given by the IV route. In recent years, the heparin

---

FIGURE 23.4

Mechanism of action of coagulation modifiers.

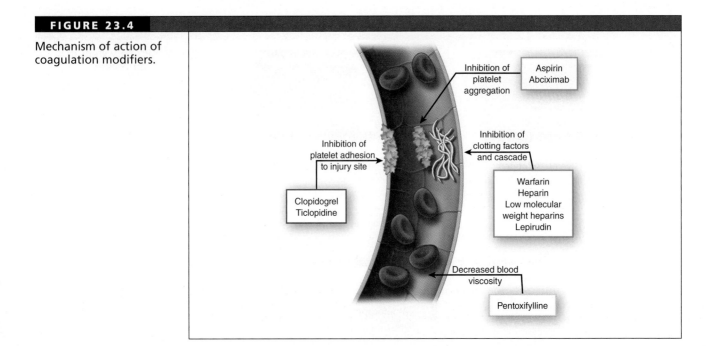

TABLE 23.2 Anticoagulants

Drug	Route and Adult Dose	Remarks
antithrombin, recombinant (ATryn)	IV infusion; dose is individualized based on the patient's pretreatment AT activity level and body weight	Thrombin inhibitor; for the prevention of perioperative and peripartum thromboembolic events in hereditary antithrombin deficient patients
apixaban (Eliquis)	PO; 2.5–5 mg bid	Factor Xa inhibitor; for prevention of stroke and pulmonary embolism in patients with atrial fibrillation
argatroban (Acova, Novastan)	IV; 2–10 mcg/kg/min	Thrombin inhibitor; for prevention of clots in patients with heparin-induced thrombocytopenia
bivalirudin (Angiomax)	IV; 0.75 mg/kg initial bolus followed by 1.75 mg/kg/hr for 4 hours	Thrombin inhibitor; used with aspirin to prevent clots during angioplasty
dabigatran (Pradaxa)	PO; 75–150 mg bid	Thrombin inhibitor; for prevention of stroke and systemic embolism in patients with atrial fibrillation
desirudin (Iprivask)	Subcutaneous; 15 mg bid for 9–12 days	Thrombin inhibitor; for DVT prophylaxis in patients undergoing hip replacement surgery
fondaparinux (Arixtra)	Subcutaneous; 2.5 mg/daily	For prevention of DVT and pulmonary embolism
(Pr) heparin	IV infusion; 5,000–40,000 units/day subcutaneously; 15,000–20,000 units/bid	For prevention and treatment of venous thrombosis and pulmonary edema; therapy begins with a higher dose, which is gradually reduced
lepirudin (Refludan)	IV; 0.4 mg/kg bolus followed by 0.15 mg/kg/hr for 2–10 days	Thrombin inhibitor; for prevention of clots in patients with heparin-induced thrombocytopenia
pentoxifylline (Trental)	PO; 400 mg tid	Reduces blood viscosity and increases the flexibility of red blood cells; for intermittent claudication (pain in legs while walking or exercising)
rivaroxaban (Xarelto)	PO; 10 mg once daily	Blocks Factor Xa; for prevention of stroke and systemic embolism in patients with atrial fibrillation
(Pr) warfarin (Coumadin)	PO; 2–15 mg/day	Same use as heparin but effect is more prolonged; IV form is available
LOW MOLECULAR WEIGHT (FRACTIONATED) HEPARINS (LMWHS)		
dalteparin (Fragmin)	Subcutaneous; 2,500–5,000 units/day	For prevention and treatment of DVT following knee or hip replacement or abdominal surgery, unstable angina, or acute coronary syndromes
enoxaparin (Lovenox)	Subcutaneous; 30 mg bid for 7–10 days	
tinzaparin (Innohep)	Subcutaneous; 175 units/kg daily for at least 6 days	

molecule has been shortened and modified to create **low molecular weight heparins (LMWHs)**, parenteral drugs that possess the same anticoagulant activity as heparin but have several advantages. They produce a more predictable anticoagulant response than heparin; therefore, less frequent laboratory monitoring is required. They also exhibit a two to four times longer duration of action than heparin that permits once daily dosing. Family members or the patient can be taught to give the necessary subcutaneous injections at home. LMWHs have become preferred drugs for many clotting disorders, including the prevention of DVT following surgery.

Other parenteral anticoagulants include the direct thrombin inhibitors such as lepirudin (Refludan). These drugs bind to the active site of thrombin, preventing the formation of fibrin clots. The thrombin inhibitors have limited therapeutic uses. Bivalirudin (Angiomax) is administered in combination with aspirin to prevent thrombi in patients undergoing angioplasty.

Argatroban (Acova, Novastan) and lepirudin are indicated for prevention or treatment of low platelet counts induced by heparin therapy. Desirudin (Iprivask) is given subcutaneously 15 minutes prior to hip replacement surgery for prophylaxis of DVT. Dabigatran (Pradaxa) is an oral drug in this class approved to reduce the risk of stroke and embolism in patients with atrial fibrillation.

To avoid serious adverse effects, drug therapy with coagulation modifier drugs is individualized to each patient and must be carefully monitored. For heparin, the **activated partial thromboplastin time (aPTT)** test is used to monitor the extent of anticoagulation. Baseline values of aPTT range from 25 to 40 seconds. During heparin therapy, the aPTT is maintained at 1.5 to 2 times the baseline level. If the aPTT rises above 80 seconds, the heparin dosage should be reduced. During the first few days of heparin therapy, aPTT is measured every four to six hours to avoid abnormal bleeding.

Oral Anticoagulants

The most frequently prescribed oral anticoagulant is warfarin (Coumadin). Often, patients begin anticoagulation therapy with heparin and are switched to warfarin when their condition stabilizes. When transitioning, the two drugs are administered concurrently for two to three days because warfarin takes several days of therapy before it achieves optimum anticoagulation effects.

Warfarin inhibits two enzymes involved in the formation of activated vitamin K, which is required for the synthesis of several clotting factor. Warfarin inhibits the synthesis of *new* clotting factors but does not affect clotting factors that are already circulating in the blood. The result is slowed clot formation and increased bleeding time.

Oral alternatives to warfarin include pentoxifylline, rivaroxaban, and apixaban. Although not a true anticoagulant, pentoxifylline (Trental) reduces the viscosity of red blood cells and increases their flexibility. It is given to increase the microcirculation in patients with intermittent claudication. In 2011, rivaroxaban (Xarelto) became the first anticoagulant available by the oral route to directly inhibit Factor X in the clotting cascade. Rivaroxaban is indicated for the prophylaxis of DVT in patients undergoing knee or hip replacement surgery and to reduce the risk of stroke and systemic embolism in patients with atrial fibrillation. In 2013, apixaban (Eliquis) was approved as an oral medication to reduce the incidence of stroke and pulmonary embolism in patients with atrial fibrillation. Patients with artial fibrillation are at increased risk for thrombus formation.

The laboratory test used during therapy with the oral anticoagulants is **prothrombin time (PT)**. Although the normal range for PT is 12 to 15 seconds, this value becomes prolonged with anticoagulant treatment. Daily PT tests may be conducted at the start of pharmacotherapy to ensure optimum dose levels. The frequency of PT tests is decreased to weekly or monthly as therapy progresses and the patient's condition stabilizes. Because the method of performing PT tests varies from laboratory to laboratory, clotting time is sometimes reported as an **international normalized ratio (INR)**, which is the PT multiplied by a correction factor. Recommended post-treatment INR values range from 2 to 4.

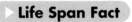
▶ Life Span Fact

Bleeding complications are more likely to occur in older adults. Prescribed doses of anticoagulants are generally lower for older patients, and this group receives more frequent assessments and laboratory testing to avoid serious complications.

Drug Prototype: ℗ *Heparin*
Therapeutic Class: Anticoagulant   **Pharmacologic Class: Indirect thrombin inhibitor**

Actions and Uses: Heparin is a natural substance found in the lining of blood vessels. Its normal function is to prevent excessive clotting within blood vessels. When given as a drug, heparin provides immediate anticoagulant activity. The binding of heparin to a substance called antithrombin III results in an inactivation of some of the clotting factors and an inhibition of thrombin activity. Heparin must be given either subcutaneously or through IV infusion. The onset of action for IV heparin is immediate, whereas subcutaneous heparin may take up to an hour for maximum therapeutic effect.

Adverse Effects and Interactions: Abnormal bleeding is common during heparin therapy. If aPTT becomes prolonged or toxicity is observed, stopping the heparin infusion will result in loss of anticoagulant activity within hours. If serious hemorrhage occurs, a specific blocker, protamine sulfate, may be administered to neutralize the anticoagulant activity of heparin. Protamine sulfate has an onset time of five minutes and is also a blocker of the LMWHs.

Heparin-induced thrombocytopenia (HIT) is a serious complication that occurs in up to 30% of patients taking the drug.

The patient may experience serious and even life-threatening thrombosis. Although the half-life of heparin is short, it may take a week after the drug is discontinued for platelets to completely recover.

Oral anticoagulants, including warfarin, increase the action of heparin. Ibuprofen, ASA, and other drugs that inhibit platelet aggregation may induce bleeding. Nicotine, digoxin, tetracyclines, or antihistamines may inhibit anticoagulation. Herbal supplements that may affect coagulation, such as ginger, garlic, green tea, feverfew, or ginkgo, should be avoided because they may increase the risk of bleeding.

> **BLACK BOX WARNING:**
> Epidural or spinal hematomas may occur when heparin or LMWHs are used in patients receiving spinal anesthesia or lumbar puncture. Because these can result in long-term or permanent paralysis, frequent monitoring for neurologic impairment is essential.

Drug Prototype: Ⓟ *Warfarin (Coumadin)*

Therapeutic Class: Anticoagulant   Pharmacologic Class: Vitamin K antagonist

Actions and Uses: Warfarin is used to prevent thrombi and emboli formation. Thus it is administered to patients at high risk for stroke, MI, DVT, and pulmonary embolism. This includes patients undergoing hip or knee surgery, those with long-term indwelling central venous catheters or prosthetic heart valves, and those who have experienced a recent MI.

Unlike heparin, the anticoagulant activity of warfarin can take several days to reach its maximum effect. This explains why heparin and warfarin therapy are overlapped. Warfarin inhibits the action of vitamin K that is essential for the synthesis of several clotting factors. Because these clotting factors are normally circulating in the blood, it takes several days for them to clear the plasma and for the anticoagulant effect of warfarin to appear. Another reason for the slow onset is that 99% of warfarin binds to plasma proteins and is unavailable to produce its effect. This high level of protein binding is responsible for a significant number of drug–drug interactions that may occur during warfarin therapy.

Adverse Effects and Interactions: Like all anticoagulants, the most serious adverse effect of warfarin is abnormal bleeding. On discontinuation of therapy, the activity of warfarin can take up to 10 days to diminish. If life-threatening bleeding occurs during therapy, the anticoagulant effects of warfarin can be reduced in six hours through the IM or subcutaneous administration of its blocker, vitamin K. The therapeutic range of serum warfarin levels varies from 1 to 10 mcg/mL to achieve an INR value of 2–3.

Extensive protein binding is responsible for numerous drug interactions, some of which occur with NSAIDs, diuretics, selective serotonin reuptake inhibitors (SSRIs) and other antidepressants, steroids, antibiotics and vaccines, and vitamins (e.g., vitamin K). Use with NSAIDs may increase bleeding risk. During warfarin therapy, the patient should not take any other prescription or over-the-counter (OTC) drugs unless approved by the healthcare provider. Use of warfarin with herbal supplements such as green tea, ginkgo, feverfew, garlic, cranberry, chamomile, and ginger may increase the risk of bleeding.

> **BLACK BOX WARNING:**
> Warfarin can cause major or fatal bleeding. Regular monitoring of INR is required. Patients should be instructed about prevention measures to minimize bleeding risk and to immediately notify healthcare providers of signs and symptoms of bleeding.

NURSING PROCESS FOCUS Patients Receiving Anticoagulant and Antiplatelet Therapy

ASSESSMENT	POTENTIAL NURSING DIAGNOSES
Prior to administration: ■ Obtain complete health history, including cardiovascular and renal conditions, surgeries or trauma, allergies, drug history, and possible drug interactions. ■ Acquire the results of a complete physical examination, including vital signs, height, and weight. ■ Evaluate laboratory blood findings: CBC, electrolytes, lipid panel, clotting factors, and renal and liver function studies.	■ *Risk for Injury (bleeding)* related to adverse effects of anticoagulant therapy ■ *Ineffective Tissue Perfusion* related to altered blood flow ■ *Deficient Knowledge* related to a lack of information about drug therapy ■ *Noncompliance* related to adverse effects of medications ■ *Ineffective Self-Health Maintenance* related to insufficient knowledge of seriousness of disease and drug therapy regimen

PLANNING: PATIENT GOALS AND EXPECTED OUTCOMES

The patient will:
■ Experience therapeutic effects (a decrease in blood coagulability).
■ Be free from or experience minimal adverse effects from drug therapy.
■ Verbalize an understanding of the drug's use, adverse effects, and required precautions.

IMPLEMENTATION

Interventions and (Rationales)	Patient Education/Discharge Planning
■ Administer medication correctly and evaluate the patient knowledge of proper administration. (Proper medication administration will increase effectiveness and help reduce complications and adverse effects.)	Instruct patient and caregivers that: ■ Correct self-administration of medication is extremely important. ■ Injections of heparin or LMWH should be administered in the fatty layers of the abdomen. ■ Skin is drawn up (pinched) and the needle is inserted at 45-90 degree angle. ■ Injections are done without aspirating for blood return. ■ Oral medications should be taken at the same time every day.

NURSING PROCESS FOCUS *(continued)*

Interventions and (Rationales)	Patient Education/Discharge Planning
Monitor for adverse clotting reaction(s): ■ Observe for skin necrosis, blue or purple mottling of the feet that blanches with pressure or fades when the legs are elevated. (Patients on anticoagulant therapy remain at risk for developing emboli resulting in cerebrovascular accident or pulmonary embolism. Coumadin may cause cholesterol microemboli, which result in gangrene, localized vasculitis, or "purple toes syndrome." Heparin can cause thrombus formation with thrombocytopenia, or "white clot syndrome.")	Instruct the patient to: ■ Immediately report to healthcare provider any sudden dyspnea or chest pain, and if temperature or color change occurs in the hands, arms, legs, and feet. (Gangrene may occur between days 3 and 8 of warfarin therapy. Purple toes syndrome usually occurs within weeks 3–10 or later.) ■ Feel pedal pulses daily to check circulation. ■ Protect feet from injury by wearing loose-fitting socks; avoid going barefoot.
■ Use with caution in patients with GI, renal, and/or liver disease, alcoholism, diabetes, hypertension, hyperlipidemia, and in older adult patients and premenopausal women. (Patients with CAD risk factors are at increased risk of developing cholesterol microemboli.)	■ Advise older adult patients; menstruating women; and those with peptic ulcer disease, alcoholism, or kidney or liver disease that they have an increased risk of bleeding. ■ Advise patients with diabetes and those with high blood pressure or high cholesterol that they are at risk of developing microscopic clots, despite anticoagulant therapy.
■ Monitor for signs of bleeding: flu-like symptoms, excessive bruising, pallor, epistaxis, hemoptysis, hematemesis, menorrhagia, hematuria, melena, frank rectal bleeding, or excessive bleeding from wounds or in the mouth. (Bleeding is a sign of anticoagulant overdose.)	Instruct the patient to: ■ Immediately report to healthcare provider flu-like symptoms (dizziness, chills, weakness, pale skin), blood coming from a cough, the nose, mouth or rectum; menstrual "flooding," "coffee grounds" vomit; tarry stools, excessive bruising; bleeding from wounds that cannot be stopped within 10 minutes, and all physical injuries. ■ Avoid all contact sports and amusement park rides that cause intense or violent bumping or jostling. ■ Use a soft toothbrush and electric shaver. ■ Keep a "pad count" during menstrual periods to estimate blood losses.
■ Monitor vital signs. (Increase in heart rate accompanied by low blood pressure or subnormal temperature may signal bleeding.)	■ Instruct the patient to immediately report palpitations, fatigue, or feeling faint, which may signal low blood pressure related to bleeding.
■ Monitor laboratory values: CBC, especially in premenopausal women; liver function studies, platelets, aPTT, PT, and/or INR for therapeutic values. (The aPTT and PT are usually 1.5–2.5 the normal control values. The value for INR is usually 2–4. Values below the norm indicate below-therapeutic levels. Values above the norm indicate a high potential for bleeding. CBC and platelet levels should remain within normal limits.) Heparin may also cause significant elevations of liver function tests because the drug is metabolized by the liver.)	Instruct the patient: ■ About the importance and need of regular laboratory testing. ■ To always inform laboratory and dental personnel of anticoagulant therapy when providing samples. ■ To carry a wallet card or wear medical ID jewelry indicating anticoagulant therapy.
■ Monitor the use of other medications or herbal supplements.	■ Instruct the patient to consult a healthcare provider before taking any other drugs, including OTC or herbal supplements. Many drugs decrease the action of anticoagulants.
■ Maintain normal diet, avoiding alcohol and increases in vitamin-K rich foods. (Vitamin K is used in the formation of clots; therefore, ingesting high amounts may decrease the effectiveness of warfarin. Alcohol may also alter the effectiveness of anticoagulants.)	■ Inform the patient to avoid alcohol and increases in vitamin K-rich foods such as broccoli, cabbage, dark leafy greens, and asparagus.

EVALUATION OF OUTCOME CRITERIA

Evaluate the effectiveness of drug therapy by confirming that patient goals and expected outcomes have been met (see "Planning"). *See Tables 23.2 and 23.3 for a list of drugs to which these nursing actions apply.*

CORE CONCEPT 23.5

Antiplatelet drugs prolong bleeding time by interfering with platelet aggregation.

Antiplatelet medications produce an anticoagulant effect by interfering with platelet aggregation. Unlike the anticoagulants, which are used primarily to prevent thrombosis in *veins*, antiplatelet drugs are used to prevent clot formation in *arteries*. Doses for antiplatelet medications are listed in Table 23.3 ◆.

Platelets are a key component of hemostasis. Too few platelets or diminished platelet function can profoundly increase bleeding time. The three primary classes of antiplatelet drugs include the following:

■ Aspirin

■ Adenosine diphosphate (ADP) receptor blockers

■ Glycoprotein IIb/IIIa receptor blockers

TABLE 23.3 Antiplatelet Drugs

Drug	Route and Adult Dose	Remarks
anagrelide (Agrylin)	PO; 0.5 mg qid or 1 mg bid (max: 10 mg/day)	Inhibits the production of platelets; for essential thrombocythemia (production of too many platelets)
aspirin (acetylsalicylic acid, ASA) (see page 208 for the Drug Prototype box)	PO; 80 mg/day–650 mg bid	Inhibits platelet aggregation; available without a prescription; higher doses are used to treat inflammation or pain
cilostazol (Pletal)	PO; 100 mg bid	Inhibits platelet aggregation; for intermittent claudication
dipyridamole (Persantine)	PO; 75–100 mg qid	Platelet inhibitor used to prevent embolism in cardiac valve replacement; usually used with warfarin
ADP RECEPTOR BLOCKERS		
Pr clopidogrel (Plavix)	PO; 75 mg daily (300 mg loading dose for patients with acute coronary syndrome)	Platelet aggregation inhibitor; for prevention of MI and stroke
prasugrel (Effient)	PO; 60 mg loading dose followed by 10 mg/day	Platelet aggregation inhibitor; for prevention of thrombotic events in patients undergoing PCI
ticagrelor (Brilinta)	PO; 90 mg bid	Newer drug for prevention of thrombosis in patients with acute coronary syndrome; given concurrently with 75–100 mg aspirin
ticlopidine (Ticlid)	PO; 250 mg bid	Platelet aggregation inhibitor; for stroke prevention
GLYCOPROTEIN IIB/IIIA BLOCKERS		
abciximab (ReoPro)	IV; 0.25 mg/kg initial bolus over 5 minutes; then 10 mcg/min for 12 hours	For prevention of cardiac ischemia during coronary angioplasty; effects continue up to 48 hours after infusion is stopped
eptifibatide (Integrilin)	IV; 180 mcg/kg initial bolus over 1–2 minutes; then 2 mcg/kg/min for 24–72 hours	For unstable angina and other acute coronary syndromes; effects continue up to 8 hours after infusion is stopped
tirofiban (Aggrastat)	IV; 0.4 mcg/kg/min for 30 minutes; then 0.1 mcg/kg/min for 12–24 hours	Similar to eptifibatide; effects continue up to 8 hours after infusion is stopped

Aspirin deserves special mention as an antiplatelet drug. Because it is available over-the-counter (OTC), patients may not consider aspirin a strong medication. However, its anticoagulant activity is well documented. Aspirin acts by inhibiting thromboxane$_2$, a powerful inducer of platelet aggregation. The anticoagulant effect of a single dose of aspirin may last for as long as a week. Use of aspirin with other coagulation modifiers should be avoided unless approved by the prescriber. The primary actions and adverse effects of aspirin are described in a Drug Prototype feature in Chapter 14.

The ADP receptor blockers are a small group of drugs that irreversibly alter the plasma membrane of platelets, preventing them from aggregating. Both ticlopidine (Ticlid) and clopidogrel (Plavix) are

CAM THERAPY

Garlic for Cardiovascular Health

Garlic (*Allium sativum*) is one of the best-studied herbs. Several substances have been isolated from garlic and shown to have pharmacologic activity. Dosage forms include eating prepared garlic oil or the fresh bulbs from the plant.

Modern claims for garlic uses have focused on the cardiovascular system: treatment of high blood lipid levels, atherosclerosis, and hypertension. Other modern claims are that garlic reduces blood glucose levels and has antibacterial and antineoplastic activity.

Like many other supplements, garlic likely has some health benefits, but controlled, scientific studies are often lacking and the results are mixed. Garlic has been shown to decrease the aggregation or "stickiness" of platelets, thus producing an anticoagulant effect. There is some research to show that the herb has a small effect on lowering blood cholesterol, although the effects seem to be short term.

Garlic is safe for consumption in moderate amounts. Patients taking anticoagulant medications should limit their intake of garlic to avoid bleeding complications. Patients with diabetes should monitor their blood glucose levels closely if taking high doses of garlic.

Drug Prototype: Clopidogrel (Plavix)

Therapeutic Class: **Antiplatelet drug**   Pharmacologic Class: **ADP receptor blocker**

Actions and Uses: Clopidogrel prolongs bleeding time by inhibiting platelet aggregation. It is given orally. Although its only approved use is to reduce the risk of stroke due to thrombi, it may be given off-label to prevent thrombi formation in patients with coronary artery stents and to prevent postoperative deep venous thrombosis. Because it is expensive, it is usually prescribed only for patients unable to tolerate aspirin, which has similar anticoagulant activity. Ticlopidine (Ticlid) acts by the same mechanism as clopidogrel but causes more adverse effects.

Adverse Effects and Interactions: Clopidogrel has approximately the same tolerability as aspirin. The incidence of GI bleeding is less than that for aspirin. Frequent adverse effects include a flu-like syndrome, headache, diarrhea, dizziness, bruising, upper respiratory tract infection, and rash or pruritus. Excessive bleeding is a potential adverse effect, although it only occurs in about 1% of patients. The other drug in this class, ticlopidine, can

cause an acute blood disorder known as thrombotic thrombocytopenia purpura, which can be fatal in up to 30% of patients who develop the disorder.

Use with anticoagulants, other antiplatelet drugs, thrombolytics, or NSAIDS, including aspirin, will increase the risk of bleeding. Barbiturates, rifampin, or carbamazepine may increase the anticoagulant activity of clopidogrel. The azole antifungals, protease inhibitors, erythromycin, verapamil, or zafirlukast may diminish the antiplatelet actions of clopidogrel.

BLACK BOX WARNING:
Because the effectiveness of clopidogrel is dependent on its metabolic activation by hepatic enzymes, poor metabolizers will exhibit less therapeutic effect and more adverse cardiovascular events.

given orally to prevent thrombi formation in patients who have experienced a recent thromboembolic event such as a stroke or MI. Clopidogrel is considerably safer and much more widely prescribed, having adverse effects comparable to those of aspirin. Prasugrel (Effient) and ticagrelor (Brilinta) are newer drugs in this class, approved to reduce thrombotic events in patients undergoing percutaneous coronary intervention (PCI).

Glycoprotein IIb/IIIa inhibitors are relatively new additions to the treatment of thromboembolic disease. **Glycoprotein IIb/IIIa** is a receptor on the surface of platelets that is necessary for platelet aggregation. Blocking this receptor has the effect of preventing thrombus formation in patients experiencing a recent MI, stroke, or PCI. These drugs are quite expensive and must be administered by the IV route.

CORE CONCEPT 23.6

Thrombolytics are used to dissolve existing clots.

It is often mistakenly believed that the purpose of anticoagulants such as heparin and warfarin is to digest and remove preexisting clots. This is not the case: A totally different type of drug is needed for this purpose. These drugs, called thrombolytics, are administered quite differently than the anticoagulants and produce their effects by different mechanisms. Thrombolytics are prescribed for situations in which a clot has already formed, including the following:

- Acute MI
- Pulmonary embolism
- Stroke
- DVT
- Arterial or coronary thrombosis
- Clearing thrombi in arteriovenous cannulas and blocked IV catheters

The goal of thrombolytic therapy is to restore blood flow quickly to essential tissues served by the blocked vessel. Delays in reestablishing circulation may result in permanent tissue damage. The therapeutic effect of thrombolytics is greater when they are administered as soon as possible after clot formation occurs, preferably within four hours. The role of the thrombolytics in treating MI, and a Nursing Process for this drug class, is presented in Chapter 20.

Thrombolytics have a narrow margin of safety between dissolving normal and abnormal clots. Vital signs must be monitored continuously, and signs of bleeding usually call for discontinuation of therapy. Because these medications are rapidly destroyed in the bloodstream, discontinuation

Drug Prototype: 🅿️ *Alteplase (Activase)*
Therapeutic Class: **Drug for dissolving clots**   Pharmacologic Class: **Thrombolytic**

Actions and Uses: Produced through recombinant DNA technology, alteplase is identical to the enzyme human tPA. Like other thrombolytics, the primary action of alteplase is to convert plasminogen to plasmin, which then dissolves clots. Alteplase should be given within six hours of the onset of symptoms of MI and within three hours of thrombotic stroke to be effective. Peak effect occurs in 5–10 minutes. Alteplase is a preferred drug for the treatment of acute MI and thrombotic stroke. It is occasionally used to reopen occluded IV catheters.

Adverse Effects and Interactions: Thrombolytics such as alteplase are contraindicated in patients with active bleeding or with a history of recent trauma. The patient must be monitored carefully for signs of bleeding every 15 minutes for the first hour of therapy and every 30 minutes thereafter. Signs of bleeding such as bruising, hematomas, or nosebleeds should be reported to the healthcare provider immediately.

Concurrent use with anticoagulants, antiplatelet drugs, or NSAIDs, including aspirin, may increase the risk of bleeding. Use with supplements that affect coagulation, such as feverfew, green tea, ginkgo, fish oil, ginger, or garlic, should be avoided because they may increase the risk of bleeding.

normally results in the immediate end of thrombolytic activity. After the clot is successfully removed by the thrombolytic medication, coagulation modifier therapy is initiated to prevent the reformation of clots.

Concept Review 23.2

■ Both warfarin and heparin are effective anticoagulants. Why would a physician choose heparin over warfarin?

Hemostatics are used to promote the formation of clots.

CORE CONCEPT 23.7

Hemostatics, also called *antifibrinolytics*, have an action opposite to that of anticoagulants: to shorten bleeding time. The name *hemostatics* comes from their ability to slow blood flow. They are used to prevent and treat excessive bleeding following surgical procedures.

All of the hemostatics have very specific indications for use, and none are commonly prescribed. Aminocaproic acid is administered IV to prevent bleeding in patients who have systemic clotting disorders. A PO form of tranexamic acid (Lysteda) was approved in 2009 for the treatment of heavy menstrual bleeding. Thrombin (Evithrom, Recothrom, Thrombinar) is approved as a topical drug to prevent minor oozing and bleeding from surgical sites. Although their mechanisms differ, all drugs in this class prevent fibrin from dissolving, thus enhancing the stability of the clot. The hemostatics are listed in Table 23.4 ◆.

TABLE 23.4   Hemostatics

Drug	Route and Adult Dose	Remarks
🅿️ aminocaproic acid (Amicar)	IV; 4–5 g for 1 hour, then 1–1.25 g/hr until bleeding is controlled	For control of excessive bleeding where fibrinolysis contributes to bleeding such as a pathologic condition known as systemic hyperfibrinolysis or surgical complications following heart surgery; oral form available
thrombin (Evithrom, Reothrom, Thrombinar)	Topical; dose varies based on the size of the treated area	Used to prevent blood loss following cardiopulmonary bypass surgery; considered an investigational new drug
tranexamic acid (Cyklokapron, Lysteda)	IV; 10 mg/kg, 3–4 times daily for 2–8 days PO; two 650 mg tablets, three times daily for a maximum of 5 days	Used just prior to and following dental surgery in patients with hemophilia and for women with heavy menstrual bleeding

Drug Prototype: ℗ *Aminocaproic Acid (Amicar)*

Therapeutic Class: Clot stabilizer   **Pharmacologic Class: Hemostatic/Antifibrinolytic**

Actions and Uses: Aminocaproic acid is prescribed in situations in which there is excessive bleeding as a result of clots being dissolved prematurely. The drug acts by inactivating plasminogen, the precursor of the enzyme plasmin, which dissolves the fibrin clot. During acute hemorrhages, it can be given IV to reduce bleeding in one to two hours. It is most commonly prescribed following surgery to reduce postoperative bleeding.

Adverse Effects and Interactions: Because aminocaproic acid tends to stabilize clots, it should be used cautiously in patients with a history of thromboembolic disease. Adverse effects are generally mild. The therapeutic serum level is 100–400 mcg/mL.

Drug interactions include hypercoagulation when used with estrogens and oral contraceptives.

PATIENTS NEED TO KNOW

Patients treated for coagulation disorders need to know the following:

1. Keep all scheduled appointments for PT, aPTT, and INR laboratory tests. Test results are used in making decisions about drug dose adjustments.
2. Report unusual bruising or bleeding, such as nosebleeds, bleeding gums, black or red stool, heavy menstrual periods, or spitting up blood, to healthcare providers.
3. Inform dental hygienists and dentists about the use of anticoagulant medication.
4. Use caution when engaged in activities that can cause bleeding, such as shaving, brushing teeth, trimming nails, and using kitchen knives. A soft toothbrush and an electric razor are safe choices. Contact sports, with their high risk for injury, should be avoided.
5. Take medications on time and as directed. Do not skip a dose, double up on doses, or discontinue taking medication without guidance from a healthcare provider.
6. Do not eat large or inconsistent amounts of foods high in vitamin K when taking warfarin because it interferes with clotting time.
7. Speak with the healthcare provider before taking any other drugs, including OTC drugs or herbal supplements. Many drugs increase or decrease the action of anticoagulants.

SAFETY ALERT

Medication Label Confusion: Heparin

Medication errors have occurred because of a nurse's failure to read the information provided on medication labels properly, such as when the strength of heparin was labeled only on a per-milliliter basis, and the volume of the vial was stated in another location. To help prevent these types of errors, the FDA now requires that heparin labels express the strength of the entire container and milliliters together. However, nurses should not rely on safety organizations alone to prevent medication errors. It is ultimately the responsibility of the nurse to read and understand the entire label before preparing and administering any medication.

CHAPTER REVIEW

CORE CONCEPTS SUMMARY

23.1 **Hemostasis is a complex process involving multiple steps and many clotting factors.**

Hemostasis is an essential mechanism protecting the body from both external and internal injury; it occurs in a sequential series of steps known as the coagulation cascade. The final result of coagulation is the formation of a fibrin clot that protects the body from excessive blood loss.

23.2 **Removing a blood clot is essential to restoring normal circulation.**

Blood clots are removed by fibrinolysis. Plasmin digests the fibrin strands, thus restoring circulation to the injured area.

23.3 **Drugs are used to modify the coagulation process.**

Anticoagulants prevent the formation of clots, thrombolytics dissolve existing clots, and hemostatics promote the formation of clots. Coagulation is always carefully monitored through the use of PT or aPTT laboratory tests.

23.4 **Anticoagulants prevent the formation and enlargement of clots.**

Anticoagulants prolong coagulation time by inhibiting platelets or a specific clotting factor in the coagulation cascade. Heparin is given IV or subcutaneously to provide immediate anticoagulation activity, and warfarin is given orally to offer more prolonged action. Protamine sulfate can reverse the anticoagulant activity of heparin, and vitamin K can reverse the effects of warfarin.

23.5 **Antiplatelet drugs prolong bleeding time by interfering with platelet aggregation.**

Aspirin, ADP receptor blockers, and glycoprotein IIb/IIIa receptor blockers prolong bleeding time by interfering with platelet function. They are used to prevent thrombus formation in arteries.

23.6 **Thrombolytics are used to dissolve existing clots.**

By dissolving existing clots, thrombolytics restore circulation to an injured area. For maximum effectiveness, they should be given as soon as possible after the thrombus is diagnosed.

23.7 **Hemostatics are used to promote the formation of clots.**

Hemostatics inhibit fibrin in a clot from dissolving and are used primarily to prevent excessive bleeding from surgical sites.

REVIEW QUESTIONS

The following questions are written in NCLEX-PN® style. Answer these questions to assess your knowledge of the chapter material, and go back and review any material that is not clear to you.

1. The patient's INR is 5.5. The nurse will:

1. Recheck the lab value.
2. Notify the physician.
3. Administer warfarin (Coumadin).
4. Hold the warfarin (Coumadin) and notify the physician.

2. The patient has been started on warfarin (Coumadin) for DVT. The patient asks when the medication will break up the clots. The nurse's best response would be:

1. "It will take 7 to 10 days for the clot to break down."
2. "This medication will not break down clots but will make it less likely that the clot will get larger."
3. "It will break down the clot within 8 to 12 hours of administration."
4. "You will need to be on this medication for a long time before it will break down the clot."

3. The patient is on IV heparin, but the nurse informs the patient that the physician has also ordered warfarin (Coumadin) to be started because:

1. Additional medication is needed.
2. Warfarin is much more effective than heparin.
3. Warfarin is not totally effective for several days after the administration of the first dose.
4. Heparin has a low molecular weight and is effective only for a short time.

4. The patient is receiving enoxaparin (Lovenox) subcutaneously every 12 hours following knee replacement surgery. The nurse monitors the patient for:

1. Gingival hyperplasia
2. Signs and symptoms of bruising and bleeding
3. Clotting at the incision site
4. Increased pain

5. The physician prescribes clopidogrel (Plavix) for a patient at risk for a MI. While instructing the patient about the adverse effects and precautions associated with this drug, the nurse tells him that the following drugs should not be used while on clopidogrel unless the doctor is consulted. (Select all that apply.)

1. Coumadin
2. Ibuprofen
3. Tissue plasminogen activator
4. Aspirin

6. The patient is receiving warfarin (Coumadin). Which of the following laboratory tests should the nurse check to ensure that clotting time stays within the therapeutic level?

1. Prothrombin time (PT)
2. International normalized ratio (INR) and PT
3. Activated partial thromboplastin time (aPTT)
4. INR

7. The physician has ordered that a patient be placed on a hemostatic drug during surgery to prevent blood loss. Which of the following medications will the nurse plan to give in this situation?

1. Aminocaproic acid (Amicar)
2. Aspirin
3. Trombin (Evithrom)
4. Tranexamic acid (Cyklokapron)

8. The patient on intermittent heparin is found to have hematuria and bleeding from old IV sites. The nurse anticipates what being ordered?

1. Protamine sulfate
2. Vitamin K
3. Pentoxifylline (Trental)
4. Ardeparin (Normiflo)

9. The physician orders 35,000 units of heparin to be given subcutaneously daily after the patient's aPTT has been checked. The label on the vial states 10,000 units/mL. How many units should the patient receive daily should the aPTT be in the recommended range?

1. 3.2 mL
2. 3.3 mL
3. 3 mL
4. 3.5 mL

10. A patient is receiving alteplase (Activase), a thrombolytic drug. The nurse monitors the patient for which of the following possible adverse effects?

1. Temperature of 100.8°F
2. Bruising and epistaxis
3. Skin rash with urticaria
4. Wheezing with labored breathing

CASE STUDY QUESTIONS

Remember Mr. Hawkins, the patient introduced at the beginning of the chapter? Now read the remainder of the case study. Based on the information you have learned in this chapter, answer the questions that follow.

Mr. Thomas Hawkins was recently admitted to the hospital with chest pain and suspected pulmonary embolism. He was immediately placed on heparin for two days and then switched to warfarin. He is now leaving the hospital with instructions to have laboratory testing every other day for the next two weeks.

1. The nurse understands that the goal of initially placing Mr. Hawkins on heparin was to:

1. Dissolve pulmonary emboli.
2. Prevent excessive bleeding.
3. Reduce blood viscosity.
4. Prevent additional thrombi from forming.

2. Mr. Hawkins is taught by the nurse that the most common adverse effect of heparin therapy is:

1. Nausea/vomiting
2. MI
3. Bleeding
4. Sedation

3. In planning for Mr. Hawkins' discharge from the hospital, he was switched from heparin to warfarin. When he inquired why his drug was switched, the nurse informed him that:

1. Warfarin is more effective.
2. Warfarin is given orally.
3. Warfarin causes less risk of hemorrhage.
4. Warfarin is less expensive.

4. As part of the discharge instructions, Mr. Hawkins is told that he will need to have blood drawn and which of the following laboratory tests need to be performed during the two weeks after his discharge?

1. PT/INR
2. Complete blood count (CBC)
3. aPTT
4. White blood cell count

NOTE: Answers to the Review and Case Study Questions appear in Appendix B. The complete rationales and answers are located on the textbook's website.

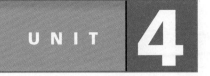

UNIT 4

The Immune System

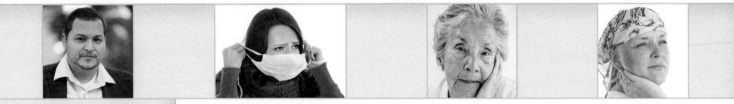

Unit Contents

Chapter 24 Drugs for Inflammation and Fever / 362

Chapter 25 Drugs for Immune System Modulation / 373

Chapter 26 Drugs for Bacterial Infections / 387

Chapter 27 Drugs for Fungal, Viral, and Parasitic Diseases / 412

Chapter 28 Drugs for Neoplasia / 430

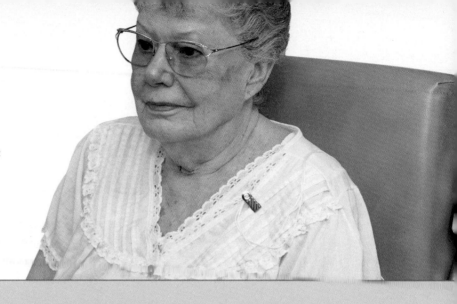

"It's so depressing. My hands are swollen all the time; and the gardening I love so much, I can't even do anymore. It's just too painful."

Mrs. Emma Greene

24 Drugs for Inflammation and Fever

CORE CONCEPTS

24.1 Inflammation is a body defense that limits the spread of invading microorganisms and injury.

24.2 The body reacts to injury by releasing chemical mediators that cause inflammation.

24.3 Inflammation may be treated with nonpharmacologic and pharmacologic therapies.

24.4 Nonsteroidal anti-inflammatory drugs (NSAIDs) are the primary drugs for the treatment of mild inflammation.

24.5 Corticosteroids are effective in treating severe inflammation.

24.6 Antipyretics are drugs used to reduce fever.

DRUG SNAPSHOT

The following drugs are discussed in this chapter:

DRUG CLASSES	DRUG PROTOTYPES
NSAIDs	**Pr** naproxen (Naprosyn) and naproxen sodium (Aleve, Anaprox) *366*
Corticosteroids	**Pr** prednisone *369*
Antipyretics	**Pr** acetaminophen (Tylenol) *369*

LEARNING OUTCOMES

After reading this chapter, the student should be able to:

1. Identify the function of inflammation as part of the body's normal defenses.

2. Outline the basic steps in the acute inflammatory response.

3. Explain the role of chemical mediators in inflammation.

4. Outline the general strategies for treating inflammation.

5. Explain the pharmacotherapy of fever.

6. Categorize drugs used in the treatment of inflammation and fever based on their classifications and mechanisms of action.

7. For each of the classes in the Drug Snapshot, identify representative drugs and explain their mechanisms of drug action, primary actions, and important adverse effects.

KEY TERMS

alternate-day therapy *368*
anaphylaxis (ANN-ah-fah-LAX-iss) *364*
antipyretics *369*
Cushing's syndrome (KUSH-ings) *368*

cyclooxygenase (COX) (SYE-klo-OK-sah-jen-ays) *366*
histamine (HISS-tuh-meen) *363*
Inflammation (IN-flah-MAY-shun) *363*

mast cells *363*
salicylism (sal-IH-sill-izm) *366*

The pain and redness of inflammation following minor abrasions and cuts is something everyone has experienced. Although there may be discomfort from such scrapes, inflammation is a normal and expected part of our body's defense against injury. For some diseases, however, inflammation can rage out of control, producing severe pain, fever, and other distressing symptoms. The purpose of this chapter is to examine these sorts of inflammatory conditions for which drug therapy may be needed.

Fast Facts Inflammatory Disorders

- Osteoarthritis affects about 27 million people and is the leading cause of disability in the United States.
- Inflammatory bowel disease has a peak onset of age 30 and affects about 1.4 million Americans each year.
- In the United States, approximately 70 million NSAID prescriptions are written, and 30 billion over-the-counter (OTC) NSAID tablets are sold each year.
- More than 1% of the U.S. population uses NSAIDs on a daily basis.
- It is estimated that NSAIDs cause about 16,000 deaths in the United States annually, largely as a result of gastrointestinal (GI) complications. This has more mortality than is caused from gastric cancer.

INFLAMMATION

Inflammation is a body defense that limits the spread of invading microorganisms and injury.

CORE CONCEPT 24.1

The human body has developed complex ways to defend itself against physical injury and invasion by microorganisms. Inflammation is one of these defense mechanisms. **Inflammation** is a nonspecific process that occurs in response to many different stimuli, including physical injury; exposure to toxic chemicals, extreme heat, or invading microorganisms; or death of cells. The central purpose of inflammation is to contain the injury or destroy the microorganism. By removing cellular debris and dead cells, repair of the injured area can move at a faster pace. Inflammation proceeds the same regardless of the cause that triggered it. Signs of inflammation include swelling, pain, warmth, and redness of the affected area.

Inflammation may be classified as *acute* or *chronic*. Acute inflammation has an immediate onset and lasts one to two weeks. During acute inflammation, 8–10 days are normally needed for the symptoms to resolve and for repair to begin. If the body cannot destroy or neutralize the damaging agent, inflammation may continue for long periods and become chronic. In chronic diseases such as lupus and rheumatoid arthritis, inflammation may persist for years, with symptoms becoming progressively worse over time. Other disorders such as seasonal allergy arise at predictable times each year, and inflammation may produce only minor, annoying symptoms.

The body reacts to injury by releasing chemical mediators that cause inflammation.

CORE CONCEPT 24.2

Whether the injury is due to an infection, chemicals, or physical trauma, the damaged tissue releases chemical mediators that act as "alarms" that notify the surrounding area of the injury. These chemical mediators initiate the processes and steps of inflammation. Chemical mediators include histamine, leukotrienes, bradykinin, complement, and prostaglandins. Table 24.1 ◆ describes the sources and actions of these mediators.

Histamine is a key chemical mediator of inflammation. It is primarily stored within **mast cells** located in tissue spaces under epithelial membranes such as the skin, in the bronchial tree and digestive tract, and along blood vessels. Mast cells detect invading microorganisms or injury and respond by releasing histamine, which initiates the inflammatory response within seconds. In addition, histamine directly stimulates pain receptors.

When released at an injury site, histamine and other mediators dilate nearby blood vessels, causing the capillaries to become more permeable or leaky. Plasma and components such as complement

TABLE 24.1	Chemical Mediators of Inflammation
Bradykinin	Vasodilator that causes pain; effects are similar to those of histamine
Complement	Series of at least 20 proteins that combine in a cascade fashion to neutralize or destroy an antigen
Histamine	Stored and released by mast cells; causes dilation of blood vessels, smooth muscle constriction, tissue swelling, and itching
Leukotrienes	Stored and released by mast cells; effects are similar to those of histamine
Prostaglandins	Present in most tissues; stored and released by mast cells; increase capillary permeability, attract white blood cells to site of inflammation, and cause pain

proteins and phagocytes can then enter the area to neutralize foreign agents. The affected area may become congested with blood, which can lead to significant swelling and pain. Thrombosis or blood clotting may result. Figure 24.1 ■ shows the basic steps in acute inflammation.

Rapid release of histamine on a larger scale throughout the body is responsible for **anaphylaxis**, a life-threatening allergic response that may result in shock and death. A number of chemicals, insect stings, foods, and some therapeutic drugs can cause this widespread release of histamine from mast cells. Drug therapy of anaphylactic shock is discussed in Chapter 21.

CORE CONCEPT 24.3

Inflammation may be treated with nonpharmacologic and pharmacologic therapies.

Because inflammation is a nonspecific process and may be caused by such a diverse variety of causes, it may occur in nearly any tissue or organ system. When treating inflammation, the following general principles apply:

- Inflammation is not a disease but a symptom of an underlying disorder. Whenever possible, the *cause* of the inflammation is identified and treated.

FIGURE 24.1

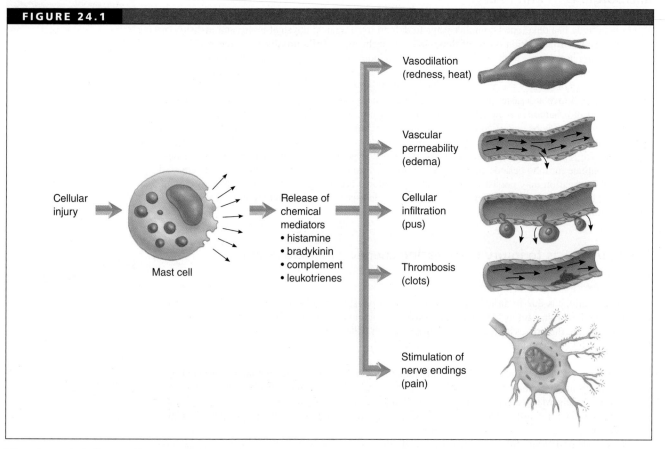

Steps in acute inflammation.

- Inflammation is a natural process for ridding the body of foreign agents, and it is usually self-limiting. For mild symptoms, nonpharmacologic therapies such as ice packs and rest should be used, as appropriate for the condition.

- When pharmacotherapy is necessary, topical drugs are used when applicable because they cause fewer adverse effects. Topical sprays, ointments, and creams are often the most effective drugs for treating inflammation of the skin and mucous membranes of the mouth, nose, rectum, and vagina. Many of these are available OTC.

The goal of pharmacotherapy with anti-inflammatory drugs is to prevent or decrease the intensity of the inflammatory response and reduce fever, if present. Most anti-inflammatory medications are nonspecific; the drug will exhibit the same inhibitory actions regardless of the cause of the inflammation. Diseases that benefit from anti-inflammatory drugs include allergic rhinitis, anaphylaxis, ankylosing spondylitis, contact dermatitis, Crohn's disease, glomerulonephritis, Hashimoto's thyroiditis, peptic ulcer disease, rheumatoid arthritis, systemic lupus erythematosus, and ulcerative colitis. If the inflammation is the result of an infection, antibiotic therapy may be necessary.

rhin = *nose*
itis = *inflammation*

The two primary drug classes used for inflammation are the NSAIDs and the corticosteroids (also called glucocorticoids). For mild to moderate pain and inflammation, NSAIDs are the preferred drugs. Should inflammation become severe, oral corticosteroid therapy is begun. Due to their serious long-term adverse effects, oral corticosteroids are usually used for only one to three weeks to bring inflammation under control, and then the patient is switched to NSAIDs.

NSAIDs are the primary drugs for the treatment of mild inflammation.

CORE CONCEPT **24.4**

NSAIDs such as aspirin and ibuprofen have analgesic, antipyretic, and anti-inflammatory effects. They are preferred drugs for the treatment of mild to moderate inflammation in most patients. Some of the specific NSAIDs used for inflammation are listed in Table 24.2 ◆.

TABLE 24.2 Selected Nonsteroidal Anti-Inflammatory Drugs (NSAIDs)

Drug	Route and Adult Dose	Remarks
aspirin (acetylsalicylic acid [ASA], others) (see page 208 for the Drug Prototype box)	PO; 350–650 mg every 4 hours (max: 4 g/day) PO; 3.6–5.4 g/day in 4–6 divided doses for arthritic conditions	Inhibits the formation of prostaglandins; also for fever, pain, and prevention of stroke and myocardial infarction (MI)
celecoxib (Celebrex)	PO; 100–200 mg bid (max: 200 mg/day)	Selective COX-2 inhibitor
diclofenac (Cataflam, Solaraze, Voltaren)	PO; 50 mg bid–qid (max: 200 mg/day)	Sustained-release and transdermal forms available
diflunisal	PO; 250–500 mg bid (max: 1,500 mg/day)	Similar to ibuprofen
etodolac	PO; 200–400 mg tid–qid (max: 1,200 mg/day)	Extended-release form available
fenoprofen (Nalfon)	PO; 300–600 mg tid–qid (max: 3,200 mg/day)	Similar to ibuprofen
flurbiprofen (Ansaid)	PO; 50–100 tid–qid (max: 300 mg/day)	Similar to ibuprofen
ibuprofen (Advil, Motrin, others)	PO; 400–800 mg tid–qid (max: 3,200 mg/day)	Blocks prostaglandin synthesis as well as modulates T-cell function; also for dysmenorrhea
ketoprofen	PO; 75 mg tid or 50 mg qid (max: 300 mg/day)	Extended-release form available; similar to ibuprofen; also for dysmenorrhea
meloxicam (Mobic)	PO: 7.5–15 mg once daily (max: 15 mg/day)	Similar to ibuprofen
nabumetone (Relafen)	PO; 1,000 mg daily (max: 2,000 mg/day)	Similar to ibuprofen
℗ naproxen (Naprosyn) and naproxen sodium (Aleve, Anaprox)	PO; 250–500 mg bid (max: 1,000 mg/day)	Also for dysmenorrhea
oxaprozin (Daypro)	PO; 600–1,200 mg daily (max: 1,800 mg/day)	Similar to naproxen; once-a-day dosage
piroxicam (Feldene)	PO; 10–20 mg once or twice a day (max: 20 mg/day)	Has prolonged half-life
tolmetin (Tolectin)	PO; 400 mg tid (max: 2 g/day)	Similar to ibuprofen

The analgesic action of NSAIDs is discussed in Chapter 14. Because they are inexpensive and readily available OTC, NSAIDs such as aspirin and ibuprofen are some of the most widely used drugs. Acetaminophen has no anti-inflammatory action and is thus not classified as an NSAID. It is, however, an effective analgesic and antipyretic (see Section 24.5).

Aspirin is useful in treating inflammation because it inhibits **cyclooxygenase (COX)**, a key enzyme in the pathway of prostaglandin synthesis that is found in every tissue. Aspirin causes irreversible inhibition of both forms of cyclooxygenase, COX-1 and COX-2. Because it is readily available, inexpensive, and effective, aspirin is sometimes a drug of first choice for treating mild inflammation. The basic pharmacology and a drug profile of aspirin are presented in Chapter 14.

Unfortunately, large doses of aspirin are necessary to suppress severe inflammation, and these doses result in a greater incidence of serious adverse effects. The most common adverse effects observed during high dose therapy relate to the digestive system. By increasing gastric acid secretion and irritating the stomach lining, aspirin may cause pain, heartburn, and even bleeding due to ulceration. In some patients, even small doses may cause GI bleeding. Some aspirin formulations are buffered or given an enteric coating to minimize GI adverse effects. Because aspirin also has an antiplatelet effect (see Chapter 23), the potential for bleeding must be carefully monitored by the healthcare provider. High doses may produce **salicylism**, a syndrome that includes symptoms such as ringing in the ears, dizziness, headache, and sweating. Patients with preexisting kidney disease should be monitored carefully because aspirin and other NSAIDs may affect kidney function.

Ibuprofen and ibuprofen-like drugs such as naproxen are available as alternatives to aspirin. Like aspirin, they exhibit their effects through inhibition of COX-1 and COX-2. Because of their similar mechanisms, they all have similar pharmacologic properties and a relatively low incidence of adverse effects. The most common adverse effects of these drugs are nausea and vomiting. Although the incidence of gastric ulceration and bleeding is less than that of aspirin, this can still be a serious problem in patients with peptic ulcers who are taking high doses of these medications. Most have only a small or insignificant effect on blood coagulation and are safer to use than aspirin in patients who may be at risk for bleeding.

Selective inhibition of COX-2 produces the analgesic, anti-inflammatory, and antipyretic effects seen with the NSAIDs without causing some of the serious adverse effects of the older NSAIDs. Because they have no adverse GI effects and do not affect blood coagulation, these drugs quickly became the treatment of choice for moderate to severe inflammation.

However, in 2004, research data revealed that one NSAID, rofecoxib (Vioxx), doubled the risk of heart attack and stroke in patients taking it for extended periods. Based on these reports, the drug manufacturer voluntarily removed the drug from the market. Shortly afterward, a second COX-2 inhibitor, valdecoxib (Bextra), was also voluntarily withdrawn, leaving celecoxib (Celebrex) the sole drug in this class.

Drug Prototype: Ⓟ *Naproxen (Naprosyn) and Naproxen Sodium (Aleve, Anaprox)*

Therapeutic Class: **Analgesic, anti-inflammatory drug, antipyretic** Pharmacologic Class: **Nonsteroidal anti-inflammatory drug (NSAID)**

Actions and Uses: Naproxen is an older NSAID that is prescribed for the treatment of mild to moderate pain, fever, and inflammation. Its efficacy at relieving pain and inflammation is similar to that of aspirin. Common indications include treating the pain associated with rheumatoid arthritis and osteoarthritis, gout, and bursitis. In treating rheumatoid arthritis, the therapeutic effects may take three to four weeks to appear.

Naproxen inhibits prostaglandin synthesis through the nonselective inhibition of cyclooxygenase type-1 and type-2 enzymes. It also inhibits platelet aggregation and prolongs bleeding time.

Adverse Effects and Interactions: Adverse effects of naproxen are generally not serious and include GI upset, dizziness, and drowsiness. Administration with food will decrease the incidence of stomach upset, which is the most common adverse effect. Because naproxen may prolong bleeding time, the drug should be administered with caution to those with bleeding disorders. Patients taking naproxen should notify their dental hygienist before dental procedures are performed.

Using naproxen concurrently with oral anticoagulants can prolong bleeding time. Lithium levels may be increased. Bleeding potential increases when used with herbal supplements such as feverfew, garlic, ginger, and ginkgo biloba.

> **BLACK BOX WARNING (PRESCRIPTION FORMS):**
> NSAIDs may cause an increased risk of MI, and stroke, which may increase with duration of use. Patients with cardiovascular disease may be at greater risk. NSAIDs are contraindicated for the treatment of perioperative pain in those undergoing coronary artery bypass graft surgery. NSAIDs increase the risk of bleeding, ulceration, and perforation of the stomach or intestines, which can be fatal. These events occur more frequently in older adults and can occur at any time during use or without warning symptoms.

ASSESSMENT	POTENTIAL NURSING DIAGNOSES
Prior to administration: ■ Obtain a complete health history, including musculoskeletal, GI, renal and liver conditions, infectious diseases, allergies, drug history, and possible drug interactions. ■ Evaluate laboratory blood findings: CBC, electrolytes, and renal and liver function studies. ■ Determine reasons for analgesic use and patterns of medication usage. ■ Acquire the results of a complete physical examination, including vital signs, height, and weight.	■ *Acute Pain* related to injury, disorder, or surgical procedure ■ *Chronic Pain* related to tissue damage ■ *Deficient Knowledge* related to a lack of information about drug therapy ■ *Ineffective Health Maintenance* related to chronic pain

PLANNING: PATIENT GOALS AND EXPECTED OUTCOMES

The patient will:
■ Experience therapeutic effects (pain relief or a reduction in pain intensity).
■ Be free from or experience minimal adverse effects from drug therapy.
■ Verbalize an understanding of the drug's use, adverse effects, and required precautions.

IMPLEMENTATION

Interventions and (Rationales)	Patient Education/Discharge Planning
■ Determine need for medication. Record the character, duration, location, and intensity of pain and the presence of inflammation. (NSAIDs are usually given to patients who have inflammatory conditions that cause pain. Monitoring pain and medication use helps to determine medication effectiveness.)	■ Instruct the patient to report to the healthcare provider any pain and/or inflammation that remains unresolved.
■ Administer NSAIDs correctly and evaluate the patient's knowledge of proper administration. (May be administered PO or topical/transdermal. Overuse may cause severe adverse effects.)	Inform the patient to: ■ Take only the prescribed amount of NSAIDs to decrease the potential for adverse effects. ■ Not cut or crush enteric-coated tablets. Regular tablets may be broken or pulverized and mixed with food. ■ Take liquid aspirin (ASA) products immediately after mixing because they break down rapidly. ■ Not take different drugs and formulations, such as ibuprofen and naproxen, concurrently. Consult the healthcare provider regarding appropriate OTC analgesics for specific types of pain. ■ Consult the healthcare provider regarding aspirin therapy following surgery. (ASA also has antiplatelet properties. The body needs time to manufacture new platelets to make clots that promote wound healing.) ■ Advise laboratory personnel of aspirin therapy when providing urine samples.
■ Monitor vital signs, especially temperature. (Increased temperature may indicate infection. Increased pulse and blood pressure may indicate discomfort; if accompanied by pallor and/or dizziness, may indicate bleeding.)	Instruct the patient to: ■ Immediately report the occurrence of a rapid heartbeat, palpitations, dizziness, or pallor to the healthcare provider. ■ Monitor blood pressure and temperature, ensuring proper use of home equipment.
■ Monitor for signs of GI bleeding, GI elimination, or hepatic toxicity. Conduct guaiac stool testing for occult blood and monitor CBC for anemia-related blood loss. (NSAIDs can be a local irritant to the GI tract with anticoagulant action that is metabolized in the liver.)	Instruct the patient to: ■ Report any bleeding, abdominal pain, anorexia, heartburn, nausea, vomiting, jaundice, or change in the color or character of stools to the healthcare provider. ■ Know the proper method of obtaining stool samples and home testing for occult blood. ■ Adhere to a regimen of laboratory testing as ordered by the healthcare provider. ■ Take NSAIDs with food to reduce stomach upset.
■ Monitor for hypersensitivity reaction.	■ Advise the patient to monitor for shortness of breath, wheezing, throat tightness, itching, or hives. If these occur, stop taking ASA immediately and inform the healthcare provider.
■ Monitor urinary output and edema in feet/ankles. (Medication is excreted through the kidneys. Long-term use may lead to renal dysfunction.)	■ Instruct the patient to report changes in urination, flank pain, or pitting edema.
■ Monitor serum levels of salicylate. (Monitoring serum levels helps to monitor for possible toxicity).	■ Advise the patient to return to the healthcare provider for prescribed follow-up appointments.
■ Monitor for sensory changes indicative of drug toxicity. (Signs and symptoms of toxicity include tinnitus and blurred vision.)	■ Inform patient to immediately report any sensory changes in sight or hearing, especially blurred vision or ringing in the ears, to the healthcare provider.

EVALUATION OF OUTCOME CRITERIA

Evaluate the effectiveness of drug therapy by confirming that patient goals and expected outcomes have been met (see "Planning"). *See Table 24.2 for a list of drugs to which these nursing actions apply.*

Corticosteroids are effective in treating severe inflammation.

Corticosteroids or glucocorticoids are natural hormones released by the cortex of the adrenal gland that have powerful effects on nearly every cell in the body. One of their most useful actions is the ability to suppress severe inflammation. When used to treat inflammatory disorders, the drug doses are many times higher than those naturally present in the blood. Corticosteroids have numerous therapeutic applications. The uses of these drugs in treating hormonal imbalances are presented in detail in Chapter 32. Doses of the corticosteroids used to treat severe inflammatory disease are listed in Table 24.3 ◆.

Corticosteroids affect inflammation in multiple ways. They suppress the actions of chemical mediators of inflammation such as histamine and prostaglandins. In addition, they inhibit the immune system by suppressing certain functions of phagocytes and lymphocytes. These multiple effects have the ability to markedly reduce inflammation, making corticosteroids the most effective medications for the treatment of severe inflammatory disorders.

Unfortunately, medications in the corticosteroid class have several potentially serious adverse effects that limit their therapeutic usefulness when they are given by the oral or parenteral routes. These include suppression of the normal functions of the adrenal gland (adrenal insufficiency), elevated blood glucose, mood changes, cataracts, peptic ulcers, electrolyte imbalances, and osteoporosis. Because of their effectiveness at reducing the signs and symptoms of inflammation, corticosteroids can mask infections that may be present in the patient. This combination of masking inflammation and suppressing the immune system creates a potential for existing infections to grow rapidly and undetected. An active infection is usually a contraindication for corticosteroids therapy.

Because the appearance of these adverse effects is a function of the dose and duration of therapy, treatment is often limited to the short-term control of acute disease. When longer therapy is indicated, doses are kept as low as possible and **alternate-day therapy** is sometimes used; the medication is taken every other day to encourage the patient's adrenal glands to function on the days when no drug is taken. During long-term therapy, the healthcare provider must be alert for signs of overtreatment, a condition called **Cushing's syndrome**. Signs include bruising and a characteristic pattern of fat deposits in the cheeks (moon face), shoulders (buffalo hump), and abdomen. The body becomes accustomed to the high doses of corticosteroids, and patients must discontinue the drug gradually because abrupt withdrawal can result in lack of adrenal function.

The serious adverse effects of the corticosteroids may be prevented by giving the drugs by the intranasal, topical, or intravaginal routes. Although small amounts of the drug are absorbed across the skin and mucous membranes, the amount reaching the blood is generally small and too low to cause serious systemic effects.

TABLE 24.3   Selected Corticosteroids for Severe Inflammation

Drug	Route and Adult Dose	Remarks
betamethasone (Celestone, Diprolene, others)	PO; 0.6–7.2 mg/day	Topical, intra-articular, IM, and IV forms available
cortisone	PO; 20–300 mg/day in divided doses	IM form available; also for adrenal insufficiency
dexamethasone	PO; 0.25–4 mg bid–qid	IM and IV forms available; also for adrenal insufficiency and immunosuppression
hydrocortisone (Cortef, Hydrocortone, Solu-Cortef, others) (see page 522 for the Drug Prototype box)	Topical; 0.5% cream applied 1–4 times daily PO; 10–320 mg tid–qid	Used widely for skin inflammation; IM, PO, rectal, and IV forms available; may be injected intra-articular
methylprednisolone (Depo-Medrol, Medrol)	PO; 4–48 mg/day in divided doses	Available in IM, IV, and rectal forms; also for neoplasia and adrenal insufficiency
prednisolone (Prelone)	PO; 5–60 mg 1–4 times daily	Available in IM and IV forms; also for neoplasia and adrenal insufficiency
(Pr) prednisone	PO; 5–60 mg 1–4 times daily	Available in oral form only; also for neoplasia
triamcinolone (Aristospan, Kenalog)	PO; 4–48 mg 1–4 times daily	Available in IM, subcutaneous, intradermal, intra-articular, and aerosol forms

Drug Prototype: (Pr) *Prednisone*
Therapeutic Class: Anti-inflammatory drug   **Pharmacologic Class: Corticosteroid**

Actions and Uses: Prednisone is a synthetic corticosteroid. Its actions are the result of being metabolized to an active form, which is also available as a drug called prednisolone. When used for inflammation, a 4- to 10-day duration for therapy is common. Alternate-day dosing is used for long-term therapy. Prednisone is occasionally used to terminate acute bronchospasm in patients with asthma (see Chapter 29) and for patients with certain cancers such as Hodgkin's disease, acute leukemia, and lymphomas (see Chapter 28).

Adverse Effects and Interactions: When used for short-term therapy, prednisone has few adverse effects. Long-term therapy may result in Cushing's syndrome, a condition that includes elevated blood glucose, fat redistribution to the shoulders and face, muscle weakness, bruising, and bones that easily fracture. Corticosteroids can raise blood glucose levels. Patients with diabetes may require an adjustment in insulin dose. Gastric ulcers may occur with long-term therapy, and an antiulcer medication may be prescribed prophylactically. Patients must report any potential infections immediately. This drug should be discontinued gradually.

Barbiturates, phenytoin, and rifampin increase the metabolism of prednisone: Increased doses of prednisone may be needed. Amphotericin B and diuretics together with prednisone can increase potassium loss. Prednisone may inhibit antibody response to vaccines and toxoids. In patients with myasthenia gravis, use of prednisone with ambenonium, neostigmine, or pyridostigmine can cause severe muscle weakness.

FEVER

Antipyretics are drugs used to reduce fever.

CORE CONCEPT 24.6

Like inflammation, fever is a natural defense mechanism for neutralizing foreign substances. Many species of bacteria are killed by high fever. Often, the healthcare provider must determine whether the fever needs to be dealt with aggressively or allowed to run its course without drug therapy. Drugs used to treat fever are called **antipyretics**.

Drug Prototype: (Pr) *Acetaminophen (Tylenol)*
Therapeutic Class: Antipyretic, nonopioid analgesic
Pharmacologic Class: Centrally acting prostaglandin inhibitor

Actions and Uses: Acetaminophen reduces fever by direct action at the level of the hypothalamus and causes dilation of peripheral blood vessels, enabling sweating and dissipation of heat. Acetaminophen and aspirin have equal efficacy in relieving pain and reducing fever. Acetaminophen is administered as a substitute for aspirin when NSAIDs are contraindicated due to age, allergy, or gastric irritation. It is not linked with Reye's syndrome, as is aspirin; thus it is safe to administer to infants, children, and adolescents who have flu-like symptoms or chickenpox.

Acetaminophen has no peripheral anti-inflammatory action; therefore, it is not effective in treating arthritis or pain caused by tissue swelling following injury. Acetaminophen is pregnancy category B.

Adverse Effects and Interactions: At recommended doses, acetaminophen is well tolerated and serious adverse effects are rare. The risk for adverse effects is dose related and increases with long-term use. Acute acetaminophen poisoning is very serious, and symptoms include anorexia, nausea, vomiting, dizziness, lethargy, diaphoresis, chills, abdominal pain, and diarrhea. Excessive acetaminophen use is the number one cause of acute hepatic failure in the United States.

Acetaminophen inhibits warfarin metabolism, causing warfarin to accumulate to toxic levels. High-dose or long-term acetaminophen usage may result in elevated warfarin levels and bleeding. Ingestion of this drug with alcohol is not recommended due to the possibility of liver failure from hepatic necrosis.

The patient should avoid taking herbs that have the potential for liver toxicity, including comfrey, coltsfoot, and chaparral.

BLACK BOX WARNING:
In 2011, the FDA issued a warning that acetaminophen has the potential to cause severe liver injury and may cause serious allergic reactions with symptoms of angioedema, difficulty breathing, itching, or rash.

In most patients, fever is more of a discomfort than a life-threatening problem. Prolonged, high fever (usually above 102°F or 38.9°C), however, can become dangerous, especially in young children in whom fever can stimulate seizures. In adults, excessively high fever can break down body tissues, reduce mental acuity, and lead to delirium or coma, particularly among elderly patients. In rare instances, an elevated body temperature may be fatal.

The goal of antipyretic therapy is to lower body temperature while identifying and treating the underlying cause of the fever, which is often an infection. Aspirin, ibuprofen, and acetaminophen are safe, inexpensive, and effective drugs for reducing fever. Many of these antipyretics are marketed for different age groups, including special, flavored brands for infants and children. For fast delivery and effectiveness, drugs may come in various forms including gels, caplets, enteric-coated tablets, and suspensions. Aspirin and acetaminophen are also available as suppositories.

PATIENTS NEED TO KNOW

Patients treated for inflammatory disorders or fever need to know the following:

Regarding Anti-Inflammatory Medications and Antipyretics

1. Take NSAIDs with food to decrease stomach irritation.
2. Avoid drinking alcohol when taking high doses of NSAIDs or aspirin because it increases stomach irritation.
3. If ringing in the ears, dizziness, headache, or signs of bleeding or bruising occur, discontinue aspirin use immediately and report the incident to the healthcare provider.
4. Take corticosteroids exactly as prescribed because improper use may lead to serious adverse effects.
5. Acetaminophen may be found in many OTC cold and flu products. Be careful not to take multiple products containing this drug, because additive toxicity may result.

CHAPTER REVIEW

CORE CONCEPTS SUMMARY

24.1 Inflammation is a body defense that limits the spread of invading microorganisms and injury.

Inflammation is a nonspecific response designed to rid the body of invading pathogens or to contain the spread of injury. Acute inflammation occurs over a period of several days, whereas chronic inflammation may continue for months or years.

24.2 The body reacts to injury by releasing chemical mediators that cause inflammation.

Inflammation is initiated by chemical mediators, the most important of which is histamine. Release of these meditators causes vasodilation, allowing capillaries to become leaky, thus causing tissue swelling. Extremely rapid release of histamine throughout the body can trigger anaphylaxis.

24.3 Inflammation may be treated with nonpharmacologic and pharmacologic therapies.

When possible, topical drugs are used because they produce fewer adverse effects than oral or parenteral drugs. The two primary drug classes used for inflammation are the NSAIDs and corticosteroids.

24.4 NSAIDs are the primary drugs for the treatment of mild inflammation.

NSAIDs are drugs that inhibit the enzyme cyclooxygenase. Nonselective cyclooxygenase inhibitors, including aspirin, are effective at reducing inflammation and pain but cause significant GI adverse effects in some patients.

24.5 Corticosteroids are effective in treating severe inflammation.

Corticosteroids are hormones that are extremely effective at reducing inflammation. Because overtreatment with these drugs can cause Cushing's syndrome, corticosteroid therapy for inflammation is generally short term.

24.6 Antipyretics are drugs used to reduce fever.

Fever is often self-limiting but when it is elevated or prolonged, pharmacotherapy is indicated. Acetaminophen is often a preferred drug for fever, although ibuprofen is equally effective.

REVIEW QUESTIONS

The following questions are written in NCLEX-PN® style. Answer these questions to assess your knowledge of the chapter material, and go back and review any material that is not clear to you.

1. A patient is getting ready to go home from the hospital and the nurse and patient are discussing the types of OTC NSAID medications that are available. The nurse states that an OTC medication that is not classified as an NSAID is:

1. Aspirin
2. Ibuprofen
3. Acetaminophen
4. Motrin

2. The patient has been taking aspirin for several days for a headache. While collecting information from the patient, the nurse discovers that the patient is experiencing ringing in the ears and dizziness. The most appropriate action by the nurse is:

1. To question the patient about history of sinus infection
2. To determine if the patient has mixed the aspirin with other medications
3. To tell the patient to hold off on taking any more aspirin until seen by the physician
4. To tell the patient to take the aspirin with food or milk

3. The nurse informs the patient that the most common adverse effect of NSAIDs is:

1. Edema
2. Rash
3. GI irritation
4. Bleeding

4. The patient is taking corticosteroids, so the nurse monitors for:

1. Bleeding
2. Respiratory distress
3. Dehydration
4. Infection

5. A patient with diabetes taking prednisone states that his blood sugar is higher than normal. The nurse's most appropriate response would be:

1. "You must not be following your diet for diabetes."
2. "Prednisone can cause blood sugar levels to increase."
3. "You must be developing an illness."
4. "Your diabetes must be getting worse."

6. The nurse is to administer 10 grains of aspirin by mouth. Available are 325 mg tablets. How many tablets will the nurse administer?

1. One-half tablet
2. One tablet
3. One and one-half tablets
4. Two tablets

7. While educating a patient about acetaminophen, the nurse instructs the patient to report to the healthcare provider if the following should occur: (Select all that apply.)

1. Lethargy
2. Anorexia
3. Tearing of the eyes
4. Difficulty breathing

8. The nurse is examining a patient with rheumatoid arthritis. The patient has been taking prednisone for an extended period of time. During the examination, the nurse observes that the patient has a very round moon-shaped face, bruising, and shoulder hump. What does the nurse suspect based on these findings?

1. These are normal reactions based on these findings.
2. These are probably birth defects.
3. These are the symptoms of myasthenia gravis.
4. These are the symptoms of adverse drug effects from prednisone.

9. A patient has been taking acetaminophen fairly regularly for headaches but has questions regarding food and beverage restrictions while taking this medication. The nurse informs the patient that taking this drug while regularly drinking alcohol may cause:

1. Liver failure
2. Renal damage
3. Thrombosis
4. Pulmonary damage

10. A mother of a 5-year-old asks the nurse why aspirin is not good for her to give to her child when she has a fever. The nurse responds that:

1. It is not as good an antipyretic as acetaminophen.
2. It may increase fever in children under 10 years.
3. It may produce nausea and vomiting.
4. It increases the risk of Reye's syndrome when flu-like symptoms are present.

CASE STUDY QUESTIONS

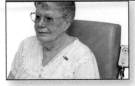

Remember Mrs. Greene, the patient introduced at the beginning of the chapter? Now read the remainder of the case study. Based on the information you have learned in this chapter, answer the questions that follow.

Mrs. Emma Greene, 62 years old, has been experiencing a gradual increase in pain and swelling of her hands. Her knuckles have also become red and warm to the touch. She enjoys gardening and sewing, but over the past six months she has not been able to participate in these activities because it is "too painful." Mrs. Greene has been treating herself with NSAIDs, specifically ibuprofen and naproxen.

1. Regarding Mrs. Greene's use of NSAIDs, what question should you ask to determine potential adverse effects?

1. "Have you experienced excessive drowsiness?"
2. "Have you experienced GI upset?"
3. "Have you experienced excessive dryness or stinging sensations in your nose?"
4. "Have you experienced any rashes or dryness of the skin?"

2. To help Mrs. Greene alleviate the adverse effects of NSAIDs, the nurse advises her to:

1. Take NSAIDs with food.
2. Take NSAIDs on an empty stomach.
3. Take both types of NSAIDs at the same time. It is okay.
4. There are no adverse effects of most NSAIDs.

3. Mrs. Greene is diagnosed with rheumatoid arthritis. She experiences a "flare-up" (acute exacerbation) of her disease. Because Mrs. Greene has experienced a "flare-up" of her condition, which of the following drug classes would likely be prescribed over a 10-day period?

1. Biologic response modifiers
2. Intranasal corticosteroids
3. Systemic corticosteroids
4. Sympathomimetics

4. Her healthcare practitioner prescribes prednisone. Mrs. Greene asks why she was given this medication. The office nurse tells her that:

1. He just wanted to try something different
2. Prednisone markedly reduces inflammation and is beneficial for short-term use
3. Prednisone is used only for pain control
4. Prednisone has very few adverse effects, even when used for long periods

NOTE: Answers to the Review and Case Study Questions appear in Appendix B. The complete rationales and answers are located on the textbook's website.

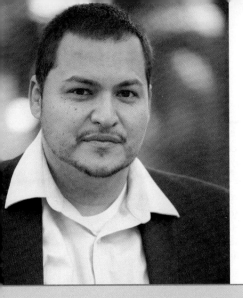

C
H
A
P
T
E
R

"Since I work directly with so many people, I thought it might be a good idea to get the hepatitis B vaccine series."

Mr. Jose Martel

Drugs for Immune System Modulation

25

CORE CONCEPTS

25.1 The human body has both innate and adaptive body defenses.

25.2 The immune response results from activation of the humoral and cell-mediated immune systems.

25.3 Vaccines are biologic agents used to prevent illness.

25.4 Biologic response modifiers are used to boost the immune response.

25.5 Immunosuppressants are used to prevent transplant rejection and to treat autoimmune disorders.

DRUG SNAPSHOT

The following drugs are discussed in this chapter:

DRUG CLASSES	DRUG PROTOTYPES
Vaccines	**Pr** hepatitis B vaccine (Energix-B, Recombivax HB) *378*
Biologic response modifiers	**Pr** interferon alfa-2b (Intron a) *380*
Immunosuppressants	**Pr** cyclosporine (Gengraf, Neoral, Sandimmune) *382*

LEARNING OUTCOMES

After reading this chapter, the student should be able to:

1. Compare and contrast innate and adaptive body defenses.

2. Compare and contrast the humoral and cell-mediated immune responses.

3. For each of the major vaccines, give the recommended dosage schedule.

4. Identify indications for pharmacotherapy with biologic response modifiers.

5. Explain the need for immunosuppressant medications following organ and tissue transplants.

6. Categorize drugs used for immunomodulation based on

their classifications and mechanisms of action.

7. For each of the classes in the Drug Snapshot, identify representative drugs and explain their mechanisms of drug action, primary actions, and important adverse effects.

KEY TERMS

active immunity *376*
adaptive body defenses *375*
antibodies (ANN-tee-BOD-ee) *375*
antigen (ANN-tih-jen) *374*
B cell *375*
biologic response modifiers *379*
boosters *376*
cytokines (SYE-toh-kines) *375*
cytotoxic T cells *375*
helper T cells *375*

humoral immunity (HYOU-mor-ul eh-MEWN-uh-tee) *375*
immune response *375*
immunoglobulins (Ig) (ih-MEW-noh-GLOB-you-lin) *375*
immunomodulators (ih-mew-no-MOF-you-layter) *374*
immunosuppressants (ih-MEW-noh-suh-PRESS-ent) *380*
innate body defenses *374*

passive immunity *376*
plasma cells *375*
T cells *375*
titer (TIE-ter) *376*
toxoid vaccine (TOX-oid vaks-EEN) *376*
transplant rejection *380*
vaccination (immunization) (VAK-sin-AYE-shun/IH-mewn-ize-AYE-shun) *376*
vaccines (vaks-EEN) *374*

O ur bodies come under continuous attack from a host of foreign invaders that include viruses, bacteria, fungi, and even multicellular organisms. In defending the body, our immune system is capable of mounting a rapid and effective response against many of these pathogens.

Immunomodulator is a general term referring to any drug that affects body defenses. In some patients, immunomodulators are used to *stimulate* body defenses so that microbes or cancer cells can be more effectively attacked. For example, **vaccines** (substances given to stimulate the body's defense so that disease can be prevented or controlled) are given at various times throughout the lifespan to prevent major illnesses. On other occasions, it is desirable to *suppress* body defenses to prevent a transplanted organ from being rejected by the immune system. The purpose of this chapter is to examine the pharmacotherapy of drugs that are used to modulate the body's immune response to disease.

CORE CONCEPT 25.1 The human body has both innate and adaptive body defenses.

anti = *against*
gen = *formation*

A foreign substance that is detected by body defenses and elicits a response is called an **antigen**. Proteins such as those present on the surfaces of pollen grains, bacteria, and viruses are the strongest antigens. When normal cells become damaged, injured, or cancerous, they too can be viewed as antigens by body defenses. The human body has an elaborate set of body defenses that is able to respond to virtually any antigen it may encounter. Dozens of different cells and processes are used to battle disease and internal threats such as cancer cells. These disease-fighting cells and processes are classified into two groups: innate defenses or adaptive defenses.

The first line of protection from pathogens consists of the **innate body defenses**, which serve as general barriers to microbes or environmental hazards. The innate defenses are called nonspecific because they are unable to distinguish one type of threat from another; the response or protection is the same regardless of the pathogen. These defenses include physical barriers, such as the skin and the lining of the respiratory and gastrointestinal tracts, which are potential entry points for pathogens. Other innate defenses are phagocytes, natural killer (NK) cells, the complement system, fever, and interferons. The purposes of the innate body defenses are to neutralize or destroy the antigen and to alert other components of body defenses that a threat has arrived. From a pharmacologic perspective, one of the most important of the innate defenses is inflammation, which was presented in Chapter 24, along with fever, another type of innate body defense.

Fast Facts Vaccines and Immune Disorders

- Vaccines lowered the number of measles cases in the United States from more than 503,000 in 1962 to only 100–130 cases annually. Most cases of measles in the United States are due to importation from other countries.

- About one-third of the girls in the United States receive the three-dose recommended vaccine for human papillomavirus (HPV).

- Severe combined immunodeficiency (SCID) is a very rare disorder, occurring in less than 1,100 births annually in the United States.

- Over 23 million Americans suffer from autoimmune disorders, and the frequency is rising.

- The most common organ transplant is kidney, with over 30,000 people annually waiting for a transplant.

FIGURE 25.1

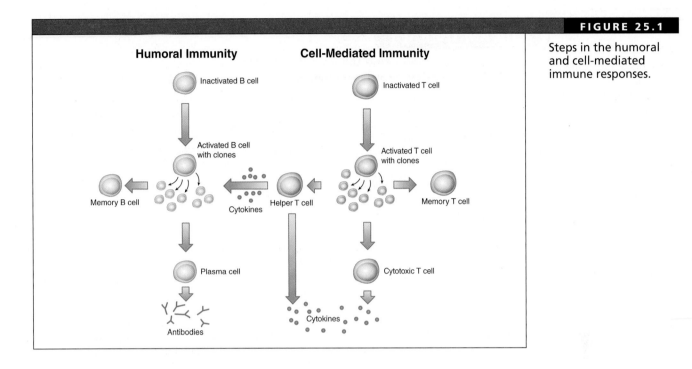

Steps in the humoral and cell-mediated immune responses.

The body also has the ability to mount a *second* line of defense known as **adaptive body defenses**, which are specific to particular threats. For example, a specific defense may act against only a single species of bacteria and be ineffective against all others. Adaptive body defenses are commonly called the **immune response**. The primary cells that accomplish most of the functions of the immune response are the *lymphocytes*. The two primary divisions of the immune response are antibody-mediated (humoral) immunity and cell-mediated immunity. These are illustrated in Figure 25.1 ■.

The immune response results from activation of the humoral and cell-mediated immune systems.

CORE CONCEPT 25.2

Humoral immunity is initiated when an antigen encounters a type of lymphocyte known as a **B cell**. The antigen activates the B cell, which then divides rapidly to form many copies, or clones, of itself. Most cells in this clone are called **plasma cells**. The primary function of the plasma cells is to secrete **antibodies**, also called **immunoglobulins (Ig)**, which are specific to the antigen that initiated the immune response. As they circulate through the body, antibodies physically interact with the antigens to neutralize or target them for destruction by other cells of the immune response. Peak production of antibodies occurs about 10 days after an immune response.

After the antigen challenge, *memory B cells* are formed that will remember the specific antigen–antibody interaction. Should the body be exposed to the same antigen in the future, the body will be able to manufacture even higher levels of antibodies in a shorter period, approximately two to three days. For some antigens, such as those for measles, mumps, or chickenpox, memory can be retained for an entire lifetime. Vaccines, discussed later in this chapter, are sometimes administered to produce these memory cells in advance of exposure to the antigen, so that when the body is exposed to the real organism it can mount a fast, effective response.

The second branch of the immune response involves lymphocytes called **T cells**. When they encounter their specific antigen, T cells become activated and rapidly form clones. Unlike B cells, however, T cells do not produce antibodies. Instead, T cells produce huge amounts of **cytokines**, which are chemicals that regulate important aspects of the immune response. Some cytokines kill foreign organisms directly, whereas others act as messengers to the immune system, stimulating T cells, B cells, and other body defenses to rid the body of the foreign agent. Specific cytokines released by activated T cells include several interleukins, interferon, colony stimulating factor, and tumor necrosis factor (TNF). Some of these cytokines have been used to treat certain immune disorders and cancers. This class of medications, called *biologic response modifiers*, is discussed later in this chapter. Drugs that *block* cytokine release are used in the pharmacotherapy of cancer and rheumatoid arthritis.

The two major types of T cells are **helper T cells** and **cytotoxic T cells**. These cells are often named after a protein receptor on their plasma membrane; the helper T cells have a CD4 receptor, and the cytotoxic T cells have a CD8 receptor. Helper T cells are particularly important because they are responsible

cyto = *cell*
kine(sis) = *movement*

> ### CAM THERAPY
>
> **Echinacea for Boosting the Immune System**
>
> *Echinacea purpurea*, or purple coneflower, is one of the most popular medicinal botanicals. This plant is native to the midwestern United States and central Canada; its flowers, leaves, and stems are harvested and dried. Preparations include dried powder, tinctures, fluid extracts, and teas. No single ingredient seems to be responsible for the herb's activity; many active chemicals have been identified from the extracts.
>
> Echinacea was used by Native Americans to treat various wounds and injuries. Echinacea is claimed to boost the immune system by increasing phagocytosis and inhibiting bacterial enzymes. Some substances in echinacea appear to have antiviral activity; the herb is sometimes taken to prevent and treat the common cold and influenza, an indication for which it has received official approval in Germany. In general, it is used as a supportive treatment for any disease involving inflammation and to enhance the immune system.

for activating most other immune cells, including B cells. Cytotoxic T cells travel throughout the body, secreting cytokines that directly kill bacteria, parasites, virus-infected cells, and cancer cells.

Like B cells, some of the activated T cells become memory cells. If the person encounters the same antigen in the future, the memory T cells will assist in mounting a more rapid immune response.

IMMUNOSTIMULANTS

Drugs that enhance the immune response are called *immunostimulants*. These types of immunomodulators include vaccines and biologic response modifiers such as interferons and interleukins.

CORE CONCEPT 25.3

Vaccines are biological agents used to prevent illness.

Vaccination (immunization) is the process of introducing a foreign substance (a vaccine) into the body to trigger immune activation *before* the patient is exposed to the real pathogen. As a result of the vaccination, memory B cells are formed. When later exposed to the actual infectious organism, these cells will react quickly by producing large quantities of antibodies that will help to neutralize or destroy the pathogen. Some immunizations require follow-up doses, called **boosters**, to provide sustained protection. The effectiveness of most vaccines can be assessed by measuring the amount of antibody produced after the vaccine has been administered, a quantity called **titer**. If the titer falls below a specified protective level over time, a booster is indicated.

The goal of vaccine administration is to induce long-lasting immunity to a pathogen *without* producing an illness in an otherwise healthy person. Therefore, the microorganisms and other substances used as vaccines must be able to strongly trigger the immune response but be modified to pose no significant risk of disease development. The four methods of producing safe and effective vaccines include the following:

- Attenuated (live) vaccines contain microbes that are alive but weakened so they are unable to produce disease. Some attenuated vaccines cause mild symptoms of the disease. An example of a live attenuated vaccine is the measles, mumps, and rubella (MMR) vaccine.

- Inactivated (killed) vaccines contain microbes that have been inactivated by heat or chemicals and are unable to replicate or cause disease. Examples of inactivated vaccines include the influenza and hepatitis A vaccines.

- **Toxoid vaccines** contain bacterial toxins that have been chemically modified to be incapable of causing disease. When injected, toxoid vaccines induce the formation of antibodies that are capable of neutralizing the real toxins. Examples include diphtheria and tetanus toxoids.

- Recombinant technology vaccines are those that contain partial organisms or bacterial proteins that are generated in the laboratory using biotechnology. The best example of this type is the hepatitis B vaccine.

The widespread use of vaccines has prevented illness in millions of patients, particularly children. One disease—smallpox—has been virtually eliminated from the planet through immunization, and others, such as polio, have diminished to extremely low levels. Table 25.1 ◆ identifies some common vaccines and their recommended schedules.

Common side effects of vaccine administration include redness and discomfort at the site of injection, minor aches, and fever. Although severe reactions are rare, anaphylaxis is possible. In the vast majority of cases, the benefits of disease prevention far outweigh the small risk of adverse effects from the vaccine. Vaccinations are contraindicated for patients who have a weakened immune system or who are currently experiencing symptoms such as diarrhea, vomiting, or fever. Most vaccines are pregnancy category C, so vaccinations are often delayed in pregnant patients until after delivery to avoid any potential harm to the fetus.

There are two types of immunity that can be obtained through the administration of pharmacologic agents, as illustrated in Figure 25.2 ■. The type of response induced by the real pathogen, or its vaccine, is called **active immunity**: The body produces its own antibodies in response to exposure. The active immunity induced by vaccines closely resembles that caused by natural exposure to the antigen, including the generation of memory cells.

Passive immunity occurs when preformed antibodies are transferred or "donated" from one person to another. Drugs for passive immunity are usually administered when the patient has already been exposed to a pathogen or is at very high risk to exposure, and there is not sufficient time to develop active immunity. Patients with weakened immune systems may receive these antibodies to *prevent* infections. Types of drugs used to provide passive immunity include:

- Gamma globulin infused to counteract recent exposure to hepatitis or chickenpox
- Antivenoms administered to treat snake bites
- Sera used to treat botulism, tetanus, and rabies

Because these medications do not stimulate the patient's immune system, their protective effects will disappear within several weeks to several months after the infusions are discontinued.

TABLE 25.1   Selected Vaccines and Their Schedules

Vaccine	Schedule and Age
Adacel and Boostrix (combination of tetanus toxoid and DTaP)	IM; single dose as an active booster after age 10 (Boostrix) or between ages 11 and 64 (Adacel)
Comvax (combination of haemophilus and hepatitis B vaccines)	IM; 3 doses at 2, 4, and 2–15 months of age
Diphtheria, tetanus, and pertussis (Daptacel, DTaP, Infanrix, Tripedia)	IM; Ages 2 months, 4 months, 6 months, 15–18 months, and 4–6 years
Haemophilus influenza type B conjugate (ActHIB, Hiberix, PedvaxHIB)	IM; Ages 2 months, 4 months, 6 months, and 12–15 months
Hepatitis A (Havrix, VAQTA)	Children: IM; Age 12 months, followed by a booster 6–12 months later; Adults: 1 mL followed by a booster 6 months to 12 months later
Pr Hepatitis B (Engerix-B, Recombivax HB)	Children/Adults: IM; three doses with the second dose 1 month after the first and the third dose 6 months after the first
Human papilloma virus (Cervarix, Gardasil)	Age 9–26 years: IM; with the second dose 2 months after the first and the third dose 6 months after the first
Influenza vaccine (Afluria, Fluarix, FluLaval, FluMist, Fluvirin, Fluzone): includes H1N1 influenza protection	Children: IM; two doses 1 month apart; then annual dose; Adults: IM; single annual dose or intranasal (FluMist)
Measles, mumps, and rubella (MMR II)	Subcutaneous; Single dose at ages 12–15 months; second dose at ages 4–6 years
Meningococcal conjugate vaccine (Menactra, Menomune, Menveo)	IM; First dose at age 11–12 years and second dose at age 16 years
Pneumococcal, polyvalent (Pneumovax 23), or 7-valent (Prevnar)	Adults (Pneumovax 23 or Pnu-Immune 23): subcutaneous or IM; single dose; Children (Prevnar): IM; four doses at ages 2 months, 4 months, 6 months, and 12–15 months
Poliovirus, inactivated (IPOL, poliovax)	Children: subcutaneous; at ages 2 months, 4 months, 6–18 months, and 4–6 years
Proquad (combination of MMR and varicella vaccines)	Subcutaneous; First dose at ages 12–15 months, second dose at ages 4–6 years
Rotavirus (Rotarix, RotaTeq)	PO; three doses at ages 2 months, 4 months, and 6 months (Rotarix does not require a dose at 6 months)
Tetanus toxoid	IM; (primary immunization, age 7 or older): three doses; the second dose is given 4–8 weeks after the first dose; the third dose is given 6–12 months after the second dose
Twinrix (combination of hepatitis A and hepatitis B vaccines)	Over age 18: three doses, with the second dose 1 month after the first, and the third dose 6 months after the first
Varicella (Varivax, Zostavax)	Subcutaneous (Varivax); at ages 12–15 months and 4–6 years, Subcutaneous (Zostavax); single dose at age 50 or older

FIGURE 25.2

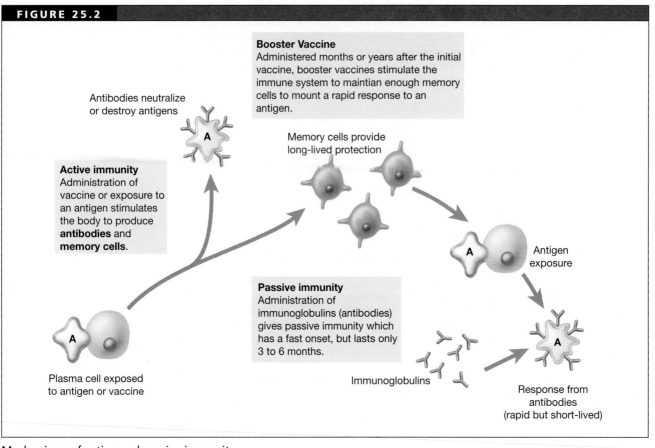

Booster Vaccine
Administered months or years after the initial vaccine, booster vaccines stimulate the immune system to maintian enough memory cells to mount a rapid response to an antigen.

Antibodies neutralize or destroy antigens

Memory cells provide long-lived protection

Active immunity
Administration of vaccine or exposure to an antigen stimulates the body to produce **antibodies** and **memory cells**.

Antigen exposure

Passive immunity
Administration of immunoglobulins (antibodies) gives passive immunity which has a fast onset, but lasts only 3 to 6 months.

Plasma cell exposed to antigen or vaccine

Immunoglobulins

Response from antibodies (rapid but short-lived)

Mechanisms of active and passive immunity.

Drug Prototype: ℗ *Hepatitis B Vaccine (Energix-B, Recombivax HB)*
Therapeutic class: Vaccine   Pharmacologic class: Vaccine

Actions and Uses: Hepatitis B vaccine is administered IM to provide prophylaxis against exposure to the hepatitis B virus (HBV). Following injection, the body produces antibodies against the virus. It is indicated for infants born to HBV-positive mothers, and those at high risk for exposure to HBV-infected blood, including nurses, physicians, dentists, dental hygienists, morticians, and paramedics. Because HBV infection is extremely difficult to treat, it is prudent for all healthcare workers to receive HBV vaccine before beginning their clinical education, unless contraindicated. The vaccine is also indicated for all persons who engage in high-risk sexual practices, such as heterosexual activity with multiple partners, prostitution, or homosexual or bisexual practices, or for persons who repeatedly contract sexually transmitted infections. The regimen involves three doses of the vaccine, usually followed by a titer to confirm that active immunity has been achieved.

Hepatitis B vaccine is sometimes given to patients *after* they have been exposed to the virus. In this case, it is often combined with hepatitis B immune globulin (HBIG), which will provide passive immunity while the body is building its own antibodies to the virus. Once a hepatitis B infection is acquired, it is difficult to eliminate; therefore, prevention is the best treatment.

Adverse Effects and Interactions: The adverse effects of hepatitis B vaccine are similar to those of other vaccines. Pain and inflammation may appear at the injection site. A fever may develop, and the patient may feel tired and lethargic. Although anaphylaxis is rare, epinephrine should be kept available. The vaccine should be given to pregnant or lactating women only if clearly needed to protect the health of the mother or child.

Biologic response modifiers are used to boost the immune response.

When challenged by antigens, certain cells in the immune system secrete cytokines that help fight the invading organism. Several of these natural chemicals are now available as medications. Drugs in this class, the **biologic response modifiers**, are administered to boost certain functions of the immune system and are shown in Table 25.2 ◆.

Interferons (IFNs) are cytokines secreted by lymphocytes and macrophages that have been infected with a virus. IFNs slow the spread of viral infections and enhance the activity of existing leukocytes. In addition to antiviral properties, these drugs exhibit anticancer and anti-inflammatory actions. Alpha IFNs have the widest therapeutic application (when used as medications, the spelling is changed to *alfa*). Indications for IFN alpha therapy include cancers, such as hairy cell leukemia and AIDS-related Kaposi's sarcoma, and chronic hepatitis virus B or C infections. Interferon alfa-2b (Intron A) is one of the most common IFNs used in therapy and is featured as a prototype drug. IFN beta is primarily used for treatment of severe multiple sclerosis (see Chapter 12). Patients receiving IFN therapy must be closely monitored because drugs in this class can cause serious adverse effects including depression, suicidal ideation, psychosis, cardiovascular disease (including myocardial infarction), pulmonary impairment, hepatic or renal failure, and a number of other life-threatening disorders.

Interleukins are another class of cytokines secreted by lymphocytes, monocytes, and macrophages. Although 30 different interleukins have been identified, only a few are available as medications. The interleukins have widespread effects on immune function, and all of them boost the activity of natural defense mechanisms. Interleukin-2 is available as aldesleukin (Proleukin), which is approved for the treatment of metastatic renal carcinoma. Interleukin-11, which is derived from bone marrow cells, is a growth factor with multiple hematopoietic effects. It is marketed as oprelvekin (Neumega) for its ability to stimulate platelet production in patients with weakened immune systems.

In addition to IFNs and interleukins, a few additional biologic response modifiers are available to enhance the immune system. Bacillus Calmette–Guérin (BCG) vaccine (Tice, TheraCys) is an attenuated strain of *Mycobacterium bovis* used for the pharmacotherapy of certain types of bladder cancer. Colony-stimulating factors such as filgrastim (Neupogen) and sargramostim (Leukine) promote the production of white blood cells (WBCs). These drugs are used to shorten the length of neutropenia (reduced leukocyte count) in patients with cancer and in those who have had a bone marrow transplant.

TABLE 25.2	Selected Biologic Response Modifiers	
Drug	**Route and Adult Dose**	**Remarks**
aldesleukin (Proleukin): interleukin-2	IV; 600,000 units/kg (0.037 mg/kg) every 8 hours by a 15-minute IV infusion for a total of 14 doses	For metastatic renal cell carcinoma and metastatic melanoma
Bacillus Calmette–Guérin (BCG) vaccine (Tice, TheraCys)	Intradermal (Tice); 0.1 mL as vaccine Intravesical (TheraCys); bladder instillation	For bladder cancer
INTERFERONS		
interferon alfa-2b (Intron-A)	IM/subcutaneous; highly variable depending upon indication	For hairy cell leukemia, malignant melanoma, follicular lymphoma, condylomata acuminata, Kaposi's sarcoma, chronic hepatitis B, and chronic hepatitis C
interferon alfacon-1 (Infergen)	Subcutaneous; 9 mcg three times per week	For chronic hepatitis C (usually in combination with ribavirin)
interferon alfa-n3 (Alferon N)	Intralesion: 0.05 mL (250,000 international units) per wart twice per week for up to 8 weeks	For treatment of genital warts
interferon beta-1a (Avonex, Rebif)	IM (Avonex); 30 mcg/wk Subcutaneous (Rebif; 44 mcg three times per week	For multiple sclerosis
interferon beta-1b (Betaseron, Extavia)	Subcutaneous; 0.25 mg (8 million units) every other day	For multiple sclerosis
peginterferon alfa-2a (Pegasys)	Subcutaneous; 180 mcg/wk for 48 weeks	For chronic hepatitis B and chronic hepatitis C

Drug Prototype: 🅟 *Interferon alfa-2b (Intron-A)*

Therapeutic Class: Immunostimulant **Pharmacologic Class: Interferon, biologic response modifier**

Actions and Uses: Interferon alfa-2b is a biologic response modifier that is prepared by recombinant DNA technology and is approved to treat cancers (hairy cell leukemia, melanoma, non-Hodgkin's lymphoma, AIDS-related Kaposi's sarcoma), as well as viral infections (HPV, chronic hepatitis virus B and C). It is available for IV, IM, and subcutaneous administration.

Rebetron is a combination drug containing interferon alfa-2b and ribavirin, an antiviral agent. Rebetron is indicated for pharmacotherapy of hepatitis C infection. Peginterferon alfa-2b (PegIntron) has a molecule of polyethylene glycol (PEG) attached to the IFN molecule, which gives the drug an extended half-life. Peginterferon alfa-2b is approved to treat chronic hepatitis C virus infections.

Adverse Effects and Interactions: A flu-like syndrome of fever, chills, dizziness, and fatigue occurs in 50% of patients, although this usually diminishes as therapy progresses. Headache, nausea, vomiting, diarrhea, and anorexia are relatively common. Depression and suicidal ideation have been reported and may be severe enough to require discontinuation of the drug. With prolonged therapy, immunosuppression, and serious toxicity such as hepatotoxicity and neurotoxicity may be observed.

Use with ethanol may cause excessive drowsiness and dehydration. Zidovudine may increase hematologic toxicity.

> **BLACK BOX WARNING:**
> IFNs may cause or aggravate fatal or life-threatening neuropsychiatric, autoimmune ischemic, or infectious disorders. Therapy should be discontinued in patients with persistently severe or worsening signs or symptoms of these conditions.

CORE CONCEPT 25.5

Immunosuppressants are used to prevent transplant rejection and to treat autoimmune disorders.

The immune system is normally viewed as a lifesaver that protects us from pathogens in the environment. For those receiving organ or tissue transplants, however, the immune system is the enemy. Despite careful tissue matching and typing, donated organs and tissues always contain some antigens that trigger the recipient's immune response. This response, called **transplant rejection**, is sometimes acute, with antibodies rushing to destroy the transplanted tissue within a few days. The cell-mediated immune system reacts more slowly to the transplant, attacking it about two weeks following surgery. Even if the organ survives these challenges, chronic rejection of the transplant may occur months or even years after surgery.

Immunosuppressants are medications given to lessen the immune response. One or more of these drugs are administered at the time of transplantation and continued for several months following surgery. In some cases, they are continued indefinitely at low doses. Transplantation would be impossible without the use of effective immunosuppressant drugs.

In addition, these drugs may be prescribed to treat the symptoms of autoimmune disorders, conditions in which the body creates antibodies against its own cells. Over a hundred different disorders have been found to have some degree of autoimmune involvement. Examples of common autoimmune disease include diabetes mellitus (Type I), psoriasis, rheumatoid arthritis, systemic lupus erythematosus (SLE), myasthenia gravis, and Hashimoto's thyroiditis. Although these disorders affect different organs, most have in common a hypersensitive immune system that causes symptoms of acute inflammation. When the disease becomes acute, immunosuppressant pharmacotherapy may be initiated. Unlike transplant recipients who may receive immunosuppressants indefinitely, patients with acute inflammation from an autoimmune disorder usually are given these drugs only for brief periods to control relapses.

Although the various immunosuppressant drugs act by different mechanisms, all suppress some aspect of lymphocyte function. Some act nonselectively by inhibiting all aspects of the immune system. Other, newer drugs suppress only a limited aspect of the immune response. The nonselective agents provide more widespread immunosuppression but carry a greater risk of adverse effects.

Nearly all the immunosuppressants are toxic to bone marrow. Because the immune system is suppressed, infections are common and the patient must be protected from situations in which exposure to pathogens is likely. Long-term survivors of transplants are also at increased risk of developing cancers, especially lymphoma, skin cancer, cervical cancer, and Kaposi's sarcoma. Doses for these drugs are listed in Table 25.3 ◆.

TABLE 25.3   Selected Immunosuppressants

Drug	Route and Adult Dose	Remarks
anakinra (Kineret)	Subcutaneous; 100 mg once daily	For rheumatoid arthritis that has not responded to safer drugs
azathioprine (Azasan, Imuran)	PO/IV; 3–5 mg/kg daily	Inhibits DNA, RNA, and protein synthesis; also for severe rheumatoid arthritis
basiliximab (Simulect)	IV; 20 mg times two doses (first dose 2 hours before surgery; second dose 4 days after transplant)	Antibody against the CD25 receptor on T cells; approved for use in patients with kidney transplant
belatacept (Nulojix)	IV; 5–10 mg/kg	For prophylaxis of rejection following a kidney transplant
(Pr) cyclosporine (Gengraf, Neoral, Sandimmune)	PO; initial dose 14–18 mg/kg just prior to surgery; after 2 weeks, then 5–10 mg/kg/day	IV form available; inhibits T cells; also for rheumatoid arthritis, severe psoriasis, and other severe inflammatory disorders
lymphocyte immune globulin or antithymocyte globulin (Atgam)	IV; 10–30 mg/kg daily for 1–2 weeks	Polyclonal antibodies that reduce T cell numbers; for prevention of renal transplant rejection
methotrexate (Rheumatrex, Trexall) (see page 440 for the Drug Prototype box)	PO; 15–30 mg/day for 5 days; repeat every 12 weeks for three courses	IV, IM, and intrathecal forms available; blocks metabolism of folic acid; also for neoplasia, severe psoriasis, and severe rheumatoid arthritis
muromonab-CD3 (Orthoclone OKT 3)	IV; 5 mg/day administered for 10–14 days	Antibodies against the CD3 receptor on T cells; often a treatment of choice to prevent renal transplant rejection
mycophenolate (CellCept, Myfortic)	PO/IV; 720 mg bid	IV form available; inhibits B cells, T cells, and antibody formation; for prevention of kidney, liver or heart transplant rejection
sirolimus (Rapamune)	PO; 6 mg loading dose, then 2 mg/day	Suppresses antibody production; for prevention of renal transplant rejection
tacrolimus (Prograf)	PO; 0.15–0.3 mg/kg/day in two divided doses every 12 hours	IV form available; inhibits T cells; for prevention of kidney, liver, or heart transplant rejection; ointment is approved to treat atopic dermatitis

Drug classes that have immunosuppressant activity include corticosteroids (glucocorticoids), antimetabolites, antibodies, and calcineurin inhibitors. The corticosteroids are potent inhibitors of inflammation and are often drugs of choice in the short-term therapy of severe inflammation (see Chapter 24). Antimetabolites such as sirolimus (Rapamune) and azathioprine (Imuran) inhibit aspects of lymphocyte replication. By binding to the intracellular messenger calcineurin, cyclosporine (Gengraf, Sandimmune, Neoral), and tacrolimus (Prograf) disrupt T-cell function. The calcineurin inhibitors are of value in treating psoriasis, an inflammatory disorder of the skin (see Chapter 36).

The final group of immunosuppressants, and the most recently developed, are monoclonal antibodies. Monoclonal antibodies have been designed that attack very specific targets, usually receptors on T cells. For example, muromonab-CD3 (Orthoclone OKT3) blocks the function of the CD3 receptor, which is present on T cells that attack transplanted tissue. Muromonab-CD3 is administered to prevent rejection of kidney, heart, and liver transplants, and to deplete the bone marrow of T cells prior to marrow transplant. Basiliximab (Simulect), belatacept (Nulojix), and daclizumab (Zenapax) are given to prevent acute rejection of kidney transplants. Infliximab (Remicade) is used to suppress the severe inflammation that often accompanies autoimmune disorders such as Crohn's disease and rheumatoid arthritis. Belimumab (Benlysta) reduces abnormal B cells that are a problem in people with severe SLE. Because many drugs in this monoclonal antibody class are used as antineoplastics, the student should refer to Chapter 28 for additional information.

Concept Review   25.1

- Why are oral glucocorticoids usually used concurrently with immunosuppressant drugs following a transplant operation?

Drug Prototype: 🅟 *Cyclosporine (Gengraf, Neoral, Sandimmune)*

Therapeutic Class: Immunosuppressant **Pharmacologic Class: Calcineurin inhibitor**

Actions and Uses: Cyclosporine is a complex chemical obtained from a soil fungus that inhibits helper T cells. It is approved for the prophylaxis of kidney, heart, and liver transplant rejection, psoriasis, and xerophthalmia, an eye condition of diminished tear production caused by ocular inflammation. Cyclosporine is normally administered by the oral route but an IV form is available for severe cases of ulcerative colitis or Crohn's disease. When prescribed for transplant recipients, it is usually administered in combination with high doses of corticosteroids such as prednisone.

Adverse Effects and Interactions: The primary adverse effect of cyclosporine occurs in the kidney, with up to 75% of patients experiencing reduction in urine output. Frequent laboratory tests of kidney function, such as BUN and creatinine, are necessary. Other common adverse effects are tremor, hypertension, and elevated hepatic enzyme values. Although opportunistic infections are common during cyclosporine therapy, they are fewer than with other immunosuppressants. Periodic blood counts are necessary to be certain that WBCs do not fall below 4,000 or platelets below 75,000.

Because cyclosporine is extensively metabolized in the liver, many drug interactions are possible. The following drugs increase the metabolism of cyclosporine, making the drug *less effective:* phenytoin, carbamazepine, TMP–SMZ, and phenobarbital. The following drugs decrease the metabolism of cyclosporine, causing the drug to build high concentrations and become *potentially toxic:* macrolide antibiotics, azole antifungals, and amphotericin B. Because cyclosporine can damage the kidneys, other nephrotoxic drugs such as amphotericin B, NSAIDs, or aminoglycosides should be administered with great caution.

> **BLACK BOX WARNING:**
> Therapy with cyclosporine may result in serious infections and increases the risk of malignancies.

NURSING PROCESS FOCUS   Patients Receiving Immunosuppressants

ASSESSMENT	POTENTIAL NURSING DIAGNOSES
Prior to administration: ■ Obtain a complete health history, including cardiovascular, neurological, immune, oral, renal and liver conditions, allergies, drug history, and possible drug interactions. ■ Evaluate laboratory blood findings: CBC, electrolytes, lipid panel, and renal and liver function studies. ■ Attain history or current cases of cancer, fever, or active infections (such as herpes and HIV). ■ Acquire the results of a complete physical examination, including vital signs, height, and weight.	■ *Risk for Infection* related to adverse effects of drug therapy ■ *Risk for Injury* related to adverse effects of drug therapy ■ *Risk for Impaired Mucous Membrane* related to adverse effects of drug therapy ■ *Deficient Knowledge* related to a lack of information about drug therapy

PLANNING: PATIENT GOALS AND EXPECTED OUTCOMES

The patient will:
■ Experience therapeutic effects (depending on the reason the drug is being given).
■ Be free from or experience minimal adverse effects from drug therapy.
■ Verbalize an understanding of the drug's use, adverse effects, and required precautions.

IMPLEMENTATION

Interventions and (Rationales)	Patient Education/Discharge Planning
■ Administer medications correctly and evaluate the patient's knowledge of proper administration. (Most immunosuppressants are administered either po and/or IV and require specific instructions.)	Inform the patient to: ■ Use enclosed equipment to mix the drug. ■ Use glass; not paper or plastic cups unless package directions indicate they are to be used. ■ Mix drug with milk, chocolate milk or orange juice, stirring well. Take additional liquid to ensure the drug is taken.
■ Monitor all vital signs and observe for signs and symptoms of infection such as fever, elevated pulse, respiration and BP, fatigue, cough, white patches on mucous membranes, vaginal discharge, itchy blister-like vesicles on skin. (Immunosuppressants increase the risk of infection, especially opportunistic infections such as herpes and yeast infections.)	Advise the patient: ■ To immediately report any signs and symptoms of infection such as wounds with redness or drainage, increasing cough, fatigue, and fever to the healthcare provider. ■ To use proper hand washing techniques. ■ To avoid large crowds and people with known infections or young children who have higher risk of infection. ■ To cook food thoroughly, allowing others to prepare raw foods and clean up afterward.
■ Monitor changes in level of consciousness, disorientation/confusion or tremors. (Neurological changes may indicate adverse effects of drug therapy.)	■ Instruct the patient to report increasing lethargy, disorientation, confusion, changes in behavior or mood, slurred speech, or tremors to the healthcare provider.

NURSING PROCESS FOCUS *(continued)*

IMPLEMENTATION

■ Continue to monitor serum and urine laboratory tests, specifically noting: CBC, platelets, electrolytes, glucose, liver and renal studies, and lipid levels. (Depending on drug, immunosuppressants may cause leukopenia, anemia, thrombocytopenia, hyperglycemia, hyperkalemia, and renal failure.)	Instruct the patient: ■ That it is extremely important to keep scheduled laboratory and doctor appointments. ■ To carry a wallet identification or wear medical ID jewelry indicating immunosuppressant therapy.
■ Inspect oral mucous membrane and dental health. (Immunospressants increase the risk of oral candidiasis and gingivitis. Oral antifungal medications may be needed.)	Instruct the patient to: ■ Maintain excellent oral hygiene, inspecting the mouth daily. ■ Keep regular dental visits and consult with dentist about frequency.
■ Determine the patient's diet and consumption of grapefruit juice. (Grapefruit juice significantly increases cyclosporine levels and should be avoided while on immunosuppressant therapy.)	■ Advise the patient to avoid/eliminate grapefruit and grapefruit juice from diet while on drug.
■ Collect information about pregnancy status. (Pregnancy should be avoided for up to four months after discontinuing immunosuppressive therapy.)	■ Explain the effects of medications on pregnancy and breastfeeding and the need to delay pregnancy. ■ Discuss options for family planning; alternative contraception methods may be necessary.
■ Monitor for the development of hirsutism or alopecia. (Hirsutism is reversible when drug is discontinued. Alopecia indicates significant immunosuppression.)	■ Advise patient to notify healthcare provider of changes to hair growth or texture.

EVALUATION OF OUTCOME CRITERIA

Evaluate the effectiveness of drug therapy by confirming that patient goals and expected outcomes have been met (see "Planning"). *See Table 25.3 for a list of drugs to which these nursing actions apply.*

PATIENTS NEED TO KNOW

Patients treated for inflammatory or immune disorders need to know the following:

Regarding Vaccines

1. Maintain an accurate, written record of vaccinations, including the date of the vaccination, route and site of vaccination, type of vaccine (including manufacturer and lot number), and the address of the physician's office where the vaccination occurred.
2. Keep immunizations up to date to prevent illness. Because recommendations can change, seek current information from a healthcare provider periodically.
3. Vaccines may contain a number of additives, including antibiotics, formaldehyde, thimersol, and monosodium glutamate. If an allergy is known or suspected to any of these additives, notify a healthcare provider before getting a vaccination.

Regarding Biologic Response Modifiers

4. Regular laboratory testing is extremely important, especially monitoring complete blood count (CBC).
5. Immediately report neurological symptoms (depression, suicidal ideations) and cardiovascular effects to healthcare provider.

Regarding Immunosuppressants

6. Never take cyclosporine with grapefruit juice; blood levels of the drug are increased by this combination.
7. Reduce risk of illness by avoiding crowds, avoiding those with colds/infections, and washing hands frequently.
8. Keep scheduled laboratory and doctor appointments. Regular laboratory testing is extremely important, especially monitoring CBC, electrolytes, hormone levels, and urine studies.
9. Immediately report an elevation in temperature, sore throat, mouth ulcers, and fatigue to the healthcare provider.

CHAPTER REVIEW

CORE CONCEPTS SUMMARY

25.1 The human body has both innate and adaptive body defenses.

Innate body defenses are nonspecific, general barriers to disease, such as the skin, inflammation, and phagocytes. Adaptive body defenses, known as the immune response, involve lymphocytes and are specific to the particular threats.

25.2 The immune response results from activation of the humoral and cell-mediated immune systems.

B cells become plasma cells and secrete large quantities of antibodies. The antibodies are specific to the antigen and neutralize the foreign agent or destroy it. Some B cells remember the antigen for many years. T cells also recognize specific antigens, but instead of producing antibodies, they produce cytokines, some of which rid the body of the foreign agent. Memory B and T cells remember the antigen for many years and mount a faster immune response on subsequent exposures.

25.3 Vaccines are biologic agents used to prevent illness.

Vaccines are usually given to prevent a serious infectious disease. Vaccines may be live, attenuated, or toxoids. They are effective when taken according to schedule and rarely produce serious adverse effects.

25.4 Biologic response modifiers are used to boost the immune response.

Several drugs are available to boost a patient's immune function. Interleukins, interferons, and other agents enhance the body's natural defenses, primarily in the pharmacotherapy of cancer.

25.5 Immunosuppressants are used to prevent transplant rejection and to treat autoimmune disorders.

For an organ or tissue transplant to be successful, the patient's immune system must be suppressed following surgery. Immunosuppressants are effective in lessening the immune response but must be monitored carefully because loss of immune function can lead to infections and cancer.

REVIEW QUESTIONS

The following questions are written in NCLEX-PN® style. Answer these questions to assess your knowledge of the chapter material, and go back and review any material that is not clear to you.

1. The nurse is evaluating drug effects in a patient who has been given interferon alfa-2b (Intron A) for MS. Which of the following are common adverse effects? (Select all that apply.)

1. Thoughts of suicide
2. Hepatotoxicity
3. Hypotension
4. Depression

2. The nurse would question an order for aldesleukin (Proleukin) if the patient had which of the following conditions? (Select all that apply.)

1. Liver disease
2. Metastatic lung cancer
3. Metastatic renal cancer
4. Metastatic melanoma

3. The physician has ordered oprelvekin (Neumega) for a patient who has just had chemotherapy. The patient asks the nurse why she needs this drug. The nurse responds:

1. "You are being given this drug to suppress your immune system because you are having a hypersensitivity reaction."
2. "You are being given this drug to help reduce any inflammation response you may develop."
3. "You are being given this drug because it acts as an antiviral, helping to reduce infection."
4. "You are being given this drug to stimulate platelet production."

4. While receiving filgrastim (Neupogen), the nurse should monitor for a(n):

1. Increase in the production of WBC
2. Increase in the production of platelets
3. Increase in the production of red blood cells (RBCs)
4. Decrease in the production of RBCs

5. A patient who is pregnant with her first child is at the clinic for a checkup and an infant care class. An informational pamphlet on immunizations has been provided and the nurse begins to review the information with the patient. She informs the patient that the DTaP vaccine should be given at ages:

1. 1 months, 4 months, 12 months, 15–18 months, and 4–6 years
2. 2 months, 6 months, 15–18 months, and 4–6 years
3. 2 months, 4 months, 6 months, 15–18 months, and 4–6 years
4. 2 months, 4 months, 6 months, and 15–18 months

6. A patient comes to the physician's office immediately after a suspected exposure to hepatitis B. He is to start the hepatitis B vaccine series and also receive the hepatitis B immune globulin (HBIG) vaccine injection. He tells the nurse that he understands how the hepatitis B vaccine series works but wants to know why he also needs to have the HBIG vaccine. The nurse responds the HIBG vaccine is given to:

1. Enhance the ability of the hepatitis B (Engerix-B) series of vaccines to provide permanent immunity.
2. Ensure that the hepatitis B (Engerix-B) series eliminates the virus.
3. Provide temporary immunity while the body is building its own antibodies to the virus.
4. Provide active immunity by causing the immune system to form antibodies.

7. The nurse evaluates the patient on immunosuppressants for:

1. Hypotension
2. Infection
3. Hypoglycemia
4. Bleeding

8. A patient is to receive tacrolimus (Prograf) 0.15 mg/kg/day to be given in two doses (every 12 hours). She weighs 100 pounds. How many milligrams will the patient receive per dose?

1. 6.82 mg
2. 6.60 mg
3. 3.30 mg
4. 3.41 mg

9. Which of the following statements by a patient taking cyclosporine (Neoral, Sandimmune) would indicate the need for more information?

1. "I will report any reduction in urine output to my health-care provider."
2. "I will wash my hands frequently."
3. "I will take my blood pressure at home every day."
4. "I will take my cyclosporine at breakfast with a glass of grapefruit juice."

10. The nurse should monitor a transplant patient for the primary adverse effect of cyclosporine (Neoral, Sandimmune) therapy by collecting information on which of the following laboratory tests?

1. CBC
2. BUN and creatinine
3. Liver enzymes
4. Electrolytes

CASE STUDY QUESTIONS

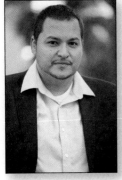

Remember Mr. Martel, the patient introduced at the beginning of the chapter? Now read the remainder of the case study. Based on the information you have learned in this chapter, answer the questions that follow.

Mr. Jose Martel, a 32-year-old night club manager, arrives at the office for his annual check-up. While being interviewed by the nurse, he tells her he had called the office in advance and made arrangements to begin the hepatitis B vaccine series. He states, "Since I work directly with so many people, I thought it might be a good idea." He has read about the vaccine from some online sites but still has some questions.

1. Mr. Martel asks the nurse how the hepatitis B vaccine works. The nurse responds that the vaccine stimulates the immune system to produce antibodies after exposure to components of the vaccine. This type of vaccine provides _____ immunity.

1. Passive
2. Attenuated
3. Live
4. Active

2. While providing information about the hepatitis B vaccine series, the nurse informs Mr. Martel that:

1. It is a series of three shots: the first one today, the second one a month from now, and the last shot six months after the first shot.
2. It is a series of two shots: the first one today and then the last one a month from now.
3. It is a series of three shots: the first one today, the second one a month from now, and the last shot six months after the second shot.
4. It is a series of four shots: the first one today, the second one a month from now, the third one six months after the first shot, and the last one a year after the first one.

3. The nurse and Mr. Martel are reviewing his health history. Which of the following information would cause the nurse to withhold the vaccine and check with the healthcare practitioner?

1. Mr. Martel smokes cigarettes, one-half pack a day.
2. Mr. Martel is frightened by needles and injections.
3. Mr. Martel is allergic to yeast and yeast products.
4. Mr. Martel drinks several glasses of wine on the weekends.

4. Just prior to administering the first injection of the series, the nurse tells Mr. Martel that he might expect which adverse effect(s) to occur? (Select all that apply.)

1. Pain or inflammation at the injection site
2. Nausea
3. Fatigue
4. Fever

NOTE: Answers to the Review and Case Study Questions appear in Appendix B. The complete rationales and answers are located on the textbook's website.

Pearson Nursing Student Resources Find additional review materials at **nursing.pearsonhighered.com.**

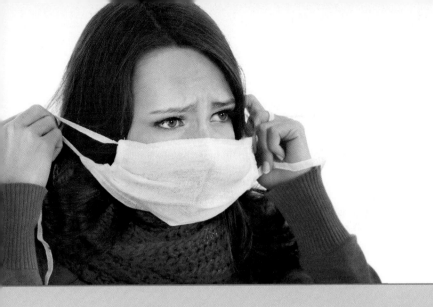

"I don't know what is going on. Ever since I had my kidney transplant, I've been experiencing repeated bacterial infections and now I have to wear this mask when I'm around people."

Ms. Shelly Jackson

Drugs for Bacterial Infections

26

CORE CONCEPTS

26.1 Pathogens are organisms that cause disease by invading tissues or secreting toxins.

26.2 Anti-infective drugs are classified by their chemical structures or by their mechanisms of action.

26.3 Anti-infective drugs act by selectively targeting a pathogen's metabolism or life cycle.

26.4 Acquired resistance is a major clinical problem that is worsened by improper use of anti-infectives.

26.5 Careful selection of the correct antibiotic is essential for effective pharmacotherapy and to limit adverse effects.

26.6 The penicillins are one of the oldest and safest groups of anti-infectives.

26.7 The cephalosporins are similar in structure and function to the penicillins and are one of the most widely prescribed anti-infective classes.

26.8 The tetracyclines have broad spectrums but are drugs of choice for few diseases.

26.9 The macrolides are safe alternatives to penicillin for many infections.

26.10 The aminoglycosides are narrow-spectrum drugs that have the potential to cause serious toxicity.

26.11 Fluoroquinolones have wide clinical applications because of their broad spectrum of activity and relative safety.

26.12 Sulfonamides and urinary antiseptics are traditional drugs for urinary tract infections.

26.13 A number of additional anti-infectives have distinct mechanisms of action and specific indications.

26.14 The pharmacotherapy of tuberculosis requires special dosing regimens and schedules.

DRUG SNAPSHOT

The following drugs are discussed in this chapter:

DRUG CLASSES	DRUG PROTOTYPES
Penicillins	**Pr** penicillin G Sodium/Potassium *395*
Cephalosporins	**Pr** cefotaxime (Claforan) *396*
Tetracyclines	**Pr** tetracycline (Sumycin, others) *397*
Macrolides	**Pr** erythromycin (E-Mycin, Erythrocin) *398*
Aminoglycosides	**Pr** gentamicin (Garamycin) *400*

DRUG CLASSES	DRUG PROTOTYPES
Fluoroquinolones	**Pr** ciprofloxacin (Cipro) *401*
Sulfonamides	**Pr** trimethoprim–sulfamethoxazole (Bactrim, Septra) *402*
Miscellaneous antibacterials	**Pr** vancomycin (Vancocin) *403*
Antitubercular drugs	**Pr** isoniazid (INH) *406*

LEARNING OUTCOMES

After reading this chapter, the student should be able to:

1. Distinguish between the terms *pathogenicity* and *virulence*.

2. Explain how bacteria are described and classified.

3. Compare and contrast the terms *bacteriostatic* and *bacteriocidal*.

4. Using an example, explain how resistance can develop to an anti-infective drug.

5. Explain the importance of culture and sensitivity testing to anti-infective chemotherapy.

6. Identify the mechanism of development and symptoms of superinfections caused by anti-infective therapy.

7. Explain how the pharmacotherapy of tuberculosis differs from that of other infections.

8. For each of the classes in the Drug Snapshot, identify representative drugs and explain their mechanisms of drug action, primary actions, and important adverse effects.

KEY TERMS

acquired resistance *392*
antagonism *393*
antibiotic (ann-tie-bye-OT-ik) *390*
anti-infective (ann-tie-in-FEK-tive) *390*
bacteriocidal (bak-teer-ee-oh-SY-dall) *391*
bacteriostatic (bak-teer-ee-oh-STAT-ik) *391*
beta-lactam ring (bay-tuh LAK-tam) *393*
beta-lactamase/penicillinase (bay-tuh-LAK-tam-ace/pen-uh-SILL-in-ace) *393*
broad-spectrum antibiotic *393*
chemoprophylaxis (kee-moh-pro-fill-AX-is) *392*

culture and sensitivity (C&S) testing *393*
directly observed therapy (DOT) *408*
host flora (host FLOR-uh) *393*
mutations (myou-TAY-shuns) *391*
narrow-spectrum antibiotic *393*
nephrotoxicity (NEF-row-toks-ISS-ih-tee) *400*
nosocomial infections (noh-soh-KOH-mee-ul) *392*
ototoxicity (OH-toh-toks-ISS-ih-tee) *400*
pathogen (PATH-oh-jen) *389*

pathogenicity (path-oh-jen-ISS-ih-tee) *389*
photosensitivity *398*
plasmids (PLAZ-midz) *392*
red-man syndrome *403*
superinfections *393*
toxins (TOX-in) *389*
tubercles (TOO-burr-kyouls) *406*
urinary antiseptics *403*
virulence (VEER-you-lens) *389*

The human body has adapted quite well to living in a world teeming with microorganisms (microbes). Present in the air, water, food, and soil, microbes are an essential component to life on the planet. In some cases, microorganisms, such as those in the colon, play a beneficial role in human health. When in an unnatural environment or when present in unusually high numbers, however, microorganisms can cause a variety of ailments ranging from mildly annoying to fatal. The development of the first anti-infective drugs in the mid-1900s was a milestone in the field of medicine. In the past 60 years, pharmacologists have attempted to keep pace with microbes that rapidly become resistant to therapeutic drugs. This chapter examines two groups of anti-infectives: the antibacterial drugs and the specialized medications used to treat tuberculosis (TB).

Fast Facts Bacterial Infections

- Infectious diseases are the third most common cause of death in the United States and the most common cause of death worldwide.

- Foodborne illness is responsible for 76 million illnesses, 300,000 hospitalizations, and 5,000 deaths each year. About 500 people die of food poisoning each year in the United States.

- Urinary tract infections (UTIs) are the most common infection acquired in hospitals. Nearly all are associated with the insertion of a urinary catheter. Hospital-acquired urinary infections add an average of 3.8 days to a hospital stay and can cost over $3,800 per infection.

- More than 2 million nosocomial infections are acquired each year. These infections add 1 day to a hospital stay for UTI, 7–8 days for surgical site infections, and 6–30 days for pneumonia.

- Up to 30% of all *Streptococcus pneumoniae* found in some areas of the United States are resistant to penicillin.

- Nearly all strains of *Staphylococcus aureus* in the United States are resistant to penicillin.

- About 73,000 cases of *Escherichia coli* (*E. coli*) poisoning are reported annually in the United States, with the most common source being ground beef.

Pathogens are organisms that cause disease by invading tissues or secreting toxins.

path = *disease*
gen = *producing*

An organism that can cause disease in humans is called a **pathogen**. Human pathogens include viruses, bacteria, fungi, unicellular organisms (protozoans), and multicellular animals. Examples of these pathogens are illustrated in Figure 26.1 ■. To infect humans, pathogens must bypass a number of elaborate body defenses, such as those described in Chapter 25. Pathogens may enter through broken skin, or by ingestion, inhalation, or contact with a mucous membrane such as the nasal, urinary, or vaginal mucosas.

Some pathogens are extremely infectious and life threatening to humans, whereas others simply cause annoying symptoms or none at all. The ability of an organism to cause infection is called its **pathogenicity**. Pathogenicity depends on an organism's ability to bypass or overcome the body's immune system. Fortunately for us, only a few dozen pathogens commonly cause disease in humans. Some of these are listed in Table 26.1 ◆. Another common word used to describe a pathogen is **virulence**. A highly virulent organism is one that can produce disease when present in very small numbers.

After gaining entry, pathogens generally cause disease by one of two basic mechanisms. Invasiveness is the ability of a pathogen to grow extremely rapidly and damage surrounding tissues by their sheer numbers. Because a week or more may be needed to mount an immune response against the organism, this rapid growth can easily overwhelm body defenses. A second mechanism is the production of **toxins**. Even very small amounts of some bacterial toxins may disrupt normal cellular activity and, in extreme cases, result in death of the individual.

Several methods are used to describe and classify the millions of species of bacteria on the planet. The three most common methods are shown in Table 26.2 ◆. Healthcare providers must learn these organizational schemes because anti-infective drugs are often effective only for a specific type of bacteria, such as gram-positive bacilli or gram-negative anaerobes.

FIGURE 26.1

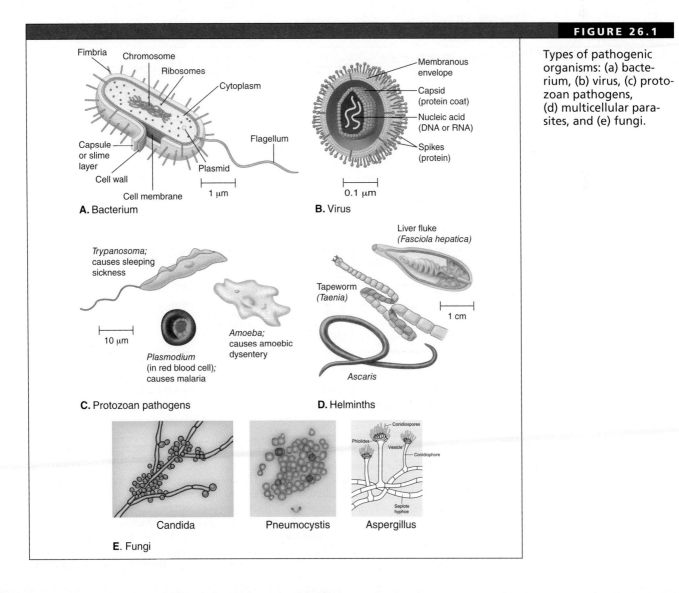

A. Bacterium

B. Virus

C. Protozoan pathogens

D. Helminths

E. Fungi

Types of pathogenic organisms: (a) bacterium, (b) virus, (c) protozoan pathogens, (d) multicellular parasites, and (e) fungi.

TABLE 26.1 Common Bacterial Pathogens

Name of Organism	Disease(s)	Remarks
Bacillus anthracis	Anthrax	Appears in cutaneous and respiratory forms
Borrelia burgdorferi	Lyme disease	Acquired from tick bites
Chlamydia trachomatis	Venereal disease, eye infection	Most common cause of sexually transmitted disease in the United States
Enterococcus	Wounds, urinary tract infections (UTI), endocarditis, bacteremia	Common opportunistic microbe, part of normal flora of the urogenital and intestinal tracts
Escherichia coli	Traveler's diarrhea, UTI, bacteremia, meningitis in children	Part of normal flora of the intestinal tract
Haemophilus	Pneumonia, meningitis in children, bacteremia, otitis media, sinusitis	Some species are part of the normal host flora of the upper respiratory tract
Klebsiella	Pneumonia, UTI	Common opportunistic microbe
Mycobacterium tuberculosis	Tuberculosis	Incidence very high in patients infected with HIV
Mycoplasma pneumoniae	Pneumonia	Most common cause of pneumonia in patients ages 5 to 35
Neisseria gonorrhoeae	Gonorrhea and other sexually transmitted diseases, endometriosis, neonatal eye infection	Can be part of the normal host flora
Neisseria meningitidis	Meningitis in children	Can be part of the normal host flora
Pneumococcus	Pneumonia, otitis media, meningitis, bacteremia, endocarditis	Part of normal flora in upper respiratory tract
Proteus mirabilis	UTI, skin infections	Part of normal flora in the gastrointestinal (GI) tract
Pseudomonas aeruginosa	UTI, skin infections, septicemia	Common opportunistic microbe
Rickettsia rickettsii	Rocky Mountain spotted fever	Acquired from tick bites
Salmonella enteritidis	Food poisoning	From infected animal products, raw eggs, or undercooked meat or chicken
Staphylococcus aureus	Pneumonia, food poisoning, impetigo, wounds, bacteremia, endocarditis, toxic shock syndrome, osteomyelitis, UTI	Can be part of the normal host flora on the skin and mucous membranes
Streptococcus	Pharyngitis, pneumonia, skin infections, septicemia, endocarditis, otitis media	Some species are part of the normal host flora of the respiratory, genital, and intestinal tracts

TABLE 26.2 Methods of Describing and Classifying Bacteria

Method	Description
Staining	Gram positive or gram negative
Shape	Bacilli (rods), cocci (spheres), and spirilla (spirals)
Ability to use O_2	Aerobic (uses O_2) or anaerobic (without O_2)

CORE CONCEPT 26.2

Anti-infective drugs are classified by their chemical structures or by their mechanisms of action.

anti = against
bio = life
ic = pertaining to

Anti-infective is a general term that applies to any drug that is effective against pathogens. In its broadest sense, an anti-infective drug may be used to treat bacterial, fungal, viral, or parasitic infections. The most frequent term used to describe an anti-infective drug is *antibiotic*. Technically, **antibiotic** refers to a natural substance produced by bacteria that can kill other bacteria. In clinical practice, however, the terms *antibacterial*, *anti-infective*, *antimicrobial*, and *antibiotic* are often used interchangeably.

With more than 300 anti-infective drugs available, it is helpful to group these drugs into classes that have similar properties. Two means of grouping are widely used: chemical classes and pharmacologic classes.

Chemical class names such as aminoglycosides, fluoroquinolones, and sulfonamides refer to the fundamental chemical structure of the anti-infectives. Anti-infectives belonging to the same chemical class usually share similar antibacterial properties and adverse effects. Although chemical names are often long and difficult to pronounce, placing drugs into chemical classes will assist the student in mentally organizing these drugs into distinct therapeutic groups.

Pharmacologic classes are used to group anti-infectives by their *mechanism of action*. Examples include cell wall inhibitors, protein synthesis inhibitors, folic acid inhibitors, and reverse trancriptase inhibitors. These classifications are used in this text, where appropriate.

Anti-infective drugs act by selectively targeting a pathogen's metabolism or life cycle.

The primary goal of antimicrobial therapy is to assist the body's defenses in eliminating a pathogen. Drugs that accomplish this goal by *killing* bacteria are called **bacteriocidal**. Some medications do not kill the bacteria but instead *slow their growth*, allowing the body's natural defenses to eliminate the microorganisms. These growth-slowing drugs are called **bacteriostatic**.

Bacterial cells are quite different from human cells. Bacteria have cell walls and contain certain enzymes that human cells lack. Antibiotics exert selective toxicity on bacterial cells by targeting these unique differences. Through this selective action, pathogens can be killed or their growth severely hampered without major effects on human cells. Of course, there are limits to this selective toxicity, depending on the specific antibiotic and the dose used, and adverse effects can be expected from all the anti-infectives. The basic mechanisms of action of antimicrobial drugs are shown in Figure 26.2 ■.

bacterio = *bacteria*
cidal = *killing*
static = *staying the same*

Acquired resistance is a major clinical problem that is worsened by improper use of anti-infectives.

Microorganisms have the ability to replicate extremely rapidly. For example, under ideal conditions, *E. coli* can produce a million cells every 20 minutes. During this rapid replication, bacteria make frequent errors, or **mutations**, while duplicating their genetic code. These mutations occur spontaneously and randomly in the bacterial cell. Although most mutations are harmful to the organism, mutations occasionally result in a bacterial cell that has reproductive advantages over its neighbors. The mutated bacterium may be able to survive in harsher conditions or perhaps grow faster than surrounding cells. One such mutation of particular importance to medicine is that which confers drug resistance on a microorganism.

FIGURE 26.2

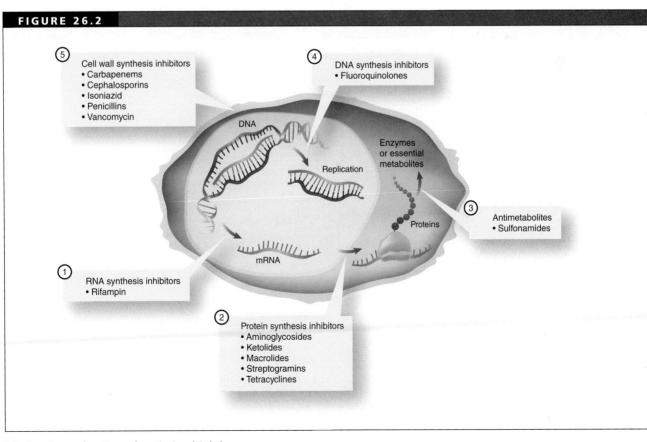

Mechanisms of action of antimicrobial drugs.

Antibiotics help promote the appearance of drug-resistant bacterial strains by killing the masses of bacteria that are sensitive to the drug. Consequently, the only bacteria remaining are those microbes that possess mutations that make them *insensitive* to the effects of the antibiotic. These drug-resistant bacteria are then free to grow faster because they are no longer competing for food with neighboring bacteria that were killed by the antibiotic. Soon the patient develops an infection that is resistant to conventional drug therapy. This phenomenon, called **acquired resistance**, is illustrated in Figure 26.3 ■. Bacteria may pass the resistance gene to other bacteria by transferring small pieces of circular DNA called **plasmids**.

The widespread and sometimes unwarranted use of antibiotics has led to many resistant strains. For example, 60% of all *Staphylococcus* bacteria are now resistant to penicillin. The longer an antibiotic is used in the population and the more often it is prescribed, the larger will be the percentage of resistant strains. Infections acquired in a hospital or other healthcare setting, called **nosocomial infections**, are often resistant to common antibiotics. Two particularly serious resistant infections are those caused by methicillin-resistant *Staphylococcus aureus* (MRSA) and vancomycin-resistant enterococci (VRE).

Healthcare providers play important roles in delaying the emergence of resistance. The following are four principles recommended by the Centers for Disease Control and Prevention (CDC):

- Prevent infections whenever possible. It is always easier to prevent an infection than to treat one. This includes teaching the patient the importance of getting immunizations.

- Restrict the use of antibiotics to those conditions deemed medically necessary. Antibiotics should be prescribed only when there is a clear rationale for their use.

- Advise the patient to take anti-infectives for the full length of therapy, even if symptoms disappear before the regimen is finished. Prematurely stopping antibiotic therapy allows some pathogens to survive, thus promoting the development of resistant strains.

- Prevent transmission of the pathogen by using proper infection control procedures. This includes the use of standard precautions and teaching patients the methods of proper hygiene for preventing transmission in the home and community settings.

In most cases, antibiotics are given when there is clear evidence of bacterial infection. Some patients, however, receive antibiotics to *prevent* an infection, a practice called *prophylactic use*, or **chemoprophylaxis**. Examples of patients who might receive prophylactic antibiotics include those who have suppressed immune systems, have experienced deep puncture wounds such as dog bites, and have prosthetic heart valves and are about to undergo medical or dental surgery.

FIGURE 26.3

Acquired resistance.

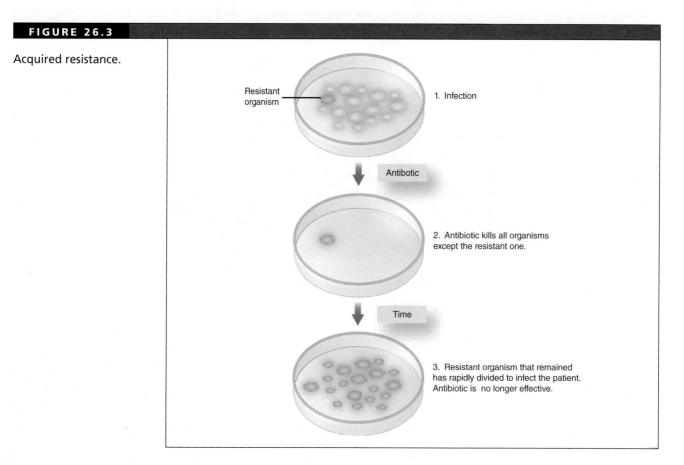

Resistant organism

1. Infection

Antibotic

2. Antibiotic kills all organisms except the resistant one.

Time

3. Resistant organism that remained has rapidly divided to infect the patient. Antibiotic is no longer effective.

Careful selection of the correct antibiotic is essential for effective pharmacotherapy and to limit adverse effects.

Selection of an antibiotic that will be effective against a specific pathogen is an important task of the healthcare provider. Selecting an incorrect drug will delay proper treatment, giving the microorganisms more time to invade. Prescribing ineffective antibiotics also promotes the development of resistance and may cause unnecessary adverse effects in the patient.

Ideally, laboratory tests should be conducted to identify the organism prior to beginning anti-infective therapy. Laboratory tests may include examination of body specimens such as urine, sputum, blood, or pus for microorganisms. Organisms isolated from the specimens are grown in the laboratory and identified. The laboratory then tests several antibiotics to determine which is most effective against the identified pathogen. This process of growing the organism and identifying the effective antibiotic is called **culture and sensitivity (C&S) testing**.

Ideally, the pathogen should be identified *before* anti-infective therapy is begun. However, laboratory testing and identification may take several days and, in the case of viruses, several weeks. If the infection is severe, therapy is often begun with a **broad-spectrum antibiotic**, one that is effective against a wide variety of different microbial species. After laboratory testing is completed, the drug may be changed to a **narrow-spectrum antibiotic**, one that is effective against a smaller group of microbes or only the isolated species. In general, narrow-spectrum antibiotics have less effect on normal host flora, thus causing fewer adverse effects.

In most cases, anti-infective therapy uses a single drug, because combining two antibiotics may actually decrease each drug's effectiveness. This phenomenon is known as **antagonism**. Use of multiple antibiotics also has the potential to promote resistance. However, multidrug therapy is warranted if the patient's infection is caused by different organisms or if therapy must be started before C&S testing has been completed. Multidrug therapy is common in the treatment of TB and HIV infection.

One common adverse effect of anti-infective therapy is the appearance of secondary infections, called **superinfections**, which occur when microorganisms normally present in the body are killed by the drug. These normal microorganisms, or **host flora**, inhabit the skin and the upper respiratory, urogenital, and intestinal tracts. Some of these organisms serve a useful purpose by producing antibacterial substances and by competing with pathogenic organisms for space and nutrients. Removal of host flora by an antibiotic gives pathogenic microorganisms space to grow or allows for overgrowth of nonaffected normal flora. Appearance of a new infection while receiving anti-infective therapy is suspicious of a superinfection. Signs and symptoms of a superinfection may include diarrhea, bladder pain, painful urination, or abnormal vaginal discharges. Broad-spectrum antibiotics are more likely to cause superinfections because they kill so many different species of microorganisms. Figure 26.3 illustrates the production of a superinfection.

The penicillins are one of the oldest and safest groups of anti-infectives.

Although not the first anti-infective discovered, penicillin was the first *mass-produced* antibiotic. Isolated from the fungus *Penicillium* in 1941, penicillin quickly became a miracle drug by preventing thousands of deaths from what are now considered to be minor infections. The penicillins are listed in Table 26.3 ◆.

Penicillins kill bacteria by disrupting their cell walls. The chemical structure of penicillin that is responsible for its antibacterial activity is called the **beta-lactam ring**. However, some bacteria secrete an enzyme, called **beta-lactamase/penicillinase**, which splits the beta-lactam ring. This structural change allows these bacteria to become resistant to the effects of most penicillins. The action of penicillinase is illustrated in Figure 26.4 ■. Since their discovery, large numbers of resistant bacterial strains that limit the therapeutic usefulness of the penicillins have emerged.

Chemical modifications to the natural penicillin molecule produced drugs offering several advantages.

- *Penicillinase-resistant penicillins* Oxacillin and cloxacillin (Cloxapen) are examples of drugs that are effective against penicillinase-producing bacteria. These are sometimes called antistaphylococcal penicillins.

- *Broad-spectrum penicillins* Ampicillin (Principen) and amoxicillin (Amoxil, Trimox) are effective against a wide range of microorganisms and are called *broad-spectrum* penicillins. These are sometimes referred to as aminopenicillins.

- *Extended-spectrum penicillins* Carbenicillin (Geocillin) and piperacillin are effective against even more microbial species than the aminopenicillins, including *Pseudomonas, Enterobacter, Klebsiella*, and *Bacteroides fragilis*.

Several drugs are available that inhibit the bacterial beta-lactamase enzyme. When combined with penicillin, these drugs protect the penicillin molecule from destruction, extending its spectrum of activity.

TABLE 26.3 Penicillins

Drug	Route and Adult Dose	Remarks
amoxicillin (Amoxil, Trimox)	PO; 250–500 mg tid	Broad-spectrum penicillin
amoxicillin–clavulanate (Augmentin)	PO; 250–500 mg every 8–12 hours	Broad-spectrum penicillin with a beta-lactamase inhibitor
ampicillin (Principen)	PO; 250–500 mg qid	Broad-spectrum penicillin; IM and IV forms available
ampicillin–sulbactam (Unasyn)	IV/IM; 1.5–3 g qid	Broad-spectrum penicillin
dicloxacillin	PO; 125–300 mg qid	Penicillinase resistant
nafcillin	IV/IM; 500 mg–1 g qid (max: 12 g/day)	Penicillinase resistant; IM and IV forms available
oxacillin	IV; 250 mg–1 g every 4–6 hours (max: 12 g/day)	Penicillinase resistant; IV and IM forms available
penicillin G benzathine (Bicillin)	IM; 1.2 million units as a single dose	Prolonged duration of action
Pr penicillin G potassium	IV/IM; 2–24 million units divided every 4–6 hours	Ineffective against most forms of *S. aureus*
penicillin G procaine (Wycillin)	IM; 600,000–1.2 million units daily	Prolonged duration of action
penicillin V (Pen-Vee K, Veetids, others)	PO; 125–500 mg qid	Acid stable
piperacillin	IM; 2–4 g tid–qid (max: 24 g/day)	Extended-spectrum penicillin
piperacillin–tazobactam (Zosyn)	IV; 3.375–4.5 g qid over 30 minutes	Extended-spectrum penicillin with a beta-lactamase inhibitor
ticarcillin–clavulanate (Timentin)	IV; 3.1 g qid	Extended-spectrum penicillin with a beta-lactamase inhibitor

FIGURE 26.4

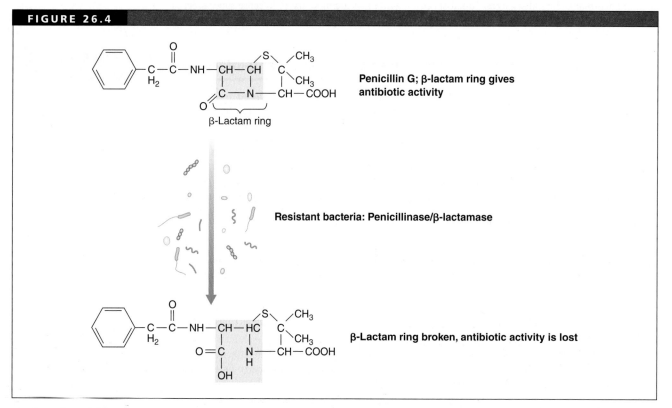

Penicillin G; β-lactam ring gives antibiotic activity

Resistant bacteria: Penicillinase/β-lactamase

β-Lactam ring broken, antibiotic activity is lost

Action of penicillinase.

CAM THERAPY

The Antibacterial Properties of Goldenseal

Goldenseal (*Hydrastis canadensis*) was once a common plant found in woods in the eastern and midwestern United States. As word spread of its medicinal properties, the plant was harvested to near extinction. In particular, goldenseal was reported to mask the appearance of drugs in the urine of patients wanting to hide their drug abuse. This claim has been proven false.

The roots and leaves of goldenseal are dried and available as capsules, tablets, salves, and tinctures. One of the primary ingredients in goldenseal is hydrastine, which is reported to have antibacterial and antifungal properties. When used topically or locally, it is claimed to be of value in treating bacterial and fungal skin infections and oral conditions such as gingivitis and thrush. Other possible indications include hypertension, duodenal ulcers, and conjunctivitis.

Drug Prototype: 🅟 *Penicillin G Sodium/Potassium*
Therapeutic Class: Antibacterial   **Pharmacologic Class: Cell wall inhibitor, natural penicillin**

Actions and Uses: Similar to penicillin V, penicillin G is sometimes a drug of first choice against *streptococcal, pneumococci*, and *staphylococcal* organisms that do not produce penicillinase and are shown to be susceptible by C&S testing. It is also a preferred drug for gonorrhea and syphilis caused by susceptible strains. Penicillin V is more acid stable; over 70% is absorbed after an oral dose compared to the 15% to 30% from penicillin G. Because of its low oral absorption, penicillin G is often given by the IV or IM routes. Penicillinase-producing organisms inactivate both penicillin G and penicillin V.

Adverse Effects and Interactions: Penicillin G has few adverse effects. Although not serious, diarrhea, nausea, and vomiting are the most common adverse effects. Anaphylaxis is the most serious adverse effect, although its incidence is very low. Pain at the injection site may occur, and superinfections are possible.

Penicillin G may decrease the effectiveness of oral contraceptives. Colestipol decreases absorption of penicillin G. Potassium-sparing diuretics may cause hyperkalemia with penicillin G. Food increases the breakdown of penicillin in the stomach. Probenecid decreases renal excretion of penicillin G.

The three beta-lactamase inhibitors—clavulanate, sulbactam, and tazobactam—are only available in fixed-dose combinations with specific penicillins. These include Augmentin (amoxicillin plus clavulanate), Timentin (ticarcillin plus clavulanate), Unasyn (ampicillin plus sulbactam), and Zosyn (piperacillin plus tazobactam).

In general, the adverse effects of penicillins are minor, and this has contributed to their widespread use for more than 60 years. Allergy is the most common adverse effect. Symptoms of penicillin allergy may include rash, fever, and anaphylaxis. The incidence of anaphylaxis is quite low, ranging from 0.04% to 2%. Allergy to one penicillin increases the risk of allergy to other drugs in the same class. Other less common adverse effects of the penicillins include skin rashes and lowered red blood cell, white blood cell, or platelet counts.

Concept Review   26.1

■ Why does antibiotic resistance become more of a problem when antibiotics are prescribed too often?

The cephalosporins are similar in structure and function to the penicillins and are one of the most widely prescribed anti-infective classes.

CORE CONCEPT 26.7

Isolated shortly after the penicillins, the four generations of cephalosporins comprise the largest antibiotic class. Like the penicillins, the cephalosporins contain a beta-lactam ring that is primarily responsible for their antimicrobial activity. The cephalosporins are bacteriocidal and inhibit bacterial cell wall synthesis. Table 26.4 ◆ lists the cephalosporins and their dosages.

TABLE 26.4   Selected Cephalosporins

Drug	Route and Adult Dose	Remarks
FIRST GENERATION		
cefadroxil (Duricef)	PO; 500 mg–1 g once or twice daily (max: 2 g/day)	Binds to bacterial cell walls; bacteriocidal
cefazolin (Ancef, Kefzol)	IM; 250 mg–2 g tid (max: 12 g/day)	IV form available
cephalexin (Keflex)	PO; 250–500 mg qid	Binds to bacterial cell walls; bacteriocidal; broad spectrum
SECOND GENERATION		
cefaclor (Ceclor)	PO; 250–500 mg tid	Binds to bacterial cell walls; extended-release form available; bacteriocidal
cefotetan (Cefotan)	IM; 1–2 g every 12 hours	IV form available
cefprozil (Cefzil)	PO; 250–500 mg once or twice daily	Binds to bacterial cell walls; bacteriocidal
cefuroxime (Ceftin, Zinacef)	PO; 250–500 mg bid	Binds to bacterial cell walls; IM and IV forms available; bacteriocidal
THIRD TO FIFTH GENERATIONS		
cefdinir (Omnicef)	PO; 300 mg bid	Third generation; broad spectrum
cefditoren (Spectracef)	PO; 400 mg bid for 10 days	Third generation
cefepime (Maxipime)	IM; 0.5–1 g bid (max: 3 g/day)	Fourth generation; IV form available
cefixime (Suprax)	PO; 400 mg daily or 200 mg bid	Third generation; binds to bacterial cell walls; bacteriocidal
Pr cefotaxime (Claforan)	IM; 1–2 g bid–tid (max: 12 g/day)	Third generation; binds to bacterial cell walls; bacteriocidal; IV form available
ceftaroline (Teflaro)	IV; 600 mg every 12 hours for 5–14 days	Fifth generation; broad spectrum effective against MRSA
ceftriaxone (Rocephin)	IM; 1–2 g once or twice daily (max: 4 g/day)	Third generation; binds to bacterial cell walls; IV form also available; bacteriocidal

More than 20 cephalosporins are available, all having similar sounding names that can challenge even the best memory. They are classified by their "generation." The first-generation drugs contain a beta-lactam ring, and bacteria that produce beta-lactamase will normally be resistant to these medications. The second-generation cephalosporins are more potent and more resistant to beta-lactamase and exhibit a broader spectrum than the first-generation drugs. The third-generation cephalosporins generally have a longer duration of action, an even broader spectrum, and are resistant to beta-lactamases. Third-generation cephalosporins are preferred drugs against infections by *Pseudomonas, Klebsiella, Neisseria, Salmonella,*

Drug Prototype: Pr *Cefotaxime (Claforan)*

Therapeutic Class: Antibacterial   **Pharmacologic Class: Cell wall inhibitor; third-generation cephalosporin**

Actions and Uses: Cefotaxime is a third-generation cephalosporin with a broad spectrum of activity against gram-negative organisms. It is effective against many organisms that have developed resistance to earlier generation cephalosporins and to other classes of anti-infectives. Cefotaxime exhibits bacteriocidal activity by inhibiting cell wall synthesis. It is prescribed for serious infections of the lower respiratory tract, central nervous system (CNS), urogenital system, bones, and joints. It may also be used for blood infections such as bacteremia or septicemia. Like many of the cephalosporins, cefotaxime is not absorbed from the GI tract and must be given by the IM or IV routes.

Adverse Effects and Interactions: For most patients, cefotaxime and the other cephalosporins are safe medications. Hypersensitivity is the most common adverse effect, although symptoms may include only a minor rash and itching. Anaphylaxis is possible; thus, the healthcare provider should be alert for this reaction. GI-related adverse effects such as diarrhea, vomiting, and nausea may occur. Some patients experience considerable pain at the injection site.

Probenecid decreases elimination by the kidneys. Alcohol interacts with cefotaxime to produce a disulfiram-like reaction. Cefotaxime interacts with nonsteroidal anti-inflammatory drugs (NSAIDs) to cause an increase in platelet inhibition.

Proteus, and *Haemophilus influenzae*. Newer, fourth- and fifth-generation drugs are more effective against organisms that have developed resistance to earlier cephalosporins. There are not always clear distinctions between the generations.

The primary therapeutic use of the cephalosporins is for gram-negative infections and for patients who cannot tolerate the less expensive penicillins. Like the penicillins, allergic reactions are the most common adverse effect. Skin rashes are a common sign of allergy and may appear several days following the initiation of therapy. GI complaints are common. Earlier generation cephalosporins exhibited kidney toxicity, but this is diminished with the newer drugs. The nurse must be aware that some patients (5% to 10%) who are allergic to penicillin will also be allergic to cephalosporins. Despite this small incidence of cross allergy, cephalosporins offer a reasonable alternative for *most* patients who are unable to take penicillins. However, cephalosporins are contraindicated if the patient has previously experienced a *severe* allergic reaction to a penicillin.

The tetracyclines have broad spectrums but are drugs of choice for few diseases.

CORE CONCEPT 26.8

The first tetracyclines were extracted from *Streptomyces* soil microorganisms in 1948. Their widespread use in the 1950s and 1960s has resulted in a large number of resistant bacterial strains that now limits their therapeutic usefulness. Table 26.5 ◆ lists the tetracyclines and their dosages.

Tetracyclines exert a bacteriostatic effect by inhibiting bacterial protein synthesis. They are effective against a wide range of gram-negative and gram-positive organisms and have one of the broadest spectrums of any class of antibiotics. They are drugs of first choice for relatively few diseases, including Rocky Mountain spotted fever, typhus, cholera, Lyme disease, ulcers caused by *Helicobacter pylori*, and *Chlamydia* infections. Drugs in this class are occasionally used for the treatment of acne vulgaris, for which they are given topically or PO at low doses. Minocycline (Arestin) and doxycycline (Atridox, Periostat) are used to treat periodontal disease. The newest tetracycline, tigecycline (Tygacil) is approved to treat drug-resistant intra-abdominal infections and complicated skin infections, especially those caused by MRSA.

TABLE 26.5   Tetracyclines

Drug	Route and Adult Dose	Remarks
demeclocycline (Declomycin)	PO; 150–300 mg bid–qid (max: 2.4 g/day)	Intermediate duration of action; broad spectrum
doxycycline (Vibramycin, others)	PO; 100 mg bid on day 1, then 100 mg daily (max: 200 mg/day)	Long duration of action; IV form available; subgingival form available for periodontitis
minocycline (Minocin, others)	PO; 200 mg as one dose followed by 100 mg bid	Long duration of action; IV form available; available as microsphere powder for periodontitis and as extended-release tablet for acne
℞ tetracycline (Sumycin)	PO; 250–500 mg bid–qid (max: 2 g/day)	Short acting; inhibits protein synthesis; bacteriostatic; IM and topical forms available
tigecycline (Tygacil)	IV; 100 mg, followed by 50 mg every 12 hours	Newest tetracycline; very limited indications

Drug Prototype: ℞ *Tetracycline (Sumycin, Others)*

Therapeutic Class: Antibacterial   Pharmacologic Class: Tetracycline, protein synthesis inhibitor

Actions and Uses: Tetracycline is effective against many different microorganisms, including some protozoans. Its use has increased over the past decade due to its effectiveness against *H. pylori* in the treatment of peptic ulcer disease. It is given orally and has a short half-life. A topical preparation is available for treating acne. When given PO, it should be administered at least one hour before or two hours after a meal to avoid drug interactions.

Adverse Effects and Interactions: As a broad-spectrum antibiotic, tetracycline has a tendency to affect vaginal, oral, and intestinal flora and cause superinfections. Diarrhea may be severe enough to cause discontinuation of therapy. Other common adverse effects include nausea, vomiting, and photosensitivity.

Tetracycline can decrease the effectiveness of oral contraceptives, and thus alternative precautions should be taken during therapy to prevent pregnancy. Pregnant patients and those who are breastfeeding should not take tetracyclines because they are pregnancy category D medications.

The tetracyclines cause few serious adverse effects. Gastric distress is relatively common with tetracyclines, so patients tend to take tetracyclines with food. Patients should be urged *not* to drink milk with these medications because tetracyclines bind ions such as calcium and iron, thereby decreasing the drug's absorption by as much as 50%. Patients should be advised to avoid direct exposure to sunlight because tetracyclines can cause **photosensitivity**, which makes the skin particularly susceptible to sunburn. Unless suffering from a life-threatening infection, patients younger than 9 years are not given tetracyclines because these drugs may cause permanent yellow-brown teeth discoloration in young children. These drugs are pregnancy category D drugs; tetracyclines should not be used during pregnancy. Because of their broad spectrum, the risk for superinfection is relatively high, and nurses should always be observant for signs of a secondary infection. Outdated tetracycline may deteriorate and become nephrotoxic; therefore, unused prescriptions should be discarded promptly.

The macrolides are safe alternatives to penicillin for many infections.

CORE CONCEPT 26.9

Erythromycin (E-Mycin, Erythrocin), the first macrolide antibiotic, was isolated from *Streptomcyes* in a soil sample in 1952. Macrolides are prescribed for infections that are resistant to penicillins. Commonly prescribed macrolides are listed in Table 26.6 ◆.

TABLE 26.6 Macrolides

Drug	Route and Adult Dose	Remarks
azithromycin (Zithromax, Zmax)	PO (Zithromax); 500 mg for one dose, then 250 mg daily for 4 days PO (Zmax): 1–2 g single dose	Inhibits protein synthesis; bacteriostatic; IV form available
clarithromycin (Biaxin)	PO; 250–500 mg bid	Inhibits protein synthesis; bacteriostatic; part of regimen for *Helicobacter pylori* infections
℗ erythromycin (E-Mycin, Erythrocin)	PO; 250–500 mg qid or 333 mg tid	Bacteriostatic or bacteriocidal depending on nature of organism and drug concentration; IV form available
fidaxomicin (Dificid)	PO; 200 mg bid	Newer drug in this class for treatment of pseudomembranous colitis or *Clostridium difficile*–associated diarrhea

Drug Prototype: ℗ *Erythromycin (E-Mycin, Erythrocin)*
Therapeutic Class: **Antibacterial**   Pharmacologic Class: **Macrolide protein synthesis inhibitor**

Actions and Uses: Erythromycin is inactivated by stomach acid and is thus administered as coated tablets or capsules that dissolve in the small intestine. The drug's main application is for patients who are allergic to penicillins or who may have a penicillin-resistant infection. It is a preferred drug for infections by *Bordetella pertussis* (whooping cough), *Legionella pneumophila* (Legionnaire's disease), *Mycoplasma pneumoniae*, and *Corynebacterium diphtheriae*.

Adverse Effects and Interactions: The most common adverse effects from erythromycin are nausea, abdominal cramping, and vomiting, although these are rarely serious enough to cause discontinuation of therapy. Concurrent administration with food reduces these symptoms. Its spectrum of activity is similar to that of the penicillins.

Anesthetics and anticonvulsant drugs may interact to cause serum drug levels to rise and result in toxicity. This drug interacts with cyclosporine, increasing the risk for kidney toxicity. It may increase the effects of warfarin. The concurrent use of erythromycin with lovastatin or simvastatin is not recommended because it may increase the risk of muscle toxicity.

The macrolide antibiotics inhibit bacterial protein synthesis and may be either bacteriocidal or bacteriostatic, depending on the dose and the target organism. Macrolides are considered safe alternatives to penicillin, although they are drugs of first choice for relatively few infections. Common uses of macrolides include the treatment of whooping cough, Legionnaire's disease, and infections by *Streptococcus*, *H. influenzae*, *M. pneumoniae*, and *Chlamydia*. Clarithromycin is one of several antibiotics used to treat peptic ulcer disease.

The macrolides exhibit no serious adverse effects. Mild GI upset, diarrhea, and abdominal pain are the most common adverse effects. Because macrolides are broad-spectrum drugs, patients should be observed for signs of superinfection. Like most of the older antibiotics, macrolide-resistant strains are becoming more common. Other than prior allergic reactions to macrolides, there are no contraindications to therapy.

The newer macrolides have a longer half-life and cause less GI irritation than erythromycin. For example, azithromycin (Zithromax) has such an extended half-life that it can be administered for only 5 days, rather the 10 days required for most antibiotics. Even shorter durations, often a single dose, are sometimes used when azithromycin (Zmax) is administered to treat gonorrhea, otitis media, or acute bacterial sinusitis. The shorter duration of therapy is thought to increase patient adherence.

Concept Review 26.2

■ If penicillins are inexpensive, why might a healthcare provider prescribe a more expensive cephalosporin or macrolide antibiotic?

The aminoglycosides are narrow-spectrum drugs that have the potential to cause serious toxicity.

CORE CONCEPT **26.10**

The aminoglycosides, first isolated from soil organisms in 1942, share a common chemical structure of an amino group (NH_2) and a sugar group. Although more toxic than most other antibiotic classes, they have important therapeutic applications for the treatment of a number of aerobic gram-negative bacteria, mycobacteria, and some protozoans. Table 26.7 ◆ lists the aminoglycosides and their dosages.

Aminoglycosides are bacteriocidal and act by inhibiting bacterial protein synthesis. They are normally reserved for serious aerobic gram-negative infections, including those caused by *E. coli*, *Serratia*, *Proteus*, *Klebsiella*, and *Pseudomonas*. When used for systemic bacterial infections, they are given parenterally because they are poorly absorbed from the GI tract. They are occasionally given orally to sterilize the bowel before intestinal surgery. Neomycin is available for topical infections of the skin, eyes, and ears. Paromomycin (Humatin) is given orally for the treatment of parasitic infections. The first aminoglycoside, streptomycin, was once widely prescribed, but its use is now limited to the treatment of TB due to the development of a large number of resistant strains. The student should note the differences in spelling of some of these drugs, from *-mycin* to *-micin*, which reflects the different organisms from which the drugs were originally isolated.

TABLE 26.7 Aminoglycosides

Drug	Route and Adult Dose	Remarks
amikacin (Amikin)	IM; 5–7.5 mg/kg as a loading dose, then 7.5 mg/kg bid	Broader spectrum than others in this class; usually bacteriocidal; IV form available
💊 gentamicin (Garamycin)	IM; 1.5–2 mg/kg as a loading dose, then 1–2 mg/kg bid–tid	IV, topical, and ophthalmic forms available
kanamycin (Kantrex)	IM; 5–7.5 mg/kg bid–tid	Also used to sterilize the bowel prior to colon surgery; oral, inhalation, and IV forms available
neomycin	PO; 4–12 g/day in divided doses	Oral, topical, and IV forms available
paromomycin (Humatin)	PO; 7.5–12.5 mg/kg tid	For parasitic infections of the intestine; also used to treat hepatic coma
streptomycin	IM; 15 mg/kg up to 1 g as a single dose	For tuberculosis, tularemia, and plague
tobramycin (Tobrex)	IM/IV; 3 mg/kg tid (max: 5 mg/kg/day)	Most effective aminoglycoside against *P. aeruginosa*

Drug Prototype: Ⓟ *Gentamicin (Garamycin)*

Therapeutic Class: Antibacterial **Pharmacologic Class: Aminoglycoside, protein synthesis inhibitor**

Actions and Uses: Gentamicin is a broad-spectrum, bacteriocidal antibiotic usually prescribed for serious urinary, respiratory, nervous, or GI infections. Activity includes *Enterobacter, E. coli, Klebsiella, Citrobacter, Pseudomonas,* and *Serratia.* It is often used in combination with other antibiotics or when other antibiotics have proven ineffective. A topical formulation (Genoptic) is available for infections of the external eye.

Adverse Effects and Interactions: As with other aminoglycosides, adverse effects from gentamicin may be severe. Ototoxicity is possible and may become permanent with continued use. Ringing in the ears, dizziness, and persistent headaches are early signs of ototoxicity. Frequent hearing tests should be conducted so that gentamicin may be discontinued if early signs of ototoxicity are detected. The healthcare provider must also

be alert for signs of nephrotoxicity because this may limit drug therapy with gentamicin.

Using this drug together with amphotericin B, capreomycin, cisplatin, polymyxin B, or vancomycin increases the risk of nephrotoxicity. The risk of ototoxicity increases if the patient is currently taking amphotericin B, furosemide, aspirin, bumetanide, ethacrynic acid, cisplatin, or paromomycin.

> **BLACK BOX WARNING:**
> Adverse effects from parenteral gentamicin may be severe and include neurotoxicity, neuromuscular blockade, and nephrotoxicity.

oto = *ear*
toxicity = *poison*

nephron = *kidney*

The clinical applications of the aminoglycosides are limited by their potential to cause serious adverse effects. The degree and types of potential toxicity are similar for all drugs in this class. Of greatest concern are their effects on the inner ear and the kidney. Damage to the inner ear, or **ototoxicity**, causes hearing impairment, dizziness, loss of balance, persistent headache, and ringing in the ears. Because permanent deafness may occur, aminoglycosides are usually discontinued when symptoms of hearing impairment first appear. Kidney damage, or **nephrotoxicity**, is recognized by abnormal urinary function tests, such as elevated serum creatinine or blood urea nitrogen (BUN). Nephrotoxicity caused by aminoglycosides is usually reversible. Serum drug levels are sometimes monitored during therapy to prevent toxic doses of these antibiotics.

CORE CONCEPT 26.11

Fluoroquinolones have wide clinical applications because of their broad spectrum of activity and relative safety.

The fluoroquinolones were once reserved only for urinary tract infections (UTIs) because of their toxicity. However, the newer fluoroquinolones are safer, have a broader spectrum of activity, and are used for a variety of infections. The fluoroquinolones are listed in Table 26.8 ◆.

TABLE 26.8 Fluoroquinolones		
Drug	**Route and Adult Dose**	**Remarks**
Ⓟ ciprofloxacin (Cipro)	PO; 250–750 mg bid	For lung, skin, bone, and joint infections, and for anthrax; broad spectrum; IV form available
gatifloxacin (Zymar)	PO; 400 mg tid	For respiratory infections, UTI, and gonorrhea; IV form available
gemifloxacin (Factive)	PO; 320 mg daily	For respiratory infections
levofloxacin (Levaquin)	PO; 250–500 mg daily	For respiratory tract and skin infections; IV form available
moxifloxacin (Avelox, Moxeza, Vigamox)	PO/IV; 400 mg daily	For sinus and respiratory tract infections; otic drops available
nalidixic acid (NegGram)	PO; acute therapy: 1 g qid; PO; chronic therapy: 500 mg qid	For UTI
norfloxacin (Noroxin)	PO; 400 mg bid	For UTI; ophthalmic form available
ofloxacin (Floxin)	PO; 200–400 mg bid	For UTI, respiratory tract infections, and gonorrhea; otic drops available

Drug Prototype: ℗ *Ciprofloxacin (Cipro)*

Therapeutic Class: Antibacterial   Pharmacologic Class: Fluoroquinolone, bacterial DNA synthesis inhibitor

Actions and Uses: Ciprofloxacin (Cipro), a second-generation fluoroquinolone, is the most widely used drug in this class. Ciprofloxacin inhibits bacterial replication and DNA repair and is more effective against gram-negative than gram-positive organisms. It is prescribed for respiratory infections, bone and joint infections, GI infections, ophthalmic infections, sinusitis, and prostatitis. It is rapidly absorbed after oral administration, and an IV form is available for severe infections. An extended-release form of the drug, Proquin XR, is administered for only three days and is approved for bladder infections.

Adverse Effects and Interactions: Ciprofloxacin is well tolerated by most patients, and serious adverse effects are uncommon. Nausea, vomiting, and diarrhea may occur in as many as 20% of patients. Ciprofloxacin may be administered with food to lessen adverse GI effects; however, it should not be taken with antacids or mineral supplements because drug absorption will be diminished. Some patients report headache and dizziness.

Using this drug with warfarin may increase warfarin's anticoagulant effects and result in bleeding. Antacids, ferrous sulfate, and sucralfate decrease the absorption of ciprofloxacin. Caffeine should be restricted to avoid excessive nervousness, anxiety, or tachycardia.

> **BLACK BOX WARNING:**
> Tendinitis and tendon rupture may occur, especially in patients over age 60; in kidney, heart, and lung transplant recipients; and in those receiving concurrent corticosteroid therapy. Fluoroquinolones may cause extreme muscle weakness in patients with myasthenia gravis.

The first drug in this class, nalidixic acid (NegGram), was approved in 1962, but its use is restricted to UTIs. Four generations of fluoroquinolones have since become available. All fluoroquinolones have activity against gram-negative pathogens; the newer ones are significantly more effective against gram-positive microbes.

The fluoroquinolones are bacteriocidal and act by inhibiting bacterial DNA synthesis. These antibiotics are extensively used as alternatives to other antibiotics. Clinical applications include infections of the respiratory, GI, and gynecologic tracts, and some skin and soft-tissue infections.

The most widely used drug in this class, ciprofloxacin (Cipro), is a preferred drug for exposure to anthrax (*Bacillus anthracis*), a potential bioterrorist threat. If exposure to anthrax is *suspected*, 500 mg of ciprofloxacin is administered by the oral route every 12 hours for 60 days. If exposure is *confirmed*, ciprofloxacin is immediately administered IV, 400 mg every 12 hours. Other antibiotics are also effective against anthrax, including penicillin, vancomycin, ampicillin, erythromycin, tetracycline, and doxycycline.

A major advantage of the fluoroquinolones is that most are well absorbed orally and may be administered either once or twice daily. They should not be taken together with multivitamins or mineral supplements because these interact to reduce the absorption of some fluoroquinolones by as much as 90%.

Fluoroquinolones are safe for most patients, with nausea, vomiting, and diarrhea being the most frequent adverse effects. The most serious adverse effects are dysrhythmias (for gatifloxacin and moxifloxacin) and potential hepatotoxicity. Fluoroquinolones have been shown to exhibit cartilage toxicity, resulting in an increased risk of tendonitis and tendon rupture, particularly of the Achilles tendon. The risk of tendon rupture is especially increased in patients over age 60 and those receiving concurrent corticosteroids. Because they may affect cartilage development, these drugs are not approved for children under age 18. Fluoroquinolones are pregnancy category C and their use should be avoided during pregnancy or in lactating patients.

Sulfonamides and urinary antiseptics are traditional drugs for urinary tract infections.

CORE CONCEPT 26.12

The discovery of the sulfonamides in the 1930s heralded a new era in the treatment of infectious disease. With their wide spectrum of activity, the sulfonamides significantly reduced deaths due to infections and earned their discoverer a Nobel Prize in medicine. The sulfonamides are listed in Table 26.9 ◆. Sulfonamides suppress bacterial growth by inhibiting folic acid, an essential substance in cellular metabolism.

TABLE 26.9 Sulfonamides and Urinary Antiseptics		
Drug	**Route and Adult Dose**	**Remarks**
SULFONAMIDES		
silver sulfadiazine	Topical; Apply cream 1–2 times per day to thickness of 1.5 mm	For prevention of sepsis in patients with serious burns
sulfadiazine	PO; 2–4 g daily in 4–6 divided doses	Also for malaria, toxoplasmosis, and prophylaxis of rheumatic fever
sulfadoxine–pyrimethamine (Fansidar)	PO; 1 tablet weekly (500 mg sulfadoxine, 25 mg pyrimethamine)	Also for prevention and treatment of malaria
sulfasalazine (Azulfidine)	PO; 1–2 g/day in four divided doses (max: 8 g/day)	Also for ulcerative colitis and rheumatoid arthritis
sulfisoxazole (Gantrisin)	PO; 2–4 g initially, followed by 1–2 g qid	For UTI; short acting; vaginal form available
(Pr) trimethoprim-sulfamethoxazole (Bactrim, Septra)	PO; 160 mg TMP/800 mg SMZ bid	Combination drug; for UTI, *Pneumocystis*, and ear infections; IV form available
URINARY ANTISEPTICS		
fosfomycin (Monurol)	PO; 3 g sachet dissolved in 3–4 oz of water as a single dose	Bactericidal; for UTI
methenamine (Mandelamine, Hiprex, Urex)	PO; hippurate 1 g bid; mandelate 1 g qid	For chronic UTI; broad spectrum
nalidixic acid (NegGram)	PO; acute therapy: 1 g qid; PO; chronic therapy: 500 mg qid	Urinary antiseptic; similar to the fluoroquinolones
nitrofurantoin (Furadantin, Macrobid, Macrodantin)	PO; 50–100 mg qid	For UTI; extended-release form available; interferes with bacterial enzymes

Although initially very effective, several factors led to a significant decline in the use of sulfonamides. Their widespread availability over 70 years produced a substantial number of resistant bacterial strains. The development of the penicillins, cephalosporins, and macrolides gave healthcare providers greater choices of safer drugs. Approval of the combination antibiotic trimethoprim–sulfamethoxazole (Bactrim, Septra) marked a resurgence in the use of sulfonamides in treating UTIs. In communities with high resistance rates, trimethoprim–sulfamethoxazole is no longer a first-line drug, unless C&S testing determines it to be the most effective drug for the specific pathogen.

Drug Prototype: (Pr) *Trimethoprim–Sulfamethoxazole (Bactrim, Septra)*

Therapeutic Class: Antibacterial   Pharmacologic Class: Sulfonamide, folic acid inhibitor

Actions and Uses: The combination of sulfamethoxazole (SMZ), a sulfonamide, with the anti-infective trimethoprim (TMP) is most frequently used in the pharmacotherapy of UTIs. It is also approved for the treatment of *Pneumocystis carinii* pneumonia, *Shigella* infections of the small bowel, and acute episodes of bronchitis.

Both SMZ and TMP are inhibitors of the bacterial metabolism of folic acid. Combining the two drugs produces a greater bacterial kill than would be achieved with either drug used separately. Another advantage of the combination is that development of resistance is lower than is observed when either of the drugs is used alone.

Adverse Effects and Interactions: Nausea and vomiting are the most frequent adverse effects of TMP–SMZ therapy. Hypersensitivity is relatively common and usually manifests as skin rash, itching, and fever. This medication should be used cautiously in patients with preexisting kidney disease, because sulfonamides can adversely affect renal function. Periodic laboratory evaluations are usually performed to identify early signs of adverse blood effects.

TMP and SMZ may increase the effects of oral anticoagulants. These drugs may also increase methotrexate toxicity. Potassium supplements should not be taken during therapy, unless directed by the healthcare provider.

Sulfonamides are classified by their route of administration: systemic or topical. Systemic medications, such as sulfisoxazole (Gantrisin) and trimethoprim–sulfamethoxazole, are readily absorbed when given PO and excreted rapidly by the kidney. Other sulfonamides such as silver sulfadiazine (Silvadene) are used only for topical infections. The topical sulfonamides are rarely used because many patients are allergic to substances containing sulfur. One drug in this class, sulfadoxine–pyrimethamine (Fansidar), has an exceptionally long half-life and is occasionally prescribed for malarial prophylaxis.

In general, the sulfonamides are safe medications; however, some adverse effects may be serious. Adverse effects include the formation of crystals in the urine, allergic reactions, nausea, and vomiting. Although not common, potentially fatal blood abnormalities, such as aplastic anemia, acute hemolytic anemia, and agranulocytosis, can occur.

Urinary antiseptics are drugs given by the PO route for their antibacterial action in the urinary tract. The kidney concentrates the drugs; thus, their actions are specific to the urinary system. Urinary antiseptics reach therapeutic levels in the kidney tubules, and their anti-infective action continues as they travel to the urinary bladder. Although not considered first-line drugs for UTI, they serve important roles as secondary medications, especially in patients who present with infections resistant to TMP–SMZ or the fluoroquinolones.

A number of additional anti-infectives have distinct mechanisms of action and specific indications.

CORE CONCEPT 26.13

Some anti-infectives cannot be grouped into classes, or the class is too small to warrant separate discussion. That is not to diminish their importance in medicine; some of these miscellaneous anti-infectives are critical drugs for specific infections. For example, clindamycin (Cleocin) is sometimes the drug of choice for oral infections caused by *Bacteroides* species. It is considered to be appropriate treatment when less toxic alternatives are not effective. Vancomycin (Vancocin) is an antibiotic usually reserved for severe infections from gram-positive organisms such as *S. aureus* and *Streptococcus pneumoniae*. It is often used after bacteria have become resistant to other, safer antibiotics. Vancomycin is the most effective drug for treating MRSA infections.

Several miscellaneous drugs represent newer classes of antibiotics. Linezolid (Zyvox) is the first drug in a class called the oxazolidinones. This drug is effective against MRSA infections. Quinupristin–dalfopristin (Synercid) is a combination drug that is the first in an antibiotic class called streptogramins. This drug is primarily indicated for treatment of vancomycin-resistant *Enterococcus faecalis* infections. Daptomycin (Cubicin) is the first in a newer class of antibiotics called the cyclic lipopeptides. It is approved for the treatment of serious skin and skin-structure infections such as major abscesses, postsurgical skin-wound infections, and infected ulcers. Table 26.10 ◆ lists some of these miscellaneous antibiotics and their dosages.

Drug Prototype: 🅟 *Vancomycin (Vancocin)*
Therapeutic Class: **Antibiotic**   Pharmacologic Class: **Bacterial cell wall synthesis inhibitor**

Actions and Uses: Vancomycin is usually reserved for severe infections from gram-positive organisms such as *S. aureus* and *Streptococcus pneumoniae*. It is often used after bacteria have become resistant to other safer antibiotics. It is bacteriocidal, inhibiting bacterial cell wall synthesis. Because vancomycin was not used frequently during the first 30 years following its discovery, the incidence of vancomycin-resistant organisms is smaller than with other antibiotics. Vancomycin is the most effective drug for treating MRSA infections. Vancomycin-resistant strains of *S. aureus*, however, have begun to appear in recent years. Vancomycin is normally given IV because it is not absorbed from the GI tract.

Adverse Effects and Interactions: Frequent, minor side effects include flushing, hypotension, and rash on the upper body, sometimes called **red-man syndrome**. More serious adverse effects are possible with higher doses, including nephrotoxicity and ototoxicity. Some patients experience an acute allergic reaction and even anaphylaxis.

Vancomycin adds to toxicity of aminoglycosides, amphotericin B, cisplatin, cyclosporine, polymyxin B, and other ototoxic and nephrotoxic medications. Cholestyramine and colestipol can decrease the absorption of vancomycin.

TABLE 26.10 Miscellaneous Anti-infectives

Drug	Route and Adult Dose	Remarks
aztreonam (Azactam)	IM; 0.5–2 g bid–qid (max: 8 g/day)	Monobactam class; for gram-negative aerobic bacteria; IV form available
chloramphenicol	PO; 50 mg/kg qid	Broad spectrum; for typhoid fever and meningitis; IV form available
clindamycin (Cleocin)	PO; 150–450 mg qid	Bacteriostatic; effective against anaerobic organisms; topical, IM, and IV forms available
daptomycin (Cubicin)	IV; 4 mg/kg once every 24 hours for 7–14 days	Bacteriocidal; for serious skin infections
doripenem (Doribax)	IV; 500 mg every 8 hours for 5–14 days IV; 500 mg every 8 h for 5–14 days (max: 500 mg every 8 h)	Carbapenum class; newer drug approved for the treatment of serious abdominopelvic and skin infections, pneumonia, and complicated UTI
ertapenem (Invanz)	IV/IM: 1 g/day	Carbapenem class; very broad spectrum
imipenem-cilastatin (Primaxin)	IV; 250–500 mg tid–qid (max: 4 g/day)	Carbapenum class; combination drug; IM form available; one of the broadest spectrums of any anti-infective
lincomycin (Lincocin)	PO; 500 mg tid–qid (max: 8 g/day)	Bacteriostatic; effective against anaerobic organisms; IM form available
linezolid (Zyvox)	PO; 600 mg bid (max: 1,200 mg/day)	For vancomycin-resistant *Enterococcus*; IV form available
meropenem (Merrem IV)	IV; 1–2 g tid	Carbapenum class; for intra-abdominal infections, bacterial meningitis
metronidazole (Flagyl) (see page 427 for the Drug Prototype box)	PO; 7.5 mg/kg qid	For serious infections with anaerobic bacteria; also for protozoan infections; IV form available
quinupristin-dalfopristin (Synercid)	IV; 7.5 mg/kg infused over 50 minutes every 8 hours	Streptogamins class; for serious infections resistant to vancomycin
spectinomycin (Trobicin)	IM; 2 g as single dose	Bacteriostatic; for gonorrhea
telavancin (Vibativ)	IV; 10 mg/kg over 60 minutes for 24 hours	Approved for treatment of hospital-acquired pneumonia from gram-positive microbes
telithromycin (Ketek)	PO; 800 mg daily	Ketolide class; for community-acquired respiratory tract infections
(Pr) vancomycin (Vancocin)	IV; 500 mg qid–1 g bid	For *S.aureus*-resistant infections

Imipenem (Primaxin), ertapenem (Invanz), and meropenem (Merrem IV) belong to a newer class of antibiotics called *carbapenems*. These drugs are bacteriocidal and have some of the broadest antimicrobial spectrums of any class of antibiotics. Imipenem, the most widely prescribed drug in this small class, is administered in a fixed-dose combination with cilastatin, which increases the serum levels of the antibiotic. Meropenem is approved only for peritonitis and bacterial meningitis. Ertapenem is approved for the treatment of serious abdominopelvic and skin infections, community-acquired pneumonia, and complicated UTI. Diarrhea, nausea, rashes, and thrombophlebitis at injection sites are the most frequent adverse effects of the carbapenems.

NURSING PROCESS FOCUS | Patients Receiving Antibacterial Therapy

ASSESSMENT

Prior to administration:
■ Obtain a complete health history, including neurological, GI, renal and liver conditions, past infections, allergies, drug history, and possible drug interactions.
■ Acquire the results of a complete physical examination, including vital signs, height, weight, and any signs or symptoms of infection.
■ Evaluate laboratory blood findings: CBC, electrolytes, lipid panel, and renal and liver function studies.
■ Obtain specimens for C&S before initiating therapy.

POTENTIAL NURSING DIAGNOSES

■ *Infection* related to inadequate primary defenses
■ *Acute Pain* related to tissue damage secondary to infection
■ *Risk for Injury* related to tissue destruction and adverse effects of drug therapy
■ *Deficient Knowledge* related to a lack of information about disease process, transmission and drug therapy

NURSING PROCESS FOCUS *(continued)*

PLANNING: PATIENT GOALS AND EXPECTED OUTCOMES

The patient will:
- Experience therapeutic effects (reduction in symptoms related to the diagnosed infection).
- Be free from or experience minimal adverse effects from drug therapy.
- Verbalize an understanding of the drug's use, adverse effects, and required precautions.

IMPLEMENTATION

Interventions and (Rationales)	Patient Education/Discharge Planning
Monitor signs and symptoms of infection, including vital signs. (Monitoring of patient signs and symptoms is used to determine antibacterial effectiveness or worsening of infection. Another drug or different dosage may be required.)	Instruct the patient to notify the healthcare provider if there are changes in LOC, if the fever does not return to normal parameters (under 100 ºF), or if other symptoms persist or worsen.
Administer medication correctly and evaluate the patient's knowledge of proper administration, especially monitoring for compliance with antibiotic therapy. (Partial doses, skipped doses, and shortened length of treatment encourage the recurrence of infection or development of resistant organisms.)	Instruct the patient to: • Take the medication on schedule. • Complete the entire prescription even if feeling better to prevent development of resistant bacteria. • Follow-up with the healthcare provider after antibiotic therapy is completed.
If drug is being given intravenously, monitor the IV site for signs and symptoms of tissue irritation, severe pain, and extravasation.	Instruct the patient to immediately report pain or other symptoms of discomfort to the healthcare provider during intravenous infusion.
Monitor for hypersensitivity reaction. (Immediate hypersensitivity reaction may occur within 2–30 minutes; accelerated reaction occurs in 1–72 hours; and delayed reaction after 72 hours.)	Instruct the patient to discontinue the medication and inform the healthcare provider if symptoms of hypersensitivity reaction develop such as wheezing; shortness of breath; swelling of face, tongue, or hands; or itching or rash.
Monitor for severe diarrhea. (The condition may occur due to superinfection or the possible adverse effect of specific antibiotics.)	Instruct the patient to: • Report any diarrhea that increases in frequency or amount, or that contains mucus or blood, to the healthcare provider. • Consult the healthcare provider before taking antidiarrheal drugs, which could cause retention of harmful bacteria. • Consume cultured dairy products with live active cultures, such as kefir, yogurt, or buttermilk, to help maintain normal intestinal flora.
Monitor for superinfection, especially in elderly, debilitated, or immunosuppressed patients. (Increased risk for superinfections is due to elimination of normal flora.)	Instruct the patient to: • Report signs and symptoms of superinfection, such as fever; white patches in the mouth; itchy rash; loose, foul-smelling stools or whitish thick vaginal discharge to the healthcare provider. • Use infection control measures such as frequent hand washing.
Monitor intake of over-the-counter (OTC) products such as antacids, calcium supplements, iron products, and laxatives containing magnesium. (These products interfere with absorption of many antibiotics.)	Advise the patient to consult with the healthcare provider before using OTC medications or herbal products.
Monitor for photosensitivity and sensitivity of the skin to the sun. (Tetracyclines, fluoroquinolones, and sulfonamides can increase the patient's sensitivity to ultraviolet light and increase risk of sunburn.)	Encourage the patient to: • Avoid exposure to direct sunlight during and after therapy. • Wear protective clothing, sunglasses, and sunscreen when outdoors.
Determine the interactions of the prescribed antibiotics with various foods and beverages. (Many antibiotics are associated with significant GI effects. Food or milk may impair absorption of some antibiotics such as macrolides.)	Instruct the patient regarding foods and beverages that should be avoided with specific antibiotic therapies: • No acidic fruit juices with penicillins • No alcohol intake with cephalosporins • No dairy product/calcium products with tetracyclines
Monitor for other adverse effects specific to various antibiotic therapies. (See each Core Concept for each antibiotic classification in this chapter.)	Instruct the patient to report adverse effects specific to the antibiotic therapy prescribed.
Continue to monitor periodic laboratory work: CBC, liver and renal function studies, C & S, peak and trough drug levels as applicable and possibly a urinalysis. (Many antibiotics are renal or hepatic toxic. Periodic C & S are done to confirm effectiveness of therapy. Drug levels will be monitored with some drugs.)	Inform the patient: • About the importance and purpose of required laboratory tests. • To schedule follow-ups with the healthcare provider. • To help with renal function, increase fluid intake to 2,000–3,000 mL/day.
Monitor for symptoms of ototoxicity. (Some antibiotics, such as the aminoglycosides and vancomycin, may cause vestibular or auditory nerve damage.)	Instruct the patient to notify the healthcare provider of: • Changes in hearing, ringing in the ears, or full feeling in the ears. • Nausea and vomiting with motion, ataxia, nystagmus, or dizziness.
Monitor for symptoms of neurotoxicity. (Penicillins, cephalosporins, sulfonamides, aminoglycosides, and fluoroquinolones have an increased risk of neurotoxicity.)	Instruct the patient to notify the healthcare provider if dizziness, drowsiness, severe headache changes in LOC, or seizures occur.

EVALUATION OF OUTCOME CRITERIA

Evaluate the effectiveness of drug therapy by confirming that patient goals and expected outcomes have been met (see "Planning"). *See Tables 26.3 through 26.10 for lists of drugs to which these nursing actions apply.*

TUBERCULOSIS

TB is a highly contagious infection caused by the organism *Mycobacterium tuberculosis*. Although *M. tuberculosis* typically invades the lungs, it may travel to other body systems, particularly bone. The slow-growing mycobacteria activate cells of the immune response, which attempt to isolate the pathogens by creating a wall around them. The mycobacteria usually become dormant, lying inside cavities called **tubercles**. They may remain dormant during an entire lifetime, or they may become reactivated if the immune system becomes suppressed. When active, TB can be quite infectious, being spread by contaminated sputum. With the immune suppression characteristic of AIDS, the incidence of TB has greatly increased: As many as 20% of all patients with AIDS develop active TB.

Two other types of mycobacteria infect humans. *Mycobacterium leprae* is responsible for leprosy, a disease rarely seen in the United States and Canada. *M. leprae* is treated with multiple drugs, usually beginning with rifampin. *Mycobacterium avium* complex (MAC) causes an infection of the lungs, most commonly observed in patients with AIDS. The most effective drugs against MAC are the macrolides azithromycin (Zithromax) and clarithromycin (Biaxin).

CORE CONCEPT 26.14

The pharmacotherapy of tuberculosis requires special dosing regimens and schedules.

Drug therapy of TB differs from that of most other infections. Mycobacteria have a cell wall that is resistant to penetration by anti-infective drugs. For medications to reach the microorganisms isolated in the tubercles, therapy must continue for 6–12 months. Although the patient may not be infectious this entire time and have no symptoms, it is critical that therapy continue the entire period. Some patients develop multidrug-resistant infections and require therapy for as long as 24 months.

A second feature of the pharmacotherapy of TB is that at least two—and sometimes four or more—antibiotics must be administered concurrently. During the 6- to 12-month treatment period, different combinations of drugs may be used. Multidrug therapy is necessary because the mycobacteria grow slowly, and resistance is common. Using multiple drugs and switching the combinations during the long treatment period lowers the potential for resistance and increases therapeutic success. Although many different drug combinations are used, a typical regimen for patients with no complicating factors includes the following:

- *Initial phase* two months of daily therapy with isoniazid (INH), rifampin (Rifadin, Rimactane), pyrazinamide (PZA), and ethambutol (Myambutol). If laboratory test results show that the strain is sensitive to the first three drugs, ethambutol is dropped from the regimen.

- *Continuation phase* four months of therapy with isoniazid and rifampin, two to three times per week.

There are two broad categories of antitubercular drugs. One category consists of first-line drugs, which are safer and generally the most effective. Second-line medications, more toxic and less effective than the first-line drugs, are used when resistance develops. Table 26.11 ◆ lists the first-line drugs for therapy of TB.

Drug Prototype: 🅟 *Isoniazid (INH, Nydrazid)*
Therapeutic Class: Antituberculosis drug   **Pharmacologic Class: Mycolic acid inhibitor**

Actions and Uses: Isoniazid is a drug of choice for the treatment of *M. tuberculosis* because decades of experience have shown it to have a superior safety profile and to be the most effective single drug for the disease. Isoniazid acts by inhibiting the synthesis of mycolic acid, an essential cell wall component of mycobacteria. It is bacteriocidal for actively growing organisms but bacteriostatic for dormant mycobacteria. It is selective for *M. tuberculosis*. Isoniazid is used alone for chemoprophylaxis, or in combination with other antitubercular drugs for treating active disease.

Adverse Effects and Interactions: The most common adverse effects of isoniazid are numbness of the hands and feet, rash, and fever.

Aluminum-containing antacids should not be administered concurrently because they can decrease the absorption of isoniazid. When disulfiram is taken with INH, lack of coordination or psychotic reactions may result.

BLACK BOX WARNING:
Although rare, hepatotoxicity is a serious and sometimes fatal adverse effect; thus, the patient should be monitored carefully for jaundice, fatigue, elevated hepatic enzymes, or loss of appetite. Liver enzyme tests are usually performed monthly during therapy. Hepatotoxicity usually appears in the first 1–3 months of therapy but may occur at any time during treatment. Older adults and those with daily alcohol consumption are at greater risk of developing hepatotoxicity.

TABLE 26.11   First-Line Antitubercular Drugs

Drug	Route and Adult Dose	Remarks
ethambutol (Myambutol)	PO; 15–25 mg/kg daily	Used in combination with other antituberculars
(Pr) isoniazid (INH, Nydrazid)	PO; 15 mg/kg daily	Used in combination with other antituberculars; IM form available
pyrazinamide (PZA)	PO; 5–15 mg/kg tid–qid	Rifater is a fixed-dose combination of pyrazinamide with isoniazid and rifampin
rifabutin (Mycobutin)	PO; 300 mg once daily (for prophylaxis) or 5 mg/kg/day (for active TB) (max: 300 mg/day)	Very similar to rifampin and rifapentine
rifampin (Rifadin, Rimactane)	PO; 600 mg daily as a single dose or 900 mg twice weekly for 4 months	Used in combination with other antituberculars; IV form available; also for leprosy, *H. influenzae*, and meningococcus infections
rifapentine (Priftin)	PO; 600 mg twice a week for 2 months, then once a week for 4 months	Used in combination with other antituberculars

NURSING PROCESS FOCUS Patients Receiving Antitubercular Drugs

ASSESSMENT

Prior to administration:
- Obtain a complete health history, including respiratory, neurological, renal and liver conditions, allergies, drug history, past infections, and possible drug interactions.
- Evaluate laboratory blood findings: CBC, electrolytes, and renal and liver function studies.
- Acquire the results of a complete physical examination, including vital signs and any signs or symptoms of infection.
- Collect information on the presence or history of the following: positive tuberculin skin test, sputum culture, or smear; close contact with person recently infected with TB; HIV infection, or AIDS; immunosuppressant drug therapy; alcohol abuse; cognitive ability to comply with long-term therapy.

POTENTIAL NURSING DIAGNOSES

- *Infection* related to inadequate primary defenses, environmental exposure
- *Risk for Injury* related to tissue destruction and adverse effects of drug therapy
- *Fatigue* related to presence of infection; adverse effects of drug therapy
- *Deficient Knowledge* related to a lack of information about drug therapy
- *Noncompliance* related to adverse drug effects, deficient knowledge, length of treatment or cost of medication

PLANNING: PATIENT GOALS AND EXPECTED OUTCOMES

The patient will:
- Experience therapeutic effects (an absence or reduction in TB symptoms).
- Be free from or experience minimal adverse effects from drug therapy.
- Verbalize an understanding of the drug's use, adverse effects, and required precautions.

IMPLEMENTATION

Interventions and (Rationales)	Patient Education/Discharge Planning
- Administer medication correctly and evaluate the patient's knowledge of proper administration, especially monitoring the patient's ability and motivation to comply with therapeutic regimen. (Treatment must continue for the full-length of therapy to eliminate all *M. tuberculosis* organisms.)	Explain the importance of complying with the entire therapeutic plan, including: - Taking all medications as directed by the healthcare provider. - Not discontinuing medication until so instructed. - Wearing a medical alert bracelet. - Keeping all appointments for follow-up care.
- Monitor for hepatic adverse effects. (Antituberculosis drugs, such as isoniazid and rifampin, cause hepatic impairment.)	- Instruct the patient to report yellow eyes and skin, loss of appetite, dark urine, and unusual tiredness.

continued . . .

Interventions and (Rationales)	Patient Education/Discharge Planning
■ Monitor for neurologic adverse effects such as numbness and tingling of the extremities. (Antituberculosis drugs, such as isoniazid, cause peripheral neuropathy and depletion of vitamin B_6.)	Instruct the patient to: ■ Report numbness and tingling of extremities. ■ Take supplemental vitamin B_6 as ordered to reduce risk of adverse effects.
■ Monitor for dietary compliance when patient is taking isoniazid. (Foods high in tyramine can interact with the drug and cause palpitations, flushing, and hypertension.)	■ Advise patients taking isoniazid to avoid foods containing tyramine, such as aged cheese, smoked and pickled fish, beer and red wine, bananas, and chocolate.
■ Monitor for other adverse effects specific to various antituberculosis drugs.	Instruct the patient to report to the healthcare provider any adverse effects specific to the antituberculosis therapy prescribed, such as: ■ Blurred vision or changes in color or vision field (ethambutol). ■ Difficulty in voiding (pyrazinamide). ■ Fever, yellowing of skin, weakness, dark urine (isoniazid, rifampin). ■ GI system disturbances (rifampin). ■ Changes in hearing (streptomycin). ■ Numbness and tingling of extremities (isoniazid). ■ Red discoloration of body fluids (rifampin). ■ Dark concentrated urine, weight gain, edema (streptomycin).
■ Establish therapeutic environment to ensure adequate rest, nutrition, hydration, and relaxation. (Symptoms of TB are manifested when the immune system is suppressed.)	Instruct the patient: ■ About infection control measures, such as frequent handwashing, covering the mouth when coughing or sneezing, and proper disposal of soiled tissues. ■ To incorporate health-enhancing activities, such as adequate rest and sleep, intake of essential vitamins and nutrients, and intake of six to eight glasses of water/day.
■ Collect sputum specimens as directed by the healthcare provider. (This will determine the effectiveness of the antituberculosis drug.)	■ Instruct the patient in technique needed to collect a quality sputum specimen.

EVALUATION OF OUTCOME CRITERIA

Evaluate the effectiveness of drug therapy by confirming that patient goals and expected outcomes have been met (see "Planning"). *See Table 26.11 for a list of drugs to which these nursing actions apply.*

A third feature of anti-TB therapy is that drugs are used extensively for *preventing* the disease in addition to treating it. Chemoprophylaxis is common for close contacts or family members of patients recently infected with TB. Therapy usually begins immediately after a patient receives a positive tuberculin test. Patients with immunosuppression, such as those with AIDS or those receiving immunosuppressant drugs, may receive preventive treatment with anti-TB drugs. A short-term therapy of two months, consisting of a combination treatment with isoniazid and pyrazinamide, is approved for TB prophylaxis in patients positive for HIV.

Treatment guidelines strongly recommend that **directly observed therapy (DOT)** be used in the treatment of TB (CDC, 2010). DOT means that a healthcare worker or other trained individual administer the medications and watch the patient swallow the dose. This ensures that the medication is taken exactly as prescribed and decreases the risk for relapse, limits the spread of the infection in the community, and reduces the development of drug resistance that could result from erratic or partial treatment.

Concept Review **26.3**

■ How does drug therapy of TB differ from that of conventional anti-infective chemotherapy? What are the rationales for these differences?

PATIENTS NEED TO KNOW

Patients treated for bacterial infections need to know the following:

In General

1. Take the entire prescription of anti-infective medication exactly as directed because partial doses, skipped doses, and shortened length of treatment encourage the development of resistant organisms.
2. Some antibiotics may cause GI upset. If this occurs, take the drug with food or milk as directed. Check prescription label for specific directions.
3. Eating active-culture yogurt or buttermilk may decrease the risks for diarrhea and vaginitis associated with antibiotic destruction of normal flora.
4. Antibiotics are most effective if taken around the clock, rather than just during normal waking hours.

Regarding Penicillins

5. It may be necessary to stay in the office for at least 30 minutes after receiving an injection of penicillin so the healthcare providers can monitor for possible allergic reactions.
6. Avoid intake of caffeinated beverages, citrus fruits, and fruit juices for at least one hour before and two hours after taking oral penicillin to maximize the drug's absorption.

Regarding Sulfonamides and Tetracyclines

7. Take oral cephalosporins and oral lincomycin with food, and oral sulfonamides with food or milk, to decrease GI upset. Drink a glass of water with each dose of sulfonamide, tetracycline, lincomycin, or fluoroquinolone, and drink a total of 2–3 L of fluid a day.
8. Avoid sun/tanning exposure while taking sulfonamides and tetracyclines because these drugs cause photosensitivity.
9. Antacids, dairy products, iron, baking soda, and kaolin-pectin bind and inactivate tetracycline. Separate intake by two to three hours for full antibiotic effectiveness.
10. Sulfonamides, tetracycline, and other antibiotics may interfere with the effectiveness of oral contraceptives. Ask a healthcare provider about the advisability of using an additional form of contraception.

SAFETY ALERT

Allergic Reactions and Antibiotics

After receiving the medication her first dose of levofloxacin (Levaquin), Mrs. Jones reported itching and a slight swelling of the tongue and lips (angioedema). However, later that day she had no discomfort or presence of the previous symptoms. Prior to the initial administration of the drug, the nurse checked Mrs. Jones' chart for the presence of allergies, but it is imperative that the nurse now monitor her for an allergic reaction. Hypersensitivity reactions can worsen with each exposure to an antigen (the antibiotic). The next dose could cause a life-threatening anaphylactic response.

CHAPTER REVIEW

CORE CONCEPTS SUMMARY

26.1 Pathogens are organisms that cause disease by invading tissues or secreting toxins.

Pathogens can overwhelm natural immune defenses by growing extremely rapidly and invading normal tissues or by producing potent toxins. Bacteria are classified on the basis of their staining ability and structural and functional characteristics.

26.2 Anti-infective drugs are classified by their chemical structures or by their mechanisms of action.

Because of the large number of anti-infectives available, it is advantageous for the student to understand how to classify these drugs because medications in the same class exhibit similar pharmacologic activity. Anti-infective drugs are classified based on similarities in their chemical structures or by their mechanisms of action.

26.3 Anti-infective drugs act by selectively targeting a pathogen's metabolism or life cycle.

Bacteria multiply rapidly, and drugs have been designed to take advantage of this characteristic. Anti-infectives may be bacteriocidal or bacteriostatic, or both, depending on the organism and dose.

26.4   Acquired resistance is a major clinical problem that is worsened by improper use of anti-infectives.

Errors during replication result in random mutations of the bacterial DNA. Although rare, an occasional mutation may confer antibiotic resistance to a bacterium. Therapy with antibiotics kills the affected bacteria, leaving the resistant ones to multiply and spread within the patient. To limit this problem, antibiotics should be prescribed only when medically necessary.

26.5   Careful selection of the correct antibiotic is essential for effective pharmacotherapy and to limit adverse effects.

Culture and sensitivity tests are used to identify the type of bacteria present and determine which antibiotics are most effective. Until test results are obtained, the patient may be started on a broad-spectrum antibiotic. Because broad-spectrum drugs are more likely to affect the patient's normal flora, a narrow-spectrum drug may be prescribed after the organism is identified.

26.6   The penicillins are one of the oldest and safest groups of anti-infectives.

Penicillins have been widely used because of their high margin of safety and effectiveness. Some patients are allergic to this class of drugs, and many bacterial species have become resistant to penicillins, thus limiting their use.

26.7   The cephalosporins are similar in structure and function to the penicillins and are one of the most widely prescribed anti-infective classes.

The cephalosporins consist of a large class of antibiotics, classified by generation, that are considered alternatives to penicillin. In general, they are used for serious gram-negative infections and for patients who are resistant to or cannot tolerate the penicillins.

26.8   The tetracyclines have broad spectrums but are drugs of choice for few diseases.

The tetracyclines have a broader spectrum of action and produce more adverse effects than the penicillins. Their use is limited to a small number of diseases such as Rocky Mountain spotted fever, typhus, cholera, Lyme disease, and chlamydial infections.

26.9   The macrolides are safe alternatives to penicillin for many infections.

The macrolides are generally prescribed when a patient is allergic to penicillin or has a penicillin-resistant infection. They produce few adverse effects.

26.10   The aminoglycosides are narrow-spectrum drugs that have the potential to cause serious toxicity.

The aminoglycosides are usually reserved for severe gram-negative infections of the urinary tract because they have the potential to cause serious adverse effects. Most of them are poorly absorbed from the GI tract and must be given parenterally.

26.11   Fluoroquinolones have wide clinical applications because of their broad spectrum of activity and relative safety.

Although fluoroquinolones are an older class of antibacterials, newer drugs in this class have been developed to greatly expand their use. They are effective oral alternatives to other antibiotics for both gram-negative and gram-positive organisms. Ciprofloxacin (Cipro) is one of the few drugs approved for the treatment of anthrax.

26.12   Sulfonamides and urinary antiseptics are traditional drugs for urinary tract infections.

In the 1930s, the sulfonamides revolutionized the treatment of infectious disease. Present-day use of these medications is limited by bacterial resistance. The fixed combination of trimethoprim–sulfamethoxazole (Bactrim, Septra) is an important drug in the pharmacotherapy of UTIs.

26.13   A number of additional anti-infectives have distinct mechanisms of action and specific indications.

A number of important antibiotics do not belong to any of the previous classes. The streptogramins and oxazolidinones are small groups of drugs having specific applications. Vancomycin is known as the "last chance" antibiotic for use when resistance has developed to most other anti-infectives.

26.14   The pharmacotherapy of tuberculosis requires special dosing regimens and schedules.

Drug therapy of TB involves taking multiple drugs for prolonged periods. Patients exhibiting a new, positive TB test are often given these drugs prophylactically, even if no signs of the disease are apparent.

REVIEW QUESTIONS

The following questions are written in NCLEX-PN® style. Answer these questions to assess your knowledge of the chapter material, and go back and review any material that is not clear to you.

1. The patient is taking amoxicillin (Amoxil). Which of the following statements by the patient demonstrates that she needs additional instruction?

1. "I will take this medication until it is gone."
2. "I will call my doctor if I develop a fever or a rash."
3. "Before I take my medication, I will avoid orange juice."
4. "I will take the medication until I feel better."

2. Before administering cefotaxime (Claforan), the nurse checks for a previous allergic reaction to:

1. Yeasts
2. Penicillins
3. Sulfonamides
4. Macrolides

3. When assisting with the development of a patient care plan, the nurse needs to include what information about tetracyclines?

1. To take it with food or milk
2. They are safe for use during pregnancy
3. To take it one to two hours before or after meals
4. That it has no adverse effects

4. The nurse monitors the patient on aminoglycosides for:

1. Nephrotoxicity
2. Hepatic failure
3. Superinfection
4. Hypertension and rash

5. A nurse is instructing a patient about ciprofloxin (Cipro). The nurse tells him that if this antibiotic is taken with antacids, absorption is:

1. Increased
2. Decreased
3. Not affected
4. Delayed

6. A patient has been diagnosed with MRSA and is prescribed vancomycin. While the patient is on this medication, what information should be provided to the patient about possible adverse effects?

1. Vancomycin may cause flushing.
2. Adverse effects are infrequent.
3. Vacomycin does not cause rashes.
4. During therapy, hypertension may occur.

7. The patient with tuberculosis is now on isoniazid (INH). Which laboratory test should the nurse monitor?

1. PT and PTT
2. CBC
3. BUN
4. Liver enzymes

8. The nurse tells the patient that the most common adverse effects of penicillin G include(s): (Select all that apply)

1. Diarrhea
2. Nausea and vomiting
3. Pain at the injection site
4. Rash

9. A patient at a rehabilitation center is prescribed erythromycin. The nurse is reviewing the patient's medication list, checking to see if there are medications that should not be taken with this antibiotic. One medication is found. What medication should not be taken with erythromycin?

1. Lisinopril
2. Ibuprofen
3. Lasix
4. Lovastatin

10. A patient is to receive Cipro 500 mg po four times a day, for a week. The pharmacy sends Cipro 250 mg tablets. How many tablet(s) will the patient receive in 24 hours?

1. Two tablets
2. Four tablets
3. Six tablets
4. Eight tablets

CASE STUDY QUESTIONS

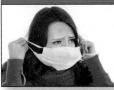

Remember Ms. Jackson, the patient introduced at the beginning of the chapter? Now read the remainder of the case study. Based on the information you have learned in this chapter, answer the questions that follow.

Ms. Shelly Jackson is a new patient at your clinic. Six months ago, she had a kidney transplant and is taking immunosuppressant drugs. Recently, she has been experiencing repeated bacterial infections due to resistant strains and has been switched to different antibiotics throughout the past six months. The physician suspects a kidney infection.

1. Ms. Jackson is admitted to the hospital and is administered gentamicin 300 mg daily by IV infusion. The nurse monitors which of the following tests?

1. Input and output ratio
2. Serum transaminase levels
3. Visual acuity tests
4. Fasting blood glucose levels

2. When speaking with Ms. Jackson about gentamicin, the nurse tells her that gentamicin can cause:

1. Anemia
2. Hearing impairment
3. Nausea and vomiting
4. Liver failure

3. Ms. Jackson is showing signs of hearing loss due to gentamicin therapy and the physician is going to switch her antibiotic. The nurse anticipates which of the following medications being ordered?

1. Sulfacetamide (Klaron)
2. Silver sulfadiazine
3. Trimethoprim–sulfamethoxazole (Septra)
4. Vancomycin (Vancocin)

4. The nurse is educating Ms. Jackson about the adverse effects of sulfonamides and tells her that this includes: (Select all that apply.)

1. Increased sensitivity of skin to sunlight
2. Liver failure
3. Nausea and vomiting
4. Hypotension

NOTE: Answers to the Review and Case Study Questions appear in Appendix B. The complete rationales and answers are located on the textbook's website.

"I'm at the office for my annual checkup. If it's not one thing it's another. Earlier in the year, I had pneumonia. Now I'm having problems with itching and discharge."

Mrs. Martha Davis, 70-year-old retired auto worker

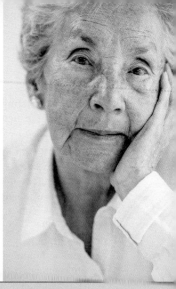

27 Drugs for Fungal, Viral, and Parasitic Diseases

CORE CONCEPTS

27.1 Fungal infections are classified as superficial or systemic.

27.2 Systemic antifungal drugs are used for serious infections of internal organs.

27.3 Superficial infections of the skin, nails, and mucous membranes are effectively treated with topical and oral antifungal drugs.

27.4 Viruses are infectious agents that require a host to replicate.

27.5 Antiretroviral drugs do not cure HIV-AIDS, but they do help many patients live longer.

27.6 Antiviral drugs are available to treat herpes simplex, influenza, and viral hepatitis infections.

27.7 Infections caused by helminths and protozoans cause significant disease worldwide.

DRUG SNAPSHOT

The following drugs are discussed in this chapter:

DRUG CLASSES	DRUG PROTOTYPES
Antifungal drugs for systemic infections	**Pr** amphotericin B (AmBisome, Fungizone, others) *416*
Antifungal drugs for superficial infections	**Pr** nystatin (Mycostatin, Nystop, others) *416*
Antiretroviral drugs for HIV-AIDS	**Pr** zidovudine (AZT, Retrovir) *421*
Antiviral drugs for herpes simplex and influenza	**Pr** acyclovir (Zovirax) *425*
Antiprotozoans and antihelminthics	**Pr** metronidazole (Flagyl) *427*

LEARNING OUTCOMES

After reading this chapter, the student should be able to:

1. Compare and contrast the pharmacotherapy of superficial and systemic fungal infections.

2. Identify the types of patients most likely to acquire serious fungal infections.

3. Describe the basic structure of a virus.

4. Identify specific viral infections that benefit from pharmacotherapy.

5. Explain the purpose and expected outcomes of HIV pharmacotherapy.

6. Define HAART, and explain why it is commonly used in the pharmacotherapy of HIV infection.

7. Identify protozoan and helminth infections that may benefit from pharmacotherapy.

8. Categorize drugs used in the treatment of fungal, viral, protozoan, and helminth infections based on their classifications and mechanisms of action.

9. For each of the classes listed in the Drug Snapshot, identify representative drugs and explain their mechanisms of drug action, primary actions, and important adverse effects.

KEY TERMS

antiretroviral (an-tie-RET-roh-veye-ral) *420*

capsid (CAP-sid) *417*

dysentery (DISS-en-tare-ee) *426*

fungi (FUN-jeye) *413*

helminths (HELL-minthz) *427*

highly active antiretroviral therapy (HAART) *420*

host *418*

influenza (in-flew-EN-zah) *424*

intracellular parasites *418*

malaria (mah-LARE-ee-ah) *426*

mycoses (my-KOH-sees) *413*

protozoans (PRO-toh-ZOH-enz) *425*

reverse transcriptase (ree-VERS trans-CRIP-tace) *420*

superficial mycoses *413*

systemic mycoses *414*

viruses *417*

yeasts (YEESTz) *413*

F ungi, protozoans, and multicellular parasites are exceedingly more complex than bacteria. Most antibacterial drugs are ineffective against these organisms because their structure and biochemistry are so different from that of bacteria. Although there are fewer medications to treat these diseases, the available medications are usually effective.

Viruses, on the other hand, are nonliving particles that infect by entering a host cell and using the host's internal machinery to replicate itself. Antiviral drugs are the least effective of all the anti-infective classes. Although the number of antiviral medications has increased dramatically in recent years, they are relatively ineffective at preventing or treating viral infections.

ANTIFUNGAL DRUGS

Fungal infections are classified as superficial or systemic.

CORE CONCEPT **27.1**

Fungi are single-celled or multicellular organisms that are much more complex than bacteria. Several species of fungi grow on skin and mucosal surfaces and are part of the normal host flora. The human body is remarkably resistant to infection by these organisms; people with healthy immune systems rarely experience serious fungal diseases. Those with a weakened immune system, however, such as patients infected with HIV, may acquire frequent fungal infections, some of which may require intensive drug therapy.

Fungal infections are called **mycoses**. Most exposure to pathogenic fungi occurs through inhalation of fungal spores or by handling contaminated soil. Thus, many fungal infections involve the respiratory tract, skin, hair, and nails. An additional common source of fungal infections, especially of the mouth or vagina, is overgrowth of normal host flora. **Yeasts**, which include the common pathogen *Candida albicans*, are single-celled fungi. Table 27.1 ◆ lists the most common fungal pathogens.

myc = *fungus*
oses = *conditions*

A simple and useful method of classifying fungal infections is to consider them as either superficial or systemic. **Superficial mycoses** typically affect the scalp, skin, nails, and mucous membranes such as the oral cavity and vagina. Mycoses of this type are often treated with topical drugs because the incidence of adverse effects is much lower by using this route of administration.

Fast Facts Fungal, Viral, and Parasitic Diseases

- Ninety percent of human fungal infections are caused by just a few dozen species.

- Of all human fungal infections, 86% are caused by *Candida albicans*. The second most common, about one to two cases per 100,000 people is caused by *Aspergillus*.

- About one of every six Americans age 14–49 years are infected with genital herpes.

- More than 1.1 million Americans are currently living with HIV infections; about 49,000 new infections occur each year.

- Approximately 63% of new HIV infections occur in men, with the largest risk category being men who have sex with other men.

- Of the new HIV infections in women, 84% are acquired through heterosexual contact.

- Since the beginning of the AIDS epidemic, more than 636,000 Americans have died of AIDS.

- About 219 million cases of malaria occur worldwide each year; about 1,500 travelers develop malaria abroad and return to the United States with the infection.

TABLE 27.1	Fungal Pathogens
Name of Fungus	**Disease and Primary Organ System**
SYSTEMIC	
Aspergillus fumigatus and others	Aspergillosis: opportunistic; most commonly affects the lungs but can spread to other organs
Blastomyces dermatitidis	Blastomycosis: begins in the lungs and spreads to other organs
Candida albicans and others	Candidiasis: most common opportunistic fungal infection; may occur in mucous membranes and nearly any organ
Coccidioides immitis	Coccidioidomycosis: begins in the lungs and spreads to the skin and other organs
Cryptococcus neoformans	Cryptococcosis: opportunistic; begins in the lungs but is the most common cause of meningitis in patients with AIDS
Histoplasma capsulatum	Histoplasmosis: begins in the lungs and spreads to other organs
Pneumocystis jiroveci	Pneumocystis pneumonia: opportunistic; primarily causes pneumonia but can spread to other organs
SUPERFICIAL	
Candida albicans and others	Candidiasis: affects the skin, nails, oral cavity (thrush), vagina
Epidermophyton floccosum	Athlete's foot (tinea pedis), jock itch (tinea cruris), and other skin disorders
Microsporum species	Ringworm of the scalp (tinea capitus)
Sporothrix schenckii	Sporotrichosis: affects primarily the skin and superficial lymph nodes
Trichophyton species	Affects the scalp, skin, and nails

Systemic mycoses are those affecting internal organs, typically the lungs, brain, and digestive organs. Although much less common than superficial mycoses, systemic fungal infections often affect multiple body systems and are sometimes fatal to patients with suppressed immune systems. Mycoses of this type require aggressive oral or parenteral medications that produce more adverse effects than the topical drugs.

CORE CONCEPT 27.2

Systemic antifungal drugs are used for serious infections of internal organs.

Systemic or invasive fungal infections require intensive pharmacotherapy for extended periods. Amphotericin B and fluconazole are the most frequently prescribed drugs for these types of infections. Table 27.2 ◆ lists the primary antifungal drugs.

Serious opportunistic fungal disease can occur in patients whose immune systems are compromised, such as those with HIV-AIDS. Others who may experience systemic infections include patients receiving prolonged therapy with corticosteroids (see Chapter 24 and Chapter 32), those with extensive burns, those receiving antineoplastic drugs (see Chapter 28), and those who have recently received organ transplants (see Chapter 25). Pharmacotherapy of systemic mycoses may continue for several months to ensure complete removal of the pathogen.

Amphotericin B (AmBisome, Fungizone, others) has been the gold standard for treating systemic fungal infections since the 1960s. However, the newer *azole* drugs such as fluconazole (Diflucan) and itraconazole (Sporanox) are safer and have become preferred drugs for the treatment of some systemic infections. Ketoconazole has also become a preferred drug for less severe systemic mycoses or for the prophylaxis of fungal infections. The azole drugs have a spectrum of activity similar to that of amphotericin B, are considerably less toxic, and have the major advantage that they can be administered orally. Several are available for both superficial and systemic mycoses.

Several other antifungals are available as treatment options for systemic mycoses. These include caspofungin (Cancidas) for aspergillosis and anidulafungin (Eraxis) and micafungin (Mycamine) for invasive candidiasis. These drugs are usually prescribed when amphotericin B and the systemic azoles have failed to produce an adequate response.

Concept Review 27.1

■ Why has the number of antifungal and antiviral drugs increased significantly over the past 20 years?

TABLE 27.2   Selected Antifungal Drugs

Drug	Route and Adult Dose	Remarks
Pr amphotericin B (AmBisome, Fungizone, others)	IV; 0.3–1.5 mg/kg/day, infused over 2–4 hours (max: 1.5 mg/kg/day)	Cream, lotion, and PO suspension forms available for topical mycoses; must infuse a test dose first; has potential for severe adverse effects
butenafine (Mentax)	Topical; apply daily for 4 weeks	For athlete's foot
anidulafungin (Eraxis)	IV; Loading dose 100 mg on day 1 followed by 50 mg/day	Newer drug for advanced *Candida* infections
caspofungin acetate (Cancidas)	IV; 70 mg infused over 1 hour on day 1, followed by 50 mg infused over 1 hour qid for 30 days	Newer drug for invasive *Candida* and *Aspergillus* infections
ciclopirox cream, gel, shampoo (Loprox) or nail lacquer (Penlac)	Topical; apply bid for 4 weeks	For skin and nail mycoses
flucytosine (Ancobon)	PO; 50–150 mg/kg in divided doses	For severe systemic infections such as candidiasis or cryptococcosis; IV form available
griseofulvin (Fulvicin)	PO; 500 mg microsize or 330–375 mg ultramicrosize daily	For ringworm and other skin and nail infections
micafungin (Mycamine)	IV; 50–150 mg/kg/day	Newer drug for advanced *Candida* infections
naftifine (Naftin)	Topical; apply cream daily or gel bid for 4 weeks	For skin mycoses
Pr nystatin (Mycostatin, Nystop, others)	PO; 500,000–1,000,000 units tid	For candidiasis; vaginal tablet form available
terbinafine (Lamisil)	Topical; apply daily or bid for 7 weeks; PO; 250 mg daily for 6–13 weeks	For skin and nail mycoses
tolnaftate (Aftate, Tinactin)	Topical; apply bid for 4–6 weeks	For skin mycoses, ringworm, athlete's foot
undecylenic acid (Fungi-Nail, Gordochom)	Topical; apply once or twice daily	For athlete's foot, diaper rash
AZOLE ANTIFUNGALS		
butoconazole (Femstat, Gynazole)	Topical; one applicator intravaginally at bedtime for 3 days	For vaginal mycoses
clotrimazole (Gyne-Lotrimin, Mycelex,)	Topical; for skin mycoses apply bid for 4 weeks; for vaginal mycoses, insert one applicatorful intravaginally at bedtime for 7 days	For vaginal and skin mycoses, athlete's foot, and candidiasis; oral troche also available for oral candidiasis
econazole (Spectazole)	Topical; apply bid for 4 weeks	For skin mycoses
fluconazole (Diflucan)	PO; 200–400 mg on day 1, then 100–200 mg daily for 2–4 weeks	For both systemic and superficial mycoses; IV form available for severe mycoses
itraconazole (Sporanox)	PO; 200 mg daily; may increase to 200 mg bid (max: 400 mg/day)	For severe systemic lung mycoses and superficial nail mycoses
ketoconazole (Nizoral)	PO; 200–400 mg daily	For severe systemic mycoses; topical form available for superficial mycoses
miconazole (Micatin, Monistat-3)	Topical; apply bid for 2–4 weeks	For vaginal and skin mycoses; also available as vaginal suppositories and tampons
oxiconazole (Oxistat)	Topical; apply daily in the evening for 2 months	For skin mycoses
posaconazole (Noxafil)	PO; 100–200 mg tid	Newer azole; for prevention of invasive *Aspergillus* and *Candida* infections
sertaconazole (Ertaczo)	Topical; 2% cream bid for 4 weeks	For tinea pedis
sulconazole (Exelderm)	Topical; apply once or twice daily for 2–6 weeks	Newer azole for skin infections
terconazole (Terazol)	Topical; insert one applicator intravaginally at bedtime for 3–7 days	For vulvovaginal candidiasis; vaginal suppository form available
tioconazole (Vagistat)	Topical; insert one applicator intravaginally at bedtime for 1 day	For vulvovaginal candidiasis
voriconazole (Vfend)	IV; 6 mg/kg every 12 hours on day 1, then 3–4 mg/kg every 12 hours	For systemic aspergillosis and esophageal candidiasis; oral form available

Drug Prototype 🅟 *Amphotericin B (AmBisome, Fungizone, Others)*
Therapeutic Class: **Antifungal (systemic type)**   Pharmacologic Class: **Polyene**

Actions and Uses: Amphotericin B has a wide spectrum of activity and is effective against most of the fungi pathogenic to humans; thus, it is a preferred drug for many severe systemic mycoses. It acts by binding to fungal cell membranes and causing them to become permeable or leaky. Because amphotericin B is not absorbed from the gastrointestinal (GI) tract, it is normally given by IV infusion. Topical preparations are available for superficial mycoses. Several months of pharmacotherapy may be required for a complete cure. Unlike antibiotics, resistance to amphotericin B is not common.

To reduce the toxicity of amphotericin B, the original drug molecule has been formulated with several lipid molecules. These include liposomal amphotericin B (AmBisome), amphotericin B lipid complex (Abelcet), and amphotericin B cholesteryl sulfate complex (Amphotec). These newer forms are very expensive and usually reserved for serious fungal infections.

Adverse Effects and Interactions: Amphotericin B can cause a number of serious adverse effects. Many patients develop fever and chills at the beginning of therapy, which subside as treatment continues. Phlebitis, or inflammation of the veins, is common during IV therapy. Some degree of nephrotoxicity is observed in most patients, and laboratory tests of kidney function are normally performed throughout the treatment period.

Amphotericin B interacts with many drugs. For example, therapy with aminoglycosides, vancomycin, carboplatin, and furosemide, which reduce renal function, is not recommended. Use with corticosteroids, skeletal muscle relaxants, and thiazole may cause hypokalemia. Use with digoxin increases the risk of digoxin toxicity in patients with preexisting hypokalemia.

CORE CONCEPT 27.3

Superficial infections of the skin, nails, and mucous membranes are effectively treated with topical and oral antifungal drugs.

Superficial fungal infections of the hair, scalp, nails, and the mucous membranes of the mouth and vagina are rarely medical emergencies. Infections of the nails and skin, for example, may be ongoing for months or even years before a patient seeks treatment. Unlike systemic fungal infections, superficial infections may occur in any patient, not just those who have suppressed immune systems.

Antifungal medications applied topically are much safer than their systemic counterparts because only small amounts are absorbed into the circulation. Many are available as over-the-counter (OTC) creams, gels, solutions, and ointments. Although a fungal infection may be diagnosed as superficial, oral antifungal drugs are occasionally prescribed along with topical medications to be certain that the infection is completely eliminated from the deeper skin layers. The length of pharmacotherapy varies widely among the different types of superficial mycoses. Vaginal infections are sometimes treated successfully with a single vaginal tablet of clotrimazole, whereas nail mycoses may require several months of therapy with itraconazole or terbinafine.

Adverse effects from topical antifungal therapy are generally minor. If applied to the skin, irritation, redness, and itching may be experienced. Vaginal administration may result in burning, itching, or irritation. Antifungal drugs should not be applied to open sores or severely abraded skin because this may result in undesirable absorption of the drug and additional adverse effects. When applying topical antifungal medication, gloves should be worn to prevent transmission.

Drug Prototype 🅟 *Nystatin (Mycostatin, Nystop, Others)*
Therapeutic Class: **Topical antifungal**   Pharmacologic Class: **Polyene**

Actions and Uses: Although it belongs to the same chemical class as amphotericin B, nystatin is available in a wider variety of formulations, including cream, ointment, powder, tablets, and lozenges. It is used as a topical drug against *Candida* infections of the vagina, skin, and mouth. It may also be used orally to treat candidiasis of the intestine because it travels through the GI tract without being absorbed. In topical forms, nystatin is often combined with triamcinolone, a corticosteroid that helps to reduce inflammation.

Adverse Effects and Interactions: When given topically, nystatin produces few adverse effects other than minor skin irritation. When given orally, it may cause diarrhea, nausea, and vomiting.

NURSING PROCESS FOCUS   Patients Receiving Superficial Antifungal Therapy

ASSESSMENT	POTENTIAL NURSING DIAGNOSES
Prior to administration: ■ Obtain a complete health history, including skin, GI, renal and liver conditions, past infections, allergies, drug history, and possible drug interactions. ■ Acquire the results of a complete physical examination, including vital signs and any signs or symptoms of infection. ■ Evaluate laboratory blood findings: CBC, electrolytes, and renal and liver function studies.	■ *Acute Pain* related to tissue damage secondary to infection ■ *Risk for Injury* related to adverse effect of drug therapy ■ *Deficient Knowledge* related to a lack of information about drug therapy ■ *Impaired Skin Integrity* related to tissue damage and adverse effects of drug therapy

PLANNING: PATIENT GOALS AND EXPECTED OUTCOMES

The patient will:
■ Experience therapeutic effects (healing of fungal infection).
■ Be free from or experience minimal adverse effects from drug therapy.
■ Verbalize an understanding of the drug's use, adverse effects, and required precautions.

IMPLEMENTATION

Interventions and (Rationales)	Patient Education/Discharge Planning
■ Administer oral medication correctly and evaluate the patient's knowledge of proper administration. (Proper administration increases medication effectiveness.)	Instruct the patient to: ■ Complete all medication as prescribed. ■ Swish the oral suspension to coat all mucous membranes, and then swallow the medication. ■ Spit out the medication instead of swallowing if GI irritation occurs. ■ Allow troche to dissolve completely, rather than chewing or swallowing; it may take 30 minutes for it to dissolve completely. ■ Avoid food or drink for 30 minutes following administration. ■ Remove dentures prior to using the oral suspension. ■ Take ketoconazole with water, fruit juice, coffee, or tea to enhance dissolution and absorption.
■ Administer topical medication correctly and evaluate the patient's knowledge of proper administration. (Proper administration increases medication effectiveness.)	Instruct the patient to: ■ Use gloves when applying medication. ■ Avoid wearing tight-fitting undergarments if using ointment in the vaginal or groin area. ■ Avoid occlusive dressings. (Dressings increase moisture in the infected areas and encourage development of additional yeast infections.)
■ Monitor for possible adverse effects or hypersensitivity.	Instruct the patient to report any of the following to the healthcare provider: ■ Burning, stinging, dryness, itching, erythema, urticaria, angioedema, and local irritation (for superficial drugs). ■ Symptoms of hepatic toxicity—jaundice, dark urine, light-colored stools, and pruritus. ■ Nausea, vomiting, and diarrhea. ■ Signs and symptoms of hypo- or hyperglycemia.
■ Monitor for contact dermatitis with topical formulations. (This is related to the preservatives found in many of the formulations.)	■ Instruct the patient to report any redness or skin rash.
■ Encourage infection control practices. Ensure that the patient, family members, and other visitors also practice infection control techniques such as handwashing and avoiding the affected area (to prevent the spread of infection).	Instruct the patient to: ■ Clean the affected area daily. ■ Apply medication while wearing a glove. ■ Wash hands properly before and after application. ■ Change socks daily if rash is on the feet. ■ Avoid sharing personal care items with family members/guests.

EVALUATION OF OUTCOME CRITERIA

Evaluate the effectiveness of drug therapy by confirming that patient goals and expected outcomes have been met (see "Planning"). *See Table 27.2 for a list of drugs to which these nursing actions apply.*

ANTIVIRAL DRUGS

Viruses are infectious agents that require a host to replicate.

CORE CONCEPT 27.4

Viruses are nonliving agents that infect bacteria, plants, and animals. Viruses contain none of the vital organelles that are present in the cells of living organisms. In fact, the structure of viruses is primitive compared to even the simplest cell. Surrounded by a protective protein coat or **capsid**, a virus contains only a few dozen

FIGURE 27.1

Structure of the human immunodeficiency virus (HIV).

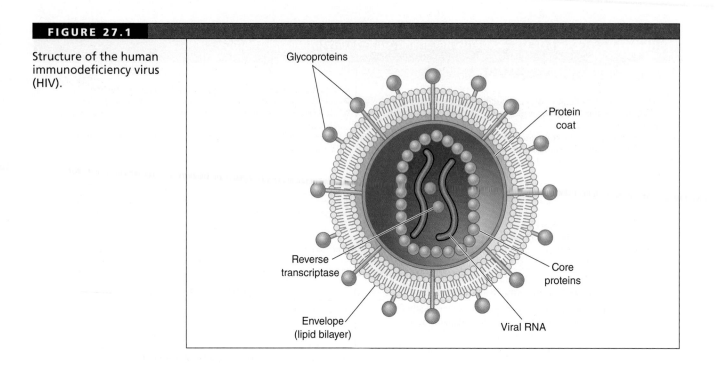

genes—either in the form of ribonucleic acid (RNA) or deoxyribonucleic acid (DNA)—that contain the information needed for viral replication. Figure 27.1 ■ shows the basic structure of one important virus: HIV.

Although nonliving and structurally simple, viruses are capable of remarkable feats. They infect an organism (the **host**), by entering a target cell and using the enzymes inside that cell to replicate. Thus, viruses are called **intracellular parasites**, meaning that they must be inside a host cell to cause infection. The host organism and cell are often very specific: It may be a single species of plant, bacteria, or animal, or even a single type of cell within that species. Most often, viruses that infect one species do not affect others, although cases have been documented in which viruses can mutate and cross species, as is likely the case for HIV.

intra = *within*
cellular = *cell*

Many viral infections, such as the rhinoviruses that cause the common cold, are self-limiting and require no medical treatment. Although symptoms may be annoying, the virus disappears in 7–10 days and causes no permanent damage if the patient is otherwise healthy. Other viruses, such as HIV, can cause serious and ultimately fatal disease and require aggressive drug therapy. Antiviral therapy is extremely challenging because of the rapid mutation rate of viruses, which can quickly render drugs ineffective. Also complicating therapy is the intracellular nature of the virus, which makes it difficult for medications to find their targets without giving excessively high doses that injure normal cells. The antiviral medications are listed in Tables 27.3 ◆ and 27.4 ◆. Each of the antiviral drugs is specific to one particular virus. The three basic strategies used for antiviral pharmacotherapy are as follows:

- Prevent viral infections through the administration of vaccines (see Chapter 25).

- Treat active infections with drugs that interrupt an aspect of the virus's replication cycle, such as acyclovir (Zovirax).

- For long-term infections, use drugs that boost the patient's immune response (immunostimulants) so that the virus remains in latency and the patient symptom free.

Antiretroviral drugs do not cure HIV-AIDS, but they do help many patients live longer.

CORE CONCEPT 27.5

Drugs for viral infections may be classified into those used to treat HIV-AIDS and those used for other viral disorders such as herpes and influenza. Antiviral medications for HIV-AIDS have been developed that slow the growth of HIV by different mechanisms.

The widespread appearance of HIV infection in 1981 created enormous challenges for public health and for the development of new antiviral drugs. HIV-AIDS is unlike any other infectious disease because it is uniformly fatal and demands a continuous supply of new drugs for the patients' survival. The challenges of HIV-AIDS have been met by the development of more than 20 antiviral drugs. Unfortunately, the initial hope of curing HIV-AIDS through antiviral therapy or vaccines has not been realized; none of these medications produces a cure for this disease. Once begun, antiretroviral therapy continues for the life of the patient because stopping the therapy results in a rapid rebound in HIV replication. HIV mutates extremely

TABLE 27.3 Antiretroviral Drugs for HIV-AIDS

Drug	Route and Adult Dose	Remarks
NONNUCLEOSIDE REVERSE TRANSCRIPTASE INHIBITORS (NNRTI)		
delavirdine (Rescriptor)	PO; 400 mg tid	Used in combination with other antivirals
efavirenz (Sustiva)	PO; 600 mg daily	Used in combination with other antivirals; a once-daily form is available
etravirine (Intelence)	PO; 200 mg bid	Less central nervous system (CNS) toxicity and hepatotoxicity than others
nevirapine (Viramune)	PO; 200 mg daily for 14 days, then increase to bid	Used in combination with other antivirals
rilpivirine (Edurant)	PO; 25 mg once daily	Newer drug in this class that offers convenience of once daily dosing
NUCLEOSIDE AND NUCLEOTIDE REVERSE TRANSCRIPTASE INHIBITORS (NRTI)		
abacavir (Ziagen)	PO; 300 mg bid	A first-line drug for HIV therapy in combination with other drugs
didanosine (Videx EC)	PO; 125–300 mg bid	For use in patients who are intolerant to AZT
emtricitabine (Emtriva)	PO; 200 mg daily	A first-line drug for HIV therapy in combination with other drugs
lamivudine (Epivir)	PO; 150 mg bid	Also used to treat chronic hepatitis B (Epivir-HBV).
stavudine (Zerit)	PO; 40 mg bid	Usually reserved for advanced HIV infections
tenofovir (Viread)	PO; 300 mg/day	A nucleotide reverse transcriptase inhibitor; a first-line drug for HIV therapy in combination with other drugs
Pr zidovudine (AZT, Retrovir)	PO; 200 mg every 4 hours for 1 month, then 100 mg every 4 hours	For symptomatic or asymptomatic HIV; off-label use: postexposure chemoprophylaxis; IV form available
PROTEASE INHIBITORS		
atazanavir (Reyataz)	PO; 400 mg/day	A first-line drug for HIV therapy in combination with other drugs
darunavir (Prezista)	PO; 600 mg taken with ritonavir 100 mg bid	Usually reserved for advanced HIV infections
fosamprenavir (Lexiva)	PO; 700–1400 mg bid in combination with 100–200 mg ritonavir bid	A first-line drug for HIV therapy in combination with other drugs
idinavir (Crixivan)	PO; 800 mg tid	Has short half-life; administer with a high-fat meal to increase absorption
lopinavir/ritonavir (Kaletra)	PO; 400/100 mg (three capsules or 5 mL of suspension) bid	A first-line drug for HIV therapy in combination with other drugs
nelfinavir (Viracept)	PO; 750 mg tid	Infrequently used due to adverse effects and three doses per day
ritonavir (Norvir)	PO; 600 mg bid	Always used in small doses to boost the effectiveness of other PIs
saquinavir (Invirase)	PO; 1,000 mg bid	Usually a second-line drug
tipranavir (Aptivus)	PO; 500 mg taken with 200 mg of ritonavir bid	Usually a second-line drug; administer with a high-fat meal to increase absorption
MISCELLANEOUS DRUGS FOR HIV		
enfuvirtide (Fuzeon)	Subcutaneous; 90 mg bid	Fusion inhibitor; usually reserved for advanced HIV infections
maraviroc (Selzentry)	PO; 150–600 mg bid	CCR5 receptor inhibitor; newer drug usually reserved for advanced HIV infections
raltegravir (Isentress)	PO; 400 mg bid	Integrase inhibitor; newer drug usually reserved for advanced HIV infections

rapidly, and resistant strains develop so quickly that the creation of novel approaches to antiretroviral drug therapy must remain an ongoing process.

After initial exposure, HIV may remain dormant for several months to many years. During this *latent phase,* patients are asymptomatic and may not even realize they are infected. Once diagnosis is established, however, a decision must be made as to when to begin pharmacotherapy. The advantage of beginning the therapy during the latent stage is that early treatment may delay the onset of acute symptoms and the development of AIDS.

Unfortunately, the decision to begin treatment during the latent phase has some negative consequences. Medications for HIV-AIDS are expensive; treatment with some of the newer drugs may cost more than $30,000 per year. These drugs produce uncomfortable and potentially serious adverse effects. Therapy over many years promotes viral resistance; when the acute stage eventually develops, the medications may no longer be effective.

The decision to begin therapy during the acute phase is much easier because the severe symptoms of AIDS can rapidly lead to death. Thus, therapy is nearly always initiated during this phase, when the CD4 T-cell count falls below 200 cells/mcL or when AIDS-defining symptoms become apparent.

The therapeutic goals for the pharmacotherapy of HIV-AIDS include the following:

- Reduce HIV-related morbidity and prolong survival
- Improve the quality of life
- Restore and preserve natural functions of the immune system
- Suppress the viral load to the extent possible
- Prevent the transmission from mother to child in pregnant patients infected with HIV

Although drug therapy for HIV-AIDS has not produced a cure, it has resulted in a number of therapeutic successes. For example, many patients with HIV are able to live symptom free with their disease for a much longer time because of antiviral therapy. Furthermore, the transmission of the virus from a mother infected with HIV to her offspring has been reduced dramatically because of drug therapy of the mother prior to delivery and of the baby immediately following birth. These two factors have resulted in a significant decline in the death rate due to HIV-AIDS in the United States.

Antiviral medications used for HIV-AIDS are called **antiretrovirals** because they block the replication cycle of HIV, which is classified as a retrovirus. The standard treatment for HIV-AIDS includes aggressive treatment with three to four drugs at a time, a regimen called **highly active antiretroviral therapy (HAART)**. The goal of HAART is to reduce the amount of HIV in the plasma to its lowest possible level. It must be understood, however, that HIV is harbored in locations other than the blood, such as in lymph nodes; therefore, elimination of the virus from the blood is not a cure.

The replication of HIV is illustrated in Figure 27.2 ■. Antiretroviral drugs are classified into groups based on how they inhibit HIV replication.

- *Nucleoside and nucleotide reverse transcriptase inhibitors (NRTIs and NtRTIs)* The oldest antiretroviral drug, zidovudine, belongs to the NRTI class. Drugs in this group are structurally similar to nucleosides, the building blocks of DNA. NRTIs inhibit the action of **reverse transcriptase**, the viral enzyme that converts viral RNA into viral DNA.

- *Nonnucleoside reverse transcriptase inhibitors (NNRTIs)* This class also inhibits the viral enzyme reverse transcriptase, but these drugs are not structurally similar to the building blocks of DNA. Instead, these drugs bind directly to the reverse transcriptase molecule and inhibit its ability to build viral DNA.

- *Protease inhibitors* These drugs block the final assembly of the HIV particle. They are effective at reducing plasma HIV to very low levels, although resistance develops quickly.

- *Miscellaneous drugs for HIV infection* Newer drugs are being developed as scientists discover more about the HIV replication cycle. Enfuvirtide (Fuzeon) blocks the fusion of HIV to the CD4 receptor on the lymphocyte. Raltegravir (Isentress) is classified as an integrase inhibitor. This drug prevents HIV from inserting its genes into the human chromosome.

Research into HIV-AIDS is constantly evolving as clinicians strive to determine the most effective combinations of antiretroviral drugs. In current clinical practice, the following regimens have been shown to be the most successful choices for the initial therapy of HIV infection (Panel on Antiretroviral Guidelines for Adults and Adolescents, 2011):

- *NNRTI-based regimen:* efavirenz +tenofovir+emtricitabine
- *PI-based regimens*
  - atazanavir (ritonavir-boosted) + tenofovir+emtricitabine
  - darunavir (ritonavir-boosted) + tenofovir+emtricitabine
- *Integrase inhibitor–based regimen:* raltegravir + tenofovir + emtricitabine

FIGURE 27.2

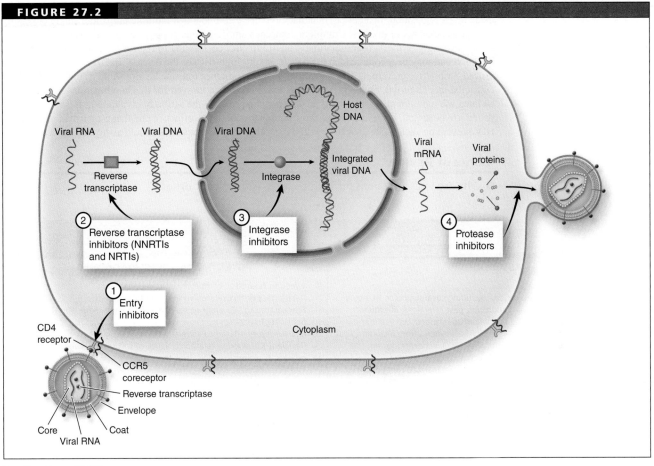

Replication of HIV.

Drug Prototype 🅟 *Zidovudine (AZT, Retrovir)*

Therapeutic Class: Antiretroviral   **Pharmacologic Class: Nucleoside reverse transcriptase inhibitor (NRTI)**

Actions and Uses: Zidovudine was first discovered in the 1960s, and its antiviral activity was demonstrated prior to the AIDS epidemic. As the HIV reverse transcriptase enzyme begins to synthesize viral DNA, it mistakenly uses zidovudine as one of the building blocks, thus creating a defective DNA strand. Once incorporated, zidovudine slows synthesis of HIV, thereby reducing symptoms associated with this infection.

Because of its widespread use over the past 25 years, strains of HIV resistant to zidovudine are common. It is usually used in combination with other antiretrovirals because this slows the development of resistance and allows HIV to be attacked by several mechanisms. Combination products containing zidovudine include Combivir (zidovudine and lamivudine) and Trizivir (zidovudine, lamivudine, and abacavir).

Zidovudine is one of the few HIV-AIDS drugs that can prevent HIV infection. By administering zidovudine to a mother infected with HIV starting at 14 weeks of gestation and to the newborn for six weeks following delivery, the risk of transmission of the virus to the child can be significantly reduced. Zidovudine is also administered as prophylaxis to healthcare providers following an accidental needlestick or other exposure to HIV.

Adverse Effects and Interactions: Zidovudine can result in severe toxicity to blood cells at high doses. Many patients report GI symptoms such as anorexia, nausea, and diarrhea. Patients may experience fatigue and report generalized weakness. Headache will occur in the majority of patients taking zidovudine, and more serious CNS effects have been reported.

Zidovudine interacts with many drugs. Acetaminophen and ganciclovir may worsen bone marrow suppression. The following drugs may increase the risk of AZT toxicity: atovaquone, amphotericin B, aspirin, doxorubicin, fluconazole, methadone, and valproic acid.

Use with caution with herbal supplements such as St. John's wort, which may cause a decrease in antiretroviral activity.

BLACK BOX WARNING:

Rare cases of fatal lactic acidosis with hepatomegaly and steatosis have been reported with zidovudine use. Bone marrow suppression may result in neutropenia or severe anemia. Myopathy may occur with long-term use.

Although no drug or drug combination has yet been found to cure HIV-AIDS, some progress has been made on its prevention. In addition, manufacturers have compounded multiple drugs into single tablets for ease of use. Approved in 2011, Complera combines emtricitabine, rilpirivine, and tenofovir into a tablet taken once daily. Truvada (emtricitabine + tenofovir) has been found to reduce the risk of acquiring HIV infection and may be recommended for people at very high risk for the disease. In 2012, the FDA also approved Stribild for preventing HIV infection. Stribild combines four medications into a single daily tablet: emtricitabine, tenofovir, elvitegravir, and cobicistat. Newly approved for this combination, elvitegravir is an integrase inhibitor and cobicistat is an enzyme that prolongs the action of elvitegravir. It is important for patients to be taught, however, that no drug combination is 100% effective and that established methods for HIV prevention such as abstinence, condoms, or other safe sex measures should always be implemented.

Concept Review 27.2

■ Why are viral infections difficult to treat with current drugs?

NURSING PROCESS FOCUS Patients Receiving Pharmacotherapy for HIV-AIDS

ASSESSMENT	POTENTIAL NURSING DIAGNOSES
Prior to administration: ■ Obtain a complete health history, including cardiovascular, GI, neurological, skin, renal and liver conditions, past infections, allergies, sexual and drug history, and possible drug interactions. ■ Acquire the results of a complete physical examination, including vital signs, height, weight, lung sounds, LOC, ECG, echocardiogram, and any signs of a current infection. ■ Evaluate laboratory blood findings: CBC, electrolytes, renal and liver function studies, amylase, glucose, and HIV viral load/CD4 count. ■ Obtain specimens for C&S before initiating therapy for possible bacterial infections.	■ *Infection* related to compromised immune system ■ *Decisional Conflict* related to therapeutic regimen ■ *Fear* related to HIV diagnosis and a lack of knowledge about therapeutic regimen ■ *Risk for Injury* related to adverse effects of drug therapy ■ *Deficient Knowledge* related to a lack of information about disease process, transmission, and drug therapy ■ *Ineffective Therapeutic Regimen Management* related to the complexity of therapies (medications, counseling, diet)

PLANNING: PATIENT GOALS AND EXPECTED OUTCOMES

The patient will:
■ Experience therapeutic effects (a decrease in viral load and an increase in CD4 counts).
■ Be free from or experience minimal adverse effects from drug therapy.
■ Verbalize an understanding of the drug's use, adverse effects, and required precautions.
■ Adhere to recommended treatment regimen.

IMPLEMENTATION

Interventions and (Rationales)	Patient Education/Discharge Planning
■ Administer medication correctly and evaluate the patient's knowledge of proper administration, especially monitoring the patient's ability and motivation to comply with treatment regimen. (Antiretroviral therapy continues for the life of the patient. Stopping the therapy results in a rapid rebound in HIV replication.)	Inform the patient: ■ That treatment for HIV-AIDS is a life-long, ongoing process. Stopping therapy will result in a rebound in the HIV viral replication. ■ Not to stop taking the drug regimen when "feeling better." ■ To take according to drug schedule. ■ Not to share doses with others. ■ To return to healthcare provider if adverse effects make adherence to therapy difficult to continue.
■ Monitor for symptoms of hypersensitivity reactions. (Zalcitabine may cause anaphylactic reaction.)	■ Instruct the patient to discontinue the medication and inform the healthcare provider if symptoms of hypersensitivity reaction develop, such as wheezing; shortness of breath; swelling of face, tongue, or hands; or itching or rash.
■ Monitor vital signs, especially temperature, and for symptoms of infection. Monitor white blood cell count. (Antiretroviral drugs such as delavirdine may cause neutropenia.)	Instruct the patient: ■ To report symptoms of infections such as fever, chills, sore throat, and cough to the healthcare provider. ■ On methods to minimize exposure to infection, such as frequent handwashing; avoiding crowds and people with colds, flu, and other infections; limiting exposure to children and animals; increasing fluid intake; emptying the bladder frequently; and coughing and deep breathing several times per day.
■ Monitor the patient for signs of stomatitis. (Immunosuppression may result in the proliferation of oral bacteria.)	■ Inform the patient to be alert for mouth ulcers and to report their appearance to the healthcare provider.
■ Monitor blood pressure. (Antiviral drugs such as abacavir may cause significant decrease in blood pressure.)	Instruct the patient to: ■ Rise slowly from lying or sitting position to minimize effects of postural hypotension. ■ Report changes in blood pressure.

NURSING PROCESS FOCUS *(continued)*

Interventions and (Rationales)	Patient Education/Discharge Planning
■ Monitor HIV RNA assay, CD4 counts, liver function, kidney function, CBC, blood glucose, and serum amylase and triglyceride levels. (Monitoring labs will aid in determining effectiveness and/or drug toxicity.)	Instruct the patient: ■ On the purpose of required laboratory tests and scheduled follow-ups with the healthcare provider. ■ To monitor weight and presence of swelling. ■ To keep all appointments for laboratory tests.
■ Determine potential drug–drug and drug–food interactions. (Antiretroviral medications have multiple drug–drug interactions and must be taken as prescribed.)	Instruct the patient: ■ When to take the specific medication in relationship to food intake. ■ About foods or beverages to avoid when taking medication; some antiretrovirals should not be taken with acidic fruit juice. ■ To take medication exactly as directed; do not skip any doses. ■ To consult with the healthcare provider before taking any OTC medications or herbal supplements.
■ Monitor for symptoms of pancreatitis, including severe abdominal pain, nausea, vomiting, and abdominal distention. (Antiretroviral drugs such as didanosine may cause pancreatitis.)	■ Instruct the patient to report the following immediately: fever, severe abdominal pain, nausea/vomiting, and abdominal distention.
■ Monitor the skin for rash; withhold medication and notify the physician at the first sign of rash. (Several antiretroviral drugs may cause Stevens–Johnson syndrome, which may be fatal.)	■ Advise the patient to check the skin frequently and to notify the healthcare provider at the first sign of any rash.
■ Establish therapeutic environment to ensure adequate rest, nutrition, hydration, and relaxation. (Support of the immune system is essential in patients with HIV to minimize opportunistic infections.)	Advise the patient to incorporate the following health-enhancing activities: ■ Adequate rest and sleep ■ Proper nutrition that provides essential vitamins and nutrients ■ Intake of six to eight glasses of water per day
■ Monitor blood glucose levels. (Antiretroviral drugs may cause hyperglycemia, especially in patients with type 1 diabetes.)	■ Instruct the patient to report excessive thirst, hunger, and urination to the healthcare provider. ■ Instruct patients with diabetes to monitor blood glucose levels regularly.
■ Monitor for neurologic adverse effects such as numbness and tingling of the extremities. (Many NRTI drugs cause peripheral neuropathy.)	Instruct the patient to: ■ Report numbness and tingling of extremities. ■ Use caution when in contact with heat and cold due to possible peripheral neuropathy.
■ Determine the effect of the prescribed antiretroviral drugs on oral contraceptives. (Many drugs reduce the effectiveness of oral contraceptives.)	■ Instruct the patient to use an alternate form of birth control while taking antiretroviral medications.
■ Provide resources for medical and emotional support. (Medications for the treatment of HIV-AIDS can be expensive.)	■ Advise the patient on community resources and support groups.
■ Determine the patient's understanding of the effect of the medication and impact on lifestyle activities. (Antiviral medications used for HIV-AIDS do not "cure" the disease therefore patients need to understand that lifestyle changes still need to occur.)	Advise the patient: ■ That the medication may decrease the level of HIV infection in the blood but will not prevent transmission of the virus. ■ To use barrier protection during sexual activity. ■ To avoid sharing needles. ■ To not donate blood.

EVALUATION OF OUTCOME CRITERIA

Evaluate the effectiveness of drug therapy by confirming that patient goals and expected outcomes have been met (see "Planning"). *See Table 27.3 for lists of drugs to which these nursing actions apply.*

Antiviral drugs are available to treat herpes simplex, influenza, and viral hepatitis infections.

CORE CONCEPT 27.6

Other than the drugs used to treat HIV, only a few antivirals are available to treat serious viral infections. These include drugs to treat infections with the herpesviruses, the influenza virus, and the hepatitis virus.

Treatment of herpesvirus infection

Herpes simplex viruses (HSVs) are a family of viruses that cause repeated, blisterlike lesions on the skin, genitals, and other mucosal surfaces. Herpesviruses are acquired through sexual intercourse or other direct physical contact with an infected person. The herpesvirus family includes the following:

- HSV-type 1—primarily causes infections of the eye, mouth, and lips, although the incidence of genital infections is increasing
- HSV-type 2—primarily genital infections
- Cytomegalovirus (CMV)—affects multiple body systems, usually in patients with immunosuppression

- Varicella-zoster virus—shingles (zoster) and chickenpox (varicella)
- Epstein-Barr virus—infectious mononucleosis and Burkitt's lymphoma (a form of cancer)

Following its initial entrance into the human host, HSV may remain in a latent, nonreplicating state in nerve cells for many years. Immunosuppression, physical challenge, or emotional stress can activate the virus and cause the characteristic lesions to reappear. *Initial* HSV-1 and HSV-2 infections are usually treated with oral antiviral therapy for 5 to 10 days. Topical drugs are available for application on active lesions, but they are not as effective as oral medications. Although *recurrent* herpes lesions are often mild and require no drug therapy, patients who experience frequent or severe recurrences may benefit from low doses of prophylactic antiviral therapy. It should be noted that the antiviral drugs used to treat herpesviruses do not cure the patient; the virus remains in the patient for life. Drugs for treating herpesviruses are listed in Table 27.4.

Treatment of Influenza Virus Infection

Influenza is a viral infection characterized by acute symptoms that include sore throat, sneezing, coughing, fever, and chills. The virus is easily spread via airborne droplets. In patients with compromised immune systems, an influenza infection may be fatal.

The best approach to influenza infection is prevention through annual vaccination. Those who benefit greatly from vaccinations include residents of long-term care facilities, those with chronic cardiopulmonary disease, women who will be in their second or third trimester during the peak flu season, and healthy adults older than age 50. Adequate immunity is achieved about two weeks after vaccination and lasts for several months to a year. The CDC recommends that people get vaccinated as soon as the vaccine becomes available in their community. Additional details on vaccines are presented in Chapter 25.

Antivirals may be used to prevent influenza or decrease the severity of influenza symptoms. The drug amantadine (Symmetrel) has been available to prevent and treat influenza for many years. Amantadine or rimantadine is indicated for unvaccinated high-risk patients after a confirmed outbreak of influenza type A. Therapy with these antivirals is sometimes started at the same time as vaccination; the antiviral offers protection during the period before antibody titers are achieved from the vaccine. Antivirals for influenza are shown in Table 27.4.

The *neuroamidase inhibitors* are used to treat active infections. If given within 48 hours of the onset of symptoms, oseltamivir (Tamiflu) and zanamivir (Relenza) are reported to shorten the normal seven-day duration of influenza symptoms to five days. Because these influenza antivirals produce only modest benefits for patients with an active infection, prevention through vaccination remains the best alternative.

TABLE 27.4 Antiviral Drugs for Herpes and Influenza Infections

Drug	Route and Adult Dose	Remarks
HERPES VIRUS DRUGS		
🅿️ acyclovir (Zovirax)	PO; 400 mg tid	For HSV-1, HSV-2, and varicella-zoster; topical and IV forms available
cidofovir (Vistide)	IV; 5 mg/kg once weekly for 2 consecutive weeks	For cytomegalovirus retinitis in patients with AIDS; must give probenecid before and after infusion
docosanol (Abreva)	Topical; 10% cream applied to lesion up to five times/day	For herpes simplex lesions on the face and lips
famciclovir (Famvir)	PO; 500 mg tid for 7 days	For HSV-2 and varicella-zoster
foscarnet (Foscavir)	IV; 40–60 mg/kg infused over 1–2 hours tid	For cytomegalovirus retinitis; for the treatment of acyclovir-resistant herpes virus
ganciclovir (Cytovene)	PO; 1 g tid IV; 5 mg/kg infused over 1 hour bid	Preferred drug for cytomegalovirus; oral form available
penciclovir (Denavir)	Topical; 0.5 inch of ointment to each eye every 3 hours	For herpes simplex lesions on the face and lips
trifluridine (Viroptic)	Topical; one drop in each eye every 2 hours during waking hours (max: nine drops/day)	For herpes eye infections
valacyclovir (Valtrex)	PO; 1 g tid	For HSV-1, HSV-2, and varicella-zoster
INFLUENZA DRUGS		
amantadine (Symmetrel)	PO; 100 mg bid	For treatment and prevention of influenza A; also for Parkinson's disease
oseltamivir (Tamiflu)	PO; 75 mg bid for 5 days	For treatment of influenza
rimantadine (Flumadine)	PO; 100 mg bid	For treatment and prevention of influenza
zanamivir (Relenza)	Inhalation; two inhalations per day for 5 days	For treatment of influenza

Drug Prototype ℗ Acyclovir (Zovirax)
Therapeutic Class: Antiviral for herpesviruses   **Pharmacologic Class: Nucleoside analog**

Actions and Uses: The antiviral activity of acyclovir is limited to the herpesviruses, for which it is the preferred drug. It is most effective against HSV-1 and HSV-2 and effective only at high doses against CMV and varicella-zoster. By inhibiting viral DNA synthesis, acyclovir decreases the duration and severity of herpes episodes. Resistance has developed to the drug, particularly in patients with HIV-AIDS. When given for prophylaxis, it may decrease the frequency of active herpes episodes, but it does not cure the patient. It is available in topical form for placing directly on active lesions, in oral form for prophylaxis, and as an IV for particularly severe disease.

Adverse Effects and Interactions: There are few adverse effects to acyclovir when administered topically or orally. When given IV, the drug may cause painful inflammation of vessels at the site of infusion. Because nephrotoxicity is possible, especially when the drug is given by the IV route, kidney function should be carefully monitored.

Acyclovir interacts with several drugs. For example, probenecid decreases acyclovir elimination, and zidovudine may cause increased drowsiness and lethargy.

Treatment of Viral Hepatitis Infection

Viral hepatitis is a common infection caused by several different viruses: hepatitis A, hepatitis B, and hepatitis C. Although each has its own unique features, all hepatitis viruses cause inflammation and death of liver cells and produce similar symptoms. Acute symptoms include fever, chills, fatigue, anorexia, nausea, and vomiting. Chronic hepatitis may result in prolonged fatigue, jaundice, liver cirrhosis, and, ultimately, hepatic failure.

Hepatitis A Hepatitis A virus (HAV) infection in the United States is usually caused by eating food contaminated with the virus. The best treatment for HAV is prevention by the administration of HAV vaccine (Havrix, VAQTA). Because acute HAV infection is self-limiting, there is no specific therapy for the condition. Unlike the other hepatitis viruses, HAV infection is not considered to have a chronic component.

Hepatitis B Hepatitis B virus (HBV) is transmitted primarily through exposure to contaminated blood and body fluids. Major risk factors for HBV include injected drug abuse, sex with a partner infected with HBV, and sex between men. Healthcare workers are at risk because of accidental exposure to HBV-contaminated needles or body fluids.

Treatment of *acute* HBV infection is symptomatic because 90% of these infections resolve with complete recovery and do not progress to chronic disease. Symptoms of *chronic* HBV, however, may develop as long as 10 years following exposure. The final stage of the infection is hepatic cirrhosis. In addition, chronic HBV infections are associated with an increased risk of hepatocellular carcinoma.

The best treatment for HBV infection is prevention through vaccination with HBV vaccine (Recombivax HB, Engerix-B). Once chronic hepatitis becomes active, three different therapies are approved for pharmacotherapy:

- Interferon alfa-2B (Intron A) or peginterferon alfa-2A (Pegasys) or 2B (PEG-Intron): these drugs are natural proteins that suppress viral replication and enhance body defenses

- Lamivudine (Epivir): resembles a building block for DNA; inhibits viral DNA synthesis

- Adefovir (Hepsera): blocks viral DNA synthesis; primarily used for patients with viruses resistant to lamivudine.

Hepatitis C Transmitted primarily through exposure to infected blood or body fluids, hepatitis C virus (HCV) is more common than HBV. HCV is the most common cause of liver transplants. Current pharmacotherapy for chronic HCV infection includes interferon (or peginterferon) and the antiviral ribavirin. In 2011, two new antivirals boceprevir (Victrelis) and telaprevir (Incivek) were approved for chronic hepatitis C infection.

ANTIPARASITIC DRUGS

Infections caused by helminths and protozoans cause significant disease worldwide.

CORE CONCEPT 27.7

Other pathogens that may infect humans include single-celled organisms, or **protozoans**, and multicellular animals such as mites, ticks, and worms. Some of these parasites thrive in conditions in which sanitation and personal hygiene are poor and population density is high. Although many of these diseases are rare in

proto = *first*
zoans = *animals*

TABLE 27.5 Selected Drugs for Helminth and Protozoan Infections

Drug	Route and Adult Dose	Remarks
ANTIHELMINTHICS		
albendazole (Albenza)	PO; 400 mg bid (max: 800 mg/day)	Only antihelminthic drug active against all stages of the helminth life cycle
ivermectin (Stromectol)	PO; 150–200 mcg/kg for one dose	Preferred drug for many helminth infections
mebendazole (Vermox)	PO; 100 mg for one dose or 100 mg bid for 3 days	For the treatment of whipworm, roundworm, hookworm, and pinworm
praziquantel (Biltricide)	PO; 5 mg/kg for one dose or 25 mg/kg tid	For all stages of schistosomiasis; bitter tablet
pyrantel (Antiminth, Ascarel, Pin-X, Pinworm Caplets)	PO; 11 mg/kg for one dose (max: 1 g)	For the treatment of hookworm and roundworm
ANTIMALARIALS		
artemether and lumefantrine (Coartem)	Oral; 3–6 doses for 3 days (20 mg of arte-mether and 120 mg of lumefantrine per dose)	Newer drug for patients with chloroquine-resistant malaria.
atovaquone and proguanil (Malarone)	PO; for prophylaxis; one tablet/day starting 1–2 days before travel, and continuing until 7 days after return	Also for *Pneumocystis*
chloroquine (Aralen)	PO; 600 mg initial dose, then 300 mg weekly	Preferred drug for malaria; also for amebiasis and rheumatoid arthritis; IM form available; if administered IV, oral medication is ineffective
hydroxychloroquine (Plaquenil) (see page 575 for the Drug Prototype box)	PO; 620 mg initial dose, then 310 mg weekly	Also for rheumatoid arthritis and lupus erythematosus
pyrimethamine (Daraprim)	PO; 25 mg once per week for 10 weeks	Also antiprotozoan; drug of choice for toxoplasmosis
ANTIPROTOZOANS (NONMALARIAL)		
doxycycline (Vibramycin)	PO; 100 mg/day	For traveler's diarrhea; used also for malaria prophylaxis; a tetracycline antibiotic
ⓟ metronidazole (Flagyl)	PO; 250–750 mg tid	For many parasitic infections; IV form available
paromomycin (Humatin)	PO; 25–35 mg/kg divided in three doses for 5–10 days	For acute and chronic amebiasis; an aminoglycoside antibiotic
pentamidine (NebuPent, Pentam)	IV; 4 mg/kg daily for 14–21 days; infuse over 60 minutes	For *Pneumocystis* active infections and prophylaxis; IM and inhalation forms available
tinidazole (Tindamax)	PO; 2 grams per day for 3 days	Newer drug for amebiasis, giardiasis, or trichomoniasis

the United States and Canada, travelers to Africa, Asia, and South America may acquire infections overseas and return home with them. Table 27.5 ◆ lists selected antiparasitics. Scabicides and pediculicides are covered in Chapter 36.

With a few exceptions, antibiotics, antifungal, and antiviral drugs are ineffective against these complex organisms. Drugs prescribed for parasitic diseases may be classified as antimalarials, antiprotozoans (other than antimalarial drugs), antihelminthics, and scabicides/pediculicides.

Malaria is a disease caused by four species of the protozoan *Plasmodium*. Although rare in the United States and Canada, malaria is the second most common fatal infectious disease in the world, with 300 to 500 million cases occurring annually. The Centers for Disease Control and Prevention (CDC) recommends that travelers to infected areas receive prophylactic antimalarial drugs prior to and during their visit and for one week after leaving. Chloroquine (Aralen) is the traditional drug of choice, however, most regions of the world have developed chloroquine-resistant strains of *Plasmodium*. Many of the newer drugs used in high malaria regions have not been approved by the FDA. Healthcare providers planning travel to these regions should consult the CDC website for the most current information on pharmacotherapy.

Other species of protozoans that cause significant disease worldwide include *Entamoeba*, *Giardia*, *Leishmania*, *Pneumocystis*, *Toxoplasma*, and *Trypanosoma*. Amebiasis is a disease caused by *Entamoeba histolytica*, commonly found in Africa, Latin America, and Asia, where it frequently causes serious disease. Although primarily an intestinal disease, *E. histolytica* can invade the liver, where it causes abscesses. The primary sign of amebiasis is a severe form of diarrhea known as amebic **dysentery**. Drugs used to treat amebiasis include those that act directly on amebas in the intestine and those that are administered for their systemic effects on the liver and other organs.

dys = difficult or painful
enter = intestine

Helminths consist of various species of parasitic worms, including hookworms, pinworms, round-worms, tapeworms, and flukes. Many of these worms attach to the mucosa of the human intestinal tract. Helminth diseases are quite common in areas of the world lacking high standards of sanitation. Helminth infections in the United States and Canada are generally neither common nor fatal, although drug therapy may be indicated. The most common helminth disease worldwide is caused by the roundworm *Ascaris*; however, infection by the pinworm *Enterobius* is more common in the United States. For ascariasis, oral mebendazole (Vermox) for three days is the standard treatment. Pharmacotherapy of enterobiasis includes a single dose of mebendazole, albendazole (Albenza), or pyrantel (Antiminth). To prevent the spread of these parasites, good handwashing techniques must be practiced.

Concept Review   27.3

■ How do most patients in the United States and Canada acquire protozoan infections?

Drug Prototype ℗ *Metronidazole (Flagyl)*

Therapeutic Class: Anti-infective, antiprotozoan   Pharmacologic Class: Drug that disrupts nucleic acid synthesis

Actions and Uses: Metronidazole is a preferred drug for amebiasis because it is effective against amebas in the intestine and in other organs. Metronidazole is also a drug of choice for two other protozoan infections: giardiasis from *Giardia lamblia* and trichonomiasis due to *Trichomonas vaginalis*.

Metronidazole is somewhat unique in that it also has antibiotic activity against anaerobic bacteria and thus is used to treat a number of respiratory, bone, skin, and CNS infections. Topical forms are used to treat rosacea, a disease characterized by reddening of the sebaceous glands in the skin around the nose and face. It is used in combination with bismuth and tetracycline to eradicate *H. pylori* infection, which is associated with peptic ulcer disease.

Adverse Effects and Interactions: Although adverse effects are relatively common, most are not serious enough to cause discontinuation of therapy. The most common adverse effects of metronidazole are anorexia, nausea, diarrhea, dizziness, and headache. Dryness of the mouth and an unpleasant metallic taste may be experienced.

Metronidazole interacts with several drugs. For example, oral anticoagulants increase hypoprothombinemia. In combination with alcohol and medications that contain alcohol, metronidazole may cause a disulfiram reaction. It may also elevate lithium levels.

BLACK BOX WARNING:
Metronidazole (oral and injection) causes cancer in laboratory animals and should be used only for approved indications.

PATIENTS NEED TO KNOW

Patients treated for fungal, viral, or parasitic infections need to know the following:

Regarding Antifungals

1. Avoid alcohol and other drugs toxic to the liver while taking azole-type antifungals.
2. Griseofulvin, used to treat superficial mycoses, can decrease the effectiveness of oral contraceptives. An alternative method of contraception is advised.
3. Older children and adult patients should swish oral antifungal drugs around in their mouths and swallow them. Caregivers should swab the mouths of infants and toddlers. Wait at least 10 minutes after antifungal treatment to put anything else in the mouth.
4. Rinse the mouth after use of corticosteroid inhalers to avoid a decrease in local immune defenses against oral candidiasis.
5. While taking antifungal drugs for a vaginal infection, refrain from sexual intercourse until the infection is resolved.
6. Wear gloves when applying topical medications.

Regarding Antivirals

7. When taking antivirals, it is important to report symptoms of hypersensitivity reactions.
8. When taking drugs for HIV-AIDS, avoid crowds and those with infections because many of these medications will suppress your immune system.

Regarding Helminths and Protozoans

9. Course of treatment depends on the nature of the infection/infestation, and treatment plan is to be followed completely as prescribed.
10. Take showers instead of baths. Change underwear, linens, and towels daily.
11. Good handwashing practices are a must in the prevention of pinworms/roundworms.

CHAPTER REVIEW

CORE CONCEPTS SUMMARY

27.1 Fungal infections are classified as superficial or systemic.

Fungi are multicellular organisms. Because most are unaffected by antibiotics, they require different classes of medications. Fungal infections are usually a serious problem only in patients with compromised immune systems. Mycoses are classified as superficial or systemic.

27.2 Systemic antifungal drugs are used for serious infections of internal organs.

Systemic mycoses affect the internal organs and may require prolonged and aggressive drug therapy. Systemic antifungal drugs may cause serious adverse effects.

27.3 Superficial infections of the skin, nails, and mucous membranes are effectively treated with topical and oral antifungal drugs.

Superficial mycoses of the hair, skin, nails, and mucous membranes are very common, though rarely serious. Antifungals given topically as powders, troches, and ointments produce few adverse effects.

27.4 Viruses are infectious agents that require a host to replicate.

Viruses take over the cellular machinery of host cells and use it to replicate themselves. Although most viral infections require no pharmacotherapy, patients with infections by HIV, herpesviruses, and the influenza virus may benefit from drug treatment.

27.5 Antiretroviral drugs do not cure HIV-AIDS, but they do help many patients live longer.

Drugs used to treat HIV infections include the nucleoside and nonnucleoside reverse transcriptase inhibitors, protease inhibitors, and fusion inhibitors. These drugs may produce significant toxicity. Although they are not able to cure the disease, they may extend the symptom-free period.

27.6 Antiviral drugs are available to treat herpes simplex, influenza, and viral hepatitis infections.

Drug therapy is used to extend the latent period of genital herpes and to speed the recovery from active lesions. A few antivirals are available to prevent influenza, and these are most useful when combined with vaccines. New drugs have been developed to shorten the discomfort period for influenza symptoms, although these drugs have limited effectiveness.

27.7 Infections caused by helminths and protozoans cause significant disease worldwide.

Malaria is one of the most common infections in the world, and a significant number of drugs are available to disrupt the *Plasmodium* life cycle. Similarly, amebiasis is a common protozoan disease requiring intensive drug treatment. Diseases caused by helminths are common in areas of the world lacking adequate sanitation.

REVIEW QUESTIONS

The following questions are written in NCLEX-PN® style. Answer these questions to assess your knowledge of the chapter material, and go back and review any material that is not clear to you.

1. The nurse would expect that the patient on amphotericin B must be monitored for:

1. Ototoxicity
2. Hepatic toxicity
3. Nephrotoxicity
4. Anoxia

2. The patient has oral candidiasis. Which of the following medications does the nurse expect to be ordered?

1. Terbinafine (Lamisil)
2. Clotrimazole (Mycelex)
3. Ketoconazole (Nizoral)
4. Nystatin (Mycostatin)

3. The patient with a fungal infection of her toenails asks how long treatment must occur. The nurse's best response would be:

1. "Treatment is very quick, requiring only one tablet of clotrimazole."
2. "Treatment will occur daily for three days."
3. "Treatment will last for several months."
4. "You will need to speak to your physician."

4. When instructing a patient on zidovudine (AZT), the nurse would include:

1. The importance of taking the medication every four hours for a month
2. That the medication is taken daily for one month only
3. That if taken correctly, AZT will cure the disease.
4. That the medication is used to treat symptoms of influenza

5. A patient has just been diagnosed with genital herpes and has been prescribed acyclovir (Zovirax). The patient asks how this drug will help his condition. The nurse replies: (Select all that apply.)

1. "It can be given to reduce the frequency of herpes episodes."
2. "If taken correctly, this medication will cure the disease."
3. "It decreases the duration and severity of herpes episodes."
4. "In addition to treating herpes, it also can be used to treat HPV."

6. The patient complains of flu-like symptoms that started 24 hours ago. Which of the following class of medications would the nurse anticipate being ordered?

1. Protease inhibitors
2. Nonnucleoside reverse transcriptase inhibitors
3. Nucleoside reverse transcriptase inhibitors
4. Neuroamidase inhibitors

7. A patient has started taking metronidazole (Flagyl) for the treatment of *Trichomonas vaginalis*. The nurse knows to monitor her for which of the following adverse effects? (Select all that apply.)

1. Vomiting
2. Anorexia
3. A metallic taste
4. Dryness of the mouth

8. When applying topical antifungals, which of the following statements should be included in a patient teaching plan?

1. No other antifungals should be administered.
2. Gloves should be worn to prevent transmission.
3. Antifungals should not be applied to open areas.
4. Vital signs should be checked prior to administration.

9. A patient on an antiretroviral for HIV has developed anemia. The nurse suspects that this condition could indicate which of the following?

1. The patient is most likely being abused.
2. The patient is experiencing minor adverse reactions.
3. The patient is not taking the medications as ordered.
4. The patient may be experiencing severe toxicity due to high doses of the drug.

10. The nurse is providing education to a mother of a young patient about pinworms and roundworms. Which of the following should be included in this educational session?

1. Good handwashing practices are a must in preventing the spread of pinworms and roundworms.
2. Play habits do not contribute to the transmission of pinworms and roundworms.
3. It is not important that children wear shoes when playing outside.
4. Once the child has had worms, reinfection cannot occur.

CASE STUDY QUESTIONS

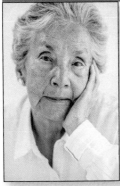

Remember Mrs. Davis, the patient introduced at the beginning of the chapter? Now read the remainder of the case study. Based on the information you have learned in this chapter, answer the questions that follow.

Mrs. Martha Davis is a 70-year-old retired auto worker who is frail and in ill health and comes to the healthcare provider's office for her annual fall check-up. Her arthritis is getting worse so she "can't get around" like she used to do. Although she is not demonstrating any respiratory difficulties at the time of the visit, she had pneumonia earlier in the year and she states she is "still tired all the time." In addition, she complains that she started having problems with itching and discharge in the vaginal area.

1. The office nurse gives her an informational pamphlet on the flu vaccine. The information contained in the pamphlet states that the best way to avoid a potential life-threatening bout with the flu is to:

1. Begin taking oseltamivir (Tamiflu) one month before the flu season begins.
2. Take zanamavir (Relenza) within 48 hours of the onset of flu symptoms.
3. Receive a flu vaccination as soon as it becomes available.
4. Take acyclovir (Zovirax) during the flu season.

2. Mrs. Davis states, "If I get the vaccine today, when will it start working?" The nurse tells her that immunity is achieved:

1. In about a day or two
2. Within a week after the vaccination
3. About two weeks after the vaccination
4. About three to four weeks after the vaccination

3. Mrs. Davis also reported vaginal itching and abnormal discharge, and the physician diagnoses vaginal candidiasis. Which of the following medications does the nurse expect to be ordered?

1. Amphotericin B (Fungizone)
2. Clotrimazole (Gyne-Lotrimin)
3. Acyclovir (Zovirax)
4. Tinidazole (Tindamax)

4. The nurse advises Mrs. Davis that she may experience what adverse effect when taking clotrimazole? (Select all that apply.)

1. Burning
2. An increase in discharge
3. Itching
4. Irritation

NOTE: Answers to the Review and Case Study Questions appear in Appendix B. The complete rationales and answers are located on the textbook's website.

Pearson Nursing Student Resources Find additional review materials at **nursing.pearsonhighered.com**.

*"I know they are helping
with my cancer, but four
different drugs? I guess it
could be worse."*

Ms. Patricia Novak

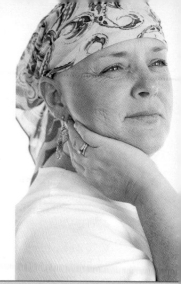

28 Drugs for Neoplasia

CORE CONCEPTS

28.1 Cancer is characterized by rapid, uncontrolled growth of cells.

28.2 The causes of cancer may be chemical, physical, or biological.

28.3 Personal risk of cancer may be lowered by a number of lifestyle factors.

28.4 The three primary goals of chemotherapy are cure, control, and palliation.

28.5 To achieve a total cure, every malignant cell must be removed or killed.

28.6 Use of multiple drugs and special dosing schedules improves the success of chemotherapy.

28.7 Serious toxicity limits therapy with most of the antineoplastic drugs.

28.8 Alkylating drugs act by changing the structure of DNA in cancer cells.

28.9 Antimetabolites disrupt critical cellular pathways in cancer cells.

28.10 A few cytotoxic antibiotics are used to treat cancer rather than infections.

28.11 Some natural products kill cancer cells by preventing cell division.

28.12 Some hormones and hormone antagonists are effective against prostate and breast cancer.

28.13 Targeted therapies and some miscellaneous antineoplastic drugs are effective against specific tumors.

28.14 Adjunct medications are sometimes necessary to treat cancer symptoms and to reduce the intensity of adverse effects from antineoplastic drugs.

DRUG SNAPSHOT

The following drugs are discussed in this chapter:

DRUG CLASSES	DRUG PROTOTYPES
Alkylating drugs	(Pr) cyclophosphamide (Cytoxan) *438*
Antimetabolites	(Pr) methotrexate (Rheumatrex, Trexall) *440*
Antitumor antibiotics	(Pr) doxorubicin (Adriamycin) *441*

DRUG CLASSES	DRUG PROTOTYPES
Natural products	(Pr) vincristine (Oncovin) *443*
Hormones and hormone antagonists	(Pr) tamoxifen *444*
Adjunct drugs for cancer patients	(Pr) epoetin alfa (Epogen, Procrit) *446*

LEARNING OUTCOMES

After reading this chapter, the student should be able to:

1. Explain differences between normal cells and cancer cells.

2. Identify the factors associated with an increased incidence of cancer.

3. Describe the lifestyle factors associated with a reduced risk of acquiring cancer.

4. Differentiate among the terms neoplasm, benign, malignant, and carcinoma.

5. Identify the three primary treatments for cancer.
6. Explain why cancer is difficult to cure.
7. Explain how combination therapy and special dosing schedules

increase the effectiveness of chemotherapy.
8. Describe the general adverse effects of antineoplastic drugs.
9. Categorize anticancer drugs based on their classifications and mechanisms of action.

10. For each of the classes listed in the Drug Snapshot, explain their mechanisms of drug action, primary actions, and important adverse effects.

KEY TERMS

adenomas (AH-den-OH-mahz) *432*
adjuvant chemotherapy (AD-ju-vent) *433*
alkylation (AL-kill-AYE-shun) *437*
alopecia (AL-oh-PEESH-ee-uh) *436*
anemia (ah-NEE-mee-ah) *446*
benign (bee-NINE) *432*
cancer (KAN-sir) *431*
carcinogens (kar-SIN-oh-jenz) *432*
chemotherapy *433*
folic acid (FOH-lik) *440*

gliomas (glee-OH-muhz) *432*
leukemia (lew-KEE-mee-ah) *432*
lipomas (lip-OH-mahz) *432*
liposomes (LIP-oh-sohms) *441*
lymphomas (lim-FOH-mahz) *432*
malignant (mah-LIG-nent) *432*
metastasis (mah-TAS-tah-sis) *432*
neoplasm (NEE-oh-PLAZ-um) *432*
nitrogen mustards *437*
palliation (PAL-ee-AYE-shun) *433*

purines (PYUR-eenz) *439*
pyrimidines (peer-IM-uh-deenz) *439*
targeted therapies *445*
taxanes (TAKS-ane) *442*
topoisomerase (TOH-poh-eye-SOM-er-ase) *442*
tumor (TOO-more) *432*
tumor suppressor genes *432*
vinca alkaloids (VIN-ka AL-kah-loids) *442*

Cancer is one of the most feared diseases for a number of valid reasons. It may be silent, producing no symptoms until it is too advanced for a complete cure. It sometimes requires painful and disfiguring surgery. It may strike at an early age—even during childhood—depriving people of a normal lifespan. Perhaps worst of all, the medical treatment of cancer often cannot offer a cure, and progression to death is sometimes psychologically difficult for patients and their loved ones.

Despite its feared status, many advances have been made in the diagnosis, understanding, and treatment of cancer. Modern treatment methods result in a cure for nearly two of every three cancer patients and the five-year survival rate has steadily increased for many types of cancer. This chapter examines the role of drugs in the treatment of cancer. Medications used to treat this disease are called anticancer drugs, antineoplastics, or cancer chemotherapeutic agents.

Cancer is characterized by rapid, uncontrolled growth of cells.

CORE CONCEPT **28.1**

Cancer is a disease characterized by abnormal, uncontrolled cell division. Cell division is a normal process occurring extensively in most body tissues from conception to late childhood. At some point in time, however, most cells stop dividing at such a rapid rate. Indeed, some adult cells such as muscle cells and brain cells have a total lack of ability to divide. In other cells, the genes controlling growth can be turned back on whenever it is necessary to replace worn-out cells, as is the case for blood cells and cells lining the digestive tract.

Fast Facts Cancer

- It is estimated that more than 1,660,000 new cancer cases occur each year, in the United States, with about 580,300 deaths (almost 1,600 people every day).
- Although cancer occurs most frequently in older adults, over 11,600 new cases of childhood cancer occur annually.
- Leukemia is the most common childhood cancer and is responsible for one quarter of all cancers occurring before age 20.
- Lung cancer has the highest mortality rate in both women and men, being responsible for about 29% of all cancer deaths.
- Death rates for breast cancer have steadily decreased in women since 1989, with larger decreases in younger than in older women.
- Pancreatic cancer has the lowest five-year survival rate at 6%. About 65% of patients with pancreatic cancer have either diabetes or prediabetes at the time of diagnosis.
- The highest five-year survival rates are for cancers of the prostate, testes, and thyroid. The lowest survival rates are for pancreatic, lung, and liver cancers.
- Among ethnic groups, African Americans have the highest incidence and death rates for most types of cancers.

FIGURE 28.1

Invasion and metastasis by cancer cells.

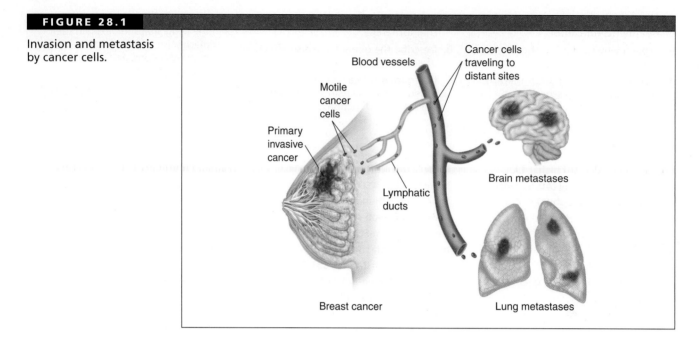

Cancer is thought to result from the damage to genes controlling cell growth. Once damaged, the cell becomes unresponsive to normal chemical signals checking its growth. The cancer cells lose their normal functions, divide rapidly, and invade surrounding cells. The abnormal cells often travel to distant sites, where they populate new tumors, a process called **metastasis**. Figure 28.1 ■ illustrates the metastasis of cancer cells.

neo = *new*
plasm = *thing formed*

The word **tumor** means swelling, abnormal enlargement, or mass. **Neoplasm** is often used interchangeably with tumor. The suffix *-oma* signifies tumor. Tumors may be either benign or malignant.

adeno = *gland*
oma = *tumor*
lip = *fat*

Benign tumors grow slowly, do not metastasize, and rarely require drug treatment. Although they do not kill patients, their growth may cause pressure on nerves, blood vessels, or other tissues. When this occurs, they may be surgically removed; they do not normally grow back. Examples include **adenomas**, which are benign tumors of glandular tissue, and **lipomas**, which are tumors of adipose tissue.

Malignant tumors are called cancer. The word **malignant** refers to a disease that grows rapidly worse, becomes resistant to treatment, and normally results in death. The two major divisions of malignant neoplasms are carcinomas and sarcomas. Other types include cancer of the blood-forming cells in bone marrow (**leukemia**), cancers of lymphatic tissue (**lymphomas**), and cancers of the central nervous system (CNS) (**gliomas**).

leuk = *white*
emia = *blood condition*

CORE CONCEPT 28.2

The causes of cancer may be chemical, physical, or biological.

A large number of factors have been found to cause cancer or to be associated with a higher risk for acquiring the disease. These factors are known as **carcinogens**.

Many chemical carcinogens have been identified. For example, chemicals in tobacco smoke are responsible for about one-third of all cancers in the United States. Some chemicals, such as asbestos and benzene, have been associated with a higher incidence of cancer in the workplace. The actual site of the cancer may be distant from the site of exposure, as is the case of bladder cancer caused by the inhalation of certain industrial chemicals.

A number of physical factors are also associated with cancer. For example, exposure to large amounts of x-rays is associated with a higher risk of leukemia. Ultraviolet (UV) light from the sun is a known cause of skin cancer.

Viruses are associated with about 15% of all human cancers. Examples include herpes simplex viruses types I and II, Epstein-Barr virus, human papillomavirus (HPV), cytomegalovirus, and human T-lymphotrophic viruses. Factors that suppress the immune system, such as HIV or drugs given after transplant surgery, may encourage the growth of cancer cells.

Some cancers have a strong genetic component. The fact that close relatives may acquire the same type of cancer suggests that the patient may have certain genes that predispose him or her to the condition. These abnormal genes interact with chemical, physical, and biological agents to promote cancer formation in the patient. Other genes, called **tumor suppressor genes**, may *inhibit* the formation of tumors. The *BRCA* gene is an example of a tumor suppressor gene that, once damaged, results in a significantly higher incidence of breast cancer. About 40% to 65% of women who have the BRCA mutation will develop breast cancer before age 70.

Concept Review   28.1

■ What is the fundamental feature that makes a cancer cell different from a normal cell?

Personal risk of cancer may be lowered by a number of lifestyle factors.

CORE CONCEPT 28.3

Fortunately, adopting healthy lifestyle habits such as those shown in the following list may reduce the risk of acquiring cancer. Eliminating tobacco use is the most important means of reducing cancer risk. Limiting exposure to exhaled, or secondhand, smoke is also thought to be important. Intake of alcoholic beverages and saturated fats should be limited, and body weight kept within medically recommended ranges. The following list indicates some actions that healthcare providers can recommend to their patients to reduce their risk of cancer:

- Eliminate tobacco use and exposure to secondhand tobacco smoke.
- Maintain a healthy diet low in fat and high in fresh vegetables and fruit.
- Choose most of the foods from plant sources; increase fiber in the diet.
- Exercise regularly and keep body weight within optimum guidelines.
- Self-examine your body monthly for abnormal lumps and skin lesions.
- Avoid chronic or prolonged exposure to direct sunlight and/or wear protective clothing or sunscreen.
- For women, have periodic mammograms, according to the schedule recommended by their healthcare provider.
- For men, receive prostate screening, as recommended by their healthcare provider.
- Receive screening colonoscopy, as recommended by the healthcare provider.
- For women who are sexually active or have reached age 18, have an annual Pap test and pelvic examination.
- For girls, receive the HPV vaccine (Cervarix, Gardasil) according to the schedule recommended by the Centers for Disease Control and Prevention.

The three primary goals of chemotherapy are cure, control, and palliation.

CORE CONCEPT 28.4

Pharmacotherapy of cancer is sometimes simply referred to as **chemotherapy**. Because oral and parenteral drugs are transported through the blood, chemotherapy has the potential to reach cancer cells in virtually any location. Chemotherapy has three general goals: cure, control, or palliation.

When diagnosed with cancer, the primary goal desired by most patients is to achieve a complete cure: permanent removal of all cancer cells from the body. The possibility for cure is much greater if a cancer is identified and treated in its early stages, when the tumor is small and localized to a well-defined region. Examples in which chemotherapy has been used successfully as curative treatments include Hodgkin's lymphoma, certain leukemias, and choriocarcinoma.

When cancer has progressed and cure is not possible, a second goal of chemotherapy is to control or manage the disease. Although the cancer is not eliminated, preventing the growth and spread of the tumor may extend the patient's life. Essentially, the cancer is managed as a chronic disease, as is hypertension or diabetes.

In its advanced stages, cure or control of the cancer may not be achievable. For these patients, chemotherapy is used as **palliation**. Chemotherapy drugs are administered to reduce the size of the tumor, easing the severity of pain and other tumor symptoms, thus improving the quality of life.

Chemotherapy may be used alone or in combination with surgery or radiation therapy. Surgery is especially useful for removing solid tumors that are localized. Surgery lowers the number of cancer cells in the body so that radiation therapy and pharmacotherapy can be more successful. Surgery is not an option for tumors of blood cells or when it would not be expected to extend a patient's life span or to improve the quality of life.

Approximately 50% of patients with cancer receive radiation therapy as part of their treatment. Radiation therapy is most successful for cancers that are localized. Radiation treatments are frequently prescribed postoperatively to kill cancer cells that may remain following an operation. Radiation is sometimes given as palliation for inoperable cancers to shrink the size of a tumor that may be pressing on vital organs and to relieve pain, difficulty breathing, or difficulty swallowing.

Adjuvant chemotherapy is the administration of antineoplastic drugs *after* surgery or radiation therapy. The purpose of adjuvant chemotherapy is to rid the body of any cancerous cells that were not removed during the surgery or to treat any microscopic metastases that may be developing. In a few cases, drugs are given as *chemoprophylaxis* with the goal of preventing cancer from occurring. For example, some patients who have had a primary breast cancer removed may receive tamoxifen, even if there is no evidence of metastases, because there is a high likelihood that the disease will recur. Chemoprophylaxis of cancer is uncommon, because most of these drugs have potentially serious adverse effects.

<table>
<tr><td>**CORE CONCEPT** 28.5</td></tr>
</table>

To achieve a total cure, every malignant cell must be removed or killed.

To cure a patient, it is believed that every single cancer cell must be eliminated from the body. Leaving even a single malignant cell could result in regrowth of the tumor. Eliminating every cancer cell, however, is a very difficult task.

Consider that a 1-cm breast tumor may contain 1 billion cancer cells before it is detected. A drug that kills 99% of these cells would be considered a very effective drug. Yet even with this fantastic achievement, 10 million cancer cells would still remain, any one of which could cause the tumor to return and kill the patient. The relationship between cell kill and chemotherapy is shown in Figure 28.2 ■.

It is likely that no antineoplastic drug (or combination of drugs) will kill 100% of the tumor cells. The large burden of cancer cells, however, may be lowered sufficiently to permit the patient's immune system to control or eliminate the remaining cancer cells. Because the immune system is able to eliminate only a relatively small number of cancer cells, it is important that as many cancerous cells as possible be eliminated during treatment. This example reinforces the need to diagnose and treat tumors at an *early* stage, when the number of cancer cells is smaller.

FIGURE 28.2

Cell kill and chemotherapy.

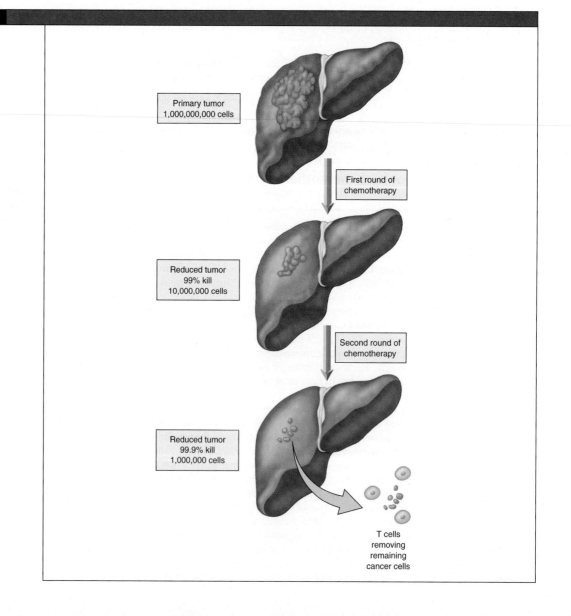

Primary tumor
1,000,000,000 cells

First round of chemotherapy

Reduced tumor
99% kill
10,000,000 cells

Second round of chemotherapy

Reduced tumor
99.9% kill
1,000,000 cells

T cells removing remaining cancer cells

Selenium's Role in Cancer Prevention

Selenium is an essential trace element that is necessary to maintain healthy immune function. It is a vital antioxidant, especially when combined with vitamin E. It protects the immune system by preventing the formation of free radicals, which can damage cells.

Selenium can be found in meat and grains, Brazil nuts, brewer's yeast, broccoli, brown rice, dairy products, garlic, molasses, and onions. The amount of selenium in food, however, has a direct correlation to the selenium content of the soil. The soil of much American farmland is low in selenium, resulting in selenium-deficient produce. Low dietary intake of selenium is associated with increased incidence of several cancers, including lung, colorectal, skin, and prostate cancers. Selenium supplementation has resulted in increased natural killer cell activity, and studies have shown its promise as protection against prostate and colorectal cancers, especially among smokers.

Use of multiple drugs and special dosing schedules improve the success of chemotherapy.

CORE CONCEPT 28.6

Because of their rapid cell division, tumor cells express a high mutation rate. This causes the tumor to change its genetic make-up as it grows, resulting in hundreds of different clones with different growth rates and physiologic properties. An antineoplastic drug may kill only a small portion of the tumor, leaving some clones unaffected. Complicating the chances for a cure is that cancer cells often develop resistance to antineoplastic drugs. Thus a therapy that was very successful in reducing the tumor mass at the start of chemotherapy may become less effective over time.

A number of treatment strategies have been found to increase the effectiveness of anticancer drugs. In most cases, multiple medications from different antineoplastic classes are given concurrently during a course of chemotherapy. Multiple classes will affect different stages of the cancer cell's life cycle, as illustrated in Figure 28.3 ■. This allows the tumor to be attacked through several mechanisms of action, thus increasing the cell kill percentage. Using multiple drugs also allows the dosages of each individual medication to be lowered, thereby reducing toxicity and slowing the development of resistance. Examples of common therapies include cyclophosphamide-methotrexate-fluorouracil (CMF)

FIGURE 28.3

Antineoplastic drugs and the cell cycle.

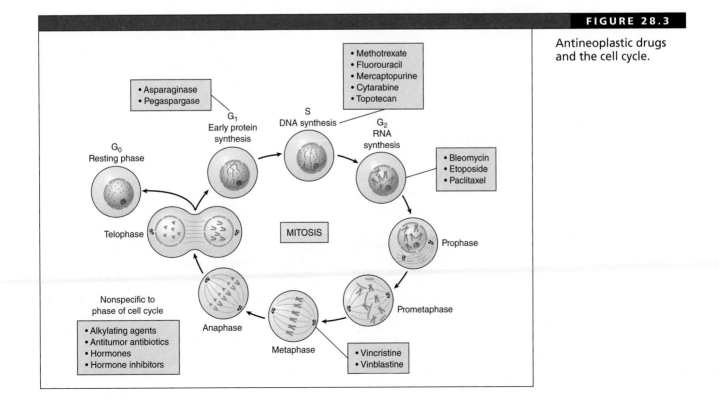

for breast cancer, cyclophosphamide-doxorubicin-vincristine (CAV) for lung cancer, and cyclo-phosphamide-doxorubicin-vincristine-prednisone (CHOP) for non-Hodgkin's lymphoma. Each type of cancer requires its own individual protocol, which is continually being revised based on recent research.

Specific dosing schedules or cycles have been found to increase the effectiveness of antineoplastic drugs. For example, some anticancer drugs are given as single doses or perhaps a couple of doses over a few days. Several weeks may pass before the next series of doses. This gives normal cells time to recover from the adverse effects of the drugs, especially bone marrow suppression. It also allows tumor cells that may not have been replicating at the time of the first dose to begin dividing and become more sensitive to the next round of chemotherapy. The specific dosing schedule depends on the type of tumor, stage of the disease, and the patient's overall condition.

Concept Review 28.2

■ Why is it important to kill or remove 100% of the cancer cells to achieve a cure?

CORE CONCEPT 28.7

Serious toxicity limits therapy with most of the antineoplastic drugs.

Almost all anticancer drugs have the potential to cause serious toxicity. These drugs are often pushed to their maximum possible dosages so that the greatest cell kill can be obtained. Such high dosages always result in adverse effects in the patient. A list of typical adverse effects of anticancer drugs is given in Table 28.1 ◆.

Normal tissues that are rapidly dividing in the adult are most susceptible to adverse effects. Hair follicles are damaged, resulting in hair loss or **alopecia**. The lining of the digestive tract is affected, sometimes resulting in bleeding, difficulty eating, or severe diarrhea. The vomiting center in the medulla is triggered by many antineoplastics, resulting in severe nausea and vomiting. Vomiting is often so severe that patients may be treated with antiemetic drugs such as prochlorperazine (Compazine) or odansetron (Zofran) just prior to the start of antineoplastic therapy. Blood cells in the bone marrow may be destroyed, causing a reduction in the number of red blood cells (RBCs), white blood cells (WBCs), and platelets. Severe effects on blood cells often cause discontinuation of chemotherapy. Efforts to minimize this toxicity may include therapy with growth factors such as filgrastim (Neupogen) or sargramostim (Leukine). These drugs stimulate the production of WBCs within the bone marrow.

Antineoplastic drugs act by many mechanisms, most of which involve cell killing, or cytotoxicity. Classification is quite variable because some drugs kill cancer cells by several mechanisms and have characteristics from more than one class. Furthermore, the mechanisms by which some of these medications act are not completely understood. A simple method of classifying this complex class of drugs includes the following groups:

- Alkylating drugs
- Antimetabolites
- Antitumor antibiotics
- Natural products
- Hormones and hormone blockers
- Targeted therapies and miscellaneous drugs

TABLE 28.1 Adverse Effects of Anticancer Drugs		
Blood Toxicity	**GI Toxicity**	**Other Effects**
Anemia (low red blood cell count)	Anorexia (loss of appetite)	Alopecia (loss of hair)
Leukopenia (low white blood cell count)	Bleeding	Fatigue
Thrombocytopenia (low platelet count)	Diarrhea	Fetal birth defects
	Nausea and vomiting	Opportunistic infections
		Ulceration and bleeding of the lips and gums

Alkylating drugs act by changing the structure of DNA in cancer cells.

Alkylating drugs act by chemically binding to DNA and inhibiting cell division. They are some of the most widely used antineoplastic drugs. Table 28.2 ◆ lists the alkylating drugs and their dosages.

The first alkylating drugs, the **nitrogen mustards**, were developed in secrecy as chemical warfare agents during World War II. Although the drugs in this class have very different chemical structures, all have the common characteristic of being able to form bonds or linkages with DNA. These agents physically attach to DNA, a process called **alkylation**. Alkylation changes the shape of DNA and prevents it from functioning normally. Although each alkylating drug attaches to DNA in a different manner, collectively they have the effect of inducing cell death, or at least slowing the replication of tumor cells. The alkylation may occur in any cancer cell; however, the killing action does not occur until the affected cell attempts to divide. Figure 28.4 ■ illustrates the process of alkylation.

Because blood cells are particularly sensitive to alkylating drugs, bone marrow suppression is the primary dose-limiting toxicity of these drugs. Within days of administration, the numbers of RBCs, WBCs, and platelets begin to decline. Cells lining the gastrointestinal (GI) tract are also damaged, resulting in nausea, vomiting, and diarrhea. Alopecia is expected from most of the alkylating drugs. As a delayed adverse effect, some patients treated with alkylating agents will develop acute leukemia four years or more after chemotherapy has been completed.

TABLE 28.2   Alkylating Drugs

Drug	Route and Adult Dose	Remarks
NITROGEN MUSTARDS		
bendamustine (Treanda)	IV; 90–120 mg/m^2 (variable schedule)	Newer antineoplastic drug; for chronic lymphocytic leukemia and non-Hodgkin's lymphoma
busulfan (Busulflex, Myleran)	PO; 4–8 mg daily	For chronic myelogenous leukemia; also available IV, prior to stem cell transplant
chlorambucil (Leukeran)	PO; initial dose 0.1–0.2 mg/kg daily; maintenance dose 4–10 mg daily	For chronic lymphocytic leukemia; non-Hodgkin's lymphoma, and cancer of the breast and ovary
ⓟ cyclophosphamide (Cytoxan)	PO; initial dose 1–5 mg/kg daily; maintenance dose 1–5 mg/kg every 7–10 days	For Hodgkin's disease, non-Hodgkin's lymphoma, leukemias, multiple myeloma, and cancer of the breast, ovary, and lung; IV form available
estramustine (Emcyt)	PO; 14 mg/kg/day in 3–4 divided doses	For palliative treatment of advanced prostate cancer
ifosfamide (Ifex)	IV; 1.2 g/m^2 daily for five consecutive days	For testicular cancer
mechlorethamine (Mustargen)	IV; 6 mg/m^2 on days 1 and 8 of a 28-day cycle	For Hodgkin's disease, non-Hodgkin's lymphoma, and lung cancer
melphalan (Alkeran)	PO; 6 mg daily for 2–3 weeks	For multiple myeloma
NITROSOUREAS		
carmustine (BiCNU, Gliadel)	IV; 200 mg/m^2 every 6 weeks	For Hodgkin's disease, malignant melanoma, multiple myeloma, and brain cancer
lomustine (CeeNU)	PO; 130 mg/m^2 as a single dose	For Hodgkin's disease and brain cancer
streptozocin (Zanosar)	IV; 500 mg/m^2 for five consecutive days	For pancreatic cancer
OTHER ALKYLATING DRUGS		
carboplatin (Paraplatin)	IV; 360 mg/m^2 every 4 weeks	For cancer of the ovary
cisplatin (Platinol)	IV; 20 mg/m^2 daily for 5 days	For testicular, bladder, ovarian, uterine, head, and neck carcinomas
dacarbazine (DTIC-Dome)	IV; 2–4.5 mg/kg daily for 10 days	For Hodgkin's disease and malignant melanoma
oxaliplatin (Eloxatin)	IV; 85 mg/m^2 infused over 120 minutes once every 2 weeks	For metastatic colorectal cancer
temozolomide (Temodar)	PO; 150 mg/m^2 daily for five consecutive days	For brain cancer
thiotepa (Thioplex)	IV; 0.3–0.4 mg/kg every 1–4 weeks	For Hodgkin's disease and breast and ovarian cancer

FIGURE 28.4

Mechanism of action of alkylating drugs.

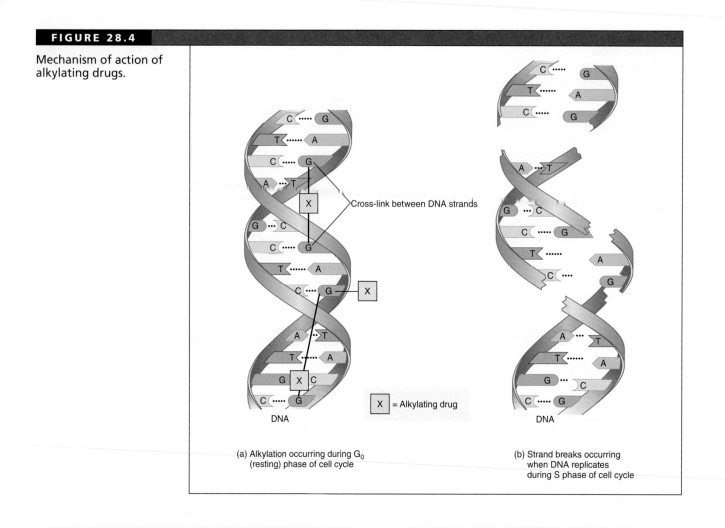

Cross-link between DNA strands

X = Alkylating drug

DNA

DNA

(a) Alkylation occurring during G₀ (resting) phase of cell cycle

(b) Strand breaks occurring when DNA replicates during S phase of cell cycle

Drug Prototype: 🅟 *Cyclophosphamide (Cytoxan)*
Therapeutic Class: Antineoplastic **Pharmacologic Class: Alkylating drug**

Actions and Uses: Cyclophosphamide is a commonly prescribed nitrogen mustard. It is used alone or in combination with other drugs against a wide variety of cancers, including Hodgkin's disease, lymphoma, multiple myeloma, breast cancer, and ovarian cancer. Cyclophosphamide acts by attaching to DNA and disrupting cell replication, particularly in rapidly dividing cells. It is one of only a few anticancer drugs that are well absorbed when given orally.

Cyclophosphamide is a powerful immunosuppressant. Although this is considered an adverse effect during cancer chemotherapy, the drug is sometimes used to *intentionally* cause immunosuppression for the prophylaxis of organ transplant rejection and to treat severe rheumatoid arthritis and systemic lupus erythematosus (SLE).

Adverse Effects and Interactions: Bone marrow suppression is a potentially life-threatening adverse reaction that occurs during days 9–14 of therapy; the patient is at dangerous risk for severe infection and sepsis during this period. Thrombocytopenia is common; thus bleeding and bruising may be observed. Nausea, vomiting, and diarrhea are frequently experienced. Fifty percent of patients will develop total baldness, although this effect is usually reversible. Unlike other nitrogen mustards, cyclophosphamide causes little neurotoxicity.

Cyclophosphamide interacts with many drugs. For example, immunosuppressant agents may increase the risk of infections and promote the development of neoplasms. There is an increased chance of bone marrow toxicity if cyclophosphamide is used together with allopurinol. There is an increased risk of bleeding if given with anticoagulants.

If used with digoxin, decreased serum levels of digoxin occur. Using it with insulin may lead to increased hypoglycemia. Phenobarbital, phenytoin, or glucocorticoids may lead to an increased rate of cyclophosphamide metabolism by the liver. Thiazide diuretic use with cyclophosphamide may lead to leukopenia.

St. John's wort may increase the toxic effects of cyclophosphamide.

Antimetabolites disrupt critical cellular pathways in cancer cells.

Rapidly growing cancer cells require large amounts of nutrients to build proteins and nucleic acids. Antimetabolites are drugs that chemically resemble essential building blocks of the cell. When cancer cells attempt to construct proteins or DNA, they use the antimetabolite drugs instead of the normal building blocks. By disrupting metabolic pathways in this manner, antimetabolites can kill cancer cells or slow their growth. For example, methotrexate interferes with the synthesis of folate. Folate is required for the synthesis of DNA, RNA, and protein in rapidly dividing cancer cells. The antimetabolites are listed in Table 28.3 ◆.

Several of these antimetabolites resemble **purines** and **pyrimidines**, chemicals that are the building blocks of DNA and RNA. These antimetabolites are called purine or pyrimidine analogs. For example, floxuridine (FUDR) and fluorouracil (Adrucil) are able to block the formation of thymidylate, an essential chemical needed to make DNA. After becoming activated and incorporated into DNA, cytarabine (Cytosar) blocks DNA synthesis. Figure 28.5 ■ illustrates the similarities of some of these analogs to their natural counterparts.

TABLE 28.3	Antimetabolites	
Drug	**Route and Adult Dose**	**Remarks**
FOLIC ACID ANTAGONISTS		
℗ methotrexate (Rheumatrex, Trexall)	PO; 10–30 mg/day for 5 days	For acute lymphoblastic leukemia, choriocarcinoma, lymphoma, head and neck cancer, testicular cancer, bone cancer; IV and IM forms available
pemetrexed (Alimta)	IV; 500 mg/m^2 on day 1 of each 21-day cycle	For malignant mesothelioma and non–small cell lung cancer
pralatrexate (Folotyn)	IV; 30 mg/m^2 administered over 3–5 minutes	For refractory T-cell lymphoma
PYRIMIDINE AND PURINE ANALOGS		
capecitabine (Xeloda)	PO; 2,500 mg/m^2 daily for 2 weeks	For metastatic breast cancer and colon cancer
cladribine (Leustatin)	IV; 0.09 mg/m^2	For hairy cell leukemia
clofarabine (Clolar)	IV; 52 mg/m^2 over 2 hours for five consecutive days	For childhood acute lymphoblastic leukemia
cytarabine (Cytosar, Cytosine arabinoside, Depot-Cyt)	IV; 200 mg/m^2 as a continuous infusion over 24 hours	For leukemias and lymphomas; subcutaneous and intrathecal forms available
fludarabine (Fludara)	IV; 25 mg/m^2 daily	For chronic lymphocytic leukemia
floxuridine (FUDR)	Intra-arterial; 0.1–0.6 mg/kg daily as a continuous infusion	For metastasis from the GI tract to the liver
fluorouracil (5-FU, Adrucil, Efudex, Fluorodex)	IV; 12 mg/kg daily for four consecutive days	For cancer of the breast, colon, rectum, stomach, and pancreas; topical form available for basal cell carcinoma
gemcitabine (Gemzar)	IV; 1,000 mg/m^2 every week	For advanced cancers of the pancreas, breast, ovaries, and lung
mercaptopurine (6-MP, Purinethol)	PO; 2.5 mg/kg daily	For childhood acute leukemia
nelarabine (Arranon)	IV; 1,500 mg/m^2 on days 1, 3, and 5; repeat every 21 days	For leukemias and lymphomas
pentostatin (Nipent)	IV; 4 mg/m^2 every other week	For hairy cell leukemia
thioguanine (Tabloid)	PO; 2 mg/kg daily	For remission induction in adult acute leukemia

FIGURE 28.5

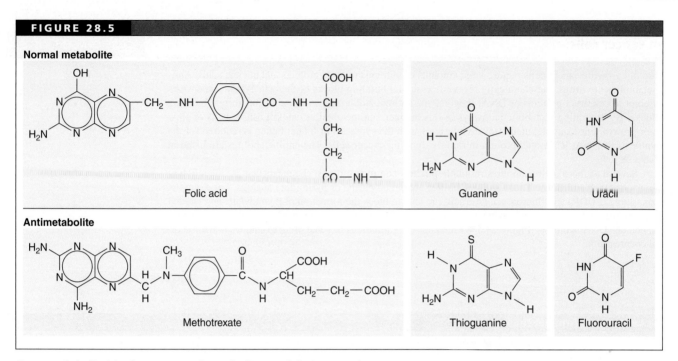

Structural similarities between antimetabolites and their natural counterparts.

Drug Prototype: ℗ *Methotrexate (Rheumatrex, Trexall)*

Therapeutic Class: Antineoplastic   **Pharmacologic Class: Antimetabolite, folic acid analog**

Actions and Uses: Methotrexate blocks folic acid metabolism in rapidly growing tumor cells. **Folic acid** is a water-soluble vitamin found in eggs, veal, liver, whole grains, and dark green vegetables. Folic acid is part of a coenzyme essential to the synthesis of nucleic acids.

Methotrexate is prescribed alone or in combination with other drugs for choriocarcinoma, bone cancers, leukemias, head and neck cancers, breast carcinoma, and lung carcinoma. It is occasionally used to treat non-neoplastic disorders such as severe psoriasis, rheumatoid arthritis, and lupus that are unresponsive to safer medications.

Adverse Effects and Interactions: Methotrexate has many adverse effects, some of which can be life threatening and which are described in the black box warning. In addition, hemorrhage and bruising due to low platelet counts are often observed. Nausea, vomiting, and anorexia are common. Methotrexate is a pregnancy category X drug.

Methotrexate interacts with several drugs. Bone marrow suppressants such as other antineoplastic drugs may cause increased effects; the patient will require a lower dose of methotrexate. When used with NSAIDs, severe methotrexate toxicity may occur.

Aspirin may interfere with excretion of methotrexate, leading to increased serum levels and toxicity. Administration with live oral vaccine may result in decreased antibody response and increased adverse reactions to the vaccine. Use with caution with herbal supplements, such as echinacea, which may interfere with the drug's immunosuppressant effects.

BLACK BOX WARNINGS:
Methotrexate combined with nonsteroidal anti-inflammatory drugs (NSAIDs) may cause severe and sometimes fatal bone marrow suppression, which is the primary dose-limiting toxicity of this drug. The drug is hepatotoxic and may cause liver cirrhosis. Ulcerative stomatitis and diarrhea require suspension of therapy because they may lead to intestinal bleeding or perforation. Potentially fatal opportunistic infections may occur during therapy. Pulmonary toxicity may result in acute or chronic interstitial pneumonitis at any dose level. Severe, sometimes fatal, dermatologic reactions such as toxic epidermal necrolysis and Stevens–Johnson syndrome (SJS) have been reported.

CORE CONCEPT 28.10

A few cytotoxic antibiotics are used to treat cancer rather than infections.

Antitumor antibiotics are drugs obtained from bacteria that have the ability to kill cancer cells. Although they are not widely prescribed, they are very effective against certain tumors. Table 28.4 ◆ lists the primary antitumor antibiotics.

TABLE 28.4   Antitumor Antibiotics

Drug	Route and Adult Dose	Remarks
bleomycin (Blenoxane)	IV; 0.25–0.5 units/kg every 4–7 days	For squamous cell carcinoma, Hodgkin's disease, lymphomas, and testicular cancer
dactinomycin (Cosmegen)	IV; 500 mcg/day for a maximum of 5 days	For Wilms' tumor and rhabdomyosarcoma
daunorubicin (Cerubidine)	IV; 30–60 mg/m^2 daily for 3–5 days	For leukemias and lymphomas
daunorubicin liposomal (DaunoXome)	IV; 40 mg/m^2 every 2 weeks	For Kaposi's sarcoma
Pr doxorubicin (Adriamycin)	IV; 60–75 mg/m^2 as a single dose	For lymphomas, sarcomas, acute leukemia, and cancer of the breast, lung, testes, thyroid, and ovary
doxorubicin liposomal (Doxil, Evacet)	IV; 20 mg/m^2 every 3 weeks	For Kaposi's sarcoma, refractory ovarian cancer and refractory multiple myeloma
epirubicin (Ellence)	IV; 100–120 mg/m^2 as a single dose	For breast cancer
idarubicin (Idamycin)	IV; 8–12 mg/m^2 daily for 3 days	For acute myelogenous leukemia
mitomycin (Mutamycin)	IV; 2 mg/m^2 as a single dose	For cancer of the colon, stomach, lung, head and neck, rectum, bladder, pancreas, and breast; also for malignant melanoma
mitoxantrone (Novantrone)	IV; 12 mg/m^2 daily for 3 days	For acute nonlymphocytic leukemia

Several substances isolated from bacteria have been found to possess antitumor properties. These chemicals are more toxic than the traditional antibiotics; thus, their use is restricted to treating specific cancers. All the antitumor antibiotics interact with DNA in a manner similar to the alkylating drugs. Because of this, their general actions and adverse effects are similar to those of the alkylating drugs. Unlike the alkylating drugs, however, all the antitumor antibiotics must be administered intravenously or through direct instillation into a body cavity using a catheter. A major dose-limiting adverse effect of drugs in this class is bone marrow suppression.

Drug Prototype: Pr *Doxorubicin (Adriamycin)*
Therapeutic Class: Antineoplastic   Pharmacologic Class: Antitumor antibiotic

Actions and Uses: Doxorubicin attaches to DNA, causing the double strands to be distorted, thus preventing cancer cell division. It is prescribed for solid tumors of the lung, breast, ovary, and bladder, and for certain types of leukemias and lymphomas. It is structurally similar to daunorubicin (Cerubidine). Doxorubicin is one of the most effective single drugs against solid tumors.

A novel delivery method has been developed for both doxorubicin and daunorubicin. The drug is enclosed in small sacs, or vesicles, of lipids called **liposomes**. The liposomal vesicle opens and releases the antitumor antibiotic when it reaches a cancer cell. The goal is to deliver a higher concentration of drug directly to the cancer cells, thus sparing normal cells. Doxorubicin liposomal is approved for use in patients with Kaposi's sarcoma, refractory ovarian tumors, and relapsed multiple myeloma.

Adverse Effects and Interactions: Doxorubicin has many adverse effects, some of which can be life threatening and which are described in the black box warning. In addition, nausea, vomiting, diarrhea, and hair loss are common.

Doxorubicin interacts with many drugs. If digoxin is taken at the same time, the patient will have decreased serum digoxin levels. Phenobarbital leads to increased plasma clearance of doxorubicin and decreased effectiveness. Using doxorubicin with phenytoin may lead to decreased phenytoin levels and possible seizure activity. Liver toxicity may occur if mercaptopurine is taken at the same time. Using with verapamil may increase serum doxorubicin levels, leading to doxorubicin toxicity.

BLACK BOX WARNING:
Severe bone marrow suppression may occur, which is the major dose-limiting toxicity with doxorubicin. It may manifest as seriously low blood cell counts. Doxorubicin exhibits significant cardiotoxicity, which may be either acute or chronic. Cardiac adverse effects can be life threatening and may include sinus tachycardia, bradycardia, delayed heart failure, acute left ventricular failure, and myocarditis. Heart failure may occur months or years after the termination of therapy. Acute, IV infusion–related reactions may occur, including anaphylaxis. Severe local necrosis may result if extravasation occurs. Secondary malignancies, especially acute myelogenous leukemia, may occur one to three years following therapy.

Some natural products kill cancer cells by preventing cell division.

Natural products are substances with anticancer properties that have been extracted from plants. The natural products used as antineoplastics are listed in Table 28.5 ◆.

Chemicals with antineoplastic activity have been isolated from a number of plants, including the common periwinkle (*Vinca rosea*), the Pacific yew, the mandrake plant (May apple), and the shrub *Campothecus acuminata*. Although structurally very different, drugs in this class have the common ability to arrest cell division; thus they are sometimes called *mitotic inhibitors*.

The **vinca alkaloids**, vincristine (Oncovin) and vinblastine (Velban), are older medications derived from the periwinkle plant. Their biological properties were described in folklore for many years in various parts of the world prior to their use as anticancer drugs.

Native Americans described uses of the May apple long before teniposide (Vumon) and etoposide (VePesid) were isolated from this plant and used for chemotherapy. These drugs are called **topoisomerase** inhibitors because they block the enzyme topoisomerase, whose natural function is to help repair DNA damage. Bone marrow suppression is a serious adverse effect of most natural product drugs. More recently isolated topoisomerase inhibitors include topotecan (Hycamtin), which is used to treat metastatic ovarian cancer and lung cancer, and irinotecan (Camptosar), which is indicated for metastatic cancer of the colon.

The **taxanes**, which include cabazitaxel (Jevtana), paclitaxel (Abraxane, Taxol), and docetaxel (Taxotere), were isolated from the Pacific yew, an evergreen found throughout the Western United States. Paclitaxel is approved for metastatic ovarian and breast cancer and for Kaposi's sarcoma; however, off-label uses include many other cancers. Bone marrow toxicity is usually the dose-limiting factor for the taxanes.

TABLE 28.5 Natural Products

Drug	Route and Adult Dose	Remarks
VINCA ALKALOIDS		
vinblastine (Velban)	IV; 3.7–18.5 mg/m² every week	For cancer of the breast and testes; Hodgkin's disease
Pr vincristine (Oncovin, Vincasar)	IV; 1.4 mg/m² every week (max: 2 mg/m²)	For acute leukemias, Hodgkin's disease, lymphosarcoma, neuroblastoma, Wilms' tumor, lung and breast cancer, reticular cell carcinoma, and osteogenic sarcomas
vincristine liposome (Marquibo)	IV; 2.25 mg/m² once every week	For acute lymphoblastic leukemia
vinorelbine (Navelbine)	IV; 30 mg/m² every week	For lung cancer
TAXANES		
cabazitaxel (Jevtana)	IV: 25 mg/m² every 3 weeks	For prostate cancer
docetaxel (Taxotere)	IV; 60–100 mg/m² every 3 weeks	For ovarian cancer, metastatic breast and prostate cancer, advanced stomach cancer, and lung cancer
paclitaxel (Abraxane, Taxol)	IV; 135–175 mg/m² every 3 weeks	For Kaposi's sarcoma, ovarian cancer, metastatic breast cancer, lung cancer, and certain other solid tumors
TOPOISOMERASE INHIBITORS AND OTHER NATURAL PRODUCTS		
eribulin (Halaven)	IV; 1.4 mg/m² on days 1 and 8 of a 21-day cycle	For metastatic breast cancer
etoposide (VePesid)	IV; 50–100 mg/m² daily for 5 days	For testicular and lung cancer; choriocarcinomas; PO form available
irinotecan (Camptosar)	IV; 125 mg/m² every week for 4 weeks	For colorectal cancer
teniposide (Vumon)	IV; 165 mg/m² every 3–4 days for 4 weeks	For acute lymphocytic leukemia
topotecan (Hycamtin)	IV; 1.5 mg/m² daily for 5 days	For ovarian cancer

Drug Prototype: ⓟ *Vincristine (Oncovin)*
Therapeutic Class: Antineoplastic   **Pharmacologic Class: Vinca alkaloid, plant extract**

Actions and Uses: Vincristine affects rapidly growing cells by inhibiting their ability to complete mitosis. Although it must be given IV, a major advantage of vincristine is that it causes minimal immunosuppression. It is usually prescribed in combination with other antineoplastics for the treatment of lymphoma, leukemias, Kaposi's sarcoma, Wilms' tumor, bladder carcinoma, and breast carcinoma. A newer form of vincristine (Marquibo), encased in a liposomal carrier, was approved in 2012 for acute lymphoblastic leukemia.

Adverse Effects and Interactions: Vincristine has many adverse effects, some of which can be life threatening and which are described in the black box warning. In addition, the major dose-limiting adverse effect of vincristine is neurotoxicity. Symptoms include numbness and tingling in the limbs, muscular weakness, loss of neural reflexes, and pain. CNS effects may include seizures, depression, hallucinations, and coma. Severe constipation is common. Reversible alopecia occurs in most patients.

Vincristine interacts with many drugs. Asparaginase used together with or before vincristine may cause increased neurotoxicity secondary to decreased liver clearance of vincristine. Doxorubicin or prednisone may increase bone marrow suppression. Calcium channel blockers may increase vincristine accumulation in cells. When used with digoxin, the patient may need an increased digoxin dose. When vincristine is given with methotrexate, the patient may need lower doses of methotrexate. Vincristine may decrease serum phenytoin levels, leading to increased seizure activity.

BLACK BOX WARNINGS:
Myelosuppression may be severe and predispose to opportunistic infections. Extravasation can cause intense pain, inflammation, and tissue necrosis. If extravasation occurs, treatment with warm compresses and hyaluronidase is recommended; cold compresses will significantly increase the toxicity of vinca alkaloids.

Some hormones and hormone antagonists are effective against prostate and breast cancer.

CORE CONCEPT 28.12

Use of hormones or hormone antagonists is a strategy used to slow the growth of hormone-dependent tumors. Most hormone therapies are limited to treating hormone-sensitive tumors of the breast or prostate. The major hormones and hormone antagonists prescribed for cancer are given in Table 28.6 ◆.

The growth of certain tumors of reproductive tissues is greatly stimulated by natural hormones. Administering high doses of specific hormones or hormone antagonists can block these receptors and slow tumor growth. For example, administering the male hormone testosterone or the antiestrogen drug tamoxifen can slow specific types of breast cancer that depend on estrogen for growth. Tamoxifen is one of the most widely used drugs for this type of cancer. Administration of the female sex hormone estrogen slows the growth of prostate cancer. The other major class of hormones used for chemotherapy is the corticosteroids. When used for chemotherapy, the doses of these hormones are much higher than the levels normally found in the body. Additional indications for hormone pharmacotherapy are discussed in Chapter 32.

As a group, hormones and hormone antagonists are the least toxic of the antineoplastic classes. They can, however, cause serious adverse effects when given at high doses for prolonged periods. Because they rarely produce cancer cures when used singly, these drugs are normally given for palliation.

Concept Review 28.3

■ Would a patient with breast cancer be given estrogen, or an estrogen antagonist? Explain your answer.

TABLE 28.6   Hormones and Hormone Antagonists

Drug	Route and Adult Dose	Remarks
HORMONES		
dexamethasone (Decadron, others)	PO; 0.25 mg bid–qid	For palliative treatment of leukemias and lymphomas
diethylstilbestrol (DES, Stilbestrol)	PO; for treatment of prostate cancer, 500 mg tid; for palliation, 1–15 mg daily	For cancer of the prostate and breast
ethinyl estradiol (Estinyl, others)	PO; for treatment of breast cancer, 1 mg tid for 2–3 months; for palliation of prostate cancer, 0.15–3 mg/day	For cancer of the prostate and breast, and contraception
fluoxymesterone (Halotestin)	PO; 10 mg tid	For breast cancer

(continued)

TABLE 28.6 Hormones and Hormone Antagonists (*continued*)

Drug	Route and Adult Dose	Remarks
methoxyprogesterone (Depo-Provera, Depo-SubQ-Provera, Provera) (see page 552 for the Drug Prototype box)	IM; 400–1,000 mg every week	For uterine and renal cancer, dysfunctional uterine bleeding, and contraception
megestrol (Megace)	PO; 40–160 mg bid–qid	For advanced cancer of the prostate and breast
prednisone (see page 369 for the Drug Prototype box)	PO; 20–100 mg/m^2 daily	For acute leukemia, Hodgkin's disease, lymphomas, and many inflammatory conditions
testolactone (Teslac)	PO, 250 mg qid	For breast cancer
testosterone (Andro 100, Histerone, Testred, Delatest)	IM; 200–400 mg every 2–4 weeks	For breast cancer and replacement therapy in men
HORMONE ANTAGONISTS		
abiraterone (Zytiga)	PO: 1 g once daily in combination with prednisone	For prostate cancer
anastrozole (Arimidex)	PO; 1 mg daily	For advanced breast cancer
bicalutamide (Casodex)	PO; 50 mg daily	For metastatic prostate cancer
degarelix (Firmagon)	Subcutaneous; 240 mg loading dose followed by 80 mg every 28 days	For advanced prostate cancer
enzalutamide (Xtandi)	PO; 160 mg once daily	For metastatic prostate cancer
exemestane (Aromasin)	PO; 25 mg daily after a meal	For advanced breast cancer
flutamide (Eulexin)	PO; 250 mg tid	For prostate cancer
goserelin (Zoladex)	Subcutaneous; 3.6 mg every 28 days	For prostate and breast cancer, dysfunctional uterine bleeding, and endometriosis
histrelin (Vantas)	Implant; one implant every 12 months (50 mg)	For palliation of advanced prostate cancer
letrozole (Femara)	PO; 2.5 mg daily	For advanced breast cancer
leuprolide (Eligard, Lupron, Viadur)	Subcutaneous; 1 mg daily	For palliation of advanced prostate cancer, endometriosis, and precocious puberty; IM depot form available
nilutamide (Nilandron)	PO; 300 mg/daily for 30 days, then 150 mg daily	For metastatic prostate cancer
raloxifene (Evista) (see page 571 for the Drug Prototype box)	PO; 60 mg once daily	For prophylaxis of breast cancer; treatment of osteoporosis in postmenopausal women;
Ⓟ tamoxifen	PO; 10–20 mg bid	For breast cancer
toremifene (Fareston)	PO; 60 mg daily	For metastatic breast cancer
triptorelin (Trelstar)	IM; 3.75 mg once monthly	For palliation of advanced prostate cancer

Drug Prototype: Ⓟ *Tamoxifen*

Therapeutic Class: Antineoplastic **Pharmacologic Class: Hormone, estrogen receptor blocker**

Actions and Uses: Because it blocks estrogen receptors in cancer cells, tamoxifen is sometimes classified as an antiestrogenic. Tamoxifen is effective against breast tumors that require estrogen for their growth. These susceptible cancer cells are known as estrogen receptor (ER)-positive cells. Tamoxifen is given orally and is a preferred drug for treating breast cancer.

A unique feature of tamoxifen is that it is the only antineoplastic that is approved for prophylaxis of breast cancer—for high-risk patients who are at risk of developing the disease. In addition, it is approved as adjunctive therapy in women following mastectomy to decrease the potential for cancer in the other breast.

Adverse Effects and Interactions: Other than nausea and vomiting, tamoxifen produces little of the serious toxicity observed with other antineoplastics. Hot flashes, fluid retention, venous blood clots, and abnormal vaginal bleeding are relatively common.

Tamoxifen interacts with several drugs. For example, anticoagulants may increase the risk of bleeding. Using this drug with cytotoxic drugs may increase the risk of blood clots.

BLACK BOX WARNINGS:
The most serious problem associated with tamoxifen use is the increased risk of endometrial cancer. The benefits of tamoxifen outweigh the risks in women who are taking tamoxifen to *treat* breast cancer. The benefit versus risk is not as clear in women who are taking tamoxifen to *prevent* breast cancer. There is also a slightly increased risk of thromboembolic disease, including stroke, pulmonary embolism, and deep venous thrombosis (DVT) with the use of tamoxifen. The risk of a thromboembolic event is believed to be about the same as for oral contraceptives.

Targeted therapies and some miscellaneous antineoplastic drugs are effective against specific tumors.

Although they originated from normal cells, cancer cells are clearly different. Scientists have been quite productive in finding ways that cancer cells differ, and in developing drugs that take advantage of these differences. Dozens of new antineoplastic drugs are now available that target specific aspects of cancer cell physiology. These drugs, appropriately called **targeted therapies**, were developed with the hope that they would be more selective in their cell killing than existing drugs and thus cause fewer adverse effects in normal cells. Unfortunately, this has not always been the case.

Monoclonal antibodies (MABs) are a type of targeted therapies that are engineered to attack only one *specific* type of tumor cell. Once the MAB binds to its target cell, the cancer cell dies or is marked for destruction by other cells of the immune response. For example, rituximab (Rituxan) is a MAB that binds to CD20, a surface protein present on cancerous B lymphocytes. Once bound, rituximab shatters the tumor cells. The largest group of targeted therapies attack tyrosine kinase, a key enzyme for cell growth. The development of new targeted therapies for cancer is progressing at a rapid rate. These drugs, along with some miscellaneous antineoplastics, are shown in Table 28.7 ◆.

TABLE 28.7   Selected Targeted Therapies and Miscellaneous Anticancer Drugs*

Drug	Route and Adult Dose	Remarks
alemtuzumab (Campath)	IV; 3–30 mg/day	For chronic lymphocytic leukemia
altretamine (Hexalen)	PO; 65 mg/m^2/day	For ovarian cancer
arsenic trioxide (Trisenox)	IV; 0.15 mg/kg/day	For acute promyelocytic leukemia
axitinib (Inlyta)	PO; 5 mg bid	For advanced renal cancer
bevacizumab (Avastin)	IV; 5 mg/kg every 14 days	For metastatic colorectal cancer
cetuximab (Erbitux)	IV; 400 mg/m^2 over 2 hours, then 250 mg/m^2 over 1 hour weekly	For metastatic colorectal cancer
erlotinib (Tarceva)	PO; 150 mg once daily	For metastatic non–small cell lung cancer
gefitinib (Iressa)	PO; 250–500 mg/day	For advanced or metastatic lung cancer
gemtuzumab (Mylotarg)	IV; 9 mg/m^2 for 2 hours	For acute myeloid leukemia
imatinib (Gleevec)	PO; 400–600 mg daily	For chronic myeloid leukemia after failure with interferon alfa therapy
Pr interferon alfa-2 (Intron A)	Subcutaneous or IM; 2–3 million units daily for leukemia; 36 million units daily for Kaposi's sarcoma	For hairy cell leukemia, Kaposi's sarcoma non-Hodgkin's lymphoma, and malignant melanoma; also for chronic hepatitis B and C viral infections
levamisole (Ergamisol)	PO; 50 mg tid for 3 days	For colon cancer
mitotane (Lysodren)	PO; 3–4 mg tid–qid	For adrenal cortex cancer
ofatumumab (Arzerra)	IV; 300 mg initial dose followed by 2,000 mg weekly for 7 doses	Newer antineoplastic drug; for chronic lymphocytic leukemia
pazopanib (Votrient)	PO; 800 mg once daily	Newer antineoplastic drug; for advanced renal carcinoma
pegaspargase (Oncaspar, PEG-L-asparaginase)	IV; 2,500 international units/m^2 every 14 days	For acute lymphocytic leukemia; IM form available
pertuzumab (Perjeta)	IV; 840 mg followed every 3 weeks thereafter by 420 mg	For metastatic breast cancer
procarbazine (Matulane)	PO; 2–4 mg/kg daily	For Hodgkin's disease
rituximab (Rituxan)	IV; 375 mg/m^2 daily as a continuous infusion	For non-Hodgkin's lymphomas
scinitinib (Sutent)	PO; 50 mg once daily for 4 weeks followed by 2 weeks off	For gastrointestinal and advanced renal carcinoma
sunitinib (Sutent)	PO; 37.5–50 mg once daily for 4 weeks	For gastrointestinal, advanced renal and pancreatic tumors
trastuzumab (Herceptin) and ado-trastuzumab (Kadcycla)	IV (Herceptin); 4 mg/kg as a single dose, then 2 mg/kg every week IV (Kadcycla); 3.6 mg/kg every 3 weeks	For metastatic breast cancer
vismodegib (Erivedge)	PO; 150 mg once daily	For advanced or metastatic basal cell carcinoma
zoledronic acid (Zometa)	IV; 4 mg over at least 15 minutes	For multiple myeloma, severe hypercalcemia caused by malignancy, and Paget's disease

*This table includes a selected sample of drugs in this class. For a complete listing, see Adams & Urban, *Pharmacology: Connections to Nursing Practice*, 2nd ed., 2013. Upper Saddle River, NJ: Pearson.

All targeted therapies, including the MABs, are very specific: They are designed to affect only cells with certain antibodies or proteins. The key point about targeted therapies is that the tumor cells must possess the specific antibody or protein; otherwise, the drug will be ineffective.

Adjunct medications are sometimes necessary to treat cancer symptoms and to reduce the intensity of adverse effects from antineoplastic drugs.

CORE CONCEPT 28.14

Antineoplastic drugs are only part of the arsenal of medications used to treat cancer patients. Adjunctive medications are those used to supplement the primary therapies. The three primary groups of drugs used as adjunctive therapy are opioid analgesics, antiemetics, and hematopoietic drugs.

Many types of cancer produce extreme pain, which affects the patient's quality of life. Indeed, pain management is one of the primary concerns of both patients and healthcare providers. Pain management proceeds up a ladder, starting with NSAIDs to the weak opioid analgesics (codeine, tramadol) and eventually to the strongest opioids (morphine, fentanyl, hydromorphone). Drug combinations may be used to achieve optimum pain control. At high levels, opioids produce significant adverse effects (see Chapter 14).

Chemotherapy-induced nausea and vomiting (CINV) can be debilitating for patients. CINV can occur in the first few hours after the initiation of chemotherapy, or be delayed more than 24 hours. Antineoplastics are classified as their emetogenic potential and those with the highest potential require adjunctive therapy with antiemetics. The most effective drug class used for this purpose are called serotonin receptor antagonists. Examples include palonosetron (Alxi) and ondansetron (Zofran, Zuplenz), which can be given as an orally disintegrating tablet. The antiemetic drugs are presented in Chapter 30.

Many antineoplastic drugs are toxic to bone marrow and can produce serious blood abnormalities. Some drugs are given during chemotherapy to limit or counteract this toxicity. Oprelvekin (Neumega) stimulates platelet production and helps to prevent severe thrombocytopenia. Epoetin alfa (Epogen, Procrit) stimulates RBC production and is used to limit **anemia**, the loss of RBCs, caused by certain antineoplastics. Administration of filgrastim (Neupogen) increases neutrophil production in patients with cancer whose bone marrow has been suppressed by antineoplastic drugs. Low WBC counts (neutropenia) often result in severe bacterial and fungal infections in patients during chemotherapy or following organ transplants.

Drug Prototype: Ⓟ *Epoetin Alfa (Epogen, Procrit)*
Therapeutic Class: **Drug for anemia**   Pharmacologic Class: **Hematopoietic growth factor, erythropoietin**

Actions and Uses: Epoetin alfa is made through recombinant DNA technology and functions like human erythropoietin. Because of its ability to stimulate red blood cell formation, epoetin alfa is effective in treating specific disorders caused by a deficiency in the number of red blood cells. Patients with chronic renal failure often cannot secrete enough erythropoietin and thus will benefit from epoetin administration. Epoetin is sometimes given to patients undergoing cancer chemotherapy to counteract the anemia caused by antineoplastic drugs. It is occasionally prescribed for patients prior to blood transfusions or surgery and to treat anemia in patients infected with HIV. Epoetin alfa is usually administered three times per week until a therapeutic response is achieved.

Adverse Effects and Interactions: Epoetin alfa has some serious adverse effects which are described in the black box warning. The most common adverse effect of epoetin alfa is hypertension, which may occur in as many as 30% of patients receiving the drug. Blood pressure should be monitored during therapy, and an antihypertensive drug may be indicated.

The effectiveness of epoetin alfa will be greatly reduced in patients with iron deficiency or other vitamin-depleted states because erythropoiesis cannot be enhanced without these vital nutrients. There are no clinically significant drug interactions with epoetin alfa.

BLACK BOX WARNING:
The risk of serious cardiovascular events is increased with epoetin alfa therapy. Transient ischemic attacks (TIAs), myocardial infarctions (MIs), and strokes have occurred in patients who are on dialysis and being treated with epoetin alfa. Epoetin increased the rate of deep venous thrombosis (DVT) in patients not receiving concurrent anticoagulation. The lowest dose possible should be used in patients with cancer because the drug can promote tumor progression and shorten overall survival in some patients.

NURSING PROCESS FOCUS Patients Receiving Antineoplastic Therapy

ASSESSMENT	POTENTIAL NURSING DIAGNOSES
Prior to administration: ■ Obtain a complete health history, including GI, renal and liver conditions, allergies, drug history, past infections, and possible drug interactions. ■ Evaluate laboratory blood findings: CBC, platelets, electrolytes, uric acid, glucose, and renal and liver function studies. ■ Acquire the results of a complete physical examination, including vital signs, height, weight, and any diagnostic test dependent on type of antineoplastic therapy (audiology, cardiac, electromyography). ■ Determine neurologic status, including level of consciousness (LOC), mood, and/or sensory impairment. ■ Collect information about previous immunization and a history or presence of herpes zoster or chickenpox.	■ *Infection* related to compromised immune system secondary to adverse effects of antineoplastic drugs and disease process ■ *Imbalanced Nutrition: Less than Body Requirements* related to nausea, vomiting, diarrhea, and anorexia secondary to adverse effects of drug therapy ■ *Impaired Skin Integrity* related to extravasation of antineoplastic drug therapy ■ *Risk for Disturbed Body Image* related to physical changes from the adverse effects of drug therapy or other treatment regimens ■ *Fatigue* related to adverse effects of drug therapy ■ *Fear* related to lack of knowledge of disease process and effects of treatment regimen ■ *Deficient Knowledge* related to a lack of information about drug therapy

PLANNING: PATIENT GOALS AND EXPECTED OUTCOMES

The patient will:
■ Experience therapeutic effects (a reduction in tumor mass and/or progression of abnormal cell growth).
■ Experience minimal adverse effects from drug therapy.
■ Verbalize an understanding of the drug's use, adverse effects, and required precautions.

IMPLEMENTATION

Interventions and (Rationales)	Patient Education/Discharge Planning
■ Monitor immune status. Observe for signs and symptoms for potential and actual infections and monitor laboratory tests such as CBC, specifically WBC and neutrophil counts. (Most antineoplastic drugs cause immunosuppression neutropenia.)	Instruct the patient to: ■ Immediately report profound fatigue, fever, sore throat, epigastric pain, coffee-grounds vomit, bruising, tarry stools, or frank bleeding to the healthcare provider. ■ Avoid crowded indoor places and persons with active infections. ■ Monitor vital signs daily, ensuring proper use of home equipment. ■ Take temperature every four hours, if symptoms indicate a need, and to notify the healthcare provider if it goes above approved parameters. ■ Not use antipyretics unless approved by oncology provider. ■ Not eat raw foods. Cook foods thoroughly, allowing family members to prepare raw foods. ■ Anticipate fatigue and balance daily activities to prevent exhaustion.
■ Monitor cardiac and respiratory status, including vital signs, heart and breath sounds, presence of edema, ECG, and laboratory testing. (Many antineoplastic agents, such as alkylating drugs, antimetabolites, and antitumor antibodies, have adverse effects that cause problems with the cardiac and respiratory systems.)	Instruct the patient: ■ To report immediately any problems with dyspnea; pain in the chest, arm, neck, or back; tachycardia; cough; frothy sputum; swelling; or activity intolerance to the healthcare provider. ■ To adhere to laboratory testing regimen for serum blood level tests (CBC, clotting factors, chemistry panel), as directed. Alert lab personnel of chemotherapy use. ■ That heart changes may be a sign of drug toxicity; heart failure may not appear for up to six months after completion of doxorubicin therapy.
■ Monitor nutritional status. Administer antiemetics 30–45 minutes prior to antineoplastic administration or at the first sign of nausea. (Profound nausea, dry heaves, and/or vomiting are common with antineoplastic therapy. Dry mouth can also occur. Dietary consultation may be needed.)	Instruct the patient to: ■ Report loss of appetite, nausea/vomiting. ■ Consume frequent small, high calorie, and nutrient dense meals. Nutritional supplements may help. ■ Avoid highly scented, spicy foods; high-roughage and very hot or cold foods. ■ Avoid carbonated and acidic beverages, alcohol, and caffeine.
■ Monitor for mucositis. (Antineoplastic drugs may cause significant mucositis because of its effects on rapidly dividing cells.)	Instruct the patient to: ■ Examine mouth daily for changes and report the presence of mouth redness, soreness, or ulcers. ■ Maintain regular dental exams. ■ Encourage frequent oral hygiene, use of lip balm, and avoid alcohol-based mouthwash, which can be drying to the mucosa. ■ Use a soft toothbrush; avoid toothpicks.

continued . . .

NURSING PROCESS FOCUS (continued)

Interventions and (Rationales)	Patient Education/Discharge Planning
■ Monitor for diarrhea and constipation. (An adverse effect of many antineoplastic drugs is diarrhea although severe constipation may occur with vincristine use, especially among older adults.)	Instruct the patient to: ■ Report changes in bowel habits to the healthcare provider. ■ Report excessive diarrhea, especially if it contains blood or mucus. ■ Increase fluid intake 2–3 L a day to prevent constipation.
■ Monitor liver function tests. (Antineoplastics are metabolized by the liver, increasing the risk of hepatotoxicity.)	Instruct the patient to: ■ Report nausea, vomiting, jaundice, abdominal pain, tenderness or bloating, or light or clay-colored stool to the healthcare provider. ■ Adhere to laboratory testing regimen for serum blood level tests of liver enzymes, as directed.
■ Monitor DTRs, neurologic/sensory status, and LOC. (Antineoplastics such as cyclophosphamide and natural product antineoplastics such as vincristine have neurological adverse effects. Such neurologic changes may be irreversible.)	Instruct the patient to: ■ Report any changes in skin color, vision, hearing; numbness or tingling; staggering gait; changes in consciousness; or depressed mood to the healthcare provider.
■ Monitor genitourinary status: intake and output, daily weights, and renal function tests. (Antineoplastic drugs may cause significant renal toxicity. Hormones, and especially tamoxifen, increase the risk of endometrial cancer and may alter menstrual cycles in women and may produce impotence in men.)	Instruct the patient: ■ To report the following immediately: diminished urinary output, changes in thirst; changes in color, quantity, and character of urine (e.g., "cloudy," with odor or sediment); joint, suprapubic, abdominal, flank, or lower back pain; difficult urination; and weight gain to the healthcare provider. ■ That doxorubicin will turn urine red-brown for one to two days after administration; blood in the urine may occur several months after cyclophosphamide has been discontinued. ■ To increase fluid intake to 2–3 L a day. ■ To report changes in menstruation, sexual functioning, and/or vaginal discharge. ■ To recognize the risk of endometrial cancer before taking tamoxifen.
■ Monitor for hypersensitivity or other adverse reactions. (Antineoplastic drugs may cause significant hypersensitivity and allergic responses.)	■ Instruct the patient to immediately report chest or throat tightness, difficulty swallowing, swelling (especially facial), abdominal pain, headache, or dizziness to the healthcare provider.
■ Monitor hair and skin status. (Alopecia is associated with most antineoplastic drugs. Alkylating and antimetabolites may cause significant skin reactions including SJS.)	Instruct the patient to: ■ Immediately report desquamation of skin on hands and feet, rash, pruritus, acne, or boils to the healthcare provider. ■ Wear a cold gel cap during chemotherapy to minimize hair loss.
■ Monitor for conjunctivitis. (Doxorubicin may cause conjunctivitis.)	■ Instruct the patient or caregiver to immediately report eye redness, stickiness, or pain or weeping.
■ Administer with caution to patients with diabetes mellitus. (Hypoglycemia may occur secondary to combination of cyclophosphamide and insulin.)	Instruct the patient to: ■ Report any signs and symptoms of hypoglycemia (e.g., sudden weakness, tremors) to the healthcare provider. ■ Monitor blood glucose daily; consult the healthcare provider regarding reportable results (e.g., less than 70 mg/dL).
■ Be aware of specific policies and procedures related to antineoplastic administration. (Intense education programs are usually required prior to administering chemotherapy drugs.)	■ Provide the patient, family, and caregiver education and support when giving antineoplastic (chemotherapy) drugs.

EVALUATION OF OUTCOME CRITERIA

Evaluate the effectiveness of drug therapy by confirming that patient goals and expected outcomes have been met (see "Planning"). See Tables 28.2–28.7 for lists of drugs to which these nursing actions apply.

PATIENTS NEED TO KNOW

Patients treated for cancer need to know the following:

1. If hair loss is expected, cut long hair and be fitted for a wig or hairpiece before starting treatment. Select hats, scarves, or turbans. Use mild shampoo and conditioner.
2. Limit sun exposure; wear sunscreen, sunglasses, and long sleeves when outdoors. When hair is lost, protect the scalp from sunburn with sunscreen or a hat.
3. Eat foods that appeal in small amounts at frequent intervals if appetite is decreased. A healthcare provider may provide an appetite stimulant such as megestrol (Megace).
4. Discuss drugs to control nausea with a healthcare provider if nausea is a problem. Drink liquids between meals rather than with food.
5. Because the mouth may become irritated or ulcerated, avoid alcohol-based mouthwash, and use plain water or mild salt solution instead. Use a soft toothbrush. Avoid spicy foods and very hot or very cold food and drink. Ask about a mouth rinse to coat, soothe, and numb, such as Benadryl, Maalox, and Xylocaine.
6. Because chemotherapy may decrease sperm production or increase the risk of genetic damage to sperm, consider sperm banking prior to receiving chemotherapy.
7. Increase fluid intake to decrease the risk of kidney damage and uric acid crystal formation.
8. Avoid exposure to crowds and individuals with infections or recent vaccinations because the immune system may be less able to protect you. Report temperatures of 101°F (38°C) or higher.
9. Follow a neutropenic diet if WBC count is significantly reduced. Avoid raw fruits and vegetables, peppercorns, and raw fish and meat.
10. Report easy bruising, blood in the stool or urine, vomiting, severe fatigue, epigastric pain, and difficulty clotting. Many chemotherapeutic drugs reduce production platelets needed for clot formation.

CHAPTER REVIEW

CORE CONCEPTS SUMMARY

28.1 Cancer is characterized by rapid, uncontrolled growth of cells.

Cancer cells grow rapidly, seemingly unaffected by their host surroundings. Cancer cells continue dividing until they invade normal tissues and eventually metastasize. Benign neoplasms grow slowly and rarely result in death. Malignant neoplasms, also known as cancer, are fast growing and often fatal.

28.2 The causes of cancer may be chemical, physical, or biological.

Many factors have been found to cause or promote cancer. These include industrial chemicals, x-rays, UV light, and viruses. The genetic make-up of the patient plays an important role in whether or not cancer will develop after exposure to carcinogens.

28.3 Personal risk of cancer may be lowered by a number of lifestyle factors.

Eliminating tobacco use and limiting the intake of saturated fats and alcohol are important factors in reducing the risk of developing cancer. Periodic self-examinations and physician checkups are important in catching cancer at an early, more treatable stage.

28.4 The three primary goals of chemotherapy are cure, control, and palliation.

Surgery, radiation, and chemotherapy are the therapies used for treating cancer. The three primary goals of chemotherapy are cure, control, and palliation. Antineoplastic drugs may also be administered as adjuvant or neoadjuvant chemotherapy, prophylaxis, or myeloablation.

28.5 To achieve a total cure, every malignant cell must be removed or killed.

A single cancer cell may be able to divide rapidly enough to kill its host. Therefore, to achieve a complete cure, every single cancer cell must be eliminated by surgery, radiation, drugs, or the patient's immune system.

28.6 Use of multiple drugs and special dosing schedules improve the success of chemotherapy.

Combinations of antineoplastic drugs are often used to attack cancer cells through several mechanisms and to allow lower doses than if a single drug were used. The schedule of drug administration is critical to the success of the chemotherapy.

28.7 Serious toxicity limits therapy with most of the antineoplastic drugs.

Antineoplastic drugs are among the most toxic medications available. Adverse effects are expected and may be severe. Whereas each drug has somewhat different toxicities, common adverse effects include thrombocytopenia, anemia, leukopenia, alopecia, severe nausea, vomiting, and diarrhea.

28.8 Alkylating drugs act by changing the structure of DNA in cancer cells.

Alkylating drugs are some of the oldest and most reliable of the antineoplastic drugs. By attaching to DNA, they prevent cancer cells from replicating.

28.9 Antimetabolites disrupt critical cellular pathways in cancer cells.

Antimetabolites block a specific step in cancer cell metabolism. By blocking the synthesis of critical cellular molecules, the drugs can slow the growth of cancer cells.

28.10 A few cytotoxic antibiotics are used to treat cancer rather than infections.

Antitumor antibiotics attach to the DNA of cancer cells, thereby inhibiting their growth. Their properties and adverse effects resemble those of the alkylating drugs.

28.11 Some natural products kill cancer cells by preventing cell division.

Natural products of the periwinkle plant and the Pacific yew have provided several important antineoplastic drugs. Drugs in this class also include the topoisomerase inhibitors.

28.12 Some hormones and hormone antagonists are effective against prostate and breast cancer.

A number of estrogens, androgens, corticosteroids, and hormone inhibitors have antitumor activity and are most often given for palliation. They are usually reserved for tumors of the breast or prostate.

28.13 Targeted therapies and some miscellaneous antineoplastic drugs are effective against specific tumors.

Targeted therapies include monoclonal antibodies that have been designed to affect some specific aspect of cancer cell physiology. While a large number of new targeted therapies have been marketed, they are only effective against specific cancers and most have significant adverse effects.

28.14 Adjunct medications are sometimes necessary to treat cancer symptoms and to reduce the intensity of adverse effects from antineoplastic drugs.

Adjunct medications are needed to reduce the intense pain, nausea, and drug adverse effects that can occur during cancer treatment. Adjuncts include opioid analgesics, antiemetics, and drugs to reduce bone marrow toxicity.

REVIEW QUESTIONS

The following questions are written in NCLEX-PN® style. Answer these questions to assess your knowledge of the chapter material, and go back and review any material that is not clear to you.

1. The nurse administers antiemetic drugs to a patient receiving chemotherapy:

1. Only when vomiting occurs
2. Once the treatment regimen is completed
3. Just prior to treatment
4. Only if the patient requests to be medicated

2. The patient with testicular cancer is receiving cisplatin (Platinol) IV. The nurse plans to monitor for:

1. Irreversible heart failure
2. Bone marrow suppression
3. Cardiac toxicity
4. Peripheral neuropathy

3. Before a patient begins drug therapy with methotrexate, the nurse collects information regarding the use of other medications. What medication(s) would be of concern if the patient were to take it along with the methotrexate? (Select all that apply.)

1. Aspirin
2. Iron supplement
3. Acetaminophen
4. Nonsteroidal anti-inflammatory drugs (NSAIDs)

4. The patient with breast cancer has been receiving IV doxorubicin (Adriamycin). The patient is now complaining of severe pain at the IV site. The nurse understands that the following most likely occurred:

1. An allergic reaction
2. Leaking at the IV site
3. Loss of neural reflexes
4. Development of a blood clot

5. A patient has started on tamoxifen as a treatment for cancer. The physician orders 20 mg, po, daily but it is only available in 10 mg tablets. How many tablets will the patient receive in a day? How many tablets in a week?

1. 1 tablet a day, 7 tablets a week
2. 2 tablets a day, 14 tablets a week
3. 2 tablets a day, 10 tablets a week
4. 4 tablets a day, 14 tablets a week

6. The patient on cyclosphosphamide (Cytoxan) is taught:

1. That alopecia is not irreversible
2. About signs and symptoms of neurotoxicity
3. About signs and symptoms of renal toxicity
4. That nausea, vomiting, and diarrhea frequently occur

7. The nurse monitors a patient taking methotrexate for which adverse effect(s)? (Select all that apply.)

1. Cardiac dysthymias
2. Bruising
3. Decreased urinary output
4. Diarrhea

8. A patient is about to start his chemotherapy treatments. He will be taking rituximab (Rituxan), a type of monoclonal antibody. He asks the nurse how it works. The nurse tells him that this type of monoclonal antibody:

1. Changes the structure of cancer cell's DNA, preventing them from replicating

2. Binds to surface proteins present on cancer cells and shatters them
3. Blocks a specific step in cancer cell metabolism
4. Attaches to the DNA of cancer cells, inhibiting their growth

9. The nurse informs a patient with a decreased white blood cell count that he should:

1. Use alcohol-based mouthwash for mouth sores.
2. Increase liquid intake with meals.
3. Avoid raw foods.
4. Ask his physician about ordering megestrol (Megace).

10. The patient on tamoxifen must be checked for:

1. Flu-like symptoms
2. Uterine cancer
3. Alopecia
4. Thrombocytopenia

CASE STUDY QUESTIONS

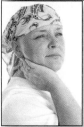

Remember Ms. Novak, the patient introduced at the beginning of the chapter? Now read the remainder of the case study. Based on the information you have learned in this chapter, answer the questions that follow.

Ms. Patricia Novak has arrived at the cancer center in her community. She is being treated for an invasive type of cancer. She is getting really tired of all the drugs she has to take, stating, "I know they are helping but four different drugs? I guess it could be worse." Ms. Novak is receiving the following drugs:

1. *vincristine (Oncovin)*
2. *interferon alfa-2b (Intron A)*
3. *tamoxifen (Soltamox)*
4. *epoetin alfa (Epogen)*

1. Ms. Novak knows that one of her medications boosts her immune system but can't remember which one. The nurse tells her that the medication she is referring to is:

1. Vincristine (Oncovin)
2. Epoetin alfa (Epogen)
3. Interferon alfa-2b (Intron A)
4. Tamoxifen

2. Asked why she is taking epoetin alfa (Epogen), the nurse responds that it is being administered to:

1. Boost Ms. Novak's immune system.
2. Boost the number of her red blood cells.
3. Reduce possible neurotoxicity.
4. Kill her cancer cells.

3. During vincristine (Oncovin) therapy, the nurse must regularly monitor for:

1. Blood glucose levels
2. Signs of peripheral neuropathy
3. Ototoxicity
4. Signs of confusion

4. Because of the type of cancer she has and the type of antineoplastic drug she is taking, Ms. Novak complains of pain. The physician orders a pain medication. Understanding the pain management protocols, the nurse may expect to use what type of medication to achieve optimum pain control for Ms. Novak?

1. Combination drugs such as an NSAID and codeine
2. A strong opioid such as fentanyl
3. A weak opioid such as codeine
4. A nonsteroidal anti-inflammatory drug

NOTE: Answers to the Review and Case Study Questions appear in Appendix B. The complete rationales and answers are located on the textbook's website.

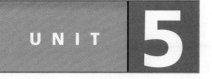

The Respiratory and Digestive Systems

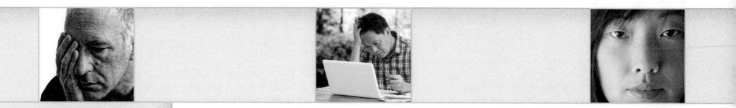

Unit Contents

Chapter 29   Drugs for Respiratory Disorders / 454

Chapter 30   Drugs for Gastrointestinal Disorders / 476

Chapter 31   Vitamins, Minerals, and Nutritional Supplements / 496

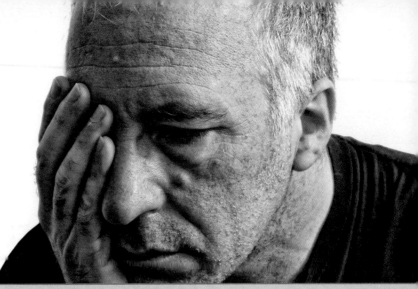

C H A P T E R

"I can't sleep at night with this cough, and I can hardly work without getting short of breath."

Mr. Michael Thomas

29 Drugs for Respiratory Disorders

CORE CONCEPTS

29.1 The respiratory system supplies oxygen for the body and provides protection against inhaled organisms.

29.2 The inhalation route of drug administration quickly delivers medications directly to their sites of action.

29.3 Allergic rhinitis is characterized by sneezing, watery eyes, and nasal congestion.

29.4 Antihistamines are widely used to treat allergic rhinitis and other minor allergies.

29.5 Intranasal corticosteroids are first-line drugs for treating allergic rhinitis.

29.6 Decongestants are used to reduce nasal congestion caused by allergic rhinitis and the common cold.

29.7 Antitussives and expectorants are used to treat symptoms of the common cold.

29.8 Asthma is a chronic inflammatory disease characterized by bronchospasm.

29.9 Beta-adrenergic agonists are the most effective drugs for relieving acute bronchospasm.

29.10 Corticosteroids are the most effective drugs for the long-term prophylaxis of asthma.

29.11 Mast cell stabilizers and leukotriene modifiers are alternative anti-inflammatory drugs for the prophylaxis of asthma.

29.12 Chronic obstructive pulmonary disease is a progressive disorder treated with multiple drugs.

DRUG SNAPSHOT

The following drugs are discussed in this chapter:

DRUG CLASSES	DRUG PROTOTYPES
Antihistamines (H₁-receptor blockers)	Pr diphenhydramine (Benadryl, others) *460*
Intranasal corticosteroids	Pr fluticasone (Flonase, Veramyst) *463*
Decongestants (sympathomimetics)	Pr oxymetazoline (Afrin, others) *464*
Antitussives, expectorants, and mucolytics	

DRUG CLASSES	DRUG PROTOTYPES
Beta-adrenergic drugs	
Anticholinergics	
Inhaled corticosteroids	
Xanthines	
Mast cell stabilizers	Pr cromolyn (Intal) *471*
Leukotriene modifiers	

LEARNING OUTCOMES

After reading this chapter, the student should be able to:

1. Identify major structures and functions associated with the respiratory system.

2. Explain why inhalation is an effective route of drug administration for respiratory medicines.

3. Describe the types of devices used to deliver medications via the inhalation route.

4. Describe some common causes and symptoms of allergic rhinitis, asthma, and chronic obstructive pulmonary disease.

5. Explain the pharmacologic management of allergic rhinitis, asthma, and chronic obstructive pulmonary disease.

6. Identify the drugs that are used to bring symptomatic relief from the common cold.

7. Categorize drugs used in the treatment of respiratory disorders based on their classifications and mechanisms of action.

8. For each of the classes in the Drug Snapshot, identify representative drugs and explain their mechanisms of drug action, primary actions, and important adverse effects.

KEY TERMS

aerosol (AIR-oh-sol) 456

allergen 458

allergic rhinitis (rye-NYE-tis) 458

alveoli (al-VEE-oh-lie) 455

antitussive (anti-TUSS-ive) 465

asthma (AZ-muh) 465

bronchi (BRON-ky) 455

bronchioles (BRON-key-oles) 455

bronchoconstriction (BRON-koh-kun-STRIK-shun) 466

bronchodilation (BRON-koh-dye-LAY-shun) 467

bronchospasm (bron-koh-SPAZ-um) 466

chronic bronchitis (KRON-ik bron-KEYE-tis) 472

dry powder inhaler (DPI) 456

dyspnea 466

emphysema (em-fuss-EE-muh) 472

expectorants (eks-PEK-tor-entz) 465

H_1-receptor blocker 458

metered-dose inhalers (MDIs) 456

mucolytics 465

nebulizers (NEB-you-lyes-urz) 456

perfusion (purr-FEW-shun) 455

rebound congestion 463

respiration (res-purr-AY-shun) 455

status asthmaticus (STAT-us az-MAT-ik-us) 467

ventilation (ven-tah-LAY-shun) 455

The respiratory system is one of the most important organ systems; a mere five to six minutes without breathing may result in death. When functioning properly, the respiratory system filters incoming air and provides the body with the oxygen critical for all cells to function. The respiratory system also provides a means by which the body can rid itself of excess acids and bases, a topic that is covered in Chapter 17. The first portion of this chapter examines drugs used to treat conditions associated with the upper respiratory tract: allergic rhinitis, nasal congestion, and cough. The second portion presents the pharmacotherapy of asthma and conditions that affect the lower respiratory tract.

The respiratory system supplies oxygen for the body and provides protection against inhaled organisms.

CORE CONCEPT 29.1

The primary function of the respiratory system is to bring oxygen into the body and to remove carbon dioxide. The process by which gases are exchanged is called **respiration**. The basic structures of the respiratory system are shown in Figure 29.1 ■. This system is sometimes divided into two anatomic divisions: the upper and lower respiratory tracts.

Upper Respiratory Tract

The upper respiratory tract (URT) consists of the nose, nasal cavity, pharynx, and paranasal sinuses. These passageways warm, humidify, and clean the air before it enters the lungs. The URT traps and removes particulate matter and many pathogens before they reach the lower portions of the lungs, where they would be able to access the capillaries of the systemic circulation.

The nasal mucosa is a dynamic structure, richly supplied with vascular tissue, under the control of the autonomic nervous system. For example, certain drugs can reduce the thickness of the mucosal layer, thus relieving nasal congestion (see Core Concept 29.5). The nasal mucosa is also the first line of immune defense. Up to a quart of nasal mucus is produced daily, and this fluid is rich with substances that are able to neutralize airborne pathogens. Unfortunately, these cells can overreact to some substances and cause symptoms typical of seasonal allergies, such as nasal congestion, watery eyes, and sneezing.

Lower Respiratory Tract

The lower respiratory tract (LRT) consists of the lungs and associated structures. Air leaving the URT travels into the trachea and **bronchi**, which divide into smaller and smaller passages called **bronchioles**. The bronchial tree ends in dilated sacs called **alveoli**. Although they have no smooth muscle, the alveoli are abundantly rich in capillaries. An extremely thin membrane in the alveoli allows gases to readily move between the internal environment of the blood and the inspired air. As oxygen crosses this membrane, it is exchanged for carbon dioxide, a cellular waste product that travels from the blood to the air. The lung is richly supplied with blood. Blood flow through the lung is called **perfusion**. The process of gas exchange is depicted in Figure 29.1.

Ventilation is the process of moving air into and out of the lungs. As the muscular diaphragm contracts and lowers in position, it creates a negative pressure that draws air into the lungs. This process, known as inspiration, requires energy to produce the contraction. During expiration, the diaphragm relaxes and air

FIGURE 29.1

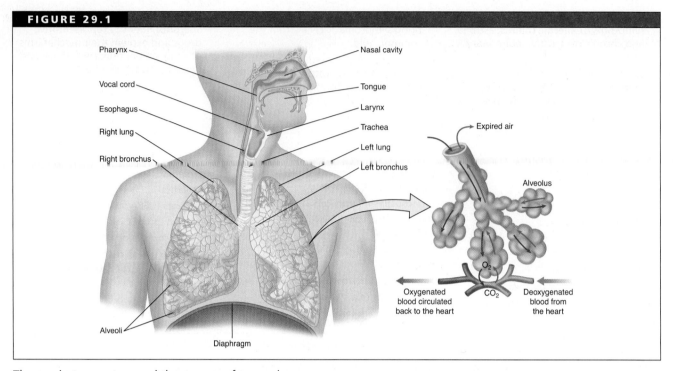

The respiratory system and the process of gas exchange.

leaves the lung passively, with no energy expenditure required. Ventilation is a purely mechanical process that occurs approximately 12–18 times per minute in adults, a rate determined by neurons in the brainstem. This rate may be modified by a number of factors, including emotions, fever, stress, and the pH of the blood.

Concept Review 29.1

■ What is the difference between ventilation and perfusion?

CORE CONCEPT 29.2

The inhalation route of drug administration quickly delivers medications directly to their sites of action.

The respiratory system offers a rapid and efficient mechanism for delivering drugs. The enormous surface area of the bronchioles and alveoli, and the rich blood supply to these areas, results in an almost instantaneous onset of action for inhaled substances.

Medications are delivered to the respiratory system by aerosol therapy. An **aerosol** is a suspension of very small liquid droplets or fine solid particles suspended within a gas. Aerosol therapy can give immediate relief for bronchospasm. Drugs may also be given to loosen thick mucus in the bronchial tree. The major advantage of aerosol therapy is that it delivers the medications to their immediate site of action, thus reducing systemic adverse effects. To produce the same therapeutic action, an oral medication would have to be given at higher doses and would be distributed to all body tissues.

It should be clearly understood that drugs delivered by inhalation can produce *systemic* effects because there is always some degree of absorption across the respiratory membrane. For example, anesthetics such as nitrous oxide and isoflurane (Forane) are delivered via the inhalation route and are rapidly distributed to cause central nervous system (CNS) depression, as presented in Chapter 15. Solvents such as paint thinners and glues are sometimes intentionally inhaled and can cause serious adverse effects on the nervous system and even death. In general, however, drugs administered by the inhalation route for respiratory conditions produce minimal systemic toxicity.

Several devices are used to deliver medications via the inhalation route. **Nebulizers** are small machines that vaporize a liquid drug into a fine mist that can be inhaled, often using a facemask. If the drug is a solid, it may be administered using a **dry powder inhaler (DPI)**. A DPI is a small device that is activated by the process of inhalation to deliver a fine powder directly to the bronchial tree. Turbohalers and rotahalers are types of DPIs. **Metered-dose inhalers (MDIs)** are a third type of device commonly used to deliver respiratory medicines. MDIs use a propellant to deliver a measured dose of drugs to the lungs during each breath. The patient times the inhalation to the puffs of drug emitted from the MDI. Patients must be carefully instructed on the correct use of these devices because drug dose depends on their correct use. Patients should be advised to rinse their mouth thoroughly following drug use to reduce the potential for absorption of the drug across the oral mucosa because swallowing medication that has been deposited

FIGURE 29.2

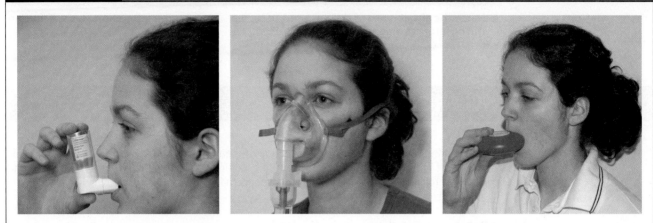

Devices used to deliver respiratory drugs.

in the oral cavity may cause the drug to be absorbed in the gastrointestinal (GI) tract, causing potential adverse effects. Devices used to deliver respiratory drugs are shown in Figure 29.2 ■.

The primary goal of drug therapy for many respiratory disorders is to keep the airways open. Drugs include bronchodilators, which directly open the airways, and anti-inflammatory drugs, which prevent their closure. Drugs may be used to act on excessive mucus blocking the airways, either by causing it to become thinner or by breaking up thick mucus plugs. These and other types of drugs used to treat respiratory disorders are illustrated in Figure 29.3 ■.

FIGURE 29.3

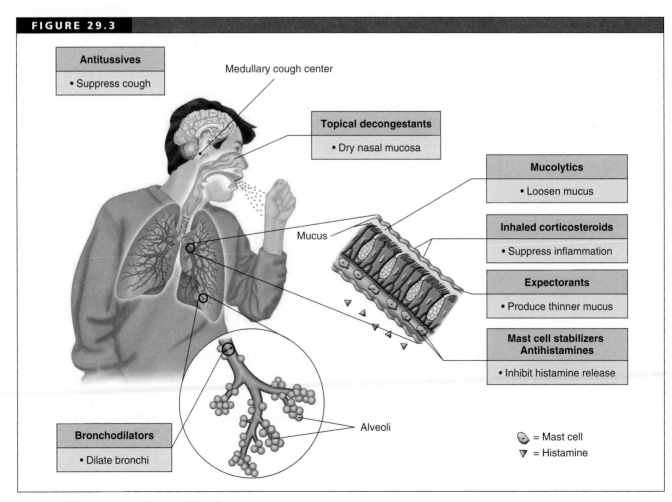

Drugs used to treat respiratory disorders.

Concept Review **29.2**

■ Name the three types of devices used to deliver drugs by the inhalation route. What are the differences among them?

ALLERGIC RHINITIS

Allergic rhinitis, or hay fever, is inflammation of the nasal mucosa due to exposure to allergens. Although not life threatening, allergic rhinitis is a condition affecting millions of patients, and pharmacotherapy is frequently necessary to control symptoms and to prevent secondary complications.

CORE CONCEPT 29.3

Allergic rhinitis is characterized by sneezing, watery eyes, and nasal congestion.

Allergic rhinitis is a common disorder affecting millions of people annually. Symptoms resemble those of the common cold: tearing eyes, sneezing, nasal congestion, postnasal drip, and itching of the throat. In addition to the acute symptoms, complications of allergic rhinitis may include loss of taste or smell, sinusitis, chronic cough, hoarseness, and middle ear infections in children.

As with other allergies, the cause of allergic rhinitis is exposure to an antigen. An antigen, or **allergen**, may be defined as anything that is recognized as foreign by the body's defense system. The specific allergen is often difficult to pinpoint; however, common agents include pollen from weeds, grasses, and trees; molds; dust mites; certain foods; and animal dander. Nonallergenic factors such as chemical fumes, tobacco smoke, or air pollutants such as ozone may contribute to the symptoms. Although some patients experience symptoms at specific times of the year, when pollen and mold are at high levels in the environment, others are bothered throughout the year.

The fundamental problem of allergic rhinitis is inflammation of the mucous membranes in the nose, throat, and airways. Chemical mediators such as histamine are released and initiate the distressing symptoms. The pathophysiology of allergic rhinitis is illustrated in Figure 29.4 ■.

The therapeutic goals of treating allergic rhinitis are to prevent its occurrence and to relieve symptoms. Drugs used to treat allergic rhinitis may thus be grouped into two basic categories: preventers and relievers. Preventers are used for prophylaxis and include antihistamines, intranasal corticosteroids, and mast cell stabilizers. Relievers are used to provide immediate, though temporary, relief for allergy symptoms once they have occurred. Relievers include the oral and intranasal sympathomimetics.

Fast Facts Allergies

■ The odds that a child with two allergic parents will develop allergies is 70%.

■ A person is more likely to have a severe allergic reaction to food if he or she also has asthma or has had a previous anaphylactic reaction.

■ Most children outgrow milk, egg, soy, and wheat allergies by the teenage years.

CORE CONCEPT 29.4

Antihistamines are widely used to treat allergic rhinitis and other minor allergies.

Antihistamines are drugs that selectively block the actions of histamine at the H_1-receptor, thus alleviating allergic symptoms. Also called **H_1-receptor blockers**, they are available over the counter (OTC) and frequently used for relief of allergy symptoms, motion sickness, and insomnia. Common H_1-receptor blockers used to treat allergies and other disorders are listed in Table 29.1 ◆.

FIGURE 29.4

Pathophysiology of allergic rhinitis.

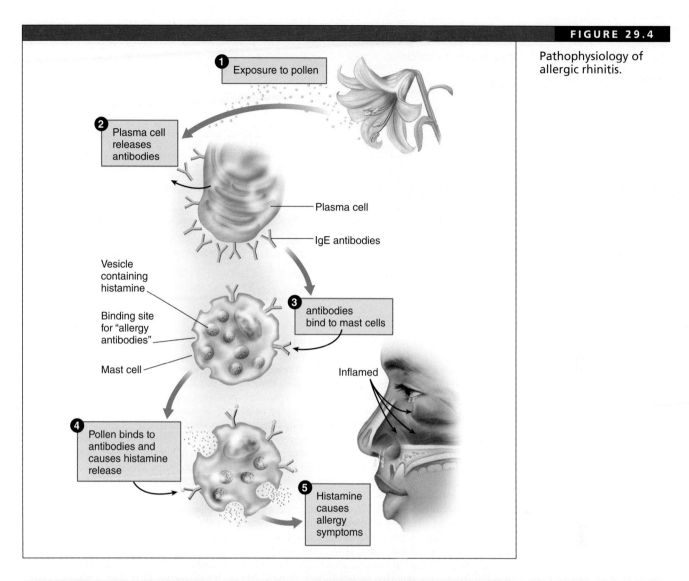

TABLE 29.1 H₁-Receptor Blockers (Antihistamines)

Drug	Route and Adult Dose	Remarks
FIRST-GENERATION DRUGS		
azelastine (Astelin, Astepro)	Intranasal; one or two sprays daily per nostril	First-generation antihistamine; for nonallergic rhinitis
brompheniramine (Dimetapp, others)	PO; 4–8 mg tid–qid (max: 40 mg/day)	Less sedative effect than diphenhydramine; combined with other drugs for OTC use
chlorpheniramine (Chlor-Trimeton, others)	PO; 2–4 mg tid–qid (max: 24 mg/day)	Usually combined with a decongestant to treat cold, flu, and allergy symptoms; available for OTC use
clemastine (Tavist)	PO; 1.34–2.68 mg bid (max: 8.04 mg/day)	Central sedative effects are generally mild
dexchlorpheniramine (Dexchlor, Poladex, others)	PO; 2 mg every 4–6 hours (max: 12 mg/day)	For seasonal rhinitis and other allergy disorders
dimenhydrinate (Dramamine)	PO; 50–100 mg every 4–6 hours	Primarily for motion sickness and treatment of nausea and vomiting; IV/IM form available
Pr diphenhydramine (Benadryl, others)	PO; 25–50 mg tid–qid (max: 300 mg/day)	Topical, IV, IM, and subcutaneous forms available; also for motion sickness, Parkinson's disease, vertigo, and as an OTC sleep aid
promethazine (Phenergan)	PO; 12.5–25 mg/day (max: 100 mg/day)	IV, IM, and rectal suppository forms available; also for preoperative sedation, motion sickness, nausea, and vertigo

(continued)

TABLE 29.1 H₁-Receptor Blockers (Antihistamines) *(continued)*

Drug	Route and Adult Dose	Remarks
SECOND-GENERATION DRUGS		
acrivastine with pseudoephedrine (Semprex-D)	PO; One capsule daily (8 mg acrivastine/ 60 mg pseudoephedrine)	For allergic rhinitis
cetirizine (Zyrtec)	PO; 5–10 mg/day (max: 10 mg/day)	Nonsedating; available OTC
desloratadine (Clarinex)	PO; 5 mg/day (max: 5 mg/day)	Nonsedating; the active metabolite of loratadine
fexofenadine (Allegra)	PO; 60 mg twice daily or 180 mg once daily	Once-a-day dosing; nonsedating
levocetirizine (Xyzal)	PO; 5 mg (1 tablet or 2 teaspoons) once daily	Very similar to cetirizine; also for chronic idiopathic urticaria
loratadine (Claritin)	PO; 10 mg daily	Nonsedating; became available OTC in 2001
olopatadine (Patanase)	Intranasal; two sprays per nostril twice daily	Newer drug, approved in 2007; the first second-generation nasal spray for allergic rhinitis

Because the term *antihistamine* is nonspecific and does not specify which of the two histamine receptors is affected, *H₁-receptor blocker* is the more accurate term. Although a large number of H₁-receptor blockers are available for use, their effectiveness, therapeutic uses, and adverse effects are similar. A simple classification of these drugs is based on their ability to cause sedation. Older, first-generation H₁-receptor blockers have the potential to cause significant drowsiness, whereas the newer, second-generation drugs lack this effect in most patients. Care must be taken to avoid alcohol and other CNS depressants when taking antihistamines because their sedating effects may be additive.

The most common therapeutic use of H₁-receptor blockers is for the treatment of allergies. These drugs provide relief from the characteristic sneezing; runny nose; and itching of the eyes, nose, and throat of allergic rhinitis. Many H₁-receptor blockers are used in OTC cold and sinus medicines, often in combination with decongestants and antitussives. Some common OTC antihistamine combinations used to treat allergies are listed in Table 29.2 ◆.

Antihistamines are most effective when taken to *prevent* allergic symptoms; their ability to treat allergy symptoms after they are present is limited. Their effectiveness may diminish with long-term use. It should be noted that during severe allergic reactions such as anaphylaxis, histamine is just one of several chemical mediators released; thus, H₁-receptor blockers are not very effective in treating this disorder.

Although most antihistamines are given orally, two are available by the intranasal route. Azelastine (Astelin, Astepro) is approved for nonallergic rhinitis. Although a first-generation drug, azelastine causes less drowsiness than others in its class because it is applied locally to the nasal mucosa, and limited systemic absorption occurs. Dymista is a newer combination that includes azelastine with fluticasone, an intranasal corticosteroid. Olopatadine (Patanase) is a newer second-generation intranasal antihistamine approved for allergic rhinitis.

Drug Prototype: 🅟 *Diphenhydramine (Benadryl, Others)*
Therapeutic Class: Drug to treat allergies **Pharmacologic Class: H₁-receptor blocker, antihistamine**

Actions and Uses: Diphenhydramine is a first-generation H₁-receptor blocker whose primary use is to treat symptoms of allergy and the common cold such as sneezing, runny nose, and tearing of the eyes. Diphenhydramine is often combined with an analgesic, a decongestant, or an expectorant in OTC cold and flu products. Diphenhydramine is also used as a topical drug to treat rashes, and IM/IV forms are available for severe allergic reactions. Other indications for diphenhydramine include Parkinson's disease, motion sickness, and insomnia.

Adverse Effects and Interactions: First-generation H₁-receptor blockers such as diphenhydramine cause significant drowsiness, although this usually diminishes with long-term use. Occasionally, a patient will exhibit CNS stimulation and excitability rather than drowsiness. Excitation is more frequent in children than in adults. Anticholinergic effects such as dry mouth, tachycardia, and mild hypotension are seen in some patients.

Use of diphenhydramine with alcohol, CNS depressants, or monoamine oxidase (MAO) inhibitors may cause additive CNS depression. Use with other OTC cold preparations may increase anticholinergic adverse effects.

TABLE 29.2   Selected OTC Antihistamine Combinations

Brand Name	Antihistamine	Decongestant	Analgesic
Actifed Cold and Allergy tablets	chlorpheniramine	phenylephrine	—
Benadryl Allergy/Cold caplets	diphenhydramine	phenylephrine	acetaminophen
Chlor-Trimeton Allergy/Decongestant tablets	chlorpheniramine	pseudoephedrine	—
Dimetapp Children's Cold and Allergy	brompheniramine	phenylephrine	—
Sudafed PE Nighttime Cold	diphenhydramine	phenylephrine	acetaminophen
Sudafed PE Sinus and Allergy tablets	chlorpheniramine	phenylephrine	—
Tavist Allergy tablets	clemastine	—	—
Triaminic Cold/Allergy	chlorpheniramine	phenylephrine	—
Tylenol Allergy Multisystem gels	chlorpheniramine	phenylephrine	acetaminophen
Tylenol PM gelcaps	diphenhydramine	—	acetaminophen

H_1-receptor blockers have been used to treat a number of other disorders. Motion sickness responds well to these medications. It is also one of the few classes of drugs available to treat vertigo, a form of dizziness that causes significant nausea. Some of the older antihistamines are marketed as OTC sleep aids, taking advantage of their ability to cause drowsiness. A few are used to treat tremors associated with Parkinson's disease.

Concept Review   29.3

■ Why are the antihistamines most effective if given *before* inflammation occurs?

NURSING PROCESS FOCUS   Patients Receiving Antihistamine Therapy

ASSESSMENT	POTENTIAL NURSING DIAGNOSES
Prior to administration: ■ Obtain a complete health history including respiratory, cardiovascular, renal, liver, thyroid, and skin conditions; experiences with anaphylaxis, asthma, or other allergies; drug history; and possible drug interactions. ■ Evaluate laboratory blood levels: CBC, renal, and liver function studies. ■ Acquire the results of a complete physical examination including vital signs, ECG, pulmonary function tests, breathing patterns, and neurological status (LOC).	■ *Ineffective Airway Clearance* related to difficulty swallowing and coughing ■ *Ineffective Breathing Pattern* related to retained secretions and discomfort ■ *Disturbed Sleep Pattern* related to somnolence or agitation ■ *Deficient Knowledge* related to a lack of information about drug therapy

PLANNING: PATIENT GOALS AND EXPECTED OUTCOMES

The patient will:
■ Experience therapeutic effects (relief from allergic symptoms such as congestion, itching, or postnasal drip).
■ Be free from or experience minimal adverse effects from drug therapy.
■ Verbalize an understanding of the drug's use, adverse effects, and required precautions.

IMPLEMENTATION

Interventions and (Rationales)	Patient Education/Discharge Planning
■ Auscultate breath sounds before administering drug therapy. Use with extreme caution in patients with asthma or chronic obstructive pulmonary disease (COPD). Keep resuscitative equipment accessible. (Anticholinergic effects of antihistamines may trigger bronchospasm.)	■ Instruct the patient to immediately report wheezing or difficulty breathing. ■ Advise patients with asthma to consult the nurse regarding the use of injectable epinephrine in emergency situations.
■ Administer medication correctly and evaluate the patient's knowledge of proper administration. (Proper administration helps increase effectiveness of drugs. Mixing antihistamines with other medication may increase adverse effects such as drowsiness.)	Instruct the patient to: ■ Begin taking antihistamines before allergy season begins or at the earliest possible appearance of symptoms for best effects. ■ Follow directions on specific medication label. ■ Avoid mixing OTC antihistamines; always consult the healthcare provider before taking any OTC drugs or herbal supplements.

continued . . .

NURSING PROCESS FOCUS *(continued)*

Interventions and (Rationales)	Patient Education/Discharge Planning
■ Monitor vital signs (including ECG) before administering drug therapy. Use with extreme caution in patients with a history of cardiovascular disease. (Anticholinergic effects can increase heart rate and lower blood pressure. Fatal dysrhythmias and cardiovascular collapse have been reported in some patients receiving antihistamines.)	Instruct the patient to: ■ Immediately report dizziness, palpitations, headache, or chest, arm, or back pain accompanied by nausea/vomiting and/or sweating to the healthcare provider. ■ Monitor vital signs daily, ensuring proper use of home equipment.
■ Monitor thyroid function. Use with caution in patients with a history of hyperthyroidism. (Antihistamines exacerbate CNS-stimulating effects of hyperthyroidism and may trigger thyroid storm.)	■ Instruct the patient to report immediately any nervousness or restlessness, insomnia, fever, profuse sweating, thirst, and mood changes to healthcare provider.
■ Monitor for vision changes. Use with caution in patients with narrow-angle glaucoma. (Antihistamines can increase intraocular pressure and cause photosensitivity.)	Instruct the patient to: ■ Report head or eye pain and visual changes immediately to healthcare provider. ■ Wear dark glasses, use sunscreen, and avoid excessive sun exposure.
■ Monitor neurologic status, especially LOC. Use with caution in patients with a history of seizure disorder. (Drugs may cause sedation, especially in older adults. Antihistamines can also lower the seizure threshold.)	Instruct the patient to: ■ Avoid driving or performing hazardous activities until the effects of the drug are known. ■ Immediately report to the healthcare provider any seizure activity, including any changes in character and pattern of seizures.
■ Observe for signs of renal toxicity. Measure intake and output. Use with caution in patients with a history of kidney or urinary tract disease. (Antihistamines promote urinary retention.)	■ Instruct the patient to immediately report flank pain, difficulty urinating, reduced urine output, and changes in the appearance of urine (cloudy, with sediment, odor, etc.) to the healthcare provider.
■ Use with caution in patients with diabetes mellitus. Monitor serum glucose levels with increased dosing frequency. (Antihistamines decrease serum glucose levels.)	Instruct the patient to: ■ Immediately report symptoms of hypoglycemia. ■ Consult the healthcare provider regarding timing of glucose monitoring and reportable results (e.g., "less than 70 mg/dL").
■ Monitor for GI adverse effects. Use with caution in patients with a history of GI disorders, especially peptic ulcers or liver disease. (Antihistamines block H_1-receptors, altering the mucosal lining of the stomach. These drugs are metabolized in the liver, increasing the risk of hepatotoxicity.)	Instruct the patient to: ■ Immediately report nausea, vomiting, anorexia, bleeding, chest or abdominal pain, heartburn, jaundice, or a change in the color or character of stools to the healthcare provider. ■ Avoid substances that irritate the stomach, such as spicy foods, alcoholic beverages, and nicotine; take drug with food to avoid stomach upset.
■ Monitor for anticholinergic-related effects such as dry mouth, thickened mucus, and nasal drying. (Mild anticholinergic effects are common and are usually treated symptomatically.)	Instruct the patient to: ■ Immediately report fever or flushing accompanied by difficulty swallowing ("cotton mouth") to the healthcare provider. ■ Suck on hard candy to relieve dry mouth and maintain adequate fluid intake.

EVALUATION OF OUTCOME CRITERIA

Evaluate the effectiveness of drug therapy by confirming that patient goals and expected outcomes have been met (see "Planning"). *See Table 29.1 for a list of drugs to which these nursing actions apply.*

CORE CONCEPT 29.5

Intranasal corticosteroids are first-line drugs for treating allergic rhinitis.

Corticosteroids, also known as glucocorticoids, are applied directly to the nasal mucosa to prevent symptoms of allergic rhinitis. When applied consistently, they decrease the secretion of inflammatory mediators, reduce tissue edema, and cause mild vasoconstriction. They have largely replaced antihistamines as preferred drugs in the treatment of chronic allergic rhinitis. The intranasal corticosteroids are listed in Table 29.3 ◆. All have equal effectiveness and can require two to three weeks of therapy before optimum benefits are attained. When delivered by oral inhalation (not intranasal) some of these medications are also used to treat asthma.

Intranasal corticosteroids are administered with a metered-spray device that delivers a consistent dose of drug per spray. One to three weeks may be required to achieve peak response. Because of this delayed effect, intranasal corticosteroids are most effective when taken *in advance* of expected allergen exposure. Intranasal corticosteroids produce none of the potentially serious adverse effects that are observed when these hormones are given orally. The most frequently reported adverse effects are an intense burning sensation in the nose immediately after spraying and drying of the nasal mucosa.

TABLE 29.3   Intranasal Corticosteroids

Drug	Route and Adult Dose	Remarks
beclomethasone (Beconase AQ, Qnasl, QVAR)	Intranasal; 1–2 sprays in each nostril bid–qid	Oral inhaler available (Beclovent) for asthma
budesonide (Rhinocort Aqua)	Intranasal; two sprays in each nostril bid	Oral inhaler available (Pulmicort) for asthma
ciclesonide (Omnaris)	Intranasal; two sprays in each nostril once daily (max: 200 mcg/day)	Newer drug approved in 2006; less likely to cause steroid adverse effects than others in this class
flunisolide (Aerospan)	Intranasal; two sprays in each nostril bid	Oral inhaler available (Aerospan) for asthma
Pr fluticasone (Flonase, Flovent, Veramyst)	Intranasal; one spray in each nostril once (Veramyst) or twice (Flonase) daily	Oral inhaler available (Flovent) for asthma; topical form available (Cutivate) for dermatologic use
mometasone (Nasonex)	Intranasal; two sprays in each nostril daily	Topical form available (Elocon) for dermatologic use
triamcinolone (Nasacort AQ)	Intranasal; 2–4 sprays in each nostril qid	Oral inhaler available (Nasacort) for asthma; also available in IM, subcutaneous, intradermal, and intra-articular forms

Drug Prototype: Pr *Fluticasone (Flonase, Veramyst)*
Therapeutic Class: Drug for allergic rhinitis   **Pharmacologic Class: Intranasal corticosteroid**

Actions and Uses: Fluticasone is typical of the intranasal corticosteroids used to treat allergic rhinitis. Therapy usually begins with two sprays in each nostril twice daily and decreases to one dose per day. Fluticasone acts to decrease local inflammation in the nasal passages, thus reducing nasal stuffiness.

Adverse Effects and Interactions: Adverse effects of fluticasone are rare. Small amounts of the intranasal corticosteroids are sometimes swallowed, which increases their potential for causing systemic adverse effects. Nasal irritation and bleeding occur in a few patients.

Decongestants are used to reduce nasal congestion caused by allergic rhinitis and the common cold.

CORE CONCEPT 29.6

Decongestants are drugs that relieve nasal congestion. They are administered by either the oral or intranasal routes and are often combined with antihistamines in the pharmacotherapy of allergies or the common cold. Most decongestants are sympathomimetics—drugs that activate the sympathetic nervous system. Doses for the decongestants are given in Table 29.4 ◆.

Sympathomimetics are effective at relieving the nasal congestion associated with allergic rhinitis and the common cold. Both oral and intranasal preparations are available. The intranasal drugs such as oxymetazoline (Afrin, others) are available OTC as sprays or drops and produce an effective response within minutes. Because of their local action, intranasal sympathomimetics produce few systemic effects. The most serious, limiting adverse effect of the intranasal preparations is **rebound congestion**, a condition characterized by hypersecretion of mucus and worsened nasal congestion once the drug effects wear off. This rebound effect sometimes leads to a cycle of increased drug use as the condition worsens. Because of rebound congestion, intranasal sympathomimetics should be used for no longer than three to five days. Patients with allergic rhinitis who develop tolerance to the effects of decongestants should be gradually switched to intranasal corticosteroids because they do not cause rebound congestion.

When administered *orally*, sympathomimetics do not produce rebound congestion. Their onset of action by this route, however, is much slower than the intranasal preparations, and they are less effective at relieving severe congestion. The possibility of systemic adverse effects is also greater with the oral drugs. Potential adverse effects include hypertension and CNS stimulation that may lead to insomnia or anxiety.

Prior to 2000, pseudoephedrine was the most common decongestant found in oral OTC cold and allergy medicines. Pseudoephedrine, however, is the starting chemical for the synthesis of illegal methamphetamine by drug traffickers. Although pseudoephedrine is still available without a prescription, pharmacists are required to monitor its distribution by keeping a log of patients' names and addresses and checking the photo identification of the buyer. Most manufacturers have reformulated their OTC cold medicines to contain phenylephrine rather than pseudoephedrine. A drug prototype feature for phenylephrine is included in Chapter 8.

TABLE 29.4 Decongestants

Drug	Route and Adult Dose	Remarks
ipratropium (Atrovent)	Nasal spray; two sprays in each nostril 3–4 times per day up to 4 days	Anticholinergic drug; also available by the inhalation route for asthma
naphazoline (Privine)	Intranasal; two drops in each nostril every 3–6 hours	Also available as spray
℗ oxymetazoline (Afrin 12 hour, Neo-Synephrine 12 hour, others)	Intranasal (0.05%); 2–3 sprays in each nostril bid for up to 3–5 days	Also available as drops
phenylephrine (Afrin 4–6 hours, Neo-Synephrine 4–6 hours, others) (see page 98 for the Drug Prototype box)	Intranasal (0.25–0.5%); one or two sprays in each nostril every 3–4 hours	Also available as drops, chewable tablets, and hemorrhoidal cream; also available by the subcutaneous, IM and IV routes for severe hypotension and shock
pseudoephedrine (Sudafed, others)	PO; 60 mg every 4–6 hours (max: 120 mg/day)	Produces little congestive rebound or irritation; also available as drops and in extended-release form
tetrahydrozoline (Tyzine)	Intranasal (0.1%); 2–4 drops in each nostril every 3 hours	Ophthalmic solution is available for allergic reactions of the eye
xylometazoline (Otrivin)	Intranasal (0.1%); one or two sprays in each nostril bid (max: 3 doses/day)	Also available as drops

Because sympathomimetics relieve only nasal congestion, they are often combined with antihistamines to control the sneezing and tearing of allergic rhinitis. It is interesting to note that some OTC drugs having the same basic name (Neo-Synephrine, Afrin, Visine) may contain different sympathomimetics. For example, Neo-Synephrine preparations with a 12-hour duration contain the drug oxymetazoline, while those with a 4- to 6-hour duration contain phenylephrine.

Ipratropium (Atrovent) is an anticholinergic drug sometimes used for the symptomatic relief of runny nose due to the common cold or allergic rhinitis. Given by the intranasal route, ipratropium has no serious adverse effects. Its actions are limited to runny nose; it does not stop the sneezing, postnasal drip, or itchy throat or eyes. A more common indication for ipratropium is for the pharmacotherapy of asthma.

Concept Review **29.4**

- The sympathomimetics are the most effective drugs for relieving nasal congestion, but physicians often prefer to prescribe antihistamines or intranasal corticosteroids. Why?

Drug Prototype: ℗ *Oxymetazoline (Afrin, Others)*
Therapeutic Class: Decongestant **Pharmacologic Class: Sympathomimetic**

Actions and Uses: Oxymetazoline activates alpha-adrenergic receptors of the sympathetic nervous system. This stimulation causes arterioles in the nasal passages to constrict, producing a drying of the mucous membranes. Relief from the symptoms of nasal congestion occurs within minutes and lasts for 10–12 hours. The drug is administered with a metered-spray device or by nose drops.

Oxymetazoline (Visine LR) is also available as eyedrops. It causes vasoconstriction of vessels in the eye and is used to relieve redness and provide relief from dryness and minor eye irritations.

Adverse Effects and Interactions: Rebound congestion is common when oxymetazoline is used for longer than three to five days. Minor stinging and dryness in the nasal mucosa may be experienced. Systemic adverse effects are unlikely, unless a considerable amount of the medicine is swallowed. Patients with thyroid disorders, hypertension, diabetes, or heart disease should use sympathomimetics only on the direction of their healthcare provider.

No clinically significant interactions have been found.

Antitussives and expectorants are used to treat symptoms of the common cold.

In addition to congestion, cough is a symptom that causes patients to take OTC remedies or to seek medical attention. Cough is a reflex mechanism controlled by neurons in the cough center, located in the medulla oblongata of the brain. In diseases such as emphysema and bronchitis, or when liquids have been aspirated into the bronchi, it is not desirable to suppress the normal cough reflex. Because cough is merely a symptom, the therapeutic goal is to identify and treat the underlying disorder whenever possible.

There are many possible causes of cough, ranging from the acute cough of an upper respiratory infection to the chronic cough of tobacco smoking. Some drugs, such as the angiotensin-converting enzyme (ACE) inhibitors and beta-adrenergic blockers, can trigger persistent cough. In many cases, keeping the throat moist with sugar-free candy, "cough drops," or frequent sips of water is sufficient to suppress cough. However, a dry, hacking, nonproductive cough can be irritating to the membranes of the throat and can deprive a patient of much-needed rest. It is these types of conditions in which therapy with drugs that control cough, or **antitussives**, may be warranted.

anti = *against*
tussive = *pertaining to a cough*

Opioids, the most effective class of antitussives, act by raising the cough threshold in the cough center, thereby decreasing both the frequency and the intensity of cough. Hydrocodone and codeine are effective opioid antitussives. Doses needed to suppress the cough reflex are low; thus there is minimal potential for dependence. Most codeine cough mixtures are classified as Schedule III, IV, or V drugs and are reserved for more serious cough conditions. The amount of codeine in cough mixtures is low and rarely causes serious adverse effects. However, care must be taken not to give these mixtures to patients allergic to codeine or other opioids. In addition, the drug must be kept secure from children because accidental overdose of opioids in infants can cause severe respiratory depression and even death. Opioids may be combined with other drugs such as antihistamines, decongestants, and nonopioid antitussives in the therapy of severe cold or flu symptoms.

The most frequently used OTC antitussive is dextromethorphan, which is included in most severe cold and flu preparations. Dextromethorphan is chemically similar to the opioids and also acts on the CNS to raise the cough threshold. Although it does not have the high abuse potential of opioids, dextromethorphan can cause slurred speech, dizziness, drowsiness, euphoria, and lack of motor coordination when taken in high amounts.

Benzonatate (Tessalon) is a nonopioid antitussive that does not act on the cough center. Instead, benzonatate has a local anesthetic-like effect on stretch receptors in the lung, which essentially interrupts the cough message. The patient must be instructed not to chew the soft capsules because they will cause numbness of the throat and tongue.

Expectorants are drugs that reduce the thickness or viscosity of bronchial secretions. They stimulate mucus flow, which thins bronchial secretions, allowing them to be removed with less forceful coughing. The most effective OTC expectorant is guaifenesin. Like dextromethorphan, guaifenesin produces few adverse effects and is a common ingredient in many OTC cold and flu preparations. Higher doses of guaifenesin are available by prescription. Nonprescription cough and cold products (including those containing guaifenesin) should not be used in children under six years of age.

Acetylcysteine (Mucomyst) is one of the few drugs available to directly loosen thick, viscous bronchial secretions by breaking down the chemical structure of mucus molecules. Drugs of this type are called **mucolytics**. Acetylcysteine is delivered by the inhalation route and is not available OTC. It is used in patients who have cystic fibrosis or other diseases that produce large amounts of thick bronchial secretions. Acetylcysteine (Acetadote) is also given as a 5% oral solution for acetaminophen overdose. When given within 24 hours of the overdose, acetylcysteine prevents acute liver damage by blocking the formation of toxic metabolites of acetaminophen.

muco = *mucus*
lytic = *destruction or disintegration*

ASTHMA

Asthma is a chronic pulmonary disease that has both inflammatory and bronchospasm components. Drugs are given to either decrease the frequency of asthmatic attacks or terminate attacks in progress. Asthma is one of the most common chronic conditions in the United States, affecting about 24 million Americans.

Asthma is a chronic inflammatory disease characterized by bronchospasm.

Asthma is characterized by chronic inflammation that occurs when potent mediators of the immune and inflammatory responses are released by mast cells lining the bronchi. The result of this inflammation is increased mucus secretion, which narrows the airways and makes breathing more difficult.

FIGURE 29.5

Changes in bronchioles during an asthma attack: (a) normal bronchiole, (b) inflammation obstructing the airway, and (c) constricted bronchiole in asthma attack.

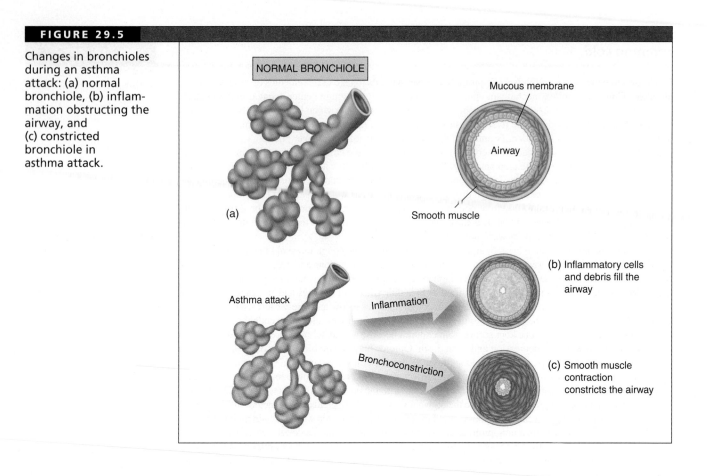

The second component of asthma is acute **bronchoconstriction** or **bronchospasm** during which bronchiolar smooth muscle contracts and the airway diameter narrows. This condition is illustrated in Figure 29.5 ■. The inflammatory conditions in the airway make the smooth muscle hyperresponsive to a variety of stimuli. Stimuli such as breathing smoke, pollutants, or cold air may trigger acute bronchospasm. Specific triggers are listed in Table 29.5 ◆. Some patients experience bronchospasm on exertion, a condition called exercise-induced asthma.

The patient with asthma will exhibit symptoms such as evening cough, **dyspnea** (shortness of breath), chest tightness, and wheezing. Intervals between symptoms may vary from days to weeks to months.

dys = *painful or difficult*
pnea = *breathing*

TABLE 29.5	Common Triggers of Asthma
Air pollutants	Tobacco smoke
	Ozone
	Nitrous and sulfur oxides
	Fumes from cleaning fluids or solvents
	Burning leaves
Allergens	Pollen from trees, grasses, and weeds
	Animal dander
	Household dust
	Mold
Chemicals and food	Drugs such as aspirin, ibuprofen, and beta blockers
	Sulfite preservatives
	Food such as nuts, monosodium glutamate (MSG), shellfish, and dairy products
Respiratory infections	Bacterial, fungal, and viral
Stress	Emotional stress or anxiety
	Exercise in dry, cold climates

FIGURE 29.6

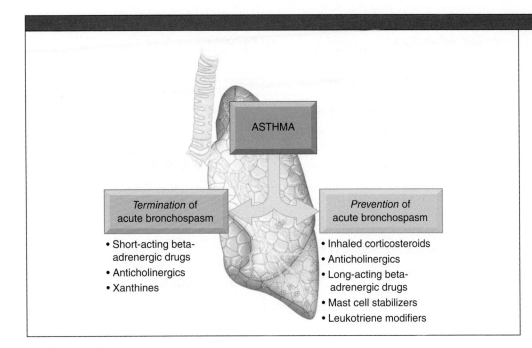

Drug classes used in the pharmacotherapy of asthma.

Status asthmaticus is a severe, prolonged form of asthma that is unresponsive to drug treatment and may lead to respiratory failure.

Because asthma has both a bronchoconstriction component and an inflammatory component, drug therapy of the disease focuses on one or both of these mechanisms. The goals of drug therapy are twofold: to terminate acute bronchospasms in progress and to reduce the frequency of acute asthma attacks. Different drugs are usually needed to achieve each of these goals. The various classes of drugs used for asthma are shown in Figure 29.6 ■.

Beta-adrenergic agonists are the most effective drugs for relieving acute bronchospasm.

Recall from Chapter 8 that the smooth muscle lining the bronchioles is under the control of the autonomic nervous system. Changes in the airway diameter are made possible by the contraction or relaxation of the bronchiolar smooth muscle. During the fight-or-flight response, beta$_2$-adrenergic receptors of the sympathetic nervous system are stimulated, the bronchiolar smooth muscle relaxes, and **bronchodilation** results. This allows more air to enter the alveoli, thus increasing the oxygen supply to the body during periods of stress or exercise. In practical terms, drugs that enhance bronchodilation will cause the patient to breathe more easily; these are some of the most common medications for treating pulmonary disorders.

Bronchodilators are medications from several drug classes that are used to rapidly relieve the acute bronchospasm characteristic of an asthmatic attack. Although the beta-adrenergic drugs are the most commonly prescribed types of bronchodilators, theophylline and ipratropium may also be used. Bronchodilators used for asthma are listed in Table 29.6 ◆.

Beta-adrenergic drugs, or sympathomimetics, are the most effective drugs for the treatment of acute bronchospasm. In most cases, the drugs used for pulmonary disease are selective for beta$_2$-receptors in the lung; thus, they produce fewer cardiac adverse effects than the nonselective beta drugs. There are two basic classes of beta-adrenergic drugs, and each has different indications.

Fast Facts Asthma

- According to the Asthma and Allergy Foundation of America, every day in America:
  - 44,000 people have an asthma attack.
  - 36,000 children miss school due to asthma.
  - 27,000 adults miss work due to asthma.
  - 4,700 people visit the emergency room due to asthma.
  - 1,200 people are admitted to the hospital due to asthma.
  - 9 people die from asthma.

TABLE 29.6 Bronchodilators

Drug	Route and Adult Dose	Remarks
BETA-ADRENERGIC DRUGS		
albuterol (Proventil, Ventolin, VoSpire)	MDI; two inhalations every 4–6 hours as needed (max: 12 inhalations/day) Nebulizer; 1.25–5 mg every 4–8 hours as needed PO; 2–4 mg tid-qid (max: 32 mg/day); Extended-release tablets: 8 mg every 12 hours (max: 32 mg/day divided)	Relaxes smooth muscle of the bronchial tree; nebulizer form available
arformoterol (Brovana)	Nebulizer; 15 mcg twice daily (max: 30 mcg/day)	Newer drug for COPD; long acting; similar to formoterol
formoterol (Foradil, Perforomist)	DPI; 12 mcg inhalation capsule every 12 hours (max: 24 mcg/day) Nebulizer; 20 mcg bid (max: 40 mcg/day)	Long acting; used for asthma prophylaxis
indacaterol (Arcapta neohaler)	Inhalation: one 75 mcg capsule daily using the Neohaler	Newer drug used as a maintenance bronchodilator for COPD
levalbuterol (Xopenex)	Nebulizer; 0.63 mg tid–qid MDI; two inhalations every 4–6 hours	Short acting; similar to albuterol
pirbuterol (Maxair)	MDI; two inhalations four times a day (max: 12 inhalations/day)	Short acting; similar to albuterol
salmeterol (Serevent)	DPI; two aerosol inhalations bid or one powder diskus bid	Long acting; used for asthma prophylaxis
terbutaline (Brethine)	PO; 2.5–5 mg tid (max: 15 mg/day) Subcutaneous; 250 mcg (may be repeated in 15 min) Inhalation; two inhalations (200 mcg/spray) every 4–6 hours	Also used to delay premature labor
XANTHINES		
aminophylline (Truphylline)	PO; 380 mg/day in divided doses every 6–8 hours (max: 928 mg/day)	IV form available
theophylline (Theo-dur)	PO; 300–600 mg/day in divided doses (max: 900 mg/day)	IV and extended-release form available
ANTICHOLINERGICS		
aclidinium (Tudorza Pressair)	Inhalation: 400 mcg bid	Newer drug for acute bronchospasm
ipratropium (Atrovent, Combivent)	MDI; two inhalations qid (max: 12 inhalations/day) Nebulizer; 500 mcg every 6–8 hours as needed	Combivent is a combination of ipratropium and albuterol
tiotropium (Spiriva)	DPI; one capsule inhaled/day	Handihaler device is used to puncture capsule

- *Short-acting beta drugs* Short-acting beta agonists are the most frequently prescribed drugs for aborting or terminating an acute asthma attack because they begin to act within minutes. Their effects, however, last only two to six hours.

- *Long-acting beta drugs* Because long-acting beta drugs take 20 to 60 minutes to act, they are not used to terminate bronchospasm. They should only be used in combination with inhaled corticosteroids for the prophylaxis of severe, persistent asthma.

Inhaled beta-adrenergic drugs produce little systemic toxicity because only small amounts of the drugs are absorbed. When given orally, a longer duration of action is achieved, but adverse effects such as tachycardia and tremor are more frequently experienced. Tolerance may develop to the therapeutic effects of the beta-adrenergic drugs; therefore, the patient must be instructed to seek medical attention if the drugs prove to be less effective with continued use.

As discussed in Chapter 8, blocking the parasympathetic nervous system produces similar effects to stimulation of the sympathetic nervous system. It is predictable then, that anticholinergic drugs would cause bronchodilation and have potential use in the pharmacotherapy of asthma and other pulmonary diseases. The most widely used drug in this class, ipratropium (Atrovent), is taken via inhalation to rapidly relieve bronchospasm. Because it is not readily absorbed from the lungs, it produces few adverse effects, although it is considered less effective than beta-adrenergic drugs. Inhaled anticholinergics are more effective when used with other bronchodilators; Combivent is a combination of ipratropium and albuterol in a single MDI canister. Tiotropium (Spiriva) is a newer anticholinergic with a long duration of action that allows for once-daily dosing.

The third class of bronchodilators is the xanthines (sometimes called methylxanthines). Chemically related to caffeine, theophylline (Theo-dur) and aminophylline (Truphylline) were drugs of choice for bronchoconstriction 20 years ago. Theophylline, however, has a narrow margin of safety and interacts with a large number of other drugs. Adverse effects such as nausea, vomiting, and CNS stimulation are relatively common, and dysrhythmias may occur at high doses. Having been largely replaced by safer and more effective drugs, theophylline is now primarily used for the long-term oral prophylaxis of persistent asthma.

NURSING PROCESS FOCUS Patients Receiving Bronchodilators

ASSESSMENT	POTENTIAL NURSING DIAGNOSES
Prior to administration: ■ Obtain a complete health history, including respiratory, cardiovascular, renal and liver conditions, drug history, and possible drug interactions. ■ Obtain information about experiences with anaphylaxis, asthma, allergies and exposure to environmental irritants; effects of respiratory difficulties on sleep, eating, and performance of ADLs. ■ Evaluate laboratory blood findings: CBC, ABGs, and renal and liver function studies. In addition, evaluate information regarding results of pulmonary function tests (peak expiratory flowmeter). ■ Acquire the results of a complete physical examination, including vital signs, pulse oximetry, and symptoms related to respiratory deficiency, such as dyspnea, orthopnea, cyanosis, nasal flaring, adventitious lung sounds (wheezing), and weakness.	■ *Impaired Gas Exchange* related to bronchial constriction ■ *Anxiety* related to difficulty in breathing ■ *Deficient Knowledge* related to a lack of information about drug therapy ■ *Ineffective Therapeutic Regimen Management* related to noncompliance with medication regimen, presence of adverse effects, and need for long-term medication use

PLANNING: PATIENT GOALS AND EXPECTED OUTCOMES

The patient will:
■ Experience therapeutic effects (adequate oxygenation, improved lung sounds, and improved pulmonary function values).
■ Be free from or experience minimal adverse effects from drug therapy.
■ Verbalize an understanding of the drug's use, adverse effects, and required precautions.

IMPLEMENTATION

Interventions and (Rationales)	Patient Education/Discharge Planning
■ Continue to monitor vital signs (including pulse and blood pressure) respiratory pattern, pulse oximetry, and lung sounds. Monitor periodic pulmonary function tests: peak expiratory flow meter and arterial blood gas. (Monitoring is necessary to determine drug effectiveness.)	Instruct the patient to: ■ Use medication as directed even if asymptomatic to prevent the onset of respiratory difficulties. ■ Instruct the patient to report symptoms of deteriorating respiratory status such as increased dyspnea, breathlessness with speech, and/or orthopnea to the healthcare provider.
■ Administer medication correctly and evaluate the patient's knowledge of proper use of the inhaler. (Proper administration techniques and use of equipment ensures correct dosage.)	Instruct the patient to: ■ Recognize the difference between long- and short-acting inhalers. ■ Use a spacer between MDI and mouth. ■ Shake or load the inhaler with tablet or powder. ■ If using a bronchodilator inhaler with a corticosteroid inhaler: Use the bronchodilator first to open the airway, wait 5 to 10 minutes, then take the corticosteroid. ■ Use the medication strictly as prescribed; do not "double up" on doses. ■ Rinse the mouth thoroughly following use. ■ Rinse inhaler and spacer with water daily.
■ Observe for adverse effects specific to the medication used. (An increase in pulse rate, changes in blood pressure or sensations of palpitations may occur with beta-adrenergic drugs.)	Instruct the patient regarding adverse effects and to report specific drug adverse effects such as palpitations or fast heart rate and respirations.
■ Maintain the environment free of respiratory contaminants such as dust, dry air, flowers, and smoke. (These substances may exacerbate bronchial constriction.)	Instruct the patient to: ■ Avoid respiratory irritants. ■ Maintain a "clean air environment." ■ Stop smoking and avoid secondhand smoke, if applicable.
■ Maintain dietary intake adequate in essential nutrients and vitamins. (Dyspnea interferes with proper nutrition.)	Instruct the patient to: ■ Maintain nutrition with foods high in essential nutrients. ■ Consume small frequent meals to prevent fatigue.
■ Ensure that the patient maintains adequate hydration of 3 to 4 L/day (to liquefy pulmonary secretions).	Instruct the patient to: ■ Consume 3 to 4 L of fluid per day if not contraindicated. ■ Avoid caffeine (increases CNS irritability).

continued . . .

NURSING PROCESS FOCUS *(continued)*

Interventions and (Rationales)	Patient Education/Discharge Planning
■ Provide emotional and psychosocial support during periods of shortness of breath. (Providing support and remaining calm helps to reduce the anxiety brought on by respiratory difficulties.)	■ Instruct the patient in relaxation techniques and controlled breathing techniques.
■ Monitor patient compliance. (Maintaining therapeutic drug levels is essential to effective therapy.)	■ Inform the patient of the importance of ongoing medication compliance and follow-up.

EVALUATION OF OUTCOME CRITERIA

Evaluate the effectiveness of drug therapy by confirming that patient goals and expected outcomes have been met (see "Planning"). See Table 29.6 for a list of drugs to which these nursing actions apply.

CORE CONCEPT 29.10

Corticosteroids are the most effective drugs for the long-term prophylaxis of asthma.

The role of intranasal corticosteroids as first-line drugs in the treatment of allergic rhinitis is discussed in Core Concept 29.5. When given by the inhalation route, corticosteroids are also prime drugs for the management of asthma.

Because asthma has a major inflammatory component, several classes of anti-inflammatory drugs are used for asthma prophylaxis. The inhaled corticosteroids are most commonly used for this purpose, although mast cell stabilizers and leukotriene inhibitors are also effective. Doses of the anti-inflammatory drugs used for asthma are given in Table 29.7 ◆.

Corticosteroids are the most effective drugs available for the *prevention* of acute asthmatic episodes. When inhaled on a daily schedule, corticosteroids suppress inflammation without producing major adverse effects. Mucus production and edema are diminished, thus reducing airway obstruction. Patients should

TABLE 29.7 Anti-Inflammatory Drugs for Asthma

Drug	Route and Adult Dose	Remarks
INHALED CORTICOSTEROIDS		
beclomethasone (Beconase AQ, Qvar)	MDI; one or two inhalations tid or qid (max: 20 inhalations/day)	Intranasal form available for allergic rhinitis
budesonide (Pulmicort Turbuhaler, Rhinocort)	DPI; one or two inhalations (200 mcg/ inhalation) daily (max: 800 mcg/day)	Intranasal form available for allergic rhinitis
ciclesonide (Alvesco)	MDI; one or two inhalations/day (max: 320–640 mcg/day)	Newer drug; for asthma prophylaxis, not for acute bronchospasm
flunisolide (Aerospan)	MDI; two or three inhalations bid or tid (max: 12 inhalations/day)	Intranasal form available for allergic rhinitis
fluticasone (Flovent)	MDI (44 mcg); two inhalations bid (max: 10 inhalations/day)	Intranasal form available for allergic rhinitis; also available in 110 and 120 mcg inhalers
mometasone (Asmanex)	DPI; one inhalation daily (max: two inhalations daily)	Intranasal form available for allergic rhinitis and topical form for skin inflammation
triamcinolone (Azmacort)	MDI; two inhalations tid or qid (max: 16 inhalations/day)	Also available in IM, subcutaneous, intradermal, topical, and oral forms
MAST CELL STABILIZERS		
cromolyn (Intal)	MDI; one inhalation qid	Intranasal form available OTC for allergic rhinitis; also for ophthalmic use
nedocromil (Tilade)	MDI; two inhalations qid	Topical form available for ophthalmic use
LEUKOTRIENE MODIFIERS		
montelukast (Singulair)	PO; 10 mg/day in evening	Not for acute bronchospasm; also for allergic rhinitis
roflumilast (Daliresp)	PO; 500 mcg once daily	Newer drug for COPD
zafirlukast (Accolate)	PO; 20 mg bid 1 hour before or 2 hours after meals	Not for acute bronchospasm; also for allergic rhinitis
zileuton (Zyflo)	PO; 1,200 mg bid	Not for acute bronchospasm

be informed that inhaled corticosteroids must be taken daily to produce their therapeutic effect and that these medications are not effective at terminating episodes in progress. Although symptoms will improve in the first one to two weeks of therapy, four to eight weeks may be required for maximum benefit. For some patients, a beta-adrenergic drug may be prescribed along with an inhaled corticosteroid because this permits the dose of the corticosteroid to be reduced by as much as 50%.

For severe, persistent asthma that is unresponsive to other treatments, oral corticosteroids may be prescribed. Treatment time is limited to the shortest length possible, usually five to seven days. If taken for longer than 10 days, oral corticosteroids may produce significant adverse effects such as adrenal gland suppression, peptic ulcers, and hyperglycemia. Other uses and adverse effects of corticosteroids are presented in Chapters 24 and 31.

Mast cell stabilizers and leukotriene modifiers are alternative anti-inflammatory drugs for the prophylaxis of asthma.

CORE CONCEPT 29.11

Two mast cell inhibitors play a limited though important role in the prophylaxis of asthma. These drugs act by inhibiting the release of histamine from mast cells.

Cromolyn (Intal) is an anti-inflammatory drug that is useful in preventing asthma attacks. When administered via an MDI or a nebulizer, cromolyn is a safe alternative to the corticosteroids. Patients must be informed that cromolyn should be taken on a daily basis and should not be used to terminate acute attacks. An intranasal form of cromolyn (Nasalcrom) is used in the treatment of seasonal allergies. The second mast cell stabilizer, nedocromil (Tilade), has actions and uses similar to cromolyn. The drug is used for asthma prophylaxis and has an unpleasant taste.

The leukotriene modifiers reduce inflammation and ease bronchoconstriction by modifying the action of leukotrienes, which are mediators of the inflammatory response in patients with asthma. Leukotriene modifiers are alternative drugs used for the management of persistent asthma that cannot be controlled with inhaled corticosteroids or short-acting beta drugs.

The leukotriene modifiers are approved for the prophylaxis of chronic asthma; they are ineffective in relieving acute bronchospasm. They are all given orally. Zileuton and roflumilast have a rapid onset of, whereas the other two leukotriene modifiers take as long as a week to provide therapeutic benefit. Adverse effects associated with the leukotriene modifiers include headache, cough, nasal congestion, GI upset, and psychiatric effects such as depression and suicidal thinking.

Concept Review   29.5

■ Distinguish the classes of drugs that *prevent* asthma attacks from those that can *terminate* an attack in progress. Name at least one drug in each class.

Drug Prototype: Pr *Cromolyn (Intal)*

Therapeutic Class: **Anti-inflammatory drug for asthma and allergic rhinitis**   Pharmacologic Class: **Mast cell stabilizer**

Actions and Uses: Cromolyn prevents the inflammation that is characteristic of asthma and COPD. For asthma therapy the drug is administered via oral inhalation. An intranasal over the counter (OTC) formulation (NasalCrom) is available for allergic rhinitis. Cromolyn is considered an alternate drug for the treatment of mild to moderate asthma when inhaled corticosteroids have not proven effective.

Cromolyn is only effective for preventing asthma and should not be used to terminate an asthma attack. Several weeks of therapy are needed for optimum benefit. An ophthalmic solution (Crolom) is used to treat allergic disorders of the conjunctiva. Gastrocrom is a PO dosage form of cromolyn that is the only FDA-approved drug to treat systemic mastocytosis, which is a rare condition in which the patient has an excessive number of mast cells.

Adverse Effects and Interactions: Adverse effects are uncommon when the drug is administered by oral inhalation. The most common effects are bronchospasm, cough, and pharyngeal irritation. Intranasal and ophthalmic administration may cause local burning and stinging. There are no significant drug interactions.

CHRONIC OBSTRUCTIVE PULMONARY DISEASE

Chronic obstructive pulmonary disease (COPD) includes progressive lung disorders primarily caused by tobacco smoking. COPD is a major cause of death and disability. Drugs may bring symptomatic relief but do not cure the disorders.

Chronic obstructive pulmonary disease is a progressive disorder treated with multiple drugs.

bronch = *bronchus*
itis = *inflammation*

The two primary disorders classified as COPD are chronic bronchitis and emphysema. Both are strongly associated with smoking tobacco products and, secondarily, air pollutants. In **chronic bronchitis**, excess mucus is produced in the respiratory tree due to inflammation and irritation from smoke or pollutants. The airway becomes partially obstructed with mucus, resulting in the classic signs of dyspnea and coughing. Because microbes enjoy the mucus-rich environment, pulmonary infections are common. Gas exchange may be impaired.

COPD is a progressive disease, with the terminal stage being **emphysema**. After years of chronic inflammation, the bronchioles lose their elasticity, and the alveoli dilate to maximum size to get more air into the lungs. The patient suffers from extreme dyspnea from even the slightest physical activity.

Patients with COPD may receive a number of pulmonary drugs for symptomatic relief of their disorder. The goal of pharmacotherapy is to control cough and bronchospasm. Typical drugs considered in COPD therapy include the following:

- Long-acting beta-adrenergic drugs such as salmeterol
- Anticholinergic bronchodilators such as ipratropium or tiotropium
- Inhaled corticosteroids such as budesonide
- Mucolytics and expectorants to reduce the thickness of the bronchial mucus and to aid in its removal
- Oxygen therapy may be used in patients with emphysema.

Patients should be taught to avoid taking any drugs that have beta-blocking activity or that otherwise cause bronchoconstriction. Respiratory depressants should be avoided. It is important to note that none of the pharmacotherapies offer a cure for COPD; they only treat the symptoms of a progressively worsening disease.

PATIENTS NEED TO KNOW

Patients treated for pulmonary disorders need to know the following:

In General

1. Because tolerance to some medications may occur, if medication is no longer effective, report this tolerance to a healthcare provider. Do not take extra medication without notifying a healthcare provider.

Regarding Inhaled Medications

2. When using MDIs or DPIs, allow an interval of at least one minute to pass between puffs.
3. When taking more than one respiratory medicine, take the bronchodilator first. This opens the airways and increases the effectiveness of the second medication.
4. Rinse the mouth thoroughly following inhaler use to reduce the oral absorption of inhaled medicines.
5. Take inhaled corticosteroids on a regular basis—not as needed. These medications are not used to stop acute asthma attacks.
6. Do not use decongestant nasal sprays for more than two or three days unless instructed to do so by a healthcare provider.

Regarding Bronchodilators

7. Avoid caffeine-containing foods and beverages
8. Immediately report any abnormalities in pulse rate, changes in blood pressure, or sensations of palpitations when taking beta-adrenergic stimulators.

Regarding Antihistamines and Decongestants

9. If taking antihistamines for the first time, avoid operating machinery or performing other tasks requiring alertness because drowsiness may occur.
10. Use hard candies, chewing gum, or ice chips to reduce the dry mouth caused by some decongestants and antihistamines.
11. Stop taking antihistamines and notify a healthcare provider if excessive sedation, wheezing, chest tightness, or bleeding/bruising occurs.
12. Do not take OTC cold or allergy medicines containing antihistamines at the same time as prescription antihistamines.

CHAPTER REVIEW

CORE CONCEPTS SUMMARY

29.1 **The respiratory system supplies oxygen for the body and provides protection against inhaled organisms.**

The URT warms the incoming air and reacts to particles or pathogens that attempt to enter the body. The LRT brings needed oxygen into the body and removes carbon dioxide through expiration. The process of moving air into and out of the lungs, or ventilation, is distinct from the process of gas exchange across the alveoli, a process known as respiration.

29.2 **The inhalation route of drug administration quickly delivers medications directly to their sites of action.**

Inhalation is frequently used as a route of drug administration for those medications targeted for the respiratory system. Nebulizers, DPIs, and MDIs are used to deliver drugs via the inhalation route.

29.3 **Allergic rhinitis is characterized by sneezing, watery eyes, and nasal congestion.**

Allergic rhinitis, also known as hay fever, is a chronic allergy triggered by a wide variety of antigens. The release of chemicals mediating the immune response can result in seasonal symptoms for some patients, and chronic, continuous symptoms for others.

29.4 **Antihistamines are widely used to treat allergic rhinitis and other minor allergies.**

The H_1-receptor blockers, or antihistamines, are used to treat allergies, motion sickness, and insomnia. Newer drugs in this class are nonsedating and offer the advantage of once-a-day dosing.

29.5 **Intranasal corticosteroids are first-line drugs for treating allergic rhinitis.**

Intranasal corticosteroids are the treatment of choice for allergic rhinitis because of their high effectiveness and wide margin of safety. When used by this route, they do not produce the serious adverse effects observed when they are given orally or parenterally.

29.6 **Decongestants are used to reduce nasal congestion caused by allergic rhinitis and the common cold.**

Oral and intranasal sympathomimetics are effective at relieving nasal congestion. The intranasal drugs act more rapidly and are more effective. Use of the intranasal preparations, however, is usually limited to three to five days because of the potential for rebound congestion.

29.7 **Antitussives and expectorants are used to treat symptoms of the common cold.**

Antitussives are effective at inhibiting the cough reflex. Although opioids are the most effective, there is some risk of physical dependence. Guaifenesin is an OTC drug used to increase bronchial secretions so that cough may be more productive. Mucolytics loosen mucus so that it may be more easily removed from the bronchial tree.

29.8 **Asthma is a chronic inflammatory disease characterized by bronchospasm.**

Asthma is a common disease characterized by bronchospasm and chronic airway inflammation. Exposure to a number of factors, including allergens, can cause an acute episode.

29.9 **Beta-adrenergic agonists are the most effective drugs for relieving acute bronchospasm.**

Inhaled beta$_2$-adrenergic drugs are preferred medications for relieving bronchospasm. Anticholinergics are sometimes used for bronchodilation, but fewer are available because of their incidence of adverse effects. Xanthines, once widely used in pulmonary medicine, are now second-choice drugs for relieving bronchospasm because of their higher potential for adverse effects.

29.10 **Corticosteroids are the most effective drugs for the long-term prophylaxis of asthma.**

Inhaled corticosteroids are the drugs of choice for asthma prophylaxis. The inhaled corticosteroids, even when used on a long-term basis, produce few adverse effects compared to oral corticosteroids.

29.11 **Mast cell stabilizers and leukotriene modifiers are alternative anti-inflammatory drugs for the prophylaxis of asthma.**

Mast cell stabilizers such as cromolyn are sometimes used for asthma prophylaxis, although they are not as effective as the corticosteroids. The leukotriene modifiers offer another option for the prophylaxis of chronic asthma.

29.12 **Chronic obstructive pulmonary disease is a progressive disorder treated with multiple drugs.**

Chronic bronchitis and emphysema are two disorders of COPD that often require multiple drug therapy. Bronchodilators, expectorants, mucolytics, antibiotics, and oxygen may offer symptomatic relief.

REVIEW QUESTIONS

The following questions are written in NCLEX-PN® style. Answer these questions to assess your knowledge of the chapter material, and go back and review any material that is not clear to you.

1. The patient is having an acute asthma attack. The nurse would expect which of the following drugs to be most appropriate?

1. Pirbuterol (Maxair)
2. Budesonide (Pulmicort)
3. Fluticasone (Flovent)
4. Zafirlukast (Accolate)

2. Salmeterol (Serevent) has been added to your patient's treatment regimen for asthma. Which of the following would be of highest priority for patients to know?

1. Nausea and vomiting may be adverse effects.
2. It is important to take this medication every day in order to prevent an asthma attack.
3. The drug causes tremors.
4. Avoid caffeine-containing foods and beverages.

3. A 24-year-old patient has just started taking Benadryl because of an allergic reaction. The nurse knows to monitor the patient for: (Select all that apply.)

1. Drowsiness
2. Dry mouth
3. Tachycardia
4. Nausea

4. The physician has ordered montelukast (Singulair). As the nurse begins to administer the medication, the patient asks how soon the medication will begin working. The nurse responds by answering:

1. "The medication has a rapid onset—within 2 hours."
2. "It will take about a week to become effective."
3. "This medication is used to treat acute bronchospasms only."
4. "Therapeutic benefits may take several weeks."

5. The patient asks what the difference is between antitussives and mucolytics. The nurse replies:

1. "Antitussives loosen bronchial secretions, and mucolytics stimulate removal of bronchial secretions."
2. "Antitussives suppress cough, whereas mucolytics loosen bronchial secretions."

3. "The terms are interchangeable."
4. "Both types of drugs work to loosen and remove secretions."

6. A patient with asthma states that it has become worse over the past few months. He continues to say that when an acute asthma attack occurs, budesonide (Pulmicort Turbuhaler) does not stop the episode. The nurse should advise the patient:

1. To use four inhalations of budesonide instead of two
2. That budesonide must be taken on a regular schedule to work
3. To request a tablet form of corticosteroid, rather than an inhaler
4. To always clear his nose gently just prior to using budesonide

7. The patient complains of numbness of the throat and tongue after taking benzonatate (Tessalon). The nurse instructs the patient:

1. To swallow, not chew, the medication
2. To decrease the dosage of medication
3. To stop taking the medication immediately
4. That this is a common adverse effect and that will subside over time

8. The healthcare practitioner ordered albuterol 4 mg, three times a day. The available concentration is 2 mg in 5 mL. How many milliliters would be given per dose?

1. 2 mL
2. 5 mL
3. 10 mL
4. 20 mL

9. The nurse informs patients taking intranasal corticosteroids that they may experience which of the following adverse effects?

1. Rebound congestion
2. Intense burning sensation
3. Drowsiness
4. Nervousness

10. While planning an educational session for patients using Afrin, the nurse would include:

1. Not to use it for longer than three to five days to prevent rebound congestion from occurring
2. The importance of monitoring for hypertension
3. To notify the physician if nervousness occurs
4. Not to take it with any other medications

CASE STUDY QUESTIONS

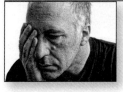

Remember Mr. Thomas, who was introduced at the beginning of the chapter? Now read the remainder of the case study. Based on the information you have learned in this chapter, answer the questions that follow.

Mr. Michael Thomas arrives at the office with what appears to be an acute upper respiratory tract infection. He tells the nurse, "I can't sleep at night with this cough, and I can hardly work without getting short of breath." Upon examination, he has low-grade *fever and shortness of breath when walking. He is 60 years old, smokes a pack of cigarettes daily, and has a history of emphysema, although he doesn't usually take any medications. For his upper respiratory infection, the physician prescribes hydrocodone, guaifenesin, acetaminophen, and an ipratropium (Atrovent) inhaler.*

1. Before leaving the doctor's office, Mr. Thomas asks the nurse which of his prescribed drugs will directly help him with his shortness of breath. The nurse tells him that it is:

1. Hydrocodone
2. Acetaminophen

3. Guaifenesin
4. Ipratropium

2. He also wants to know which of his prescriptions will help him "get the mucus up that's stuck in the back of my throat." The nurse tells him that _____ will help thin bronchial secretions, allowing them to be removed more easily.

1. Hydrocodone
2. Acetaminophen
3. Guaifenesin
4. Ipratropium

3. Mr. Thomas calls the office the next day, complaining that he is unable to drive his car because of excessive drowsiness. The nurse suspects that _____ is most likely causing this drowsiness.

1. Hydrocodone
2. Acetaminophen

3. Guaifenesin
4. Ipratropium

4. Mr. Thomas also has emphysema. The physician plans to continue him on guaifenesin and ipratropium. He also wants him to take an inhaled corticosteroid. The nurse expects that Mr. Thomas will be given a prescription for:

1. Salmeterol
2. Tiotropium
3. Budesonide
4. Olopatadine

NOTE: Answers to the Review and Case Study Questions appear in Appendix B. The complete rationales and answers are located on the textbook's website.

Pearson Nursing Student Resources   Find additional review materials at **nursing.pearsonhighered.com**.

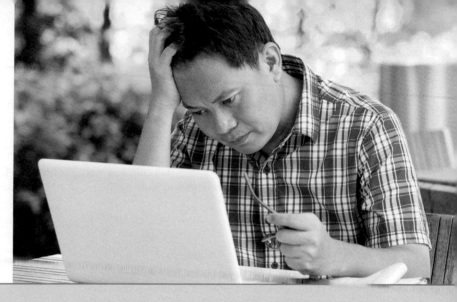

CHAPTER

"An ulcer . . . this is the last thing I need right now. My job is stressful enough."

Mr. Jeffery Han, stockbroker

30 Drugs for Gastrointestinal Disorders

CORE CONCEPTS

30.1 The digestive system breaks down food, absorbs nutrients, and eliminates wastes.

30.2 Peptic ulcer disease is caused by an erosion of the mucosal layer of the stomach or duodenum.

30.3 Peptic ulcer disease is treated by a combination of lifestyle changes and pharmacotherapy.

30.4 Proton-pump inhibitors are effective at reducing gastric acid secretion.

30.5 H_2-receptor blockers reduce the secretion of gastric acid.

30.6 Antacids rapidly neutralize stomach acid and reduce the symptoms of peptic ulcer disease and GERD.

30.7 Antibiotics are administered to eliminate *Helico-bacter pylori*, the cause of many peptic ulcers.

30.8 Several miscellaneous drugs are also beneficial in treating peptic ulcer disease.

30.9 Laxatives are used to promote defecation.

30.10 Opioids are the most effective drugs for controlling severe diarrhea.

30.11 Antiemetics are prescribed to treat nausea, vomiting, and motion sickness.

30.12 Anorexiants and lipase inhibitors are used for the short-term management of obesity.

30.13 Pancreatic enzymes are administered as replacement therapy for patients with pancreatitis or malabsorption syndromes.

DRUG SNAPSHOT

The following drugs are discussed in this chapter:

DRUG CLASSES	DRUG PROTOTYPES
Proton-pump inhibitors	**Pr** omeprazole (Prilosec) *483*
H_2-receptor blockers	**Pr** ranitidine (Zantac) *483*
Antacids	
Antibiotics for *H. pylori*	
Laxatives	**Pr** psyllium mucilloid (Metamucil, others) *487*

DRUG CLASSES	DRUG PROTOTYPES
Antidiarrheals	**Pr** diphenoxylate with atropine (Lomotil) *488*
Antiemetics	**Pr** ondansetron (Zofran, Zuplenz) *490*
Antiobesity drugs	
Pancreatic enzyme replacements	

LEARNING OUTCOMES

After reading this chapter, the student should be able to:

1. Describe the major anatomic structures of the digestive system.
2. Identify common causes, signs, and symptoms of peptic ulcer disease and gastroesophageal reflux disease (GERD).
3. Identify classes of drugs used to treat peptic ulcer disease and GERD.
4. Explain why two or more antibiotics are used concurrently in the treatment of *H. pylori*.
5. Explain the conditions in which the drug treatment of constipation is warranted.
6. Identify the major classes of laxatives.
7. Explain the conditions in which the drug treatment of diarrhea is warranted.
8. Identify the major classes of antiemetics.
9. Describe the types of drugs used in the short-term management of obesity and their effectiveness.
10. Describe the pharmacotherapy of pancreatic insufficiency.
11. Categorize drugs used in the treatment of digestive system disorders based on their classifications and mechanisms of action.
12. For each of the classes listed in the Drug Snapshot, identify representative drugs and explain their mechanisms of drug action, primary actions, and important adverse effects.

KEY TERMS

alimentary canal (AL-uh-MEN-tare-ee) *478*
anorexia (AN-oh-REX-ee-uh) *480*
anorexiant (AN-oh-REX-ee-ant) *491*
antacid (an-TASS-id) *485*
antiemetic (AN-tie-ee-MET-ik) *489*
antiflatulent (an-tie-FLAT-u-lent) *485*
cathartic (kah-THAR-tik) *486*
constipation (kon-stah-PAY-shun) *486*
Crohn's disease (KROHNS) *480*
defecation (def-ah-KAY-shun) *486*

diarrhea *488*
dietary fiber *486*
digestion (dye-JES-chun) *478*
emesis (EM-eh-sis) *489*
emetics (ee-MET-ikz) *490*
gastroesophageal reflux disease (GERD) (GAS-troh-ee-SOF-ah-JEEL REE-flux) *480*
H^+, K^+-ATPase *482*
H_2-receptor blocker *483*
Helicobacter pylori (hee-lick-oh-BAK-tur py-LOR-eye) *479*

inflammatory bowel disease (IBD) *480*
pancreatic insufficiency *492*
peptic ulcer *479*
peristalsis (pair-ih-STAL-sis) *478*
proton-pump inhibitors (PPIs) *482*
triple therapy *481*
ulcerative colitis (UL-sir-ah-tiv koh-LIE-tuss) *480*
Zollinger–Ellison syndrome (ZOLL-in-jer ELL-ih-sun) *483*

Very little of the food we eat is directly available for use as energy to our body. Food must be broken down, absorbed, and chemically modified before it is in a form useful to cells. The digestive system performs these functions and more. Some disorders of the digestive system are mechanical in nature, slowing or speeding up the transit of substances through the gastrointestinal tract. Other disorders are metabolic, affecting the secretion of digestive enzymes and fluids or the absorption of essential nutrients. Many signs and symptoms are nonspecific and may be caused by any number of different disorders. This chapter examines the drug therapy of common conditions affecting the digestive system.

Fast Facts Gastrointestinal Tract Disorders

- Sixty to seventy million Americans are affected by a digestive disease.
- Thirteen percent of all hospitalizations are for digestive disorders.
- Over a million people experience pancreatitis each year, and about 3,000 die from the disorder.
- More than 480,000 new cases of peptic ulcer disease are diagnosed each year.
- Colorectal cancer is the second leading cause of cancer deaths, killing more than 55,000 Americans annually.
- Irritable bowel syndrome affects 10% to 20% of adults.
- Americans spend more than $33 billion annually on weight-reduction products and services.

CORE CONCEPT 30.1

The digestive system breaks down food, absorbs nutrients, and eliminates wastes.

The digestive system consists of two basic anatomic divisions: the alimentary canal and the accessory organs. The **alimentary canal**, or gastrointestinal (GI) tract, is a long, continuous, hollow tube that extends from the mouth to the anus. The accessory organs of digestion include the liver, gallbladder, and pancreas. The structure of the digestive system is shown in Figure 30.1 ■.

Digestion is the process by which the body breaks down ingested food into small molecules that can be absorbed. The primary functions of the GI tract are to physically transport ingested food and to provide the necessary enzymes and surface area for chemical digestion and absorption. The inner surface is lined with a mucosa layer that secretes acids, bases, mucus, and enzymes important to digestion. The mucosa of the small intestine is lined with tiny projections called villi and microvilli that provide a huge surface area for the absorption of food and medications.

Substances are propelled along the GI tract by the contractions of several layers of smooth muscle, a process known as **peristalsis**. The speed of transit is critical to the absorption of nutrients and water and for the removal of wastes. If peristalsis is too fast, substances will not have sufficient contact with the mucosa to be absorbed. In addition, the large intestine will not have enough time to absorb water, and diarrhea may result. Abnormally slow transit times may result in constipation or even obstructions in the small or large intestine.

To chemically break down ingested food, a large number of enzymes and other substances are required. Digestive enzymes are secreted by the salivary glands, stomach, small intestine, and pancreas. The liver makes bile, which is stored in the gallbladder until needed for lipid digestion. Because these digestive substances are not common targets for drug therapy, their discussion in this chapter is limited, and the student should refer to anatomy and physiology texts for additional information.

peri = *around*
stalsis = *contraction*

FIGURE 30.1

The digestive system.

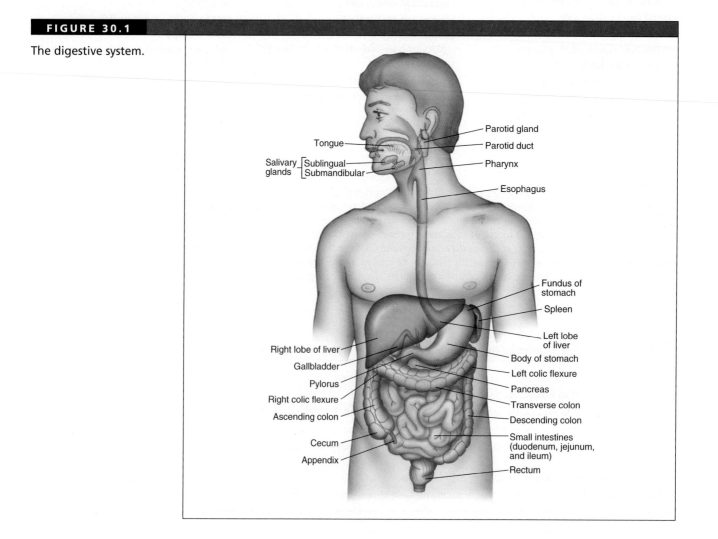

PEPTIC ULCER DISEASE

An ulcer is a sore or erosion of the mucosa of the GI tract. Although ulcers may occur in any portion of the GI tract, the duodenum is the most common site.

Peptic ulcer disease is caused by an erosion of the mucosal layer of the stomach or duodenum.

CORE CONCEPT 30.2

The term **peptic ulcer** refers to a lesion located in either the stomach (gastric) or small intestine (duodenal). The disorder is very common, affecting about 10% of the population at some point during their life span. Peptic ulcer disease (PUD) is associated with lifestyle factors such as cigarette smoking, stress, alcohol consumption, caffeine, and the use of drugs such as corticosteroids and nonsteroidal anti-inflammatory drugs (NSAIDs).

pept = to digest
ic = pertaining to

One to three liters of hydrochloric acid are secreted each day by cells in the stomach mucosa. Although this strong acid aids in the chemical breakdown of food and helps to protect the body from ingested microbes, it may be quite damaging to stomach cells. A number of natural defenses protect the stomach lining against this extremely acidic fluid. Certain cells lining the surface of the stomach secrete a thick mucus layer and bicarbonate, a basic ion that neutralizes acid and provides a protective function. On reaching the duodenum, the stomach contents are further neutralized by bicarbonate from pancreatic and biliary secretions. These natural defenses are depicted in Figure 30.2 ■.

The primary cause of peptic ulcers is infection by the bacterium *Helicobacter pylori*. In noninfected patients, the most common cause is therapy with NSAIDs. Secondary factors that contribute to ulcer and the subsequent inflammation include secretion of excess stomach acid and hyposecretion of adequate mucous protection. Figure 30.3 ■ illustrates the mechanism of peptic ulcer formation.

The characteristic symptom of duodenal ulcer is a gnawing or burning upper abdominal pain that occurs one to three hours after a meal. The pain is worse between meals when the stomach is empty and it often disappears following ingestion of food. Nighttime pain, nausea, and vomiting are uncommon. If the erosion progresses deeper into the mucosa, bleeding will occur, and this may be evident as bright red blood in vomit or black, tarry stools. Many duodenal ulcers heal spontaneously, although they often recur after months of remission.

FIGURE 30.2

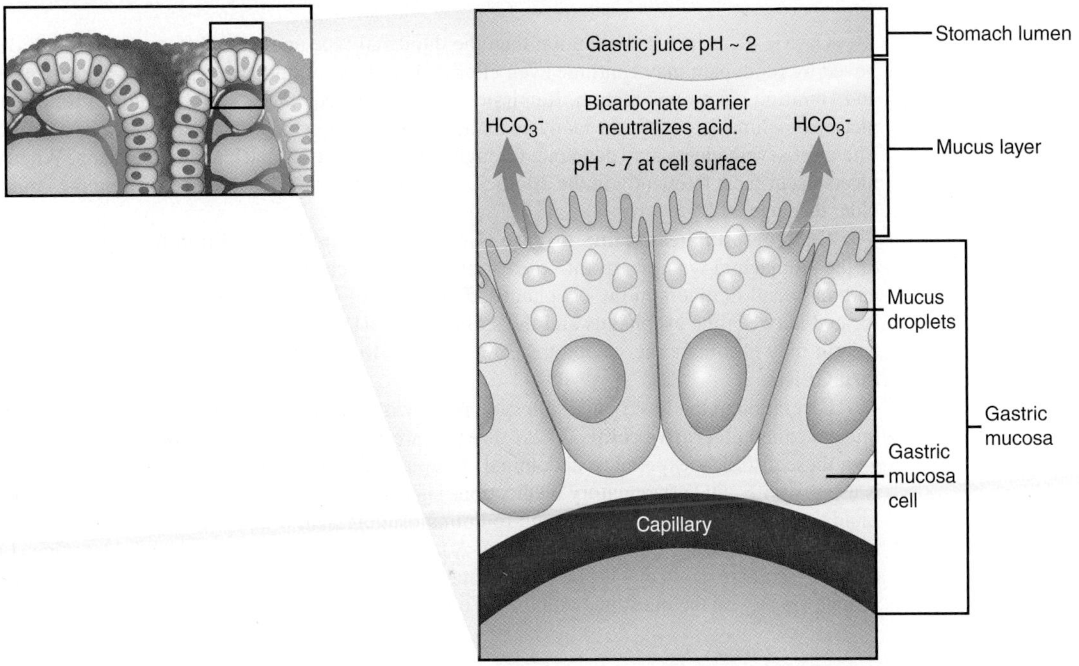

Natural defenses against stomach acid.

FIGURE 30.3

Mechanism of peptic ulcer formation.

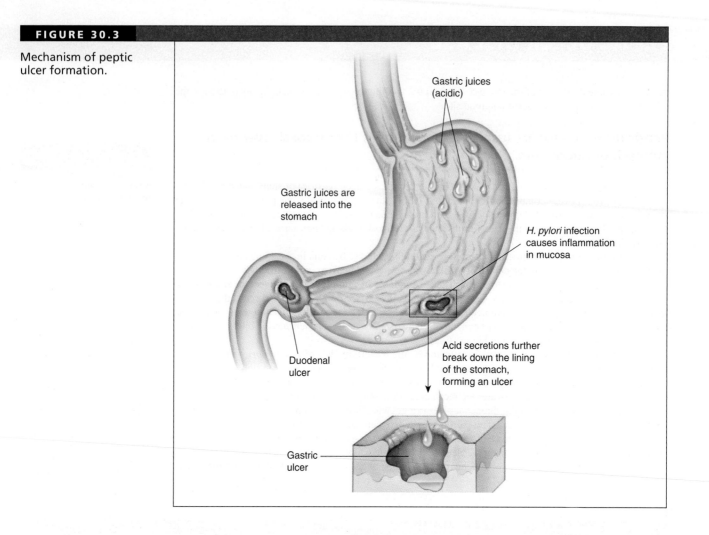

Gastric juices (acidic)

Gastric juices are released into the stomach

H. pylori infection causes inflammation in mucosa

Acid secretions further break down the lining of the stomach, forming an ulcer

Duodenal ulcer

Gastric ulcer

an = *not or without*
orexia = *appetite*

Gastric ulcers are less common than the duodenal type and have different symptoms. Although relieved by food, pain may continue even after a meal. Loss of appetite (known as **anorexia**), weight loss, and vomiting are more common. Remissions may be infrequent or absent. Medical follow-up of gastric ulcers sometimes proceeds for many years because a small percentage of the erosions become cancerous. The most severe ulcers may penetrate through the wall of the stomach and cause death. Whereas duodenal ulcers occur most frequently in the 30- to 50-year-old age group, gastric ulcers are more common in those older than age 60.

Gastroesophageal reflux disease (GERD) is a common condition in which the acidic contents of the stomach move upward into the esophagus. This causes an intense burning known as *heartburn* and may lead to ulcers in the esophagus. The cause of GERD is usually a loosening of the sphincter located between the esophagus and the stomach. GERD is strongly associated with obesity, and losing weight may eliminate the symptoms. Many of the drugs prescribed for peptic ulcers are also used to treat GERD.

Ulceration in the lower small intestine is known as **Crohn's disease**, and erosions in the large intestine are called **ulcerative colitis**. These diseases are called **inflammatory bowel disease (IBD)**. Patients with these disorders experience abdominal cramping, diarrhea, and weight loss. Pharmacotherapy of IBD is usually with anti-inflammatory medications such as sulfasalazine (Azulfidine) or mesalamine (Asacol, Lialda, others). Severe cases may require immunosuppressant drugs such as corticosteroids, or immuno-modulators such as infliximab (Remicade). A newer approach is to administer budesonide (Entocort EC, Uceris), a corticosteroid that is taken orally but is not absorbed. Budesonide produces its anti-inflammatory actions directly on the intestine, with few or no systemic side effects.

Concept Review **30.1**

■ What are the similarities and differences between duodenal ulcers and gastric ulcers?

Peptic ulcer disease is treated by a combination of lifestyle changes and pharmacotherapy.

Before starting drug therapy, patients are usually advised to change lifestyle factors that contribute to PUD. For example, eliminating tobacco, alcohol, and caffeine consumption, and reducing stress often allow healing of the ulcer, causing it to go into remission.

For patients requiring drug therapy, a wide variety of both prescription and over-the-counter (OTC) medications are available. These drugs fall into four primary classes, plus one miscellaneous group:

- Proton-pump inhibitors
- H_2-receptor blockers
- Antacids
- Antibiotics
- Miscellaneous drugs

The treatment goals for pharmacotherapy are to provide immediate relief from symptoms, promote healing of the ulcer, and prevent recurrence of the disease. The choice of medication depends on the source of the disease (infectious versus inflammatory), the severity of symptoms, and the convenience of OTC versus prescription drugs. The most common therapy for the management of PUD is a combination of a proton-pump inhibitor plus two antibiotics. This approach, referred to as **triple therapy**, eliminates the cause of most peptic ulcers (*H. pylori*) while also reducing acid secretion. The mechanisms of action of the four major classes of drugs used to treat PUD are depicted in Figure 30.4 ■.

FIGURE 30.4

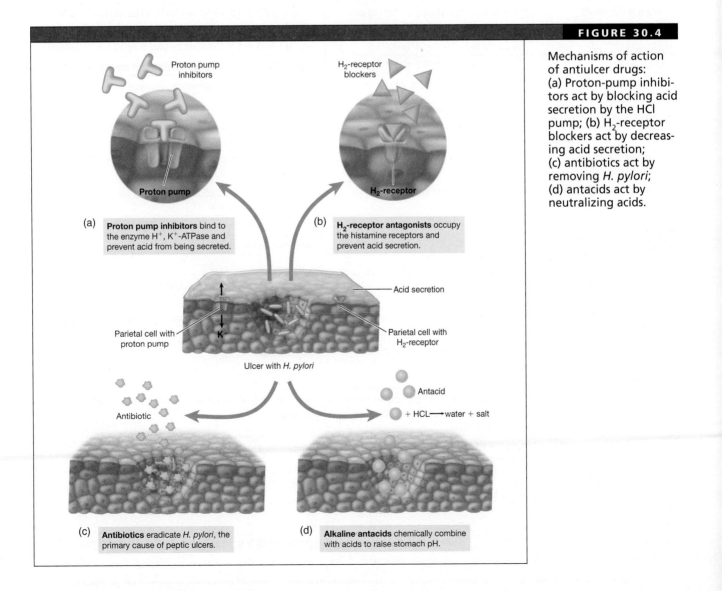

Mechanisms of action of antiulcer drugs: (a) Proton-pump inhibitors act by blocking acid secretion by the HCl pump; (b) H_2-receptor blockers act by decreasing acid secretion; (c) antibiotics act by removing *H. pylori*; (d) antacids act by neutralizing acids.

(a) **Proton pump inhibitors** bind to the enzyme H^+, K^+-ATPase and prevent acid from being secreted.

(b) **H_2-receptor antagonists** occupy the histamine receptors and prevent acid secretion.

(c) **Antibiotics** eradicate *H. pylori*, the primary cause of peptic ulcers.

(d) **Alkaline antacids** chemically combine with acids to raise stomach pH.

CORE CONCEPT 30.4

Proton-pump inhibitors are effective at reducing gastric acid secretion.

Proton-pump inhibitors act by blocking the enzyme responsible for secreting hydrochloric acid in the stomach. The proton-pump inhibitors are listed in Table 30.1 ◆.

Proton-pump inhibitors (PPIs) are the most effective medications available for reducing acid secretion and thus are preferred drugs for the treatment of PUD and GERD. These drugs reduce acid secretion by binding irreversibly to the enzyme **H+, K+-ATPase**. In the mucosal cells of the stomach, this enzyme acts as a pump to release acid (also called H+, or protons) onto the surface of the GI mucosa. PPIs reduce acid secretion to a greater extent than do the H₂-receptor blockers and have a longer duration of action.

In addition to PUD, the PPIs are also indicated for GERD and for acid hypersecretory conditions such as Zollinger–Ellison syndrome. They may also be prescribed to *prevent* PUD in patients taking high doses of NSAIDs. As a component of triple therapy, PPIs are usually continued for one to two weeks. In refractory cases, therapy may continue for four to eight weeks. The beneficial effects of PPIs last three to five days after therapy is stopped.

Adverse effects from short-term therapy with PPIs are uncommon. Headache, abdominal pain, diarrhea, nausea, and vomiting are the most frequently reported adverse effects. If taken for prolonged periods, PPIs may interfere with calcium absorption and cause osteoporosis and fractures.

TABLE 30.1	Drugs for Peptic Ulcer Disease	
Drug	**Route and Adult Dose**	**Remarks**
H₂-RECEPTOR BLOCKERS		
cimetidine (Tagamet)	PO; 300 mg every 6 hours or 800 mg at bedtime or 400 mg bid with food	Also for GERD and hypersecretory disorders; IM and IV forms available
famotidine (Pepcid)	PO; 20 mg bid or 40 mg at bedtime	Also for GERD and hypersecretory disorders; IV form available
nizatidine (Axid)	PO; 150–300 mg at bedtime	Newest drug in this class; rapid onset with few adverse effects
Pr ranitidine (Zantac)	PO; 100–150 mg bid or 300 mg at bedtime	Also for GERD and hypersecretory disorders; IM and IV forms available
PROTON-PUMP INHIBITORS		
esomeprazole (Nexium)	PO; 20–40 mg/day	Also for GERD and hypersecretory disorders; IV form available
lansoprazole (Prevacid)	PO; 15–60 mg/day	Also for GERD and hypersecretory disorders; Prevpac combines lansoprazole, amoxicillin, and clarithromycin
Pr omeprazole (Prilosec)	PO; 20–60 mg once or twice daily	Often used in combination with antibiotics for *Helicobacter* infections; also for GERD
pantoprazole (Protonix)	PO; 40 mg/day	Primarily for GERD and hypersecretory disorders; IV form available
rabeprazole (AcipHex)	PO; 20 mg/day	Also for GERD and hypersecretory disorders
ANTACIDS		
aluminum hydroxide (AlternaGEL, others)	PO; 600 mg tid–qid	Not absorbed; may cause constipation
calcium carbonate (Titralac, Tums)	PO; 1–2 g bid–tid	Also for calcium replacement therapy; may cause constipation
calcium carbonate with magnesium hydroxide (Mylanta Gel-caps, Rolaids)	PO; two to four capsules or tablets prn (max: 12 tablets/day)	Common OTC therapy
magaldrate (Riopan)	PO; 540–1080 mg (5–10 mL suspension or one or two tablets) daily (max: 20 tablets or 100 mL/day)	Lower incidence of bowel adverse effects than magnesium or aluminum antacids
magnesium hydroxide (Milk of Magnesia)	PO; 5–15 mL or two to four tablets as needed up to four times daily	Also used as a laxative; may cause diarrhea
magnesium hydroxide and aluminum hydroxide with simethicone (Mylanta, Maalox Plus)	PO; 10–20 mL prn (max: 120 mL/day) or two to four tablets prn (max: 24 tablets/day)	Common OTC therapy
sodium bicarbonate (NaHCO₃) (see page 261 for the Drug Prototype box)	PO; 325 mg–2 g one to four times per day	IV form available to treat metabolic acidosis and cardiac arrest

Drug Prototype: 🅟 *Omeprazole (Prilosec)*

Therapeutic Class: Antiulcer drug   **Pharmacologic Class: Proton-pump inhibitor**

Actions and Uses: Omeprazole was the first proton-pump inhibitor approved for PUD; both prescription and OTC forms are available. Although this drug may take 2 hours to reach therapeutic levels, its effects last up to 72 hours. It is used for the short-term therapy of peptic ulcers and GERD. Most patients are symptom-free after two weeks of therapy. It is used for longer periods in patients who have chronic hypersecretion of gastric acid, a condition known as **Zollinger–Ellison syndrome**. Omeprazole is available in oral form only. Zegerid is a combination drug containing omeprazole and the antacid sodium bicarbonate.

Adverse Effects and Interactions: Adverse effects are generally minor and include headache, nausea, diarrhea, and abdominal pain. Long-term therapy can interfere with calcium absorption and result in fractures due to weakened bones.

Omeprazole interacts with several drugs. For example, using it together with diazepam, phenytoin, and central nervous system (CNS) depressants will cause increased blood levels of these drugs. Concurrent use with warfarin may increase the risk of bleeding.

H$_2$-receptor blockers reduce the secretion of gastric acid.

CORE CONCEPT 30.5

The discovery of the H$_2$-receptor blockers in the 1970s marked a major breakthrough in the treatment of PUD. Since then they have become available OTC and are widely used in the treatment of PUD and GERD. Doses of the H$_2$-receptor blockers are given in Table 30.1.

Histamine has two types of receptors: H$_1$ and H$_2$. Activation of H$_1$-receptors produces the classic symptoms of allergy, whereas the H$_2$-receptors are responsible for increasing acid secretion in the stomach. Cimetidine (Tagamet), the first **H$_2$-receptor blocker**, and other drugs in this class are quite effective at suppressing the volume and acidity of stomach acid. These drugs are also used to treat the symptoms of GERD.

Adverse effects of the H$_2$-receptor blockers are minor and rarely cause discontinuation of therapy. Patients taking high doses, or those with renal or hepatic disease, may experience confusion, restlessness, hallucinations, or depression. Patients should be advised not to take antacids at the same time as H$_2$-receptor blockers because the absorption of these drugs will be lessened.

Concept Review   30.2

■ Explain the following statement: All H$_2$-receptor blockers are antihistamines, but not all antihistamines are H$_2$-receptor blockers.

Drug Prototype: 🅟 *Ranitidine (Zantac)*

Therapeutic Class: Antiulcer drug   **Pharmacologic Class: H$_2$-receptor blocker**

Actions and Uses: Ranitidine has become one of the most frequently used drugs in the treatment of PUD and GERD. It has a higher potency than cimetidine, which allows it to be administered once daily, usually at bedtime. Adequate healing of the ulcer takes four to eight weeks. Patients with persistent disease may continue on drug maintenance for long periods to prevent recurrence. Gastric ulcers heal more slowly than duodenal ulcers and require longer drug therapy. IV and IM forms are available for the treatment of acute stress-induced bleeding ulcers. Ranitidine is available in a dissolving tablet form (EFFERdose) for treating GERD in children and infants older than one month of age.

Adverse Effects and Interactions: Adverse effects are uncommon and mild. Ranitidine does not cross the blood–brain barrier to any appreciable extent, so the confusion and CNS depression observed with cimetidine does not occur with ranitidine. Ranitidine has fewer drug–drug interactions than cimetidine. Although rare, severe reductions in the number of red and white blood cells and platelets are possible.

Ranitidine exhibits fewer drug–drug interactions than cimetidine. Ranitidine may reduce the absorption of cefpodoxime, ketoconazole, and itraconazole. Antacids should not be given within one hour of H$_2$-receptor antagonists because effectiveness may be decreased due to reduced absorption.

NURSING PROCESS FOCUS Patients Receiving Drug Therapy for Peptic Ulcer Disease

ASSESSMENT	POTENTIAL NURSING DIAGNOSES
Prior to administration: ■ Obtain a complete health history, including GI and liver conditions, nutrition, allergies, drug history, and possible drug interactions. ■ Evaluate laboratory blood findings: CBC, electrolytes, renal, and liver function studies. ■ Acquire the results of a complete physical examination, including vital signs, height and weight, pain, signs of bleeding, and LOC.	■ *Deficient Knowledge* related to a lack of information about drug therapy ■ *Acute Pain* related to tissue damage of the gastric mucosa or gastric inflammation and/or to ineffective drug therapy ■ *Imbalanced Nutrition: Less than Body Requirements* related to adverse effects of drug

PLANNING: PATIENT GOALS AND EXPECTED OUTCOMES

The patient will:
■ Experience therapeutic effects (diminished or absent gastric pain and bloating).
■ Be free from or experience minimal adverse effects from drug therapy.
■ Verbalize an understanding of the drug's use, adverse effects, and required precautions.

IMPLEMENTATION

Interventions and (Rationales)	Patient Education/Discharge Planning
■ Administer medications correctly and evaluate the patient's knowledge of proper administration. (Following guidelines with regard to meals and other medications will result in improved outcomes.)	Inform the patient to: ■ Take PPIs before meals, preferably before breakfast. ■ Shake liquid antacids well before pouring. ■ Take H_2-receptor antagonists and other medications at least one hour before antacids. Patients taking antacids should avoid taking other medications for at least two hours.
■ Monitor level of abdominal pain or discomfort (to assess effectiveness of drug therapy; it may take days to weeks before pain is controlled).	Advise the patient: ■ That pain relief may not occur for several days after beginning therapy ■ To immediately report episodes of severe or increasing pain to the healthcare provider.
■ Monitor patient use of alcohol. (Alcohol can increase gastric irritation.)	■ Instruct the patient to avoid alcohol use.
■ Discuss and monitor for possible drug interactions, including OTC drugs like antacids. (Antacids can decrease the effectiveness of other drugs taken concurrently.)	Instruct the patient to: ■ Consult with the healthcare provider before taking other medications or herbal products. ■ Avoid drugs that may cause stomach irritation such as aspirin or NSAIDs.
■ Institute effective safety measures regarding falls. (Drowsiness may occur when starting H_2-receptor blockers.)	■ Instruct the patient to avoid driving or performing hazardous activities until drug effects are known.
■ Explain need for lifestyle changes. Provide consultation for dietitian and information on smoking cessation programs. (Smoking and certain foods increase gastric acid secretion.)	Encourage the patient to: ■ Adopt a healthy lifestyle: eliminate alcohol and smoking, increase exercise, and choose low-fat foods. ■ Keep a food diary in order to identify foods that trigger discomfort. Avoid foods that cause stomach discomfort.
■ Observe the patient for signs of GI bleeding. (Drugs used to treat PUD decrease gastric acidity making the gastric environment less favorable for ulcer development, but they do not heal existing ulcers. Blood in the stool or emesis and abdominal pain may indicate a worsening condition.)	■ Instruct the patient to immediately report to the healthcare provider any episodes of blood in the stool or vomitus, increase in abdominal discomfort, or diarrhea.
■ Monitor CBC, electrolytes, liver function, and serum gastrin during long-term use of medications for PUD. (Abnormal liver function tests may indicate adverse effect of drug therapy. Long-term therapy with PPIs can lead to decreased calcium absorption. H_2 receptors can affect CBC values. Antacids may affect electrolytes such as sodium and phosphorus.)	■ Inform the patient of the importance of keeping all scheduled doctor and laboratory visits.
■ Monitor for pregnancy or breastfeeding. (Women who are breastfeeding should not take these medications.)	■ Instruct the patient to report possible pregnancy and plans for breastfeeding to the healthcare provider.

EVALUATION OF OUTCOME CRITERIA

Evaluate the effectiveness of drug therapy by confirming that patient goals and expected outcomes have been met (see "Planning"). *See Table 30.1 for a list of drugs to which these nursing actions apply.*

Antacids rapidly neutralize stomach acid and reduce the symptoms of peptic ulcer disease and GERD.

Antacids are alkaline substances that have been used to neutralize stomach acid for hundreds of years. Doses of the antacids are listed in Table 30.1.

Prior to the development of H_2-receptor blockers and PPIs, antacids were the mainstay of peptic ulcer and GERD pharmacotherapy. Indeed, many patients still use these inexpensive and readily available OTC medications. Antacids, however, are no longer recommended as the sole medication for PUD because they do not promote healing of the ulcer.

Antacids are alkaline, inorganic compounds of aluminum, magnesium, or calcium. Combinations of aluminum hydroxide and magnesium hydroxide are the most common type. Both aluminum hydroxide and magnesium hydroxide are bases that are capable of rapidly neutralizing stomach acid. A few products combine antacids and H_2-receptor blockers into a single tablet; for example, Pepcid Complete contains calcium carbonate, magnesium hydroxide, and famotidine.

Simethicone is sometimes added to antacid preparations because it reduces gas bubbles that cause bloating and discomfort. For example, Mylanta contains simethicone, aluminum hydroxide, and magnesium hydroxide. Simethicone is classified as an **antiflatulent** because it reduces gas. It also is available by itself in OTC products such as Gas-X and Mylanta.

anti = *against*
flatus = *gas in the GI tract*

Self-medication with antacids is safe when taken in doses directed on the labels. Although they act within 10 to 15 minutes, their duration of action is only 2 hours. Therefore, they must be taken often during the day. Products containing sodium, calcium, or magnesium can result in absorption of these minerals to the general circulation. When given in high doses, aluminum compounds may interfere with phosphate metabolism and cause constipation. Magnesium compounds may cause diarrhea. Patients should follow the label instructions very carefully and not take more than the recommended dosages.

Antibiotics are administered to eliminate *Helicobacter pylori*, the cause of many peptic ulcers.

The bacterium *H. pylori* is associated with 80% of all duodenal ulcers and 70% of all gastric ulcers. This organism has adapted well as a human pathogen by devising ways to neutralize the high acidity surrounding it and by making substances that allow it to stick tightly to the GI mucosa. *H. pylori* causes inflammation of the stomach mucosa by both increasing acid secretion and reducing bicarbonate secretion.

Because *H. pylori* infections can remain active for life if not treated, treatment for this infection is a primary goal of PUD management. Elimination of this organism causes ulcers to heal more rapidly and to remain in remission longer. The following antibiotics are commonly used for this purpose:

- amoxicillin (Amoxil)
- clarithromycin (Biaxin)
- metronidazole (Flagyl)
- tetracycline (Sumycin)

Two or more antibiotics are given concurrently (usually with a PPI) to increase the effectiveness of therapy and to lower the potential for bacterial resistance. Clarithromycin and amoxicillin are the preferred drugs. Antibiotic therapy generally continues for 7 to 14 days. Bismuth compounds (Pepto-Bismol, Tritec) are sometimes added to the antibiotic regimen. Although not antibiotics, bismuth compounds do inhibit bacterial growth and prevent *H. pylori* from adhering to the surface of the gastric mucosa. Dosages and additional information for these anti-infectives can be found in Chapter 26.

Several miscellaneous drugs are also beneficial in treating peptic ulcer disease.

Three additional drugs are beneficial in treating PUD. Sucralfate (Carafate) consists of sucrose (a sugar) plus aluminum hydroxide (an antacid). The drug produces a thick, gel-like substance that coats the ulcer, protecting it against further erosion and promoting healing. Very little of the drug is absorbed from the GI tract. Other than constipation, adverse effects are minimal. A major disadvantage of sucralfate is that it must be taken four times a day.

Misoprostol (Cytotec) is a prostaglandin-like substance that inhibits gastric acid secretion and stimulates the production of protective mucus. Its primary use is for the prevention of peptic ulcers in patients taking high doses of NSAIDs. Diarrhea and abdominal cramping are relatively common. Classified as a pregnancy category X drug, misoprostol is contraindicated during pregnancy. In fact, misoprostol is sometimes used to terminate pregnancies, as discussed in Chapter 34.

Metoclopramide (Reglan) is occasionally used for the short-term therapy of PUD in patients who fail to respond to first-line drugs. It is also approved to treat nausea and vomiting associated with surgery or cancer chemotherapy. Metoclopramide is available for the oral, IM, or IV routes. CNS adverse effects such as drowsiness, fatigue, confusion, and insomnia may occur in a significant number of patients.

Concept Review 30.3

- Is peptic ulcer disease considered an infection, an inflammation, or both?

CONSTIPATION

A major function of the large intestine is to reabsorb water from stools. If the waste material remains in the colon for an extended period, however, too much water will be reabsorbed, leading to small, hard stools. The normal frequency of bowel movements varies widely among individuals, from two to three per day to as few as one per week. Difficult or infrequent bowel movements, known as **constipation**, is a common problem with a large number of different causes that include lack of exercise, insufficient food or fluid intake, and lack of sufficient insoluble **dietary fiber**. Certain medications such as opioids, antihistamines, certain antacids, and iron supplements promote constipation. Dietary adjustments and increased physical activity should be considered before drugs are used to treat constipation.

CORE CONCEPT 30.9

Laxatives are used to promote defecation.

Occasional constipation is common and does not require drug therapy. However, chronically infrequent and painful bowel movements accompanied by severe straining may justify pharmacotherapy. Also, pharmacotherapy may be indicated following surgical procedures to prevent the patient from straining or bearing down when attempting a bowel movement. Drugs are given to cleanse the bowel prior to surgery or for diagnostic procedures of the colon, such as a colonoscopy or barium enema.

laxat = *to loosen*
ive = *nature of, quality of*

Laxatives are drugs that promote emptying of the bowel, or **defecation**. **Cathartic** is a related term that implies a stronger and more complete bowel emptying. When taken in prescribed amounts, laxatives have few adverse effects. Selected medications used to treat constipation are listed in Table 30.2 ◆. These drugs are often classified into four primary groups and a miscellaneous category.

- *Bulk-forming* absorb water, thus adding size to the fecal mass. These are preferred drugs for the prevention and treatment of chronic constipation. They have a slow onset of action and are not used when a rapid and complete bowel evacuation is necessary.

- *Stimulants* promote peristalsis by irritating the bowel. Although drugs in this class are effective and act rapidly, they are more likely to cause diarrhea and cramping than the other types of laxatives. They should only be used occasionally because they may cause laxative dependence and depletion of fluid and electrolytes.

- *Saline/osmotic* cause water to be retained in the fecal mass, causing a more liquid stool. These drugs produce a bowel movement in one to six hours, and they should not be used on a regular basis because of the possibility of fluid and electrolyte depletion.

- *Stool softeners/surfactants* cause more water and fat to be absorbed into the stools. They are most often used to *prevent* constipation, especially in patients who have undergone recent surgery.

- *Miscellaneous* act by mechanisms other than those just described.

Although laxatives are safe drugs, there are several conditions and potential adverse effects that must be monitored carefully. Laxatives are contraindicated in any patient with a suspected bowel obstruction because their use could cause the bowel to perforate. If acute abdominal cramping or diarrhea occurs, laxatives should be discontinued. Patients should be advised not to overuse laxatives because the smooth muscle in the colon can lose its tone and cause chronic constipation.

Concept Review 30.4

- Bismuth compounds are used to treat several digestive disorders. Describe these drugs and their uses.

TABLE 30.2   Laxatives

Drug	Route and Adult Dose	Remarks
bisacodyl (Correctol, Dulcolax, others)	PO; 10–15 mg daily prn	Stimulant type; also available as a rectal suppository
calcium polycarbophil (Equalactin, FiberCon, others)	PO; 1 g/day	Bulk-forming type
castor oil (Emulsoil, Neoloid)	PO; 15–60 mL daily	Stimulant type; the only laxative to act on the small intestine
docusate (Colace, Surfak)	PO; 50–500 mg daily	Stool softener/surfactant type
lubiprostone (Amitiza)	PO; 24 mcg bid	Stool softener type; used for constipation-dominant irritable bowel syndrome
magnesium hydroxide (Milk of Magnesia)	PO; 20–60 mL daily	Saline type
methylcellulose (Citrucel)	PO; 5–20 mL tid in 8–10 oz water	Bulk-forming type
mineral oil	PO; 45 mL bid	Miscellaneous type; lubricates the stools
Pr psyllium mucilloid (Metamucil, others)	PO; 1–2 tsp in 8 oz water daily	Bulk-forming type; also used for diarrhea and as an aid in lowering blood cholesterol
senna (Ex Lax, Senokot, others)	PO; 8.6–17.2 mg/day	Stimulant type; considered an herbal product

Drug Prototype: Pr *Psyllium Mucilloid (Metamucil, Others)*

Therapeutic Class: Drug for constipation   Pharmacologic Class: Bulk-type laxative

Actions and Uses: Like other bulk-forming laxatives, psyllium is an insoluble fiber that is indigestible and not absorbed from the GI tract. When taken with plenty of water, psyllium swells and increases the size of the fecal mass by drawing water into the intestine. The larger the size of the fecal mass, the more the defecation reflex will be stimulated to promote bowel movements. Several doses of psyllium may be needed to produce a therapeutic effect. More frequent doses of psyllium (7 g/day) may cause a small reduction in blood cholesterol level.

Adverse Effects and Interactions: Psyllium is a safe laxative and rarely produces adverse effects. It causes less cramping than the stimulant-type laxatives and produces a more natural bowel movement. If taken with insufficient water, it may cause obstructions in the esophagus or intestine.

Psyllium may decrease absorption and the clinical effects of antibiotics, warfarin, digoxin, nitrofurantoin, and salicylates.

NURSING PROCESS FOCUS   Patients Receiving Laxative Therapy

ASSESSMENT	POTENTIAL NURSING DIAGNOSES
Prior to administration: ■ Obtain a complete health history, including GI and liver conditions, nutrition, allergies, drug history, and possible drug interactions. ■ Evaluate laboratory blood findings: CBC, electrolytes, and liver function studies. ■ Acquire the results of a complete physical examination, including vital signs, height, weight, bowel elimination patterns, and bowel sounds.	■ *Diarrhea* related to adverse effect of drug therapy ■ *Deficient Knowledge* related to a lack of information about drug therapy ■ *Acute Pain* related to intestinal irritation or adverse effect of drug therapy

PLANNING: PATIENT GOALS AND EXPECTED OUTCOMES

The patient will:
■ Experience therapeutic effects (relief from constipation).
■ Be free from or experience minimal adverse effects from drug therapy.
■ Verbalize an understanding of the drug's use, adverse effects, and required precautions.

IMPLEMENTATION

Interventions and (Rationales)	Patient Education/Discharge Planning
■ Administer medications correctly and evaluate the patient's knowledge of proper administration. (Following guidelines will result in improved outcomes.)	Instruct the patient to: ■ Take medication as prescribed. ■ Expect results from medication within two to three days of the initial dose. ■ Increase fluids and dietary fiber, such as whole grains, fibrous fruits, and vegetables.

continued . . .

NURSING PROCESS FOCUS *(continued)*

Interventions and (Rationales)	Patient Education/Discharge Planning
■ Determine the patient's ability to swallow. (Bulk laxatives can swell and cause obstruction in the esophagus.)	■ Instruct the patient to discontinue the medication and notify the healthcare provider if having difficulty swallowing.
■ Monitor the patient's fluid intake. (Adequate fluid intake helps to prevent constipation or intestinal obstruction.)	Instruct the patient to: ■ Drink six 8-oz glasses of fluid per day. ■ Mix medication in a full 8 oz of liquid. ■ Drink at least 8 oz of additional fluid.
■ Monitor frequency, volume, and consistency of bowel movements. (Changes in bowel habits can indicate a serious condition.)	Advise the patient to: ■ Discontinue laxative use if diarrhea occurs. ■ Notify the healthcare provider if constipation continues.

EVALUATION OF OUTCOME CRITERIA

Evaluate the effectiveness of drug therapy by confirming that patient goals and expected outcomes have been met (see "Planning"). *See Table 30.2 for a list of drugs to which these nursing actions apply.*

DIARRHEA

dia = *through/between*
rrhea = *flow/discharge*

Occasionally, the colon does not reabsorb enough water from the fecal mass, and stools become watery. **Diarrhea** is an increase in the frequency and fluidity of bowel movements. Like constipation, occasional diarrhea is a common, self-limiting disorder that does not require drug therapy. When prolonged or severe, especially in children, diarrhea can result in significant loss of body fluids, and medications may be indicated. Prolonged diarrhea may lead to acid–base or electrolyte disorders, as discussed in Chapter 17.

Diarrhea is not a disease; it is a symptom of an underlying disorder. Diarrhea may be caused by certain medications, infections of the bowel, inflammatory bowel disease such as Crohn's disease or ulcerative colitis, and substances such as lactate. Superinfections occurring during anti-infective therapy are common causes of diarrhea because they disrupt the normal microbial flora in the colon.

CORE CONCEPT 30.10

Opioids are the most effective drugs for controlling severe diarrhea.

Drug therapy of diarrhea depends on the severity of the condition and whether or not a specific cause can be identified. If the cause is an infectious disease, then an antibiotic or antiparasitic drug such as metronidazole (Flagyl) is indicated. If the cause is inflammatory, anti-inflammatory drugs are needed. If the cause appears to be drug induced, the medication should be discontinued and another substituted.

Antidiarrheals act by relaxing the colon's smooth muscle, thus relieving cramping. Slower transit through the large intestine allows for better-formed stools. The selection of a particular drug depends on the severity of the diarrhea. Some antidiarrheals are listed in Table 30.3 ◆.

Drug Prototype: 🅟 *Diphenoxylate with Atropine (Lomotil)*
Therapeutic Class: Antidiarrheal **Pharmacologic Class: Opioid**

Actions and Uses: The primary antidiarrheal ingredient in Lomotil is diphenoxylate. Like other opioids, diphenoxylate slows peristalsis, resulting in additional water being reabsorbed from the colon and formation of more solid stools. It is effective for moderate to severe diarrhea. The atropine in Lomotil is not added for its anticholinergic effect; it is added to discourage patients from taking too much of the drug. Diphenoxylate is discontinued as soon as the diarrhea symptoms resolve.

Adverse Effects and Interactions: Unlike most opioids, diphenoxylate has no analgesic properties and has an extremely low potential for abuse. The drug is well tolerated at normal doses. Some patients experience dizziness or drowsiness, and care should be taken not to operate machinery until the effects of the drug are known. At higher doses, the anticholinergic effects of atropine may be observed, which include drowsiness, dry mouth, and tachycardia.

Other CNS depressants, including alcohol, will cause additive CNS depressant/sedative effects. Monoamine oxidase (MAO) inhibitors may cause hypertensive crisis. Alcohol and other CNS depressants may enhance CNS effects.

TABLE 30.3   Antidiarrheals

Drug	Route and Adult Dose	Remarks
bismuth salts (Pepto-Bismol)	PO; two tablets or 30 mL prn	OTC adsorbent
camphorated opium tincture (Paregoric)	PO; 5–10 mL one to four times daily	Contains morphine: Schedule III drug; also used to prevent severe opioid withdrawal symptoms in neonates
difenoxin with atropine (Motofen)	PO; one to two mg after each diarrhea episode (max: 8 mg/day)	Opioid; Schedule IV drug
℗ diphenoxylate with atropine (Lomotil)	PO; one or two tablets or 5–10 mL tid–qid	Opioid; Schedule V drug
loperamide (Imodium)	PO; 4 mg as a single dose, then 2 mg after each diarrhea episode (max: 16 mg/day)	Opioid with no physical dependence; abuse is so low, it is not classified as a controlled substance
octreotide (Sandostatin)	Subcutaneous/IV; 100–600 mcg/day in two to four divided doses	For severe diarrhea associated with cancer

Acute or long-lasting diarrhea can lead to serious and even life-threatening conditions. The opioids are drugs of choice for this type of diarrhea because of their rapid onset and effectiveness. At doses used for diarrhea, opioids do not produce dependence or serious adverse effects. The most common opioid antidiarrheal is diphenoxylate (Lomotil), which is a Schedule V controlled substance. Loperamide (Imodium) is an opioid that carries no risk for dependence and is available OTC.

Nonopioid antidiarrheals include bismuth subsalicylate (Pepto-Bismol), which acts by binding and absorbing toxins. The psyllium and pectin preparations slow diarrhea by absorbing large amounts of fluid to form bulkier stools. Intestinal flora modifiers are supplements that help to correct the altered GI flora; a good source of healthy bacteria is yogurt with active cultures.

NAUSEA AND VOMITING

Nausea is an uncomfortable, subjective sensation that is sometimes accompanied by dizziness and an urge to vomit. Vomiting, or **emesis**, is a reflex primarily controlled by the vomiting center, which is located in the medulla oblongata of the brain. Nausea and vomiting are commonly associated with a wide variety of conditions such as food poisoning, early pregnancy, extreme pain, migraines, trauma to the head or abdominal organs, inner ear disorders, and emotional disturbances. Some drugs cause nausea or vomiting as an adverse effect. The most extreme example of this is the antineoplastic drugs, almost all of which cause some degree of nausea or vomiting. In treating nausea or vomiting, an important therapeutic goal is to remove the cause whenever feasible.

Antiemetics are prescribed to treat nausea, vomiting, and motion sickness.

CORE CONCEPT 30.11

Drugs from several pharmacologic classes are prescribed to prevent or treat nausea and vomiting. As shown in Table 30.4 ◆, Antiemetic drugs belong to a number of different classes, including the following:

- Antipsychotics
- Antihistamines
- Serotonin-receptor blockers
- Corticosteroids (glucocorticoids)
- Benzodiazepines

Therapy with antineoplastic drugs is one of the most common reasons why **antiemetic** medications are prescribed. When cancer chemotherapy is initiated, it is common for a patient to receive three or more antiemetics.

anti = against
emetic = vomit

To avoid losing antiemetic medication due to vomiting, many of these drugs are available through the IM, IV, transdermal, and suppository routes, as well as orally disintegrating tablets and soluble films. The most effective antiemetics for serious nausea and vomiting are serotonin-receptor blockers such as ondansetron (Zofran, Zuplenz).

Motion sickness is a disorder that affects a portion of the inner ear known as the vestibular apparatus that is associated with significant nausea. The most common drug used for motion sickness is scopolamine, which is administered as a transdermal patch placed behind the ear. Antihistamines such as dimenhydrinate

TABLE 30.4   Selected Antiemetics

Drug	Route and Adult Dose	Remarks
cyclizine (Marezine)	PO; 50 mg every 4 hours–qid	Antihistamine; for prevention of motion sickness and postoperative nausea and vomiting; IM form available
dexamethasone (Decadron)	IV; 10–20 mg before chemotherapy	Corticosteroid; IM, inhalation, and IV forms available; also for inflammatory disorders, severe allergies, acute asthma, and neoplasia
dimenhydrinate (Dramamine, others)	PO; 50–100 mg every 4 hours–qid (max: 400 mg/day)	Antihistamine; also used for allergies and cold/flu symptoms; IM and IV forms available
diphenhydramine (Benadryl, others) (see page 460 for the Drug Prototype box)	PO; 25–50 mg tid–qid (max: 300 mg/day)	Antihistamine; IM, IV, and topical forms available; also for allergies, Parkinson's disease, and anaphylaxis
dolasetron (Anzemet)	PO; 100 mg 1 hour before chemotherapy	Serotonin-receptor blocker; IV form available
doxylamine (Diclegis)	PO; 2 tablets daily at bedtime	Newer formulation that contains pyridoxine (vitamin B_6) for the nausea and vomiting of pregnancy
granisetron (Kytril)	IV; 10 mcg/kg 30 minutes before chemotherapy	Serotonin-receptor blocker; oral form available
hydroxyzine (Atarax, Vistaril)	PO; 25–100 mg tid or qid	Antihistamine; IM form available; also for anxiety and as a preoperative medication
meclizine (Antivert, Bonine)	PO; 25–50 mg/day, 1 hour before travel	Antihistamine; for motion sickness and nausea associated with vertigo
methylprednisolone (Medrol, Solu-Medrol)	IV; two doses of 125–500 mg 6 hours apart before chemotherapy	Corticosteroid; IM and IV forms available; also for inflammatory disorders, severe allergies, acute asthma, and neoplasia
metoclopramide (Reglan)	PO; 2 mg/kg 1 hour before chemotherapy	Phenothiazine-like; IV and IM forms available; also for GERD, facilitation of small-bowel intubation, and gastric stasis
Pr ondansetron (Zofran)	IV; 4 mg tid prn	Serotonin-receptor blocker; IM and PO forms available
perphenazine (Phenazine, Trilafon)	PO; 8–16 mg bid–qid	Phenothiazine; IM and IV forms available; also for psychoses
prochlorperazine (Compazine)	PO; 5–10 mg tid or qid	Phenothiazine; IM, IV, and suppository forms available; also for treatment of psychoses
promethazine (Phenergan)	PO; 12.5–25 mg every 4 hours–qid	Both a phenothiazine and an antihistamine; IM, IV, and suppository forms available; also for allergic disorders and as an adjunct to anesthesia and surgery
scopolamine (Isopto hyoscine, Transderm Scop)	Transdermal patch; 0.5 mg every 72 hours	Anticholinergic; oral, IV, IM, and subcutaneous forms available

(Dramamine) and meclizine (Antivert) are also effective but may cause significant drowsiness in some patients. Drugs used to treat motion sickness are most effective when taken 20 to 60 minutes before travel is expected.

On some occasions, it is desirable to *stimulate* the vomiting reflex with drugs called **emetics**. Indications for emetics include ingestion of poisons and overdoses of oral drugs. Ipecac syrup, given orally, or apomorphine, given subcutaneously, will induce vomiting in about 15 minutes. Drugs used to stimulate emesis should be used only in emergency situations under the direction of a healthcare provider.

Drug Prototype: Pr *Ondansetron (Zofran, Zuplenz)*
Therapeutic Class: Antiemetic   Pharmacologic Class: Serotonin (5-HT) receptor blocker

Actions and Uses: Ondansetron and other drugs in the serotonin-receptor blocker class have replaced other, older drugs for the treatment of serious nausea and vomiting. To prevent chemotherapy-induced nausea and vomiting the medication is started at least 30 minutes prior to chemotherapy and continued for several days after.

Ondansetron acts by blocking serotonin receptors in the chemoreceptor trigger zone, an area of the brain responsible for nausea and vomiting. It is available by the PO, IV, IM, oral disintegrating tablet, and oral soluble film routes.

Adverse Effects and Interactions: The most common adverse effects are headache, dizziness, drowsiness, and diarrhea. Caution must be used when treating patients with cardiac abnormalities because ondansetron can prolong the QT interval and cause dysrhythmias. Ondansetron exhibits few drug interactions.

WEIGHT LOSS

Hunger occurs when the hypothalamus in the brain responds to the levels of certain chemicals (glucose) or hormones (insulin) in the blood. Hunger is a normal physiologic response that drives people to seek nourishment. Appetite is somewhat different than hunger. Appetite is a psychological response that drives food intake based on associations and memory. For example, people often eat not because they are experiencing hunger, but because it is a particular time of day or they find the act of eating pleasurable or social.

Anorexiants and lipase inhibitors are used for the short-term management of obesity.

Despite the public's desire for effective drugs to promote weight loss, there are few such drugs available. The approved drugs used for the treatment of obesity produce only modest weight loss.

Obesity may be defined as being more than 20% above ideal body weight or having a body mass index of 30 kg/m^2 or higher. Because of the prevalence of obesity in society and the difficulty that most patients experience when following weight-reduction plans for extended periods, drug manufacturers have long sought to develop safe drugs that cause weight loss. In the 1970s, amphetamine and dextroamphetamine (Dexedrine) were widely prescribed as **anorexiants** to reduce appetite. These drugs, however, are addictive, and amphetamines are rarely prescribed for this purpose today. In the 1990s, the combination of fenfluramine and phenteramine, known as fen-phen, was widely prescribed until fenfluramine was removed from the market for causing heart valve defects. Sibutramine (Meridia), once the most widely prescribed *anorexiant* for the short-term control of obesity, was removed from the market in 2010 due to an increased risk for heart attacks and strokes. Current pharmacologic strategies for weight management focus on two mechanisms: lipase inhibitors and anorexiants.

Orlistat (Xenical) acts by inhibiting the enzyme lipase in the GI tract. This blocks the absorption of fats in the small intestine. Unfortunately, orlistat may also decrease absorption of other substances, including fat-soluble vitamins and warfarin (Coumadin). Orlistat produces only a small decrease in weight compared to placebos.

A second strategy to reduce weight is to block parts of the nervous system responsible for hunger with anorexiants, also called appetite suppressants. Phentermine, once part of the combination fen-phen, was approved in 2012 as a fixed dose combination with topiramate (Qysmia). Phenteramine decreases appetite but the precise mechanism of antiobesity action of topiramate (an antiepileptic) drug is unknown. Side effects of Qysmia include paresthesia, dizziness, dysgeusia, insomnia, constipation, and dry mouth.

Also approved in 2012, lorcaserin (Belviq) is one of the newest anorexiants that is believed to act by activating serotonin receptors in the hypothalamus, causing a feeling of fullness or satiety. The drug is well tolerated, with headache and upper respiratory tract infection being the most common side effects. Like other antiobesity drugs, it should be combined with a regimen of diet and exercise for optimum weight loss.

CAM THERAPY

Ginger for Nausea

Ginger is obtained from the roots of the herb *Zingiber officinale*, which grows in a wide variety of places across the world. Active ingredients include aromatic oils that give the herb its characteristic scent and antiemetic activity. Because of its widespread use as a spice in Asian cooking, ginger is widely available in a number of forms, including tincture, tea, dried and fresh root, and capsules. Commercial products that use ginger as a flavoring include ginger cookies, gingerbread, and ginger ale. Consumers should check the product ingredients to be certain that the item truly contains ginger extract, rather than artificial ginger flavoring.

Ginger has been used in Chinese medicine for thousands of years. Indications relating to the digestive system include nausea, vomiting, morning sickness, and motion sickness. Studies have shown its effectiveness to be comparable to OTC medications.

Ginger is purported to have other significant benefits. The herb is said to have anti-inflammatory properties that are of benefit to patients with arthritis. It is sometimes given to patients with flu symptoms to help coughs and lower fever. Because of a possible effect on blood clotting, patients taking anticoagulants should avoid ginger unless otherwise directed by their healthcare provider.

PANCREATIC ENZYMES

In addition to secreting insulin, the pancreas is also responsible for the producing essential digestive enzymes. Lack of secretion, or **pancreatic insufficiency**, will result in malabsorption disorders. Replacement therapy with pancreatic enzymes is sometimes necessary.

CORE CONCEPT 30.13

Pancreatic enzymes are administered as replacement therapy for patients with pancreatitis or malabsorption syndromes.

The pancreas secretes more than 1 L of pancreatic juice daily, which contains enzymes that split proteins, fats, and carbohydrates. Because these nutrients must be broken down into simpler molecules before they can be absorbed, lack of sufficient pancreatic juice can cause malabsorption syndromes. Lipase, the enzyme that digests fats, is most affected. The most common cause of pancreatic insufficiency is chronic pancreatitis, which is most often associated with alcoholism.

Symptoms of chronic pancreatitis include upper abdominal pain, loss of appetite, nausea, vomiting, and weight loss. *Steatorrhea*, the passing of bulky, foul-smelling fatty stools, occurs because dietary fats are passing through the GI tract without being broken down.

steato = *fat*
rrhea = *flow or discharge*

Pancrelipase (Cotazym, Pancrease, others) is a pancreatic enzyme supplement obtained from pigs that contains the necessary enzymes to digest fats, carbohydrates, and proteins. To avoid destruction by stomach acid, capsules are made with an enteric coating. Dosing is individualized to the degree of pancreatic insufficiency in each patient. Administration of the drug is timed to coincide with meals so that the enzymes are available when food reaches the duodenum. Overtreatment can cause nausea, vomiting, and diarrhea.

PATIENTS NEED TO KNOW

Patients treated for digestive disorders need to know the following:

Regarding Antiulcer Medications

1. Do not smoke tobacco when taking H_2-receptor blockers because this interferes with the drug action.
2. Because drowsiness may occur when starting therapy with H_2-receptor blockers or proton-pump inhibitors, monitor operating equipment and the use of alcohol or other CNS drugs carefully.
3. When taking medications for peptic ulcer, avoid drugs that may cause stomach irritation such as aspirin or NSAIDs.
4. Shake liquid antacids well before pouring. Chewable tablets should be thoroughly chewed before swallowing.

Regarding Laxatives

5. Because bulk-forming laxatives and stool softeners may take several days for results, be patient and do not take more than prescribed.
6. Take bulk-forming laxatives with at least two full glasses of water because this aids in forming larger stools.
7. If constipation is a frequent problem, try drinking more fluids and adding fiber to the diet rather than taking laxatives on a continual basis. Foods rich in fiber include all fruits and vegetables, bran cereals, and whole grain breads.

Regarding Antiemetics

8. Before taking antiemetic medications, try other methods of relieving nausea, such as drinking flat carbonated beverages or weak tea or eating small amounts of crackers or dry toast.
9. When taking phenothiazines or antihistamines as antiemetics, use sugarless candy, gum, or ice chips to minimize dry mouth.
10. Recall that medications taken to suppress hunger produce only modest weight loss and are not effective without a reduced-calorie diet. True, sustained weight loss can only be achieved by modification of exercise and dietary habits.

CHAPTER REVIEW

CORE CONCEPTS SUMMARY

30.1 The digestive system breaks down food, absorbs nutrients, and eliminates wastes.

The alimentary canal provides a large surface area for the absorption of nutrients and drugs. Substances are propelled through the GI tract by peristalsis. Abnormally fast or slow peristalsis can affect nutrient, drug, and water absorption.

30.2 Peptic ulcer disease is caused by an erosion of the mucosal layer of the stomach or duodenum.

Infection with *H. pylori* and therapy with NSAIDs are the most common causes of peptic ulcers. A gnawing pain in the upper abdomen that is relieved by eating is the most common symptom of duodenal ulcer. Though less common, gastric ulcers may be more serious and require longer treatment and follow-up. GERD has symptoms similar to those of peptic ulcers and is treated with some of the same medications.

30.3 Peptic ulcer disease is treated by a combination of lifestyle changes and pharmacotherapy.

Before beginning drug therapy, the patient should eliminate tobacco and alcohol use and reduce stress levels because these changes will favor remission of peptic ulcer disease. Goals of drug therapy include relief of symptoms, promotion of ulcer healing, and prevention of recurrences.

30.4 Proton-pump inhibitors are effective at reducing gastric acid secretion.

Proton-pump inhibitors diminish gastric acid secretion by interfering with the enzyme H^+, K^+-ATPase, which is present in the mucosal cells in the stomach. Although very effective, use is usually limited to two months because of the possibility of long-term adverse effects.

30.5 H_2-receptor blockers reduce the secretion of gastric acid.

H_2-receptor blockers reduce the volume and acidity of stomach acid. Healing of duodenal ulcers occurs in four to eight weeks, and adverse effects are uncommon.

30.6 Antacids rapidly neutralize stomach acid and reduce the symptoms of peptic ulcer disease and GERD.

Once drugs of choice for treating peptic ulcer disease, antacids are now primarily used to give immediate relief for the heartburn associated with GERD or peptic ulcers.

30.7 Antibiotics are administered to eliminate *Helicobacter pylori*, the cause of many peptic ulcers.

Elimination of *H. pylori* using combination therapy with different antibiotics has been found to promote more rapid ulcer healing and longer remissions.

30.8 Several miscellaneous drugs are also beneficial in treating peptic ulcer disease.

Sucralfate produces a gel-like substance that provides a protective coating for ulcers. Misoprostol inhibits gastric acid secretion and promotes the secretion of protective mucus. Pirenzepine inhibits acid secretion by blocking cholinergic receptors.

30.9 Laxatives are used to promote defecation.

Laxatives are given to promote emptying of the colon. Laxatives act by stimulating peristalsis or by adding more bulk or water to the fecal mass.

30.10 Opioids are the most effective drugs for controlling severe diarrhea.

Diarrhea is treated by addressing its cause, which may include anti-inflammatory drugs or anti-infectives. Opioids are the most effective drugs for relieving severe diarrhea, but they have some abuse potential. OTC bismuth compounds can help with simple diarrhea.

30.11 Antiemetics are prescribed to treat nausea, vomiting, and motion sickness.

Symptomatic treatment of nausea and vomiting involves drugs from many different classes, including phenothiazines, antihistamines, corticosteroids, benzodiazepines, and serotonin-receptor blockers. Motion sickness can be controlled through medications such as transdermal scopolamine or dimenhydrinate (Dramamine).

30.12 Anorexiants and lipase inhibitors are used for the short-term management of obesity.

Only a few drugs are available for the short-term management of obesity, and these drugs produce only modest weight loss. The anorexiant sibutramine and the lipase inhibitor orlistat are used to help obese patients lose weight.

30.13 Pancreatic enzymes are administered as replacement therapy for patients with pancreatitis or malabsorption syndromes.

Pancreatic insufficiency leads to lack of breakdown and absorption of sufficient quantities of fats, carbohydrates, and proteins. This can lead to malabsorption syndromes. Pancrelipase and pancreatin are used to restore the deficient enzymes.

REVIEW QUESTIONS

The following questions are written in NCLEX-PN® style. Answer these questions to assess your knowledge of the chapter material, and go back and review any material that is not clear to you.

1. A nurse is providing information about peptic ulcers to a group at a senior residential facility. She tells them that the primary cause of peptic ulcers is:

1. Stress
2. Smoking
3. *H. pylori* bacteria
4. Family history

2. The patient with a gastric ulcer has been started on ranitidine (Zantac). The nurse should include what instructions: (Select all that apply.)

1. Drug therapy will extend over several weeks or months.
2. Information about the signs and symptoms of CNS depression.
3. Drug therapy will extend over a few days.
4. Antacids should not be given within one hour of taking H_2-receptor antagonists.

3. A patient has been experiencing acute diarrhea. In order to control this condition, the physician initially orders Lomotil 10 mL (2 teaspoons), four times a day. Every 5 mL (1 teaspoon) contains 2.5 mg of medication. How many milligrams of medication will the patient receive a day?

1. 20 mg
2. 15 mg
3. 10 mg
4. 2.5 mg

4. The nurse understands that it is important that the teaching plan for a patient on omeprazole (Prilosec) should include which of the following?

1. This drug is safe for long-term use.
2. This drug should not be taken for a prolonged period of time.
3. Therapeutic effects may take weeks.
4. This drug must be used with antacids to be effective.

5. After administering magnesium hydroxide (Mylanta) to a patient, the nurse monitors for:

1. Diarrhea
2. Peripheral disease
3. Neuropathy
4. Respiratory disorders

6. The nurse instructs patients using laxatives to:

1. Use daily for best results.
2. Not overuse them because they can cause chronic constipation
3. Decrease fluid intake.
4. Decrease food intake.

7. A patient about ready to receive chemotherapy has an order for ondansetron (Zofran). When should the nurse administer the ondansetron?

1. Every time the patient complains of nausea
2. Thirty to sixty minutes before starting chemotherapy
3. Only if the patient complains of nausea
4. When the patient begins to experience vomiting during the chemotherapy

8. A patient, newly diagnosed with a peptic ulcer, needs more education when he states:

1. "It's OK for me take aspirin if I get a headache."
2. "Good thing I can eat raw foods. I love to go to the salad bar."
3. "If I need to take an appetite suppressant, I should be able to."
4. "Right now, I'm not feeling sick but if I do feel nauseous, I can take an antiemetic."

9. The patient on topiramate (Qysmia) must be monitored for: (Select all that apply.)

1. Constipation
2. Dizziness
3. Hypertension
4. Diarrhea

10. The patient demonstrates understanding about the medication pancrelipase (Cotazym) when she states:

1. "I will take this medication with meals."
2. "I will take this medication on an empty stomach."
3. "I will only take this medication when I am eating carbohydrates."
4. "If I develop nausea, vomiting, or diarrhea, I will increase my dosage."

CASE STUDY QUESTIONS

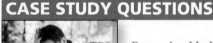

Remember Mr. Han, who was introduced at the beginning of the chapter? Now read the remainder of the case study. Based on the information you have learned in this chapter, answer the questions that follow.

Mr. Jeffery Han is a 32-year-old stockbroker with a very stressful job. He has just been diagnosed with a peptic ulcer. Although he is relieved to find out what has been causing "all this pain," *he is not happy to learn he has an ulcer and states,* "This is the last thing I need right now. My job is stressful enough." *The physician prescribed omeprazole (Prilosec), clarithromycin, and amoxicillin, with OTC antacids as needed.*

1. Mr. Han is a little confused about the function of each one of his new drugs. He asks the nurse about how each drug is going to help him "overcome" the ulcer. The nurse begins by explaining that part of the pain he is experiencing is due to inflammation caused by both the hydrochloric acid produced in his stomach and the presence of *H. pylori*, a bacteria. She also tells him that the medication responsible for blocking acid secretion is:

1. Omeprazole
2. Antacid
3. Clarithromycin
4. Amoxicillin

2. The nurse explains to Mr. Han that _____ was prescribed to eradicate the bacteria *H. pylori*. (Select all that apply.)

1. Omeprazole
2. Clarithromycin
3. Amoxicillin
4. Antacid

3. In the treatment of *H. pylori*, the nurse explains that the use of two or more antibiotics is essential to: (Select all that apply.)

1. Lower the potential for bacterial resistance
2. Increase the effectiveness of therapy
3. Guarantee that the bacteria will be totally destroyed
4. Decrease the cost of future drug therapy

4. Mr. Han had already been taking aluminum-based antacids for his pain but explains that he has started to experience constipation. In order to promote bowel movements, which of the following OTC medications would be beneficial for Mr. Han?

1. Methylcellulose (Citrucel)
2. Famotidine (Pepcid)
3. Omeprazole (Prilosec)
4. Bismuth salts (Pepto-Bismol)

NOTE: Answers to the Review and Case Study Questions appear in Appendix B. The complete rationales and answers are located on the textbook's website.

Pearson Nursing Student Resources   Find additional review materials at **nursing.pearsonhighered.com**.

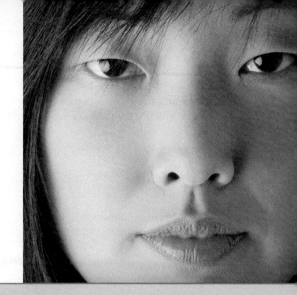

C H A P T E R

"I'm so busy, I don't eat very much so I take lots of vitamins and minerals. I figure it's better to take more than not enough."

Ms. Mei Chin

31

Vitamins, Minerals, and Nutritional Supplements

CORE CONCEPTS

31.1 Vitamins are needed to promote growth and maintain health.

31.2 Vitamins are classified as fat soluble or water soluble.

31.3 Recommended dietary allowances (RDAs) for vitamins have been established for the average healthy adult.

31.4 Vitamin therapy is indicated for specific conditions.

31.5 Minerals are inorganic substances needed in very small amounts to maintain normal body metabolism.

31.6 Enteral and total parenteral nutrition are therapies that deliver essential nutrients to patients with deficiencies.

DRUG SNAPSHOT

The following drugs are discussed in this chapter:

DRUG CLASSES	DRUG PROTOTYPES
Vitamins	**Pr** cyanocobalamin (Crystamine, others) *499*
Minerals	**Pr** ferrous sulfate (Feosol, Feostat, others) *501*
Enteral nutrition	
Total parenteral nutrition	

LEARNING OUTCOMES

After reading this chapter, the student should be able to:

1. Identify the characteristics that differentiate vitamins from other nutrients.

2. Describe the functions of vitamins and minerals.

3. Explain the rationale behind recommended dietary allowances (RDAs).

4. Describe the role of vitamin and mineral therapies in the treatment of deficiency disorders.

5. Identify drug–vitamin and drug–mineral interactions.

6. Compare and contrast the functions of major minerals and trace minerals.

7. Compare and contrast the enteral and parenteral methods of providing nutrition.

KEY TERMS

enteral nutrition *504*
hypervitaminosis *499*
intrinsic factor *499*
major mineral (macromineral) *500*

pernicious (megaloblastic) anemia
  (pur-NISH-us ah-NEE-mee-ah) *499*
provitamin *497*
recommended dietary allowance (RDA) *498*

total parenteral nutrition (TPN) *505*
trace mineral *500*
undernutrition *504*
vitamins *497*

Most people are able to obtain all necessary nutrients their body requires through a balanced diet. There are some conditions, however, in which dietary supplementation is necessary and will benefit the patient's health. This chapter focuses on these conditions and explores the role of vitamins, minerals, and nutritional supplements in pharmacology.

Vitamins are needed to promote growth and maintain health.

CORE CONCEPT **31.1**

Vitamins are organic compounds required by the body in small amounts for growth and for the maintenance of normal metabolic processes. Since the discovery of thiamine in 1911, over a dozen vitamins have been identified. Because scientists did not know the chemical structures of the vitamins when they were discovered, they were assigned letters and numbers such as A, B_{12}, and C. These names are still widely used today.

An important characteristic of vitamins is that, with the exception of vitamin D, human cells cannot synthesize them. They or their precursors—known as **provitamins**—must be supplied in the diet. A second important characteristic is that if the vitamin is not present in adequate amounts, the body's metabolism will be disrupted and disease will result. Furthermore, the symptoms of the deficiency can be reversed by the administration of the missing vitamin.

Vitamins serve diverse and important roles in human physiology. For example, the B complex vitamins are coenzymes essential to many metabolic pathways. Vitamin A is a precursor of retinal, a pigment needed for normal vision. Calcium metabolism is regulated by a hormone that is derived from vitamin D. Without vitamin K, abnormal prothrombin is produced, and blood clotting is affected. Patients having a low or unbalanced dietary intake, those who are pregnant, and those experiencing a chronic disease may benefit from vitamin therapy.

pro = *before*
vitamin = *essential substance*

Fast Facts Vitamins, Minerals, and Dietary Supplements

- About 33% of Americans take a multivitamin supplement daily.
- There is no difference between the chemical structure of a natural vitamin and a synthetic vitamin, yet consumers pay much more for the natural type.
- Because vitamin B_{12} is present only in animal products, vegetarians must obtain this vitamin in fortified cereals, nutritional supplements, or yeast.
- Administration of folic acid during pregnancy has been found to reduce birth defects in the nervous system of the baby.
- Patients who never receive sun exposure may need vitamin D supplements.
- Heavy menstrual periods may result in considerable iron loss.
- Technically, vitamins and minerals cannot increase a patient's energy levels. Energy can be provided only by adding calories in carbohydrates, proteins, and fats.

Vitamins are classified as fat soluble or water soluble.

CORE CONCEPT **31.2**

A simple way to classify vitamins is by their ability to mix with water. Those that dissolve easily in water are called water-soluble vitamins. Examples include vitamin C and the B vitamins. Those that dissolve in lipids are called fat soluble or lipid soluble and include vitamins A, D, E, and K.

The difference in solubility affects the way the vitamins are absorbed by the gastrointestinal (GI) tract and stored in the body. The water-soluble vitamins are absorbed along with water in the digestive tract and readily dissolve in blood and body fluids. When excess water-soluble vitamins are ingested, they cannot be stored for later use and are simply excreted in the urine. Because they are not stored to any significant degree, they must be ingested daily; otherwise deficiencies will quickly develop.

Fat-soluble vitamins, however, cannot be absorbed in sufficient quantity in the small intestine unless they are ingested with other fats. These vitamins can be stored in large quantities in the liver and fat.

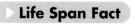 **Life Span Fact**

Infancy and childhood are times of potential vitamin deficiency due to the high growth demands placed on the body.

Should the patient not ingest sufficient quantities, fat-soluble vitamins are removed from storage depots in the body as needed. Unfortunately, this storage can lead to dangerously high levels of the fat-soluble vitamins if they are taken in excessive amounts.

CORE CONCEPT 31.3

Recommended dietary allowances (RDAs) for vitamins have been established for the average healthy adult.

Based on scientific research on humans and animals, the Food and Nutrition Board of the National Academy of Sciences has established levels for the intake of vitamins and minerals, called **recommended dietary allowances (RDAs)**. The RDA values represent the *minimum* amount of a vitamin or mineral needed to prevent a deficiency in a healthy adult. The RDAs are revised periodically to reflect the latest scientific research. Current RDAs for vitamins are listed in Table 31.1 ◆ A newer standard, the Dietary Reference Index (DRI), is sometimes used to represent the *optimum* level of nutrient needed to ensure wellness.

Vitamin, mineral, or nutritional supplements should never substitute for a balanced diet. Sufficient intake of proteins, carbohydrates, and fats is needed for proper health. Furthermore, although the label on a vitamin supplement may indicate that it contains 100% of the RDA for a particular vitamin, the body may absorb as little as 10% to 15% of the amount ingested. With the exception of vitamins A and D,

TABLE 31.1 Vitamins

Vitamin	Function(s)	RDA Men	RDA Women	Common Cause(s) of Deficiency
A	Visual pigments, epithelial cells	1,000 RE*	800 RE	Prolonged dietary deprivation, particularly when rice is the main food source; pancreatic disease; cirrhosis
B complex: Biotin (B₇)	Coenzyme in metabolic reactions	30 mcg	30 mcg	Deficiencies are rare.
ⓟ Cyanocobalamin (B₁₂)	Coenzyme in nucleic acid metabolism	2 mcg	2 mcg	Lack of intrinsic factor, inadequate intake of foods from animal origin
Folic acid/folate (B₉)	Coenzyme in amino acid and nucleic acid metabolism	200 mcg	160–180 mcg	Pregnancy, alcoholism, cancer, oral contraceptive use
Niacin (B₃)	Coenzyme in metabolic reactions	15–20 mg	13–15 mg	Prolonged dietary deprivation, particularly when Indian corn (maize) or millet is the main food source; chronic diarrhea; liver disease; alcoholism
Pantothenic acid (B₅)	Coenzyme in metabolic reactions	5 mg	5 mg	Deficiencies are rare.
Pyridoxine (B₆)	Coenzyme in amino acid metabolism	2 mg	1.5–1.6 mg	Alcoholism; oral contraceptive use; malabsorption diseases
Riboflavin (B₂)	Coenzyme in metabolic reactions	1.4–1.8 mg	1.2–1.3 mg	Inadequate consumption of milk or animal products; chronic diarrhea; liver disease; alcoholism
Thiamine (B₁)	Coenzyme in metabolic reactions	1.2–1.5 mg	1.0–1.1 mg	Prolonged dietary deprivation, particularly when rice is the main food source; hyperthyroidism, pregnancy, liver disease; alcoholism
C	Coenzyme and antioxidant	60 mg	60 mg	Inadequate intake of fruits and vegetables; pregnancy; chronic inflammatory disease; burns; diarrhea; alcoholism
D	Calcium and phosphate metabolism	5–10 mcg	5–10 mcg	Low dietary intake; inadequate exposure to sunlight
E	Antioxidant	10 TE**	8 TE	Premature infants; malabsorption diseases
K	Cofactor in blood clotting	65–80 mcg	55–65 mcg	Newborns; liver disease; long-term parenteral nutrition; certain drugs such as cephalosporins and salicylates

*RE = retinoid equivalents
**TE = alpha-tocopherol equivalents

it is not harmful for most patients to consume two to three times the recommended levels of vitamins. In cases where there is an increase in dietary needs, such as during pregnancy and growth periods, the RDAs will need adjustment and supplements may be needed to achieve optimum wellness.

Vitamin therapy is indicated for specific conditions.

CORE CONCEPT **31.4**

Most people who eat a normal, balanced diet obtain all the necessary nutrients without vitamin supplementation. Indeed, megavitamin therapy is not only expensive but may be harmful to health if taken for long periods. **Hypervitaminosis**, or toxic levels of vitamins, has been reported for vitamins A, C, D, E, B₆, niacin, and folic acid. In the United States, it is actually more common to observe syndromes of vitamin *excess* than those of vitamin *deficiency*. Most patients are unaware that taking too much of a vitamin or mineral can cause serious adverse effects.

hyper = *above*
vitamin = *vitamin*
osis = *condition*

Vitamin deficiencies may have a number of causes. Table 31.1 lists the functions of the vitamins and some common causes of deficiencies. In the United States, deficiencies are most often the result of poverty, fad diets, chronic alcoholism, or prolonged parenteral feeding. Infants, pregnant women, nursing mothers, older adults, and those eating a vegan or vegetarian diet often require larger amounts of vitamins and minerals to maintain optimal health. Men and women can have different vitamin and mineral needs, as do persons who participate in vigorous exercise. Vitamin deficiencies in patients with chronic liver and kidney disease are well documented. Patients with alcohol or serious drug dependency are often deficient in the quality and quantity of their nutritional intake. In cases in which dietary needs are increased, the RDAs will need adjustment, and supplements are indicated to achieve optimum wellness.

Certain drugs affect vitamin metabolism. Alcohol is well known for its ability to inhibit the absorption of thiamine and folic acid; alcohol abuse is the most common cause of thiamine deficiency in the United States. Folic acid levels may be reduced in patients taking phenothiazines, oral contraceptives, phenytoin (Dilantin), or barbiturates. Vitamin D deficiency can be caused by therapy with certain anticonvulsants. Inhibition of vitamin B₁₂ absorption has been reported with a number of drugs, including trifluoperazine, alcohol, and oral contraceptives.

One of the most common and clinically important vitamin syndromes is deficiency of vitamin B₁₂. The most obvious consequence of B₁₂ deficiency is a type of anemia called **pernicious or megaloblastic anemia**. Insufficient vitamin B₁₂ creates a lack of activated folic acid, which is essential for DNA synthesis and cell division. Lack of vitamin B₁₂ also affects the nervous system, causing tingling or numbness in the limbs, mood disturbances, and even hallucinations in severe deficiencies.

megalo = *large*
blastic = *embryonic state*
an = *lack of*
emia = *blood condition*

Treatment of vitamin B₁₂ deficiency is most often accomplished by weekly or biweekly intramuscular (IM) or subcutaneous injections. Although oral supplements are available, they are effective only in patients who have sufficient intrinsic factor and normal absorption in the small intestine (see Drug Prototype for cyanocobalamin). Parenteral administration rapidly reverses most signs and symptoms of B₁₂ deficiency. If the disease has been prolonged, symptoms may take longer to resolve, and some neurologic damage may be permanent. Treatment may need to continue for the remainder of the patient's life.

Vitamins are indicated for several additional conditions. Vitamin K is administered to patients with certain clotting disorders and as an antidote to warfarin (Coumadin) overdose. B complex vitamins such as folic acid, thiamine, and riboflavin are commonly administered to patients with chronic alcoholism. The role of vitamin D therapy in the pharmacotherapy of bone disorders is discussed in Chapter 33.

> **Life Span Fact**

Elderly patients who have less exposure to direct sunlight may need vitamin D supplements.

> **Life Span Fact**

Infants fed only breast milk receive insufficient amounts of vitamin D, which can result in rickets.

Drug Prototype: Pr *Cyanocobalamin (Crystamine, Others)*
Therapeutic Class: Drug for anemia **Pharmacologic Class: Vitamin supplement**

Actions and Uses: Cyanocobalamin is a purified form of vitamin B₁₂ that is administered in deficiency states. Vitamin B₁₂ is not synthesized by either plants or animals; only bacteria perform this function. Because only miniscule amounts of vitamin B₁₂ are required, deficiency of this vitamin is not usually caused by insufficient dietary intake. The most common cause of vitamin B₁₂ deficiency is lack of **intrinsic factor**, which is secreted by stomach cells. Intrinsic factor is required for vitamin B₁₂ to be absorbed from the intestine. Figure 31.1 ■ illustrates the metabolism of vitamin B₁₂. Inflammatory diseases of the stomach or surgical removal of the stomach may result in deficiency of intrinsic factor.

Cyanocobalamin is available by the PO, IM, and intranasal routes. The intranasal spray and gel formulations (Nascobal) provide for once-weekly dosage. Intranasal formulations are used for *maintenance therapy* after normal vitamin B₁₂ levels have been restored by IM preparations.

Adverse Effects and Interactions: Adverse effects from cyanocobalamin are uncommon. Hypokalemia is possible; thus, serum potassium levels are monitored periodically.

Alcohol, aminosalicylic acid, neomycin, and colchicine may decrease absorption of oral cyanocobalamin. Chloramphenicol may interfere with therapeutic response to cyanocobalamin.

FIGURE 31.1

Metabolism of vitamin B$_{12}$.

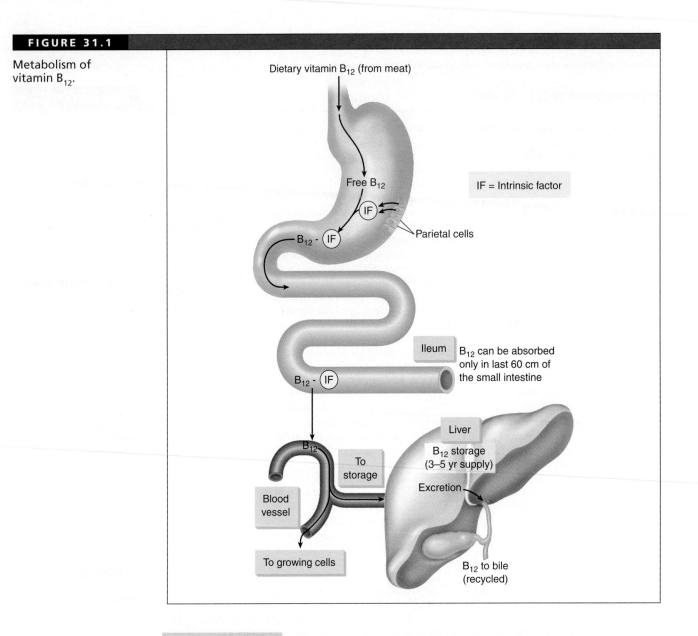

Concept Review 31.1

■ What are some conditions in which the RDA for a vitamin may not be sufficient?

CORE CONCEPT 31.5

Minerals are inorganic substances needed in very small amounts to maintain normal body metabolism.

Minerals are inorganic substances that constitute about 4% of body weight. The most common minerals are the bone salts, calcium and phosphorus, which make up about 75% of the total mineral content in the body. Minerals are classified as **major minerals (macrominerals)** or **trace minerals**, depending on how much is needed in the diet. The seven major minerals must be obtained daily from dietary sources in amounts of 100 mg or higher. Required daily amounts of the nine trace minerals are 20 mg or less. These minerals are listed in Table 31.2 ◆.

Minerals serve many important and diverse functions in the body. Some minerals, such as sodium and magnesium, appear primarily as ions in body fluids. Others, such as iron and cobalt, are usually bound to organic molecules. The functions of many of the minerals in human physiology, such as calcium, sodium, and potassium, are well known. The functions of some of the trace minerals, such as aluminum, silicon, arsenic, and nickel, are less understood.

Because minerals are needed in very small amounts for human metabolism, a balanced diet will supply the necessary quantities for most patients. Like vitamins, excess amounts of minerals can lead to toxicity, and patients should be advised not to exceed recommended doses. For example, arsenic,

▶ **Life Span Fact**

For each decade after age 40, bone mass decreases approximately 3% to 5%. To avoid bone fractures, older adults must ensure a substantial dietary intake of calcium or take calcium supplements.

TABLE 31.2 Minerals

Major Minerals	Recommended Daily Intake	Trace Minerals	Recommended Daily Intake
Calcium	800–1,200 mg	Chromium	0.05–2 mg
Chloride	750 mg	Cobalt	0.1 mcg
Magnesium	Men: 350–400 mg	Copper	1.5–3 mg
	Women: 280–300 mg		
Phosphorus	700 mg	Fluoride	1.5–4 mg
Potassium	2 g	Iodide	150 mcg
Sodium	500 mg	Iron	Men: 10–12 mg
Sulfur	Not established		Women: 10–15 mg
		Manganese	2–5 mg
		Molybdenum	75–250 mg
		Selenium	Men: 50–70 mcg
			Women: 50–55 mcg
		Zinc	12–15 mg

chromium, and nickel have been implicated as human carcinogens, and excess sodium intake can lead to water retention and hypertension.

Mineral therapy is indicated for certain disorders. Iron-deficiency anemia is the most common nutritional deficiency in the world and is a primary indication for iron supplements. Women at high risk for osteoporosis are advised to consume extra calcium, either in their diet or as a supplement (see Chapter 35). Magnesium deficiencies are promptly treated with oral or IV magnesium salts because lack of sufficient amounts of this electrolyte can lead to weakness, dysrhythmias, and hypertension. Iodine-based drugs serve a number of functions, including use as topical antiseptics, as contrast drugs in radiologic procedures of the urinary and cardiovascular systems, and the treatment of thyroid abnormalities (see Chapter 32). Selected minerals used in pharmacotherapy are shown in Table 31.3 ◆.

osteo = *bone*
por = *passage*
osis = *condition*

Certain drugs affect mineral metabolism. For example, loop or thiazide diuretics can cause significant urinary potassium loss. Corticosteroids, oral contraceptives, and a number of other drugs can cause sodium retention. The uptake of iodine by the thyroid gland can be impaired by certain oral hypoglycemics and lithium (Eskalith). Oral contraceptives have been reported to lower the plasma levels of zinc and increase those of copper.

Concept Review **31.2**

■ What is the difference between a vitamin and a mineral?

hemo = *blood*
globin = *protein*

Drug Prototype: Ⓟ *Ferrous Sulfate (Feosol, Feostat, Others)*
Therapeutic Class: Drug for anemia **Pharmacologic Class: Iron supplement**

Actions and Uses: Ferrous sulfate is an iron supplement. Iron is a mineral essential to the function of several biological molecules, the most significant of which is hemoglobin. Each molecule of hemoglobin in a red blood cell contains four iron atoms, each of which can bind reversibly to an oxygen atom. Sixty to eighty percent of all iron in the body is associated with hemoglobin.

After red blood cells die, nearly all of the iron in their hemoglobin is recycled for later use. Because of this recycling, very little iron is excreted; thus, dietary iron requirements in most individuals are small.

Iron deficiency is a common cause of anemia. The usual cause of iron-deficiency anemia is blood loss, such as may occur during menstruation or from peptic ulcers. Certain patients have an increased demand for iron, including those who are pregnant and those undergoing intensive athletic training. Ferrous sulfate is available in a wide variety of dosage forms to prevent or rapidly reverse symptoms of iron-deficiency anemia.

Adverse Effects and Interactions: The most common adverse effect of iron sulfate is GI upset. Although taking iron with meals will lessen GI upset, food can decrease the absorption of iron by as much as 70%. It is recommended that iron preparations be administered one hour before or two hours after a meal. However, if major gastric irritation is experienced, the iron may be taken with juice or small meals. Patients should be advised that iron preparations may darken stools and that this is a harmless adverse effect. Excessive doses of iron are very toxic, and patients should be advised to take their medication exactly as directed.

Antacids and food decrease the absorption of iron. Vitamin C increases the absorption of iron, whereas calcium (including dairy products) and bran block its absorption. Vitamin C may increase the absorption of ferrous sulfate.

TABLE 31.3 Selected Minerals Used for Pharmacotherapy

Drug	Route and Adult Dose	Remarks
potassium chloride (KCl) (see page 260 for the Drug Prototype box)	PO; 10–100 mEq/hr in divided doses IV; 10–60 mEq/hr diluted to at least 10–20 mEq/100 mL of solution (max: 200–400 mEq/day)	Drug should be discontinued immediately if hyperkalemia is suspected.
sodium bicarbonate (NaHCO₃) (see page 261 for the Drug Prototype box)	PO; 0.3–2 g once or twice daily or 1 tsp of powder in a glass of water	For treatment of metabolic acidosis, to enhance renal excretion of certain drugs, and as an antacid
CALCIUM		
calcium acetate (PhosLo)	PO; two to four tablets with each meal (each tablet contains 169 mg)	To prevent high blood phosphate levels in patients who are on dialysis
calcium carbonate (Rolaids, Tums, Os-Cal, others)	PO; 1–2 g bid–tid	For calcium supplementation and as an antacid
calcium citrate (Citracal)	PO; 1–2 g bid–tid	For calcium supplementation
calcium gluconate (Kalcinate)	PO; 1–2 g bid–qid	For calcium supplementation and to reverse cardiac signs of hyperkalemia
calcium lactate (Cal-Lac)	PO; 325 mg–1.3 g tid with meals	To correct mild hypokalemia
IRON		
ferrous fumarate (Feostat, others)	PO; 200 mg tid–qid	For iron supplementation
ferrous gluconate (Fergon, others)	PO; 325–600 mg qid; may be gradually increased to 650 mg qid as needed and tolerated	For iron supplementation
ⓟ ferrous sulfate (Feosol, others)	PO; 750–1,500 mg/day in one to three divided doses	For iron supplementation
iron dextran (Dexferrum, others)	IM/IV; dose is individualized and determined from a table in the package insert (max: 100 mg [2 mL] of iron dextran within 24 hours)	For iron supplementation when oral administration is not indicated
MAGNESIUM		
magnesium chloride (Chloromag, Slow-Mag)	PO; 270–400 mg/day	For magnesium supplementation
magnesium hydroxide (Milk of Magnesia)	PO; 5–15 mL or two to four tablets up to four times per day	For constipation, hyperacidity, or magnesium supplementation
magnesium oxide (Mag-Ox, Maox, others)	PO; 400–1,200 mg/day in divided doses	For constipation, hyperacidity, or magnesium supplementation
magnesium sulfate (Epsom salt)	IV/IM; 0.5–3 g/day	For constipation, to control seizures, or for magnesium supplementation
PHOSPHORUS		
potassium/sodium phosphates (K-Phos original, K-Phos MF, K-Phos neutral, Neutra-Phos-K, Uro-KP neutral)	PO; 250–1,000 mg /day	For correction of phosphate deficiency and to lower urinary calcium concentration
ZINC		
zinc gluconate	PO; 20–100 mg (20-mg lozenges may be taken to a max of six per day)	For correction of zinc deficiency
zinc sulfate (Orazinc, Zincate, others)	PO; 15–220 mg/day	For correction of zinc deficiency

NURSING PROCESS FOCUS Patients Receiving Iron Supplements

ASSESSMENT	POTENTIAL NURSING DIAGNOSES
Prior to administration: ■ Obtain a complete health history, including GI, renal and liver conditions; problems with anemia; prophylaxis during infancy, childhood, and pregnancy; allergies, drug history, and possible drug interactions. ■ Evaluate laboratory blood findings: CBC (specifically hematocrit and hemoglobin levels), electrolytes, and liver function studies. ■ Acquire the results of a complete physical examination including vital signs, height, and weight.	■ *Risk for Imbalanced Nutrition* related to inadequate iron intake ■ *Risk for Injury* (weakness, dizziness, syncope) related to anemia ■ *Deficient Knowledge* related to a lack of information about drug therapy

PLANNING: PATIENT GOALS AND EXPECTED OUTCOMES

The patient will:
■ Experience therapeutic effects (an increase in hematocrit level and improvement in anemia-related symptoms).
■ Be free from or experience minimal adverse effects from drug therapy.
■ Verbalize an understanding of the drug's use, adverse effects, and required precautions.

IMPLEMENTATION

Interventions and (Rationales)	Patient Education/Discharge Planning
■ Monitor vital signs, especially pulse. (Increased pulse is an indicator of decreased oxygen content in the blood.)	■ Instruct the patient to monitor pulse rate and report irregularities and changes in rhythm to the healthcare provider.
■ Monitor CBC to evaluate effectiveness of treatment. (Increases in hematocrit and hemoglobin values indicate increased red blood cell [RBC] production.)	Instruct the patient: ■ On the need for initial and continuing laboratory blood monitoring. ■ To keep all laboratory appointments.
■ Monitor changes in stool. (Supplement may cause constipation, change stool color, and cause false positives when stool is tested for occult blood.)	Instruct the patient: ■ That stool color may change, and that this is no cause for alarm. ■ On measures to relieve constipation, such as including fruits and fruit juices in the diet and increasing fluid intake and exercise.
■ Plan activities and allow for periods of rest to help the patient conserve energy. (Diminished iron levels result in decreased formation of hemoglobin, leading to weakness.)	Instruct the patient to: ■ Rest when he or she is feeling tired and avoid overexertion. ■ Plan activities to avoid fatigue.
■ Administer oral forms of ferrous sulfate (iron) one hour before or two hours after meals with a full glass of water or juice for better absorption.	Instruct the patient: ■ Not to crush or chew sustained-release preparations; take with a full glass of water or juice. ■ That medication may cause GI upset and may be taken with food if this becomes a problem.
■ Administer liquid iron preparations through a straw or place on the back of the tongue (to avoid staining the teeth).	Instruct the patient to: ■ Dilute liquid medication before using and to use a straw to take the medication. ■ Rinse the mouth after swallowing to decrease the chance of staining the teeth.
■ Monitor dietary intake to ensure adequate intake of foods high in iron.	■ Instruct the patient to increase intake of iron-rich foods such as liver, egg yolks, brewer's yeast, wheat germ, and muscle meats.
■ Monitor for potential for child access to the medication. (Iron poisoning can be fatal to young children.)	■ Advise the parent to store iron-containing vitamins out of reach of children and in childproof containers.

EVALUATION OF OUTCOME CRITERIA

Evaluate the effectiveness of drug therapy by confirming that patient goals and expected outcomes have been met (see "Planning").

> ## CAM THERAPY
>
> ### Sea Vegetables
>
> Sea vegetables, or seaweeds, are a form of marine algae that grow in the upper levels of the ocean, where sunlight can penetrate. Examples of these edible seaweeds include spirulina, kelp, chlorella, arame, and nori, many of which are used in Asian cooking. Sea vegetables are found in coastal locations throughout the world. Kelp, or Laminaria, is found in the cold waters of the North Atlantic and Pacific oceans.
>
> Sea vegetables contain a multitude of vitamins as well as protein. Their most notable nutritional aspect, however, is their mineral content. Plants from the sea contain more minerals than most other food sources, including calcium, magnesium, phosphorus, iron, potassium, and all essential trace elements. Because they are so rich in minerals, seaweeds act as alkalizers for the blood, helping to rid the body of acid conditions (acidosis). Spirulina, kelp, and chlorella are available in capsule or tablet form.

CORE CONCEPT 31.6

Enteral and total parenteral nutrition are therapies that deliver essential nutrients to patients with deficiencies.

When a patient is eating or drinking fewer nutrients than required for normal body growth and maintenance, **undernutrition** occurs. Undernutrition can also occur in certain malabsorption disorders of the intestinal tract. The two primary goals in treating undernutrition are to *identify* the specific type of deficiency and *supply* the missing nutrients. Nutritional supplements may be needed for short-term therapy or for the remainder of a patient's life.

Causes of undernutrition range from simple to complex and include the following:

- Advanced age
- HIV-AIDS
- Alcoholism
- Severe burns
- Cancer
- Chronic inflammatory bowel disease
- Eating disorders

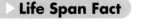

Life Span Fact

Elderly patients may have poor-fitting dentures or difficulty chewing or swallowing following a stroke.

The most obvious cause for undernutrition is low dietary intake. Reasons for the inadequate intake must be carefully assessed. Patients may have no resources to purchase food and may be suffering from starvation. Clinical depression leads many patients to shun food. Older adults may have poorly fitting dentures or difficulty chewing or swallowing after a stroke. In terminal disease, patients may be comatose or otherwise unable to take food orally. Although the causes differ, patients with insufficient intake exhibit a similar pattern of general weakness, muscle wasting, and loss of subcutaneous fat.

Many different types of nutritional supplements are available to assist patients suffering from undernutrition. Products administered via the GI tract, either orally or through a feeding tube, are called **enteral nutrition**. Oral feeding allows natural digestive processes to occur and requires less nursing care. Tube feeding is necessary when the patient has difficulty swallowing or is otherwise unable to take meals orally (Figure 31.2 ■). An advantage of tube feeding is that the amount of enteral nutrition the patient is receiving can be precisely measured and recorded.

FIGURE 31.2

Nurse administering enteral nutrition through a feeding tube.

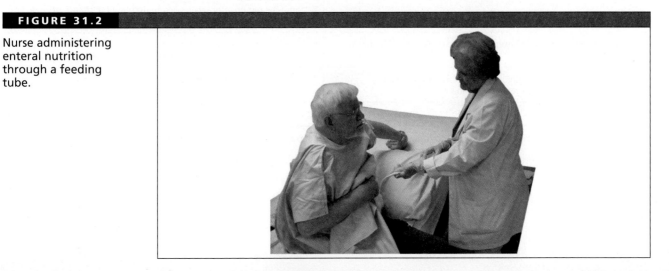

The particular enteral product is chosen to address the specific nutritional needs of the patient. For example, some contain mixtures of amino acids and protein, whereas others contain primarily carbohydrates or fats. There are many different formulations of enteral products available, each designed to meet a specific nutrient need. Examples of enteral products include Vivonex T.E.N., Peptamen, Sustacal, Ensure-Plus, Casec, Polycose, Microlipid, and MCT Oil.

Patients sometimes exhibit vomiting, nausea, or diarrhea when first receiving enteral nutrition. Therapy is often started slowly, with small quantities so that adverse effects can be assessed.

When the metabolic needs of the patient cannot be met through enteral nutrition, **total parenteral nutrition (TPN)** is indicated. For short-term therapy, peripheral vein TPN may be used. Because of the risk of phlebitis, however, long-term therapy often requires central vein TPN. Because the GI tract is not being used, patients with severe malabsorption disease may be successfully treated with TPN.

TPN is able to provide all the patient's nutritional needs with solutions containing amino acids, fats, carbohydrate (as dextrose), electrolytes, vitamins, and minerals. The particular formulation may be specific to the disease state, such as products for renal failure or hepatic failure. TPN is administered through an infusion pump so that nutrition can be precisely monitored. Patients in various settings such as acute care, long-term care, and home health care often benefit from TPN therapy.

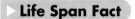

▶ Life Span Fact

The absorption of food diminishes with age, and often the quantity of ingested food is reduced, leading to vitamin deficiencies in elderly patients.

📋 PATIENTS NEED TO KNOW

Patients treated with vitamins, minerals, or herbs need to know the following:

In General

1. If receiving regular monthly injections of vitamin B_{12}, do not take additional oral supplements of vitamin B_{12} or folic acid without the advice of a healthcare provider.
2. Do not take more than the recommended doses of any vitamin or mineral without first checking with a healthcare provider. Although small amounts of these substances are beneficial, large amounts may be dangerous.
3. Ensure that diet is nutritionally adequate, adding foods that naturally supply the needed vitamins and minerals before taking supplements. See a dietician for advice, particularly for special needs such as pregnancy or diabetes.
4. Avoid foods with high zinc or oxalate content if a calcium supplement is being taken because these may interfere with absorption. These foods include nuts, peas, beans, spinach, and soy products.
5. Know that niacin, or vitamin B_3, is also effective at lowering lipid levels. The dose for lowering cholesterol, however, is 2–3 g per day, whereas the vitamin dose is only 25 mg per day.
6. When providing a medical or drug history to the physician or dentist, always report vitamins, minerals, herbs, or dietary supplements being taken. If allergies to any dietary supplements are known, be sure to report these also.
7. Because liquid iron preparations can stain teeth, dilute these solutions with juice or water and rinse the mouth after taking the medication to reduce staining.
8. Take oral forms of ferrous sulfate (iron) one hour before or two hours after meals for better absorption. Take with a full glass of water or juice.

⚠ SAFETY ALERT

Accidental Overdose of Vitamins and Other Medications

Accidental overdose of vitamins or other medications are of special concern in children. They have the ability to cause injury and death. Medications used for children, such as vitamins and cough medicine, may be appealing to children because of their candy-like appearance. To avoid tragedy, nurses should teach caregivers not to refer to any medications as "candy" and to store all medications in a secure place; out of the reach and sight of children even if the containers have child-resistant caps.

CHAPTER REVIEW

CORE CONCEPTS SUMMARY

31.1 Vitamins are needed to promote growth and maintain health.

With the exception of vitamin D, vitamins cannot be synthesized by the body and must be provided in the diet. Although only very small amounts of vitamins are needed, lack of sufficient quantity will result in disease.

31.2 Vitamins are classified as fat soluble or water soluble.

Water-soluble vitamins include vitamins C and B. Fat-soluble vitamins include vitamins A, D, E, and K. Water-soluble vitamins cannot be stored and must be ingested daily, whereas excess fat-soluble vitamins can be stored for later use.

31.3 Recommended dietary allowances (RDAs) for vitamins have been established for the average healthy adult.

RDA values represent the minimum amount of vitamin or mineral needed to prevent a deficiency in a healthy adult. These values must be adjusted for changes in health status, such as athletic training, pregnancy, or chronic disease.

31.4 Vitamin therapy is indicated for specific conditions.

Most people do not need vitamin supplementation, and excess intake may lead to hypervitaminosis. Indications for vitamin therapy include alcoholism, pregnancy or breast-feeding, chronic kidney or liver disease, therapy with certain drugs that affect vitamin metabolism, and reduced food intake in elderly patients.

31.5 Minerals are inorganic substances needed in very small amounts to maintain normal body metabolism.

Like vitamins, most people receive all the minerals they need through a balanced diet. Certain conditions, such as osteoporosis or iron-deficiency anemia, do warrant mineral therapy.

31.6 Enteral and total parenteral nutrition are therapies that deliver essential nutrients to patients with deficiencies.

Enteral nutrition supplies patients all the essential nutrients via the oral route or through feeding tube. For patients who cannot take oral supplements, nutrients are supplied parenterally by way of total parenteral nutrition.

REVIEW QUESTIONS

The following questions are written in NCLEX-PN® style. Answer these questions to assess your knowledge of the chapter material, and go back and review any material that is not clear to you.

1. The nurse knows that Vitamin B$_{12}$ is indicated for which of the following conditions?

1. Liver disease
2. Chronic inflammatory bowel disease
3. Pernicious anemia
4. Inadequate exposure to sunlight

2. The nurse administers which vitamin for a patient experiencing warfarin (Coumadin) overdose?

1. Vitamin A
2. Vitamin D
3. Vitamin E
4. Vitamin K

3. For the patient taking ferrous sulfate, the nurse will provide what instructions?

1. Do not take antacids with this medication.
2. This medication can cause severe diarrhea.

3. This medication should never be taken on an empty stomach.
4. Blood pressure must be monitored closely.

4. The nurse monitors patients with a history of alcohol abuse for a _____ deficiency.

1. Biotin
2. Thiamine
3. Niacin
4. Riboflavin

5. The patient on a thiazide or loop diuretic, such as Lasix, is monitored for which electrolyte?

1. Selenium
2. Calcium
3. Potassium
4. Magnesium

6. The nurse instructs the patient taking liquid iron to:

1. Swish medication in his mouth for one minute.
2. Take medication with food.
3. Avoid foods with high iron content.
4. Rinse his mouth with water after swallowing.

7. The patient is exhibiting weakness, hypertension, and dysrhythmias. Which of the following will the nurse check?

1. Calcium levels
2. Magnesium levels
3. Aluminum levels
4. Chromium levels

8. The nurse understands that which of the following is a common indication for vitamin or mineral pharmacotherapy? (Select all that apply.)

1. Chronic alcoholism
2. Liver failure
3. Anemia
4. Pregnancy

9. The patient's GI tract is not functioning. Which type of feeding technique does the nurse expect to use to ensure the patient is receiving adequate nutrition?

1. Oral
2. Enteral
3. TPN
4. GI

10. The patient has hypomagnesemia and is to receive and IV infusion of 350 mg of magnesium in 250 mL over four hours. How many milliliters per hour will the patient receive?

1. 65.5 mL
2. 50.5 mL
3. 62.5 mL
4. 55.5 mL

CASE STUDY QUESTIONS

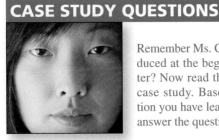

Remember Ms. Chin, who was introduced at the beginning of the chapter? Now read the remainder of the case study. Based on the information you have learned in this chapter, answer the questions that follow.

Ms. Mei Chin, a young woman, has come to the office for a routine check-up. While reviewing her medications, Ms. Chin tells the nurse that she has been taking multivitamins with minerals for the last year, and that lately, she has been taking four times the label dose because she doesn't eat very much and figures that "it's better to take more than not enough."

1. While teaching Ms. Chin about multivitamins, the nurse identifies which of the following as a water-soluble vitamin?

1. A
2. B complex
3. D
4. E

2. While continuing the discussion on the topic of multivitamins and minerals, Ms. Chin asks the nurse the meaning of RDA. The nurse responds:

1. "It is the amount of nutrient required by all people."
2. "It is the maximum amount of nutrient needed to prevent a deficiency in healthy adults."

3. "It is the amount of nutrient needed by an average person."
4. "It is the minimum amount of nutrient needed to prevent a deficiency in healthy adults."

3. Ms. Chin asks if she should be taking the multivitamins. The nurse collects what information before responding? (Select all that apply.)

1. Weight
2. Diet
3. Presence of any chronic diseases
4. Use of alcohol

4. Ms. Chin wants to continue to take the multivitamins, convinced that it is helping her. She states that sometimes she just doesn't feel like eating. The nurse tells Ms. Chin to:

1. Stop taking the multivitamins, her diet is good enough.
2. Continue taking four times the label dose until she starts to feel sick.
3. Not take more than the recommended dose until she speaks to the doctor about the problems associated with her diet
4. Discontinue taking four times the recommended dose, instead take two times the recommended dose because she hasn't been eating well.

NOTE: Answers to the Review and Case Study Questions appear in Appendix B. The complete rationales and answers are located on the textbook's website.

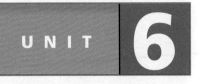

The Endocrine and Reproductive Systems

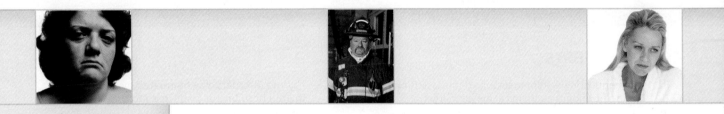

Unit Contents

Chapter 32   Drugs for Endocrine Disorders / 510

Chapter 33   Drugs for Diabetes Mellitus / 528

Chapter 34   Drugs for Disorders and Conditions of the Reproductive System / 542

"I don't know why I'm so tired all the time. I've gained a lot of weight and am cold all the time too. Maybe it's just hormones."

Mrs. Helen Brookfield

32 Drugs for Endocrine Disorders

CORE CONCEPTS

32.1 The endocrine system maintains homeostasis by using hormones as chemical messengers.

32.2 The hypothalamus and the pituitary gland secrete hormones that control other endocrine organs.

32.3 Hormones are used as replacement therapy, as antineoplastics, or as "antihormones" to block endogenous actions.

32.4 Of the many pituitary and hypothalamic hormones, several have clinical applications as drugs.

32.5 The thyroid gland controls the basal metabolic rate and affects virtually every cell in the body.

32.6 Thyroid disorders may be treated by administering thyroid hormone or by decreasing the activity of the thyroid gland.

32.7 Corticosteroids are released during periods of stress and influence carbohydrate, lipid, and protein metabolism in most cells.

32.8 Corticosteroids are prescribed for adrenocortical insufficiency and to dampen inflammatory and immune responses.

DRUG SNAPSHOT

The following drugs are discussed in this chapter:

DRUG CLASSES	DRUG PROTOTYPES
Hypothalamic and Pituitary Drugs	Pr desmopressin (DDAVP) *514*
Thyroid Drugs	Pr levothyroxine (Synthroid) *518*
Antithyroid Drugs	Pr propylthiouracil (PTU) *519*
Adrenal Drugs	Pr hydrocortisone (Cortef, Hydrocortone, Solu-Cortef, others) *522*

LEARNING OUTCOMES

After reading this chapter, the student should be able to:

1. Describe the general structure and functions of the endocrine system.

2. Explain the primary functions of the thyroid gland.

3. Identify the signs and symptoms of hypothyroidism and hyperthyroidism.

4. Explain the primary functions of the adrenal cortex.

5. Describe the signs and symptoms of Addison's disease and Cushing's syndrome.

6. Categorize drugs used in the treatment of endocrine disorders

based on their classifications and mechanisms of action.

7. For each of the drug classes listed in the Drug Snapshot, identify representative drugs and explain their mechanisms of drug action, primary actions, and important adverse effects.

KEY TERMS

Addison's disease (ADD-iss-uns) *521*

adrenal atrophy (AT-troh-fee) *521*

adrenocorticotropic hormone (ACTH) (uh-dreen-oh-kor-tik-o-TRO-pik) *520*

anterior pituitary *511*

antidiuretic hormone (ADH) (ANT-eye-DYE-yure-EH-tick) *514*

corticosteroid (KORT-ik-ko-STARE-oyd) *520*

cretinism (KREE-ten-izm) *516*

Cushing's syndrome (KUSH-ings) *522*

diabetes insipidus (die-uh-BEE-tees in-SIP-uh-dus) *514*

dwarfism *515*

follicular cells (fo-LIK-yu-lur) *516*

glucocorticoids (glu-ko-KORT-ik-oyds) *520*

gonadocorticoids (go-NAD-oh-KORT-ik-oyds) *521*

Graves' disease *516*

hormones *511*

hypothalamus (hi-po-THAL-ih-mus) *511*

mineralocorticoids (min-ur-al-oh-KORT-ik-oyds) *520*

myxedema (mix-uh-DEEM-uh) *516*

parafollicular cells (par-uh-fo-LIK-u-lur) *516*

pituitary gland (pit-TOO-it-air-ee) *511*

posterior pituitary *511*

releasing hormones *511*

somatotropin (so-mat-oh-TROH-pin) *515*

vasopressin (vaz-oh-PRESS-in) *514*

L ike the nervous system, the endocrine system is a major controller of homeostasis. Whereas a nerve may exert instantaneous control over a single muscle or gland, a hormone from the endocrine system may affect thousands of body cells and take as long as several days to produce an optimal response. Hormonal balance must be maintained within a narrow range. Too little or too much of a hormone may produce profound changes in the body. This chapter examines common endocrine disorders and their pharmacotherapy. Drugs for diabetes mellitus are covered in Chapter 33. The reproductive hormones are covered in Chapter 34

endo = *within*
crine = *to secrete*

The endocrine system maintains homeostasis by using hormones as chemical messengers.

CORE CONCEPT **32.1**

The endocrine system consists of various glands that secrete **hormones**, chemical messengers released in response to a change in the body's internal environment. For example, whenever body temperature falls, the thyroid gland secretes thyroid hormone. When levels of calcium in the bloodstream fall, the parathyroid glands secrete parathyroid hormone (PTH). The various endocrine glands and their locations in body are illustrated in Figure 32.1 ■.

In the endocrine system, it is common for one hormone to control the secretion of another hormone. In addition, it is common for the last hormone or action in the pathway to provide feedback to turn off the action of the first hormone. For example, as serum calcium level falls, PTH is released. PTH causes an increase in serum calcium level, which provides feedback to the parathyroid glands to shut off PTH secretion. This is a common feature of endocrine homeostasis known as *negative feedback*.

The hypothalamus and the pituitary gland secrete hormones that control other endocrine organs.

CORE CONCEPT **32.2**

Two endocrine structures in the brain deserve special recognition because they control many other endocrine glands. The **hypothalamus** secretes chemicals called **releasing hormones** that travel via blood vessels a short distance to an area immediately below, called the **pituitary gland**. These releasing factors tell the pituitary which hormone to release. After the pituitary releases the appropriate hormone, it travels to its target organ to cause its effect. For example, the hypothalamus secretes thyrotropin-releasing hormone, which travels to the pituitary gland with the message to secrete thyroid-stimulating hormone (TSH). TSH then travels to its target organ—the thyroid gland—to stimulate the release of thyroid hormone.

The pituitary gland comprises two distinct areas, the **anterior pituitary** or *adenohypophysis* and the **posterior pituitary** or *neurohypophysis*. The majority of hormones are released by *glandular tissue* of the adenohypophysis. Only a few hormones are released from *neural tissue* of the neurohypophysis. Selected hormones associated with the hypothalamus and pituitary gland are shown in Figure 32.2 ■.

adeno = *glandular tissue*
neuro = *neural tissue*
hypo = *under*
physis = *growth*

FIGURE 32.1

The endocrine system.

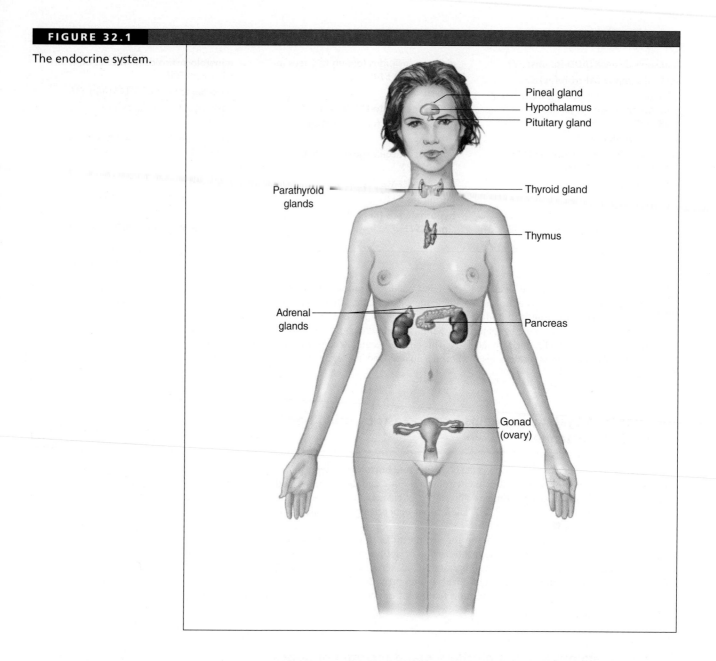

Pineal gland
Hypothalamus
Pituitary gland

Parathyroid glands

Thyroid gland

Thymus

Adrenal glands

Pancreas

Gonad (ovary)

CORE CONCEPT 32.3

Hormones are used as replacement therapy, as antineoplastics, or as "antihormones" to block endogenous actions.

endo = *within*
genous = *generated from*

The goals of hormone pharmacotherapy vary widely. In many cases, the hormone is administered simply as replacement therapy for patients who are unable to secrete sufficient quantities of their own endogenous hormones. Examples of replacement therapy include the administration of thyroid hormone after the thyroid gland has been surgically removed or supplying insulin to a patient whose pancreas is not functioning. Replacement therapy usually supplies the same physiologically low-level amounts of the hormone that would normally be present in the body. A summary of selected endocrine disorders and their drug therapy is given in Table 32.1 ◆.

Some hormones are used in cancer chemotherapy to shrink the size of hormone-sensitive tumors. Examples include testosterone for breast cancer and estrogen for testicular cancer. Exactly how these hormones produce their antineoplastic action is unknown. When used as antineoplastics, the doses of these hormones far exceed those levels normally present in the body (see Chapter 28).

Another goal of hormone therapy may be to produce an exaggerated response that is part of the normal action of the drug. Administering hydrocortisone to suppress inflammation takes advantage of the

FIGURE 32.2

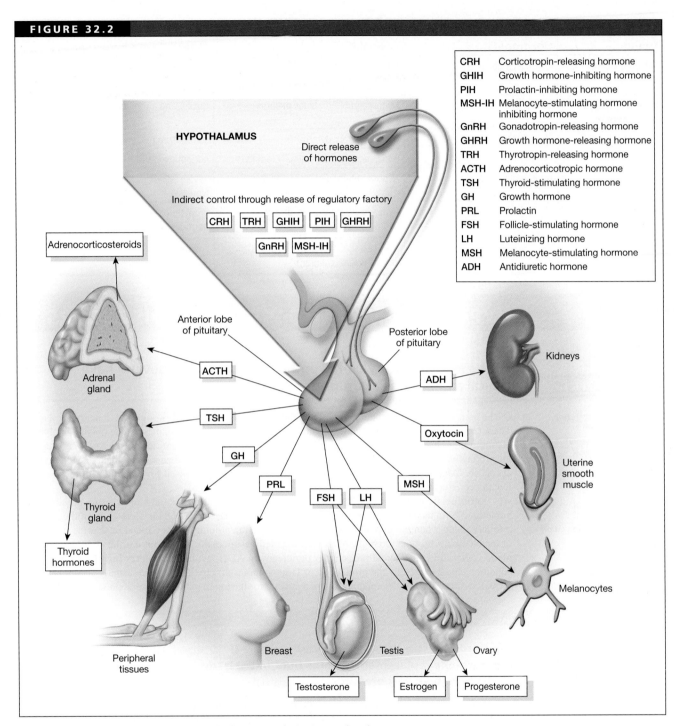

CRH	Corticotropin-releasing hormone
GHIH	Growth hormone-inhibiting hormone
PIH	Prolactin-inhibiting hormone
MSH-IH	Melanocyte-stimulating hormone inhibiting hormone
GnRH	Gonadotropin-releasing hormone
GHRH	Growth hormone-releasing hormone
TRH	Thyrotropin-releasing hormone
ACTH	Adrenocorticotropic hormone
TSH	Thyroid-stimulating hormone
GH	Growth hormone
PRL	Prolactin
FSH	Follicle-stimulating hormone
LH	Luteinizing hormone
MSH	Melanocyte-stimulating hormone
ADH	Antidiuretic hormone

Hormones associated with the hypothalamus and pituitary gland.

normal action of the corticosteroids but to a greater extent than would normally occur in the body. Supplying small amounts of estrogen or progesterone at specific times during the menstrual cycle can prevent ovulation and pregnancy.

Endocrine pharmacotherapy also involves the use of "antihormones." These hormones block the actions of endogenous hormones. For example, propylthiouracil (PTU) is given to block the effects of an overactive thyroid gland. Tamoxifen (Nolvadex) is given to block the actions of estrogens in estrogen-dependent breast cancers (see Chapter 34).

TABLE 32.1 Endocrine Disorders and Their Drug Treatment

Gland	Hormone(s)	Disorder	Drugs
Adrenal Cortex	Corticosteroids	Hypersecretion: Cushing's syndrome	Antiadrenal drugs
		Hyposecretion: Addison's disease	Corticosteroids
Pancreas (Islets of Langerhans)	Insulin	Hyposecretion: diabetes mellitus	Insulin and antidiabetic drugs
Pituitary	Growth hormone	Hyposecretion: dwarfism	somatotropin (Genotropin, others)
		Hypersecretion: acromegaly (adults)	octreotide (Sandostatin)
	Antidiuretic hormone	Hyposecretion: diabetes insipidus	vasopressin, desmopressin, and lypressin
Thyroid	Thyroid hormone (T$_3$ and T$_4$)	Hypersecretion: Graves' disease	propylthiouracil (PTU) and I-131 thyroid hormone
		Hyposecretion: myxedema (adults) and cretinism (children)	levothyroxine (T$_4$)

HYPOTHALAMIC AND PITUITARY DISORDERS

CORE CONCEPT 32.4

Of the many pituitary and hypothalamic hormones, several have clinical applications as drugs.

diabetes = siphon (urine passing through)
mellitus = sweetened
insipidus = tasteless (watered down)
en = in
uresis = to urinate

osmolality = concentration

vaso = blood vessel
pressin = tension

Of the hormones secreted by the pituitary and the hypothalamus, only a few are used in pharmacotherapy. There are valid reasons why they are not widely used. Some of these hormones can be obtained only from natural sources and can be quite expensive when used in therapeutic quantities. Furthermore, it is usually more effective to give drugs that *directly* affect secretion at the target organs. Hypothalamic and pituitary agents are listed in Table 32.2 ◆. Hypothalamic and pituitary agents used for conditions of the male and female reproductive systems are presented in Chapter 34.

Antidiuretic hormone (ADH) is one of the most important means the body uses to maintain fluid homeostasis. As its name implies, ADH conserves water in the body. ADH is secreted from the posterior pituitary gland when the hypothalamus senses that plasma volume has decreased or that the osmolality of the blood has become too high. ADH is also called **vasopressin**, because it has the ability to constrict blood vessels and raise blood pressure. A deficiency in ADH results in **diabetes insipidus (DI)**, a rare condition characterized by the production of large volumes of very dilute urine, usually accompanied by increased thirst. Two ADH preparations are available for the treatment of DI: desmopressin (DDAVP) and

Drug Prototype: ℞ *Desmopressin (DDAVP, Stimate)*
Therapeutic Class: Antidiuretic hormone replacement; retains fluid in the body
Pharmacologic Class: Antidiuretic hormone; vasopressin

Actions and Uses: Desmopressin is a synthetic analog of human ADH that acts on the kidneys to increase the reabsorption of water. It is used to control the acute symptoms of DI in patients who have insufficient ADH secretion. The oral route is preferred, although intranasal and parenteral forms are available. It has a duration of action of up to 20 hours, whereas vasopressin has a duration of only 2–8 hours. Desmopressin is available as a nasal spray (Stimate) to treat von Willebrand's disease, a disorder of blood clotting.

Adverse Effects and Interactions: Desmopressin causes contraction of smooth muscle in the vascular system, uterus, and GI tract. It also is used for the management of bleeding in patients with hemophilia A. When taken an hour prior to bedtime, desmopressin lowers the production of urine during the night and thus is useful in the management of nocturnal enuresis (bed-wetting).

Desmopressin can cause symptoms of water intoxication: edema, weight gain, hypertension, drowsiness, headache, and listlessness, progressing to convulsions and coma. Patients are advised to weigh themselves daily. Other adverse effects include transient headache, nausea, mild abdominal pain and cramping, facial flushing, hypertension (HTN), pain, or swelling at the injection site. Intranasal forms can cause nasal congestion, rhinitis, and epistaxis. Desmopressin is contraindicated in patients with DI that is caused by kidney disease because the drug can worsen fluid retention and overload. It is used with caution in patients with coronary artery disease and HTN and in patients at risk for hyponatremia or thrombi.

Increased antidiuretic action can occur with carbamazepine, chlorpropamide, clofibrate, and nonsteroidal anti-inflammatory drugs (NSAIDs). Decreased antidiuretic action can occur with lithium, alcohol, heparin, and epinephrine.

TABLE 32.2   Selected Hypothalamic and Pituitary Drugs

Drug	Route and Adult Dose	Remarks
HYPOTHALAMIC DRUG		
bromocriptine (Cycloset, Parlodel)	PO (Cycloset); 0.8 mg daily, increased weekly to achieve 1.6–4.8 mg daily PO; 1.25–2.5 mg/day for 3 days, then increase dose every 3–7 days to 30–60 mg/day	Blocks the release of prolactin; for treatment of acromegaly (overproduction of GH) and pituitary tumors; for signs and symptoms of Parkinson's disease and type 2 diabetes mellitus
PITUITARY DRUGS		
Posterior Pituitary – ADH Drugs		
(Pr) desmopressin (DDAVP, Stimate)	IV/subcutaneous; 2–4 mcg in two divided doses PO; 0.2–0.4 mg/day	To control symptoms of diabetes insipidus; in children under 6 years old, for bed-wetting (enuresis); also used to treat von Willebrand's disease
vasopressin	IM/subcutaneous; 5–10 units aqueous solution two to four times per day IV: 0.2–0.4 units/min up to 1 unit/min	Human antidiuretic hormone; reduces urine output by targeting renal collecting tubules
Anterior Pituitary – GH and TSH Drugs		
lanreotide (Somatuline Depot)	Subcutaneous; 60–100 mg every 4 weeks	For long term treatment of patients with acromegaly who cannot be treated with surgery or radiation
mecasermin (Increlex)	Subcutaneous; 0.04–0.08 mg/kg twice daily. Must be administered within 20 min of a meal or snack (max: 0.12 mg/kg given twice daily)	Synthetic version of insulin-like growth factor (IGF-1); suppresses liver glucose production and stimulates glucose uptake in the body; for long-term treatment of growth failure in children with antibodies that neutralize GH
octreotide (Sandostatin)	Subcutaneous/IV; 100–600 mcg/day in two to four divided doses; after 2 weeks may switch to IM depot, 20 mg every 4 weeks	For treatment of acromegaly due to too much GH in the body; may be used to treat severe diarrhea and other symptoms that occur with intestinal tumors or metastatic carcinoid tumors (tumors already spread in the body)
pegvisomant (Somavert)	Subcutaneous; 40 mg loading dose, then 10 mg/day (max: 30 mg/day)	Growth hormone receptor antagonist (blocker) used in the treatment of patients with acromegaly who cannot be treated with surgery or radiation
somatropin (Genotropin, Humatrope, Norditropin, Nutropin, Saizen, Serostim, Zorbtive)	Humatrope: Subcutaneous; 0.006 mg/kg daily (max: 0.0125 mg/kg/day) Serostim: Subcutaneous; Weight more than 55 kg: 6 mg at bedtime; 45–55 kg: 5 mg at bedtime; 35–45 kg: 4 mg at bedtime; less than 35 kg: 0.1 mg/kg at bedtime Child: Genotropin: Subcutaneous; 0.16–0.24 mg/kg/week in six to seven divided doses Norditropin: 0.024–0.034 mg/kg six to seven times per week	Growth hormone; protein-based peptide prescribed in human growth hormone therapy

vasopressin. Desmopressin is the most common drug for treating DI. Details regarding this drug are found in the Prototype Drug feature.

Growth hormone (GH), also called **somatotropin**, stimulates the growth and metabolism of nearly every cell in the body. Deficiency of this hormone in children can cause *short stature*, a condition characterized by significantly decreased physical height compared with the norm of a specific age group. Severe deficiency results in **dwarfism**. Short stature is caused by many conditions other than GH deficiency, and often a specific cause cannot be identified. Treatment of this condition usually involves the administration of the growth hormone. It is given subcutaneously, several times a week during periods of active growth and may continue until adulthood. The earlier the condition is treated, the better the chance that a child will grow to be a near-normal adult height. When hormone therapy is first initiated, the gain in growth is very rapid but then slows over time.

somato = *cells of the body*
tropin = *attraction toward*

dwarfism = *small stature*

acro = *extremeties*
megaly = *enlarged*

Excess secretion of GH in adults is known as acromegaly. Acromegaly is a rare disorder caused by a GH-secreting tumor of the pituitary gland. Because the epiphyseal plates are closed in adults, bones become deformed rather than elongated with this disorder. The onset is gradual, with enlargement of the small bones of the hands and feet, face, and skull; broad nose, protruding lower jaw; and slanting forehead.

Treatment of acromegaly consists of a combination of surgery, radiation therapy, and pharmacotherapy to suppress GH secretion or block GH receptors. Pharmacotherapy is generally attempted only in patients who are unable to undergo surgical removal of the tumor. Octreotide (Sandostatin) is a synthetic GH *antagonist* (blocker) structurally related to GH–inhibiting hormone (somatostatin). Other choices to treat acromegaly include pegvisomant (Somavert), bromocriptine (Cycloset, Parlodel), and lanreotide (Somatuline Depot).

THYROID DISORDERS

CORE CONCEPT 32.5

The thyroid gland controls the basal metabolic rate and affects virtually every cell in the body.

The thyroid gland secretes hormones that affect nearly every cell in the body. Thyroid hormone increases basal metabolic rate, which is the baseline speed at which cells perform their functions. By increasing cellular metabolism, this hormone increases body temperature. Adequate secretion of thyroid hormone is also necessary for the normal growth and development in infants and children. **Cretinism** is the abnormal stunting of growth due to the lack of thyroid hormone. The thyroid strongly affects cardiovascular, respiratory, gastrointestinal, and neuromuscular function.

The thyroid gland lies in the neck, just below the larynx and in front of the trachea. **Follicular cells** in the gland secrete thyroid hormone, which is actually a combination of two different hormones: thyroxine (tetraiodothyronine or T_4) and triiodothyronine (T_3). Iodine is essential for the synthesis of these hormones and is provided through the dietary intake of common iodized salt. T_3 is named for the three iodine atoms that make up its chemical structure; T_4 has four iodine atoms. **Parafollicular cells** in the thyroid gland secrete calcitonin, a hormone that is involved with calcium homeostasis (see Chapter 35).

Thyroid function is regulated in various ways. Thyroid-releasing hormone (TRH) from the hypothalamus stimulates the pituitary gland to secrete TSH. TSH then stimulates the thyroid gland to release thyroid hormone. As blood levels of thyroid hormone increase, negative feedback suppresses the secretion of TRH and TSH. High levels of iodine can also cause a temporary decrease in thyroid activity that can last for several weeks. One of the strongest stimuli for increased thyroid hormone production is exposure to cold temperatures. The negative feedback mechanism for the thyroid gland is shown in Figure 32.3 ■.

CORE CONCEPT 32.6

Thyroid disorders may be treated by administering thyroid hormone or by decreasing the activity of the thyroid gland.

Disorders of the thyroid result from *hypofunction* or *hyperfunction* of the thyroid gland. Abnormal thyroid hormone levels could occur due to disease within the thyroid gland itself or be caused by abnormalities of the pituitary gland or hypothalamus. Thyroid disorders are quite common, and drug therapy is often indicated.

Hypothyroidism is a common disease caused by insufficient secretion of either TSH or thyroid hormone. Symptoms of hypothyroidism in adults, also known as **myxedema**, include slowed body metabolism, fatigue, slurred speech, bradycardia, weight gain, low body temperature, and intolerance to cold environments. Low or absent thyroid function may be a consequence of autoimmune disease, surgical removal of the gland, or aggressive treatment with antithyroid drugs. Hypothyroidism is treated with natural or synthetic thyroid hormone.

Hypersecretion of thyroid hormone results in symptoms that are the opposite of hypothyroidism and are the result of increased body metabolism. The symptoms include nervousness, irritability, insomnia, tachycardia, palpitations, weight loss, hyperthermia, and heat intolerance. A particularly severe form of hyperthyroidism is called **Graves' disease**. If the cause of the hypersecretion is found to be a tumor, the disease is corrected through surgical removal of the thyroid gland, or thyroidectomy. In less severe conditions, the patient may receive antithyroid medications or ionizing radiation to kill or inactivate some of the hyperactive thyroid cells. Antithyroid drugs are sometimes given 10 to 14 days prior to thyroidectomy to decrease bleeding during surgery.

FIGURE 32.3

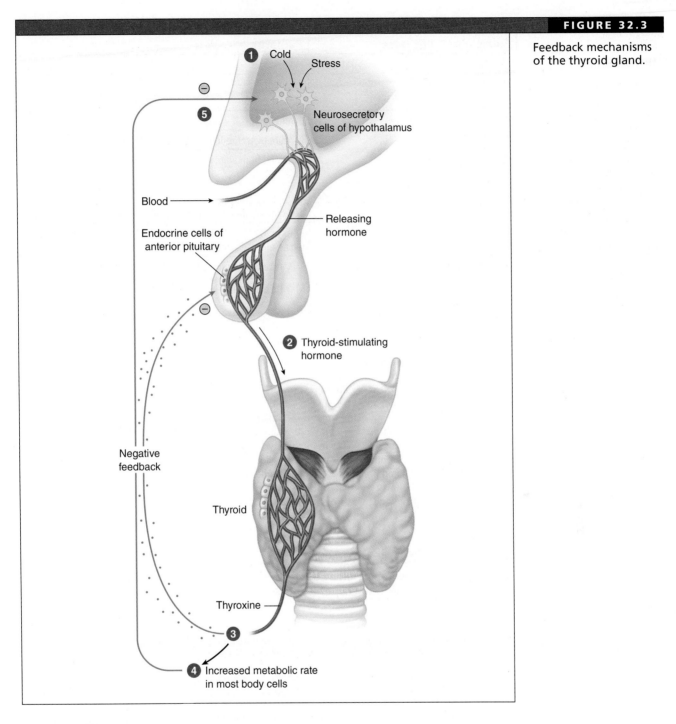

Feedback mechanisms of the thyroid gland.

Fast Facts Thyroid Disorders

- Hypothyroidism is 10 times more common in women than men; hyperthyroidism is 5–10 times more common in women.
- The two most common thyroid disorders, Graves' disease and Hashimoto's thyroiditis, are autoimmune diseases and may run in families.
- One of every five women older than age 75 has Hashimoto's thyroiditis.
- One of every 4,000 babies is born without a working thyroid gland.
- About 15,000 new cases of thyroid cancer are diagnosed each year.
- Postpartum thyroiditis occurs in 5–9% of women after giving birth and may recur in future pregnancies.
- Both hyperthyroidism and hypothyroidism can affect a woman's ability to become pregnant; both also can cause miscarriages.

TABLE 32.3 Thyroid and Antithyroid Drugs

Drug	Route and Adult Dose	Remarks
THYROID DRUGS		
(Pr) levothyroxine (Levothroid, Synthroid, others)	PO; 100–400 mcg/day	Synthetic T_4; IV form available
liothyronine (Cytomel, Triostat)	PO; 25–75 mcg/day	Synthetic T_3
liotrix (Thyrolar)	PO; 12.5–30 mcg/day	Mixture of synthetic T_3 and synthetic T_4 in a 1:4 ratio
thyroid dessicated (Armour Thyroid, Thyrar, Thyroid USP)	PO; 60–100 mg/day	Obtained from animal thyroid glands
ANTITHYROID DRUGS		
methimazole (Tapazole)	PO; 5–15 mg tid	Ten times more potent than propylthiouracil
potassium iodide and iodine (Lugol's solution, Thyro-block)	PO; 0.1–1.0 mL tid	IV form available; Lugol's is a mixture of 5% elemental iodine and 10% potassium iodide
(Pr) propylthiouracil (PTU)	PO; 100–150 mg tid	May take 6–12 months for full therapeutic effect
radioactive iodide (I-131)	PO; 0.8–150 mCi (based on radiation quantity)	May take 2–3 months for full therapeutic effect

The thyroid is the organ most susceptible to nuclear and radiation exposure (see Chapter 1). Symptoms of radiation exposure remain some of the most difficult to treat pharmacologically. Apart from the symptomatic treatment of *acute radiation syndrome*, taking potassium iodide (KI) tablets after an incident or an attack is the only recognized therapy.

Following a nuclear explosion, one of the resultant radioisotopes is iodine-131 (I-131). Because iodine is naturally concentrated in the thyroid gland, I-131 will immediately enter the thyroid and damage thyroid cells. If taken prior to, or immediately following, a nuclear incident, KI can prevent up to 100% of the radioactive iodine from entering thyroid tissue. Unfortunately, KI only protects the thyroid gland from I-131. It has no protective effects on other body tissues, and it offers no protection against the dozens of other harmful radioisotopes generated by a nuclear blast. Interestingly, I-131 is also a medication used to shrink the size of overactive thyroid glands. The thyroid and antithyroid medications are listed in Table 32.3 ◆.

Concept Review   32.1

■ If thyroid hormone is secreted by the thyroid gland, how can a deficiency in this hormone be caused by disease in the hypothalamus or pituitary gland?

Drug Prototype: (P) *Levothyroxine (Levothroid, Synthroid, Others)*
Therapeutic Class: Thyroid hormone replacement; metabolic enhancer   Pharmacologic Class: Thyroid hormone

Actions and Uses: Levothyroxine is a synthetic form of thyroxine (T_4) used for replacement therapy in patients with low thyroid function. Actions are those of thyroid hormone and include loss of weight, improved tolerance to environmental temperature, increased activity, and increased pulse rate. Blood levels of thyroid hormone are monitored carefully until the patient's symptoms stabilize. In order to closely approximate the body's own hormone level, levothyroxine should be taken in the morning, ideally at the same time each day. To achieve the proper level of thyroid function, doses may require periodic adjustments for several months or longer.

Adverse Effects and Interactions: The difference between a therapeutic dose of levothyroxine and one that produces adverse effects is quite narrow. Adverse effects of levothyroxine resemble symptoms of hyperthyroidism and include tachycardia, anxiety, insomnia, weight loss, and heat intolerance. Menstrual irregularities may occur in women. Long-term use of levothyroxine has been associated with osteoporosis in women.

Levothyroxine interacts with many other drugs; for example, cholestyramine and colestipol decrease the absorption of levothyroxine. Using it with epinephrine and norepinephrine increases the risk of cardiac insufficiency. Oral anticoagulants may increase hypoprothrombinemia.

High fiber foods may affect absorption. Herbal supplements such as lemon balm should be used cautiously. Lemon balm may interfere with thyroid hormone function.

Drug Prototype: 🅟 *Propylthiouracil (PTU)*

Therapeutic Class: Drug for hyperthyroidism   Pharmacologic Class: Antithyroid drug

Actions and Uses: Propylthiouracil is administered to patients with hyperthyroidism, sometimes prior to surgery. It acts by interfering with the synthesis of T_3 and T_4. Because it does not affect thyroid hormone that has already been secreted, its action may be delayed from several days to as long as 6 to 12 weeks. Effects include a return to normal thyroid function: weight gain, reduction in anxiety, less insomnia, and slower pulse rate.

Adverse Effects and Interactions: Overtreatment with propylthiouracil produces symptoms of hypothyroidism. In addition,

a small percentage of patients display blood changes such as decreased platelet and white blood cell counts, which may increase the risk of infection. Periodic laboratory blood counts and thyroid hormone values are necessary to establish the proper dosage.

Antithyroid medications interact with many other drugs. For example, propylthiouracil can reverse the effectiveness of drugs such as aminophylline, anticoagulants, and cardiac glycosides.

NURSING PROCESS FOCUS   Patients Receiving Thyroid Hormone Replacement

ASSESSMENT	POTENTIAL NURSING DIAGNOSES
Prior to administration: ■ Obtain a complete health history, including cardiovascular, neurological, renal and liver conditions; pregnancy, allergies, drug history, and possible drug interactions. ■ Evaluate laboratory blood findings: CBC, electrolytes, lipid panel, renal and liver function studies, T_4, T_3, and TSH levels. ■ Acquire the results of a complete physical examination, including vital signs, height, weight, and ECG.	■ *Activity Intolerance* related to decrease in levels of thyroid hormones ■ *Fatigue* related to impaired metabolic status ■ *Deficient Knowledge* related to a lack of information about drug therapy ■ *Infective Health Maintenance* related to adverse effects of drug therapy ■ *Risk for Infection* related to adverse effects of drug therapy

PLANNING: PATIENT GOALS AND EXPECTED OUTCOMES

The patient will:
■ Experience therapeutic effects of drug regimen (normal thyroid levels).
■ Be free from or experience minimal adverse effects from drug therapy.
■ Verbalize an understanding of the drug's use, adverse effects, and required precautions.

IMPLEMENTATION

Interventions and (Rationales)	Patient Education/Discharge Planning
■ Administer medication correctly and evaluate the patient's knowledge of proper administration. In addition, monitor the patient for signs of decreased compliance with therapeutic regimen. (Proper administration and compliance helps to ensure adequate thyroid hormone levels and a decrease in adverse effects.)	■ Instruct the patient about the disease, the importance of taking the medication regularly each day, and the importance of follow-up care.
■ Monitor vital signs. (Changes in metabolic rate will be manifested as changes in blood pressure, pulse, and body temperature.)	Instruct the patient to: ■ Take and record pulse rate two to three times a week. ■ Report to the healthcare provider any dizziness, palpitations, and an intolerance to temperature changes.
■ Monitor for symptoms related to hypothyroidism, such as fatigue, constipation, cold intolerance, lethargy, depression, and menstrual irregularities. (Decreasing symptoms will help determine effectiveness of hormone replacement hormone.)	■ Instruct the patient about the signs of hypothyroidism and to report symptoms to the healthcare provider.
■ Monitor for symptoms related to hyperthyroidism, such as nervousness, irritability, insomnia, tachycardia, palpitations, weight loss, hyperthermia, and heat intolerance. (Symptoms of hyperthyroidism may indicate overuse or adverse effect of hormone replacement medication.)	■ Instruct the patient about the signs of hyperthyroidism and to report symptoms to the healthcare provider.
■ Monitor T_3, T_4, and TSH levels. (This helps to determine need or effectiveness of drug therapy.)	Instruct the patient: ■ About the importance of ongoing monitoring of thyroid hormone levels. ■ To keep all laboratory appointments.

continued . . .

NURSING PROCESS FOCUS *(continued)*

Interventions and (Rationales)	Patient Education/Discharge Planning
■ Monitor blood glucose levels, especially in individuals with diabetes mellitus. (Thyroid hormones increase metabolic rate and may alter glucose utilization.)	■ Instruct the patient with diabetes to monitor blood glucose levels and adjust insulin doses as directed by the healthcare provider.
■ Provide supportive nursing care to cope with symptoms of hypothyroidism such as constipation, cold intolerance, and fatigue until the drug has achieved therapeutic effect. (Providing care will ensure patient comfort and enable the nurse to monitor sign/symptoms.)	Instruct the patient to: ■ Increase fluid and fiber intake, as well as activity, to reduce constipation. ■ Wear additional clothing and maintain a comfortable room environment for cold intolerance ■ Plan activities and include rest periods to avoid fatigue.
■ Monitor weight at least weekly. (Weight loss or gain may indicate disease process and helps to determine the effectiveness of drug therapy.)	Instruct the patient to: ■ Take and record weight weekly. ■ Report significant changes in weight to the healthcare provider.
■ Unless approved by the healthcare provider, avoid iodine-containing foods such as soy sauce, tofu, milk, eggs, yogurt, and some fish. (Increasing or decreasing normal intake of these foods may result in adverse drug effects.)	■ Provide dietary instruction on foods to avoid.

EVALUATION OF OUTCOME CRITERIA

Evaluate the effectiveness of drug therapy by confirming that patient goals and expected outcomes have been met (see "Planning"). *See Table 32.3 for a list of drugs to which these nursing actions apply.*

ADRENAL DISORDERS

CORE CONCEPT 32.7

Corticosteroids are released during periods of stress and influence carbohydrate, lipid, and protein metabolism in most cells.

mineralo = *minerals (i.e., sodium, potassium)*

cortic/cortico = *cortex*
tropin/tropic = *attraction toward*
adreno = *adrenal glands*

hyper = *elevated*
natri = *sodium*
emia = *blood levels*
tension = *blood pressure*

gluco/glyc = *sugar*
al/oid = *resembling*

neo = *new*

Though small, the adrenal glands secrete hormones that affect almost every body tissue. Adrenal disorders include those resulting from either *excess* hormone production or *deficient* hormone production. The specific pharmacotherapy depends on which portion of the adrenal gland is being affected. There are two major portions of the adrenal glands: the outer cortex and the inner medulla. The outer cortex releases three important classes of hormones: the *mineralocorticoids*, *glucocorticoids*, and *androgens*. Collectively, these hormones are referred to as **corticosteroids** or *adrenocortical hormones*.

Control of corticosteroids begins with corticotropin-releasing factor (CRF), secreted by the hypothalamus. CRF travels to the pituitary, where it causes the release of **adrenocorticotropic hormone (ACTH)**. ACTH then travels through the bloodstream and reaches the adrenal cortex, causing the adrenal gland to release cortisol and other important corticosteroids. When the level of corticosteroids in the bloodstream rises, it provides negative feedback to the hypothalamus and pituitary to shut off further release of corticosteroids. This negative feedback mechanism is shown in Figure 32.4 ■.

Aldosterone accounts for most of the **mineralocorticoids** secreted by the adrenal glands. Mineralocorticoids regulate the extracellular concentrations of mineral salts, particularly sodium and potassium, in the body. Aldosterone is the principle mineralocorticoid. The primary function of aldosterone is to regulate plasma volume by promoting sodium reabsorption and potassium secretion by the renal tubules. When plasma volume falls, the kidney secretes renin, which results in the production of angiotensin II. Angiotensin II then causes aldosterone secretion, which promotes sodium retention (*hypernatremia*) and water retention. Attempts to modify this pathway led to the development of the angiotensin-converting enzyme (ACE) inhibitor class of medications, which are often preferred drugs for treating hypertension and heart failure (see Chapters 18 and 19).

Cortisol is one of numerous **glucocorticoids** secreted from the outer portion, or cortex, of the adrenal gland. Glucocorticoids affect the metabolism of nearly every cell in the body. During long-term stress, these hormones increase the level of blood glucose (*hyperglycemia*) and promote the breakdown of proteins and lipids for energy (*gluconeogenesis*). They have a potent anti-inflammatory effect and they suppress the immune response (Chapters 24 and 29).

FIGURE 32.4

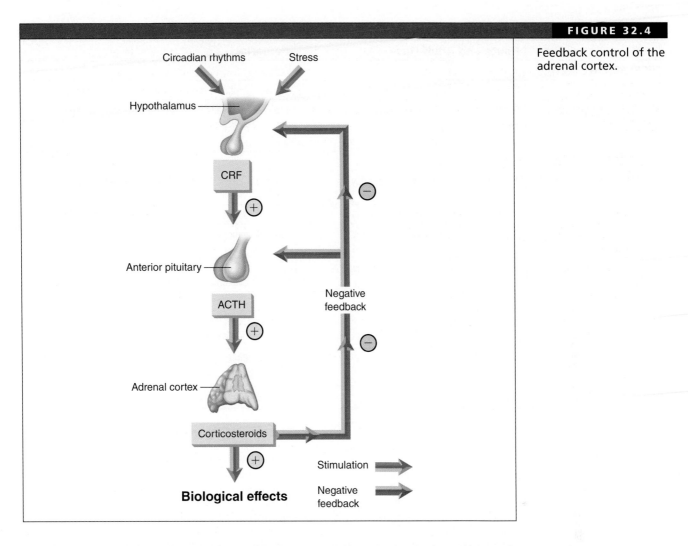

Feedback control of the adrenal cortex.

The **gonadocorticoids** secreted by the adrenal cortex are mostly androgens (male sex hormones), though small amounts of estrogens (female sex hormones) are also produced. The amounts of these hormones are far less than the levels secreted by either the testes or ovaries. The physiological effects of androgens and estrogens are detailed in Chapter 34.

gonado = *gonads (e.g., sex organs)*
andro = *male hormones*
estro = *female hormones*
gens/genesis = *synthesized*

Corticosteroids are prescribed for adrenocortical insufficiency and to dampen inflammatory and immune responses.

CORE CONCEPT 32.8

Symptoms of adrenocortical insufficiency include hypoglycemia, unusual fatigue, orthostatic hypotension, darkening skin pigmentation, joint pain, and GI disturbances such as anorexia, vomiting, and diarrhea. Low plasma levels of cortisol, accompanied by high plasma levels of ACTH indicate that the adrenal gland is not responding to ACTH stimulation. *Primary* adrenocortical insufficiency, known as **Addison's disease**, is quite rare and includes a deficiency of both glucocorticoids and mineralocorticoids. *Secondary* adrenocortical insufficiency is more common than primary and can occur when corticosteroids are suddenly withdrawn during pharmacotherapy.

When corticosteroids are taken as medications for prolonged periods, they provide negative feedback to the pituitary to stop secreting ACTH. Without stimulation by ACTH, the adrenal cortex shrinks and stops secreting endogenous corticosteroids, a condition known as **adrenal atrophy**. If the corticosteroid medication is abruptly discontinued, the shrunken adrenal glands will not be able to secrete sufficient corticosteroids, and symptoms of adrenocortical insufficiency will appear. Gradual withdrawal of corticosteroids allows adrenal glands to resume normal function. The goal of replacement therapy is to achieve the same physiologic level of corticosteroids in the blood that would be present if the adrenal glands were functioning properly. Patients requiring replacement therapy must take corticosteroids their entire lifetime, and concurrent therapy with a mineralocorticoid such as fludrocortisone (Florinef) is essential. Selected corticosteroids are listed in Table 32.4 ◆.

a = *without*
trophy = *nourishment*

TABLE 32.4 Selected Corticosteroids

Drug	Route and Adult Dose	Remarks
SHORT ACTING		
cortisone	PO; 20–300 mg/day	IM form available; has mineralocorticoid activity
℗ hydrocortisone (Cortef, Solu-Cortef)	PO; 10–320 mg/day in three to four divided doses IV/IM; 15–800 mg/day in three to four divided doses (max: 2 g/day)	Topical form available; has both glucocorticoid and mineralocorticoid activity
INTERMEDIATE ACTING		
methylprednisolone (Depo-Medrol, Medrol, others)	PO; 2–60 mg one to four times per day	IV and IM forms available; has little mineralocorticoid activity
prednisolone	PO; 5–60 mg one to four times per day	IV and IM forms available; has little mineralocorticoid activity
prednisone (see page 369 for the Prototype Drug box)	PO; 5–60 mg one to four times per day	Has little mineralocorticoid activity
triamcinolone (Aristospan, Kenalog)	PO; 4–48 mg one to two times per day	IV, intra-articular, subcutaneous, topical, inhalation, and IM forms available; has little mineralocorticoid activity
LONG ACTING		
betamethasone (Celestone, Diprolene, others)	PO; 0.6–7.2 mg/day IM; 0.5–9 mg/day	IV, topical, and IM forms available; has little mineralocorticoid activity
dexamethasone	IM; 8–16 mg bid–qid PO; 0.25–4 mg bid–qid	IV, ophthalmic, topical, intranasal, inhalation, and IM forms available; has little mineralocorticoid activity
fludrocortisone (Florinef)	PO; 0.1–0.2 mg/day	Has strong mineralocorticoid activity

In addition to treating adrenal insufficiency, corticosteroids are prescribed for a large number of nonendocrine disorders. Their ability to suppress inflammatory and immune responses quickly and effectively gives them tremendous therapeutic utility to treat a diverse set of conditions including shock, swelling, post-transplant surgery, some cancers, allergies, asthma, inflammatory bowel disease, and some rheumatic and skin disorders.

Cushing's syndrome occurs when high levels of corticosteroids are present in the body over a prolonged period. Although hypersecretion of these hormones can be due to pituitary (due to excess ACTH) or adrenal tumors, the most common cause of Cushing's syndrome is long-term therapy with high doses of systemic corticosteroids. Signs and symptoms include adrenal atrophy, behavioral changes, changes in vision, osteoporosis, hypertension, increased risk of infections, delayed wound healing, acne, peptic ulcers, fluid retention, weight gain, and a redistribution of fat around the face (moon face) and shoulders and neck (buffalo hump).

Concept Review **32.2**

■ Why does administration of corticosteroids for extended periods result in adrenal atrophy?

Drug Prototype: **℗** *Hydrocortisone (Cortef, Hydrocortone, Others)*

Therapeutic Class: Adrenal hormone replacement; drug for moderate to severe asthma and allergies, and antineoplastic therapy **Pharmacologic Class: Systemic corticosteroid**

Actions and Uses: Structurally identical to the natural hormone cortisol, hydrocortisone is a synthetic corticosteroid that is the drug of choice for treating adrenocortical insufficiency. When used for replacement therapy, it is given at physiologic doses. Once proper dosing is achieved, its therapeutic effects should mimic those of natural corticosteroids. Hydrocortisone is also available for the treatment of inflammation, allergic disorders, and many other conditions. Intra-articular injections may be given to decrease severe inflammation in affected joints.

Adverse Effects and Interactions: When used at physiologic doses for replacement therapy, adverse effects of hydrocortisone should not be evident. The patient and the healthcare professional must be vigilant, however, in observing for signs of Cushing's syndrome, which can develop with high doses. If taken for longer than two weeks, hydrocortisone should be discontinued gradually.

Hydrocortisone interacts with many drugs. For example, barbiturates, phenytoin, and rifampin may increase liver metabolism, thus decreasing hydrocortisone levels. Estrogens increase the effects of hydrocortisone. Nonsteroidal anti-inflammatory drugs (NSAIDs) increase the risk of ulcers. Cholestyramine and colestipol decrease hydrocortisone absorption. Diuretics and amphotericin B increase hypokalemia. Anticholinesterase drugs may produce severe weakness. Hydrocortisone may cause a decrease in immune response to vaccines and toxoids.

Herbal supplements, such as aloe and buckthorn (a laxative), may cause potassium deficiency.

NURSING PROCESS FOCUS Patients Receiving Systemic Corticosteroid Therapy

ASSESSMENT	POTENTIAL NURSING DIAGNOSES
Prior to administration: ■ Obtain a complete health history, including cardiovascular, respiratory, neurological, renal, and liver conditions; pregnancy, allergies, drug history, and possible drug interactions. ■ Evaluate laboratory blood findings: CBC, electrolytes, glucose, lipid panel, renal and liver function studies. ■ Acquire the results of a complete physical examination, including vital signs, height, and weight.	■ *Risk for Infection* related to immunosuppression ■ *Risk for Injury* related to adverse effects of drug therapy ■ *Deficient Knowledge* related to a lack of information about drug therapy ■ *Risk for Fluid Volume Excess* related to fluid retention properties of corticosteroids ■ *Risk for Electrolyte Imbalance* related to adverse drug effects of drug therapy ■ *Risk for Impaired Blood Glucose* related to adverse effects of drug therapy

PLANNING: PATIENT GOALS AND EXPECTED OUTCOMES

The patient will:
■ Experience therapeutic effects (decreased signs and symptoms of inflammation or allergic response).
■ Be free from or experience minimal adverse effects from drug therapy.
■ Verbalize an understanding of the drug's use, adverse effects, and required precautions.

IMPLEMENTATION

Interventions and (Rationales)	Patient Education/Discharge Planning
■ Administer medication correctly and evaluate the patient's knowledge of proper administration. Do not stop drug abruptly; tamper off over a one- to two-week period. Monitor the patient's compliance with the drug regimen. (Improper use can cause an increase in adverse effects. Sudden discontinuation of these drugs can precipitate an adrenal crisis/insufficiency.)	Instruct the patient to: ■ Not stop taking corticosteroids abruptly and to notify the healthcare provider if unable to take drug for more than one day ■ Use the self-administering tapering dose pack properly. ■ Take oral medications with food.
■ Monitor vital signs. (Corticosteroids may cause increase in blood pressure and tachycardia because of increased blood volume and potential vasoconstriction effect.)	Instruct the patient: ■ To report tachycardia, blood pressure over 140/90, dizziness, palpitations, or headaches to the healthcare provider. ■ How to use blood pressure monitoring equipment properly.
■ Monitor for infection. Protect the patient from potential infections. (Corticosteroids increase susceptibility to infections by suppressing the immune response.)	Instruct the patient to: ■ Avoid people with infections. ■ Report signs of infection: fever, cough, sore throat, joint pain, increased weakness, rash, white patches in mouth, and malaise to the healthcare provider. ■ Consult with the healthcare provider before taking any immunizations.
■ Monitor for symptoms of Cushing's syndrome, such as moon face, "buffalo hump" contour of shoulders, weight gain, muscle wasting, and increased deposits of fat in the trunk. (Symptoms may indicate excessive use of corticosteroids.)	Instruct the patient: ■ To weigh self daily. ■ That initial weight gain is expected; provide the patient with weight-gain parameters that warrant reporting. ■ That there are multiple adverse effects to therapy and that changes in health status should be reported to the healthcare provider.
■ Monitor blood glucose levels. (Corticosteroids cause an increase in glucose formation [gluconeogenesis] and a decrease in glucose utilization causing hyperglycemia.)	Instruct the patient to: ■ Report symptoms of hyperglycemia, such as excessive thirst, copious urination, and insatiable appetite to the healthcare provider. ■ Adjust insulin dose based on blood glucose level, as directed by the healthcare provider.
■ Monitor skin and mucous membranes for lacerations, abrasions, or breaks in integrity. (Corticosteroids impair wound healing.)	Instruct the patient to: ■ Examine skin daily for cuts and scrapes and to cover any injuries with sterile bandage. ■ Watch for symptoms of skin infection such as redness, swelling, and drainage. ■ Notify the healthcare provider of any nonhealing wound or symptoms of infection.
■ Monitor GI status: evidence of ulcers, GI bleeding. (Corticosteroids decrease gastric mucus production and predispose patients to peptic ulcers.)	Instruct the patient to ■ Report GI adverse effects such as heartburn, dizziness, abdominal pain, blood in emesis, or tarry stools to the healthcare provider. ■ Take drug with food or milk to decrease GI irritation. ■ Avoid or eliminate alcohol.

continued . . .

Interventions and (Rationales)	Patient Education/Discharge Planning
■ Continue to monitor periodic laboratory work: CBC, electrolytes glucose, lipid panel, liver and renal function studies. (Corticosteroids can cause hypernatremia and hypokalemia.)	Instruct the patient to: ■ Consume a diet high in protein, calcium, and potassium but low in fat and concentrated simple carbohydrates. ■ Keep all laboratory appointments.
■ Monitor changes in the musculoskeletal system. (Corticosteroids decrease bone density and strength and cause muscle atrophy and weakness.)	Instruct the patient: ■ That the drug may cause weakness in bones and muscles; avoid strenuous activity that may cause injury. ■ To participate in weight-bearing exercise or physical activity to help maintain bone and muscle strength. ■ To maintain adequate calcium in diet.
■ Monitor emotional status. (Corticosteroids may produce mood and behavior changes such as depression or feeling of invulnerability.)	■ Instruct the patient that mood changes may be expected and to report excessive mood swings or unusual changes in mood to the healthcare provider.
■ Monitor vision periodically. (Corticosteroids may cause increased intraocular pressure and an increased risk of glaucoma and cataracts.)	Inform the patient to: ■ Have regular eye exams twice a year. ■ Immediately report any eye pain, halos, inability to focus, or diminished or blurring vision to the healthcare provider.
■ Weigh patient daily and report increasing peripheral edema. (Daily weight is an accurate measure of fluid status.)	■ Instruct the patient to weigh self daily at the same time every day and to report a gain of two pounds per day or presence of or increase in edema.

EVALUATION OF OUTCOME CRITERIA

Evaluate the effectiveness of drug therapy by confirming that patient goals and expected outcomes have been met (see "Planning"). *See Table 32.4 for a list of drugs to which these nursing actions apply.*

PATIENTS NEED TO KNOW

Patients treated for endocrine disorders need to know the following:

Regarding Hypothalamic and Pituitary Drugs
1. Patients taking GH should record height and weight weekly. Records should be brought to the healthcare provider each visit.
2. A diary of nighttime sleep habits and any bed-wetting should be kept and provided to the healthcare provider.
3. Patients should be aware of drug costs, especially when taking ADH and GH drugs.

Regarding Thyroid Medications
4. Pulse rates should be taken regularly because they are a good indicator of the effectiveness of thyroid medications. If the pulse rate consistently exceeds 100 or any other significant change is noted, contact the healthcare provider.
5. Because finding the correct dosage of thyroid hormone often takes several months, do not change the prescribed dose without being advised to do so by a healthcare provider.

Regarding Corticosteroids
6. When taking oral corticosteroids for more than two weeks, do not miss doses or discontinue the drug without consulting a healthcare provider.
7. See a physician if any infections, cuts, or injuries appear to be healing too slowly while on corticosteroids.
8. If taking hydrocortisone for replacement therapy, take the medication between 6:00 a.m. and 9:00 a.m. because this is the time when natural corticosteroids are released.

CHAPTER REVIEW

CORE CONCEPTS SUMMARY

32.1 The endocrine system maintains homeostasis by using hormones as chemical messengers.

Hormones are secreted by endocrine glands in response to changes in the internal environment. The hormones act on their target cells to return the body to homeostasis. Negative feedback prevents the body from overresponding to internal changes.

32.2 The hypothalamus and the pituitary gland secrete hormones that control other endocrine organs.

The hypothalamus secretes releasing hormones that signal the anterior pituitary gland to release its hormones. Pituitary hormones travel throughout the body to affect many other organs.

32.3 Hormones are used as replacement therapy, as antineoplastics, or as "antihormones" to block endogenous actions.

Hormones are often given as replacement therapy to patients who are not able to secrete sufficient quantities of endogenous hormones. In high doses, several hormones may be used as antineoplastics. Hormones may also be used therapeutically to block natural physiologic effects.

32.4 Of the many pituitary and hypothalamic hormones, several have clinical applications as drugs.

Growth hormone, or somatotropin, is used to increase the height of children with growth hormone deficiencies. ADH, or vasopressin, increases water reabsorption in the kidney and is used to treat diabetes insipidus.

32.5 The thyroid gland controls the basal metabolic rate and affects virtually every cell in the body.

TSH released from the pituitary gland stimulates release of thyroid hormone. The thyroid gland secretes thyroid hormone, which is essential for normal growth and development. Adequate hormone levels are necessary for infants, children, and adults. Thyroid hormone is a combination of two different hormones, thyroxine and triiodothyronine, both of which require iodine for their synthesis.

32.6 Thyroid disorders may be treated by administering thyroid hormone or by decreasing the activity of the thyroid gland.

Hypothyroidism produces symptoms such as slowed body metabolism, slurred speech, bradycardia, weight gain, low body temperature, and intolerance to cold environments. Administration of thyroid hormone reverses these effects. Hyperthyroid patients exhibit the opposite symptoms. Hyperthyroidism may be treated with drugs that kill or inactivate thyroid cells.

32.7 Corticosteroids are released during periods of stress and influence carbohydrate, lipid, and protein metabolism in most cells.

The adrenal cortex secretes corticosteroids in response to stimulation by ACTH from the pituitary gland. Corticosteroids affect the metabolism of nearly every cell in the body and have potent anti-inflammatory effects.

32.8 Corticosteroids are prescribed for adrenocortical insufficiency and to dampen inflammatory and immune responses.

Corticosteroids are given to patients whose adrenal glands are unable to produce adequate amounts of these hormones and for a wide variety of other conditions. When used at high doses, oral therapy is limited because of the potential for producing Cushing's syndrome and adrenal atrophy.

REVIEW QUESTIONS

The following questions are written in NCLEX-PN® style. Answer these questions to assess your knowledge of the chapter material, and go back and review any material that is not clear to you.

1. The patient, who has been diagnosed with adrenal insufficiency, has been started on corticosteroids. The nurse explains that at high doses, and for long periods of time, these drugs may cause symptoms like those seen in _____.

1. Cushing's syndrome
2. Graves' disease
3. Diabetes insipidus
4. Diabetes mellitus

2. The nurse is assisting a patient with chronic adrenal insufficiency to make a medication plan for an upcoming camping trip. He is taking hydrocortisone (Cortef) and fludrocortisones (Florinef) as replacement therapy. Which detail does this patient need to remember?

1. Take his blood pressure once or twice a day.
2. Avoid crowded indoor areas to avoid infections.
3. Have his vision check before he leaves.
4. Make sure to carry extra medication in case there is a delay in getting home.

3. A patient is being treated with propylthiouracil (PTU) for hyperthyroidism while awaiting a thyroidectomy. While the patient is taking this drug, what symptoms will the nurse tell the patient to report to the healthcare provider?

1. Tinnitus, altered taste, thickened saliva
2. Insomnia, nightmares, night sweats
3. Sore throat, chills, low-grade fever
4. Dry eyes, decreased blinking, reddened conjunctiva

4. The physician ordered Vasopressin 5 units subcutaneously, bid, for a patient. The pharmacy has Vasopressin 20 units/mL. How many milliliters will the nurse administer per dose?

1. 0.5 mL
2. 0.25 mL
3. 0.75 mL
4. 1 mL

5. The patient has been on methylprednisolone (Medrol) for an exacerbation of asthma. Which of the following instructions to the patient is of the highest priority?

1. "This medication may cause weight gain."
2. "Do not stop taking this medication abruptly."
3. "This medication can cause sleeplessness."
4. "This medication may cause restlessness."

6. An older adult with chronic bronchitis has been taking a low dose of dexamethasone for several months. In order to reduce the risk of osteoporosis, an adverse effect, the nurse informs the patient to: (Select all that apply.)

1. Perform weight-bearing exercises at least three to four times a week.
2. Increase dietary intake of calcium and vitamin D enriched foods.
3. Remain sedentary except during periods of exercise.
4. Increase fluid intake, including carbonated sodas, but avoid alcohol.

7. A patient will be started on desmopressin (DDAVP) for treatment of diabetes insipidus. Which instruction should the nurse include in the patient teaching plan?

1. Drink plenty of fluids, especially those high in calcium.
2. Avoid close contact with children or pregnant women for one week after administration of the drug.
3. Obtain and record your weight daily.
4. Wear a mask if around children and pregnant women.

8. The patient has been started on desmopressin (DDAVP). The nurse understands the medication is effective when the patient's.

1. Urinary output increases.
2. Blood pressure falls below 90/60.
3. Blood sugar level is between 80 and 120 mg/dL.
4. Urinary output decreases.

9. The nurse will be talking with the parents of a child who has been prescribed somatropin (Humatrope). The nurse should inform the parents that:

1. The drug must be given by injection.
2. The drug must be given regularly to prevent mental deficiencies.
3. If the drug is given during late adolescence, it could add 6 to 8 inches to the child's height.
4. Daily laboratory monitoring will be required during the first weeks of therapy.

10. A nurse is helping to prepare a teaching plan for a patient who will be discharged on methylprednisolone (Medrol Dosepak) after a significant response to poison ivy. The nurse includes which of the following information about the adverse effects of this medication: (Select all that apply.)

1. Tinnitus
2. Edema
3. Visual changes
4. Lower abdominal pain

CASE STUDY QUESTIONS

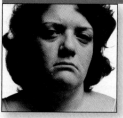

Remember Mrs. Brookfield, the patient introduced at the beginning of the chapter? Now read the remainder of the case study. Based on the information you have learned in this chapter, answer the questions that follow.

Mrs. Helen Brookfield is a 42-year-old mother of two children who works full time at a department store. She has been feeling very tired, gaining weight, and says she feels cold all the time. Because of this, she saw the doctor several weeks ago. At that visit, the physician ordered some laboratory tests including T3, T4, and TSH. She has returned to the office today to discuss her continuing symptoms and lab results. Her vital signs are 94/60, 58 (pulse), and a temperature of 36.3°C (97.4°F). Her weight has increased 30 pounds over the past 6 months, but she says that her appetite has decreased. The symptoms and lab results indicate that she has hypothyroidism. She is prescribed levothyroxine (Synthroid) 100 mcg/day.

1. The nurse explains to Mrs. Brookfield that the adverse effects of levothyroxine (Synthroid) are: (Select all that apply.)

1. Constipation
2. Weight gain
3. Tachycardia
4. Insomnia

2. The nurse also instructs Mrs. Brookfield:

1. To take the pill in the afternoon with a high fiber snack to prevent stomach upset
2. To eat plenty of fruits and vegetables to replace nutrients
3. To take the dose in the morning before breakfast, as close to the same time each day as possible
4. That the drug may be taken every other day if diarrhea occurs

3. Mrs. Brookfield has been on levothyroxine (Synthroid) 100 mcg/day. The nurse recognizes the medication is being effective when the:

1. Patient sleeps more hours per day.
2. Patient's weight increases.
3. Patient's pulse rate increases.
4. Patient states she feels tired.

4. A month later, Mrs. Brookfield reports feeling nervous and is having occasional palpations and tremors. The nurse recognizes that these symptoms may indicate that:

1. Mrs. Brookfield is still experiencing symptoms of hypothyroidism and the dose may need to be increased.
2. Mrs. Brookfield's thyroid is now functioning normally and levothyroxine is no longer needed.
3. Mrs. Brookfield has developed diabetes and needs further evaluation.
4. Mrs. Brookfield is experiencing symptoms of hyperthyroidism and the drug dosage needs to be decreased.

NOTE: Answers to the Review and Case Study Questions appear in Appendix B. The complete rationales and answers are located on the textbook's website.

Pearson Nursing Student Resources

Find additional review materials at **nursing.pearsonhighered.com**.

"I've always felt OK but recently I've been feeling sluggish. Now I learn that my sugar levels are high."

Mr. Brian Jones

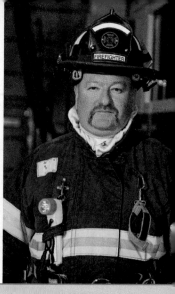

33 Drugs for Diabetes Mellitus

CORE CONCEPTS

33.1 The pancreas is responsible for the regulation of blood glucose levels.

33.2 Type 1 diabetes is caused by a deficiency in insulin.

33.3 Insulin replacement therapy is required for type 1 diabetes.

33.4 Type 2 diabetes is the most common form of the disorder.

33.5 Antidiabetic drugs are prescribed after diet and exercise have failed to reduce blood glucose to normal levels.

DRUG SNAPSHOT

The following drugs are discussed in this chapter:

DRUG CLASSES	DRUG PROTOTYPES
Insulin	**Pr** regular insulin (Humulin R, Novolin R) *532*
Antidiabetic drugs for Type 2 diabetes	**Pr** metformin (Fortamet, Glucophage, Glumetza, others) *537*

LEARNING OUTCOMES

After reading this chapter, the student should be able to:

1. Explain how blood glucose levels are maintained within narrow limits by insulin and glucagon.

2. Explain the cause of type 1 diabetes mellitus.

3. Compare and contrast types of insulin.

4. Describe the signs and symptoms of insulin overdose and underdose.

5. Explain the cause of type 2 diabetes mellitus.

6. Compare and contrast the drug classes used to treat type 2 diabetes mellitus.

7. For each of the classes listed in the Drug Snapshot, identify representative drug examples and explain their mechanisms of drug action, primary actions, and important adverse effects.

KEY TERMS

diabetic ketoacidosis (DKA) (KEY-toe-assi-doh-sis) *530*

diabetic ketoacids (KEY-toe-ass-ids) *530*

glucagon (GLUE-kah-gon) *529*

hyperglycemic effect (hi-pur-gli-SEEM-ik) *529*

hypoglycemic effect (hi-po-gli-SEEM-ik) *529*

incretin–glucose control mechanism *537*

incretins (EN-kreh-tenz) *537*

insulin (IN-sule-in) *529*

insulin analogs (ANNAH-logs) *531*

insulin resistance *534*

islets of Langerhans (EYE-lits of LANG-gur-hans) *529*

type 1 diabetes mellitus (die-uh-BEE-tees MEL-uh-tiss) *530*

type 2 diabetes mellitus *534*

Diabetes is one of the leading causes of death in the United States. Mortality due to diabetes has been steadily increasing, causing concern among public health officials and the general public. Diabetes can lead to serious complications, including heart disease, stroke, blindness, kidney failure, and amputations. Since healthcare providers frequently care for patients with diabetes, it is imperative that its treatment and possible complications are well understood.

The pancreas is responsible for the regulation of blood glucose levels.

Located behind the stomach and between the duodenum and spleen, the pancreas is an organ that is essential to function of both the digestive and the endocrine systems. It is responsible for the secretion of enzymes that assist in the chemical digestion of nutrients in the duodenum. This is the *exocrine* function of the pancreas. Clusters of cells in the pancreas, called **islets of Langerhans**, are responsible for the secretion of hormones, glucagon, and insulin. This is the pancreas' *endocrine* function (Figure 33.1 ■).

exo = *out/away from*
crine = *to secrete*

endo = *within*

Glucose is one of the body's most essential molecules. The body prefers to use glucose as its primary energy source: The brain relies almost exclusively on glucose for its energy needs. Because of this need, blood levels of glucose must remain relatively constant throughout the day. Although many factors contribute to maintaining a stable blood glucose level, the two pancreatic hormones play major roles: **insulin** acts to *decrease* blood glucose levels and **glucagon** acts to *increase* blood glucose levels (Figure 33.2 ■).

gluco = *glucose*

Following a meal, the pancreas recognizes the rising blood glucose level and releases insulin. Without insulin, glucose stays in the bloodstream and is not able to enter cells of the body. Cells may be virtually surrounded by glucose but they are unable to use it until insulin arrives. Insulin acts like a gateway for the entry of glucose into the cell. Thus, insulin is said to have a **hypoglycemic effect**, because its presence causes glucose to *leave* the bloodstream, and therefore blood glucose *falls*. Some of the glucose is stored as glycogen in the liver, where it can be converted back to glucose between meals.

hypo = *lowered*
glyc = *sugar*
emic = *blood*

The pancreas also secretes glucagon, which has the *opposite* effect of insulin. When levels of blood glucose fall, glucagon is secreted. Glucagon's primary function is to maintain adequate blood levels of glucose between meals. Thus, glucagon has a **hyperglycemic effect**, because it causes glucose in the bloodstream to *rise*. The physiological actions of glucagon are essentially opposite of insulin.

hyper = *elevated*

TYPE 1 DIABETES MELLITUS

Type 1 diabetes is caused by a deficiency in insulin.

Diabetes mellitus (DM) is a metabolic disorder in which there is deficient insulin secretion or decreased sensitivity of insulin receptors on target cells. Without insulin present, glucose is prevented from entering the cells and builds to high levels in the blood; thus, hyperglycemia is the hallmark characteristic of DM. The causes of DM include a combination of genetic and environmental factors. The recent increase in the frequency of the disease is probably the result of trends toward more inactive and stressful lifestyles and increasing consumption of foods with higher calories. According to the International Diabetes Federation, diabetes and obesity are among the biggest public health challenges of the 21st century.

FIGURE 33.1

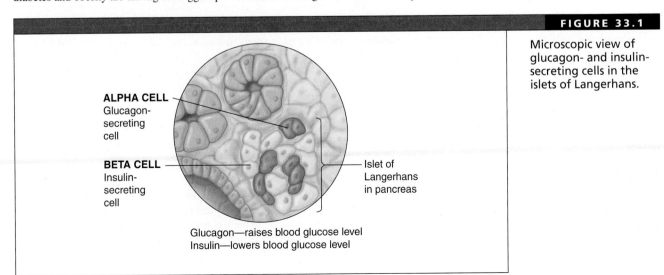

Microscopic view of glucagon- and insulin-secreting cells in the islets of Langerhans.

ALPHA CELL Glucagon-secreting cell

BETA CELL Insulin-secreting cell

Islet of Langerhans in pancreas

Glucagon—raises blood glucose level
Insulin—lowers blood glucose level

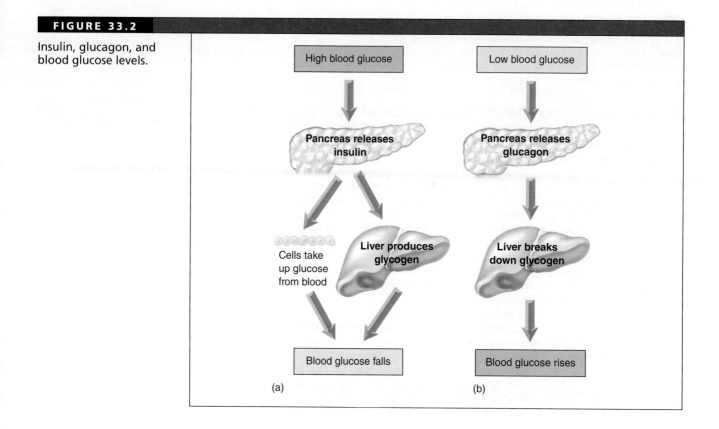

FIGURE 33.2

Insulin, glucagon, and blood glucose levels.

Fast Facts Diabetes Mellitus

- Of the 26 million Americans over age 20 who have diabetes, 7 million are unaware that they have the disease.
- Gestational diabetes affects about 5% to 10% of all pregnant women in the United States each year.
- Diabetes is the seventh leading cause of death; the risk of death among people with diabetes is twice that of people of similar age without diabetes.
- Diabetes is the leading cause of blindness in adults.
- Diabetes is responsible for 60% of nontraumatic lower-limb amputations; over 65,000 amputations are performed each year on patients with diabetes.

dia = *through (e.g., siphon)*
betes = *to go*
mellitus = *sweet*

Type 1 diabetes mellitus is one of the most common diseases of childhood. Type 1 DM was previously called *juvenile-onset diabetes*. It is often diagnosed in children between the ages of 11 and 13. Because approximately one-fourth of patients with type 1 DM develop the disease in adulthood, this is not the most accurate name for this disorder. This type of diabetes is also sometimes referred to as *insulin-dependent diabetes mellitus* because with this disorder the pancreas *does not produce insulin*.

The signs and symptoms of type 1 DM are consistent from patient to patient. The typical signs and symptoms are fasting blood glucose greater than 126 mg/dL on at least two separate occasions, polyuria (excessive urination), polyphagia (increased hunger), polydipsia (increased thirst), glucosuria (high levels of glucose in the urine), weight loss, and fatigue.

poly = *excessive*
phagia = *hunger*
dipsia = *thirst*

glucos = *glucose*
uria = *urination*

keto = *ketone chemical compound (e.g., acetone)*
acids/acidosis = *state of lowered pH*

When glucose is unable to enter cells, lipids are used as the primary energy source and **ketoacids** are produced as waste products. These ketoacids can give the patient's breath an acetone-like, fruity odor. More importantly, high levels of ketoacids lower the pH of the blood, causing **diabetic ketoacidosis (DKA)**. Untreated DM produces long-term damage to arteries, which leads to heart disease, stroke, kidney disease, and blindness. Lack of adequate circulation to the feet may cause gangrene of the toes, requiring amputation. Nerve degeneration, or neuropathy, is common, with symptoms ranging from tingling in the fingers or toes to complete loss of sensation of a limb.

Insulin replacement therapy is required for type 1 diabetes.

Patients with type 1 DM are severely deficient in insulin production; thus, insulin replacement therapy is required in normal physiological amounts. Insulin is also required for those with type 2 diabetes who are unable to manage their blood glucose levels with diet, exercise, and antidiabetic drugs.

Because normal insulin secretion varies greatly in response to daily activities such as eating and exercise, glucose monitoring and insulin administration must be carefully planned along with proper meal planning and lifestyle habits. The desired outcome of insulin therapy is to prevent the long-term consequences of the disorder by strictly maintaining blood glucose levels within the normal range. Poor compliance (not properly monitoring glucose levels or skipping insulin injections) can lead to continuing hyperglycemia and even death. Illness and stress can also cause an increase in blood glucose levels.

Many types of insulin are available, differing in their source, time of onset and peak effect, and duration of action. Until the 1980s, the source of all insulin was beef or pork pancreas. Almost all insulin today, however, is human insulin obtained through recombinant DNA technology because it is more effective, causes fewer allergies, and has a lower incidence of resistance. Pharmacologists have modified human insulin to create forms that have a more rapid onset of action or a more prolonged duration of action. These modified forms are called **insulin analogs**. All the different types of insulin are administered by the subcutaneous route and are listed in Table 33.1 ◆.

Doses of insulin are highly individualized for the precise control of blood glucose levels in each patient. Some patients require two or more injections daily for proper diabetes management. If mixing insulin, such as rapid or short acting with an intermediate acting, the rapid or short-acting insulin is always drawn into the syringe first. For ease of administration, some of these combinations are marketed in cartridges containing premixed solutions:

- Humulin 70/30 and Novolin 70/30: contain 70% NPH insulin and 30% regular insulin
- Humulin 50/50: contains 50% NPH insulin and 50% regular insulin
- NovoLog Mix 70/30: contains 70% insulin aspart protamine and 30% insulin aspart
- Humalog Mix 75/25: contains 75% insulin lispro protamine and 25% insulin lispro

Some patients may have an insulin pump (Figure 33.3 ■). This pump is usually abdominally anchored and is programmed to release small subcutaneous doses of insulin into the abdomen at predetermined intervals, with larger amounts administered manually at mealtime if necessary. Most pumps contain an alarm that sounds to remind patients to take their insulin.

Adverse effects of insulin may include allergic reactions, redness at the site of injection, and changes in fat tissue (lipodystrophy) in the areas of body where injections are given more frequently. However, the most common adverse effect of insulin therapy is overtreatment: when insulin removes too much glucose

TABLE 33.1 Types of Insulin: Actions and Administration					
Drug	**Action**	**Onset**	**Peak**	**Duration**	**Administration**
insulin aspart (NovoLog)	Rapid	15 minutes	1–3 hours	3–5 hours	Subcutaneous; 5–10 minutes before a meal
insulin lispro (Humalog)	Rapid	5–15 minutes	0.5–1 hours	3–4 hours	Subcutaneous; 5–10 minutes before a meal
insulin glulisine (Apidra)	Rapid	15–30 minutes	1 hours	3–4 hours	Subcutaneous; 15 minutes before a meal or within 20 minutes after starting a meal
insulin regular (Humulin R, Novolin R)	Short	30–60 minutes	2–4 hours	5–7 hours	Subcutaneous; 30–60 minutes before a meal; IV in emergencies
insulin isophane (NPH, Humulin N, Novolin N, ReliOn N)	Intermediate	1–2 hours	4–12 hours	18 24 hours	Subcutaneous; 30 minutes before first meal of the day and 30 minutes before evening meal, if necessary
insulin detemir (Levemir)	Long	Gradual: over 24 hours	6–8 hours	To 24 hours	Subcutaneous; with evening meal or at bedtime
insulin glargine (Lantus)	Long	Gradual; over 24 hours	N/A	To 24 hours	Subcutaneous; once daily, given at the same time each day

FIGURE 33.3

Insulin pump programmed to release insulin at predetermined intervals throughout the day.

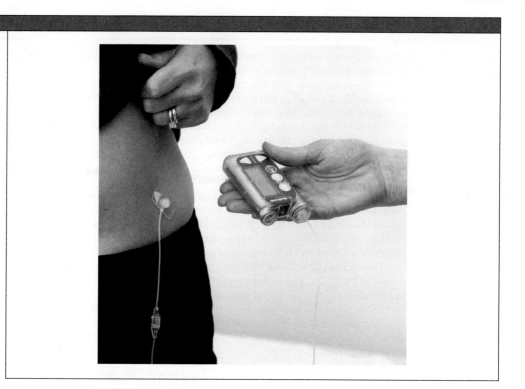

from the blood resulting in hypoglycemia. This occurs when a patient with type 1 diabetes has more insulin in the blood than is needed to balance the amount of glucose in the blood. Hypoglycemia may occur when insulin levels peak, during exercise, when the patient receives too much insulin due to medication error, or if the patient skips a meal. Signs and symptoms of hypoglycemia include the sudden onset of pale, cool, and moist skin; confusion; mild tremors; and dizziness, usually with blood glucose of less than 50 mg/dL.

Giving food or drinks containing glucose (sugar) can reverse mild to moderate hypoglycemia symptoms. Patients are encouraged to routinely carry candy or other readily absorbable carbohydrates, such as crackers, to take at the first signs of a drop in blood glucose. For serious hypoglycemia, glucose can be administered via the intravenous (IV) route. In addition, the hormone glucagon is also used in emergency treatment. Glucagon can be administered IV, IM, or subcutaneously.

Drug Prototype: ℞ *Regular Insulin (Humulin R, Novolin R)*
Therapeutic Class: Drug for diabetes mellitus   **Pharmacologic Class: Hypoglycemic drug**

Actions and Uses: Regular insulin is prepared as human insulin through recombinant DNA technology. It is classified as short-acting insulin, with an onset of action of 30 to 60 minutes, a peak effect at 2 to 3 hours, and a duration of 5 to 7 hours. Its primary action is to promote the entry of glucose into cells. For the emergency treatment of acute ketoacidosis, it may be given subcutaneously or IV. Regular insulin is also available as Humulin 70/30 (a mixture of 30% regular insulin and 70% isophane insulin) or as Humulin 50/50 (a mixture of 50% of both regular and isophane insulin).

Adverse Effects and Interactions: The most serious adverse effect from insulin therapy is hypoglycemia. Hypoglycemia may result from taking too much insulin, not properly timing the insulin injection with food intake, or skipping a meal. Dietary carbohydrates must be in the blood when insulin is injected; otherwise the drug will remove too much glucose, and signs of hypoglycemia—tachycardia, confusion, sweating, and drowsiness—will result. If severe hypoglycemia is not quickly treated with glucose, convulsions, coma, and death may follow.

Regular insulin interacts with many drugs. For example, the following substances may increase hypoglycemic effects: alcohol, salicylates, monoamine oxidase inhibitors (MAOIs), and anabolic steroids. The following substances may decrease hypoglycemic effects: corticosteroids, thyroid hormones, and epinephrine. Serum glucose levels may be increased with furosemide or thiazide diuretics. Symptoms of hypoglycemic reaction may be hidden if beta blockers are used at the same time.

Use cautiously with herbal supplements such as garlic and ginseng, which may increase the hypoglycemic effects of insulin.

NURSING PROCESS FOCUS   Patients Receiving Insulin Therapy

ASSESSMENT	POTENTIAL NURSING DIAGNOSES
Prior to administration: ■ Obtain a complete health history, including cardiovascular, vision, skin, neurological, renal, and liver conditions; allergies; drug history; and possible drug interactions. ■ Evaluate laboratory blood findings: CBC, electrolytes, lipid panel, liver and renal function studies, glucose, and HbA1$_C$. ■ Acquire the results of a complete physical examination, including vital signs, height, and weight; presence of paresthesia of hands or feet; ulceration of lower extremities; and condition of skin at insulin injection sites. ■ Obtain a dietary history including caloric intake if on ADA diet, number of meals and snacks, fluid type, and amount of intake. ■ Determine knowledge of diabetic medications, adverse effects, self-administration, and blood glucose monitoring.	■ *Risk for Unstable Blood Glucose Level* related to lack of diabetes management, unhealthy diet, inadequate glucose monitoring, or improper use of medication ■ *Risk for Injury* related to blood glucose elevations, impaired circulation, or adverse effects of drug therapy ■ *Deficient Knowledge* related to a lack of information about the disease process, medications, and need for lifestyle changes ■ *Risk for Imbalanced Nutrition* related to adverse effects of drug therapy ■ *Risk for Infection* related to blood glucose elevations and impaired circulation ■ *Ineffective Therapeutic Regimen Management* related to noncompliance with medication regimen, presence of adverse effects, and lifelong need for medication ■ *Noncompliance* related to the complexity of the medication regimen, lifestyle changes, and adverse effects of drug therapy

PLANNING: PATIENT GOALS AND EXPECTED OUTCOMES

The patient will:
■ Experience therapeutic effects (stable blood glucose levels).
■ Be free from or experience minimal adverse effects from drug therapy.
■ Verbalize an understanding of the drug's use, adverse effects, and required precautions.
■ Demonstrate an understanding of lifestyle modifications necessary for successful maintenance of drug therapy.

IMPLEMENTATION

Interventions and (Rationales)	Patient Education/Discharge Planning
■ Monitor blood glucose at least several times a day, usually before meals. Hold or provide insulin per healthcare provider's protocols. (Daily glucose levels will assist in maintaining stable blood glucose.)	■ Instruct the patient how to monitor blood glucose, including use of equipment, and when to notify the healthcare provider.
■ Administer insulin as prescribed, planning administration around meal or insulin peak times. In addition, evaluate the patient's knowledge of proper administration. (Maintaining levels of insulin with meal times or peak times will assist in maintaining stable blood glucose levels.)	Inform patient or caregivers the: ■ Correct administration techniques for type of insulin ordered. Have patient return demonstration. ■ Peak insulin levels and proper food sources needed to prevent both hyper/hypoglycemia. Provide written materials for future reference. ■ Need to rotate insulin injection sites on a weekly basis to prevent tissue damage.
■ Increase frequency of blood glucose monitoring if the patient is experiencing fever, nausea, vomiting, or diarrhea. (Illness usually requires adjustments in insulin doses.)	Instruct the patient to: ■ Increase blood glucose monitoring when experiencing fever, nausea, vomiting, or diarrhea. ■ Notify the healthcare provider if unable to eat normal meals for a possible change in insulin dose.
■ Continue to monitor periodic laboratory work: CBC, electrolytes, glucose, HbA1$_C$, lipid profile, liver and renal function studies. (Insulin can cause potassium to move into the cell and may cause hypokalemia. Periodic monitoring assists in determining glucose control, need for medication changes, and any indicators of complications.)	Inform the patient: ■ About the need to keep laboratory appointments. ■ To report to the healthcare provider the first sign of heart irregularity.
■ Monitor weight on a routine basis. (Changes in weight will alter insulin needs.)	■ Instruct the patient to weigh self on a routine basis at the same time each day and to report to the healthcare provider any significant changes (e.g., plus or minus 10 lb).
■ Monitor vital signs. (Increased pulse and blood pressure are early signs of hypoglycemia. Patients with diabetes may have circulatory problems and/or impaired kidney function that can increase blood pressure.)	■ Ensure that the patient knows how to take blood pressure and pulse and to report significant changes.
■ Check for signs of hypoglycemia, especially around the time of insulin peak activity. If symptoms occur, provide quick-acting carbohydrate source (juice or simple sugar) and then recheck blood glucose. (Using a simple sugar will raise blood sugar immediately.)	Advise the patient: ■ To always carry a quick-acting carbohydrate source in case symptoms of hypoglycemia occur. ■ If unsure whether symptoms are hypo or hyper, treat as hypoglycemia, wait 10–15 minutes then check glucose level. ■ If symptoms are not relieved or glucose is below 70 mg/dL, notify the healthcare provider.

continued . . .

NURSING PROCESS FOCUS *(continued)*

Interventions and (Rationales)	Patient Education/Discharge Planning
■ Encourage patient to increase physical activity gradually but continue to monitor blood glucose level before and after exercise. (Exercise assists muscle cells to use glucose more efficiently, lowering blood glucose. Effects may last up to 48 hours after activity, increasing risk of hypoglycemia.)	Inform the patient: ■ About the benefit of exercise. ■ To check blood glucose before and after exercise and to keep a simple sugar on his or her person while exercising. ■ To eat some form of simple sugar or complex carbohydrate before strenuous exercise as prophylaxis against hypoglycemia.
■ Ensure the proper storage of insulin to maintain potency. (Unopened vials may be stored at room temperature, avoiding direct sunlight and heat. Opened vials may be stored at room temperature for up to one month. Discard if any changes in solution are noted.)	■ Inform the patient about proper storage of insulin.

EVALUATION OF OUTCOME CRITERIA

Evaluate the effectiveness of drug therapy by confirming that patient goals and expected outcomes have been met (see "Planning"). *See Table 33.1 for a list of drugs to which these nursing actions apply.*

TYPE 2 DIABETES MELLITUS

CORE CONCEPT 33.4

Type 2 diabetes is the most common form of the disorder.

Type 2 diabetes mellitus is the more common form of the disorder. Because type 2 DM first appeared in middle-aged adults, it has been referred to as *adult-onset diabetes* or *maturity-onset diabetes*. These are inaccurate descriptions of this disorder, however, because increasing numbers of children are being diagnosed with type 2 DM. Type 2 is more common in patients who are overweight and those with low HDL-cholesterol and high triglyceride levels. Patients with type 2 DM are often asymptomatic and may have the condition for years before their diagnosis.

asymptomatic = *without having symptoms*

Unlike patients with type 1 diabetes, some patients with type 2 are capable of secreting insulin, although in amounts that are too small. However, the fundamental problem in type 2 is that insulin receptors in the target tissues have become unresponsive to the hormone, a phenomenon called **insulin resistance**. Essentially, the pancreas produces sufficient amounts of insulin, but target cells do not recognize it. Whereas patients with type 1 diabetes must take insulin, those with type 2 diabetes are usually controlled with antidiabetic drugs. In severe, unresponsive cases, insulin may also be necessary for patients with type 2 diabetes.

CAM THERAPY

Omega-3 Fatty Acids and Diabetes

Omega-3 fatty acids are unsaturated fats found in fatty fish such as salmon, mackerel, and tuna; vegetables oils such as canola and soybean; and nuts, green leafy vegetables, and beans. Omega-3 fatty acids are essential to the body and necessary for regulating muscle function, blood clotting, digestion, cell growth, and other functions.

Research has clearly shown that omega-3 fatty acids reduce inflammation and lower the risk for cardiovascular disease. The research on type 2 diabetes is not as clear. Fish oils (which contain high amounts of omega-3 fatty acids) lower triglyceride levels and decrease some inflammatory markers that signal a risk for diabetes. Some studies suggest insulin sensitivity may be increased. Other research, however, suggests that supplementation with omega-3 fatty acids does not improve the risk of developing cardiovascular disease in diabetic patients. Because fish oils have the potential to raise blood sugar levels, all diabetic patients should check with their healthcare provider before taking these supplements.

In many people as they get older, cells become more resistant to insulin, blood glucose levels rise, and the pancreas responds by secreting even more insulin. Eventually, the hypersecretion of insulin causes beta cell exhaustion and ultimately leads to beta cell death. As type 2 DM progresses, it becomes a disorder characterized by insufficient insulin levels as well as insulin resistance. The long-term consequences of untreated type 1 and type 2 diabetes are the same.

The activity of insulin receptors can be increased by physical exercise and lowering the level of circulating insulin. In fact, adhering to a healthy diet and a regular exercise program has been shown to reverse insulin resistance and delay or prevent the development of type 2 DM. Many patients with type 2 diabetes are obese and need a medically supervised plan to help them reduce weight gradually and exercise safely. This is an important lifestyle change for such patients; they will need to maintain these changes for the remainder of their lives.

Antidiabetic drugs are prescribed after diet and exercise have failed to reduce blood glucose to normal levels.

CORE CONCEPT 33.5

Type 2 DM is usually controlled with noninsulin antidiabetic drugs. These drugs are sometimes referred to as *oral hypoglycemic drugs* but this is an inaccurate name because some are given by the subcutaneous route and some do not cause hypoglycemia.

The primary groups of antidiabetic drugs for type 2 DM are classified by their chemical structures and their mechanisms of action. These include alpha-glucosidase inhibitors, biguanides, incretin enhancers, meglitinides, sulfonylureas, and thiazolidinediones (or glitazones). Therapy with type 2 antidiabetic drugs is not effective for persons with type 1 DM. Antidiabetic drugs for type 2 DM are listed in Table 33.2 ◆.

incretin = *gut-derived*

TABLE 33.2   Antidiabetic Drugs for Type 2 Diabetes

Drug	Route and Adult Dose	DRUG Class Remarks
ALPHA-GLUCOSIDASE INHIBITORS		
acarbose (Precose)	PO; 25–100 mg tid (max: 300 mg/day), taken with the first bite of each meal	These drugs block an intestinal enzyme that breaks down complex carbohydrates into simple sugars. Avoid use in patients with chronic intestinal diseases; use cautiously in patients with renal impairment.
miglitol (Glyset)	PO; 25–100 mg tid (max: 300 mg/day), taken with the first bite of each meal	
BIGUANIDE		
(Pr) metformin Immediate release (Glucophage, Riomet) Extended release (Fortamet, Glucophage XR, Glumetza)	PO; 500 mg two times per day or 850 mg once daily; increase to 1,000–2,550 mg in two to three divided doses per day (max: 2.55 g/day) Fortamet: 1,000 mg once daily (max: 2.5 g/day) Glumetza: 1,000–2,000 mg once daily (max: 2 g/day) Glucophage XR: 500 mg once daily (max: 2 g/day)	Immediate-release forms and extended-release forms are available. Lactic acidosis is a potential complication with this medication.
INCRETIN ENHANCERS		
exenatide (Byetta)	Subcutaneous; 5–10 mcg one to two times per day 60 minutes prior to a meal	These drugs target a chemical called glucagon-like peptide (GLP). Insulin release is stimulated and glucagon release is inhibited. Nausea, diarrhea, headaches, and dizziness are common symptoms due to falling blood glucose levels. These drugs decrease appetite and promote weight loss. These drugs should be taken or injected prior to meals.
linagliptin (Tradjenta)	PO: 5 mg once daily	
liraglutide (Victoza)	Subcutaneous: 0.6–1.8 mg once daily	
saxagliptin (Onglyza)	PO: 2.5–5 mg once daily	
sitagliptin (Januvia)	PO; 100 mg once daily	

(continued)

TABLE 33.2 Antidiabetic Drugs for Type 2 Diabetes *(continued)*

Drug	Route and Adult Dose	DRUG Class Remarks
MEGLITINIDES		
nateglinide (Starlix)	PO; 60–120 mg tid, 1–30 minutes prior to meals	These drugs stimulate the release of insulin from pancreatic islet cells similar to sulfonylurea drugs.
repaglinide (Prandin)	PO; 0.5–4 mg bid–qid, 1–30 minutes prior to meals (max: 16 mg/day)	
SODIUM-GLUCOSE CO-TRANSPORTER 2 (SGLT2) INHIBITOR		
canagliflozin (Invokana)	PO; 100 mg taken before the first meal of the day; for additional glycemic control, may increase to 300 mg every day (patients who have an effective glomerular filtration rate of 60 mL/min/1.73 m²)	SGLT2 is an enzyme in the kidney tubule that causes glucose to be reabsorbed from urine; this drug blocks the action of SGLT2 leading to more excretion of glucose in the urine.
SULFONYLUREAS, FIRST GENERATION		
chlorpropamide (Diabinese)	PO; 100–250 mg/day (max: 750 mg/day)	These drugs stimulate the release of insulin from pancreatic islet cells. Symptoms are hypoglycemia, weight gain, GI distress, and liver toxicity.
tolazamide (Tolinase)	PO; 100–500 mg one to two times per day (max: 1 g/day)	
tolbutamide (Orinase)	PO; 250–1,500 mg one to two times per day (max: 3 g/day)	
SULFONYLUREAS, SECOND GENERATION		
glimepiride (Amaryl)	PO; 1–4 mg/day (max: 8 mg/day)	Symptoms are similar to first-generation sulfonylureas except that there are fewer drug–drug interactions. These drugs should be taken 30 minutes before breakfast.
glipizide (Glucotrol)	PO; 2.5–20 mg one to two times per day (max: 40 mg/day)	
glyburide (DiaBeta, Micronase)	PO; 1.25–10 mg one to two times per day (max: 20 mg/day)	
glyburide micronized (Glynase)	PO; 0.75–12 mg one to two times per day (max: 12 mg/day)	
THIAZOLIDINEDIONES		
pioglitazone (Actos)	PO; 15–30 mg/day (max: 45 mg/day)	Have been under review since 2007, due to the increased risk of heart failure with drugs in this class.
rosiglitazone (Avandia)	PO; 2–4 mg one to two times per day (max: 8 mg/day)	
MISCELLANEOUS DRUG		
bromocriptine (Cycloset)	PO; 0.8–4.8 mg/day upon awakening	Approved for Parkinson's disease, pituitary adenoma, acromegaly, for women with amenorrhea, and infertility caused by prolactin secretion.

The first oral hypoglycemics available, sulfonylureas are divided into first- and second-generation categories. Although drugs from both generations are equally effective at lowering blood glucose, the second-generation drugs exhibit fewer drug–drug interactions. The sulfonylureas act by stimulating the release of insulin from pancreatic islet cells and by increasing the sensitivity of insulin receptors on target cells.

Metformin (Glucophage) is the only drug in the biguanide drug class. Information on this drug is presented in the prototype feature box in this chapter.

The alpha-glucosidase inhibitors, which include acarbose (Precose) and miglitol (Glyset), act by blocking enzymes in the small intestine that are responsible for breaking down complex carbohydrates into monosaccharides. Because carbohydrates must be in the monosaccharide form to be absorbed, digestion of glucose is delayed.

The thiazolidinediones, or glitazones, reduce blood glucose by decreasing insulin resistance and by inhibiting hepatic production of glucose. Optimal lowering of blood glucose may take three to four months of therapy. Liver function should be monitored, because thiazolidinediones may be hepatotoxic. Drugs in this class contain black box warnings. In the summer of 2013, Food and Drug Administration (FDA) panel experts voted to modify or remove measures that limited patient access to rosiglitazone. Under the FDA's risk-evaluation management strategy (REMS), this drug remains under close scrutiny due to the risk of fluid retention and heart problems observed in some patients.

The meglitinides, repaglinide (Prandin) and nateglinide (Starlix), act by stimulating the release of insulin from the pancreas in a manner similar to that of the sulfonylureas. Both drugs in this class have short durations of action of two to four hours, and they are well tolerated.

Drug Prototype: Ⓟ *Metformin (Fortamet, Glucophage, Glumetza, Others)*
Therapeutic Class: Antidiabetic drug   Pharmacologic Class: Hypoglycemic drug; biguanide

Actions and Uses: Metformin is a preferred antidiabetic drug for managing type 2 DM because of its effectiveness and safety. It is used alone or in combination with other oral hypoglycemics or insulin. It is approved for use in children age 10 or above. It is available as immediate release and extended release.

Metformin reduces glucose levels by decreasing the hepatic production of glucose and reducing insulin resistance. It does not promote insulin release from the pancreas. A major advantage of the drug is that it does not cause hypoglycemia. The drug's actions do not depend on stimulating insulin release, so it is able to lower glucose levels in patients who no longer secrete insulin. In addition to lowering blood glucose levels, it lowers triglyceride and total and low-density lipoprotein (LDL) cholesterol levels, and it promotes weight loss.

Metformin is used off-label to treat women with polycystic ovary syndrome. Women with this syndrome have insulin resistance and high serum insulin levels.

Adverse Effects and Interactions: The most common adverse effects are GI related and include nausea, vomiting, abdominal discomfort, metallic taste, diarrhea, and anorexia. It may also cause headache, dizziness, agitation, and fatigue. Unlike the sulfonylureas, metformin rarely causes hypoglycemia or weight gain.

Metformin is contraindicated in patients with impaired renal function. It is also contraindicated in patients with heart failure, liver failure, history of lactic acidosis, or concurrent serious infection. It is contraindicated for two days prior to and two days after receiving IV radiographic contrast.

Alcohol increases the risk for lactic acidosis. Captopril, furosemide, and nifedipine may increase the risk for hypoglycemia. The following drugs may decrease renal excretion of metformin: amiloride, cimetidine, digoxin, dofetilide, midodrine, morphine, procainamide, quinidine, ranitidine, triamterene, trimethoprim, and vancomycin. Acarbose may decrease blood levels of metformin. Use with other antidiabetic drugs potentiates hypoglycemic effects. Metformin decreases the absorption of vitamin B_{12} and folic acid. Garlic and ginseng may increase hypoglycemic effects.

> **BLACK BOX WARNING:**
> Lactic acidosis is a rare, though potentially fatal, adverse effect of metformin therapy. The risk for lactic acidosis is increased in patients with renal insufficiency or any condition that puts them at risk for increased lactic acid production, such as liver disease, severe infection, excessive alcohol intake, shock, or hypoxemia.

Several new drugs have been approved that act by the **incretin–glucose control mechanism. Incretins** are hormones secreted by the mucosa of the small intestine following a meal, when blood glucose is elevated. Incretins signal the pancreas to increase insulin secretion and the liver to stop producing glucagon. Both of these actions lower blood glucose levels. In addition, these drugs decrease food intake by increasing the feeling of satiety (fullness), and they also delay gastric emptying, which slows glucose absorption.

hypox = *lowered oxygen*
emia = *blood levels*

satiety = *state of fullness*

Exenatide (Byetta) and liraglutide (Victoza) are injectable incretin enhancers that accomplish their actions by activating a receptor called *GLP-1*. Activation of the GLP-1 receptor causes the same types of effects as the natural incretin hormone: lowering blood glucose by increasing the secretion of insulin, slowing the absorption of glucose, and inhibiting glucagon.

The second group of incretin enhancers are given orally. Linagliptin (Tradjenta), saxagliptin (Onglyza), and sitagliptin (Januvia) prevent the breakdown of incretins, allowing hormone levels to rise. These drugs are effective at lowering blood glucose with few adverse effects. They work well with other antidiabetic drugs and do not cause hypoglycemia.

Combinations of antidiabetic drugs have been developed to maximize the therapeutic effects and minimize adverse effects. Examples of selected drug combinations are listed below:

- ACTOplus   pioglitazone/metformin
- Avandamet   rosiglitazone/metformin
- Avandaryl   rosiglitazone/glimepiride
- Duetact   pioglitazone/glimepiride
- Glucovance   glyburide/metformin
- Janumet   sitagliptin/metformin
- Jentadueto   linagliptin/metformin
- Juvisync   sitagliptin/simvastatin
- Metaglip   glipizide/metformin
- PrandiMet   repaglinide/metformin

Concept Review 33.1

- Why are noninsulin antidiabetic drugs ineffective for treating type 1 diabetes?

NURSING PROCESS FOCUS Patients Receiving Pharmacotherapy for Type 2 Diabetes

ASSESSMENT	POTENTIAL NURSING DIAGNOSES
Same as for patients receiving insulin (see page 533), so abbreviated here. Prior to administration: ■ Obtain a complete health history. ■ Evaluate laboratory blood findings. ■ Acquire the results of a complete physical examination. ■ Obtain a dietary history. ■ Determine knowledge of diabetic medications and blood glucose monitoring.	Same as for patients receiving insulin (see page 533), so abbreviated here. ■ *Risk for Unstable Blood Glucose Level* ■ *Risk for Injury* ■ *Deficient Knowledge* ■ *Risk for Imbalanced Nutrition* ■ *Risk for Infection* ■ *Ineffective Therapeutic Regimen Management* ■ *Noncompliance*

PLANNING: PATIENT GOALS AND EXPECTED OUTCOMES

The patient will:
■ Experience therapeutic effects (stable blood glucose levels).
■ Be free from or experience minimal adverse effects from drug therapy.
■ Verbalize an understanding of the drug's use, adverse effects, and required precautions.
■ Demonstrate an understanding of lifestyle modifications necessary for successful maintenance of drug therapy.

IMPLEMENTATION

Interventions and (Rationales)	Patient Education/Discharge Planning
■ Monitor blood glucose at least daily. (Daily glucose levels will assist in maintaining stable blood glucose.)	■ Instruct the patient how to monitor blood glucose, including use of equipment, and when to notify the healthcare provider.
■ Administer medication correctly (at appropriate time according to type of medication ordered) and evaluate the patient's knowledge of proper administration. (Most oral antidiabetic medications are given at or around meal times. Maintaining levels of medication will assist in maintaining stable blood glucose levels.)	Inform patient or caregivers about: ■ Correct administration time for type of medication ordered. ■ Peak medication levels and proper food sources needed to prevent both hyperglycemia and hypoglycemia. Provide written materials for future reference.
■ Monitor for signs of lactic acidosis if the patient is receiving a biguanide. (Mitochondrial oxidation of lactic acid is inhibited, and lactic acidosis may result.)	■ Instruct the patient to report signs of lactic acidosis such as hyperventilation, muscle pain, fatigue, and increased sleeping to the healthcare provider.
■ Continue to monitor periodic laboratory work: CBC, electrolytes, glucose, HbA1$_C$, lipid profile, liver and renal function studies. (Periodic monitoring assists in determining glucose control, need for medication changes and any indicators of complications. These drugs are metabolized in the liver and may cause elevations in AST and LDH.)	Instruct the patient: ■ On sulfonylureas to immediately report any nausea, vomiting, yellow skin, pale or clay colored stools, abdominal pain, or dark urine to the healthcare provider. ■ Taking biguanides to immediately report any drowsiness, malaise, decreased respiratory rate, or general body aches to the healthcare provider. ■ About the need to keep laboratory appointments.
■ Ensure dietary needs are met based on weight and current glucose levels. Avoid alcohol. (Patients taking sulfonylurea or biguanides should avoid alcohol entirely to prevent an antabuse-like reaction.)	■ Advise the patient to abstain from alcohol and to avoid liquid over-the-counter (OTC) medications, which may contain alcohol.
■ Monitor for edema, blood pressure, and lung sounds in patients taking thiazolidiones. (These drugs may cause edema and worsening heart failure.)	■ Instruct the patient to immediately report to the healthcare provider any signs of edema of the hands or feet, dyspnea or excessive fatigue.
■ Increase frequency of blood glucose monitoring if the patient is experiencing fever, nausea, vomiting, or diarrhea. (Illness may affect blood glucose levels and usually requires adjustments in medication)	■ Instruct the patient to report the first signs of fatigue, muscle weakness, and nausea. ■ Discuss the importance of adequate rest and healthy routines.
■ Check for signs of hypoglycemia, especially around the time of insulin peak activity. If symptoms occur, provide quick-acting carbohydrate source (juice or simple sugar) and then recheck blood glucose. (Using a simple sugar will raise blood sugar immediately.) Also monitor carefully patients who also take beta blockers, because early signs of hypoglycemia may not be apparent.	Inform the patient: ■ Signs and symptoms of hypoglycemia, such as hunger, irritability, sweating. ■ At first sign of hypoglycemia, to check blood glucose and eat a simple sugar; if symptoms do not improve, call 911. ■ If necessary, to monitor blood glucose before breakfast and supper. ■ Not to skip meals and to follow a diet specified by the healthcare provider.
■ Monitor weight, weighing at the same time of day each time. (Changes in weight will affect the amount of drug needed to control blood glucose.)	■ Instruct the patient to weigh each week, at the same time of day, and report any significant loss or gain.
■ Encourage patient to increase physical activity gradually but continue to monitor blood glucose level before and after exercise. (Exercise assists muscle cells to use glucose more efficiently, lowering blood glucose.)	Inform the patient: ■ About the benefit of exercise. ■ To check blood glucose before and after exercise and to keep a simple sugar on his or her person while exercising. ■ To eat some form of simple sugar or complex carbohydrate before strenuous exercise as prophylaxis against hypoglycemia.
■ Monitor hypersensitivity and allergic reactions. (Anaphylactic reactions are possible.)	■ Advise the patient of the importance of immediately reporting symptoms such as skin rashes, itching, swelling of the tongue or face, flushing, dizziness syncope wheezing, throat tightness, or shortness of breath to the healthcare provider.

continued . . .

NURSING PROCESS FOCUS *(continued)*

Interventions and (Rationales)	Patient Education/Discharge Planning
■ Determine pregnancy status. (Some oral antidiabetic medications are category C and must be stopped during pregnancy. Due to increasing the metabolic needs of pregnancy, insulin therapy may be needed.)	■ Advise female patients of childbearing age to inform the healthcare provider if pregnancy is suspected.

EVALUATION OF OUTCOME CRITERIA

Evaluate the effectiveness of drug therapy by confirming that patient goals and expected outcomes have been met (see "Planning"). *See Table 33.2 for a list of drugs to which these nursing actions apply.*

PATIENTS NEED TO KNOW

Patients treated for DM need to know the following:

1. When administering insulin, meals should not be skipped. If self-injecting insulin, carefully follow all instructions provided by the healthcare provider to avoid injury or infection. Store unopened vials of insulin in the refrigerator. Do not use after the expiration date.

2. Check with a healthcare provider before beginning a vigorous exercise program. Often, insulin doses should be reduced or extra food should be ingested just prior to intense exercise.

3. Know the time of peak action of any insulin, because that is when the risk for hypoglycemic adverse effects is greatest.

4. The right amount of insulin must be available to cells when glucose is available in the blood. Without insulin present, glucose from a meal can build up to high levels in the blood, causing hyperglycemia and possible coma.

5. When taking antidiabetic drugs, report to your healthcare provider immediately any signs of hypoglycemia, such as weakness, sweating, dizziness, tremor, anxiety, or tachycardia. Mild symptoms may be treated with small amounts of sugar in the form of candy or fruit juice.

6. Always take antidiabetic drugs the same time each day. When self-monitoring blood glucose, recall that normal values are 80–120 mg/dL before meals and 100–140 mg/dL before bedtime.

7. Read the directions for all medications very carefully because many drug–drug interactions are possible. Medications such as corticosteroids, thiazide diuretics, and sympathomimetics can raise blood glucose levels and inhibit the effects of insulin.

SAFETY ALERT

Expiration Dates on Multidose Vials

Multidose vials, such as insulin, can be kept for a specific period of time depending institutional policy and manufacturers recommendations. When a vial is punctured, it is imperative that the nurse not forget to document either the expiration date or the date it was opened on the vial label. If this is not done, the vial may not be discarded appropriately, allowing the use of a medication that may no longer be safe or effective.

Source: Institute for Safe Medication Practices

CHAPTER REVIEW

CORE CONCEPTS SUMMARY

33.1 The pancreas is responsible for the regulation of blood glucose levels.

The pancreas is both an endocrine and an exocrine gland. The islets of Langerhans are responsible for secretion of insulin and glucagon. Insulin is released when blood glucose increases, and glucagon is released when blood glucose decreases.

33.2 Type 1 diabetes is caused by a deficiency in insulin.

Type 1 DM is caused by an absolute lack of insulin secretion due to autoimmune destruction of pancreatic islet cells. If untreated, it results in serious, chronic conditions affecting the cardiovascular and nervous systems.

33.3   Insulin replacement therapy is required for type 1 diabetes.

Type 1 DM is treated by dietary restrictions, exercise, and insulin therapy. The many types of insulin preparations vary as to their onset of action, time to peak effect, and duration. Doses of insulin are highly individualized in each patient.

33.4   Type 2 diabetes is the most common form of the disorder

Type 2 DM is caused by a lack of sensitivity of insulin receptors at the target cells and a deficiency in insulin secretion. If untreated, the same chronic conditions result as in type 1 DM. Most people with type 2 DM are older adults; more obese children and adolescents are being diagnosed.

33.5   Antidiabetic drugs are prescribed after diet and exercise have failed to reduce blood glucose to normal levels.

Type 2 DM is controlled through lifestyle changes and oral hypoglycemic drugs. Various classes of drugs are available for the pharmacotherapy of type 2 DM: alpha-glucosidase inhibitors, biguanides, incretin enhancers, meglitinides, sulfonylureas, and thiazolidinediones (or glitazones). Combinations of antidiabetic drugs maximize therapeutic effects and minimize adverse effects.

REVIEW QUESTIONS

The following questions are written in NCLEX-PN® style. Answer these questions to assess your knowledge of the chapter material, and go back and review any material that is not clear to you.

1. While collecting information from a patient, the nurse notes which of the following symptoms of type I diabetes? (Select all that apply.)

1. Polyphagia
2. Polyuria
3. Polydipsia
4. Weight gain

2. When giving insulin, the nurse plans on administering it by what route?

1. Oral
2. Intradermal
3. Subcutaneous
4. Intramuscular

3. A patient, who has just been prescribed an incretin enhancer (oral hypoglycemic medication), asks the nurse how it works. The nurse informs the patient that these types of medications:

1. Decrease the uptake of glucose by body cells.
2. Stimulate insulin release from the pancreas.
3. Increase insulin production by the pancreas.
4. Decrease the amount of insulin produced by the pancreas.

4. A patient receives NPH and regular insulin every morning. The nurse, verifying that the patient understands that there are two different peak times to be aware of for this insulin combination, questions the patient because:

1. The patient needs to plan the next insulin injection around the peak times.
2. Additional insulin may be needed at peak times to avoid hyperglycemia.
3. It is best to plan exercise or other activities around the peak insulin activity.
4. The risk for hypoglycemia is greatest around the peak of insulin activity.

5. The nurse is evaluating the patient's knowledge about the use and effects of insulin. Which of the following statements indicates that the patient needs additional information?

1. "If I experience hypoglycemia, I should drink half a cup of apple juice."
2. "My insulin needs may increase when I have an infection."
3. "I must draw the NPH insulin first if I am mixing it with regular insulin."
4. "If my blood glucose levels are above 140 mg/dL, I should notify my healthcare provider."

6. The physician starts a patient on 500 mg, po, twice a day. The pharmacy provides him or her with scored 1,000 mg tablets. How many tablets will he or she take in a day?

1. One tablet
2. Two tablets
3. One and one-half tablets
4. One-half tablet

7. The patient with diabetes has decided to start an exercise program. He remembers that the nurse told him that exercise:

1. Increases glucose in the blood thus increasing the need for insulin just after exercise.
2. Decreases glucose in the blood thus decreasing the need for more insulin just after exercise.
3. Does not affect glucose or the need for insulin.
4. Decreases glucose in the blood thus increasing the need for insulin after exercise.

8. The nurse informs a group of patients, newly diagnosed with type 1 DM, that the following factors can influence the amount of insulin needed to control blood glucose levels: (Select all that apply.)

1. Exercise
2. Diet
3. Illness
4. Sleep

9. The nurse administers glipizide (Glucotrol):

1. Subcutaneously only
2. After meals
3. At bedtime
4. Just before breakfast

10. The nurse plans to administer glargine (Lantus) to a patient with type 1 diabetes:

1. Before meals
2. With meals
3. Only at bedtime
4. Same time each day.

CASE STUDY QUESTIONS

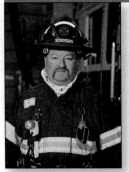

Remember Mr. Jones, the patient introduced at the beginning of the chapter? Now read the remainder of the case study. Based on the information you have learned in this chapter, answer the questions that follow.

Mr. Brian Jones is a 45-year-old fire-fighter who smokes and is somewhat overweight. Over the past five years, he has begun to develop slightly elevated blood pressure as determined by annual physical exams. He knows he should lose weight and is concerned about his energy level. He has always felt "OK" despite the fact that he smokes, but recently he has begun to feel sluggish and wonders what's going on. He thinks to himself, "Maybe I'm just getting older." At this current visit to the doctor, laboratory results reveal a fasting blood glucose level of 136 mg/dL. His blood pressure is 150/90 mmHg. Mr. Jones has not been taking medications for any reported disorders.

1. Mr. Jones is told that his blood glucose level is above the normal range, a condition known as hyperglycemia. In helping to determine factors that influenced his test results, the nurse asks him about: (Select all that apply.)

1. His daily diet
2. His level of stress
3. How long he has smoked
4. How long he has had hypertension

2. Mr. Jones is told that he has the symptoms of type 2 DM. He wants to know how it can be controlled. The nurse tells him that it can be controlled by: (Select all that apply.)

1. Regular exercise
2. Oral antidiabetic medications
3. Maintaining current weight
4. Better coping skills to deal with stress

3. Mr. Jones is started on metformin. As part of the information packet given to newly diagnosed patients with diabetes, there is a section on antidiabetic medications. Mr. Jones starts to read it but instead asks the nurse about adverse effects. The nurse states that some of the adverse effects of metformin are: (Select all that apply.)

1. Constipation
2. Diarrhea
3. Abdominal discomfort
4. Headaches

4. Mr. Jones also has high blood pressure and is going to be prescribed medication. The nurse understands that several blood pressure drugs, captopril, furosemide, and nifedipine, may cause a(n):

1. Increased risk for hypoglycemia
2. Decreased renal excretion
3. Increased renal excretion
4. Decreased risk for hypoglycemia

NOTE: Answers to the Review and Case Study Questions appear in Appendix B. The complete rationales and answers are located on the textbook's website.

Pearson Nursing Student Resources   Find additional review materials at **nursing.pearsonhighered.com**.

C
H
A
P
T
E
R

"I can't wait until all this stops. My periods hurt so bad and last so long. It just makes me tired."

Ms. Marge Philips

34 Drugs for Disorders and Conditions of the Reproductive System

CORE CONCEPTS

34.1 The hypothalamus, pituitary, and gonads control reproductive function in both men and women.

34.2 Oral contraceptives are drugs used in low doses to prevent pregnancy.

34.3 Hormone replacement therapy provides estrogen to treat postmenopausal symptoms, but benefits may not outweigh risks.

34.4 Conjugated estrogens and progestins are prescribed for dysfunctional uterine bleeding, endometrial cancer, and postmenopausal symptoms.

34.5 Oxytocin and tocolytics are drugs that influence uterine contractions and labor.

34.6 Androgens are used to treat hypogonadism in males.

34.7 Erectile dysfunction is a common disorder successfully treated with drug therapy.

34.8 In its early stages, benign prostatic hyperplasia is successfully treated.

DRUG SNAPSHOT

The following drugs are discussed in this chapter:

DRUG CLASSES	DRUG PROTOTYPES
Oral contraceptives (OCs)	**Pr** estradiol with norethindrone (Ortho-Novum, others) *547*
Hormone replacement therapy (HRT)	**Pr** estrogen, conjugated (Cenestin, Enjuvia, Premarin) *551*
Drugs for dysfunctional uterine bleeding	**Pr** methoxyprogesterone (Depo-Provera, Depo-SubQ-Provera, Provera) *552*

DRUG CLASSES	DRUG PROTOTYPES
Uterine stimulants and relaxants	**Pr** oxytocin (Pitocin) *553*
Androgens	**Pr** testosterone *554*
Drugs for erectile dysfunction	**Pr** sildenafil (Viagra) *556*
Drugs for benign prostatic hyperplasia	**Pr** finasteride (Proscar) *558*

LEARNING OUTCOMES

After reading this chapter, the student should be able to:

1. Describe the roles of the hypothalamus, pituitary, and sex organs in maintaining female and male reproductive function.

2. Explain the mechanisms by which estrogens and progestins prevent conception.

3. Describe the role of drug therapy in the treatment of menopausal and postmenopausal symptoms.

4. Discuss the uses of progestins in the therapy of dysfunctional uterine bleeding.

5. Identify the role of the female sex hormones in the treatment of endometrial cancer.

6. Compare and contrast the use of uterine stimulants and relaxants in

the treatment of patients giving birth and after delivery of the baby.

7. Identify the reasons for pharmacotherapy with androgens.

8. Describe the pharmacotherapy of erectile dysfunction.

9. Describe the pharmacotherapy of benign prostatic hyperplasia.

10. For each of the classes listed in the Drug Snapshot, identify representative drugs and explain their mechanisms of drug action, primary actions, and important adverse effects.

KEY TERMS

amenorrhea (ah-men-oh-REE-ah) *550*

androgens (AN-droh-jens) *554*

benign prostatic hyperplasia (BPH) (bee-NINE pros-TAT-ik hy-PURR-plays-she-ah) *557*

breakthrough bleeding *550*

corpora cavernosa (KORP-us kav-ver-NOH-sah) *555*

corpus luteum (KORP-us LUTE-ee-uhm) *544*

dysfunctional uterine bleeding *549*

endometrial carcinoma (en-doh-MEE-tree-ahl CAR-sin-OH-mah) *550*

endometriosis (en-doh-MEE-tree-oh-sis) *550*

estrogen (ES-troh-jen) *544*

follicle-stimulating hormone (FSH) *543*

gonadotropin-releasing hormone (GnRH) (go-NAD-oh-TROPE-en) *543*

hormone replacement therapy (HRT) *549*

hypogonadism (hy-poh-GO-nad-izm) *554*

impotence (IM-poh-tense) *555*

libido (lih-BEE-do) *554*

luteinizing hormones (LH) (LEW-ten-iz-ing) *543*

menopause (MEN-oh-paws) *549*

menorrhagia (men-oh-RAGE-ee-uh) *550*

oligomenorrhea (ol-ego-men-oh-REE-uh) *550*

ovulation (ov-you-LAY-shun) *543*

oxytocics (ox-ee-TOH-sicz) *552*

oxytocin (ox-ee-TOH-sin) *552*

postmenopausal bleeding (POST-men-oh-pause-ahl) *550*

premenstrual syndrome (PMS) (PREE-men-stroo-ahl) *550*

progesterone (pro-JESS-ter-own) *544*

prolactin (pro-LAK-tin) *552*

prostaglandins (pros-tah-GLAN-dins) *552*

testosterone (test-AHST-erh-own) *544*

tocolytics (toh-koh-LIT-ikz) *552*

virilization (veer-you-lih-ZAY-shun) *554*

H ormones from the pituitary gland and the sex organs provide for the growth and continued maintenance of the male and female reproductive systems. Reproductive hormones impact virtually every body system, including coagulation, blood vessels, bone, muscles, overall body growth, and behavior. Hormonal therapy of the female reproductive system is used to achieve a variety of therapeutic goals, ranging from replacement therapy after menopause to prevention of pregnancy to milk production. The pharmacologic treatment of reproductive disorders in men is less complex because hormonal secretion in men is relatively constant throughout the adult life span. This chapter examines hormones and drugs used to treat disorders and conditions associated with the reproductive system.

The hypothalamus, pituitary, and gonads control reproductive function in both men and women.

Regulation of the reproductive system is achieved by hormones from the hypothalamus, pituitary gland, and the sex organs. The hypothalamus secretes **gonadotropin-releasing hormone (GnRH)**, which travels a short distance to the pituitary to stimulate the secretion of **follicle-stimulating hormone (FSH)** and **luteinizing hormone (LH)**. Both of these pituitary hormones act at the levels of the reproductive organs. The hormonal changes that occur during the ovarian and uterine cycles are illustrated in Figure 34.1 ■.

During a woman's reproductive years and under the influence of FSH and LH, several ovarian follicles begin the maturation process each month. On approximately day 14 of the ovarian cycle, a surge of LH secretion causes one follicle to expel its oocyte, a process called **ovulation**. The ruptured follicle,

gonads/gonado = *sex organs*
tropin = *attraction toward*

luteum/luteinizing = *yellowing (color of developing structures)*

FIGURE 34.1

Hormonal changes
during the ovarian and
uterine cycles.

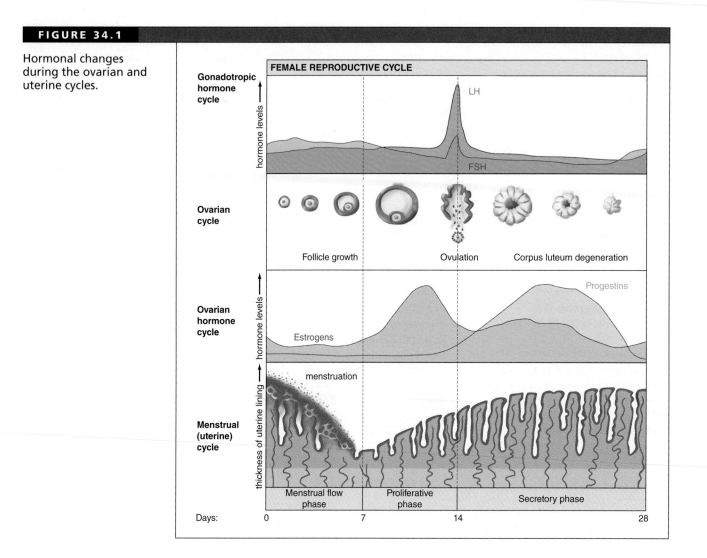

corpus = *body*

oocyte = *egg cell*

estro = *desire*
gen = *forming*

pro = *before*
gest = *gestation*

testo = *testis*
erone/sterone = *sterol
chemical compound*

minus its oocyte, remains in the ovary and is transformed into the hormone-secreting **corpus luteum**. The expelled oocyte begins its journey through the uterine tube and eventually reaches the uterus. If conception does not occur, the outer lining of the uterus degenerates and is shed to the outside during menstruation.

As ovarian follicles mature, they secrete the female sex hormones **estrogen** and **progesterone**. Estrogen is responsible for the maturation of the female reproductive organs and for the appearance of secondary sex characteristics. In addition, estrogen has numerous metabolic effects on nonreproductive tissues in the body. When women enter menopause at about age 50 to 55, the ovaries stop secreting estrogen.

In the last half of the monthly cycle, the corpus luteum secretes progesterone. In combination with estrogen, progesterone promotes breast development and regulates the monthly changes in the uterus. Under the influence of estrogen and progesterone, the uterine lining thickens in preparation for receiving a fertilized egg. High progesterone and estrogen levels in the final part of the uterine cycle provide negative feedback to shut off GnRH, FSH, and LH secretion. This negative feedback loop is illustrated in Figure 34.2 ■.

The same pituitary hormones that control reproductive function in women also affect men. FSH regulates sperm production. LH regulates the production of testosterone. If the level of testosterone in the blood rises above normal, negative feedback to the pituitary shuts off the secretion of LH and FSH.

Testosterone is the primary male sex hormone responsible for male secondary sex characteristics. Unlike the 28-day cyclic secretion of estrogen and progesterone in women, testosterone secretion is relatively constant. Beginning in puberty, testosterone production increases rapidly and is maintained at a high level until late adulthood, after which it slowly declines.

FIGURE 34.2

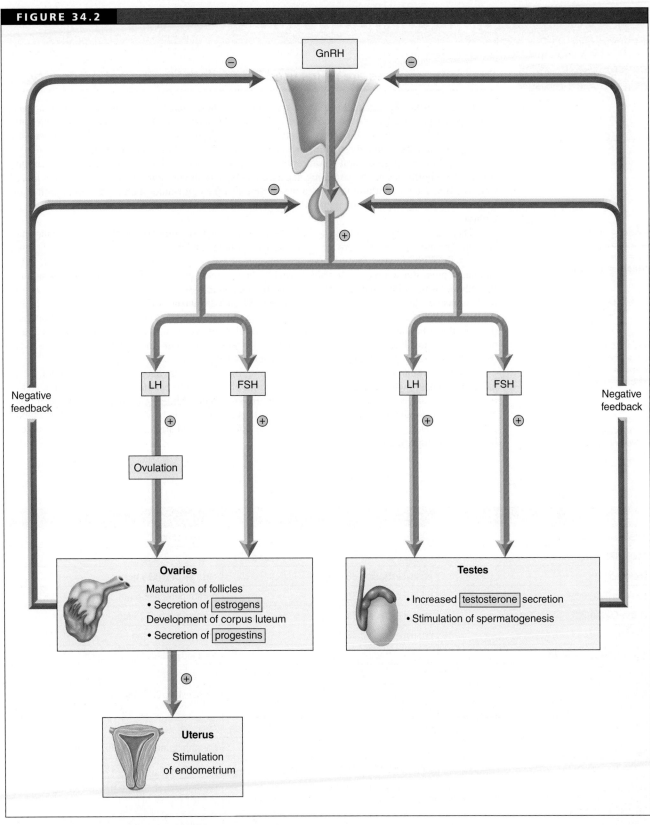

Hormonal control over male and female reproductive hormones.

ORAL CONTRACEPTIVES

CORE CONCEPT 34.2

Oral contraceptives are drugs used in low doses to prevent pregnancy.

The most widespread pharmacologic use of the female sex hormones is for the prevention of pregnancy. When used appropriately, they are nearly 100% effective. Most oral contraceptives (OCs) contain a combination of estrogen and progestin, although a few contain only progestin. The most common estrogen used in these preparations is ethinyl estradiol, and the most common progestin is norethindrone.

The estrogen–progestin oral contraceptives prevent ovulation, which is required for conception to occur. These hormones act by providing negative feedback to the pituitary gland that shuts down secretion of LH and FSH. Without these pituitary hormones, the egg cannot mature, and ovulation is prevented. The estrogen–progestin agents also make the lining of the uterus less favorable to receiving an embryo.

mono = *single*
bi = *two*
tri = *three*
phasic = *dosing level(s)*

There are four types of estrogen–progestin OCs: monophasic, biphasic, triphasic, and quadriphasic version. The monophasic delivers a constant dose of estrogen and progestin throughout the 21-day treatment cycle. With biphasic formulations, the amount of estrogen in each pill remains constant, but the amount of progestin is increased toward the end of the treatment cycle to better nourish the uterine lining. In triphasic formulations, the amounts of both estrogen and progestin vary in three distinct phases during the treatment cycle. In 2010, the first quadriphasic OC, called Natazia, was introduced. Natazia contains a synthetic estrogen called estradiol valerate and a progestin called dienogest; it is the first drug containing this specific combination. All four types of OC formulations are equally effective, although a common problem, and most likely the most common reason for treatment failure (pregnancy), is forgetting to take the medication daily. Selected OCs are listed in Table 34.1 ◆.

dys = *abnormal or unhealthy*
a = *without*
meno = *monthly*
rrhea = *flow*

thrombo = *stationary blood clot*
embolytic = *circulating blood clot*

The most common adverse effects of estrogen–progestin OCs are nausea, breast tenderness, weight gain, and breakthrough bleeding. Less common serious effects include edema, gallbladder disease, abdominal cramps, changes in urinary function, dysmenorrhea, fatigue, skin rash, headache, and vaginal candidiasis. Cardiovascular adverse effects, the most serious of all, include hypertension and thromboembolic disorders. The estrogen component of the pill can lead to venous and arterial thrombosis, which can result in pulmonary, myocardial, and thrombotic strokes.

TABLE 34.1	Selected Oral Contraceptives	
Trade Name	**Estrogen**	**Progestin**
MONOPHASIC		
Desogen	ethinyl estradiol; 30 mcg	desogestrel; 0.15 mg
Loestrin 1.5/30 Fe	ethinyl estradiol; 30 mcg	norethindrone; 1.5 mg
Ortho-Cyclen-28	ethinyl estradiol; 35 mcg	norgestimate; 0.25 mg
Yasmin	ethinyl estradiol; 30 mcg	drospirenone; 3 mg
Zovia 1/50E-21 and 28	ethinyl estradiol; 50 mcg	ethynodiol diacetate 1 mg
BIPHASIC		
Mircette	ethinyl estradiol 20 mcg for 21 days; 10 mcg for 5 days	desogestrel; 0.15 mg for 21 days
TRIPHASIC		
ⓟ Ortho-Novum 7/7/7-28	ethinyl estradiol; 35 mcg	norethindrone; 0.50, 0.75, 0.1 mg
Ortho Tri-Cyclen-28	ethinyl estradiol; 35 mcg	norgestimate; 0.18, 0.215, 0.25 mg
Trivora-28	ethinyl estradiol; 30, 40, 30 mcg	levonorgestrel; 0.05, 0.075, 0.125 mg
PROGESTIN ONLY		
Micronor	None	norethindrone; 0.35 mg
Nor-Q.D.	None	norethindrone; 0.35 mg

The progestin-only OCs, sometimes called *minipills*, prevent pregnancy primarily by producing a thick, viscous mucus at the entrance to the uterus that prevents penetration by sperm. A thicker mucosal lining inhibits implantation of a fertilized egg. Progestin-only agents are less effective than estrogen–progestin combinations and produce a higher incidence of menstrual irregularities. Because of this, they are generally reserved for women who are at high risk for adverse effects from estrogen. When women taking estrogen also smoke, they have an increased chance of developing blood clots which may be fatal.

Several long-term hormonal formulations of contraception are available. These extended-duration formulations are equally effective in preventing pregnancy and have the same basic safety profile as OCs. Examples of alternative formulations are:

- Depot injections: Depo-Provera (IM injection of medroxyprogesterone), Depo-SubQ-Provera (subcutaneous injection of medroxyprogesterone)

- Implants: Implanon (single rod containing the progestin etonogestrel inserted under the skin of the upper arm)

- Transdermal patches: Ortho Evra (transdermal patch containing ethinyl estradiol and norelgestromin), Minivelle (transdermal patch containing estradiol)

- Vaginal route: NuvaRing (2-inch-diameter ring containing estrogen and progestin inserted into the vagina)

- Intrauterine route: Mirena (polyethylene cylinder placed in the uterus and releases levonorgestrel), Skyla (levonorgestrel release may last up to three years)

- Extended-regimen OCs: Seasonale consists of tablets containing levonorgestrel and ethinyl estradiol that are taken for 84 consecutive days, followed by 7 inert tablets (without hormones).

Emergency contraception (EC) is the *prevention* of pregnancy following unprotected intercourse. The treatment goal for EC is to provide effective and immediate contraception. Two different medications are approved for EC: Levonorgestrel (Plan B) and ulipristal (Ella).

Plan B is approved for purchase over the counter (OTC). Dosing for Plan B involves taking 0.75 mg of levonorgestrel in two doses, 12 hours apart. Plan B One Step includes a single 1.5 mg dose. The drug acts in a manner similar to OCs; it prevents ovulation and also alters the lining of the uterus so that implantation does not occur. If implantation has already occurred, Plan B will not terminate the pregnancy. Plan B must be taken as soon as possible after unprotected intercourse; if taken more than 120 hours later, it becomes less effective. Adverse effects are mild and may include nausea, vomiting, abdominal pain, fatigue, headache, menstrual changes, diarrhea, dizziness, and breast tenderness. In 2010, ulipristal (Ella) was approved as a single-dose product for EC. Unlike Plan B, which is available OTC, ulipristal requires a prescription. One advantage of ulipristal is that it retains its effectiveness for five days following unprotected sex.

Drug Prototype: ℗ *Estradiol with Norethindrone (Ortho-Novum, Others)*
Therapeutic Class: **Oral Contraceptive**   Pharmacologic Class: **Estrogen/Progestin**

Actions and Uses: Ortho-Novum is typical of the monophasic oral contraceptives, containing fixed amounts of estrogen and progesterone for 21 days followed by placebo tablets for 7 days. It is nearly 100% effective at preventing conception. If a dose is missed, the patient should take the dose as soon as possible, or take two tablets the next day. If two consecutive doses are missed, conception is possible, and the patient should use other birth control methods until the regular dosing schedule is reestablished.

Adverse Effects and Interactions: Like most oral contraceptives, Ortho-Novum can increase the risks of thromboembolic disease: the potential for blood clots, hemorrhage, pulmonary embolism, or stroke. It should be used with caution in women with hypertension because it has the potential to raise blood pressure. Bleeding in the early or mid-menstrual cycle is relatively common.

Ethinyl estradiol interacts with many drugs. For example, rifampin, some antibiotics, barbiturates, anticonvulsants, and antifungals decrease efficacy of oral contraceptives, so the risks of breakthrough bleeding and pregnancy are higher

BLACK BOX WARNING:
Cigarette smoking increases the risk of serious cardiovascular adverse effects in women who are taking OCs containing estrogen.

NURSING PROCESS FOCUS Patients Receiving Oral Contraceptive Therapy

ASSESSMENT	POTENTIAL NURSING DIAGNOSES
Prior to administration: ■ Obtain a complete health history, including genitourinary (GU), sexual, cardiovascular (especially hypertension or thromboembolic), thyroid, renal and liver conditions; pregnancy (or lactating); allergies; drug history; and possible drug interactions. ■ Gather information about lifestyle such as pain, cigarette smoking, and diet. ■ Evaluate laboratory blood findings: CBC, electrolytes, lipid panel, renal and liver function studies. ■ Acquire the results of a complete physical examination, including vital signs, height, and weight.	■ *Deficient Knowledge* related to a lack of information about drug therapy ■ *Infective Health Maintenance* related to noncompliance with medication regimen or adverse drug effects ■ *Risk for Ineffective Peripheral Tissue Perfusion* related to adverse drug effects ■ *Risk of Excess Fluid Volume* related to adverse drug effects

PLANNING: PATIENT GOALS AND EXPECTED OUTCOMES

The patient will:
■ Experience therapeutic effects (effective birth control).
■ Be free from or experience minimal adverse effects from drug therapy.
■ Verbalize an understanding of the drug's use, adverse effects, and required precautions.

IMPLEMENTATION

Interventions and (Rationales)	Patient Education/Discharge Planning
■ Administer medication correctly and evaluate the patient's knowledge of proper administration. (Incorrect use may lead to pregnancy.)	Instruct the patient to: ■ Take the pill at the same time every day. ■ Not omit, increase, or decrease doses without consulting health-care provider: omitting or decreasing doses increases the chance of pregnancy. ■ Take medication according to the specific type of hormone being taken. For estrogen–progestin combinations: take a missed dose as soon as remembered. If two consecutive doses are missed, take the two missed pills on the day remembered and next two pills on the following day. Then follow the remaining schedule of pills but use additional birth control until the regular schedule is reestablished. ■ Contact the healthcare provider if two consecutive periods are missed because pregnancy may have occurred.
■ Monitor for the occurrence of breakthrough bleeding. (Spotting may occur, especially with low-dose hormone therapy, at mid-cycle. Any continuous, unusual, or heavy bleeding may indicate adverse effects, pregnancy loss, or disease and should be reported.)	■ Inform the patient that spotting may occur with low-dose hormone therapy, at mid-cycle but to report any unusual changes in the amount of bleeding or if bleeding continues.
■ Monitor for thrombophlebitis or other thromboembolic disease. (Estrogen predisposes to thromboembolic disorders by increasing levels of clotting factors.)	■ Instruct the patient to immediately report to the healthcare provider any pain in the calves, limited movement in the legs, dyspnea, sudden severe chest pain, headache, seizures, anxiety, or fear.
■ Monitor for cardiac disorders: take vital signs, especially pulse and blood pressure. (These drugs can increase blood levels of angiotensin and aldosterone, which increase blood pressure.)	Instruct the patient to: ■ Report immediately signs of possible cardiac problems such as chest pain, dyspnea, edema, tachycardia or bradycardia, and palpitations. ■ Have blood pressure monitored regularly. ■ Report to the healthcare provider any symptoms of hypertension such as headache, flushing, fatigue, dizziness, palpitations, tachycardia, and nosebleeds.
■ Encourage the patient not to smoke. (Smoking increases risk of thromboembolic disease.)	Instruct the patient to: ■ Be aware that the combination of oral contraceptives and smoking greatly increases risk of cardiovascular disease, especially MI. ■ Be aware that the risk increases with age (>35) and with number of cigarettes smoked (15 or more per day).
■ Monitor liver function tests, lipid profile studies, and thyroid studies periodically. (These drugs are associated with an increased risk of gallbladder disease and a rare risk of liver toxicity.)	Instruct the patient to: ■ Return periodically for laboratory tests. ■ Report any symptoms of abdominal or right upper quadrant discomfort, yellowing of the skin or sclera, fatigue, anorexia, darkened urine, or clay-colored stools to the healthcare provider.
■ Monitor for the development of breast or other estrogen-dependent tumors. (Estrogen may cause tumor growth or proliferation.)	■ Instruct the patient to immediately report to the healthcare provider if a first-degree relative is diagnosed with any estrogen-dependent tumor.

continued . . .

Interventions and (Rationales)	Patient Education/Discharge Planning
■ Encourage compliance with follow-up treatment. (Follow-up is necessary to avoid serious adverse effects.)	Instruct the patient to: ■ Schedule annual Pap smears. ■ Perform breast self-exams (BSEs) monthly and obtain routine mammograms as recommended by the healthcare provider.

EVALUATION OF OUTCOME CRITERIA

Evaluate the effectiveness of drug therapy by confirming that patient goals and expected outcomes have been met (see "Planning"). *See Table 34.1 for a list of drugs to which these nursing actions apply.*

CAM THERAPY

Dong Quai for Premenstrual Syndrome

Since antiquity, dong quai has been recognized as an important herb for women's health in Chinese medicine. Obtained from *Angelica sinensis*, a small plant that grows in China, dong quai, contains a number of active substances that are said to exert analgesic, antipyretic, anti-inflammatory, and antispasmodic activity. The dried root is available as capsules, tablets, teas, and tinctures.

The reproductive effects of dong quai may be due to active substances that have estrogenic activity. These estrogenic ingredients act as a "uterine tonic" to improve the overall hormonal balance of the female reproductive system. Dong quai is used to treat the symptoms of premenstrual syndrome, as well as other disorders such as irregular menstrual periods or painful menstruation.

Dong quai has also been used for its cardiovascular effects. It is claimed to increase circulation by dilating blood vessels. Because some of the active ingredients of dong quai may have anticoagulant activity, patients taking warfarin (Coumadin) or high doses of aspirin should not take the herb without notifying their healthcare practitioner.

MENOPAUSE

Hormone replacement therapy provides estrogen to treat postmenopausal symptoms, but benefits may not outweigh risks.

CORE CONCEPT 34.3

Menopause is the permanent cessation of menses, resulting in a lack of estrogen secretion by the ovaries. Menopause is neither a disease nor a disorder, but a natural consequence of aging that is often accompanied by unpleasant symptoms that include hot flashes, night sweats, irregular menstrual cycles, vaginal dryness, and bone mass loss.

post = *after*
meno = *monthly*
pause/pausal = *stopping*

Over the past 50 years, healthcare providers have commonly prescribed **hormone replacement therapy (HRT)** for menopause. HRT supplies physiological doses of estrogen, sometimes combined with a progestin, to treat unpleasant symptoms of menopause and to prevent the long-term consequences of estrogen loss.

Studies have raised questions regarding the safety of HRT for menopause. Data suggest that patients may have an increased risk of coronary artery disease, stroke, and venous thromboembolism. Women are now encouraged to discuss alternatives with their healthcare provider. Undoubtedly, research will continue to provide valuable information on the long-term effects of HRT. Until then, the choice of HRT to treat menopausal symptoms will remain a highly individualized one between the patient and her healthcare provider.

UTERINE ABNORMALITIES

Conjugated estrogens and progestins are prescribed for dysfunctional uterine bleeding, endometrial cancer, and postmenopausal symptoms.

CORE CONCEPT 34.4

Conjugated estrogens are *combined* estrogens, and these, along with progestins, treat a variety of conditions. **Dysfunctional uterine bleeding** is a condition in which hemorrhage occurs on a noncyclic basis or

hyster = *womb or uterus*
ectomy = *excision*

endo = *inside (e.g., uterus lining)*
metri/metrial = *measure*
osis = *abnormal*

oligo = *scanty*
meno = *month*
rrhagia = *excessive*
rrhea = *flow*

in abnormal amounts. It is the most frequent health problem reported by women and is a common reason for hysterectomy. Other types of uterine abnormalities include the following:

- **Amenorrhea**—absence of menstruation
- **Endometriosis**—abnormal location of endometrial tissues
- **Oligomenorrhea**—infrequent menstruation
- **Menorrhagia**—prolonged or excessive menstruation
- **Breakthrough bleeding**—hemorrhage between menstrual periods
- **Premenstrual syndrome (PMS)**—symptoms develop during the luteal phase
- **Postmenopausal bleeding**—hemorrhage following menopause
- **Endometrial carcinoma**—cancer of the endometrium

Dysfunctional uterine bleeding is often caused by a hormonal imbalance between estrogen and progesterone. Poor estrogen levels cause the uterine lining to remain thin. Progestins (progesterone-like hormones) limit and stabilize growth of the uterine lining.

The primary indication for conjugated estrogens has been to treat moderate to severe symptoms of menopause, which include irregular menstrual cycles and extreme uterine bleeding. Progestins are the drugs most commonly used for treating uterine abnormalities. Administration of a progestin in a pattern starting 5 days after the onset of menses and continuing for the next 20 days can sometimes reestablish a normal, monthly cyclic pattern. OCs may also be prescribed for this disorder. Progestins are also occasionally prescribed for the treatment of metastatic endometrial carcinoma. In cases like this, progestins are used for total patient care, usually in combination with other antineoplastics. Conjugated estrogens and selected progestins with their dosages are listed in Table 34.2 ◆.

Concept Review   34.1

osteo = *bone*
porosis = *porous condition*

- Why is a progestin usually prescribed along with estrogen in oral contraceptives and when treating postmenopausal symptoms?

TABLE 34.2 Drugs for Hormone Replacement Therapy and Uterine Abnormalities		
Drug	**Route and Adult Dose**	**Drug Class Remarks**
ESTROGENS		
estradiol (Alora, Climara, Divigel, Elestrin, Estraderm, Estrace, others)	PO (Estrace); 0.5–2 mg daily Transdermal patch; 1 patch either once weekly (Climara) or twice weekly (Alora, Estraderm) (0.025–0.1 mg/day) Topical gel (Divigel, Elestrin); 0.25–1 g/day applied to the skin of the upper thigh or arm Intravaginal cream (Estrace); Insert 2–4 g/day for 2 weeks, then reduce to one-half the initial dose for 2 weeks, then use 1 g one to three times per week	Systemic estrogens come in pill form, skin patches, gels, creams, and sprays. Low-dose vaginal preparations of estrogen are available in cream, tablet, and ring form. Estradiol valerate injection is provided as a long-acting estrogen dissolved in sterile oil solution for intramuscular use.
estradiol valerate (Delestrogen)	IM; 10–20 mg every 4 weeks	
Pr estrogen, conjugated (Cenestin, Enjuvia, Premarin)	PO; 0.3–1.25 mg/day for 21 days each month	
estropipate (Ogen)	PO; 0.75–6 mg/day for 21 days each month Intravaginal cream (Ogen): Insert 2–4 g/day	

(continued)

TABLE 34.2 Drugs for Hormone Replacement Therapy and Uterine Abnormalities (*continued*)

Drug	Route and Adult Dose	Drug Class Remarks
PROGESTINS		
(Pr) medroxyprogesterone (Depo-Provera, Depo-SubQ-Provera, Provera)	PO; 5–10 mg daily on days 1–12 of the menstrual cycle IM (Depo-Provera); 150 mg daily for 3 months. Give the first dose during the first 5 days of the menstrual period or within the first 5 days postpartum if not breastfeeding Subcutaneous (Depo-SubQ-Provera); 104 mg daily for 3 months. Give the first dose during the first 5 days of the menstrual period or at the sixth week postpartum if not breastfeeding	Synthetic versions of progestin are generally provided as high-dose pills or birth control pills. Injectable forms are also available. Treatments help restore hormonal balance.
norethindrone (Micronor, Norlutin, Nor-Q.D.)	PO (for amenorrhea); 5–20 mg/day on days 5–25 of the menstrual cycle	
progesterone (Crinone, Endometrin, Prochieve, Prometrium)	Amenorrhea or functional uterine bleeding: IM; 5–10 mg/day Assisted reproductive technology: Intravaginal; 90 mg gel once daily or 100 mg tablets two to three times per day	
ESTROGEN–PROGESTIN COMBINATIONS		
Conjugated estrogens with medroxyprogesterone (Premphase, Prempro)	PO; Premphase: estrogen 0.625 mg/daily on days 1–28; add 5 mg medroxyprogesterone daily on days 15–28 PO; Prempro: estrogen 0.3 mg and medroxyprogesterone 1.5 mg daily Intravaginal cream: insert 1/2 to 2 g daily for 3–6 months	Conjugated estrogens combined with progestins are prescribed to help women treat symptoms of menopause. Preparations are also used to treat certain menstrual disorders and to prevent osteoporosis (bone loss) in women.
estradiol with norgestimate (Prefest)	PO; 1 tablet of 1 mg estradiol for 3 days, followed by 1 tablet of 1 mg estradiol combined with 0.09 mg norgestimate for 3 days. Regimen is repeated continuously without interruption	
ethinyl estradiol with norethindrone acetate (Activella)	PO; 1 tablet daily, which contains 0.5–0.1 mg of estradiol and 0.5–1 mg norethindrone Transdermal patch; 1 patch, twice weekly	

Drug Prototype: (Pr) *Estrogen, conjugated (Cenestin, Enjuvia, Premarin)*

Therapeutic Class: Hormone replacement therapy **Pharmacologic Class: Estrogen**

Actions and Uses: Conjugated estrogens (Premarin) contain a mixture of different natural estrogens. Conjugated estrogen A (Cenestin) and conjugated estrogen B (Enjuvia) contain a mixture of 9–10 different synthetic plant estrogens. Conjugated estrogens exert several positive metabolic effects, including an increase in bone density and a reduction in LDL cholesterol. It may also lower the risk of coronary artery disease and colon cancer in some patients.

Adverse Effects and Interactions: Adverse effects of conjugated estrogens include nausea, fluid retention, edema, breast tenderness, abdominal cramps, and bloating. Conjugated estrogens are contraindicated in pregnant patients and in women with breast cancer. Caution should be used when treating patients with a history of thromboembolic disease, hepatic impairment, or abnormal uterine bleeding.

Drug interactions include a decreased effect of tamoxifen and anticoagulants. The effects of estrogen may be decreased if taken with barbiturates, and there is a possible increased effect of tricyclic antidepressants.

> **BLACK BOX WARNING:**
> Estrogens, when used alone, have been associated with a higher risk of endometrial cancer in postmenopausal women. Although adding a progestin may exert a protective effect by lowering the risk of uterine cancer, studies suggest that progestin may increase the risk of breast cancer following long-term use.

Drug Prototype: ℗ *Medroxyprogesterone (Depo-Provera, Depo-SubQ-Provera, Provera)*

Therapeutic Class: Drug for endometriosis and dysfunctional uterine bleeding and endometriosis
Pharmacologic Class: Progestin

Actions and Uses: Medroxyprogesterone is a synthetic progestin with a prolonged duration of action. As with its natural counterpart, the primary target tissue for medroxyprogesterone is the endometrium of the uterus. It inhibits the effect of estrogen on the uterus, thus restoring normal hormonal balance. Indications include dysfunctional uterine bleeding, secondary amenorrhea, and contraception.

Medroxyprogesterone may also be given by sustained release IM (Depo-Provera) or subcutaneous (Depo-SubQ-Provera) depot injection. This is available in two doses: a lower dose for contraception and a higher dose for the alleviation of inoperable metastatic uterine or renal carcinoma.

Adverse Effects and Interactions: The most frequent adverse effects of medroxyprogesterone are breast tenderness, breakthrough bleeding, and other menstrual irregularities. Weight gain, depression, hypertension, nausea, vomiting, dysmenorrhea, and vaginal candidiasis may also occur. The most serious adverse effect is an increased risk for thromboembolic disease.

Medroxyprogesterone is contraindicated during pregnancy and in women with known or suspected carcinoma of the breast. Caution should be used when treating patients with a history of thromboembolic disease, hepatic impairment, or undiagnosed vaginal bleeding.

> **BLACK BOX WARNING:**
> Progestins combined with conjugated estrogens may increase the risk of stroke, deep venous thrombosis (DVT), myocardial infarction (MI), pulmonary emboli, and invasive breast cancer.

LABOR AND BREASTFEEDING

CORE CONCEPT 34.5

Oxytocin and tocolytics are drugs that influence uterine contractions and labor.

oxytocic = *oxytocin-related*
toco = *contraction*
lytic = *arrested*

Several drugs are used to manage uterine contractions and to stimulate lactation. **Oxytocics** are drugs that *stimulate* uterine contractions to promote the induction of labor. **Tocolytics** are used to *inhibit* uterine contractions during premature labor. These drugs are listed in Table 34.3 ◆.

The most widely used oxytocic is the natural hormone **oxytocin**, which is secreted by the posterior portion of the pituitary gland. The target organs for oxytocin are the uterus and the breast. As the growing fetus distends the uterus, oxytocin is secreted in increasingly larger amounts, thus promoting labor and the delivery of the baby. This process is referred to as *positive feedback*.

post = *after*
partum = *childbirth*

In postpartum women, oxytocin is released in response to suckling, which causes milk to be *ejected* (let down) from the mammary glands. Oxytocin does not increase the *volume* of milk production. This function is provided by the pituitary hormone **prolactin**, which increases the synthesis of milk.

preterm = *before term*

Several prostaglandins including dinoprostone (Cervidil, Prepidil, Prostin E2) and carboprost (Hemabate) are also used as uterine stimulants. Unlike most hormones, which travel through the blood to affect distant tissues, **prostaglandins** are local hormones that act directly at the site where they are secreted. These drugs are used to initiate labor, dilate the cervix prior to delivery, and control hemorrhage following delivery.

Tocolytics are given as uterine relaxants to suppress preterm labor. This option is carefully weighed against harm to the mother and the baby. Risks to the baby involve an elevated heart rate, circulatory collapse, and respiratory paralysis. Risk to the mother is elevated blood pressure. Of the tocolytics listed in Table 34.3, only hydroxyprogesterone (Makena) is approved for this indication: the others are used off-label.

Concept Review **34.2**

■ What is the difference between the effects of prolactin and oxytocin on the breast?

TABLE 34.3   Uterine Stimulants and Relaxants

Drug	Route and Adult Dose	Drug Class Remarks
OXYTOCICS		
(Pr) oxytocin (Pitocin)	To control postpartum bleeding: 10–40 units per infusion pump in 1,000 mL of IV fluid To induce labor: IV 0.5–2 milliunits/min, gradually increasing the dose no greater than 1–2 milliunits/min at 30–60 minute intervals until contraction pattern is established	Rapidly causes uterine contractions and induces labor; postpartum bleeding is partially controlled due to the stimulatory effect that oxytocin has on uterine smooth muscle
ERGOT ALKALOID		
methylergonovine (Methergine)	PO; 0.2–0.4 mg bid–qid	Ergot alkaloids help to prevent and control bleeding after delivery of the baby
PROSTAGLANDINS		
carboprost (Hemabate)	IM; initial: 250 mcg (1 mL) repeated at 1½- and 3½-hour intervals if indicated by uterine response	Prostaglandins make uterine muscles contract; during the uterine cycle, they naturally help the uterus shed its lining; clinically, these drugs are for refractory postpartum uterine bleeding
dinoprostone (Cervidil, Prepidil, Prostin E$_2$)	Intravaginal; 10 mg	
TOCOLYTICS		
magnesium sulfate	IV; 1–4 g in 5% dextrose by slow infusion (initial max dose = 10–14 g/day, then no more than 30–40 g/day at a max rate of 1–2 g/hour)	These drugs inhibit uterine contractions in pregnant women at risk for preterm labor. Drugs are from different classes: magnesium sulfate (mineral supplement), hydroxyprogesterone (progestin), nifedipine (calcium channel blocker), and terbutaline (beta-adrenergic drug)
hydroxyprogesterone (Makena)	IM; 250 mg once weekly, beginning at 16 week gestation and continuing until week 37	
nifedipine (Adalat, Procardia)	PO; Initial dosage of 20 mg, followed by 20 mg orally after 30 minutes If contractions persist, therapy can be continued with 20 mg orally every 3–8 hours for 48–72 hours with a maximum dose of 160 mg/day After 72 hours, if maintenance is still required, long-acting nifedipine 30–60 mg daily can be used	
terbutaline (Brethine)	IV; 2.5–10 mcg/min; increase every 10–20 minutes; duration of infusion: 12 hours (max: 17.5–30 mcg/min) PO; maintenance dose: 2.5–10 mg every 4–6 hours	

Drug Prototype: (Pr) *Oxytocin (Pitocin)*

Therapeutic Class: Drug to induce labor; uterine stimulant   **Pharmacologic Class: Oxytocic**

Actions and Uses: Oxytocin (Pitocin), identical to the natural hormone secreted by the posterior pituitary gland, is a preferred drug for inducing labor. It is timed to the final stage of pregnancy, after the cervix has dilated, membranes have ruptured, and presentation of the fetus has occurred.

Adverse Effects and Interactions: The most common adverse effects of oxytocin are elevated blood pressure, rapid, painful uterine contractions and fetal tachycardia. Serious complications in the mother may include uterine rupture, seizures, or coma. Risk of uterine rupture increases in women who have delivered five or more children.

> **BLACK BOX WARNING:**
> Oxytocin is not indicated for the *elective* induction of labor (the initiation of labor in a pregnant patient who has no medical reason for induction).

HYPOGONADISM

Androgens are used to treat hypogonadism in males.

andro = *male*
gen = *forming*

hypo = *reduced*
gonadism = *sex hormone function*

libido = *sexual desire*

virilization = *appearance of male characteristics*

Androgens are male sex hormones. Testosterone is the primary androgen. Lack of sufficient testosterone secretion by the testes can result in male **hypogonadism**. Hypogonadism is the reduced function of gonads or sex organs in the body. Hypogonadism may be congenital or acquired later in life. When the condition is caused by a testicular disorder, it is called *primary* hypogonadism. Without sufficient FSH and LH secretion by the pituitary, the testes will lack their stimulus to produce testosterone. This condition is known as *secondary* hypogonadism. Lack of FSH and LH secretion may have a number of causes, including Cushing's syndrome (negative feedback from corticosteroids), thyroid disorders, and estrogen-secreting tumors.

Symptoms of male hypogonadism include a diminished appearance of the secondary sex characteristics of men: sparse axillary (armpit) hair, less facial and pubic hair; increased subcutaneous fat; and small testicular size. In adult men, lack of testosterone can lead to erectile dysfunction, low sperm counts, and decreased **libido** or *interest in sex*. In young men, lack of sufficient testosterone secretion may lead to delayed puberty.

Pharmacotherapy of hypogonadism includes replacement therapy with testosterone or other androgens. Within days or weeks of initiating therapy, androgens improve libido and correct erectile dysfunction resulting from low testosterone levels. Male sex characteristics reappear, a condition called *masculinization* or **virilization**. Therapy with androgens is targeted to return serum testosterone to normal levels. Above-normal levels serve no therapeutic purpose and increase the risk of adverse effects. High levels of androgens may cause abnormal growth of body hair, testicular shrinkage, altered sex drive, development of breasts, infertility, severe acne on the face and back, and possible mood swings involving rage or depression.

Testosterone is available in a variety of formulations to better meet individual patient preferences and lifestyles:

- Implantable pellets (subcutaneous): Testopel one to six pellets are implanted on the anterior abdominal wall.

- Intramuscular (IM): Testosterone cypionate (Depo-Testosterone) and testosterone enanthate (Delatestryl).

- Testosterone buccal system: Striant tablet is applied to the gum area just above the front teeth producing a continuous supply of testosterone in the bloodstream.

- Transdermal testosterone gel: Androgel, Fortesta, and Testim are applied once daily to the upper arms, shoulders, or abdomen. The drug is absorbed across the skin and into the bloodstream.

- Transdermal testosterone patch: Androgen patch is applied directly to the upper arm, thigh, back, or abdomen.

Selected androgens with indications for men are listed in Table 34.4 ◆.

Drug Prototype: Pr *Testosterone*
Therapeutic Class: Male hypogonadism drug   **Pharmacologic Class: Androgen**

Actions and Uses: The primary therapeutic use of testosterone is for the treatment of hypogonadism in men. The administration of testosterone to young men who have an abnormally delayed puberty will stimulate normal secondary sex characteristics to appear, including enlargement of the sexual organs, facial hair, and a deepening of the voice. In adult men, testosterone administration will increase interest in sexual activity, or libido, and restore masculine characteristics that may be deficient.

Adverse Effects and Interactions: An obvious adverse effect of testosterone therapy is virilization or appearance of masculine characteristics. Salt and water are often retained, causing edema. Liver damage is a rare, although potentially serious, adverse effect. Acne and skin irritation is common during therapy.

Testosterone base interacts with many drugs. For example, when taken with oral anticoagulants, testosterone base may increase hypoprothrombinemia. Insulin requirements may decrease, and the risk of liver toxicity may increase when used with echinacea.

BLACK BOX WARNING:
Virilization in women and children may occur following secondary exposure. Signs of virilization may include any of the following; deepening of the voice, hirsutism, oily skin, and male-pattern baldness.

TABLE 34.4   Selected Androgens and Anabolic Steroids

Drug	Route and Adult Dose	Remarks
danazol (Danocrine)	PO; 200–400 mg bid for 3–6 months	Prevention of attacks of angioedema of all types (cutaneous, abdominal, laryngeal)
fluoxymesterone (Halotestin)	PO; 5 mg one to four times per day	Replacement therapy for deficiency or absence of endogenous testosterone, primary and secondary hypogonadism, or delayed puberty
methyltestosterone (Android, Testred, Virilon)	PO; 10–50 mg/day Buccal: 5–25 mg/day	Primary hypogonadism, testicular failure, hypogonadotropic hypogonadism, and delayed puberty
nandrolone (Durabolin, Hybolin)	IM; 50–200 mg/week	Management of anemia due to renal insufficiency, to increase hemoglobin and red cell mass, and for patients who have had kidney surgery with symptoms of swelling and inflammation
oxandrolone (Oxandrin)	PO; 2.5–20 mg/day divided two to four times per day for 2–4 weeks	Adjunctive therapy to offset the protein breakdown associated with prolonged administration of corticosteroids, and for the relief of the bone pain accompanying osteoporosis
oxymetholone (Anadrol-50)	PO; 1–5 mg/kg/day	Treatment of anemias caused by deficient red cell production, aplastic anemias, and myelofibrosis; drugs should not replace other supportive measures such as transfusion, correction of iron, folic acid, vitamin B_{12} or pyridoxine deficiency, antibacterial therapy, and the appropriate use of corticosteroids.
(Pr) testosterone (buccal: Striant); (transdermal patch: Androderm); (topical gels: Androgel, Fortesta, Testim); (implantable pellets: Testopel)	Buccal; 30 mg/12 hours Transdermal; apply 1–2 patches daily (max: 5 mg/day) Gel; apply 5 g daily (max 10 g) IM; 50–400 mg every 2–4 weeks Pellets: 150–450 mg every 6 months (each pellet is 75 mg)	Primary therapy is for delayed puberty and hypogonadism; other indications are described in the Prototype drug feature
testosterone cypionate (Depo-Testosterone)	IM; 50–400 mg every 2–4 weeks	For replacement therapy in conditions associated with symptoms of deficiency or absence of endogenous testosterone
testosterone enanthate (Delatestryl)	IM; 50–400 mg every 2–4 weeks	For replacement therapy in conditions associated with a deficiency or absence of endogenous testosterone, primary hypogonadism, secondary hypogonadism, and delayed puberty

ERECTILE DYSFUNCTION

Erectile dysfunction is a common disorder successfully treated with drug therapy.

CORE CONCEPT 34.7

Penile erection has both neuromuscular and vascular components. Autonomic nerves dilate arterioles leading to the major erectile tissues of the penis, called the **corpora cavernosa**. The corpora have vascular spaces that fill with blood to cause rigidity. In addition, constriction of veins draining blood from the corpora allows the penis to remain rigid long enough for successful penetration. After ejaculation, the veins dilate, blood leaves the corpora, and the penis quickly loses its rigidity. Organic causes of erectile dysfunction may include damage to the nerves or blood vessels involved in the erection reflex.

corpora = bodies
cavernosa = cavernous

Erectile dysfunction, or **impotence**, is a common disorder in men. The defining characteristic of this condition is the consistent inability to either obtain an erection or to sustain an erection long enough to achieve successful intercourse.

The incidence of erectile dysfunction increases with age, although it may occur in an adult male of any age. Certain diseases, most notably atherosclerosis, diabetes, kidney disease, stroke, and hypertension, are associated with a higher incidence of the condition. Smoking increases the risk of erectile dysfunction. Psychogenic causes may include depression, fatigue, guilt, or fear of sexual failure. A number of common drugs cause impotence as an adverse effect, including thiazide diuretics, phenothiazines, selective

psycho = the mind
genic = generated from

TABLE 34.5 Drugs for Erectile Dysfunction

Drug	Route and Adult Dose	Remarks
avanafil (Stendra)	PO; 100 mg approximately 30 minutes before intercourse (max: 200 mg once per day)	The PDE-5 inhibitors do not *cause* an erection; they merely *enhance* the erection by increasing blood flow and maintaining relaxation of the smooth muscle in the penis.
℗ sildenafil (Viagra)	PO; 50 mg approximately 30–60 minutes before intercourse (max: 100 mg once per day)	These drugs alter the body's response to sexual stimulation by enhancing the effect of the nitric oxide, a chemical that is normally released during stimulation. Nitric oxide causes relaxation of the muscles in the penis, which allows for better blood flow to the penile area.
tadalafil (Cialis)	PO; 10 mg approximately 30 minutes before intercourse (max: 20 mg once per day) Once-daily dosing: 2.5–5 mg daily	
vardenafil (Levitra)	PO; 10 mg approximately 1 hour before intercourse (max: 20 mg once per day)	

serotonin reuptake inhibitors (SSRIs), tricyclic antidepressants (TCAs), beta- and alpha-adrenergic blockers, and angiotensin-converting enzyme (ACE) inhibitors. Low testosterone secretion can cause an inability to develop an erection due to loss of libido.

The development of sildenafil (Viagra), an inhibitor of the enzyme phosphodiesterase-5 (PDE-5), revolutionized the medical therapy of erectile dysfunction. The PDE-5 inhibitors do not *cause* an erection; they merely *enhance* the erection resulting from physical contact or other sexual stimuli by increasing blood flow and maintaining relaxation of the smooth muscle in the penis.

Three other PDE-5 inhibitors have been approved by the Food and Drug Administration (FDA). Vardenafil (Levitra) acts by the same mechanism as sildenafil but has a faster onset and slightly longer duration of action. Tadalafil (Cialis) acts within 30 minutes and has a prolonged duration lasting from 24 to 36 hours. In 2011, the indications for tadalafil were extended to include a daily dosing for the treatment of benign prostatic hyperplasia (BPH). The newest of the drugs in this class, avanafil (Stendra), has the same properties of the others but is claimed to have a faster onset of action. Drugs for erectile dysfunction are listed in Table 34.5 ◆.

▶ **Life Span Fact**

Erectile dysfunction affects about 1 in 4 men older than age 65.

Concept Review 34.3

■ Why do you think that sildenafil is used to treat erectile dysfunction instead of testosterone?

Drug Prototype: ℗ *Sildenafil (Viagra)*
Therapeutic Class: Drug for erectile dysfunction   **Pharmacologic Class: Phosphodiesterase-5 inhibitor**

Actions and Uses: Sildenafil acts by dilating blood vessels (vasodilation) and relaxing the erectile tissues in the penis, called the *corpora cavernosa*, which allows increased blood flow into the organ. The increased blood flow results in a firmer and longer-lasting erection in about 70% of men taking the drug.

Adverse Effects and Interactions: The most serious adverse effects with sildenafil occur in men who are concurrently taking organic nitrates, common drugs that also dilate blood vessels and are used in the therapy of angina. The combination of these drugs causes a marked increase in vasodilation, causing a drop in blood pressure and decreased blood flow to the heart, possibly causing a heart attack. Minor adverse effects include headache, flushing, and nasal congestion.

Cimetidine, erythromycin, and ketoconazole increase serum levels of sildenafil and require lower drug doses. Protease inhibitors (ritonavir, amprenavir, and others) will cause increased sildenafil levels, which may lead to toxicity. Rifampin may decrease sildenafil levels, leading to decreased effectiveness.

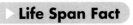

BENIGN PROSTATIC HYPERPLASIA

In its early stages, benign prostatic hyperplasia is successfully treated.

Benign prostatic hyperplasia (BPH) is the most common benign neoplasm in men. It is characterized by enlargement of the prostate gland. This decreases the outflow of urine by obstructing the urethra, causing difficult urination. Symptoms include increased urinary frequency (usually with small amounts of urine), increased urgency to urinate, excessive nighttime urination (nocturia), decreased force of the urine stream, and a sensation that the bladder is not completely empty. BPH is illustrated in Figure 34.3 ■.

Early in the course of the disease, drug therapy may relieve some symptoms. Only a few drugs are available for the treatment of BPH. These drugs are listed in Table 34.6 ◆.

benign = *mild*
hyper = *over*
plasia = *growth*

noct = *nighttime*
uria = *urine*

▶ **Life Span Fact**

BPH affects 50% of men older than age 60 and 90% of men older than age 80.

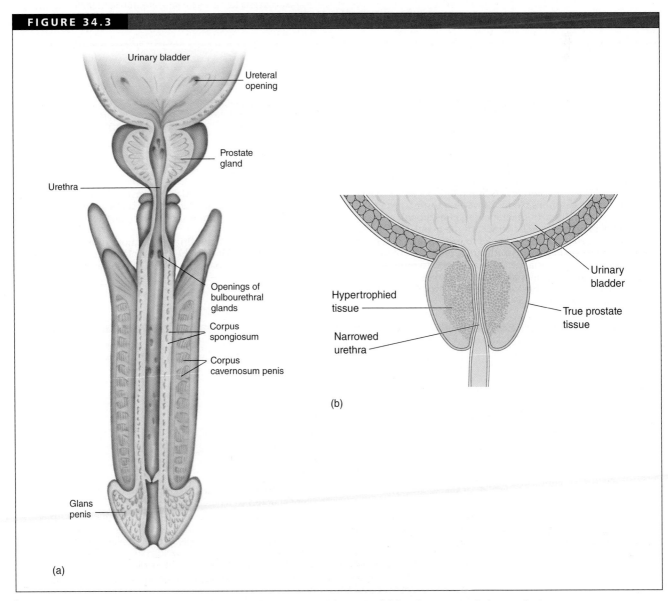

FIGURE 34.3

Benign prostatic hyperplasia (BPH): (a) normal prostate with penis; (b) benign prostatic hyperplasia.

TABLE 34.6 Drugs for Benign Prostatic Hyperplasia

Drug	Route and Adult Dose	Drug Class Remarks
ALPHA$_1$-ADRENERGIC BLOCKERS		
alfuzosin (Uroxatral)	PO; 10 mg/day (max: 10 mg/day)	When activated, the alpha$_1$-adrenergic receptors compress the urethra and provide resistance to urine outflow from the bladder. Alpha$_1$ blockers counter urethral compression.
doxazosin (Cardura)	PO (Regular-release); 1–8 mg/day (max: 8 mg/day)	
doxazosin (Cardura XL)	PO (Extended-release); 4–8 mg/day (max: 8 mg/day)	
silodosin (Rapaflo)	PO; 8 mg once daily with a meal	
tamsulosin (Flomax)	PO; 0.4 mg 30 minutes after a meal (max: 0.8 mg/day)	
terazosin (Hytrin)	PO; start with 1 mg at bedtime, then 1–5 mg/day (max: 20 mg/day)	
5-ALPHA-REDUCTASE INHIBITORS		
dutasteride (Avodart)	PO; 0.5 mg once daily	5-Alpha-reductase inhibitors block the action of the enzyme that converts testosterone into dihydrotestosterone, a promoter of prostate growth. The size of the prostate is therefore reduced.
Pr finasteride (Proscar)	PO; 5 mg once daily	

Drug Prototype: Pr *Finasteride (Proscar)*

Therapeutic Class: **Drug for benign prostatic hyperplasia (BPH)**
Pharmacologic Class: **5-Alpha-reductase enzyme inhibitor**

Actions and Uses: Finasteride acts by inhibiting 5-alpha reductase, the enzyme responsible for converting testosterone to one of its metabolites. This metabolite causes growth of prostate cells and promotes enlargement of the gland. Finasteride shrinks enlarged prostates and helps to restore urinary function. It is most effective in patients with larger prostates. This drug is also marketed as Propecia, which is prescribed to promote hair regrowth in patients with male-pattern baldness. Doses of finasteride are five times higher when prescribed for BPH than when prescribed for baldness.

Adverse Effects and Interactions: Finasteride causes various types of sexual dysfunction in some patients, including impotence, diminished libido, and ejaculatory dysfunction.

No clinically significant drug interactions have been established. Use with caution with herbal supplements. For example, saw palmetto may increase the effects of finasteride.

PATIENTS NEED TO KNOW

Patients treated for reproductive disorders need to know the following:

Regarding Oral Contraceptives

1. If taking oral contraceptives, schedule frequent medical checkups. Take blood pressure periodically and report any persistent changes to a healthcare provider.
2. Discontinue oral contraceptives, estrogen, or progestins immediately if pregnancy is suspected. Continued use may injure the fetus.
3. Be certain to inform the healthcare provider if oral contraceptives are being taken. Some drugs decrease the effectiveness of oral contraceptives and could result in pregnancy. These drugs include several common antibiotics and antiseizure medications.
4. A balanced diet is important when taking oral contraceptives, because these drugs may lower levels of folic acid and vitamin B$_6$.

Regarding Hormone Replacement Therapy

5. Before beginning HRT, a baseline mammogram should be performed. Monthly breast self-examinations should be conducted in addition to an annual exam by a healthcare provider.

Regarding Erectile Dysfunction Medications

6. If taking antihypertensive drugs, monitor blood pressure carefully when taking sildenafil. An increased risk of hypotension is possible.

Regarding Androgens

7. When taking androgens, expect virilization to occur. Prolonged erections, known as *priapisms*, should be reported to a healthcare provider immediately. This is a sign of overdose, and permanent damage to the penis may result.

CHAPTER REVIEW

CORE CONCEPTS SUMMARY

34.1 **The hypothalamus, pituitary, and gonads control reproductive function in both men and women.**

Estrogens are secreted by ovarian follicles and are responsible for maturation of the sex organs and the secondary sex characteristics of the female. Progestins are secreted by the corpus luteum and prepare the endometrium for implantation. Testosterone is secreted by the testes and is responsible for the growth and maintenance of the male reproductive system. The sex hormones are controlled by GnRH from the hypothalamus and FSH and LH from the pituitary gland.

34.2 **Oral contraceptives are drugs used in low doses to prevent pregnancy.**

OCs contain low doses of estrogens and progestins. Nearly 100% effective, these drugs prevent conception by blocking ovulation. Long-term formulations offer greater flexibility of administration. OCs are safe for the large majority of women, but they have some potentially serious adverse effects. Antibiotics, antifungals, barbiturates, and antiseizure medications can interfere with the effectiveness of OCs.

34.3 **Hormone replacement therapy provides estrogen to treat postmenopausal symptoms, but benefits may not outweigh risks.**

Estrogen–progestin combinations are used for hormone replacement therapy during and after menopause. Their long-term use may have serious adverse effects including increased risk of MI, stroke, breast cancer, and blood clots.

34.4 **Conjugated estrogens and progestins are prescribed for dysfunctional uterine bleeding, endometrial cancer, and postmenopausal symptoms.**

Dysfunctional uterine bleeding is often the result of an imbalance between progesterone and estrogen secretion. Administration of progestins may reestablish a normal cyclic menstrual pattern. Progestins are also used to treat endometrial cancer. Conjugated estrogens treat postmenopausal symptoms.

34.5 **Oxytocin and tocolytics are drugs that influence uterine contractions and labor.**

Oxytocics are drugs that stimulate uterine contractions and induce labor. Oxytocin, methylergonovine (ergot alkaloid), and prostaglandins are examples of uterine stimulants. Tocolytics slow uterine contractions to delay labor.

34.6 **Androgens are used to treat hypogonadism in males.**

Administration of testosterone promotes the appearance of masculine characteristics, a desirable action in men with hypogonadism. Anabolic steroids are testosterone-like drugs which may produce serious and permanent adverse effects.

34.7 **Erectile dysfunction is a common disorder successfully treated with drug therapy.**

Erectile dysfunction is a common disorder with many possible physiologic and psychogenic causes. Sildenafil is effective at promoting more rigid and longer-lasting erections. It is contraindicated in patients taking organic nitrates.

34.8 **In its early stages, benign prostatic hyperplasia is successfully treated.**

BPH results in urinary difficulties that may be treated by drug therapy or surgery. Alpha$_1$-blockers relax smooth muscle in the urethra to promote urine flow. 5-Alpha-reductase inhibitors reduce the size of the prostate to reduce pressure on the urethra. Goals are to minimize urinary obstruction, increase urine flow, and to minimize complications.

REVIEW QUESTIONS

The following questions are written in NCLEX-PN® style. Answer these questions to assess your knowledge of the chapter material, and go back and review any material that is not clear to you.

1. A nurse is discussing the various types of birth control with a new patient at the clinic. The nurse tells the patient that the type of birth control where the estrogen level remains constant throughout the cycle but the progestin level increases toward the end of the menstrual cycle is called:

1. Monophasic
2. Biphasic
3. Triphasic
4. Quadriphasic

2. Before a patient begins taking sildenafil (Viagra), the nurse asks which of the following questions?

1. "Are you currently taking any medications for angina?"
2. "Do you have a history of diabetes?"
3. "Have you ever had an allergic reaction to dairy products?"
4. "Have you ever been treated for migraine headaches?"

3. When planning patient care, the nurse understands that medroxyprogesterone (Prempro) would be contraindicated for which of the following patients?

1. A 37-year-old woman with dysfunctional uterine bleeding
2. A 65-year-old woman diagnosed with metastatic uterine cancer
3. A 40-year-old woman with a history of deep vein thrombosis
4. A healthy 21-year-old who needs birth control

4. The patient states she had sexual intercourse yesterday and is concerned she may be pregnant. She is requesting emergency prevention. The nurse knows that which of the following drugs may be ordered?

1. Oxytocin
2. Levonorgestrel
3. Medroxyprogesterone
4. Magnesium sulfate

5. The patient is being given oxytocin (Pitocin). The nurse evaluates her response to the drug, looking specifically for the possibility of: (Select all that apply.)

1. Uterine rupture
2. Seizures

3. Fetal dysrhythmias
4. Hypotension

6. A patient, seeking information about testosterone replacement therapy, asks the nurse about its application and possible complications. The nurse informs him that complications of testosterone therapy may include:

1. Renal failure
2. Hepatic failure
3. Decreased cholesterol levels
4. Maturation of male sex organs

7. Your patient states that she has forgotten to take her birth control pills for the last 2 days. You should instruct her to:

1. Take her missed pills immediately.
2. Get back on schedule as soon as possible.
3. Use additional birth control measures until a regular schedule is established with the birth control pills.
4. Get a home pregnancy kit.

8. The physician ordered danazol (Danocrine) 100 mg, po, twice a day. The pharmacy has 200 mg tablets. How many milligrams will the nurse administer in a day?

1. 100 mg
2. 400 mg
3. 300 mg
4. 200 mg

9. A patient states that she is experiencing menopausal symptoms and asks the nurse for advice regarding hormone replacement therapy (HRT). The nurse's best response is:

1. "HRT is dangerous and should never be prescribed."
2. "HRT is perfectly safe, with no risks."
3. "You are not a candidate for HRT."
4. "You need to discuss risks versus benefits of HRT with your physician."

10. Your patient with benign prostatic hyperplasia (BPH) is complaining of feeling like he "cannot empty his bladder." You suspect that the physician will order which of the following?

1. Finasteride (Propecia)
2. Sildenafil (Viagra)
3. Estrogen
4. Finasteride (Proscar)

CASE STUDY QUESTIONS

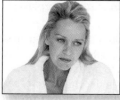

Remember Ms. Philips, the patient introduced at the beginning of the chapter? Now read the remainder of the case study. Based on the information you have learned in this chapter, answer the questions that follow.

Ms. Marge Philips, a 42-year-old female, enters the clinic with complaints of lower abdominal pain and irregular menstrual *bleeding with prolonged menstruation. Blood pressure and pulse are slightly elevated. She states that she has had problems with frequently being tired. Other than her current complaint, she has no other health problems or concerns. Ms. Philips' last physical exam was one year ago. She is diagnosed with dysfunctional uterine bleeding and is prescribed Depo-Provera.*

1. After the diagnosis is confirmed, the nurse knows that _____ is a common method of treating dysfunctional uterine bleeding.

1. Use of condoms
2. Visiting the doctor only when the pain gets really bad
3. Possible use of oral contraceptives
4. Screening of sexual partner

2. In order to determine if Ms. Philips is a good candidate for the medication, Depo-Provera, the nurse asks Ms. Philips if she:

1. Has diabetes
2. Is planning on losing weight
3. Has a diet high in protein
4. Is planning on becoming pregnant

3. Ms. Philips is to begin the oral contraceptive, Depo-Provera, as a means to control the uterine bleeding. The nurse informs her: (Select all that apply.)

1. That smoking increases the risk of serious cardiovascular adverse effects
2. That it is OK to miss taking the medication for several days in a row
3. To notify her healthcare provider if two or more consecutive periods are missed
4. That caffeine will actually be beneficial

4. The nurse also informs Ms. Philips that the adverse effects of Depo-Provera are: (Select all that apply.)

1. Weight loss
2. Breast tenderness
3. Loss of appetite
4. Breakthrough bleeding

NOTE: Answers to the Review and Case Study Questions appear in Appendix B. The complete rationales and answers are located on the textbook's website.

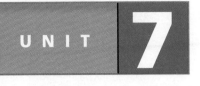

The Skeletal System, Integumentary System, and Eyes and Ears

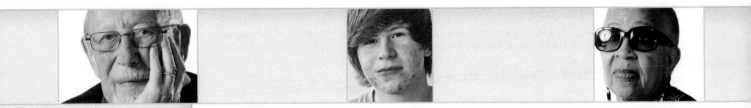

Unit Contents

Chapter 35 Drugs for Bone and Joint Disorders / 564

Chapter 36 Drugs for Skin Disorders / 582

Chapter 37 Drugs for Eye and Ear Disorders / 598

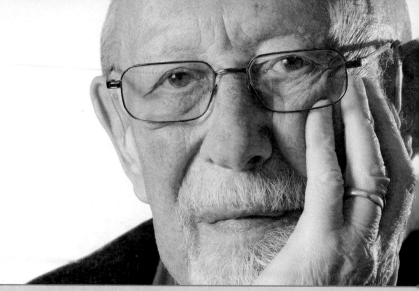

"I can't even work in the garden anymore. My joints ache so badly and I don't understand what's going on with my big toe."

Mr. Steven Hurtt

35 Drugs for Bone and Joint Disorders

CORE CONCEPTS

35.1 Adequate levels of calcium, vitamin D, parathyroid hormone, and calcitonin are necessary for bone and body homeostasis.

35.2 Hypocalcemia is a serious condition that requires immediate therapy.

35.3 Osteomalacia and rickets are successfully treated with calcium salts and vitamin D supplements.

35.4 Treatment for osteoporosis includes calcitonin, selective estrogen-receptor modulators, and bisphosphonates.

35.5 Treatment for Paget's disease includes bisphosphonates and calcitonin.

35.6 Analgesics and anti-inflammatory drugs are important components of pharmacotherapy for osteoarthritis.

35.7 Immunosuppressants and disease-modifying drugs are additional therapies used to treat rheumatoid arthritis.

35.8 Pharmacotherapy for gout requires drugs that control uric acid levels.

DRUG SNAPSHOT

The following drugs are discussed in this chapter:

DRUG CLASSES	DRUG PROTOTYPES	DRUG CLASSES	DRUG PROTOTYPES
Calcium supplements	(Pr) calcium salts **569**	Disease-modifying antirheumatic drugs (DMARDs)	(Pr) hydroxychloroquine (Plaquenil) **575**
Vitamin D therapy	(Pr) calcitriol (Calcijex, Rocaltrol) **569**	Uric acid inhibitors for gout	(Pr) allopurinol (Lopurin, Zyloprin) **578**
Selective estrogen-receptor modulators	(Pr) raloxifene (Evista) **571**		
Bisphosphonates	(Pr) alendronate (Fosamax) **572**		

LEARNING OUTCOMES

After reading this chapter, the student should be able to:

1. Identify the role of calcium and vitamin D in maintaining bone health.

2. Identify the symptoms or disorders associated with an imbalance of calcium, vitamin D, parathyroid hormone, and calcitonin.

3. Describe the pharmacologic management of disorders caused by calcium and vitamin D deficiency and disorders related directly to bones and joints.

4. Discuss drug treatments for hypocalcemia, osteomalacia, and rickets.

5. Identify important disorders characterized by weak and fragile bones.

6. Explain drug treatments for osteoarthritis, rheumatoid arthritis, and gout.

7. For each of the classes listed in the Drug Snapshot, identify representative drugs and explain their mechanisms of drug action, primary drug actions, and important adverse effects.

KEY TERMS

acute gouty arthritis (ah-CUTE GOW-ty are-THRYE-tis) *577*

autoantibodies (AW-tow-ANN-tee-BAH-dees) *575*

bisphosphonates (bis-FOSS-foh-nayts) *572*

bone deposition *565*

bone resorption (ree-SORP-shun) *565*

calcifediol (kal-SIF-eh-DYE-ol) *565*

calcitonin (kal-sih-TOH-nin) *565*

calcitriol (kal-si-TRY-ol) *565*

cholecalciferol (KOH-lee-kal-SIF-er-ol) *565*

disease-modifying antirheumatic (ANTY-roo-MAT-ik) drugs (DMARDs) *575*

gout (GOWT) *576*

osteoarthritis (OA) (OSS-tee-oh-are-THRYE-tis) *574*

osteomalacia (OSS-tee-oh-muh-LAY-shee-uh) *566*

osteoporosis (OSS-tee-oh-poh-ROH-sis) *569*

Paget's disease (PAH-jets) *573*

rheumatoid arthritis (RA) (ROO-mah-toyd are-THRYE-tis) *575*

selective estrogen-receptor modulators (SERMs) *570*

uricosurics (YOUR-ik-cose-youriks) *577*

The skeletal system and joints are at the core of movement and must be free from any defect that would destabilize the other body systems. For nerves, muscles, and bones to function well, the body needs adequate levels of calcium. Disorders associated with bones and joints affect a patient's ability to fulfill daily activities and lead to immobility.

This chapter focuses on the pharmacotherapy of skeletal disorders such as osteomalacia, osteoporosis, arthritis, and gout and stresses the importance of calcium balance and the action of vitamin D as they relate to the proper structure and function of bones and joints. Drugs are important because major mobility problems would occur without intervention.

Adequate levels of calcium, vitamin D, parathyroid hormone, and calcitonin are necessary for bone and body homeostasis.

CORE CONCEPT 35.1

As shown in Figure 35.1 ■, calcium levels in the bloodstream are controlled by two endocrine glands: the parathyroid glands and the thyroid gland. The parathyroid glands secrete parathyroid hormone (PTH), and the thyroid gland secretes calcitonin. PTH stimulates bone cells called *osteoclasts*. Osteoclasts break down bone tissue into its mineral components, a process called **bone resorption**. Once the bone is broken down, calcium is released for transport in the bloodstream and is used elsewhere in the body. The opposite of this process is **bone deposition**, or bone building. **Calcitonin** stimulates the building of bones by adding calcium to bone tissue.

Vitamin D is unique among vitamins in that the body is able to synthesize it from precursor molecules. The inactive form of vitamin D, called **cholecalciferol**, is synthesized in the skin from cholesterol. Exposure of the skin to sunlight or ultraviolet light increases the level of cholecalciferol in the bloodstream. Cholecalciferol can also be obtained from dietary products such as milk or other foods fortified with vitamin D. Figure 35.2 ■ illustrates the metabolism of vitamin D.

Once cholecalciferol is absorbed or formed in the body, it is converted to an intermediate vitamin form called **calcifediol**. Enzymes in the kidneys metabolize calcifediol to **calcitriol**, the active form of vitamin D. Patients with extensive kidney disease are unable to synthesize adequate levels of calcitriol. The primary function of calcitriol is to increase calcium absorption from the gastrointestinal (GI) tract. Dietary calcium is absorbed better in the presence of PTH and active vitamin D.

The importance of proper calcium balance in the body cannot be overstated. Calcium ions influence the excitability of all neurons. When calcium concentrations are too high (hypercalcemia), sodium permeability decreases across cell membranes. This is dangerous because nerve conduction depends on the proper influx of sodium into cells. When calcium levels in the bloodstream are too low (hypocalcemia), cell membranes become hyperexcitable. If hypocalcemia becomes severe, seizures or muscle spasms may result. Calcium is also important for the normal functioning of other body processes such as blood coagulation, neurotransmitter release, and stability of the entire skeletal system.

hyper = *elevated*

hypo = *lowered*
calc = *calcium*
emia = *blood level*

HYPOCALCEMIA

Hypocalcemia is a serious condition that requires immediate therapy.

CORE CONCEPT 35.2

Hypocalcemia, or lowered levels of calcium in the blood, is associated with a range of conditions, including poor nutrition, seizures, muscle spasms, and endocrine and bone disorders. Hypocalcemia is not a disease, but a sign of underlying pathology; therefore, diagnosis of the cause of hypocalcemia is essential. One common cause is hyposecretion of PTH, which occurs when the thyroid and parathyroid glands are

FIGURE 35.1

(a) Parathyroid hormone (PTH); (b) calcitonin action.

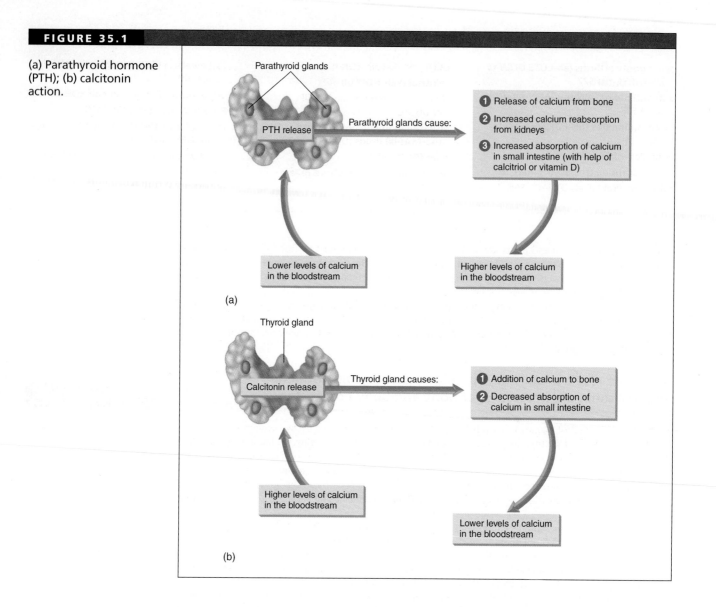

surgically removed. Digestive-related malabsorption disorders and vitamin D deficiencies also result in hypocalcemia. In cases of hypocalcemia, healthcare providers should assess for the adequate intake of calcium-containing foods. With hypocalcemia, numbness and tingling of the extremities may occur, and convulsions are possible. Symptoms of hypocalcemia are nerve and muscle excitability. Muscle twitching, tremor, or cramping may be evident. A patient may be confused or behave abnormally.

Therapies for calcium disorders involve calcium salts, vitamin D supplements, bisphosphonates, and/or miscellaneous drugs. Severe hypocalcemia requires IV administration of calcium salts, whereas less severe hypocalcemia can often be reversed with oral supplements.

OSTEOMALACIA AND RICKETS

CORE CONCEPT 35.3

Osteomalacia and rickets are successfully treated with calcium salts and vitamin D supplements.

Osteomalacia, referred to as *rickets* in children, is a disorder characterized by softening of bones without alteration of basic bone structure. The cause of osteomalacia and rickets is a lack of vitamin D and calcium in the diet, usually as a result of kidney failure or malabsorption of calcium from the GI tract.

FIGURE 35.2

Pathway for vitamin D activation.

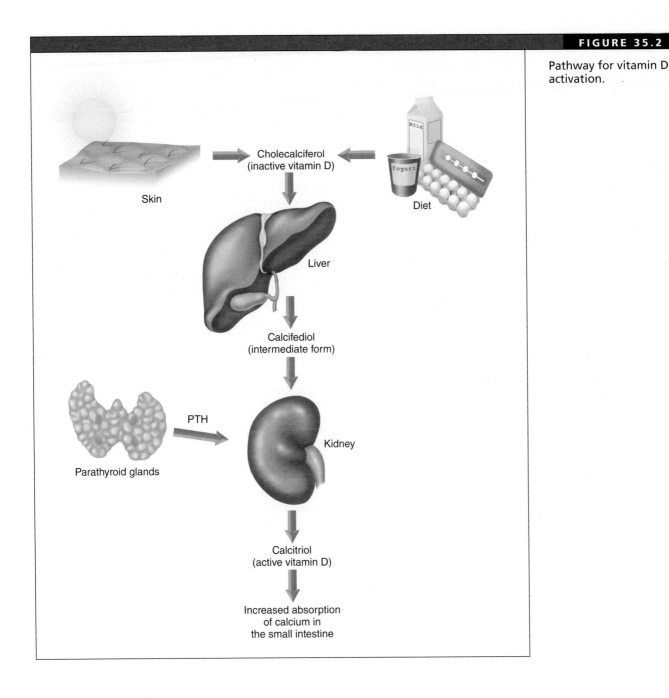

Signs and symptoms of osteomalacia include hypocalcemia, muscle weakness, muscle spasms, and diffuse bone pain, especially in the hip area. Patients may also experience pain in the arms, legs, and spinal column. Classic signs of rickets in children include bowlegs and a pigeon breast. Children may also develop a slight fever and become restless at night.

Tests performed to verify osteomalacia include bone biopsy; bone radiographs; computerized tomography (CT) scan of the vertebral column and other bone density tests; and determination of serum calcium, phosphate, and vitamin D levels. Many of these tests are routine for bone disorders and are performed as needed to determine the extent of bone health.

Drug therapy for osteomalacia consists of calcium salts and vitamin D supplements. Drugs used for treating metabolic bone disorders including hypocalcemia, osteomalacia, and rickets are shown in Table 35.1 ◆. In extreme cases, surgical correction of disfigured limbs may be required.

Most calcium salts are in the form of complexed calcium. These products are often compared on the basis of their ability to release elemental calcium into the bloodstream. The supplement is more potent when the complexed calcium has a greater ability to release elemental calcium. Milliequivalence (mEq)

TABLE 35.1 Calcium Salts and Vitamin D Therapy

Drug	Route and Adult Dose	Remarks
CALCIUM SALTS (The higher the mEq, the more potent the calcium salt)		
calcium acetate (PhosLo)	PO; 1–2 g bid–tid	One gram calcium acetate equals 250 mg (12.6 mEq) elemental calcium; phosphate binder used to treat hypophosphatemia in dialysis patients
calcium carbonate (Rolaids, Tums, others)	PO; 1–2 g bid–tid	One gram calcium carbonate equals 400 mg (20 mEq) elemental calcium
calcium chloride	IV; 0.5–1 g by slow infusion (1 mL/min)	One gram calcium chloride equals 272 mg (13.6 mEq) elemental calcium; may be irritating to body tissues
calcium citrate (Citracal)	PO; 1–2 g bid–tid	One gram calcium citrate equals 210 mg (12 mEq) elemental calcium
calcium gluconate (Kalcinate)	PO; 1–2 g bid–tid IV; 0.5–4 g by slow infusions (1 g/hour)	One gram calcium gluconate equals 90 mg (4.5 mEq) elemental calcium
calcium lactate (Cal-Lac)	PO; 100–200 mg tid with meals	One gram calcium lactate equals 130 mg (6.5 mEq) elemental calcium
calcium phosphate tribasic (Posture)	PO; 1–2 g bid–tid	One gram calcium phosphate equals 390 mg (19.3 mEq) elemental calcium
VITAMIN D SUPPLEMENTS		
℗ calcitriol (Calcijex, Rocaltrol)	PO; 0.25 mcg/day IV; 0.5 mcg three times per week at the end of dialysis	For hypocalcemia in chronic renal failure and with hypoparathyroidism
doxercalciferol (Hectorol)	PO; 10 mcg, three times per week (max: 60 mcg/week) IV; 4 mcg, three times per week at the end of dialysis (max: 18 mcg/week)	For hyperparathyroidism in patients with chronic kidney disease or in patients on dialysis
ergocalciferol (Calciferol, Drisdol)	PO; 25–125 mcg/day for 6–12 weeks	For osteomalacia; also used for vitamin D–dependent rickets and hypoparathyroidism
paricalcitol (Zemplar)	PO; 1 mcg/day or 4 mcg three times per week IV; 0.04–0.1 mcg/kg, every other day during dialysis (max: 24 mcg/kg)	For the prevention and treatment of hyperparathyroidism in patients with chronic kidney disease

is the unit used to describe the amount of electrolyte available to the bloodstream. Therefore, the higher the mEq, the more potent the calcium salt. Elemental calcium may be obtained from dietary sources such as dark green vegetables, canned salmon, and fortified products, including tofu, orange juice, and milk.

Inactive, intermediate, and active forms of vitamin D are also available. The amount of vitamin D a patient needs will often vary depending on how much he or she is exposed to sunlight. After age 70, the average recommended intake of vitamin D increases from 400 to 600 units per day. Because vitamin D is needed to absorb calcium from the GI tract, many supplements combine vitamin D and calcium into a single tablet.

Concept Review 35.1

■ Identify the major drug therapies used for hypocalcemia, osteomalacia, and rickets.

Drug Prototype: ℗ *Calcium salts*

Therapeutic Class: Calcium supplement for hypoparathyroidism, osteoporosis, and rickets

Pharmacologic Class: Reverses hypocalcemia

Actions and Uses: Calcium salts are used to correct hypocalcemia and to treat osteoporosis and rickets. The objective of calcium therapy is to return serum levels of calcium to normal. People at high risk for developing these conditions include postmenopausal women; those with little physical activity over a prolonged period; and patients taking certain medications such as corticosteroids, immunosuppressive drugs, and some antiseizure medications.

Adverse Effects and Interactions: The most common adverse effect of calcium salts is hypercalcemia, which is brought on by taking too much of these supplements. Symptoms include drowsiness, lethargy, weakness, headache, anorexia, nausea and vomiting, increased urination, and thirst. IV administration of calcium may cause hypotension, bradycardia, dysrhythmia, and cardiac arrest.

Using calcium salts with cardiac glycosides increases the risk of dysrhythmias. Magnesium antacids or supplements may compete for GI absorption. Calcium decreases the absorption of tetracyclines.

Drug Prototype: ℗ *Calcitriol (Calcijex, Rocaltrol)*

Therapeutic Class: Drug for osteoporosis, osteomalacia, and rickets

Pharmacologic Class: Vitamin D, reverses hypocalcemia

Actions and Uses: Calcitriol is the active form of vitamin D and is available in both oral and IV formulations. It promotes the intestinal absorption of calcium and elevates serum levels of calcium. This medication is used when patients have impaired kidney function or have hypoparathyroidism. Calcitriol reduces bone resorption and is useful in treating rickets. The effectiveness of calcitriol depends on the patient receiving an adequate amount of calcium; therefore, it is usually prescribed in combination with calcium supplements.

Adverse Effects and Interactions: Common adverse effects include hypercalcemia, headache, weakness, dry mouth, thirst, increased urination, and muscle or bone pain. Thiazide diuretics may increase the effects of vitamin D, causing hypercalcemia. Too much vitamin D may cause dysrhythmias in patients who are receiving cardiac glycosides. Magnesium antacids or supplements should not be given together with calcitriol because of the increased risk of hypermagnesemia.

OSTEOPOROSIS

Treatment for osteoporosis includes calcitonin, selective estrogen-receptor modulators, and bisphosphonates.

CORE CONCEPT 35.4

Osteoporosis is the most common metabolic bone disorder. This disorder is usually asymptomatic until the bones become brittle enough to fracture or a vertebra collapses. In some cases, a lack of dietary calcium and vitamin D contribute to bone deterioration. In other cases, osteoporosis is due to disrupted bone homeostasis.

Simply stated, the homeostatic imbalance with osteoporosis is that bone resorption outpaces bone deposition, and patients begin to develop weak bones. This is generally considered an aging disorder. Following are the risk factors for osteoporosis:

- Postmenopausal status
- High alcohol or caffeine consumption
- Anorexia nervosa
- Tobacco use
- Physical inactivity
- Testosterone deficiency, particularly in elderly men
- Lack of adequate vitamin D or calcium in the diet
- Drugs such as corticosteroids, some anticonvulsants, and immunosuppressants that lower calcium levels in the bloodstream

FIGURE 35.3

Calcium metabolism in osteoporosis: (a) bone deposition equals bone resorption; (b) bone resorption outpaces bone deposition).

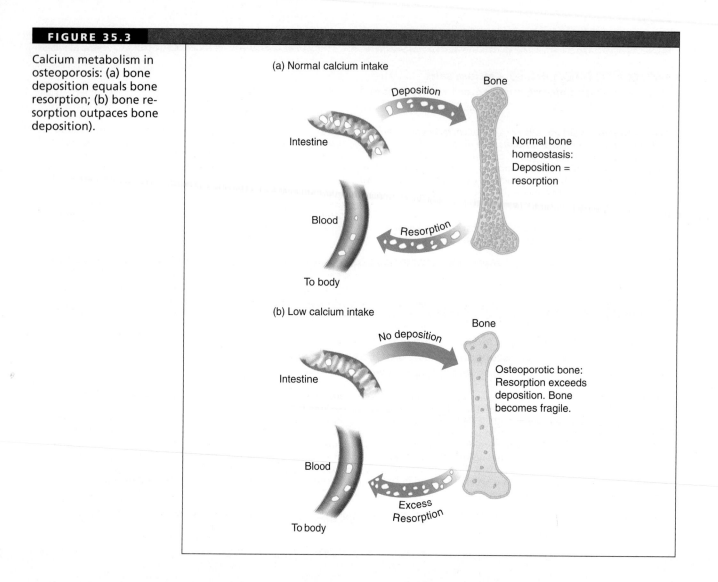

The most common risk factor associated with the development of osteoporosis is the onset of menopause. When women reach menopause, estrogen secretion declines and bones become weak and fragile. One theory to explain this occurrence is that normal levels of estrogen may limit the life span of osteoclasts, the bone cells that resorb bone. When estrogen levels become low, osteoclast activity is no longer controlled, and bone demineralization accelerates, resulting in loss of bone density. In women with osteoporosis, fractures often occur in the hips, wrists, forearms, or spine. The metabolism of calcium in osteoporosis is illustrated in Figure 35.3 ■.

Many drug therapies are available for osteoporosis. These include calcium and vitamin D therapy, hormone therapy with estrogen, estrogen-receptor modulators, calcitonin, statins, slow-release sodium fluoride, and bisphosphonates. Many of these drug classes are also used for other bone disorders or conditions unrelated to the skeletal system. Selected drugs for osteoporosis and related bone disorders are listed in Table 35.2 ◆.

Selective Estrogen-Receptor Modulators

Selective estrogen-receptor modulators (SERMs) bind to estrogen receptors and comprise a class of drugs used in the prevention and treatment of osteoporosis. SERMs may be estrogen agonists or antagonists, depending on the specific drug and the tissue involved. In the uterus and breasts, raloxifene (Evista) blocks estrogen receptors; thus, it has no estrogen-like proliferative effects on these tissues that might promote cancer. It is one of the few drugs available for the prevention of breast cancer in postmenopausal women at high risk for the disease. Evista decreases bone resorption, thus increasing bone density and making fractures less likely. Like estrogen, it has a cholesterol-lowering effect.

TABLE 35.2 Bone Resorption Inhibitors and Selected Drugs

Drug	Route and Adult Dose	Remarks
HORMONAL (BIOLOGIC) AND SELECTED DRUGS		
calcitonin–salmon (Fortical, Miacalcin)	Hypercalcemia: subcutaneous/IM; salmon, 4 units/kg bid Osteoporosis: intranasal; 1 spray/day (200 international units) in one nostril, alternating nostrils each day	Calcium regulating hormone; used commonly for hypercalcemia and postmenopausal osteoporosis
cinacalcet (Sensipar)	PO; start with 30 mg once daily; may increase every 2–4 weeks until target PTH of 150–300 mg/mL (max: 300/day)	For secondary hyperparathyroidism
denosumab (Prolia, Xgeva)	Subcutaneous (Prolia); 60 mg every 6 months	For postmenopausal osteoporosis in women at high risk for fracture (Prolia) or prevention of skeletal-related adverse events in patients with bone metastases (Xgeva)
Pr raloxifene (Evista)	PO; 60 mg daily	Selective estrogen-receptor modulator; for prevention and treatment of osteoporosis in postmenopausal women and breast cancer prophylaxis
teriparatide (Forteo)	SC; 20 mcg/day	Parathyroid hormone (rDNA origin); for osteoporosis in postmenopausal women; for male patients with high risk of fractures
BISPHOSPHONATES		
Pr alendronate (Fosamax)	Osteoporosis treatment: PO; 10 mg daily Osteoporosis prevention: PO; 5 mg daily Paget's disease: PO 40 mg daily for 6 months	For osteoporosis in men and women; for Paget's disease
etidronate (Didronel)	PO; 5–10 mg/kg daily for 6 months or 11–20 mg/kg daily for 3 months	For Paget's disease
ibandronate (Boniva)	PO; 2.5 mg daily or 150 mg once monthly	For treatment and prevention of postmenopausal osteoporosis
pamidronate (Aredia)	IV; 30–90 mg infused over 4–24 hours	For Paget's disease and hypercalcemia of malignancy
risedronate (Actonel)	PO; 5 mg daily or 35 mg once weekly or 75 mg daily for two consecutive weeks	For prevention and treatment of osteoporosis and Paget's disease
tiludronate (Skelid)	PO; 400 mg daily taken with 6–8 ounces of water 2 hours before or after food for 3 months	For Paget's disease
zoledronate (Reclast, Zometa): also called zoledronic acid	IV; 4–5 mg, may be repeated in 7 days	For hypercalcemia of malignancy; treatment of steroid-induced osteoporosis, postmenopausal osteoporosis, bone metastases, and Paget's disease

Drug Prototype: **Pr** *Raloxifene (Evista)*

Therapeutic Class: Treatment of postmenopausal osteoporosis in women
Pharmacologic Class: Bone resorption inhibitor, selective estrogen-receptor modulator

Actions and Uses: Raloxifene is a SERM. It decreases bone resorption and increases bone mass and density by acting through the estrogen receptor. Raloxifene is primarily used for the prevention of osteoporosis in postmenopausal women. It is also one of the few drugs used for the prevention of breast cancer in women at high risk for invasive breast cancer. This drug also reduces serum total cholesterol and low-density lipoprotein (LDL) without lowering high-density lipoprotein (HDL) or triglycerides.

Adverse Effects and Interactions: Common adverse effects are hot flashes, migraine headache, flu-like symptoms, endometrial disorder, breast pain, and vaginal bleeding. Patients should not take cholesterol-lowering drugs or estrogen replacement therapy concurrently with this medication.

Absorption is reduced by cholestyramine. Patients taking raloxifene, along with warfarin, should have their PT/INR tested when starting or stopping this medication

BLACK BOX WARNING:
Raloxifene increases the risk of venous thromboembolism and death from strokes. Women with a history of venous thromboembolism should not take this drug.

Calcitonin

Calcitonin is a naturally occurring hormone secreted by the thyroid gland when blood calcium becomes elevated. It is involved in the process of bone building by opposing the effects of the PTH and inhibiting osteoclast activity in the bone. As a medication, calcitonin is obtained from salmon and is approved for the treatment of osteoporosis in women who are more than five years postmenopausal. It is available by nasal spray or subcutaneous injection. Calcitonin increases bone density and reduces the risk of vertebral fractures. Adverse effects are generally minor; the nasal formulation may irritate the nasal mucosa and allergies are possible. Parenteral forms may produce nausea and vomiting. In addition to treating osteoporosis, calcitonin is indicated for Paget's disease and hypercalcemia.

Bisphosphonates

The most common drug class used to treat osteoporosis is the **bisphosphonates**. These drugs are very similar to pyrophosphate, a natural inhibitor of bone resorption. Bisphosphonates inhibit bone resorption by suppressing osteoclast activity, thereby increasing bone density and reducing the incidence of fractures. Examples include alendronate (Fosamax), etidronate (Didronel), ibandronate (Boniva), pamidronate (Aredia), risedronate (Actonel, Atelvia), tiludronate (Skelid), and zoledronate (Reclast, Zometa). Although primarily used to treat osteoporosis in postmenopausal women, drugs in this class are also used to treat Paget's disease, osteoporosis in men, hypercalcemia of malignancy and metastases due to bone cancer, multiple myeloma or breast cancer. Adverse effects include GI problems such as nausea, vomiting, abdominal pain, and esophageal irritation; therefore, patients are advised to remain in an upright position for 30 minutes after taking these medications. Because these drugs are poorly absorbed, they should be taken on an empty stomach, as tolerated by the patient. Once-weekly dosing may give the same bone-density benefits as daily dosing because of these drugs' extended duration of action.

Concept Review 35.2

- What are the major drug therapies used for the treatment of osteoporosis and related bone disorders?

Drug Prototype: Ⓟ *Alendronate (Fosamax)*

Therapeutic Class: Drug for osteoporosis   **Pharmacologic Class: Bone resorption inhibitor, bisphosphonate**

Actions and Uses: Alendronate is approved for the following indications: prevention of osteoporosis in postmenopausal women, treatment of glucocorticoid-induced osteoporosis in both women and men, to increase bone mass in men with osteoporosis, and treatment of symptomatic Paget's disease in both women and men. Alendronate is also used off-label for treating hypercalcemia due to malignancy. Therapeutic effects may take from one to three months to appear and may continue for several months after therapy is discontinued. All doses must be taken on an empty stomach, preferably in a fasting state two hours before breakfast.

Adverse Effects and Interactions: Common adverse effects of alendronate are diarrhea, nausea, vomiting, esophageal irritation, and a metallic or altered taste perception. Pathologic fractures may occur if the drug is taken longer than three months. Calcium supplements may decrease absorption of alendronate; therefore, use of these drugs together should be avoided. Food–drug interactions are common. Milk and other dairy products and medications, such as calcium, iron, antacids, and other mineral supplements, must be reviewed before beginning bisphosphonate therapy because they have the potential to decrease the effectiveness of bisphosphonates. Blood levels of the enzyme alkaline phosphatase are lowered with this drug.

NURSING PROCESS FOCUS   Patients Receiving Pharmacotherapy for Osteoporosis

ASSESSMENT	POTENTIAL NURSING DIAGNOSES
Prior to administration: ■ Obtain a complete health history, including musculoskeletal, GI, cardiovascular, neurological, thyroid/parathyroid, renal, and liver conditions; allergies; drug history; and possible drug interactions. ■ Evaluate laboratory blood findings: CBC, electrolytes, lipid panel, T_3, T_4 and TSH, and renal and liver function studies. ■ Acquire the results of a complete physical examination, including vital signs, height, and weight. ■ Collect a dietary history, noting adequacy of essential vitamins, minerals, and nutrients obtained through food sources. ■ Obtain a history of current symptoms and effect on activities of daily living (ADLs).	■ *Deficient Knowledge* related to a lack of information about drug therapy ■ *Infective Health Maintenance* related to lifestyle changes or adverse drug effects ■ *Risk for Injury* related to disease process and adverse drug effects ■ *Risk of Falls* related to disease process and adverse drug effects

continued . . .

NURSING PROCESS FOCUS *(continued)*

PLANNING: PATIENT GOALS AND EXPECTED OUTCOMES

The patient will:
- Experience therapeutic effects (a gain or maintenance of adequate bone density).
- Be free from or experience minimal adverse effects from drug therapy.
- Verbalize understanding of the drug's use, adverse effects, and required precautions.

IMPLEMENTATION

Interventions and (Rationales)	Patient Education/Discharge Planning
Administer medication correctly and evaluate the patient's knowledge of proper administration. (Incorrect use may decrease absorption of medication.)	Instruct the patient: - About the proper administration method guidelines. - Bisphosphonates should be taken on an empty stomach, and to remain in a sitting position after taking medication.
Review dietary history and discuss food source options, correcting any calcium and vitamin D deficiencies. (Adequate amounts of calcium, vitamin D and magnesium are needed for bone health. If taking bisphosphonates, a review of foods and medications should be done because calcium rich foods, medication, and supplements may decrease absorption of bisphosphonates.)	Inform the patient: - To eat adequate amounts of calcium, vitamin D, and magnesium from food. - That milk and other calcium rich foods and medications (such as ant- acids and calcium supplements) must be reviewed before beginning bisphosphonate therapy because they may decrease absorption of drug.
Monitor for adverse effects of medications. Bisphosphonates may cause GI irritation. SERMs increase the risk of venous thromboembo- lism and death from strokes. (Women with a history of thrombosis should not take this medication.)	Inform the patient: - Bisphosphonates may cause esophageal and gastric irritation, abdominal pain, and nausea; to report immediately the onset of nausea or abdominal pain to the healthcare provider. - SERMs may cause hot flashes, migraines, flu-like symptoms endome- trial problems, breast pain and increase the risk of forming blood clots. Discontinue three days prior to surgery. - That intranasal administration of calcitonin may cause nasal irritation. Allergies are also possible.
Review and monitor the use of other medications. (Concurrently using some medications with those used for osteoporosis may cause adverse effects or impact absorption.)	Instruct the patient: - Not to take cholesterol-lowering drugs or estrogen replacement therapy concurrently with SERMs. - If taking raloxifene along with warfarin, PT/INR should be tested when starting or stopping. - Calcium supplements should not be used with bisphosphonates.
Continue to monitor periodic laboratory tests, especially calcium, magnesium, phosphorus, and creatinine. Assess for sign or symptoms of hypo/hypercalcemia. (These electrolytes should remain or return to normal limits. Increased creatinine levels may require discontinuation of medication.)	Instruct the patient to: - Return periodically for laboratory tests. - Report any symptoms of hypocalcemia (muscle spasms, facial grimac- ing, irritability hyper-reflexes) or hypercalcemia (increased bone pain, anorexia, nausea, vomiting, constipation, thirst, lethargy, fatigue) to the healthcare provider.
Increase fluid intake, avoiding caffeine, soda, and alcohol. (Some kidney stones are composed of calcium; increasing fluid intake decreases the risk of kidney stones formation. Caffeine diminishes the absorption of calcium.)	Instruct the patient to: - Increase fluid intake to 2 L/day. - Avoid excessive caffeine because it diminishes the absorption of calcium. - Limit or eliminate alcohol.
Monitor for adherence to recommended lifestyle, for example, diet, exercise, and medication regimen. (Bone remodeling occurs over several months. The patient may discontinue the drug because of perceived lack of results.)	Inform the patient: - To engage in weight-bearing exercises, three to five times a week. - To acquire a limited amount of daily sun exposure (15–20 minutes) for vitamin D synthesis. - That the therapeutic effects of the medication(s) may take one to three months and to continue taking the drug as prescribed to ensure full effect.

EVALUATION OF OUTCOME CRITERIA

Evaluate the effectiveness of drug therapy by confirming that patient goals and expected outcomes have been met (see "Planning"). *See Table 35.2 for a list of drugs to which these nursing actions apply.*

PAGET'S DISEASE

Treatment for Paget's disease includes bisphosphonates and calcitonin.

CORE CONCEPT 35.5

Paget's disease, or *osteitis deformans*, is a chronic, progressive condition characterized by enlarged and abnormal bones. With this disorder, the processes of bone resorption and bone formation occur at a high rate. Excessive bone turnover causes the new bone to be weak and brittle, which may result in deformity and fractures. The patient may be asymptomatic or have only vague, nonspecific complaints for many years. Symptoms include pain of the hips and femurs, joint inflammation, headaches, facial pain, and hearing loss if bones around the ear cavity are affected. Nerves along the spinal column may be pinched in the compressed vertebrae.

Paget's disease is sometimes confused with osteoporosis because some of the symptoms are similar. In fact, medical treatments for osteoporosis are similar to those for Paget's disease. The cause of Paget's disease, however, is quite different. Blood levels of the enzyme alkaline phosphatase are elevated because of the extensive bone turnover. Detection of this enzyme in the blood often provides early confirmation of the disease. Calcium blood levels are also increased. The symptoms of Paget's disease can be treated successfully when diagnosis is made early. If the diagnosis is made late in the disease's progression, permanent skeletal abnormalities may develop, and other disorders may appear, including arthritis, kidney stones, and heart disease.

Bisphosphonates are the preferred pharmacotherapy for Paget's disease. Therapy is usually cyclic. Bisphosphonates are administered until serum alkaline phosphatase levels return to normal; then a drug-free period of several months follows. When serum alkaline phosphatase levels become elevated, therapy is begun again. The pharmacologic goals are to slow the rate of bone reabsorption and encourage the deposition of strong bone. Calcitonin nasal spray is used as an option for patients who cannot tolerate bisphosphonates. Surgery may be indicated in cases of severe bone deformity, degenerative arthritis, or fracture. Patients with Paget's disease should receive adequate daily dietary intake of calcium and vitamin D. Sufficient exposure to sunlight is also important.

Concept Review 35.3

- Identify two important disorders characterized by weak and fragile bones. What are the major drug therapies used in their treatments?

OSTEOARTHRITIS

CORE CONCEPT 35.6

Analgesics and anti-inflammatory drugs are important components of pharmacotherapy for osteoarthritis.

Arthritis is a general term meaning inflammation of a joint. There are several types of arthritis, each having somewhat different characteristics based on the etiology. Because joint pain is common to both arthritic and joint disorders, analgesics and/or anti-inflammatory drugs are important components of pharmacotherapy. A few additional drugs are specific to the particular pathologies.

osteo = *bone*
arthr = *joint*
itis = *associated disease, often linked with inflammation*

Osteoarthritis (OA) is a degenerative disease in which the cartilage at articular joint surfaces wears away. Like osteoporosis, this condition is considered to be an aging disorder. It is not accompanied by the degree of inflammation associated with other forms of arthritis. Signs are localized pain and stiffness, joint and bone enlargement, and limitations in movement. The cause of OA is thought to be excessive wear and tear of weight-bearing joints; the knee, spine, and hip are particularly affected.

The goals of pharmacotherapy for OA include reduction of pain and inflammation. The initial treatment of choice is acetaminophen. For patients whose pain is unrelieved by acetaminophen, nonsteroidal anti-inflammatory drugs (NSAIDs), including naproxen and ibuprofen-like drugs, are usually given. Tramadol (Ultram) is a non-NSAID option for the treatment of moderate to severe pain. Although classified as an opioid, tramadol does not have abuse potential and is not a scheduled drug. Opioids such as codeine may be combined with acetaminophen for severe pain.

Many patients with OA use over-the-counter (OTC) topical creams, gels, sprays, patches, or ointments that include salicylates (Aspercreme and Sportscreme), capsaicin (Capzasin), and counterirritants (Ben-Gay and Icy Hot). These therapies are well tolerated and produce few adverse effects. Pennsaid is a prescription, topical form of the NSAID diclofenac that is rubbed on the knee for symptoms of OA.

A newer approach to treating patients with moderate OA who do not respond adequately to analgesics includes sodium hyaluronate (Hyalgan), a chemical normally found in high amounts within synovial fluid. Administered by injection directly into the knee joint, this drug replaces or supplements the body's natural hyaluronic acid that deteriorated because of the inflammation of OA. By coating the articulating cartilage surface, Hyalgan helps provide a barrier that prevents friction and further inflammation of the joint.

RHEUMATOID ARTHRITIS

Immunosuppressants and disease-modifying drugs are additional therapies used to treat rheumatoid arthritis.

Rheumatoid arthritis (RA) is a systemic autoimmune disorder that causes disfigurement and inflammation of multiple joints and usually occurs at an earlier age than OA. RA is the second most common form of arthritis and has an autoimmune etiology. In RA, **autoantibodies**, called rheumatoid factors, activate other inflammatory substances called complement proteins and draw leukocytes into an area where they attack normal cells. This results in ongoing injury and formation of inflammatory fluid within the joints. Joint capsules, tendons, ligaments, and skeletal muscles may also be affected. Unlike OA, which causes local pain in affected joints, patients with RA may develop systemic manifestations that include infections, pulmonary disease, pericarditis, abnormal numbers of blood cells, and symptoms of metabolic dysfunction such as fatigue, anorexia, and weakness.

The goals for the pharmacotherapy of RA include management of pain and inflammation and slowing the progress of the disease. The same classes of analgesics and anti-inflammatory drugs used to treat OA are used to manage RA. If inflammation is especially severe, short-term therapy with corticosteroids may be indicated (see Chapter 32).

Additional drugs are sometimes prescribed to manage the immune aspects of RA. Research has shown that the progression of tissue damage can be slowed by the use of **disease-modifying antirheumatic drugs (DMARDs)**. DMARDs may require several months of treatment before maximum therapeutic effects are achieved. Because many of these drugs can be toxic, patients should be closely monitored. Adverse effects vary depending on the type of drug. There are many DMARDs available, and these drugs are listed in Table 35.3 ◆.

The newest types of DMARDs are called biologic therapies. These drugs are used to block specific steps in the inflammatory process. Examples of biologic agents include adalimumab (Humira), etanercept (Enbrel), and golimumab (Simponi). Biologic agents are very effective and some are also prescribed to treat other disease with inflammatory components, such as Crohn's disease, psoriasis, ulcerative colitis, and ankylosing spondylitis.

rheuma = *watery discharge*
toid = *associated*

auto = *self-directed*
anti = *against*
bodies = *things*

Concept Review   35.4

■ Identify the major types of arthritis. What are the general differences between these disorders?

Drug Prototype: 🅟 *Hydroxychloroquine (Plaquenil)*

Therapeutic Class: Disease-modifying antirheumatic drug (DMARD)
Pharmacologic Class: Protein synthesis inhibitor, inhibitor of DNA and RNA polymerase, rheumatoid drug

Actions and Uses: Hydroxychloroquine is prescribed for RA and lupus erythematosus in patients who have not responded well to other anti-inflammatory drugs. This drug relieves the severe inflammation characteristic of these disorders. For full effectiveness, hydroxychloroquine is most often prescribed with salicylates and glucocorticoids. This drug has also been used for prophylaxis and treatment of malaria.

Adverse Effects and Interactions: Adverse symptoms include blurred vision, GI disturbances, loss of hair, headache, and mood and mental changes. Hydroxychloroquine has possible ocular effects that include blurred vision, photophobia, diminished ability to read, and blacked out areas in the visual field.

Antacids with aluminum and magnesium may prevent absorption. This drug interferes with the patient's response to the rabies vaccine. Hydroxychloroquine may increase the risk of liver toxicity when administered with drugs that are toxic to the liver. Alcohol use should be eliminated during therapy. It also may lead to increased digoxin levels.

Fast Facts Arthritis and Joint Disorders

■ Between 20 million and 40 million patients in the United States are affected by OA.

■ After age 40, more than 90% of the population has symptoms of OA in major weight-bearing joints. After 70 years of age, almost all patients have symptoms of OA.

■ Of the world's population, 1% has RA, which most often affects patients between 30 and 50 years of age. Women are three to five times more likely to develop RA than men.

■ Between 1% and 3% of the U.S. population is affected by gout. Most of the patients are men between the ages of 30 and 60. Women are more likely to be affected after menopause.

TABLE 35.3 Disease-Modifying Antirheumatic Drugs (DMARDs) and Biologic Therapies

Drug	Route and Adult Dose	Remarks
abatacept (Orencia)	IV; 500–1,000 mg given on 0, 2, and 4 weeks, then every 4 weeks thereafter	Immune modulating drug; inhibits T lymphocyte activation
adalimumab (Humira)	Subcutaneous; 40 mg every other week; without methotrexate, dose can be increased up to 40 mg every week	Tumor necrosis factor blocker
anakinra (Kineret)	Subcutaneous; 100 mg per day	Interleukin-1 receptor blocker
azathioprine (Azasan, Imuran)	PO; 1 mg/kg/day once or in divided doses bid for 6–8 weeks (max. 2.5 mg/kg/day); maintenance dose: 1–2.5 mg/kg/day as a single dose or divided	Immunosuppressant and anti-inflammatory; may cause bone marrow depression
certolizumab pegol (Cimzia)	Subcutaneous; 400 mg initially and at weeks 2 and 4, followed by 200 mg every other week	Tumor necrosis factor blocker
etanercept (Enbrel)	Subcutaneous; 25 mg twice weekly; or 0.08 mg/kg or 50 mg once weekly	Tumor necrosis factor blocker
golimumab (Simponi)	Subcutaneous; 50 mg once monthly	Injectable man-made protein that binds to tumor necrosis factor and blocks its action
(Pr) hydroxychloroquine (Plaquenil)	PO; 400–600 mg/day for 4–12 weeks, then 200–400 mg once daily; maintenance dose: 10–20 mg/day	Has been used for acute malaria and malaria suppression
infliximab (Remicade)	IV; 3 mg/kg followed by 3 mg/kg 2 weeks and 6 weeks after initial dose and then every 8 weeks	Tumor necrosis factor-alpha blocker, used in combination with methotrexate
leflunomide (Arava)	PO; loading dose: 100 mg/day for 3 days; maintenance dose: 10–20 mg daily	Immunomodulator with anti-inflammatory effects; may cause Stevens–Johnson syndrome
methotrexate (Rheumatrex, Trexall) (see page 440 for the Drug Prototype box)	PO; 7.5 mg once/wk or 2.5–5 mg every 12 hours for three doses each week (max 20 mg/week)	Folic acid blocker; antineoplastic and immunosuppressant; may cause liver toxicity, sudden death, and pulmonary fibrosis
rituximab (Rituxan)	IV; 1,000 mg every 2 weeks for a total of two doses (give a corticosteroid 30 minutes prior to treatment)	Also indicated for the treatment of non-Hodgkin's lymphoma (NHL)
sulfasalazine (Azulfidine)	PO; 1–2 g daily in four divided doses (max: 8 g/day)	Also for ulcerative colitis
tocilizumab (Actemra)	IV; 4–8 mg/kg every other week	Interleukin-6 receptor blocker

GOUT

CORE CONCEPT 35.8

Pharmacotherapy for gout requires drugs that control uric acid levels.

Gout, a form of acute arthritis, is a metabolic disorder caused by the accumulation of uric acid in the bloodstream or joint cavities. This disorder is extremely painful. Gout occurs when excretion of uric acid by the kidneys is reduced. One metabolic step important to the pharmacotherapy of this disease is the conversion of hypoxanthine (part of the chemical structure of the genes found with the body's cells) to uric acid by the enzyme xanthine oxidase. An elevated blood level of uric acid is called *hyperuricemia*.

Gout may be classified as primary or secondary. *Primary gout*, caused by genetic errors in uric acid metabolism, is most commonly observed in Pacific Islanders. *Secondary gout* is caused by diseases or drugs that increase the metabolic turnover of nucleic acids or that interfere with uric acid excretion.

hyper = *elevated*
uric = *uric acid*
emia = *blood level*

Examples of drugs that may cause gout include thiazide diuretics, aspirin, cyclosporine, and alcohol (when ingested on a chronic basis). Conditions that can cause secondary gout include diabetic ketoacidosis, kidney failure, and diseases associated with a rapid cell turnover, such as leukemia, hemolytic anemia, and polycythemia.

Acute gouty arthritis occurs when needle-shaped uric acid crystals accumulate in joints, resulting in red, swollen, and inflamed tissue. Attacks have a sudden onset; often occur at night; and may be triggered by diet, injury, or other stresses. Gouty arthritis most often occurs in the big toes, heels, ankles, wrists, fingers, knees, and elbows. About 90% of patients with gout are men.

NSAIDs are the preferred drugs for treating the pain and inflammation associated with acute gout attacks (Table 35.4 ◆). The use of colchicine (Colcrys) has declined, although it may still be prescribed for patients whose symptoms cannot be controlled with NSAIDs. Low doses may be prescribed for gout prophylaxis.

Most patients with acute gout will experience subsequent attacks within one to two years after the first attack. Thus, long-term prophylactic therapy with drugs that lower serum uric acid is often initiated. This can be accomplished through three strategies.

One strategy to prevent hyperuricemia is to use **uricosurics**, drugs that increase the excretion of uric acid by blocking its reabsorption in the kidney. The uricosuric drugs used for gout prophylaxis include probenecid (Probalan) and sulfinpyrazone (Anturane).

uricos = *uric acid excretion*
urics = *impact on urination*

A second strategy for preventing hyperuricemia is to reduce the formation of uric acid. The traditional drug for gout prophylaxis, allopurinol (Lopurin, Zyloprim), blocks the enzyme xanthine oxidase, thus reducing the formation of uric acid. A newer antigout drug, febuxostat (Uloric), acts by the same mechanism as allopurinol but is safer for patients with renal impairment because it is not excreted by the kidneys.

A third strategy for preventing hyperuricemia is to convert uric acid to a less toxic form. Two drugs are available that act by this mechanism. Rasburicase (Elitek) is an enzyme produced through recombinant DNA technology that is used to reduce uric acid levels in patients who are receiving cancer chemotherapy. Approved in 2010, pegloticase (Krystexxa) is a synthetic enzyme that metabolizes uric acid to an inert substance. It is used to lower uric acid levels in patients with chronic gout who have not responded to conventional therapies.

Concept Review 35.5

■ Identify drug therapies used to treat the major arthritic and joint disorders.

TABLE 35.4 Uric Acid–Inhibiting Drugs for Gout and Gouty Arthritis

Drug	Route and Adult Dose	Remarks
(Pr) allopurinol (Lopurin, Zyloprim)	PO (primary); 100 mg daily; may increase by 100 mg/week (max: 800 mg/day) PO (secondary); 200–800 mg daily for 2–3 days or longer	For primary hyperuricemia, secondary hyperuricemia, and prevention of gout flare-up
colchicine (Colcrys)	PO; 0.5–1.2 mg followed by 0.5–0.6 mg every 1–2 hours until pain relief (max: 1.2 mg/day)	For acute gouty attack; may cause gastric upset at higher doses; IV form available
febuxostat (Uloric)	PO; 40–80 mg once daily	For chronic management of hyperuricemia in patients with gout
pegloticase (Krystexxa)	IV; 8 mg every 2 weeks by IV infusion	For chronic gout; enzyme that metabolizes uric acid
probenecid (Benemid, Probalan)	PO; 250 mg bid for 1 week; then 500 mg bid (max: 3 g/day)	For gout; also used as an adjunctive drug for penicillin or cephalosporin therapy
rasburicase (Elitek)	IV; 0.2 mg/kg over 30 minutes for up to 5 days	For management of plasma uric acid levels in pediatric patients with leukemia; recombinant urate-oxidase produced by a genetically modified *Saccharomyces cerevisiae* (yeast) strain; may cause hypersensitivity reactions
sulfinpyrazone (Anturane)	PO; 100–200 mg bid for 1 week; then increase to 200–400 mg bid	For gout; also used for inhibition of platelet aggregation

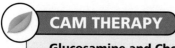

CAM THERAPY

Glucosamine and Chondroitin for Osteoarthritis

Glucosamine sulfate is a natural substance that is an important building block of cartilage. With aging, glucosamine is lost with the natural thinning of cartilage. As cartilage wears down, joints lose their normal cushioning ability, resulting in the pain and inflammation of OA. Glucosamine sulfate is available as an OTC dietary supplement. Some studies have shown it to be more effective than a placebo in reducing mild arthritis and joint pain. It is claimed to promote cartilage repair in the joints. Although reliable long-term studies are not available, glucosamine is marketed as a safe and inexpensive alternative to prescription anti-inflammatory drugs.

Chondroitin sulfate is another dietary supplement claimed to promote cartilage repair. It is a natural substance that forms part of the matrix between cartilage cells. Chondroitin is usually combined with glucosamine in specific arthritis formulas.

Drug Prototype: Ⓟ *Allopurinol (Lopurin, Zyloprim)*

Therapeutic Class: **Antigout drug**   Pharmacologic Class: **Inhibitor of uric acid formation, xanthine oxidase blocker**

Actions and Uses: Allopurinol reduces the production of uric acid, controlling the buildup of uric acid that causes severe gout and it reduces the risk of acute gout attacks. It is also approved to prevent recurrent kidney stones in patients with elevated uric acid levels. It may be used prophylactically to reduce the severity of the elevated uric acid blood levels associated with antineoplastic and radiation therapies, both of which increase blood uric acid levels by promoting nucleic acid degradation. This drug takes one to three weeks to bring blood uric acid levels to within the normal range.

Adverse Effects and Interactions: The most frequent and serious adverse effects are skin rash and rare cases of fatal toxic epidermal necrolysis and Stevens–Johnson syndrome. Other possible adverse effects include drowsiness, headache, vertigo, nausea, vomiting, abdominal discomfort, malaise, diarrhea, retinopathy, and thrombocytopenia.

Alcohol may inhibit the renal excretion of uric acid. Ampicillin and amoxicillin may increase the risk of skin rashes. An enhanced anticoagulant effect may be seen with the use of warfarin. The risk of ototoxicity is increased when allopurinol is used with thiazides and angiotensin-converting enzyme (ACE) inhibitors. Aluminum antacids taken concurrently with allopurinol may decrease its effects. An increased effect may be seen with phenytoin and anticancer drugs, necessitating the need for altered doses of these medications.

PATIENTS NEED TO KNOW

Patients taking drugs for bone or joint disorders need to know the following:

In General

1. When receiving treatment for problems with mobility, it often takes several weeks for effectiveness to begin. Follow the advice of a healthcare provider in order to achieve full therapeutic effect.

Regarding Calcium and Bone-Regulating Medications

2. When taking calcium or vitamin D supplements, be aware of the signs and symptoms of hypercalcemia. Check with the healthcare provider or pharmacist before taking supplements of any kind. In some cases, only proper diet and sunshine are needed for successful therapy.
3. Calcium may react with some foods or interfere with the absorption of iron and bisphosphonates.
4. Be familiar with the risks and long-term effects of vitamin D therapy, corticosteroids, hormone therapy involving estrogen, and estrogen-receptor modulators. Major undesirable adverse effects could occur in some cases.
5. Know how to use a nasal pump if taking calcitonin by this method.
6. Be aware that some vitamins may interfere with the pharmacologic effects of calcitonin.
7. Some medications cause GI discomfort. Most drugs like these can be taken after meals or with milk to minimize discomfort.

Regarding Arthritic and Joint-Related Medications

8. Report any unfavorable symptoms such as bone pain, restricted mobility, inflammation, or fracture to a healthcare provider. Report any muscle pain because muscles that have not been moved for a while may feel stiff and tender.
9. When taking some antigout medications, drink plenty of fluids to avoid kidney stones. To ensure proper fluid balance, monitor intake and output of fluids.
10. When taking probenecid, avoid taking aspirin for pain because it interferes with the drug's action. Take acetaminophen instead.

> ### SAFETY ALERT
>
> **Soundalike Drug Names**
>
> Nurses need to counsel patients about ways to avoid a self-medication error when taking medications that are "soundalike" drugs, such as Celebrex and Celexa. Confusing drugs with similar names accounts for about approximately 10% of all medication errors, according to the U.S. Food and Drug Administration (FDA). Patients could ask the pharmacist to package the "soundalikes" in distinctly different containers or to label the bottles with large letters describing the drug's use, like PAIN PILL and ANTIDEPRESSANT.

CHAPTER REVIEW

CORE CONCEPTS SUMMARY

35.1 Adequate levels of calcium, vitamin D, parathyroid hormone, and calcitonin are necessary for bone and body homeostasis.

One of the most important minerals in the body responsible for proper nerve conduction, muscle contractions, and bone formation is calcium. Calcium homeostasis is controlled by two important hormones, PTH and calcitonin. These hormones influence major body targets: the bones, kidneys, and GI tract. They direct the processes of bone resorption and bone deposition. Active vitamin D increases calcium absorption from the GI tract and helps to keep proper calcium balance in the body.

35.2 Hypocalcemia is a serious condition that requires immediate therapy.

Hypocalcemia, or lowered calcium levels in the bloodstream, is a sign of an underlying disorder; therefore, identifying its cause is essential. Signs of hypocalcemia are nerve and muscle excitability, muscle twitching, tremor, or cramping. These conditions are often reversed with calcium salts. Calcium salts consist of complexed and elemental calcium. Elemental calcium is also obtained from dietary sources.

35.3 Osteomalacia and rickets are successfully treated with calcium salts and vitamin D supplements.

Osteomalacia, called rickets in children, is a disorder characterized by softening of bones without alteration of basic bone structure. Drug therapy for children and adults consists of calcium supplements and vitamin D.

35.4 Treatment for osteoporosis includes calcitonin, selective estrogen-receptor modulators, and bisphosphonates.

Osteoporosis, or weak bones caused by disrupted bone homeostasis, is the most common metabolic bone disease. The onset of menopause is the most frequent risk factor. Many drug therapies are available for this disorder, including calcium and vitamin D therapy, estrogen therapy, estrogen-receptor modulators, statins, slow-release sodium fluoride, bisphosphonates, and calcitonin.

35.5 Treatment for Paget's disease includes bisphosphonates and calcitonin.

Paget's disease is a chronic progressive condition characterized by enlarged and abnormal bones. Although the cause of Paget's disease is different from that of osteoporosis, medical treatments are similar. Bisphosphonates are drugs of choice for the pharmacotherapy of Paget's disease.

35.6 Analgesics and anti-inflammatory drugs are important components of pharmacotherapy for osteoarthritis.

Arthritis is a general term meaning inflammation of the joints. The initial pharmacotherapy goals for osteoarthritis are to reduce pain and inflammation.

35.7 Immunosuppressants and disease-modifying drugs are additional therapies used to treat rheumatoid arthritis.

Rheumatoid arthritis (RA) is the second most common form of arthritis and has an autoimmune etiology. Pharmacotherapy for RA includes the same classes of analgesics and anti-inflammatory drugs, plus disease-modifying antirheumatic drugs (DMARDs), immunosuppressants, and biologic drugs.

35.8 Pharmacotherapy for gout requires drugs that control uric acid levels.

Gout is caused by an accumulation of uric acid in the bloodstream. Gout may be classified as a primary or secondary condition. Acute gouty arthritis occurs when needle-shaped uric acid crystals accumulate in the joints. The goals of gout pharmacotherapy include termination of acute attacks and prevention of future attacks with several approaches to control uric acid levels.

REVIEW QUESTIONS

The following questions are written in NCLEX-PN® style. Answer these questions to assess your knowledge of the chapter material, and go back and review any material that is not clear to you.

1. The nurse is explaining to a group of women that there are many brand names of certain medications. The brand name of a medication that lowers serum alkaline phosphatase is:

1. Azulfidine
2. Fosamax
3. Colchicine
4. Benemid

2. The patient on raloxifene (Evista) has had warfarin (Coumadin) ordered. The nurse incorporates what laboratory test into the plan of care?

1. Platelets
2. WBC
3. Sodium
4. INR/PT

3. The patient taking calcitriol should be monitored for:

1. Dysrhythmias
2. Hypercalcemia
3. Fluid overload
4. Flu-like symptoms

4. For the patient diagnosed with gout, the nurse would most likely administer which medication?

1. Calcitriol (Calcijex, Rocaltrol)
2. Azathioprine (Imuran)
3. Allopurinol (Lopurin, Zyloprim)
4. Raloxifene (Evista)

5. Because esophageal irritation can occur, the nurse instructs the patient to remain in an upright position for 30 minutes after what medication?

1. Allopurinol (Lopurin)
2. Calcitonin
3. Alendronate (Fosamax)
4. Raloxifene (Evista)

6. A patient is about to begin taking calcitonin and asks the nurse if this drug has any adverse effects. The nurse tells the patient that it may cause:

1. Nasal irritation
2. Headaches
3. Watery eyes
4. Sinus infection

7. A patient has been taking hydroxychloroquine (Plaquenil) for rheumatoid arthritis. Which of the following symptoms may alert the nurse to an adverse effect?

1. Cardiac dysrhythmias
2. Joint stiffness
3. Blurred vision
4. Decreased muscle strength

8. The nurse is speaking with a group of women at the local community center about vitamin and mineral supplements. She tells them that milliequivalence (mEq) is the unit used to describe the amount of electrolyte available to the bloodstream; the higher the mEq, the more potent the calcium salt. To demonstrate their new knowledge, the nurse has the group choose the calcium salts with the greatest potency. Which do they choose?

1. Calcium chloride
2. Calcium citrate
3. Calcium phosphate
4. Calcium gluconate

9. The nurse would include calcitonin in the plan of care for patients with: (Select all that apply.)

1. Paget's disease
2. Hypercalcemia
3. Hypocalcemia
4. Osteoporosis

10. The doctor has ordered tocilizumab (Actemra), 5 mg/kg of weight, to be given IV. The patient weighs 121 pounds and is to receive 275 mg in a 250 mL bag of solution to be delivered over 4 hours. How many milliliters will the patient receive in one hour?

1. 60 mL
2. 62 mL
3. 61.5 mL
4. 62.5 mL

CASE STUDY QUESTIONS

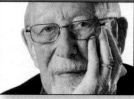

Remember Mr. Hurtt, the patient introduced at the beginning of the chapter? Now read the remainder of the case study. Based on the information you have learned in this chapter, answer the questions that follow.

Mr. Steven Hurtt is a 67-year-old white male. In an office visit, Mr. Hurtt complains of joint pain in the knees, ankles, toes, and shoulders. Over the last several years, he has taken aspirin for overall pain. Laboratory and physical examination yield the following information: small nodules found sporadically under the skin, acute swelling of the knees, redness of the big toe and elevated uric acid and white blood cell (WBC) count in the blood. Mr. Hurtt is diagnosed with gouty arthritis and is prescribed allopurinol (Lopurin).

1. Mr. Hurtt asks how allopurinol works. The nurse explains that it works by:

1. Decreasing the deposits of uric acid in the joint spaces
2. Reducing the pain associated with joint inflammation by uric acid crystals
3. Increasing renal excretion of uric acid
4. Reducing the production of uric acid

2. Since Mr. Hurtt is starting on allopurinol, the nurse informs him that this medication has several possible adverse effects that he needs to know about. These effects include: (Select all that apply.)

1. Headache
2. Vertigo

3. Toxic epidermal necrolysis
4. Skin rash

3. Mr. Hurtt asks why he should avoid drinking alcohol while he is taking allopurinol. The nurse responds by telling him that alcohol:

1. Significantly increases the drug levels of allopurinol
2. Interferes with the absorption of antigout medications
3. Raises uric acid levels
4. Causes the urine to become more alkaline

4. Which of the following statements demonstrates that Mr. Hurtt needs additional instructions?

1. "I will take my allopurinol as prescribed by my physician."
2. "I will stop having alcoholic beverages."
3. "I will avoid high purine foods."
4. "I will continue taking my aspirin."

NOTE: Answers to the Review and Case Study Questions appear in Appendix B. The complete rationales and answers are located on the textbook's website.

Pearson Nursing Student Resources Find additional review materials at **nursing.pearsonhighered.com**.

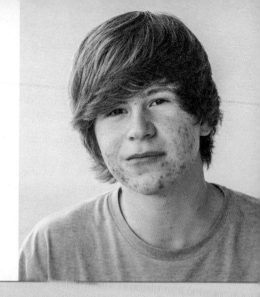

CHAPTER

*"I don't think I can go to
the game this weekend. Can
anything be done to get rid
of these zits by Friday?"*

Burt Nicholson

36 Drugs for Skin Disorders

CORE CONCEPTS

36.1 Layers of skin provide protection to the body.

36.2 The major causes of skin disorders are injury, aging, inherited factors, and other medical conditions.

36.3 Scabicides and pediculicides treat parasitic mite and lice infestations.

36.4 The goal of drug therapy for sunburn is to eliminate discomfort until healing occurs.

36.5 Acne and rosacea are treated by a combination of over-the-counter (OTC) and prescription drugs.

36.6 Topical corticosteroids are used mainly to treat dermatitis and related symptoms.

36.7 Several topical and systemic medications are used to treat psoriatic symptoms.

DRUG SNAPSHOT

The following drugs are discussed in this chapter:

DRUG CLASSES	DRUG PROTOTYPES
Drugs for skin parasites	
Scabicides and pediculicides	(Pr) permethrin (Acticin, Elimite, Nix) *587*
Drugs for sunburn and minor skin irritations	(Pr) benzocaine (Americaine, Anbesol, others) *589*
Drugs for acne and rosacea	(Pr) tretinoin (Avita, Retin-A, Tretin-X) *591*
Drugs for dermatitis and eczema	
Drugs for psoriasis	

LEARNING OUTCOMES

After reading this chapter, the student should be able to:

1. Identify important skin layers and explain how superficial skin cells must be replaced after they become damaged or lost.

2. Describe major symptoms associated with stress and injury to the skin versus those associated with a patient's changing age or health.

3. Identify the major actions of the following types of drugs as they pertain to treatment of skin disorders: scabicides, pediculicides, topical anesthetics, antibiotics, retinoids, keratolytic agents, corticosteroids, emollients, and psoralens.

4. Describe popular treatments used in conjunction with available drug therapies for skin disorders.

5. For each of the classes in the Drug Snapshot, identify representative drugs and explain their mechanisms of drug action, primary actions, and important adverse effects.

KEY TERMS

closed comedones (KOME-eh-dones) *589*

dermatitis (dur-mah-TIE-tiss) *591*

eczema (ECK-zih-mah) *591*

emollients *593*

erythema (ear-ih-THEE-mah) *584*

keratinization (keh-RAT-en-eye-zay-shun) *589*

keratolytic agents (keh-RAT-oh-lih-tik) *590*

open comedones *589*

papules (PAP-yools) *589*

pediculicides (puh-DIK-you-lih-sides) *587*

pruritus (proo-RYE-tus) *583*

psoralens (SOR-uh-lenz) *594*

psoriasis *593*

pustules (PUSS-chools) *589*

retinoids (RETT-ih-noydz) *590*

retinol (RETT-in-nall) *591*

rosacea (roh-ZAY-shee-uh) *589*

scabicides (SKAY-bih-sides) *587*

scabies (SKAY-beez) *586*

seborrhea (seb-oh-REE-ah) *589*

urticaria (EHR-tik-air-ee-ah) *583*

The integumentary system consists of the skin, hair, nails, sweat glands, and oil glands. The largest of all organs in the body is the skin. Because of its large surface area, the skin provides an effective barrier between extreme conditions in the outside environment and the body's internal tissues. At times, however, changes in external and internal conditions can damage the skin. When this happens, drug therapy may be provided to improve the skin's condition. The relationship between the integumentary system and other systems in the body is shown in Figure 36.1 ■.

The purpose of this chapter is to examine the broad scope of skin disorders and the medications used for skin therapy. Particular attention is given to drugs that are of direct benefit to lice and mite infestations, sunburn, acne, inflammation, and dry, scaly skin.

Layers of skin provide protection to the body.

CORE CONCEPT 36.1

The integument has three major layers: the epidermis, dermis, and a subcutaneous layer called the hypodermis. Studies in healthcare often describe the skin as having two major layers with the hypodermis underneath. Each layer of the integument is distinct in form and function and determines how drugs are injected or applied to the surface of the skin (see Chapter 3).

epi = *on top of*
hypo = *below*
dermis = *the skin*

sub = *underneath*
cutaneous = *skin-related*

The most superficial skin layer is the epidermis. Depending on its thickness, the epidermis has either four or five sublayers. The strongest and outermost sublayer is the stratum corneum, or horny layer. It is called this because of the abundance of the protein keratin, also found in the hair, hooves, and horns of many vertebrate mammals. Not every part of the skin has a large amount of keratin—only those areas that are subject to mechanical stress—for example, the soles of the feet and the palms of the hands.

The deepest sublayer of the epidermis is the stratum germinativum. It supplies the epidermis with new cells after older superficial cells have been damaged or lost by normal wear. Cells must migrate over their lifetime to the outermost layers of the skin, where they eventually fall off. As these cells are pushed to the surface, they are flattened and covered with a water-insoluble material, forming a protective seal. The average time it takes for a cell to move from the germinativum layer to the outer body surface is about three weeks. Specialized cells called *melanocytes* within the deeper layers of the epidermis secrete the dark pigment melanin, which offers a degree of protection from the sun's ultraviolet rays.

The next major layer of skin, the dermis, is made up of dense, irregular connective tissue, named this way because of its irregular arrangement of thick collagen fibers. The dermis provides a foundation for the epidermis and appendages such as hair and nails. Most receptor nerve endings, sweat glands, oil glands, and blood vessels are found within the dermis.

Below the dermis is the subcutaneous layer, or hypodermis. This layer is composed mainly of adipose tissue or fat that cushions, insulates, and provides a source of energy for the body. The hypodermis is involved with the maintenance of body homeostasis, temperature regulation, and metabolism.

The major causes of skin disorders are injury, aging, inherited factors, and other medical conditions.

CORE CONCEPT 36.2

Skin that is dry, cracked, scaly, or inflamed represents a disturbance in the outermost skin layer. **Pruritus**, or itching, is a general symptom often associated with dry, scaly skin, or it may be a symptom of infestation with mites and lice. **Urticaria**, commonly referred to as *hives*, is recognized as raised, red, itchy bumps. Most commonly, urticaria is caused by an allergic reaction. Many drugs, especially antibiotics, can cause urticaria and pruritus as side effects. Although most drug allergies of the skin require only symptomatic treatment with over-the-counter (OTC) medications, some are severe. Toxic epidermal necrolysis (TEN) is a life-threatening drug reaction that results in massive death of skin cells and separation of the epidermis from the dermis.

prur = *itching*
itus = *condition*

Burns are a unique type of stress that may affect all layers of the skin. They are classified according to the degree of skin damage. First-degree burns affect only the outer layers of the epidermis, are characterized by redness, and are analogous to sunburn. Second-degree burns affect most of the epidermis and part of the

FIGURE 36.1

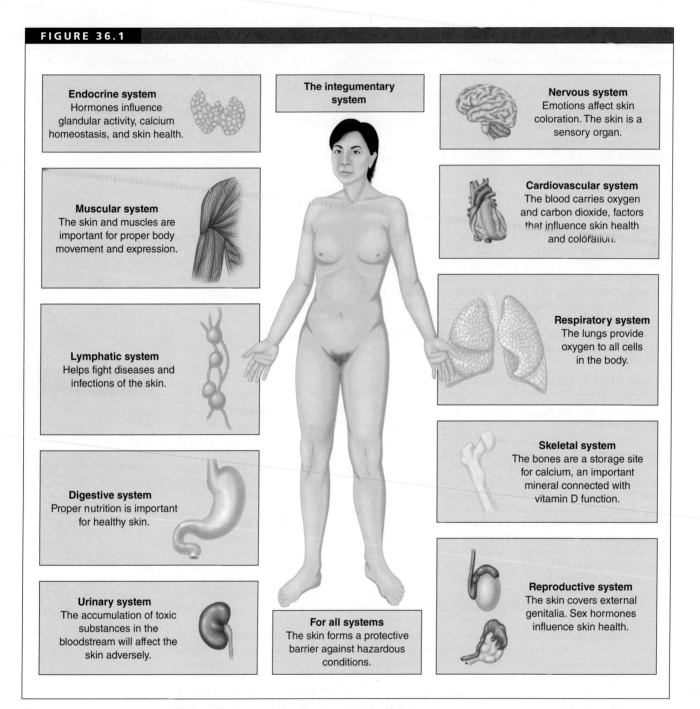

The integumentary system (skin) and how the other body systems affect it.

dermis, resulting in inflammation and blisters. Third-degree burns are full-thickness burns; all layers of the skin are damaged. With full-thickness burns, the skin cannot regenerate, and skin grafting is required.

Inflammation, a characteristic of burns and other traumatic disorders, occurs when damage to the skin is extensive. Signs accompanying inflammation include **erythema** or redness, irritation, and pain. Symptoms including bleeding, bruises, and infections may accompany trauma to deeper tissues.

Not all skin disorders are associated with injury or infection. Many common skin disorders are related to inherited factors or the normal aging process. Sometimes the skin may appear unhealthy because of a disease process occurring in a different organ system, such as yellowing of the skin (jaundice) that occurs from liver damage. In many cases, the cause of the skin condition may be unknown. Common symptoms associated with a range of conditions are presented in Table 36.1 ◆. Although the causes and symptoms of skin conditions are very diverse, a simple method of classifying them is shown in Table 36.2 ◆.

Most skin conditions are not debilitating and require only intermittent drug therapy. A few irritating disorders are of particular importance to patients who require treatment on an outpatient basis. Examples

eryth = *red*
ema = *appears*

TABLE 36.1 Signs and Symptoms of Skin Conditions Associated with a Patient's Changing Health, Age, or Weakened Immune System

Symptom	Description
Delicate skin, wrinkles, and hair loss	Many degenerative changes occur in the skin; some are found in elderly patients; others are genetically related (fragile epidermis, wrinkles, reduced activity of oil and sweat glands, male pattern baldness, poor blood circulation); hair loss may also be linked to some medical procedures, such as radiation and chemotherapy.
Discoloration of the skin	Discoloration is often a useful sign of another medical disorder (for example, anemia, cyanosis, fever, jaundice, or Addison's disease); some medications have photosensitive properties, making a patient's skin sensitive to the sun and causing erythema.
Scales, patches, and itchy areas	Some symptoms may be related to a combination of genetics, stress, and immunity; other symptoms may be related to a fast turnover of skin cells; some symptoms develop for unknown reasons.
Seborrhea/oily skin and bumps	This condition is usually associated with a younger age group; examples include cradle cap in infants and an oily face, chest, arms, and back in teenagers and young adults; pustules, cysts, papules, and nodules represent lesions connected with oily skin.
Tumors	Tumors may be genetic or may occur because of exposure to harmful agents or conditions.
Warts, skin marks, and moles	Some skin marks are congenital; others are acquired or may be linked to environmental factors.

TABLE 36.2 Classification of Skin Disorders

Disorder	Example
Infectious disorders	Bacterial infections: boils, impetigo, and infected hair follicles
	Fungal infections: ringworm, athlete's foot, jock itch, and nail infections
	Parasitic infections: ticks, mites, and lice
	Viral infections: cold sores, fever blisters (herpes simplex), chickenpox, warts, shingles (herpes zoster), measles (rubeola), and German measles (rubella)
Inflammatory disorders	Injury and exposure to the sun
	Combination of overactive glands, increased hormone production, or infection such as acne and rosacea
	Disorders marked by itching, cracking, and discomfort, such as atopic dermatitis, contact dermatitis, seborrheic dermatitis, stasis dermatitis, and psoriasis.
Neoplastic	Malignant skin cancers: squamous cell carcinoma, basal cell carcinoma, and malignant melanoma.
	Malignant melanoma is the most dangerous. Benign neoplasms include keratosis and keratoacanthoma.

include lice infestation, minor sunburn, and acne. Eczema, dermatitis, and psoriasis are more serious disorders requiring therapy for a longer time. Figure 36.2 ■ shows examples of regions of the body where irritating symptoms most likely appear.

Concept Review 36.1

■ Identify the skin layers protecting the body. Give examples of layers specifically affected by minor or major external stresses. What skin disorders are not related to the external environment? How would you categorize most skin disorders?

FIGURE 36.2

Anatomical distribution of common skin disorders: (a) contact dermatitis due to footwear, (b) cosmetics, (c) seborrheic dermatitis, (d) acne, (e) scabies, (f) sunburn.

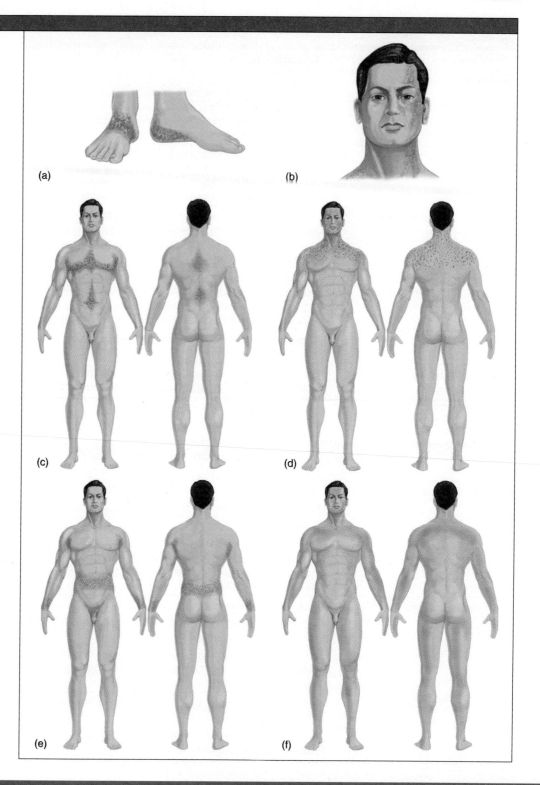

(a)

(b)

(c)

(d)

(e)

(f)

SKIN PARASITES

Common skin parasites include mites and lice. Mites cause a skin disorder called **scabies**, based on their scientific name, *Sarcoptes scabiei*. Scabies is an eruption of the skin caused by the female mite burrowing into the skin and laying eggs. This causes intense itching, most commonly between the fingers, extremities, and around the trunk and pubic area. Scabies is readily spread among family members and sexual partners.

Lice, scientific name *Pediculus*, are another type of skin parasite readily passed on by infected clothing or close personal contact. Lice often infest the pubic area or the scalp and lay eggs that attach to body hairs.

Fast Facts Skin Disorders

- An estimated three million people with new cases of lice infestation are treated each year in the United States.
- Nearly 17 million people in the United States have acne, making it the most common skin disease.
- More than 15 million people in the United States have symptoms of dermatitis.
- Ten percent of infants and young children experience symptoms of dermatitis. Roughly 60% of these infants continue to have symptoms into adulthood.
- Psoriasis affects 1% to 2% of the U.S. population. This disorder occurs in all age groups—adults mainly—affecting about the same number of men as women.

Scabicides and pediculicides treat parasitic mite and lice infestations.

Scabicides are pharmacologic agents that kill mites; **pediculicides** kill lice. Either treatment may be effective for both types of parasites. The preferred drug often depends on where the infestation has occurred.

The preferred drug for lice infestation is permethrin, a chemical derived from chrysanthemum flowers and formulated as a 1% liquid (Nix). This drug is considered the safest agent, especially for infants and children. Pyrethrin (RID, others) is a related product also obtained from the chrysanthemum plant. Permethrin and pyrethrins, which are also widely used as insecticides on crops and livestock, kill lice and their eggs on contact. Malathion (Ovide) is an alternative for resistant organisms.

Permethrin is also a preferred drug for scabies. The 5% permethrin cream (Elimite) is applied to the entire skin surface and allowed to remain for 8 to 14 hours before bathing. Itching may continue for several weeks as the dead mites are removed from the skin. Crotamiton (Eurax) is an alternative scabicide available by prescription as a 10% cream. Approved in 2012, ivermectin (Sklice) is a lotion that is left on the scalp for 10 minutes and does not require a nit comb following treatment. Because lindane (Kwell) has the potential to cause serious nervous system toxicity, it is now prescribed only after other less toxic drugs have failed to produce a therapeutic response.

All scabicides and pediculicides must be used strictly as directed, because excessive use has the potential to cause serious systemic effects and skin irritation. Drugs for the treatment of lice or mites must not be applied to the mouth, open skin lesions, or eyes, because this will cause severe irritation.

Lice lay eggs called *nits*. Fine-toothed nit combs are useful in removing nits after the lice have been killed. Patients should comb the infested area after the hair has been dried. To ensure that drug therapy is effective, patients should inspect hair shafts daily for at least 1 week after treatment. Because nits may be present in bedding and other upholstery material, all material coming in close contact with the patient should be washed or treated with the medication.

Concept Review 36.2

- Name examples of medications used to treat mite and lice infestations. What precautions should be taken when using these medications?

Drug Prototype: ℗ *Permethrin (Acticin, Elimite, Nix)*

Therapeutic Class: Antiparasitic drug   **Pharmacologic Class: Scabicide, pediculicide**

Actions and Uses: Nix is marketed as a cream or shampoo to kill head and crab lice. It will also kill mites and eradicate their ova. A 1% lotion is approved for lice and 5% lotion for mites. The medication should be allowed to remain on the hair and scalp 10 minutes before removal. Patients should be aware that itching may last up to two or three weeks even after parasites have been killed. Successful elimination of parasitic infestations should include removing the nits with a comb, washing bedding, and cleaning or removing objects that have been in contact with the head or hair.

Adverse Effects and Interactions: Permethrin causes few systemic effects. Local reactions may occur and include pruritus, rash, transient tingling, burning, stinging, erythema, and edema of the infested area.

Contraindications include hypersensitivity to pyrethrins, chrysanthemums, sulfites, or other preservatives. Permethrin should be used cautiously on inflamed skin, in those with asthma, or in lactating women. No significant clinical drug interactions have been documented.

NURSING PROCESS FOCUS Patients Receiving Pharmacotherapy for Lice or Mite Infestation

ASSESSMENT	POTENTIAL NURSING DIAGNOSES
Prior to drug administration: ■ Obtain a complete health history, including age, dermatological conditions, social history and close contacts, allergies, drug history, and possible drug interactions. ■ Examine skin areas to be treated for signs of infestation (e.g., lice or nits in hair, reddened track areas between web of fingers, around the belt or elastic lines), irritation, excoriation, or drainage.	■ *Deficient Knowledge* related to a lack of information about condition and drug therapy regimen ■ *Impaired Health Maintenance* related to treatment regimen ■ *Risk for Impaired Skin Integrity* related to infestation or adverse effects of drug therapy ■ *Risk for Poisoning* related to adverse effects of drug therapy

PLANNING: PATIENT GOALS AND EXPECTED OUTCOMES

The patient will:
■ Experience therapeutic effects (free of lice or mites).
■ Be free from or experience minimal adverse effects from drug therapy.
■ Verbalize an understanding of how lice and mites are spread; proper administration of medication; necessary household hygiene; and the need to notify household members, sexual partners, and other close contacts (such as classmates) about infestation.

IMPLEMENTATION

Interventions and (Rationales)	Patient Education/Discharge Planning
■ Apply medication correctly and evaluate the patient and caregiver's knowledge of proper administration. (Everyone in the household with mites or lice should be treated at the same time. Proper application is critical to elimination of infestation.)	Instruct the patient and family members: ■ That all skin lotions, creams, and oil-based hair products should be removed completely before applying medication. ■ To apply the drug per package directions and allow it to remain in the hair or on the skin for the prescribed length of time (approximately 10 minutes). ■ To use a fine-toothed comb to comb affected hair to remove any remaining dead lice or mites. ■ That eyelashes can be treated with the application of petroleum jelly once a day for one week. Use a fine-toothed comb to remove mites. ■ To recheck affected hair or skin daily for at least one to two weeks after treatment.
■ Monitor the skin/head areas for infestation over the next 1 to 2 weeks. Reinfestations may reappear within 1 week and retreatment may be necessary. (Monitoring helps to determine proper medication administration technique and adherence to prevention protocols.)	Instruct the patient and family members to: ■ Monitor for nits on hair shafts; lice on skin or clothes, inner thigh areas, and seams of clothes that come in contact with axilla, neckline, or beltline. ■ Monitor for mites between the fingers, on the extremities, in the axillary and gluteal folds, around the trunk, and in the pubic area.
■ Monitor household for signs of infestation. Inform the patient and others living in the home about proper care of clothing and equipment. (Contaminated articles can cause reinfestation.)	Instruct the patient and family members to: ■ Wash all bedding and clothing in hot water, and to dry-clean all nonwashable items that came in close contact with the patient. ■ Vacuum furniture or fabric that cannot be cleaned and seal children's toys in plastic bags for two weeks. ■ Not share personal care items such as combs, brushes, and towels ■ Clean combs and brushes and rinse thoroughly after every use.

EVALUATION OF OUTCOME CRITERIA

Evaluate the effectiveness of drug therapy by confirming that patient goals and expected outcomes have been met (see "Planning").

SUNBURN AND MINOR SKIN IRRITATION

CORE CONCEPT 36.4

The goal of drug therapy for sunburn is to eliminate discomfort until healing occurs.

Sunburn, a common problem among the general public, is associated with factors such as light skin complexion and lack of proper sun protection. Nonpharmacologic approaches to sun protection include the appropriate use of sunscreens, sunglasses, and sufficient clothing. Limiting the amount of time spent directly in the sun is essential to avoiding sunburn. Many dangers result from sun exposure, including eye injury and skin cancer. Some of these disorders may not appear until years after the exposure.

Pharmacologic treatments for sunburn may not be necessary. Remaining calm until the minor irritation passes is one common approach to mild sunburn. In cases in which pharmacologic intervention is necessary, drugs for sunburn and minor irritation include mild lotions and topical anesthetics such as

Drug Prototype: ℗ *Benzocaine (Americaine, Anbesol, Others)*

Therapeutic Class: Agent for sunburn pain and minor skin irritations
Pharmacologic Class: Local anesthetic, sodium channel blocker

Actions and Uses: Benzocaine provides temporary relief for pain and discomfort in cases of sunburn, pruritus, minor wounds, and insect bites. Its pharmacologic action is caused by local anesthesia of skin receptor nerve endings. Preparations are also available to treat the skin and other areas such as the ear, mouth, throat, rectal, and genital areas.

Adverse Effects and Interactions: Benzocaine should not be used for treatment of patients with open lesions, traumatized mucosal areas, or a history of drug sensitivity. Benzocaine may interfere with the activity of some antibacterial sulfonamides. Patients should use preparations only in areas of the body for which the medication is intended.

benzocaine (Solarcaine, others), dibucaine (Nupercainal), and tetracaine (Pontocaine). These are used to provide temporary relief of painful symptoms. Some of these medications may also provide minor relief from insect bites and pruritus. In cases of more lengthy sun exposure, more potent pain medications may be administered (see Chapters 14 and 24), or tetanus toxoid might be administered to prevent infection (see Chapter 26).

Concept Review 36.3

■ What is the major purpose of drugs used to treat sunburn, insect bites, and related injuries? What major class of drugs would be used for this purpose?

ACNE AND ROSACEA

Acne, sometimes called *acne vulgaris*, is a common condition found most often in adolescents and young adults. The disorder usually begins one or two years before puberty and is caused by overproductive oil glands or **seborrhea**. Acne is also caused by abnormal **keratinization** or development of the horny layer of the epithelial tissue of skin. This activity results in blocked oil glands. Administration of androgens or testosterone-like hormones may cause extensive acne by increasing keratinization and the production of sebum (oil). Following this, the bacterium *Propionibacterium acnes* grows within gland openings and modifies the sebum into an acidic and irritating substance. As a result, small inflamed bumps appear on the surface of the skin.

sebor = *oil*
rhea = *flow*

Blackheads, or **open comedones**, are a type of acne in which sebum has plugged the oil gland, causing it to become black because of the presence of melanin granules. Whiteheads, or **closed comedones**, are a type of acne that develops just beneath the surface of the skin and appears white rather than black. In more severe cases of acne, deeper bumps called *nodules* may appear and become very painful because of the intense inflammation and pus found within pore pockets.

Another skin disorder characterized by inflammation but without pus is **rosacea**. Unlike pimples or **pustules**—the technical name given to pus-filled bumps—rosacea is characterized by small **papules** or inflammatory bumps that swell, thicken, and become very painful. Characteristic of rosacea is its swelling just beneath the surface of the skin. The face of a patient with rosacea may take on a flushed appearance, particularly around the nose and cheek area. Rosacea is exacerbated by many factors, including sunlight, stress, increased temperature, and agents that dilate facial blood vessels such as alcohol, spicy foods, and warm beverages.

Acne and rosacea are treated by a combination of OTC and prescription drugs.

CORE CONCEPT 36.5

Most acne drugs slow down the turnover of skin cells, especially those surrounding pore openings. Some inhibit bacterial growth because they are combined with antibiotics such as doxycycline and tetracycline (see Chapter 26). Some drugs must be used carefully because of their ability to dramatically reduce oil gland activity and skin cell turnover. Important medications for acne and rosacea are summarized in Table 36.3 ◆.

TABLE 36.3 Drugs for Acne and Rosacea	
Drug	**Remarks**
OTC MEDICATION—TOPICAL PREPARATION	
benzoyl peroxide (Clearasil, Fostex, others)	Often combined with erythromycin or clindamycin to fight bacterial infection (see Chapter 26)
PRESCRIPTION MEDICATIONS—TOPICAL	
adapalene (Differin)	Retinoid-like compound used to treat acne formation
azelaic acid (Azelex, Finacea, others)	For mild to moderate inflammatory acne and rosacea
metronidazole (Metrogel, MetroCream)	For inflammatory papules and pustules of rosacea
sulfacetamide sodium (Cetamide, Klaron, others)	For sensitive skin; sometimes combined with sulfur to promote peeling, as in rosacea; also used for conjunctivitis
tazarotene (Avage, Tazorac)	A retinoid drug that may also be used for plaque psoriasis; has antiproliferative and anti-inflammatory effects
Pr tretinoin (Avita, Retin-A, others)	A retinoid used to prevent clogging of pore follicles associated with acne; the oral form (Vesanoid) is used for the treatment of acute promyelocytic leukemia and wrinkles
PRESCRIPTION MEDICATIONS—ORAL	
doxycycline (Vibramycin, others)	Antibiotic (see Chapter 26)
ethinyl estradiol	Oral contraceptives are sometimes used for acne treatment; combination drugs may be helpful, for example, ethinyl estradiol plus norgestimate (see Chapter 34)
isotretinoin (Accutane)	A retinoid used for severe acne with cysts or acne formed in small, rounded masses; pregnancy category X
minocycline (Minocin, others)	Antibiotic (see Chapter 26)
tetracycline (Sumycin, others) (see page 397 for the Drug Prototype box)	Antibiotic (see Chapter 26)

Benzoyl peroxide (Clearasil, Fostex, others) is one of the primary OTC medications used to treat acne. This medication may be dispensed as a lotion, cream, or gel and is available in various concentrations. Benzoyl peroxide decreases symptoms of acne by inhibiting bacterial growth and suppressing the turnover of skin cells at the pore's opening. Applied directly to affected skin, it is relatively safe, with redness, irritation, and drying being the most common adverse effects. Patients usually see some improvement with the first week but it make take weeks even a month, or longer to notice the full effect. Sometimes benzoyl peroxide is combined with antibiotics to directly fight bacterial infections. When acne is particularly severe, resorcinol, salicylic acid, or sulfur may be used as additional treatments to promote shedding of old skin. These are called **keratolytic agents**.

kerato = *horny layer*
lytic = *loosening*

Retinoids are vitamin A–like compounds used for acne. Vitamin A provides improved resistance to bacterial infection by reducing oil production and the occurrence of clogged pores. Retinoids are not recommended during pregnancy because of possible harmful effects to the fetus. A common reaction to retinoids is sensitivity to sunlight.

Some drugs may be taken in combination with or in lieu of other acne medications, including doxycycline, tetracycline, and ethinyl estradiol. Doxycycline and tetracycline are antibiotics used to inhibit bacterial growth (see Chapter 26). Oral contraceptive medications containing ethinyl estradiol may be used to help clear the skin of acne by suppressing oil production (see Chapter 34).

The two most effective treatments for rosacea are topical metronidazole (Metrogel, MetroCream) and azelaic acid (Azelex, Finacea). Alternative medications include topical clindamycin (Cleocin-T, ClindaMax) and sulfacetamide. Tetracycline antibiotics are beneficial to patients with rosacea with multiple pustules or with ocular involvement. Severe, resistant cases may respond to isotretinoin (Accutane).

Concept Review 36.4

■ What is the major purpose of drugs used to treat acne and related skin conditions? Give examples of both topical and systemic medications. Which medications are OTC, and which are prescription medications?

Drug Prototype: ℗ *Tretinoin (Avita, Retin-A, Others)*

Therapeutic Class: Antiacne drug   Pharmacologic Class: Retinoid receptor drug, vitamin derivative

Actions and Uses: This drug is indicated for the early treatment and control of mild to moderate acne vulgaris. Symptoms take 4 to 8 weeks to improve, and maximum therapeutic benefit may take up to 5 or 6 months. This drug is most often reserved for cystic acne or severe keratinization disorders.

The principal action of tretinoin is regulation of skin growth and cell turnover. As cells from the germinativum grow toward the skin's surface, skin cells are lost from the pore openings, and their replacement is slowed down. Tretinoin also decreases oil production by reducing the size and number of oil glands.

Adverse Effects and Interactions: Tretinoin is a natural derivative of **retinol** or vitamin A. Thus, vitamin A supplements, which increase toxicity, should be avoided.

Common adverse effects are skin irritation (such as a burning or stinging sensation, redness, and crusting), conjunctivitis (visual disturbance), dry mouth, inflammation of the lip, dry nose, increased serum concentrations of triglycerides, bone and joint pain, and photosensitivity. Additive phototoxicity can occur if tretinoin is used concurrently with other phototoxic drugs such as tetracyclines, fluoroquinolones, or sulfonamides.

Using tretinoin together with hypoglycemic agents may lead to loss of glycemic control as well as increased risk of cardiovascular disease due to elevated triglyceride levels.

> **BLACK BOX WARNING:**
> Patients with acute promyelocytic leukemia (APL) are at high risk for serious adverse effects: fever, weakness, fatigue, dyspnea, weight gain, peripheral edema, respiratory insufficiency, pneumonia, and rapidly evolving leukocytosis, which is associated with a high risk of life-threatening complications. There is a high risk that infants will be severely deformed if this drug is administered during pregnancy.

DERMATITIS AND ECZEMA

Dermatitis is a general term that refers to superficial inflammatory disorders of the skin. **Eczema**, also called *atopic dermatitis*, is a skin disorder with symptoms resembling an allergic reaction, including inflammation, itching, and rash. Long-term itching and scaling may cause the skin to appear thickened and leathery. Exposure to environmental irritants may make these symptoms worse. Other conditions, including stress, too little or too much moisture, and extreme temperature fluctuations, may worsen symptoms. Blisters and other lesions may also develop. In infants and small children, lesions usually begin on the face and progress to other parts of the body. The skin may become raw and infected from scratching.

dermat = *skin*
itis = *inflammation*

atopic = *out of place*

Contact dermatitis is a delayed type of allergic reaction resulting from exposure to specific allergens— for example, perfume, cosmetics, detergents, latex, or jewelry. Accompanying the allergic reaction may be various degrees of cracking, bleeding, or small blisters.

Seborrheic dermatitis is a disorder caused by overactive oil glands. This condition is sometimes seen in newborns and in teenagers after puberty. Oily and scaly patches of skin appear in areas of the face, scalp, chest, back, or pubic area. Bacterial infection or dandruff may accompany these symptoms.

Stasis dermatitis is seen more commonly in older women. It is found primarily in the lower extremities. Redness and scaling may be observed in areas where venous circulation is impaired or where deep venous blood clots have formed.

Topical corticosteroids are used mainly to treat dermatitis and related symptoms.

CORE CONCEPT 36.6

Topical corticosteroids are used in cases of dermatitis and eczema to treat symptoms of inflammation, burning, and pruritus. In conjunction with other medical therapies, topical corticosteroids are also used for the treatment of psoriasis.

Topical corticosteroids are the most effective treatment for dermatitis. As seen in Table 36.4 ◆, there are many varieties of corticosteroids supplied at different levels of potency. Creams, lotions, solutions, gels, and pads are specially formulated to cross skin membranes. These medications are especially intended for the relief of local inflammation and itching. In cases of long-term use, however, adverse effects such as irritation, redness, and thinning of the skin membranes may occur. If absorption occurs, topical corticosteroids may produce undesirable systemic effects, including adrenal insufficiency, mood changes, serum imbalances, and bone defects, as discussed in Chapter 24.

TABLE 36.4 Selected Topical Corticosteroids for Dermatitis and Related Symptoms

Generic Name	Trade Names
HIGHEST POTENCY	
betamethasone dipropionate	Diprolene
clobetasol	Temovate
diflorasone	Maxiflor
halobetasol	Ultravate
HIGH POTENCY	
amcinonide	Cyclocort
fluocinonide	Lidex
halcinonide	Halog
MEDIUM POTENCY	
betamethasone benzoate	Uticort
betamethasone valerate	Valisone
clocortolone	Cloderm
desoximetasone, cream	Topicort
fluocinolone acetonide	Synalar
flurandrenolide, cream	Cordran
fluticasone propionate, cream	Cutivate
hydrocortisone valerate	Westcort
mometasone furoate	Elocon
prednicarbate	Dermatop
triamcinolone acetonide	Aristocort, Kenalog
betamethasone benzoate	Uticort
LOWER POTENCY	
alclometasone dipropionate	Aclovate
desonide	Desonate, DesOwen, Verdeso
dexamethasone	Decaspray
hydrocortisone	Cortizone, Hycort

CAM THERAPY

Aloe Vera for Skin Conditions

Aloe vera is derived from the gel inside the leaf of the aloe plant, which is a member of the lily family. Used medicinally for thousands of years aloe vera contains over 70 active substances, including amino acids, minerals, vitamins, and enzymes. Aloe vera is best known for its ability to sooth and heal minor skin irritations, cuts, and burns. For the most part, scientific studies have confirmed its benefit for these conditions. It can be found as an ingredient in many products, including soaps, lotions, creams, and sunblocks. Some evidence suggests it may be useful in treating genital herpes lesions and moderate plaque psoriasis. Although oral formulations can be found, these are not recommended because they can cause serious gastrointestinal (GI) side effects.

PSORIASIS

Psoriasis is a chronic, noninfectious inflammatory skin disorder that affects 1% to 2% of the population. Psoriasis is characterized by red patches of skin covered with flaky, silver-colored scales called *plaques*. The reason for the appearance of plaques is an extremely fast skin turnover rate. The skin reacts as if it has been injured, but skin cells reach the surface much more quickly than usual, in about four days, or six to seven times faster than usual. The reason for this kind of reaction is not known, although scientists believe that it may be a genetic immune reaction. Plaques are ultimately shed from the skin's surface, while the underlying skin becomes inflamed and irritated.

Several topical and systemic medications are used to treat psoriatic symptoms.

CORE CONCEPT 36.7

Because psoriatic symptoms may be extreme, numerous drugs are employed to soothe the patient's symptoms, including **emollients**, topical corticosteroids, and immunosuppressant medications. Drugs used in the treatment of psoriasis are provided in Table 36.5 ◆.

emolli = *to soften*
ent = *causing*

TABLE 36.5   Drugs for Psoriasis and Related Disorders

Drug	Route and Adult Dose	Remarks
TOPICAL MEDICATIONS		
anthralin	Topical; apply to lesions daily or as directed	Second-line therapy after tolerance to corticosteroids has developed
calcipotriene (Dovonex)	Topical; apply to lesions once or twice daily up to 8 weeks	Synthetic form of vitamin D_3; may raise the level of calcium in the body to unhealthy levels
coal tar (Balnetar, Cutar, others)	Topical; apply to lesions daily or as directed	Second-line therapy after tolerance to corticosteroids has developed
salicylic acid (Salax, Neutrogena, others)	Topical; apply to lesions (concentrations ranging from 2–10%) as directed	Wide range of delivery: creams, foams, gels, lotions, ointments, pads, plasters, shampoos, soaps, and skin solutions
tazarotene (Tazorac)	Acne: topical; apply thin film to clean, dry area daily Plaque psoriasis: topical; apply a thin film daily in the evening	Topical retinoid; less toxic than corticosteroids; also approved for facial wrinkles and acne
SYSTEMIC MEDICATIONS		
acitretin (Soriatane)	PO; 10–50 mg/day with the main meal	Retinoid; pregnancy category X drug
adalimumab (Humira)	Subcutaneous; 40–80 mg every other week	Tumor necrosis factor blocker; also for rheumatoid arthritis and Crohn's disease
alefacept (Amevive)	IM; 15 mg once weekly for 12 weeks	Engineered immunosuppressant drug
cyclosporine (Gengraf, Neoral, Sandimmune) (see page 382 for Drug Prototype box)	PO; 1.25 mg/kg bid (max: 4 mg/kg/day)	Immunosuppressant drug; also to prevent transplant rejection and rheumatoid arthritis
etanercept (Enbrel)	Subcutaneous; 50 mg twice weekly (given 3–4 days apart); maintenance dose 50 mg/week	Also for rheumatoid arthritis
infliximab (Remicade)	IV; 5 mg/kg with additional doses 2 and 6 weeks after the initial infusion, then every 8 weeks thereafter	Tumor necrosis factor blocker; also for rheumatoid arthritis, Crohn's disease and ulcerative colitis
hydroxyurea (Hydrea)	PO; 80 mg/kg every 3 days or 20–30 mg/kg daily	Off-label use for psoriasis; also used for sickle cell anemia
methotrexate (Rheumatrx, Trexall) (see page 440 for the Drug Prototype box)	PO; 2.5–5 mg bid × 3 doses each week (max: 25–30 mg/week)	For rheumatoid arthritis and neoplasia
ustekinumab (Stelara)	Subcutaneous; 45–90 mg initially and 4 weeks later, followed by 45–90 mg every 12 weeks	Interleukin blocker

Topical corticosteroids, such as betamethasone or hydrocortisone, are the primary, initial treatment for psoriasis because they are effective, safe, and inexpensive. Topical corticosteroids reduce the inflammation associated with fast skin turnover. Therapy usually begins with the high potency corticosteroids and switches to moderate- and low-potency agents after the initial symptoms have been controlled.

Other topical drugs are retinoid-like compounds such as calcipotriene (Dovonex) and tazarotene (Tazorac). These drugs provide the same benefits as topical corticosteroids, but they exhibit fewer side effects. Calcipotriene produces elevated levels of calcium in the bloodstream, so this medication is not used on an extended basis.

Some patients have severe psoriasis that is resistant to topical drugs, so systemic therapy must be used. Systemic medications for psoriasis include acitretin (Soriatane), adalimumab (Humira), alefacept (Amevive), etanercept (Enbrel), infliximab (Remicade), and ustekinumab (Stelara). These drugs are taken orally to inhibit skin cell growth. Methotrexate (Rheumatrex, Trexall), an anticancer drug taken in tablet form, produces similar effects in the body (see Chapter 28). Other medications that have been used for different disorders but may provide relief of severe psoriatic symptoms are hydroxyurea (Hydrea) and cyclosporine (Sandimmune, Neoral). Cyclosporine is an immunosuppressive agent, discussed in Chapter 24.

Other skin therapy techniques may be used with or without psoriasis medications. These include various forms of tar treatment (coal tar) and a material called anthralin. Both substances are applied to the skin's surface and are not considered first-line therapies. Tar and anthralin inhibit DNA synthesis and arrest abnormal cell growth.

Ultraviolet B (UVB) and ultraviolet A (UVA) phototherapy are techniques used in cases of severe psoriasis. UVB therapy is less hazardous than UVA therapy. UVB light has a wavelength similar to sunlight; it reduces widespread lesions that normally resist topical treatments. With close supervision, this type of phototherapy can be administered at home. Keratolytic pastes are often applied between treatments. The second type of phototherapy is often referred to as PUVA (psoralen plus ultraviolet light) therapy because **psoralens** are often administered in conjunction with phototherapy. Psoralens are oral or topical agents that, when exposed to UV light, produce a photosensitive reaction. This reaction seems to provide benefit to the patient by reducing the number of lesions, but unpleasant adverse effects such as headache, nausea, and skin sensitivity may occur, limiting the effectiveness of this therapy. Immunosuppressant drugs such as cyclosporine are not used in conjunction with PUVA therapy because they increase the risk of skin cancer.

Concept Review 36.5

■ In most cases, which drug category is used to treat symptoms of dermatitis and psoriasis? What other drug therapies and techniques are used to provide a measure of relief for these symptoms?

PATIENTS NEED TO KNOW

Patients taking medications for skin disorders need to know the following:
1. Inform family members, sexual partners, school personnel, and any other persons with whom close contact has occurred about skin infestations. Treat clothes, bed linens, and personal items properly to avoid reinfestation.
2. Be informed and understand the proper way to apply medication or to remove nits if necessary. Scabicides and pediculicides should not be applied to the face, mouth, open skin lesions, or the eyes.
3. For acne and related disorders, apply medication only to areas where it is supposed to be applied. Follow instructions in package inserts and do not deviate from the precautions communicated by the healthcare provider.
4. Do not share skin medications with family or friends. Be familiar with medication adverse effects, especially those of retinoids, retinoid-like products, or medications used to treat severe skin disorders.
5. Use medications only during the time for which they are intended. With extended use, some medications (e.g., corticosteroids) may cause adverse effects. Take a medication suitable for the disorder; avoid those that are too potent or not potent enough.
6. Give medications a chance to work. Some systemic medications must be taken exactly as prescribed without skipping or stopping early.
7. Avoid contact with objects or drugs that are known to cause allergy or dermatitis. Try to avoid scratching, if possible. For severe skin disorders, see a dermatologist.

CHAPTER REVIEW

CORE CONCEPTS SUMMARY

36.1 **Layers of skin provide protection to the body.**

Two layers of skin and one underlying layer protect the body: the epidermis, dermis, and hypodermis. The most superficial layer is the epidermis, in which skin cells are replenished every three weeks. New cells arise from the bottom layer of the epidermis, called the germinativum, and are pushed to the outermost layer.

36.2 **The major causes of skin disorders are injury, aging, inherited factors, and other medical conditions.**

Many symptoms are associated with skin stress and injury. Others are associated with a patient's changing age or health. Skin disorders fit into three main categories: infectious, inflammatory, and cancerous disorders.

36.3 **Scabicides and pediculicides treat parasitic mite and lice infestations.**

Mites affect the skin and hair, whereas lice remain localized in hairy regions of the body. Both conditions are treatable with medications. Scabicides kill mites; pediculicides kill lice.

36.4 **The goal of drug therapy for sunburn is to eliminate discomfort until healing occurs.**

Local anesthetics are the primary medication used to treat mild sunburn and irritation. Often drugs are used for temporary relief of minor discomfort; in some cases, drugs may not be needed at all.

36.5 **Acne and rosacea are treated by a combination of OTC and prescription drugs.**

Blackheads, whiteheads, and rosacea are disorders in which pores become blocked, inflamed, or infected because of accelerated skin processes. Topical drugs for acne are those that inhibit bacterial growth (antibiotics) or promote shedding of old skin (keratolytic agents). Vitamin A–like compounds (retinoids) provide an improved resistance to bacterial infections by reducing oil production and the occurrence of clogged pores.

36.6 **Topical corticosteroids are used mainly to treat dermatitis and related symptoms.**

Dermatitis is treated by agents that reduce symptoms of inflammation, itchiness, flaking, cracking, bleeding, and lesions. Topical corticosteroids are the primary drug treatment for dermatitis. Potency depends on the type of drug formulation and whether it is packaged as a cream, lotion, solution, gel, or pad.

36.7 **Several topical and systemic medications are used to treat psoriatic symptoms.**

Psoriasis is a chronic disorder characterized by extreme discomfort and flaky areas called plaques. The treatments for psoriasis include topical corticosteroids, retinoid-like compounds, drugs that arrest skin cell growth, and immunosuppressants. Skin therapy techniques are also used, including keratolytic agents, coal tar, anthralin, psoralens, and phototherapy.

REVIEW QUESTIONS

The following questions are written in NCLEX-PN® style. Answer these questions to assess your knowledge of the chapter material, and go back and review any material that is not clear to you.

1. The nurse informs a patient taking benzocaine for a minor skin irritation that benzocaine:

1. Cannot be used for sunburns
2. Should not be used on open lesions
3. Causes blisters
4. Can be used on open sores

2. The nurse is helping to create a teaching plan for a patient prescribed desoximetasone (Topicort) for atopic dermatitis. The nurse will include which adverse effect in that plan?

1. Localized pruritus and hives
2. Hair loss in the application area

3. Worsening of acne
4. Skin irritation and redness in the application area

3. The nurse and a patient are discussing how to eliminate lice. The patient is given a shampoo-like medication that is applied and rinsed from the body within 10 minutes after application. This medication is:

1. Lindane
2. Crotamiton
3. Cortizone
4. Permethrin

4. The patient is complaining of discomfort related to minor sunburn. Which of the following medications would be included in a plan of care for someone who has minor sunburn?

1. Benzocaine (Solarcaine)
2. Cortizone

3. Benzoyl peroxide
4. Doxycycline

5. The nurse is providing information at a high school health fair. Many of the students ask for information on acne treatment. The nurse tells them that _____ is available but it is extremely important that women who are pregnant should not take this medication.

1. Hydrocortisone
2. Tretinoin
3. Benzoyl peroxide
4. Benzocaine

6. The patient is using topical corticosteroids. The nurse will need to monitor for which of the following systemic effects of the medication? (Select all that apply.)

1. Mood changes
2. Bone defects
3. Liver toxicity
4. Adrenal insufficiency

7. A patient with rosacea is being seen at the doctor's office with concerns about her skin. She has been trying to deal with her condition by using over-the-counter medications, but they seemed to have made her condition worse. The nurse understands the patient may need:

1. Calcipotriene (Dovonex)
2. Metronidazole (Metrogel)

3. Acitretin (Soriatane)
4. Cyclosporine (Sandimmune, Neoral)

8. Some patients with acne may need medications that promote the shedding of old skin. These medications are known as:

1. Pediculicides
2. Keratolytic agents
3. Retinoids
4. Corticosteroids

9. A nurse is caring for a newly diagnosed patient with psoriasis. The skin on her elbow is covered with red plaques and scales. She finds it very embarrassing. Even though she doesn't have much money, she wants to know what medication can help her. The nurse understands that the initial and inexpensive medication is:

1. Betamethasone
2. Doxycycline
3. Cyclosporine
4. Benzocaine

10. A patient is to receive the initial infused dose of infliximab (Remicade), 5 mg/kg. The patient weighs 198 pounds. How many milligrams will the patient receive?

1. 40 mg
2. 90 mg
3. 450 mg
4. 990 mg

CASE STUDY QUESTIONS

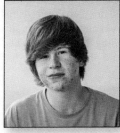

Remember Burt Nicholson, the patient introduced at the beginning of the chapter? Now read the remainder of the case study. Based on the information you have learned in this chapter, answer the questions that follow.

Burt Nicholson is a 16-year-old white male with a family history of various allergy disorders. He is complaining of general irritation and sores around the face, neck, and upper back. Upon examination, a severe case of acne and moderate erythema are observed on the chin, cheeks, and forehead. No excessive oil is noted. Although areas around the neck and upper back are inflamed, these do not appear to be infected. Burt states that he is so embarrassed about his skin, it's impacting his social life. He also says that he has tried a lot of different over-the-counter medications to help his acne but nothing seems to work. Burt is diagnosed with acne vulgaris.

1. Burt said that he had tried a lot of over-the-counter medications so the nurse asks him what medications he tried. He says that he can't remember all of them but he's sure he tried benzoyl peroxide but stopped using it after a week because his acne was still visible. The nurse responds by saying:

1. "The cream should have worked within that first week."
2. "Improvements begin in the first week but the full effects may take several weeks to a month or longer."
3. "Acne is very difficult to treat. It may take several months before you see improvements."
4. "If your acne isn't gone by now, you may need an antibiotic."

2. Right now the physician wants Burt to try the benzoyl peroxide again, but because Burt's skin is red and inflamed, the nurse suspects that a(n) _____ will also be prescribed.

1. Metronidazole
2. Benzocaine
3. Corticosteroid
4. Antibiotic

3. Other medication options are discussed. Burt is informed that he could also take tretinoin, a retinoid antiacne medication. When asked how the medication works, the nurse responds that tretinoin:

1. Sheds the outer layer of the skin
2. Decreases oil production by reducing the size and number of oil glands
3. Inhibits bacterial growth
4. Reduces inflammation

4. The nurse continues to tell Burt that tretinoin may cause the following adverse effects: (Select all that apply.)

1. Swelling around the lips
2. Dry mouth and nose
3. Photosensitivity (sensitivity to light)
4. Skin irritation such as burning and redness

NOTE: Answers to the Review and Case Study Questions appear in Appendix B. The complete rationales and answers are located on the textbook's website.

Pearson Nursing Student Resource   Find additional review materials at **nursing.pearsonhighered.com.**

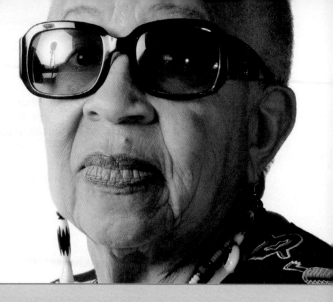

CHAPTER

"Moving is so stressful, and it's worse because I haven't had any help. I'm not even sure where I packed my medication so I've been having problems seeing."

Ms. Mary Saunders

37 Drugs for Eye and Ear Disorders

CORE CONCEPTS

37.1 Knowledge of basic eye anatomy is essential for an understanding of eye disorders and drug therapy.

37.2 Glaucoma is one of the leading causes of blindness.

37.3 Glaucoma therapy focuses on adjusting the circulation of aqueous humor.

37.4 Some antiglaucoma medications increase the outflow of aqueous humor.

37.5 Other antiglaucoma medications decrease the formation of aqueous humor.

37.6 Drugs provide relief for minor eye conditions and are used for eye exams.

37.7 Otic preparations treat infections, inflammation, and earwax buildup.

DRUG SNAPSHOT

The following drugs are discussed in this chapter:

DRUG CLASSES	DRUG PROTOTYPES
Drugs for glaucoma that increase the outflow of aqueous humor	**Pr** latanoprost (Xalatan) *601*
Drugs for glaucoma that decrease the formation of aqueous humor	**Pr** timolol (Betimol, Timoptic, others) *604*
Drugs for eye examinations and minor eye conditions	
Drugs for ear conditions	

LEARNING OUTCOMES

After reading this chapter, the student should be able to:

1. Describe important eye anatomy relevant to glaucoma development.

2. Identify the major risk factors associated with glaucoma.

3. Explain how intraocular pressure is related to nerve damage in the eye.

4. Compare and contrast the two principal types of glaucoma, and explain their reasons for development.

5. Explain the two major mechanisms by which drugs reduce intraocular pressure.

6. Identify examples of important drugs for treating glaucoma, and explain their basic actions and adverse effects.

7. Identify examples of drugs that dilate or constrict pupils, relax ciliary muscles, constrict ocular blood vessels, or moisten eye membranes.

8. Identify examples of drugs for treating ear infections, earaches, or a buildup of earwax.

9. For each of the classes listed in the Drug Snapshot, identify representative drugs and explain their mechanisms of drug action, primary actions, and important adverse effects.

KEY TERMS

closed-angle glaucoma (glaw-KOH-mah)
  601
cycloplegia (sy-kloh-PLEE-jee-ah) *602*
cycloplegic drugs (sy-kloh-PLEE-jik) *605*
external otitis (oh-TYE-tiss) *606*

mastoiditis (mass-toy-DYE-tuss) *606*
miosis (my-OH-sis) *601*
mydriasis (mih-DRY-uh-siss) *601*
mydriatic drugs (mih-
  DRY-atik) *605*

open-angle glaucoma
  (glaw-KOH-mah) *601*
otitis media (oh-TYE-tuss
  MEE-dee-ah) *606*
tonometry (toh-NAHM-uh-tree) *601*

The senses of vision and hearing provide the primary means for us to communicate with the world around us. Disorders affecting the eye and ear can result in problems with self-care, mobility, safety, and communication. The eye is vulnerable to a variety of conditions, many of which can be prevented, controlled, or reversed with proper pharmacotherapy. The first part of this chapter covers drugs used for the treatment of glaucoma and those used routinely by ophthalmic healthcare providers. The remaining part of the chapter presents drugs used for treatment of common ear disorders, including infections, inflammation, and the buildup of earwax.

Knowledge of basic eye anatomy is essential for an understanding of eye disorders and drug therapy.

CORE CONCEPT 37.1

To understand eye disorders and drug action, a firm knowledge of basic ocular anatomy is required. As shown in Figure 37.1 ■, a watery fluid called *aqueous humor* is found in the anterior cavity of the eye. The anterior cavity has two divisions: the anterior chamber and the posterior chamber. In the posterior chamber (Figure 37.2 ■), aqueous humor originates from an important muscle structure called the *ciliary body*. From there, aqueous humor flows through the pupil and into the anterior chamber. Within the anterior chamber and around the periphery is a network of spongy connective tissue called *trabecular meshwork*. Connected with trabecular meshwork is an opening called the canal of Schlemm, the location where aqueous humor drains from the anterior cavity.

trabecular = *strut-like*

FIGURE 37.1

Internal structures
of the eye.

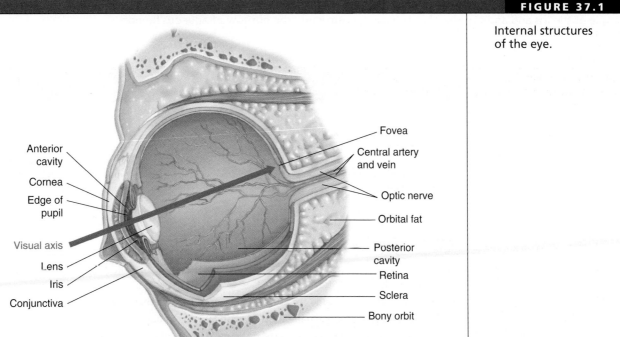

FIGURE 37.2

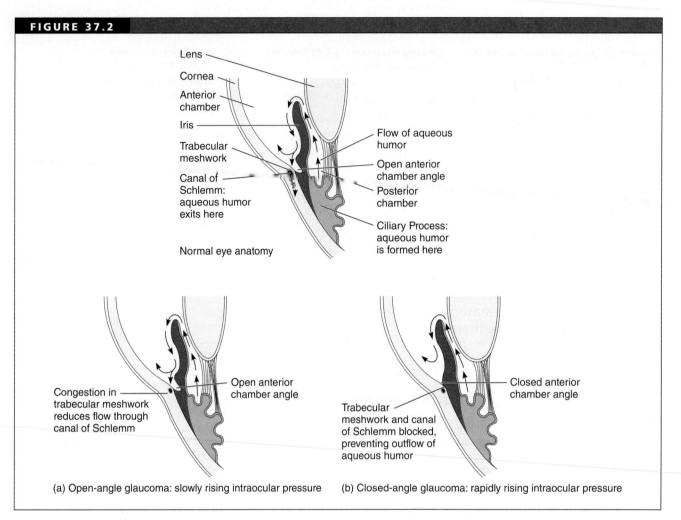

Lens

Cornea

Anterior chamber

Iris

Trabecular meshwork

Canal of Schlemm: aqueous humor exits here

Flow of aqueous humor

Open anterior chamber angle

Posterior chamber

Ciliary Process: aqueous humor is formed here

Normal eye anatomy

Congestion in trabecular meshwork reduces flow through canal of Schlemm

Open anterior chamber angle

Closed anterior chamber angle

Trabecular meshwork and canal of Schlemm blocked, preventing outflow of aqueous humor

(a) Open-angle glaucoma: slowly rising intraocular pressure

(b) Closed-angle glaucoma: rapidly rising intraocular pressure

Forms of primary adult glaucoma: (a) in chronic, open-angle glaucoma, the anterior chamber angle remains open, but drainage of aqueous humor through the canal of Schlemm is impaired; (b) in acute, narrow closed-angle glaucoma, the angle of the iris and anterior chamber is smaller, obstructing the outflow of aqueous humor.

GLAUCOMA

Glaucoma is one of the most dreaded eye disorders. In some cases, glaucoma is genetic; in other cases, glaucoma may be caused by eye trauma or disease. Some medications may contribute to the development of glaucoma, including long-term use of topical corticosteroids, some antihypertensives, antihistamines, and antidepressants. The major risk factors associated with glaucoma include high blood pressure, migraine headaches, high levels of nearsightedness or farsightedness, and older age.

Fast Facts Glaucoma

- Worldwide, more than five million people have lost their vision as a result of glaucoma. More than 50,000 are in the United States.
- Individuals of African heritage are affected more by glaucoma than any other ethnic group.
- Glaucoma is most common in patients older than 60 years of age.
- Acute glaucoma is often caused by head trauma, cataracts, tumors, or hemorrhage.
- Chronic simple glaucoma accounts for 90% of all glaucoma cases.

Glaucoma is one of the leading causes of blindness.

The presence of glaucoma may be detected by **tonometry,** an ophthalmic technique for measuring increased pressure inside the eye. Other routine refractory and visual field tests may uncover glaucoma signs. One problem with diagnosis is that patients with glaucoma typically do not experience symptoms and, therefore, do not seek medical attention. In some cases, glaucoma occurs so gradually that patients do not experience symptoms until late in the disease process.

tono = *pressure*
metry = *measurement*

Glaucoma is characterized by increased pressure inside the eyeball, termed *intraocular pressure* (IOP). The reason why IOP develops is because the normal flow of aqueous humor in the eye becomes blocked. Over time, pressure around the optic nerve can build, leading to blindness. In some cases, eye injury from the elevated IOP may be sudden, but in most cases it is gradual.

intra = *inside*
ocular = *eye*

As shown in Figure 37.2, the two principal types of glaucoma are **closed-angle glaucoma** and **open-angle glaucoma**. Both disorders result from the same problem: Pressure inside the eyeball leads to progressive damage of the optic nerve. The differences between these two disorders include how quickly the IOP develops.

Open-angle, or *chronic simple glaucoma,* is the most common type of glaucoma, accounting for more than 90% of all cases. With this disorder, IOP develops more slowly. It is called "open angle" because the iris does not cover the trabecular meshwork (Figure 37.2a). If discovered early, open-angle glaucoma can be treated successfully with medications.

Closed-angle glaucoma, sometimes referred to as *acute glaucoma,* is usually caused by stress, impact injury, or medications. Pressure inside the anterior chamber increases suddenly because the iris is pushed over the area where the aqueous fluid normally drains (Figure 37.2b). Symptoms include intense headaches, difficulty concentrating, bloodshot eyes, and blurred vision. Closed-angle glaucoma requires immediate intervention (usually surgical).

Glaucoma therapy focuses on adjusting the circulation of aqueous humor.

There are several approaches to glaucoma therapy. In cases of acute glaucoma, conventional or laser surgery might be performed to return the iris to its original position. Most therapies focus on reducing the amount of aqueous humor formed or unblocking its drainage. Generally, drug therapy for glaucoma functions by either *increasing the outflow of aqueous humor* (canal of Schlemm location) or by *decreasing the formation of aqueous humor* (ciliary body location).

Concept Review   37.1

■ Which components of the eye are specifically affected by glaucoma? Why is glaucoma such a dreaded eye disease? Drug therapy for glaucoma centers around which major approach?

Some antiglaucoma medications increase the outflow of aqueous humor.

Drugs increasing the outflow of aqueous humor include miotics, sympathomimetics, and prostaglandins. These drugs are summarized in Table 37.1 ◆.

miotic = *constricting pupil*

Although antiglaucoma drugs are not designed to directly alter pupil diameter, they often produce this effect because of their physiologic properties. Cholinergic direct- and indirect-acting drugs cause *constriction* of pupils or **miosis**. Sympathomimetics are drugs that activate the sympathetic nervous system and cause *dilation* of pupils or **mydriasis** (see Chapter 8). Prostaglandins do not affect pupil diameter, but instead they directly dilate trabecular meshwork within the anterior chamber of the eye.

Drug Prototype: ℗ *Latanoprost (Xalatan)*

Therapeutic Class: Antiglaucoma drug   **Pharmacologic Class: Prostaglandin, reducer of IOP**

Actions and Uses: Latanoprost is a prostaglandin analog believed to reduce IOP by increasing the outflow of aqueous humor. The recommended dose is one drop in the affected eye(s) in the evening. It is metabolized to its active form in the cornea, reaching its peak effect in about 12 hours. It is used to treat open-angle glaucoma and elevated IOP.

Adverse Effects and Interactions: Adverse effects include ocular symptoms such as conjunctival edema, tearing, dryness,

burning, pain, irritation, itching, sensation of a foreign body in the eye, photophobia, and visual disturbances. The eyelashes on the treated eye may grow, thicken, and darken. Changes may occur in pigmentation of the iris of the treated eye and in the periocular skin. The most common systemic adverse effect is a flu-like upper respiratory infection. Rash, asthenia, or headache may occur.

Latanoprost interacts with thimerosal: If mixed with eyedrops containing thimerosal, precipitation may occur.

TABLE 37.1 Antiglaucoma Drugs That Increase the Outflow of Aqueous Humor

Drug	Route and Adult Dose	Remarks
DIRECT- AND INDIRECT-ACTING CHOLINERGICS (MIOTIC DRUGS)		
carbachol (Miostat)	One or two drops 0.75–3% solution in the lower conjunctival sac every 4 hours three times a day	Ophthalmic solution; cholinergic drug; less useful in glaucoma than other drugs; causes stinging of the eyes
echothiophate (Phospholine Iodide)	One drop of 0.03–0.25% solution one to two times per day Acute glaucoma: 1 drop of 1–2% solution every 5–10 min for three to six doses Chronic glaucoma: 1 drop of 0.5–4% solution every 4–12 hours	Ophthalmic solution; irreversible acetylcholinesterase inhibitor; should be used cautiously due to an intense and persistent miosis and ciliary-muscle contraction that may occur
pilocarpine (Isopto Carpine, Pilopine)	Acute glaucoma: one drop 1–2% solution every 5–10 minutes for 3–6 doses Chronic glaucoma: one drop 0.5–4% solution every 4–12 hours	Ophthalmic solution; cholinergic drug; may be prescribed as an ocular therapeutic system, a slow release delivery method (Ocusert Pilo-20)
NONSELECTIVE SYMPATHOMIMETICS (MYDRIATIC DRUGS)		
dipivefrin HCl (Propine)	One drop 0.1% solution bid	Ophthalmic solution; converted to epinephrine in the eye
PROSTAGLANDINS		
bimatoprost (Lumigan)	One drop 0.03% solution daily in the evening	Ophthalmic solution
Pr latanoprost (Xalatan)	One drop (1.5 mg) solution daily in the evening	Ophthalmic solution
tafluprost (Zioptan)	One drop of 0.0015% solution in the evening	Ophthalmic solution; for reducing elevated intraocular pressure in patients with open-angle glaucoma or ocular hypertension
travoprost (Travatan)	One drop 0.004% solution daily in the evening	Ophthalmic solution; maximum effect after about 12 hours

Prostaglandins

Prostaglandins are the preferred drugs for glaucoma therapy because they have long durations of action and produce fewer side effects than drugs from other classes. In resistant cases, they may be combined with drugs from other classes. Drugs in this class increase aqueous humor outflow by reducing congestion in trabecular meshwork. Their main side effect is a change in pigmentation, usually a change to a brown iris color in patients with lighter colored eyes. These medications cause **cycloplegia** (blurred vision), local irritation, and stinging of the eyes. Because of these effects, prostaglandins are normally administered just before the patient goes to bed. Although prostaglandins can be irritating to the eyes, they usually do not prevent the patient from falling asleep.

cyclop = *round eye*
plegia = *paralysis*

Direct- and Indirect-Acting Cholinergics (Miotic Drugs)

Carbachol (Miostat), and pilocarpine (Isopto Carpine, Pilopine HS) are cholinergic drugs. These drugs directly activate the cholinergic receptors, producing various responses in the eye, including dilation of trabecular meshwork, so that the canal of Schlemm can absorb more aqueous humor. When more aqueous humor is absorbed, IOP is reduced. Thus, draining of the aqueous humor has an impact on eye pressure. Adverse effects include temporary cycloplegia. Cholinergic drugs are generally used in patients with open-angle glaucoma who have not responded to other medications. Echothiophate iodide (Phospholine iodide) is an indirect-acting cholinergic drug. It produces the same effects as direct-acting drugs, except that it blocks cholinesterase, the enzyme responsible for breaking down the natural neurotransmitter acetylcholine.

Nonselective Sympathomimetics (Mydriatic Drugs)

Dipivefrin (Propine) is a sympathomimetic drug. Dipivefrin is converted to epinephrine; epinephrine produces mydriasis, increased outflow of aqueous humor, and the subsequent fall of IOP. As discussed in Chapter 21, when epinephrine is released into the general circulation, it increases blood pressure and heart rate. Because of the potential for systemic adverse effects, this drug is rarely prescribed for the treatment of glaucoma.

Other antiglaucoma medications decrease the formation of aqueous humor.

Although prostaglandins are preferred drugs for glaucoma, other medications may be needed to bring IOP to normal levels. Beta-adrenergic blockers, alpha$_2$-adrenergic drugs, carbonic-anhydride inhibitors, and osmotic diuretics are drug classes that decrease the formation of aqueous humor. These are summarized in Table 37.2 ◆.

Beta Adrenergic Blockers

Beta-blocking drugs include betaxolol (Betaoptic), carteolol (Ocupress), levobunolol (Betagan), metipranolol (OptiPranolol), and timolol (Betimol, Timoptic, others). The exact mechanism by which these drugs produce their effects is not fully understood. However, they all reduce IOP effectively without the ocular adverse effects of other autonomic drugs. Beta blockers do not alter pupil diameter or produce cycloplegic effects. The doses of ophthalmic beta blockers are generally not high enough to enter the general circulation. Systemic adverse effects, if they occur, include bronchoconstriction, bradycardia, and hypotension.

Alpha$_2$-Adrenergic Drugs

Alpha$_2$-adrenergic drugs are less frequently prescribed than the other antiglaucoma medications. These medications include apraclonidine (Iopidine) and brimonidine (Alphagan). The most significant adverse effects are headache, drowsiness, dry mucosal membranes, blurred vision, and irritated eyelids.

Carbonic Anhydrase Inhibitors

Carbonic anhydrase inhibitors may be administered topically or PO to reduce IOP. Usually these medications are used as a second choice if beta blockers are not effective. Examples include acetazolamide (Diamox), brinzolamide (Azopt), dichlorphenamide (Daranide, Oratrol), dorzolamide (Trusopt), and methazolamide (Neptazane). These medications are more effective in cases of open-angle glaucoma. Patients must be cautioned when taking these medications because they are sulfonamides—drugs that may cause an allergic reaction. All of these drugs are diuretics, which means they can reduce IOP rather quickly and dramatically, altering serum electrolytes with continuous treatment.

TABLE 37.2 Antiglaucoma Drugs That Decrease the Formation of Aqueous Humor

Drug	Route and Adult Dose	Remarks
BETA-ADRENERGIC BLOCKERS		
betaxolol (Betaoptic)	One drop 0.5% solution bid	Ophthalmic solution; beta$_1$-blocker; reduces blood pressure, heart rate
carteolol (Ocupress)	One drop 1% solution bid	Ophthalmic solution; nonspecific beta blocker; causes bronchoconstriction
levobunolol (Betagan)	One or two drops 0.25–0.5% solution once or twice daily	Ophthalmic solution; nonspecific beta blocker
metipranolol (OptiPranolol)	One drop 0.3% solution bid	Ophthalmic solution; nonspecific beta blocker
ⓟ timolol (Betimol, Timoptic, others)	One or two drops of 0.25–0.5% solution once or twice daily; gel (salve): apply daily	Ophthalmic solution; nonspecific beta blocker
ALPHA$_2$-ADRENERGIC DRUGS		
apraclonidine (Iopidine)	One drop 0.5% solution bid	Ophthalmic solution
brimonidine tartrate (Alphagan)	One drop 0.2% solution tid	Ophthalmic solution
CARBONIC ANHYDRASE INHIBITORS		
acetazolamide (Diamox)	PO; 250 mg one to four times per day	Oral diuretic; sulfonamide; also for seizures, high altitude sickness, and renal impairment
brinzolamide (Azopt)	One drop 1% solution tid	Ophthalmic solution; sulfonamide
dorzolamide (Trusopt)	One drop 2% solution tid	Ophthalmic solution; sulfonamide
methazolamide (Neptazane)	PO; 50–100 mg bid or tid	Oral sulfonamide; less diuretic activity than acetazolamide
OSMOTIC DIURETICS		
isosorbide (Ismotic)	PO; 1–3 g/kg bid–qid	Used before and after eye surgery
mannitol (Osmitrol)	IV; 1.5–2 mg/kg as a 15–25% solution over 30–60 minutes	Raises osmotic pressure, causing diuresis; IV medication

Drug Prototype: 🅿 *Timolol (Betimol, Timoptic, Others)*

Therapeutic Class: **Antiglaucoma drug**   Pharmacologic Class: **Beta-adrenergic blocker, reducer of IOP, ocular hypotensive drug**

Actions and Uses: Timolol is a nonselective beta-adrenergic blocker available as a 0.25% or 0.5% ophthalmic solution. Timolol reduces elevated IOP in chronic open-angle glaucoma by reducing the formation of aqueous humor. The usual dose is one drop in the affected eye(s) twice a day. Timoptic XE allows for once-a-day dosing. Treatment may require two to four weeks for maximum therapeutic effect. It is also available in tablets, which are prescribed to treat mild hypertension.

Cosopt PF is a solution of timolol with dorzolamide, a carbonic-anhydrase inhibitor. Combigan combines timolol with brimonidine, an alpha adrenergic agonist.

Adverse Effects and Interactions: The most common adverse effects are local burning and stinging on instillation. In most patients there is no significant systemic absorption to cause adverse effects as long as timolol is applied correctly. If significant systemic absorption occurs, however, drug interactions could occur. Anticholinergics, nitrates, reserpine, methyldopa, and/or verapamil use could lead to increased hypotension and bradycardia. Indomethacin and thyroid hormone use could lead to decreased antihypertensive effects of timolol. Epinephrine use could lead to hypertension followed by severe bradycardia. Theophylline use could lead to decreased bronchodilation.

---

hypo = *reduced*
tensive = *tension*

thrombo = *clot*
phleb = *vein*
itis = *inflammation*

Osmotic Diuretics

Osmotic diuretics are used in cases of eye surgery or acute closed-angle glaucoma. Examples include isosorbide (Ismotic) and mannitol (Osmitrol). Because they have an ability to reduce plasma volume very quickly (see Chapter 18), they may produce unpleasant adverse effects, including headache, tremors, dizziness, dry mouth, fluid and electrolyte imbalance, and thrombophlebitis (venous clot formation) near the site of IV administration.

Concept Review   37.2

■ Describe two major approaches for controlling IOP in patients with glaucoma. What major drug classes are used in each case?

NURSING PROCESS FOCUS Patients Receiving Pharmacotherapy for Glaucoma

ASSESSMENT	POTENTIAL NURSING DIAGNOSES
Prior to drug administration: ■ Obtain a complete health history, including cardiovascular, respiratory, thyroid, and renal conditions; eye trauma or infection; allergies; drug history; and possible drug interactions. ■ Acquire the results of physical examination focusing on vital signs, visual acuity, visual fields (peripheral and central), presence of halos, blurred vision, and ocular pain.	■ *Disturbed Sensory Perception* related to disease process ■ *Risk for Injury* related to visual acuity deficits or adverse drug effects ■ *Self-Care Deficit* related to impaired vision ■ *Acute Pain* related to disease process or adverse drug effects ■ *Deficient Knowledge* related to a lack of information about drug therapy

PLANNING: PATIENT GOALS AND EXPECTED OUTCOMES

The patient will:
■ Experience therapeutic effects (normal eye pressure and no progression of visual impairment).
■ Be free from or experience minimal adverse effects from drug therapy.
■ Verbalize understanding of the drug's use, adverse effects, and required precautions.

IMPLEMENTATION

Interventions and (Rationales)	Patient Education/Discharge Planning
■ Administer ophthalmic solutions correctly and evaluate patient's knowledge of correct administration. (Using proper technique ensures that medication stays within the eye and helps to prevent complications.).	Instruct the patient in the proper administration of eye drops to: ■ Remove contact lenses prior to administering eye drops and wait 15 minutes before reinsertion. ■ Wash hands prior to eye drop administration. ■ Avoid touching the tip of the container to the eye, which may contaminate the solution. ■ Administer the eye drop in the conjunctival sac. ■ Apply pressure over the lacrimal sac for 1 minute. ■ Wait five minutes before administering other ophthalmic solutions. ■ Schedule glaucoma medications around daily routines such as waking, mealtimes, and bedtime to lessen the chance of missed doses.
■ Monitor visual acuity, blurred vision, papillary reactions, extraocular movements, and ocular pain. (Periodic monitoring helps to determine the effectiveness of drug therapy.)	■ Instruct the patient to report to the healthcare provider any changes in vision, eye pain, light sensitivity, halos around lights, or headache.

(continued)

Interventions and (Rationales)	Patient Education/Discharge Planning
■ Monitor the patient for specific contraindications for the prescribed drug. (There are many physiologic conditions for which ophthalmic solutions may be contraindicated.)	■ Instruct the patient to inform the healthcare provider of all health-related problems and prescribed and OTC medications.
■ Provide for eye comfort such as an adequately lighted room. (Ophthalmic drugs such as beta blockers used in the treatment of glaucoma can cause miosis and difficulty seeing in low-level lighting.)	■ Caution patient about driving or other activities in low-lighting conditions or at night until the effects of the drug are known.
■ Monitor for ocular reaction to the drug such as conjunctivitis and lid reactions. (These reactions may indicate adverse reactions or infection due to improper administration.)	■ Review with the patient the correct medication administration technique. ■ Instruct the patient to report itching, drainage, edema, ocular pain, sensation of a foreign body in the eye, photophobia, and visual disturbances to the healthcare provider.
■ Monitor the color of the iris and periorbital tissue of the treated eye. (Prostaglandins can change the color of the iris over time.)	Inform the patient that: ■ More brown color may appear in the iris and in the periorbital tissue of the treated eye only. ■ Any pigmentation changes develop over months to years.
■ Monitor vital signs periodically for systemic absorption of ophthalmic preparations. (Systemic ophthalmic drugs such as beta blockers and cholinergic drugs may cause serious cardiovascular complications such as hypertension, or bradycardia.)	Instruct the patient to: ■ Take and record vital signs weekly. ■ Immediately report palpitations, chest pain, shortness of breath, and irregularities in pulse and blood pressure to the healthcare provider.
■ Monitor and adjust environmental lighting to aid in patient's comfort. (People who have glaucoma are sensitive to excessive light, especially extreme sunlight.)	Instruct the patient to: ■ Adjust environmental lighting as needed to enhance vision or reduce ocular pain. ■ Wear darkened glasses as needed.
■ Encourage compliance with the treatment regimen. (Nonadherence may result in total loss of vision.)	Instruct the patient: ■ To adhere to medication schedule for eyedrop administration. ■ About the importance of regular follow-up care with the ophthalmologist. ■ That IOP readings should be done prior to beginning treatment and periodically during treatment.

EVALUATION OF OUTCOME CRITERIA

Evaluate the effectiveness of drug therapy by confirming that patient goals and expected outcomes have been met (see "Planning"). *See Tables 37.1 and 37.2 for lists of drugs to which these nursing actions apply.*

EYE EXAMINATIONS AND MINOR EYE CONDITIONS

Drugs provide relief for minor eye conditions and are used for eye exams.

CORE CONCEPT 37.6

Drugs for minor irritation and injury come from a broad range of classes, including antimicrobials, local anesthetics, corticosteroids, and nonsteroidal anti-inflammatory drugs (NSAIDs). A range of drug preparations may be used, including drops, salves, optical inserts, and injectable formulations. Some drugs only provide moisture to the eye's surface. For example, approved in 2009, bepotastine (Bepreve) is an antihistamine approved for twice daily dosing for itching associated with allergic conjunctivitis. Others penetrate and affect a specific area of the eye.

Some drugs are specifically designed for ophthalmic examinations. These include **cycloplegic drugs** to relax ciliary muscles and **mydriatic drugs** to dilate the pupils. Caution must be used when administering anticholinergic mydriatics because these drugs can increase IOP and worsen glaucoma. In addition, anticholinergic drugs have the potential for producing adverse effects of the central nervous system such as confusion, unsteadiness, or drowsiness in adults. Children generally become restless and spastic. Examples of cycloplegic, mydriatic, lubricant, and corneal edema drugs are listed in Table 37.3 ◆.

mydriatic = *dilating pupil*

Concept Review   **37.3**

■ List examples of commonly used drugs for minor eye irritation and injury. What are the major actions of cycloplegic and mydriatic drugs?

TABLE 37.3 Drugs for Eye Examinations and for Moistening Eye Membranes

Drug	Route and Adult Dose	Remarks
MYDRIATICS: SYMPATHOMIMETICS		
phenylephrine (Neo-Synephrine) (see page 98 for the Prototype Drug Box)	One drop 2.5% or 10% solution before eye exam	Decongestant and vasoconstriction properties; smaller doses provide temporary relief of eye redness; also for pupil dilation in closed-angle glaucoma
CYCLOPLEGICS: ANTICHOLINERGICS		
atropine (Atro-Pen) (see page 95 for the Prototype Drug Box)	One drop 0.5% solution daily	Also provided as ointment; should not be administered to patients with glaucoma; effects may be prolonged
cyclopentolate (Cyclogyl, Pentalair)	One drop 0.5–2% solution 40–50 minutes before procedure	Not for patients with glaucoma; cause burning and irritation; possible central adverse effects with higher doses
homatropine (Isopto Homatropine, others)	One or two drops 2 % or 5% solution before eye exam	Not for patients with glaucoma; effects may be prolonged after treatment
scopolamine hydrobromide (Isopto Hyoscine)	One or two drops 0.25% solution 1 hour before eye exam	Not for patients with glaucoma; effects may be prolonged after treatment; possible central adverse effects with higher doses
tropicamide (Mydriacyl, Tropicacyl)	One or two drops 0.5–1% solution before eye exam	Not for patients with glaucoma; central adverse effects with higher doses
LUBRICANTS CAUSING VASOCONSTRICTION		
naphazoline (Albalon, Allerest, ClearEyes, others)	One to three drops 0.1% solution every 3–4 hours prn	Over-the-counter (OTC) and prescription medications available
oxymetazoline (OcuClear, Visine LR)	One or two drops 0.025% solution qid	OTC and prescription medications available
tetrahydrozoline (Murine Plus, Visine, others)	One or two drops 0.05% solution bid–tid	Primarily OTC medication
GENERAL PURPOSE LUBRICANTS		
lanolin alcohol (Lacri-lube)	Apply a thin film to the inside of the eyelid	Mixed with mineral oil and petroleum jelly as a salve
polyvinyl alcohol (Liquifilm, others)	One or two drops prn	Artificial tear solution
DRUGS FOR CORNEAL EDEMA AND ITCHING		
sodium chloride hypertonicity ointment (Muro 128 5% Ointment)	Apply a thin film to the inside of the eyelid; instill one drop into the affected eye(s) twice a day (bid)	Ophthalmic ointment for corneal edema; mixed with lanolin, mineral oil, purified water, and white petrolatum as a salve; for itching associated with allergic conjunctivitis

EAR CONDITIONS

The ear has two major sensory functions: hearing and maintenance of equilibrium and balance. Three important structural areas—the outer ear, middle ear, and inner ear—carry out these functions (Figure 37.3 ■).

Otitis, inflammation of the ear, most often occurs in the outer and middle ear compartments. **External otitis** or *otitis externa,* commonly referred to as *swimmer's ear,* is inflammation of the outer ear; **otitis media** is inflammation of the middle ear. Outer ear infections most often occur with water exposure. Middle ear infections most often occur with upper respiratory infections, allergies, or auditory tube irritation. Of all ear infections, the most difficult ones to treat are infections of the inner ear (*otitis interna*). **Mastoiditis,** or inflammation of the mastoid sinus, can be a serious problem because if left untreated, it can result in hearing loss.

externa = *outside*
ot = *ear*
itis = *inflammation*
media = *middle*

interna = *inside*

FIGURE 37.3

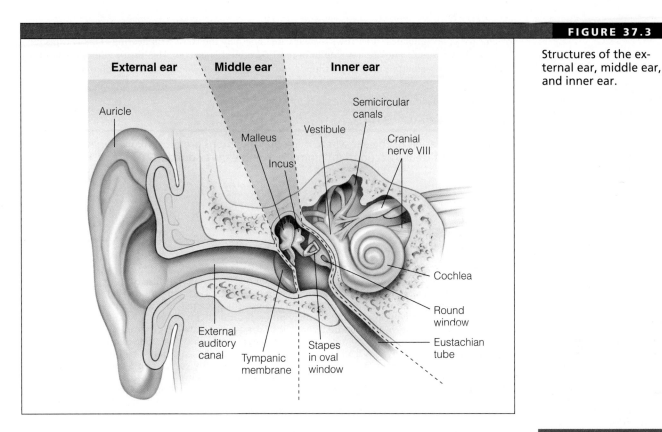

Structures of the external ear, middle ear, and inner ear.

Otic preparations treat infections, inflammation, and earwax buildup.

CORE CONCEPT **37.7**

Combination drugs effectively treat many different types of ear conditions, including infections, earaches, edema, and earwax.

The basic treatment for ear infection is essentially the same as in all places of the body: antibiotics. Topical antibiotics in the form of eardrops may be administered for external ear infections. Ciprofloxacin (Cipro HC otic, Cetraxal) is a very common topical antibiotic used for ear infections. Adverse reactions can occur with this medication. These include rashes; white patches in the mouth; vaginal itching or discharge; and itching, pain, or mild irritation within the ear.

Systemic antibiotics (see Chapter 26) may be needed in cases in which outer ear infections are extensive or in cases of middle or inner ear infections. Medications for pain, edema, and itching may also be necessary. Corticosteroids are often combined with antibiotics or with other drugs when inflammation is present. Examples of these drugs are listed in Table 37.4 ◆.

TABLE 37.4 Otic Preparations

Drug	Route and Adult Dose	Remarks
acetic acid and hydrocortisone (Vosol HC)	Three to five drops in the affected ear every 4–6 hours for 24 hours, then five drops tid–qid	Combination of acetic acid and glucocorticoid; for general ear infections and inflammation
benzocaine and antipyrine (Auralgan)	Fill the ear canal with solution tid for 2–3 days	For acute otitis media and the removal of earwax; reduces earache associated with the infection
carbamide peroxide (Debrox)	One to five drops 6.5% solution bid for 4 days	To soften, loosen, and remove excessive earwax; OTC medication
ciprofloxacin and dexamethasone (CiproDex)	Four drops of the suspension instilled into the affected ear bid for 7 days	Combination of fluoroquinolone antibiotic and corticosteroid; for ear infections and inflammation
ciprofloxacin and hydrocortisone (Cipro HC)	Three drops of the suspension instilled into the affected ear bid for 7 days	Combination of fluoroquinolone antibiotic and corticosteroid; for ear infections and inflammation
polymyxin B, neomycin, and hydrocortisone (Cortisporin)	Four drops in the ear tid–qid	Combination of antibiotics and glucocorticoid; for general ear or mastoid infections and inflammation; some patients may develop dermatitis as a result of sensitivity to neomycin

Mineral oil, earwax softeners, and commercial products are also used for proper ear health. When earwax accumulates, it narrows the ear canal and may interfere with hearing. This is especially true for older patients who are not able to properly groom themselves. Healthcare providers working with younger and elderly patients are trained to take appropriate measures when removing impacted earwax.

Concept Review 37.4

■ Identify the areas of the ear where microbial infections are most likely. What kind of otic preparations treat infections, inflammation, and earwax buildup?

Cam Therapy

Aloe Vera for Improving Eye and Ear Health

For centuries, Aloe vera has been hailed as the "medicine plant" because of its ability to treat burns, cuts, scrapes, rashes, and abrasions. It has a reputation for treating inflammation and acid indigestion, and even lowering blood cholesterol. *Aloe* may be able to treat eye irritation and conjunctivitis in addition to many other disorders.

One does not have to put aloe directly into the eyes to obtain its therapeutic effect. The benefit comes from treating areas around the eyes, including the bridge of the nose and the outside of the eyelids and cheeks. The skin around the ears may also be treated. The antiseptic properties of aloe probably come from the many components found within its sap and leaves. Some components have a reputation for killing microorganisms, including salicylic acid, urea nitrogen, cinnamonic acid, phenols, sulphur, and lupeol. Other components including plant sterols, immune modulating peptides, anti-inflammatory fatty acids, and viscous-like polysaccharides qualify as healing agents.

PATIENTS NEED TO KNOW

Patients taking medications for eye and ear disorders need to know the following:

Regarding Eye Medications

1. Have regular eye exams after the age of 40.
2. Do not strain or lift heavy objects if risk for glaucoma is present. Any effort that might produce eyestrain should be avoided.
3. Make sure that all allergies or sensitivities, including those to sulfa drugs, are known to the healthcare providers.
4. Do not take OTC medications that "get the red out" for longer than 24 hours. Use eye lubricants instead. Persistent irritation should be reported immediately.
5. Keep eye solutions clear and sterile; do not actually touch the eye when instilling drops.

Regarding Ear Medications

6. Take precautions to keep the ear canal dry when in or around water for an extensive time. Use appropriate earplugs or a bathing cap.
7. Apply 2% acetic acid to the ear canal after swimming. Acetic acid acts as a drying agent and restores the ear canal to its normal acidic condition.
8. Antibiotics (with or without steroids) may be needed to treat swimmer's ear. Consult a healthcare practitioner.
9. Do not place objects like cotton swabs in the ear canal, use a bulb syringe approved for removing debris and warm water. Use any cerumen dissolving agent responsibly.

CHAPTER REVIEW

CORE CONCEPTS SUMMARY

37.1 Knowledge of basic eye anatomy is essential for an understanding of eye disorders and drug therapy.

The anterior cavity of the eye is the place where aqueous humor is circulated. Aqueous humor originates from the ciliary body located in the posterior chamber and drains into the canal of Schlemm found in the anterior chamber.

37.2 Glaucoma is one of the leading causes of blindness.

Glaucoma develops because the flow of aqueous humor in the anterior eye cavity becomes disrupted, leading to increasing intraocular pressure (IOP). Two principal types of glaucoma are closed-angle glaucoma and open-angle glaucoma.

37.3 Glaucoma therapy focuses on adjusting the circulation of aqueous humor.

Glaucoma therapy generally works by increasing the outflow of aqueous humor or decreasing aqueous humor formation.

37.4 Some antiglaucoma medications increase the outflow of aqueous humor.

Drugs that increase the outflow of aqueous humor include miotics, sympathomimetics, prostaglandins,

and prostamides. Prostaglandins are the preferred class of drugs for glaucoma treatment.

37.5 Other antiglaucoma medications decrease the formation of aqueous humor.

Medications that decrease the formation of aqueous humor include beta blockers, alpha$_2$-adrenergic drugs, carbonic-anhydrase inhibitors, and osmotic diuretics.

37.6 Drugs provide relief for minor eye conditions and are used for eye exams.

Mydriatic or pupil-dilating drugs and cyclopegic or ciliary-muscle relaxing drugs are routinely used for eye examinations. Some drugs constrict local blood vessels. Others lubricate the eyes.

37.7 Otic preparations treat infections, inflammation, and earwax buildup.

Combination drugs provide relief of conditions associated with the outer, middle, and inner ear. Drugs include antibiotics, corticosteroids, and earwax dissolving drugs.

REVIEW QUESTIONS

The following questions are written in NCLEX-PN® style. Answer these questions to assess your knowledge of the chapter material, and go back and review any material that is not clear to you.

1. A patient is at the optometric office to have her eyes examined. She is told that the doctor will have to dilate her pupils with _____ eye drops so he can see the back of the eye.

1. Miotic
2. Mydriatic
3. Constricting
4. Corticosteroids

2. In a plan of care, a patient is to receive a drug that relieves pressure in the eye by increasing the outflow of aqueous humor. This drug would be:

1. Timolol (Timoptic)
2. Betaxolol (Betaoptic)
3. Pilocarpine (Ocusert)
4. Ciprofloxacin (Cipro)

3. The patient is informed that the medication used to relieve the pressure in her eye by decreasing production of aqueous humor is:

1. Timolol (Timoptic)
2. Atropine sulfate
3. Pilocarpine (Ocusert)
4. Ciprofloxacin (Cipro)

4. The patient has been given a prescription for acetazolamide (Diamox) 250 mg PO three times a day. What is the total amount of Diamox the patient will take in a 24-hour period?

1. 250 mg
2. 500 mg
3. 750 mg
4. 1,000 mg

5. A patient has an ear infection and is taking Cipro. If he also had inflammation, which of the following class of drug would be added?

1. Corticosteroids
2. Aluminum sulfate and calcium acetate (Domeboro)
3. Osmotic diuretics
4. Carbonic-anhydrase inhibitors

6. Prior to administering eardrops, the nurse should inform the patient that:

1. The solution should stay in the ear for one hour
2. The solution will be removed within one hour.
3. There may be a decrease in hearing for a few minutes.
4. The medication will take effect immediately.

7. A patient has just been prescribed ciprofloxacin for an ear infection. He asks the nurse if there is anything he should know about. The nurse tells him that the drug can cause adverse reactions. The symptoms can include: (Select all that apply.)

1. Rash
2. White patches in the mouth
3. Pain within the ear
4. Total loss of hearing

8. In the plan of care for patients with glaucoma, the rationale for giving antiglaucoma medications would be to reduce the pressure within the eye by:

1. Decreasing aqueous humor production and increasing outflow of aqueous humor
2. Increasing aqueous humor production and decreasing outflow of aqueous humor
3. Decreasing aqueous humor production and decreasing outflow of aqueous humor
4. Increasing aqueous humor production and increasing outflow of aqueous humor

9. The patient started on travoprost (Travatan) is instructed that:

1. This medication is administered in the morning only.
2. Due to pupil constriction, visual acuity may be affected.
3. This medication may change the pigmentation of the iris.
4. Due to dilation of the pupils, visual acuity may be affected.

10. If the patient is allergic to sulfonamides, the nurse understands that he should not take:

1. Methazolamide (Neptazane)
2. Betaxolol (Betaoptic)
3. Carteolol (Ocupress)
4. Beta blockers

CASE STUDY QUESTIONS

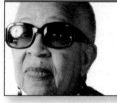

Remember Ms. Saunders, the patient introduced at the beginning of the chapter? Now read the remainder of the case study. Based on the information you have learned in this chapter, answer the questions that follow.

Ms. Mary Saunders is a 65-year-old African American female presenting with severe pain in the right eye, headache, and blurred vision. She has a history of primary hypertension and glaucoma. Her blood pressure is 140/90 mmHg. No other obvious signs are noted. In the course of the examination, she mentions that she has recently relocated. It has been a particularly stressful time because she has not had much help from her family. She has not been taking her antiglaucoma medication, the beta blocker, timolol (Timoptic).

1. The nurse and Ms. Saunders begin to discuss the importance of taking the glaucoma medication. The nurse explains that if left untreated pharmacologically, glaucoma could lead to:

1. Mydriasis
2. Cycloplegia
3. Blindness
4. Vertigo

2. Ms. Saunders states she knows that she should be taking her medications but has some concerns. She asks the nurse if timolol can cause any problems. The nurse responds that the most common adverse effect of timolol (Timoptic) is:

1. Burning and stinging
2. Sinus irritation
3. Bronchoconstriction
4. Edema around the eyes

3. In addition to the discussion about adverse effects, the nurse tells Ms. Saunders that it is not advisable to take the following drugs with timolol (Timoptic): (Select all that apply.)

1. Epinephrine
2. Ciprofloxacin
3. Nitrates
4. Corticosteroids

4. Ms. Saunders wants to know how long it would be before she could tell if the medication was working. The nurse tells her it would take about:

1. One week
2. Up to two weeks
3. Two to four weeks
4. One to two months

NOTE: Answers to the Review and Case Study Questions appear in Appendix B. The complete rationales and answers are located on the textbook's website.

CHAPTER 1
Introduction to Pharmacology: Drug Regulation and Approval

Consumers Union. (May 2009). *To err is human—To delay is deadly.* Retrieved from http://www.safepatientproject.org/safepatientproject.org/pdf/safepatientproject.org-ToDelayIsDeadly.pdf.

Jones, J. H., Treiber, L. A. (2012, October 4). When nurses become the "second" victim. *Nursing Forum, 4:* 4286–4291. doi: 10.1111/j.1744-6198.2012.00284.x

Mangoni, A. A. (2012). Predicting and detecting adverse drug reactions in old age: Challenges and opportunities. *Expert Opinion on Drug Metabolism and Toxicology, 5:* 527–530.

Moore, T. J., Cohen, M. R., Furberg, C. D. (2008). *Quarter watch.* Retrieved from http://www.ismp.org/QuarterWatch/200901.pdf.

Stosic, R., Dunagan, F., Palmer, H., Fowler, T., Adams, I. (2011). Responsible self-medication: Perceived risks and benefits of over-the-counter analgesic use. *International Journal of Pharmacy Practice, 4:* 236–245. doi: 10.1111/j.2042-7174.2011.00097.x

Szefler, S. J., Whelan, G. J., Leung, D. Y. (2006). "Black box" warning: Wake-up call or overreaction?" *Journal of Allergy and Clinical Immunology, 117:* 26–29.

U.S. Food and Drug Administration. (January 2006). *Guidance for industry. Warnings and precautions, contraindications, and boxed warning sections of labeling for human prescription drug and biological products—Content and format.* Retrieved from http://www.fda.gov/downloads/Drugs/GuidanceComplianceRegulatoryInformation/Guidances/ucm075096.pdf.

Yood, M. U., Campbell, U. B., Rothman, K. J., Jick, S. S., Lang, J., Wells, K. E., Jick, H., Johnson, C. C. (2007). Using prescription claims data for drugs available over-the-counter (OTC). *Pharmacoepidemiology and Drug Safety, 16*(9): 961–968.

CHAPTER 2
Drug Classes, Schedules, and Categories

Congressional Budget Office. (2009). *How increased competition from generic drugs has affected prices and returns in the pharmaceutical industry.* Retrieved from http://www.cbo.gov/ftpdocs/6xx/doc655/pharm.pdf.

Drug Enforcement Agency. (2005). *Drugs of abuse.* Retrieved from http://www.usdoj.gov/dea/pubs/abuse/doa-p.pdf.

Duncan, D. (2010). Generic prescribing and substitution: The big issues. *British Journal of Community Nursing, 15*(5): 248–249.

Howland, R. H. (2010). Are generic medications safe and effective? *Journal of Psychosocial Nursing Mental Health Services, 48*(3): 13–16.

Force, M. V., Deering, L., Hubbe, J., Andersen, M., Hagemann, B., Cooper-Hahn, M., & Peters, W. (2006). Effective strategies to increase reporting of medication errors in hospitals. *Journal of Nursing Administration, 36*(1): 34–41.

Keenum, A. J., Devoe, J. E., Chisolm D. J., & Wallace, L. S. (2012). Generic medications for you, but brand-name medications for me. *Research in Social and Administrative Pharmacy, 8*(6), 574–578.

Rashidee, A., Hart, J., Chen, J., & Kumar, S. (2009). High-alert medications: Error prevalence and severity. *Patient Safety & Quality Healthcare.* Retrieved from http://www.psqh.com/julyaugust-2009/164-data-trends-july-august-2009.html.

Smith, S. F., Duell, D. J., & Martin, B. C. (2011). *Clinical nursing skills* (8th ed.). Upper Saddle River, NJ: Prentice Hall. http://www.nlm.nih.gov/medlineplus/druginfo/meds/ and the AHFS® Consumer Medication Information. © Copyright, 2012. The American Society of Health-System Pharmacists, Inc.

CHAPTER 3
Methods of Drug Administration

Berman, A. J., Snyder, S., Kozier, B., & Erb, G. (2012). *Kozier & Erb's fundamentals of nursing concepts, process, and practice* (9th ed.). Upper Saddle River, NJ: Prentice Hall.

Institute for Safe Medical Practices. (2013). *List of error-prone abbreviations, symbols, and dose designations.* Retrieved from http://www.ismp.org/.

Joint Commission on Accreditation of Healthcare Organizations. (2010). *The official "do not use" list.* Retrieved from http://www.jointcommission.org/topics/patient_safety.aspx.

Olsen, J. L., Giangrasso, A. P., & Shrimpton, D. M. (2011). *Medical dosage calculations* (10th ed.). Upper Saddle River, NJ: Prentice Hall.

Smith, S. F., Duell, D. J., & Martin, B. C. (2002). *PhotoGuide of nursing skills.* Upper Saddle River, NJ: Prentice Hall.

U. S. Department of Health and Human Services, Food and Drug Administration, Center for Drug Evaluation and Research (CDER). (2008). *Guidance for industry: Orally disintegrating tablets.* Retrieved from http://www.fda.gov/cder/guidance/index.htm.

CHAPTER 4
What Happens After a Drug Has Been Administered

Bauer, L. A. (2011). Clinical pharmacokinetics and pharmacodynamics. In J. T. Dipro (Ed.), *Pharmacotherapy: A pathophysiologic approach* (8th ed., pp. 12–35). New York: McGraw-Hill.

Blumenthal, D. K., & Garrison, J. C. (2011). Pharmacodynamics: Molecular mechanisms of drug action. In B. A. Chabner, L. L. Brunton, & B. C. Knollman (Eds.), *Goodman and Gilman's the pharmacological basis of therapeutics* (12th ed.). New York: McGraw-Hill.

Buxton, I. L., & Benet, L. Z. (2011). Pharmacokinetics: The dynamics of drug absorption, distribution, metabolism, and elimination. In B. A. Chabner, L. L. Brunton, & B. C. Knollman (Eds.), *Goodman and Gilman's the pharmacological basis of therapeutics* (12th ed.). New York: McGraw-Hill.

Rosenbaum, S. E. (2011). *Basic pharmacokinetics and pharmacodynamics: An integrated textbook and computer simulations.* Hoboken, NJ: John Wiley & Sons.

CHAPTER 5
The Nursing Process in Pharmacology

American Nurses Association (ANA). (2007). *Scope of nursing informatics practice.* Retrieved from http://nursingworld.org/practice/niworkgroup/ANA.

Berman, A., & Snyder, S. (2012). *Kozier & Erb's fundamentals of nursing: Concepts, process, and practice* (9th ed.). Upper Saddle River, NJ: Pearson Education.

Huckabay, L. M. (2009). Clinical reasoned judgement and the nursing process. *Nursing Forum 44*(2), 72–78. doi:10.1111/j.1744-6198.2009.00130.x

Larson, L. (2009). Word for word, culture to culture. *Hospitals & Health Networks/AHA, 83*(7), 44–45.

LeMone, P., & Burke, K. (2011). *Medical-surgical nursing: Critical thinking in patient care* (5th ed.). Upper Saddle River, NJ: Pearson Education.

NANDA International. (2012). *Glossary of terms: Nursing diagnosis.* Retrieved from http://www.nanda.org/DiagnosisDevelopment/DiagnosisSubmission/PreparingYourSubmission.

North Carolina Concept-Based Learning Editorial Board. (2011). *Nursing: A concept-based approach to learning.* Upper Saddle River, NJ: Pearson Education.

Wilkinson, J. M., & Ahern, N. (2009). *Nursing diagnosis handbook with NIC interventions and NOC outcomes* (9th ed.). Upper Saddle River, NJ: Prentice Hall Health.

CHAPTER 6
Herbs and Dietary Supplements

Anastasi, J. K., Chang, M., & Capilli, B. (2011). Herbal supplements: Talking with your patients. *The Journal for Nurse Practitioners, 7*(1): 29–35. doi:10.1016/j.nurpra.2010.06.004

Anderson, E. (2009). Complementary therapies and older adults. *Topics in Geriatric Rehabilitation, 25*(4): 320–328.

Barnes, P. M., Bloom, B., & Nahin, R. L. (2008). Complementary and alternative medicine use among adults and children: United States, 2007 (National Health Statistics Reports No. 12). Hyattsville, MD: National Center for Health Statistics.

Blumenthal, M., Lindstrom, A. & Lynch, M.E. (2011). Herbal sales continue growth – up 3.3% in 2010. *HerbalGram: The Journal of the American Botanical Council, 90:* 64–67. Retrieved from http://cms.herbalgram.org/herbalgram/issue90/MarketReport.html.

DerMarderosian, A., Liberti, L., Beutler, J. A., Grauds, C., Tatro, D. S., Cirigliano, M., & DeSilva, D. (2010). *The review of natural products* (6th ed.). St. Louis, MO: Wolters Kluwer Health.

Fontaine, K. L. (2009). *Complementary and alternative therapies for nursing practice* (3rd ed.). Upper Saddle River, NJ: Prentice Hall.

Gagnier, J. J., van Tulder, M., Berman, B., & Bombardier, C. (2007). Herbal medicine for low back pain: A Cochrane review. *Spine, 32*(1): 82–92.

Hung, S. K., & Ernst, E. (2010). Herbal medicine: An overview of the literature from three decades. *Journal of Dietary Supplements, 7*(3): 217–226. doi:10.3109/19390211.2010.487818

Medical Economics Staff (Ed.). (2007). *PDR for herbal medicines* (4th ed.). Montvale, NJ: Thomson Healthcare.

National Center for Complementary and Alternative Medicine (NCCAM). (2010). *Complementary and alternative medicine use and children.* Retrieved from http://nccam.nih.gov/health/children.

Shen, J. & Oraka, E. (2012). Complementary and alternative medicine (CAM) use among children with current asthma. *Preventative Medicine, 54*(1): 27–31. doi:10.1016/j.ypmed.2011.10.007

CHAPTER 7
Substance Abuse

Centers for Disease Control and Prevention. (2011). Quitting smoking among adults—United States, 2001–2010. *Morbidity and Mortality Weekly Report, 60*(44): 1513–1519.

D'Apolito, K. (2013). Breastfeeding and substance abuse. *Clinical Obstetric Gynecology, 56:* 202–211.

Fiellin, L. E., Tetrault, J. M., Becker, W. C., Fiellin, D. A., Hoff, R. A. (2012). Previous use of alcohol, cigarettes, and marijuana and subsequent abuse of prescription opioids in young adults. *Journal of Adolescent Health, 52*(2): 158–163.

Fiore, M. C., Jaén, C. R., Baker, T. B., Bailey, W. C., Benowitz, N. L., Curry, S. J., Dorfman, S. F., Froelicher, E. S., Goldstein, M. G., Froelicher, E. S., Healton, C. G., et al. (2008). Treating Tobacco Use and Dependence: 2008 Update—Clinical Practice Guidelines. Rockville (MD): U.S. Department of Health and Human Services, Public Health Service, Agency for Healthcare Research and Quality.

Heinzerling, K. G., Gadzhyan, J., van Oudheusden, H., Rodriguez, F., McCracken, J., Shoptaw, S. (2013). Pilot randomized trial of Bupropion for adolescent methamphetamine. Abuse/dependence. *Journal of Adolescent Health,* Jan 16.

Leece, P., Rajaram, N., Woolhouse, S., Millson ,M. (2012). Acute and chronic respiratory symptoms among primary care patients who smoke crack cocaine. *Journal of Urban Health,* X: 542–551.

O'Brien, C. P. (2006). Drug addiction and drug abuse. In L. L. Brunton, J. S. Lazo, and K. L. Parker (Eds.), *The pharmacological basis of therapeutics* (11th ed., pp. 607–627). New York: McGraw-Hill.

CHAPTER 8
Drugs Affecting Functions of the Autonomic Nervous System

Cazzola, M., Matera, M. G. (2011). Tremor and β(2)-adrenergic agents: Is it a real clinical problem? *Pulmonary Pharmacology and Therapeutics.* Dec 24.

Hanoch, Y., Gummerum, M., Miron-Shatz, T., Himmelstein, M. (2010). Parents' decision following the Food and Drug Administration recommendation: The case of over-the-counter cough and cold medication. *Child Care Health Development,* Nov; 36(6):795–804.

Madhuvrata, P., Cody, J. D., Ellis, G., Herbison, G. P., Hay-Smith, E. J. (2012). Which anticholinergic drug for overactive bladder symptoms in adults. *Cochrane Database of Systematic Reviews.* Jan 18; 1.

Nunn, N., Womack, M., Dart, C., Barrett-Jolley, R. (2011). Function and pharmacology of spinally-projecting sympathetic pre-autonomic neurones in the paraventricular nucleus of the hypothalamus. *Current Neuropharmacology,* Jun; 9(2):262–277.

Sellers, D. J., Chess-Williams, R. (2012). Muscarinic agonists and antagonists: Effects on the urinary bladder. *Handbook of Experimental Pharmacology,* 208:375–400.

Serra, A., Ruff, R., Kaminski, H., Leigh, R. J. (2011). Factors contributing to failure of neuromuscular transmission in myasthenia gravis and the special case of the extraocular muscles. *Annals of the New York Academy of Sciences,* Sep; 1233:26–33.

van Gestel, A. J., Steier, J. (2010). Autonomic dysfunction in patients with chronic obstructive pulmonary disease (COPD). *Journal of Thoracic Disorders,* Dec; 2(4):215–222.

Westfall, T. C., Westfall, D. P. (2006). Neurotransmission: The autonomic and somatic nervous systems. In L. L. Brunton, J. S. Lazo, & K. L. Parker (Eds.), *The pharmacological basis of therapeutics* (11th ed., pp. 137–181). New York: McGraw-Hill.

CHAPTER 9
Drugs for Anxiety and Insomnia

Andai-Otlong, D. (2006). Patient education guide: Anxiety disorders. *Nursing, 36*(3): 48–49.

Baldessarini, R. J. (2006). Drug therapy of depression and anxiety disorders. In L. L. Brunton, J. S. Lazo, & K. L. Parker (Eds.), *The pharmacological basis of therapeutics* (11th ed., pp. 429–460). New York: McGraw-Hill.

Boelen, P. A, & Carleton, R. N. (2012). Intolerance of uncertainty, hypochondriacal concerns, obsessive-compulsive symptoms, and worry. *Journal of Nervous and Mental Disease,* Mar; 200(3): 208–213.

Charney, D. S., Mihic, J., & Harris, A. (2006). Hypnotics and sedatives. In L. L. Brunton, J. S. Lazo, & K. L. Parker (Eds.),*The pharmacological basis of therapeutics* (11th ed., pp. 401–438). New York: McGraw-Hill.

Chhangani, B., Greydanus, D. E., Patel, D. R., & Feucht, C. (2011). Pharmacology of sleep disorders in children and adolescents. *Pediatric Clinics of North America, 58*(1): 273–291. doi:10.1016/j.pcl.2010.11.003

Ernst, E. (2006). Herbal remedies for anxiety—a systematic review of controlled clinical trials. *Phytomedicine, 13*(3): 205–208.

Ghafoori, B., Barragan, B., Tohidian, N., & Palinkas, L. (2012). Racial and ethnic differences in symptom severity of PTSD, GAD, and depression in trauma-exposed, urban, treatment-seeking adults. *Journal of Traumatic Stress,* Feb; 25(1): 106–110.

Grandner, M. A., Martin, J. L., Patel, N. P., Jackson, N. J., Gehrman, P. R., Pien, G., Perlis, M. L., Xie, D., Sha, D., Weaver, T., & Gooneratne, N. S. (2012). Age and sleep disturbances among American men and women: Data from the U.S. Behavioral risk factor surveillance system. *Sleep,* Mar 1; 35(3): 395–406.

Kennedy, D. O., Little,W., Haskell, & C. F., Schoey, A. B. (2006). Anxiolytic effects of a combination of *Melissa officinalis* and *Valerian officinalis* during laboratory induced stress. *Phytotherapy Research,* 20(2): 96–102.

McCurry, S.M., Pike, K.C., Logsdon, R.G., Teri, L. & Vitiello, M.V. (2010a). Subjective versus objective sleep outcomes: Does the caregiver always know best? *The Gerontologist, 50*, Special Issue 1; 313.

McCurry, S.M., Pike, K.C., Logsdon, R.G., Vitiello, M.V., Larson, E.B. & Teri, L. (2010b). Walking, bright light, and combination intervention all improve sleep in community-dwelling persons with Alzheimer's disease and caregivers: Results of a randomized, controlled trial. *Sleep*, 33; A353.

National Institute for Drug Abuse (NIDA). (2010). *Prescription medications*. Retrieved from http://www.nida.nih.gov/drugpages/prescription.html.

National Institutes of Mental Health website: http://www.nimh.nih.gov/. *Anxiety disorders*.

Office of Dietary Supplements, National Institutes of Health. (2008). Retrieved from http://ods.od.nih.gov/factsheets/valerian-Health-Professional/.

The Nurse Practitioner: The American Journal of Primary Health Care (2005).*Medication update; FDA: Antidepressants a risk for kids*. Retrieved from http://www.tnpj.com

Titler, M. G., Shever, L. L., Kanak, M. F., Picone, D. M., & Qin, R. (2011). Factors associated with falls during hospitalization in an older adult population. *Research and Theory for Nursing Practice, 25*(2): 127–152. doi:10.1891/1541-6577.25.2.127

United States Drug Enforcement Agency (DEA). (2011). *Benzodiazepines*. Retrieved from http://www.usdoj.gov/dea.

United States Drug Enforcement Agency (DEA). (2011). *Depressants*. Retrieved from http://www.usdoj.gov/dea.

Vitiello, M. V. Treating Insomnia in Older Adults. In: Treating Sleep Disorders in Aging, State-of-the-Art: Should Sleep Be a Vital Sign? (Symposium), Vitiello M. V. and Bernard, M. A. (Chairs). (2007). *The Gerontologist, 47*, Special Issue 1; 751–752.

CHAPTER 10
Drugs for Emotional and Mood Disorders

Baldessarini, R. J. (2006). Drug therapy of depression and anxiety disorders. In L. L. Brunton, J. S. Lazo, & K. L. Parker (Eds.), *Goodman & Gilman's The pharmacological basis of therapeutics* (11th ed., pp. 429–460). New York, NY: McGraw-Hill.

Berlim M. T, Van den Eynde F, Daskalakis Z. J. (2013, Feb). High-frequency repetitive transcranial magnetic stimulation accelerates and enhances the clinical response to antidepressants in major depression: A meta-analysis of randomized, double-blind, and sham-controlled trials. *Journal of Clinical Psychiatry, 74*(2): e122–129. doi: 10.4088/JCP.12r07996

Biederman, J., Melmed, R. D., Patel, A., McBurnett, K., Konow, J., Lyne, A., & Scherer, N.; SPD503 Study Group. (2008, January). A randomized, double-blind, placebo-controlled study of guanfacine extended release in children and adolescents with attention-deficit/hyperactivity disorder. *Pediatrics, 121*(1): e73–84.

Boellner, S. W., Pennick, M., Fiske, K., Lyne, A., & Shojaei, A. (2007, September). Pharmacokinetics of a guanfacine extended-release formulation in children and adolescents with attention-deficit-hyperactivity disorder. *Pharmacotherapy, 27*(9): 1253–1262.

DeJesus, S. A., Diaz, V. A., Gonsalves, W. C., & Carek, P. J. (2011). Identification and treatment of depression in minority populations. *International Journal of Psychiatry in Medicine, 42*(1): 69–83.

Elia, J., & Vetter, V. L. (2010). Cardiovascular effects for the treatment of attention-deficit hyperactivity disorder: What is known and how should it influence prescribing in children? *Paediatric Drugs, 12*(3): 165–175. doi:10.2165/11532570-000000000-00000

Huang, Y. S., & Tsai, M. H. (2011, July). Long-term outcomes with medications for attention-deficit hyperactivity disorder: Current status of knowledge. *CNS Drugs, 25*(7): 539–554.

Karaosmanoğlu AD, Butros SR, Arellano R. (2013, Feb 21). Imaging findings of renal toxicity in patients on chronic lithium therapy. *Diagnostic and Interventional Radiology*. doi: 10.5152.dir.2013.097

Krasowski, M. D., & Blau, J. L. (2011). Drug interactions with St. John's wort. In A. Dasgupta & C. A. Hammett-Stabler (Eds.), *Herbal supplements: Efficacy, toxicity, interactions with Western drugs, and effects on clinical laboratory tests*. Hoboken, NJ: John Wiley & Sons. doi: 10.1002/9780470910108.ch12

Sallee, F. R., Lyne, A., Wigal, T., & McGough, J. J. (2009, June). Long-term safety and efficacy of guanfacine extended release in children and adolescents with attention-deficit/hyperactivity disorder. *Journal of Child and Adolescent Psychopharmacology, 19*(3): 215–226.

CHAPTER 11
Drugs for Psychoses

Bailey, K. (2003). Aripiprazole: The newest antipsychotic agent for the treatment of schizophrenia. *Pyschological Nursing and Mental Health Services, 41*(2): 14–18.

Baldessarini, R. J., & Tarazi, F. I. (2006). Pharmacotherapy of psychosis and mania. In L. L. Brunton, J. S. Lazo, & K. L. Parker (Eds.), *The pharmacological basis of therapeutics* (11th ed., pp. 461–500). New York: McGraw-Hill.

Correll, C. U., Manu, P., Olshanskiy, V., Napolitano, B., Kane, J. M., & Malhotra, A. K. (2009). Cardiometabolic risk of second-generation antipsychotic medications during first-time use in children and adolescents. *Journal of the American Medical Association, 302*(2): 1765–1773. doi:10.1011/jama.2009.1549

de Araújo, A. N., de Sena, E. P., de Oliveira, I. R., & Juruena, M. F. (2012). Antipsychotic agents: Efficacy and safety in schizophrenia. *Drug Healthcare Patient Safety Journal*. 4:173–180. doi: 10.2147/DHPS.S37429

Maher, A. R., & Theodore, G. (2012). Summary of the comparative effectiveness review on off-label use of atypical antipsychotics. *Journal of Managed Care Pharmacy*, Jun;18(5 Suppl B):S1–20.

National Mental Health Association. *Mental Health Issues: Schizophrenia*. Retrieved from http://www.nmha.org/.

Steinberg M, & Lyketsos C. G. (2012) Atypical antipsychotic use in patients with dementia: Managing safety concerns. *American Journal of Psychiatry*, Sep;169(9):900–906. doi:10.1176/appi.ajp.2012.12030342

CHAPTER 12
Drugs for Degenerative Diseases and Muscles

Birks, J., & Grimley, Evans J. (2009). *Ginkgo biloba* for cognitive impairment and dementia. *Cochrane Database of Systematic Reviews*, Issue 1.

Breitner, J. C., Baker, L. D., Montine, T. J., Meinert, C. L., Lyketsos, C. G., Ashe, K. H., et al. (2011). Extended results of the Alzheimer's disease anti-inflammatory prevention trial. *Alzheimer's & Dementia, 7*(4): 402–411.

Carbidopa and levodopa. Drugs.com. Retrieved from http://www.drugs.com/pro/carbidopa-and-levodopa.html.

DeKosky, S. T., Williamson, J. D., Fitzpatrick, A. L., Kronmal, R. A., Ives, D. G., Saxton, J. A., & Furberg, C. D. (2008). *Ginkgo biloba* for prevention of dementia: A randomized controlled trial. *Journal of the American Medical Association, 300*(19): 2253–2262.

Hoozemans, J. J., Veerhusi, R., Rozemuller, J. M., & Eikelenboom, P. (2011). Soothing the inflamed brain: Effect of non-steroidal anti-inflammatory drugs on Alzheimer's disease. *CNS & Neurological Disorders Drug Targets, 10*(1): 57–67.

Jaturapatpom, D., Isaac, M. G., McCleery, J., & Tabet, N. (2012). Aspirin, steroidal and non-steroidal anti-inflammatory drugs for the treatment of Alzheimer's disease. *Cochrane Database of Systematic Reviews, 2012*(2): 1–115. doi:10.1002/14651858.CD006378.pub2

National Parkinson Foundation. *Improving care. Improving lives*. Retrieved from http://www.parkinson.org/Parkinson-s-Disease/Treatment/Medications-for-Motor-Symptoms-of-PD/Carbidopa-levodopa.

Standaert, D. G., & Young, A. B. (2006). Treatment of central nervous system degenerative disorders. In L. L. Brunton, J. S. Lazo, & K. L. Parker (Eds.), *Goodman & Gilman's The pharmacological basis of therapeutics* (11th ed., pp. 527–546). New York, NY: McGraw-Hill.

Watts, R. L., Lyons, K. E., Pahwa, R., Sethi, K., Stern, M., Hauser, R. A., et al. (2010). Onset of dyskinesia with adjunct ropinirole prolonged-release or additional levodopa in early Parkinson's disease. *Movement Disorders, 25*(7): 858–866.

Weinmann, S., Roll, S., Schwarzbach, C., Vauth, C., & Willich, S. (2010). Effects of *Ginkgo biloba* in dementia: A systematic review and meta-analysis. *Biomed Central Geriatrics, 10*(14). doi:10.1186/1471-2318-10-14

CHAPTER 13
Drugs for Seizures

Borthen, I., & Gilhus, N. E. (2012, February 9). Pregnancy complications in patients with epilepsy. *Current Opinion in Obstetrics and Gynecology 24*(2): 78–83.

Brodie, M. J., H. Lerche, et al. (2010). Efficacy and safety of adjunctive ezogabine (retigabine) in refractory partial epilepsy. *Neurology, 75*(20): 1817–1824.

Chen, J. W. Y., Ruff, R. L., Eavey, R., & Wasterlain, C. G. (2009). Posttraumatic epilepsy and treatment. *Journal of Rehabilitation Research & Development, 46*(6): 685–695. doi:10.1682/JRRD.2008.09.0130

Chung, S., Ben-Menachem, E., Sperling, M. R., Rosenfeld, W., Fountain, N. B., Benbadis, S., & Doty, P. (2010, December). Examining the clinical utility of lacosamide: Pooled analyses of three phase II/III clinical trials. *CNS Drugs, 24*(12): 1041–1054.

Cross, J. H. (2009). The ketogenic diet. *Advances in Clinical Neurosciences & Rehabilitation, 8*(6): 8–10.

Dalkara, S., & Karakurt, A. (2012, February 21). Recent progress in anticonvulsant drug research: Strategies for anticonvulsant drug development and applications of antiepileptic drugs for non-epileptic central nervous system disorders. *Current Topics in Medicinal Chemistry, 12*(9): 1033–1071.

DiFilippo, T., Parisi, L., & Roccella, M. (2012, February). Evaluation of creative thinking in children with idiopathic epilepsy (absence epilepsy). *Minerva Pediatrica, 64*(1): 7–14.

Faught, E. (2011). Ezogabine: a new angle on potassium gates, *Epilepsy Currents, 11*(3): 75–78.

Foreman, B., & Hirsch, L. J. (2012, February). Epilepsy emergencies: Diagnosis and management. *Neurologic Clinics, 30*(1): 11–41.

Hirsch, L. J. (2012, February 16). Intramuscular versus intravenous benzodiazepines for prehospital treatment of status epilepticus. *New England Journal of Medicine, 366*(7): 659–660.

McDonagh, M., Peterson, K., Lee, N., et al. (2008, October). *Drug class review: Antiepileptic drugs for indications other than epilepsy: Final report update 2* [Internet]. Portland, OR: Oregon Health & Science University. Retrieved from http://www.ncbi.nlm.nih.gov/books/NBK10371/.

McNamara, J. O. (2006). Pharmacotherapy of the epilepsies. In L. L. Brunton, J. S. Lazo, and K. L. Parker (Eds.), *The pharmacological basis of therapeutics* (11th ed., pp. 501–526). New York: McGraw-Hill.

Pack, A. M., & Morrell, M. J. (2003). Treatment of women with epilepsy. *Seminars in Neurology, 22*(3): 289–298.

Pizzol, A. D., Martin, K. C, Mattiello, C. M., de Souza, A. C., Torres, C. M., Bragatti, J. A., & Bianchin, M. M. (2012, February 25). Impact of the chronic use of benzodiazepines prescribed for seizure control on the anxiety levels of patients with epilepsy.*Epilepsy and Behavior, 23*(3): 373-376.

Veiby, G., Daltveit, A. K., Schjølberg, S., Stoltenberg, C., Øyen A., Vollset, S. E., Engelsen, B. A., and Gilhus, N. E. (2013, July 18). Exposure to antiepileptic drugs in utero and child development—A prospective population-based study. *Epilepsia*; Published Online. doi: 10.1111/epi.12226

Wang, Y., & Khanna, R. (2011, March). Voltage-gated calcium channels are not affected by the novel anti-epileptic drug lacosamide.*Translational Neuroscience, 2*(1): 13–22.

CHAPTER 14
Drugs for Pain Management

Agius, A. M., Jones, N. S., Muscat, R. (2013, June). A randomized controlled trial comparing the efficacy of low-dose amitriptyline, amitriptyline with pindolol and surrogate placebo in the treatment of chronic tension-type facial pain. *Rhinology, 51*(2):143–153.

Fornasari, D. (2012, February). Pain mechanisms in patients with chronic pain. *Clinical Drug Investigation, 32* (Suppl 1).45–52.

Frost, J., Okun, S., Vaughan, T., Heywood, J., Wicks, P. (2011). Patient-reported outcomes as a source of evidence in off-label prescribing: Analysis of data from patientslikeme. *Journal of Medical Internet Research, 13*(1): e6.

Gunstein, H. B., & Akil, H. (2006). Opioid analgesics. In L. L. Brunton, J. S. Lazo, and K. L. Parker (Eds.), *The pharmacological basis of therapeutics* (11th ed., pp. 547–590). New York: McGraw-Hill.

Holland, L. N. & Goldstein, B. D. (1994). Examination of tonic nociceptive behavior using a method of substance P receptor desensitization in the dorsal horn. *Pain, 56*: 339–346.

Jensen, T. S., Finnerup, N. B. (2007, August). Management of neuropathic pain. *Current Opinion in Supportive and Palliative Care, 1*(2): 126–31.

Largent, E. A., Miller, F. G., Pearson, S. D. (2009). Going off-label without venturing off-course: Evidence and ethical off-label prescribing. *Archives of Internal Medicine, 169*: 1745–1747.

Mack, A. (2003, November-December). Examination of the evidence for off-label use of gabapentin. *Journal of Managed Care Pharmacy, 9*(6): 559–68.

National Center for Complementary and Alternative Medicine. (2010). *Evening primrose oil.* Retrieved from http://nccam.nih.gov/health/eveningprimrose.

Reddy, D. S. (2013, May). The pathophysiological and pharmacological basis of current drug treatment of migraine headache. *Expert Review of Clinical Pharmacology, 6*(3): 271–88.

Torpy, J. M., Livingston, E. H. (2013, April 17). JAMA patient page. Aspirin therapy. *Journal of the American Medical Association, 309*(15): 1645.

Whelan, A. M., Jurgens, T. M., & Naylor, H. (2009). Herbs, vitamins and minerals in the treatment of premenstrual syndrome: A systematic review. *Canadian Journal of Pharmacology, 16*(3): e407–429.

CHAPTER 15
Drugs for Anesthesia

Catterall, W. A. & Mackie, K. (2006). Local anesthetics. In L. L. Brunton, J. S. Lazo, and K. L. Parker (Eds.), *The pharmacological basis of therapeutics* (11th ed., pp. 369–386). New York: McGraw-Hill.

Evers, A. S., Crowder, C. M., & Balser, J. R. (2006). General anesthetics. In L. L. Brunton, J. S. Lazo, and K. L. Parker (Eds.), *The pharmacological basis of therapeutics* (11th ed., pp. 341–368). New York: McGraw-Hill.

Kye, Y. C., Rhee, J. E., Kim, K., Kim, T., Jo, Y. H., Jeong, J. H., & Lee, J. H. (2012, November). Clinical effects of adjunctive atropine during ketamine sedation in pediatric emergency patients. *The American Journal of Emergency Medicine, 30*(9): 1981–1985. doi: 10.1016/j.ajem.2012.04.030

Monk, T. G., Weldon, B. C., Garvan, C. W., Dede, D. E., van der Aa, M. T., Hellman, K. M., & Gravenstein, J. S. (2008). Predictors of cognitive dysfunction after major noncardiac surgery. *Anesthesia, 108*(1): 18–30. doi:0000296071.19434.1e

Persson, J. (2013, May 11). Ketamine in Pain Management. *CNS Neuroscience & Therapeutics*. doi: 10.1111/cns.12111

Stoelting, R. K. (2006). *Pharmacology and physiology in anesthetic practice* (4th ed.). Philadelphia: Lippincott Williams & Wilkins.

CHAPTER 16
Drugs for Lipid Disorders

American Heart Association. (n.d.). *Youth and cardiovascular diseases—statistics*. Retrieved from http://www.americanheart.org/downloadable/heart/1059110431975FS11YTH3REV7-03.pdf.

Bersot, T. P. (2011). Drug therapy for hypercholesterolemia and dyslipidemia. In L. L. Brunton, B. A. Chabner, & B. C. Knollman (Eds.), *The pharmacological basis of therapeutics* (12th ed., pp. 877–908). New York: McGraw-Hill.

Centers for Disease Control and Prevention. (2012). *Cholesterol: Facts*. Retrieved from http://www.cdc.gov/cholesterol/facts.htm.

Citkowitz, E. (2011). *Familial hypercholesterolemia. Medscape reference*. Retrieved from http://emedicine.medscape.com/article/121298-overview.

Eiland, L. S., & Luttrell, P. K. (2010). Use of statins for dyslipidemia in the pediatric population. *Journal of Pediatric Pharmacology and Therapeutics, 15*(3), 160–172.

Malloy, M. J., & Kane, J. P. (2012). Hyperlipidemia and cardiovascular disease. *Current Opinion in Lipidology, 23*(6), 591–592.

National Institute of Health. (2011). *Coenzyme Q10*. Retrieved from http://www.nlm.nih.gov/medlineplus/druginfo/natural/938.html.

Oldways. (n.d.). *Traditional diets and Oldways' four pyramids*. Retrieved from http://www.oldwayspt.org/eating-well/introduction-traditional-diet-pyramids.

Ray, K. K., Seshasai, S. R. K., Jukema, W., & Sattar, N. (2010). Statins and all-cause mortality in high-risk primary prevention: A meta-analysis of 11 randomized controlled trials involving 65,229 participants. *Archives of Internal Medicine, 170*(12), 1024–1031. doi:10.1001/archinternmed.2010.182

Sargent, G. M., Forrest, L. E., & Parker, R. M. (2012). Nurse delivered lifestyle interventions in primary health care to treat chronic disease risk factors associated with obesity: A systematic review. *Obesity Reviews, 13*(12), 1148–1171.

Spratt, K. A. (2010). Treating dyslipidemia: Reevaluating the data using evidence-based medicine. *Journal of the American Osteopathic Association, 110*(4), 6–11.

Taylor, F., Ward, K., Moore, T. H. M., Burke, M., Davey-Smith, G., Casas J-P., & Ebrahim, S. (2011). Statins for the primary prevention of cardiovascular disease. *Cochrane Database of Systematic Reviews, 2011*(1). Art. No.: CD004816. doi:10.1002/14651858.CD004816.pub4

CHAPTER 17
Diuretics and Drugs for Electrolyte and Acid-Base Disorders

Brandimarte, F., Mureddu, G. F., Boccanelli, A., Cacciatore, G., Brandimarte, C., Fedele, F., & Gheorghiade, M. (2010). Diuretic therapy in heart failure: Current controversies and new approaches for fluid removal. *Journal of Cardiovascular Medicine, 11*(8), 563–570. doi:10.2459/JCM.0b013e3283376bfa

Gardner, J., Mooney, J., & Forester, A. (2013). HEAL: A strategy for advanced practitioner assessment of reduced urine output in hospital inpatients. *Journal of Clinical Nursing*.doi:10.1111/jocn.12254

Martin, R. K. (2010). Acute kidney injury: Advances in definition, pathophysiology, and diagnosis. *AACN Advanced Critical Care, 21*(4), 350–356. doi:10.1097/NCI.0b013e3181f9574b

Moser, M., & Feig, P. U. (2009). Fifty years of thiazide diuretic therapy for hypertension. *Archives of Internal Medicine, 169*(20), 1851–1856. doi:10.1001/archinternmed.2009.342

National Kidney Foundation. (2009). *End stage renal disease in the United States*. Retrieved December 13, 2009, from http://www.kidney.org/news/newsroom/fs_new/esrdinUS.cfm.

Reilly, R. F., & Jackson, E. K. (2011). Diuretics. In L. L. Brunton, B. A. Chabner, & B. C. Knollman (Eds.), *The pharmacological basis of therapeutics* (12th ed., pp. 671–720). New York: McGraw-Hill.

Saccomano, S. J., & DeLuca, D. A. (2012). Living with chronic kidney disease: Related issues and treatment. *The Nurse Practitioner, 37*(8), 32–38. doi:10.1097/01.NPR.0000415873.61843.68.

St. Peter, W. (2010). Improving medication safety in chronic kidney disease patients on dialysis through medication reconciliation. *Advances in Chronic Kidney Disease, 17*(5), 413–419. doi:10.1053/j.ackd.2010.06.001

Williams, H. (2013). An Update on Hypertension for Nurse Prescribers. *Nurse Prescribing, 11*(2). 70–75.

CHAPTER 18
Drugs for Hypertension

American Heart Association. (2013). *High blood pressure, 2013 statistical fact sheet*. Retrieved from http://www.heart.org/idc/groups/heart-public/@wcm/@sop/@smd/documents/downloadable/ucm_319587.pdf.

Carter, B. L., Bosworth, H. B. & Green, B. B. (2012). The hypertension team: The role of the pharmacist, nurse, and teamwork in hypertension therapy. *The Journal of Clinical Hypertension, 14*(1): 51–65. doi:10.1111/j.1751-7176.2011.00542.x

Centers for Disease Control and Prevention. (2012). *High blood pressure facts*. Retrieved from http://www.cdc.gov/bloodpressure/facts.htm

Clark, C. E., Smith, L. F., Taylor, R. S., & Campbell, J. L. (2010). Nurse led interventions to improve control of blood pressure in people with hypertension: Systematic review and meta-analysis. *British Medical Journal, 341*, 491 doi:10.1136/bmj.c3995.

Colbert, B. J., & Mason, B. J. (2012). *Integrated cardiopulmonary pharmacology* (3rd ed.). Upper Saddle River, NJ: Pearson Prentice Hall.

Gupta, A. K., Poulter, N. R., Dobson, J., Eldridge, S., Cappuccio, F. P., Caulfield, M., & Feder. G. (2010). Ethnic differences in blood pressure response to first and second-line antihypertensive therapies in patients randomized in the ASCOT Trial. *American Journal of Hypertension, 23*(9): 1023–1030. doi:10.1038/ajh.2010.105.

Hill, M. N., Miller, N. H., & DeGeest, S. (2010). Adherence and persistence with taking medication to control high blood pressure. *Journal of the American Society of Hypertension, 5*(1): 56–63. doi:10.1016/j.jash.2011.01.001.

Hopkins, C. H. (2011). *Hypertensive emergencies in emergency medicine. Medscape Reference*. Retrieved from http://emedicine.medscape.com/article/1952052-overview. http://www.heart.org/idc/groups/heart-public/@wcm/@sop/@smd/documents/downloadable/ucm_319587.pdf.

Jayasinghe, J. (2009). Non-adherence in the hypertensive patient: Can nursing play a role in assessing and improving compliance? *Canadian Journal of Cardiovascular Nursing, 19*(1): 7–12.

Kotchen, T. A. (2010). The search for strategies to control hypertension. *Circulation, 122*: 1141–1143. doi:10.1161/CIRCULATIONAHA.110.978759.

Michel, T., & Hoffman, B. B. (2011). Treatment of myocardial ischemia and hypertension. In L. L. Brunton, B. A. Chabner, & B. C. Knollman (Eds.), *The pharmacological basis of therapeutics* (12th ed., pp. 745–788). New York: McGraw-Hill.

National Center for Complementary and Alternative Medicine (NCCAM). (2010). *Herbs at a glance: Grape Seed Extract*. Retrieved at http://nccam.nih.gov/health/grapeseed/ataglance.htm.

National Institutes of Health, National Heart, Lung, and Blood Institute, National High Blood Pressure Education Program Coordinating Committee. (2003). *JNC-7 express: The seventh report of the Joint National Committee on Prevention, Detection Evaluation and Treatment of High Blood Pressure*. Bethesda, MD: Author. Retrieved from http://www.nhlbi.nih.gov/guidelines/hypertension/express.pdf.

Seguin, B., Hardy, B., Singer, P. A., & Daar, A. S. (2008). BiDil: Reconceptualizing the race debate. *The Pharmacogenomics Journal, 8*(3): 169–173. doi:10.1038/sj.tpj.6500489.

Touyz, R. M. (2011). Advancement in hypertension pathogenesis: Some new concepts. *Current Opinion in Nephrology & Hypertension, 20*(2): 105–106. doi:10.1097/MNH.0b013e328343f526M37_

Townsend, R. R. (2011). Essential hypertension. Physicians information and education resource. Accessed at http://pier.acponline.org/physicians/diseases/d226/d226.html.

University of Maryland Medical Center. (2010). *Grape seed.* Retrieved from http://www.umm.edu/altmed/articles/grape-seed-000254.htm.

CHAPTER 19
Drugs for Heart Failure

Allen, L. A., Stevenson, L. W., Grady, K. L., Goldstein, N. E., Matlock, D. D., Arnold, R. M., . . . & Spertus, J. A. (2012). Decision making in advanced heart failure: A scientific statement from the American Heart Association. *Circulation, 125*(15): 1928–1952. doi: 10.1161/CIR.0b013e31824f2173.

American College of Cardiology/American Heart Association Task Force on Practice Guidelines. (2005). ACC/AHA 2005 guideline update for the diagnosis and management of chronic heart failure in the adult. A report of the (Writing Committee to Update the 2001 Guidelines for the Evaluation and Management of Heart Failure). *Circulation, 112:* e154–e235.

Demo, E. M., Skrzynia, C., & Baxter, S. (2009). Genetic counseling and testing for hypertrophic cardiomyopathy: The pediatric perspective. *Journal of Cardiovascular Translational Research, 2*(4): 500–507. doi:10.1007/s12265-009-9126-5

Kantor, P. F., Abraham, J. R., Dipchand, A. I., Benson, L. N., & Redington, A. N. (2010). The impact of changing medical therapy on transplantation-free survival in pediatric dilated cardiomyopathy. *Journal of the American College of Cardiology, 55*(13): 1377–1384. doi:10.1016/j.jacc.2009.11.059.

McCarthy, P. M., & Young, J. B. (Eds.). (2007). *Heart failure: A combined medical and surgical approach.* Malden, MA: Blackwell.

National Coalition for Women With Heart Disease. (2008). *Women and heart disease fact sheet.* Retrieved December 11, 2009, from http://womenheart.org/resources/cvdfactsheet.cfm.

Pahl, E., Sleeper, L. A., Canter, C. E., Hsu, D. T., Lu, M., Webber, S. A., . . . Lipshultz, S. E. (2012). Incidence of and risk factors for sudden cardiac death in children with dilated cardiomyopathy. *Journal of the American College of Cardiology, 59*(6): 607–615. doi:10.1016/jack.2011.10.878

Shah, A. M., & Mann, D. L. (2011). In search of new therapeutic targets and strategies for heart failure: Recent advances in basic science. *The Lancet, 378*(9792), 704–712. doi:10.1016/S0140-6736(11)60894-5.

Silva, J. N. A., & Canter, C. E. (2010). Current management of pediatric dilated cardiomyopathy. *Current Opinions in Cardiology, 25*(2): 80–87. doi:10.1097/HCO.0b013e328335b220.

Torpy, J. M., Lynm, C., & Glass, R. M. (2007). Heart failure. *Journal of the American Medical Association, 297*(22): 2548.

CHAPTER 20
Drugs for Angina Pectoris, Myocardial Infarction, and Stroke

Alaeddini, J. (2012). *Angina Pectoris.* Retrieved from http://emedicine.medscape.com/article/150215-overview.

Amsterdam, E. A., Kirk, J. D., Bluemke, D. A., Diercks, D., Farkouh, M. E., Garvey, J. L., et al. (2010). Testing of low-risk patients presenting to the emergency department with chest pain: A scientific statement from the American Heart Association. *Circulation, 122*(17): 1756–1776. doi:10.1161/CIR.0b013e3181ec61df

Cucherat, M., & Borer, J. S. (2012). Reduction of resting heart rate with antianginal drugs: Review and meta-analysis. *American Journal of Therapeutics, 19*(4): 269–280. doi: 10.1097/MJT.0b013e3182246a49

Geng, J., Dong, J., Ni, H., Lee, M. S., Wu, T., Jiang, K., et al. (2010). Ginseng for cognition. *Cochrane Database of Systematic Reviews, 2010*(12). Art. No.: CD007769. doi: 10.1002/14651858. CD007769.pub2

Hermida, R. C., Ayala, D. E., Mojón, A., & Fernández, J. R. (2011). Bedtime dosing of antihypertensive medications reduces cardiovascular risk in CKD. *Journal of the American Society of Nephrology, 22*(12): 2313–2321. doi:10.1681/ASN.2011040361

Parker, J. D., & Parker, J. O. (2012). Stable angina pectoris: The medical management of symptomatic myocardial ischemia. *Canadian Journal of Cardiology, 28*(2): S70–S80. doi.org/10.1016/j.cjca.2011.11.002

Potts, K. (2012). Preventing thromboembolic events and stroke. *Nursing & Residential Care, 14*(4). 179–103.

Seida, J. K., Durec, T., & Kuhle, S. (2011). North American (*Panax quinquefolius*) and Asian ginseng (*Panax ginseng*) preparations for prevention of the common cold in healthy adults: A systematic review. *Evidence-Based Complementary and Alternative Medicine, 2011* (282151). doi:10.1093/ecam/nep068

Sharma, V., Bell, R. M., & Yellon, D. M. (2012). Targeting reperfusion injury in acute myocardial infarction: A review of reperfusion injury pharmacotherapy. *Expert Opinion on Pharmacotherapy, 13*(8): 1153–1175. doi:10.1517/14656566.2012.685163

Wood, J., & Gordon, P. (2012). Preventing CVD in women: The NP's role. *The Nurse Practitioner, 37*(2): 26–33. doi: 10.1097/01. NPR.0000410275.21998.b5

Zafari, A. M. (2012). *Myocardial Infarction.* Retrieved from http://emedicine.medscape.com/article/155919-overview.

CHAPTER 21
Drugs for Shock and Anaphylaxis

Bockenstedt, T. L., Baker, S. N., & Weant, K. A. (2012). Review of vasopressor therapy in the setting of vasodilatory shock. *Advanced Emergency Nursing Journal 34*(1): 16–23. doi: 10.1097/TME.0b013e31824371d3

Bracht, H., Calzia, E., Georgieff, M., Singer, J., Radermacher, P., & Russell, J. A. (2012). Inotropes and vasopressors: More than haemodynamics! *British Journal of Pharmacology, 165*: 2009–2011. doi: 10.1111/j.1476-5381.2011.01776.x

Bunn, F., Trivedi, D., & Ashraf, S. (2008). Colloid solutions for fluid resuscitation. *Cochrane Database of Systematic Reviews*, Issue 1. Art. No.: CD001319. DOI: 10.1002/14651858.CD001319.pub2.

De Backer, D., Aldecoa, C., Njimi, H., & Vincent, J. L. (2012). Dopamine versus norepinephrine in the treatment of septic shock: A meta-analysis. *Critical Care Medicine, 40*(3): 725–730. doi: 10.1097/CCM.0b013e31823778ee

Delaney, A. P., Dan, A., McCaffrey, J., & Finfer, S. (2011). The role of albumin as a resuscitation fluid for patients with sepsis: A systematic review and meta-analysis. *Critical Care Medicine, 39*(2): 386–391. doi: 10.1097/CCM.0b013e3181ffe217

Han, J. & Martin, G.S.(2011). Does albumin fluid resuscitation in sepsis save lives? *Critical Care Medicine, 39*(2): 418–419. doi: 10.1097/CCM.0b013e318206b0ff

Havel, C., Arrich, J., Losert, H., Gamper, G., Müllner, M., & Herkner, H. (2011). Vasopressors for hypotensive shock. *Cochrane Database of Systematic Reviews,* Issue 5. Art. No.: CD003709. DOI: 10.1002/14651858.CD003709.pub3

Leone, M., & Martin, C. (2008). Vasopressor use in septic shock: An update. *Current Opinion in Anaesthesiology, 21*(2): 141–147.

Mustafa, S.S. (2012). *Anaphylaxis.* Retrieved from http://emedicine.medscape.com/article/135065-overview.

Pinsky, M. R. (2012). *Septic shock.* Retrieved from http://emedicine.medscape.com/article/168402-overview.

Xiushui, M. (2012). *Cardiogenic shock.* Retrieved from http://emedicine.medscape.com/article/152191-overview.

Younker, J. & Soar, J. (2010), Recognition and treatment of anaphylaxis. *Nursing in Critical Care,* 15: 94–98. doi: 10.1111/j.1478-5153.2010.00366.x

CHAPTER 22
Drugs for Dysrhythmias

Antzelevitch, C., & Burashnikov, A. (2011). Overview of basic mechanisms of cardiac arrhythmia. *Cardiac Electrophysiology Clinics, 3*(1): 23–45. doi:10.1016/j.ccep.2010.10.012

Marrouche, N. F., McMullan, L. L., & Gaston, V. (2010). Atrial fibrillation in the failing heart—A clinical review. *US Cardiology, 7*(1): 52–56.

National Heart, Lung, and Blood Institute. (2009). Long QT syndrome. Retrieved from http://www.nhlbi.nih.gov/health/dci/Diseases/qt/qt_whatis.html.

National Heart, Lung, and Blood Institute. (2011). Sudden cardiac arrest. Retrieved from http://www.nhlbi.nih.gov/health/dci/Diseases/scda/scda_whatis.html

Rivero, A., & Curtis, A. B. (2010). Sex differences in arrhythmias. *Current Opinion in Cardiology, 25*(1): 8–15. doi:10.1097/HCO.0b013e328333f95f

Sampson, K. J., & Kaas, R. S. (2011). Antiarrhythmic drugs. In L. L. Brunton, B. A. Chabner, & B. C. Knollman (Eds.), *The pharmacological basis of therapeutics* (12th ed., pp. 815–848). New York, NY: McGraw-Hill.

Tsiperfall, A., Ottoboni, L. K., Beheiry, S., Al-Ahmad, A., Natale, A., & Wang, P. (2011). Cardiac arrhythmia management: A practical guide for nurses and allied professionals. Ames, IA: Wiley-Blackwell.

Zevitz, M. E. (2010). Ventricular fibrillation. Medscape Reference. Retrieved from http://emedicine.medscape.com/article/158712-overview.

CHAPTER 23
Drugs for Coagulation Disorders

Abad, R., Pitarch, J., & Rocha, E. (2010). Overview of venous thromboembolism. *Drugs, 70* (Suppl 2): 3–10. doi:10.2165/1158583-S0-000000000-00000

Centers for Disease Control (2011a). Hemophilia: Data and Statistics. Retrieved from http://www.cdc.gov/ncbddd/hemophilia/data.html.

Centers for Disease Control (2011b). Von Willebrand Disease. Retrieved from http://www.cdc.gov/ncbddd/vwd/facts.html.

Centers for Disease Control (2012). Deep Vein Thrombosis/Pulmonary Embolism – Blood Clot Forming in a Vein. Retrieved from http://www.cdc.gov/ncbddd/dvt/data.html

Gay, S. (2010). An inside view of venous thromboembolism. *Nurse Practitioner, 35*(9): 32–39. doi:10.1097/01.NPR.0000387141.02789.c5

Gentilomo, C., Huang, Y.-S., & Raffini, L. (2011). Significant increase in colpidogrel use across U.S. children's hospitals. *Pediatric Cardiology, 32*(2): 167–175. doi:10.1007/s00246-010-9836-0

Heit, J.A. (2008). The epidemiology of venous thromboembolism in the community. *Arteriosclerosis, Thrombosis and Vascular Biology, 28*(3): 370–372.

Hirsh, J., Guyatt, G., Albers, G. W., Harrington, R., & Shünemann, H. J. (2008). Antithrombotic and thrombolytic therapy: American College of Chest Physicians Guidelines (8th ed.). *Chest, 133*: 110S–112S.

Lissiman, E., Bhasale, A. L., & Cohen, M. (2012). Garlic for the common cold. *Cochrane Database of Systematic Reviews, 2012*(3). Art. No.: CD006206. doi: 10.1002/14651858.CD006206.pub3.

National Center for Complementary and Alternative Medicine. (2010). Herbs at a glance: Garlic. Retrieved from http://nccam.nih.gov/health/garlic/ataglance.htm.

Weltz, D. S., & Weltz, J. I. (2010). Update on heparin: What do we need to know? *Journal of Thrombosis and Thrombolysis, 29*(2):199–207. doi:10.1007/s11239-009-0411-6

CHAPTER 24
Drugs for Inflammation and Fever

Kramer, L. C., Richards, P. A., Thompson, A. M., Harper, D. P., & Fairchok, M. P. (2008). Alternating antipyretics: Antipyretic efficacy of acetaminophen versus acetaminophen alternated with ibuprofen in children. *Clinical Pediatrics, 47*(9): 907–911. doi:10.1177/0009922808319967

Paul, I. M., Sturgis, S. A., Yang, C., Engle, L., Watts, H., & Berlin, C. M. (2010). Efficacy of standard doses of ibuprofen alone, alternating, and combined with acetaminophen for the treatment of febrile children. *Clinical Therapeutics, 32*(14): 2433–2440. doi:10.1016/j.clinthera.2011.01.006

Sherman, J. M., Sood, S. K. (2012, June). Current challenges in the diagnosis and management of fever. *Current Opinion in Pediatrics, 24*(3): 400–406. doi: 10.1097/MOP.0b013e32835333e3

Sullivan, J. E., Farrar, H. C., & Section on Clinical Pharmacology and Therapeutics; Committee on Drugs. (2011). Clinical report—fever and antipyretic use in children. *Pediatrics, 127*(3): 580–587. doi:10.1542/peds.2010.3852Trelle, S., Reichenbach, S., Wandel, S., Hildebrand, P., Tschannen, B., Villiger, PM., Egger, M., & Juni, P. (2011). Cardiovascular safety of non-steroidal anti-inflammatory drugs: Network meta-analysis. *British Medical Journal, 342*: c7086.

University of Rochester Medical Center. (2013). Arthritis and Other Rheumatic Diseases Statistics. Retrieved from https://www.urmc.rochester.edu/Encyclopedia/Content.aspx?ContentTypeID=85&ContentID=P00068.

Wiegand, T. J. (2012). Nonsteroidal Anti-inflammatory Agent Toxicity. Retrieved from http://emedicine.medscape.com/article/816117-overview.

CHAPTER 25
Drugs for Inflammation and Immune Modulation

Basu, A., Tan, H. P., & Shapiro, R. (2007). Current thinking on calcineurin inhibition in kidney transplantation. *Medscape Education*. Retrieved from http://www.medscape.com/viewprogram/8075.

Breslin, S. (2007). Cytokine-release syndrome: Overview and nursing implications. *Clinical Journal of Oncology Nursing, 11*(1): 1092–1095.

Denhaerynck, K., Burkhalter, F., Schäfer-Keller, P., Steiger, J., Bock, A., & DeGeest-Duncan, S. (2009). Clinical consequences of nonadherence to immunosuppressive medication in kidney transplant patients. *Transplant International, 22*(4): 441–446. doi:10.1111/j.1432-2277.2008.00820.x

Kaufman, C. (2011). The secret life of lymphocytes. *Nursing, 41*(6): 50–54. doi:10.1097/01.NURSE.0000396267.88998.f9

Krensky, A. M., Bennett, W. M., & Vincenti, E. (2011). Immunosuppressants, tolerogens, and immunostimulants. In L. L. Brunton, B. A. Chabner, & B. C. Knollman (Eds.), *The pharmacological basis of therapeutics* (12th ed., pp. 1005–1030). New York, NY: McGraw-Hill.

Linde, K., Barrett, B., Bauer, R., Melchart, D., & Woelkart, K. (2006). Echinacea for preventing and treating the common cold. *Cochrane Database of Systematic Reviews, 1*, CD000530. doi:10.1002/14651858. CD000530.pub2

Maggi, E., Vultaggio, A., & Matucci, A. (2011). Acute infusion reactions induced by monoclonal antibody therapy. *Expert Review of Clinical Immunology, 7*(1): 55–63. doi:10.1586/eci.10.90

Pelligrino, B. (2011). Immunosuppression. *Medscape Reference*. Retrieved from http://emedicine.medscape.com/article/432316-overview.

Shah, S. A., Sander, S., White, C. M., Rinaldi, M., & Coleman, C. I. (2007). Evaluation of echinacea for the prevention and treatment of the common cold: A meta-analysis. *The Lancet Infectious Diseases, 7*(7): 473–480. doi:10.1016/S1473-3099(07)70160-3

CHAPTER 26
Drugs for Bacterial Infections

Barnes, B. E., & Sampson, D., A. (2011). A literature review on community-acquired methicillin-resistant *Staphylococcus aureus* in the United States: Clinical information for primary care nurse practitioners. *Journal of the American Academy of Nurse Practitioners, 23*(1): 23–32. doi:10.1111/j.1745-7599.2010.00571.x

Centers for Disease Control and Prevention. (2010a). Self-study modules on tuberculosis: Module 9 Patient adherence to tuberculosis treatment. Retrieved from http://www.cdc.gov/tb/education/ssmodules/module9/ss9reading2.htm.

Centers for Disease Control and Prevention. (2010b). Sexually transmitted diseases: Treatment guidelines 2010. *Morbidity and Mortality Weekly Report, 59.* Retrieved from http://www.uphs.upenn.edu/bugdrug/antibiotic_manual/cdcstdrx2010.pdf.

Centers for Disease Control and Prevention. (2013). Get smart: Know when antibiotics work. Retrieved from http://www.cdc.gov/getsmart/.

Chen, L. F., Chopra, T., & Kaye, K. S. (2010). Pathogens resistant to antibacterial agents. *Medical Clinics of North America, 95*(4): 647–676. doi:10.1016/j.mcna.2011.03.005.

Cole, L. M. (2010). Prophylactic antibiotics: What's your game plan? *Nursing Management, 41*(4): 46–47. doi:10.1097/01.NUMA.0000370879.55842.ae

Estes, K. (2010). Methicillin-resistant *Staphylococcus aureus* skin and soft tissue infections. *Critical Care Nursing Quarterly, 34*(2): 101–109. doi:10.1097/CNQ.0b013e31820f6f9e

Furtado, G. H., & Nicolau, D. P. (2010). Overview perspective of bacterial resistance. *Expert Opinion on Therapeutic Patents, 20*(10): 1273–1276. doi:10.1517/13543776.2010.507193

Guilbeau, J. R., & Fordham, P. N. (2010). Evidence-based management and treatment of outpatient community-associated MRSA.*Journal for Nurse Practitioners, 6*(2): 140–145. doi:10.1016/j.nurpra.2009.07.011

Gumbo, T. (2011). General principles of antimicrobial therapy. In L. L. Brunton, B. A. Chabner, & B. C. Knollman (Eds.), *The pharmacological basis of therapeutics* (12th ed., pp. 1365–1382). New York, NY: McGraw-Hill.

Herchline, T.E. (2013). Medscape Reference. *Tuberculosis.* Retrieved from http://emedicine.medscape.com/article/230802-overview.

Madigan, M. T., Martinko, J. M., Stahl, A. A., & Clark, D. P. (2012). *Brock biology of microorganisms* (13th ed.). San Francisco, CA: Benjamin Cummings.

Matteo, B., Ginocchio, F., Giacobbe, D. R., & Malgorzata, M. (2011). Development of antibiotics for gram-negatives: Where now? *Clinical Investigation, 1*(2): 221–227. doi:10.4155/cli.10.31

Moonan, P. K., Quitugua, T. N., Pogoda, J. M., Woo, G., Drewyer, G., Sahbazian, B., & Weis, S. E. (2011). Does Directly Observed Therapy (DOT) Reduce Drug Resistant Tuberculosis? *BioMed Central (BMC) public health, 11*(1), 19. doi:10.1186/1471-2458-11-19

CHAPTER 27
Drugs for Fungal, Viral, and Parasitic Diseases

Bennet, J. E. (2011). Antifungal agents. In L. L. Brunton, B. A. Chabner, & B. C. Knollman (Eds.). *The pharmacological basis of therapeutics* (12th ed.). New York, NY: McGraw-Hill.

Buggs, A.M. (2012). Viral hepatitis. *Medscape Reference.* Retrieved from http://emedicine.medscape.com/article/775507-overview.

Centers for Disease Control and Prevention. (2008). Prevention and control of influenza: Recommendations of the Advisory Committee on Immunization Practices (ACIP), *Morbidity and Mortality Weekly Report, 57*(Early Release), 1–60.

Centers for Disease Control and Prevention (CDC) (2012a). Fungal Diseases. Retrieved from http://www.cdc.gov/fungal/.

Centers for Disease Control and Prevention (CDC) (2012b). HIV in the United States: At a Glance. Retrieved from http://www.cdc.gov/hiv/statistics/basics/ataglance.html.

Centers for Disease Control and Prevention. (2012c). Hepatitis B FAQs for health professionals. Retrieved from http://www.cdc.gov/hepatitis/HBV/HBVfaq.htm.

Centers for Disease Control and Prevention. (2013a). Genital herpes—CDC fact sheet. Retrieved from http://www.cdc.gov/std/herpes/stdfact-herpes.htm.

Centers for Disease Control and Prevention. (2013b) Seasonal Influenza (Flu). Retrieved from http://www.cdc.gov/flu/protect/keyfacts.html.

Perfect, J. R. & Andes, D. (2013). Antifungal therapy: Current concepts and evidence-based management. *Current Medical Research and Opinion, 29*(3): 289–290 (doi: 10.1185/03007995.2012.761136)

Derlet, R. W. (2013). Influenza. *Medscape Reference.* Retrieved from http://emedicine.medscape.com/article/219557-overview.

Hidalgo, J. A. (2013). Candidiasis. Retrieved from http://emedicine.medscape.com/article/213853-overview.

Lowes, R. (2010). Peril, progress and promise: 30 years of HIV/AIDS. *Medscape Medical News.* Retrieved from http://www.medscape.com/viewarticle/743927.

Panel on Treatment of HIV-Infected Pregnant Women and Prevention of Perinatal Transmission. (2010). Recommendations for use of antiretroviral drugs in pregnant HIV-1-infected women for maternal health and interventions to reduce perinatal HIV transmission in the United States. Retrieved from http://aidsinfo.nih.gov/contentfiles/PerinatalGL.pdf.

Panel on Antiretroviral Guidelines for Adults and Adolescents. (2011). Guidelines for the use of antiretroviral agents in HIV-1-infected adults and adolescents. *U.S. Department of Health and Human Services.* Retrieved from http://aidsinfo.nih.gov/contentfiles/lvguidelines/Adultand AdolescentGL.pdf.

Salvaggio, M. R. (2012). Herpes simplex. *Medscape Reference.* Retrieved from http://emedicine.medscape.com/article/218580-overview.

CHAPTER 28
Drugs for Neoplasia

Amaral, A. F., Cantor, K. P., Silverman, D. T. & Malats, N. (2010). Selenium and bladder cancer risk: A meta-analysis. *Cancer Epidemiology, Biomarkers & Prevention, 19*(9): 2407–2415. doi: 10.1158/1055-9965.EPI-10-0544

American Cancer Society. Cancer Facts & Figures 2013. Atlanta: American Cancer Society; 2013. Retrieved from http://www.cancer.org/acs/groups/content/@epidemiologysurveilance/documents/document/acspc-036845.pdf.

Given, B. A., Spoelstra, S. L., & Grant, M. (2011). The challenges of oral agents as antineoplastic treatments. *Seminars in Oncology Nursing, 27*(2): 93–103. doi:10.1016/j.soncn.2011.02.003

Maloney, K. W. & Kagan, S.H. (2011). Adherence and oral agents with older patients. *Seminars in Oncology Nursing, 27*(2): 154–160. doi:10.1016/j.soncn.2011.02.007Simmons, C.C. (2010). Oral chemotherapeutic drugs: Handle with care. *Nursing* 2013. *40*(7): 44–47. doi: 10.1097/01.NURSE.0000383452.55906.e7

Yarbro, C. H., Wujcik, D., & Gobel, B. H. (2011). *Cancer nursing: Principles and practice* (7th ed.). Sudbury, MA: Jones-Bartlett.

CHAPTER 29
Drugs for Respiratory Disorders

Akinbami, L. (2010). Asthma prevalence, healthcare use and mortality: United States 2003–2005 . Retrieved from http://www.cdc.gov/nchs/data/hestat/asthma03-05/asthma03-05.htm.

American Lung Association. (2010a). Trends in asthma: Morbidity and mortality. Retrieved from http://www.lungusa.org/finding-cures/our-research/trend-reports/asthma-trend-report.pdf.

American Lung Association. (2010b). Trends in COPD (chronic bronchitis and emphysema): Morbidity and mortality. Retrieved from http://www.lungusa.org/finding-cures/our-research/trend-reports/copd-trendreport.pdf.

Asthma and Allergy Foundation of America. (n.d.). Asthma facts and figures. Retrieved from http://www.aafa.org/.

Banasiak, N. (2007). Childhood asthma part one: Initial assessment, diagnosis, and education. *Journal of Pediatric Health Care, 21*(1): 44–48.

Centers for Disease Control and Prevention. (2010). Asthma. Retrieved from http://www.cdc.gov/nchs/fastats/asthma.htm.

D'Amatol, G., Perticone, M., Bucchioni, E., Salzillo1, A., D'Amato, M., & Liccardi, G. (2010). Treating moderate-to-severe allergic asthma with anti-IgE monoclonal antibody (omalizumab). An update. *European Annals of Allergy and Clinical Immunology, 42*(4): 135–140.

Hurst, J. R., & Wedzicha, J. A. (2009). Management and prevention of chronic obstructive pulmonary disease exacerbations: A state of the art review. *Biomed Central Medicine*, 7: 40. doi:10.1186/1741-7015-7-40.

Kelly-Shanovich, K., Pulvermacher, A., Sorkness, C., Bhattacharya, A., & Gustafson, B. (2007). The integration of web-based asthma education with nurse case management. *Journal of Allergy and Clinical Immunology, 119*(1): S80.

Lemanske, R. F., & Busse, W. W. (2010). The U.S. Food and Drug Administration and long-acting ß 2 agonists: The importance of striking the right balance between risks and benefits of therapy? *Journal of Allergy and Clinical Immunology, 126*(3): 449–452.

McIvor, A. R. (2011). Inhaler blues? CMAJ, 183 (4), 464. doi:10.1503/cmaj.111-2025.

National Institute of Allergy and Infectious diseases (2012). Food Allergies: Quick facts. Retrieved from http://www.niaid.nih.gov/topics/foodallergy/understanding/pages/quickfacts.aspx.

Smith, S. M., Schroeder, K., & Fahey, T. (2008). Over-the-counter medications for acute cough in children and adults in ambulatory settings. Cochrane Database of Systematic Reviews 2007, 3. Art. No.: CD001831. doi: 10.1002/14651858.CD001831.pub3

CHAPTER 30
Drugs for Gastrointestinal Disorders

Anand, B. S. (2012). Peptic Ulcer Disease Treatment and Management. Retrieved from http://emedicine.medscape.com/article/181753-treatment.

Basch, E., Prestrud, A. A., Hesketh, P. J., Kris, M. G., Feyer, P. C., Somerfield, M. R., et al. (2011). Antiemetics: American Society of Clinical Oncology clinical practice guideline update. *Journal of Clinical Oncology, 29*(31): 4189–4198.

DuPont, H. L., Ericsson, C. D., Farthing, M. J., Gorbach, S., Pickering, L. K., Rombo, L., ... & Weinke, T. (2009). Expert review of the evidence base for self-therapy of travelers' diarrhea. *Journal of Travel Medicine, 16*(3): 161–171.

Hamilton, K. (2011). Ginger and chemotherapy: A literature review [online]. *Shadows: The New Zealand Journal of Medical Radiation Technology, 54*(2): 23–28.

Herrstedt, J. (2008). Antiemetics: An update and the MASCC guidelines applied to clinical practice. *Nature Clinical Practice Oncology, 5*(1): 32–43.

Leontiadis, G. I., Sharma, V. K., & Howden, C. W. (2010). Proton pump inhibitor treatment for acute peptic ulcer bleeding. The Cochrane Library.

Makic, M. B. F. (2011). Management of Nausea, Vomiting, and Diarrhea During Critical Illness. *AACN Advanced Critical Care, 22*(3): 265–274.

Malfertheiner, P., Chan, F. K., & McColl, K. E. (2009). Peptic ulcer disease. *The Lancet, 374*(9699): 1449–1461.

Spiller, R. (2008). Review article: Probiotics and prebiotics in irritable bowel syndrome. *Alimentary Pharmacology and Therapeutics, 28*(4): 385–396.

Talley, N. J., Abreu, M. T., Achkar, J. P., Bernstein, C. N., Dubinsky, M. C., Hanauer, S. B., Kane, S.V., Sandborn, W. J., Ullman, T. A., & Moayyedi, P. (2011). An evidence-based systematic review on medical therapies for inflammatory bowel disease.*The American Journal of Gastroenterology 106*: S2–S25. doi:10.1038/ajg.2011.58

CHAPTER 31
Vitamins, Minerals, and Nutritional Supplements

Dawodu, S. T. (2011). Nutritional management in the rehabilitation setting. Retrieved from http://emedicine.medscape.com/article/318180-overview#a1.

Hitt, E., & Barclay, L. (2011). Updated USDA dietary guidelines released. Retrieved from http://www.medscape.org/viewarticle/736605.

Howes, R. M. (2011). Mythology of antioxidant vitamins? *Journal of Evidence-Based Complementary and Alternative Medicine, 16* (2): 149–159. doi:10.1177/15332101.10392995

Rollins, C. J. (2010). Drug–nutrient interactions in patients receiving enteral nutrition. In J. I. Boullata & V. T. Armenti (Eds.), *Handbook of drug–nutrient interactions*. New York, NY: Humana Press.

Soni, M. G., Thurmond, T. S., Miller, E. R., Spriggs, T., Bendich, A., & Omaye, S. T. (2010). Safety of vitamins and minerals: Controversies and perspective. *Toxicology Sciences, 118* (2): 348–355. doi:10.1093/toxsci/kfq293

Tucker, S., & Dauffenbach, V. (2011). *Nutrition and diet therapy*. Upper Saddle River, NJ: Pearson Education.

U.S. Department of Agriculture, Food and Nutrition Information Center. (2013). Dietary reference intakes. Retrieved from http://fnic.nal.usda.gov/dietary-guidance/dietary-reference-intakes/dri-tables.

U.S. Department of Agriculture and United States Department of Health and Human Services. (2010, December). *Dietary guidelines for Americans 2010* (7th ed.). Retrieved from http://www.cnpp.usda.gov/publications/dietaryguidelines/2010/policydoc/policydoc.pdf.

Williams, N. T. (2008). Medication administration through enteral feeding tubes. *American Journal of Health-System Pharmacists, 65*(24): 2347–2357. doi:10.2146/ajhp080155

CHAPTER 32
Drugs for Endocrine Disorders

Adler, G. K. (2011). Cushing syndrome. *Medscape Reference*. Retrieved from http://emedicine.medscape.com/article/117365-overview.

Brent, G. A., & Koenig, R. J. (2011). Thyroid and antithyroid drugs. In L. L. Brunton, B. A. Chabner, & B. C. Knollman (Eds.), *The pharmacological basis of therapeutics* (12th ed., pp. 1129–1162). New York, NY: McGraw-Hill.

Chernausek, S. D. (2010). Growth and development: How safe is growth hormone therapy for children? *Nature Reviews Endocrinology, 6*(5): 251–253. doi:10.1038/nrendo.2010.43

Colbert, J. B., Ankney, J., & Lee, K. T. (2011). *Anatomy and physiology for health professionals: An interactive journey* (2nd ed.). Upper Saddle River, NJ: Pearson Education.

Cooperman, M. (2011). Diabetes insipidus. *Medscape Reference*. Retrieved from http://emedicine.medscape.com/article/117648-overview.

Marieb, E. N., & Hoehn, K. (2013). *Human anatomy and physiology* (9th ed.). San Francisco, CA: Benjamin Cummings.

Simmons, S. (2010). A delicate balance: Detecting thyroid disease. *Nursing, 40*(7): 22–29. doi:10.1097/01.NURSE.0000383445.23626.82

Weetman, A. (2010). Current drug management of hypo- and hyperthyroidism. *Prescriber, 21*(21), 23–37. doi:10.1002/psb.688

CHAPTER 33
Drugs for Diabetes Mellitus

American Diabetes Association. (2011a). Standards of medical care in diabetes—2011. *Diabetes Care, 34*(Suppl. 1): S11–S60. doi:10.2337/dc11-S011

Centers for Disease Control and Prevention. (2011). *2011 Diabetes fact sheet*. Retrieved from http://www.cdc.gov/diabetes/pubs/estimates11.htm#8.

International Diabetes Federation (2008). The challenge to movers and shakers: Broad strategies to prevent obesity and diabetes. Retrieved from http://www.idf.org.

Meetoo, D., & Allen, G. (2010). Understanding diabetes mellitus and its management: An overview. *Nurse Prescribing, 8*(7): 320–326.

National Diabetes Information Clearinghouse. (2009). *Complementary and alternative medical therapies for diabetes.* Retrieved from http://diabetes.niddk.nih.gov/dm/pubs/alternativetherapies.

Powers, A. C., & D'Alessio, D. (2011). Endocrine pancreas and pharmacotherapy of diabetes mellitus and hypoglycemia. In L. L. Brunton, B. A. Chabner, & B. C. Knollman (Eds.), *The pharmacological basis of therapeutics* (12th ed., pp. 1237–1274). New York, NY: McGraw-Hill.

Phung, O. J., Sood, N. A., Sill, B. E., & Coleman, C. I. (2011). Oral anti-diabetic drugs for the prevention of type 2 diabetes. *Diabetic Medicine, 28*: 948–964. doi:10.1111/j.1464-5491.2011.03303.x

Rotenstein, L. S., Shivers, J. P., Yarchoan M. Close, J., & Close, K. L. (2012). The ideal diabetes therapy: What will it look like? How close are we? *Clinical Diabetes, 30*(option 2): 44–53. doi:10.2337/diaclin.30.2.44

CHAPTER 34
Drugs for Disorders and Conditions of the Reproductive System

Corona, G., Mondaini, N., Ungar, A., Razzoli, E., Rossi, A., & Fusco, F. (2011). Phosphodiesterase type 5 (PDE5) inhibitors in erectile dysfunction: The proper drug for the proper patient. *Journal of Sexual Medicine, 8:* 3418–3432. doi:10.1111/j.1743-6109.2011.02473.x

Estephan, A. (2010). *Dysfunctional uterine bleeding.* Retrieved from http://emedicine.medscape.com/article/795587-overview#a0104.

Freeman, S., & Schulman, L. P. (2010). Considerations for the use of progestin-only contraceptives. *Journal of the American Academy of Nurse Practitioners, 22*(2): 81–91. doi:10.1111/j.1745-7599.2009.00473.x

Kring, D. (2012). Benign prostatic hyperplasia. *Nursing 2012, 42*(5): 37. doi: 10.1097/01.NURSE.0000413610.36683.b3

Levin, E. R., & Hammes, S. R. (2011). Estrogens and progestins. In L. L. Brunton, B. A. Chabner, & B. C. Knollman (Eds.),*The pharmacological basis of therapeutics* (12th ed., pp. 1163–1194). New York, NY: McGraw-Hill.

Mao, A. J., & Anastasi, J. K. (2010). Diagnosis and management of endometriosis: The role of the advanced practice nurse in primary care. *Journal of the American Academy of Nurse Practitioners, 22*(2): 109–116. doi:10.1111/j.1745-7599.2009.00475.x

National Heart, Lung and Blood Institute. (2010). *Women's health initiative.* Retrieved from http://www.nhlbi.nih.gov/whi.

Porche, D. J., & Jeanfreau, S. G. (2010). Testosterone deficiency. Common in midlife and beyond. *Advanced Nurse Practitioner, 18*(6): 16.

Schimmer, B. P., & Parker, K. L. (2011). Contraception and the pharmacotherapy of obstetrical and gynecological disorders. In L. L. Brunton, B. A. Chabner, & B. C. Knollman (Eds.), *The pharmacological basis of therapeutics* (12th ed., pp. 1833–1852). New York, NY: McGraw-Hill.

Schreiber, C. A., Pentlicky, S., & Barnhart, K. (2010). *Female reproductive endocrinology, Chapter 8: Contraception.* Retrieved from http://www.endotext.org/female/female8/index.html.

Taylor, H. S., & Manson, J. E. (2011). Update in hormone therapy use in menopause. *Journal of Clinical Endocrinology and Metabolism, 96*(2): 255–264. doi:10.1210/jc.2010-0536

CHAPTER 35
Drugs for Bone and Joint Disorders

Allaat, C. F., & Huizinga, T. (2011). Treatment strategies in recent onset rheumatoid arthritis. *Current Opinion in Rheumatology, 23*(3): 241–244. doi:10.1097/BOR.0b013e3283454111

Buch, M. H., & Emery, P. (2011). New therapies in the management of rheumatoid arthritis. *Current Opinion in Rheumatology, 23*(3): 245–251.

Burke, A., Smyth, E. M., & Fitzgerald, G. A. (2006). Analgesic-antipyretic agents: Pharmacotherapy of gout. In L. L. Brunton, J. S. Lazo, & K. L. Parker (Eds.), *The pharmacological basis of therapeutics* (11th ed., pp. 671–716). New York: McGraw-Hill.

Committee to Review Dietary Reference Intakes for Vitamin D and Calcium, Food and Nutrition Board, Institute of Medicine. (2010). *Dietary reference intakes for calcium and vitamin D.* Washington, DC: National Academy Press.

Friedman, P. A. (2006). Agents affecting mineral ion homeostasis and bone turnover. In L. L. Brunton, J. S. Lazo, & K. L. Parker (Eds.), *The pharmacological basis of therapeutics* (11th ed., pp. 1647–1677). New York: McGraw-Hill.

Jacobs-Kosmin, D. (2011). *Osteoporosis.* Retrieved from http://emedicine.medscape.com/article/330598-overview.

National Osteoporosis Foundation. (2011). *About osteoporosis: Bone health basics.* Retrieved from http://www.nof.org/aboutosteoporosis/bonebasics/whybonehealth.

CHAPTER 36
Drugs for Skin Disorders

American Academy of Dermatology. (2011). *What is psoriasis?* Retrieved from http://www.skincarephysicians.com/psoriasisnet/whatis.html.

Edelstein, J. A. (2011). Atopic dermatitis in emergency medicine. Retrieved from http://emedicine.medscape.com/article/762045-overview#a0199.

Fulton, Jr., J. (2011). Acne vulgaris. Retrieved from http://emedicine.medscape.com/article/1069804-overview#a0101.

Guenther, L. (2012). Pediculosis (lice). Retrieved from http://emedicine.medscape.com/article/225013-overview#a0156.

Hall, B. J., & Hall, J. C. (2010). *Sauer's manual of skin diseases* (10th ed.). Philadelphia, PA: Lippincott, Williams & Wilkins.

Ingram, J. R., Gridlay, D., & Williams, H. C. (2009). Management of acne vulgaris: An evidence-based update. *Clinical and Experimental Dermatology, 35*(4): 351–354. doi:10.1111/j.1365-2230.2009.03683.x

Laws, P. M., & Young, H. S. (2010). Update of the management of chronic psoriasis: New approaches and emerging treatment options.*Clinical, Cosmetic and Investigational Dermatology, 3*: 25–37.

Meffert, J. (2012). Psoriasis. Retrieved from http://emedicine.medscape.com/article/1943419-overview.

Roebuck, H. (2011). Treatment options for rosacea with concomitant conditions. *Nurse Practitioner, 36*(2): 24–31. doi:10.1097/01.NPR.0000392794.17007

CHAPTER 37
Drugs for Eye and Ear Disorders

Clark, M. P. A., Pangilinan, L., Wang, A., Doyle, P., & Westerberg, B. D. (2010). The shelf life of antimicrobial ear drops.*Laryngoscope, 120*(3): 565–569. doi:10.1002/lary.20766

Glaucoma Research Foundation. (2011). *Are you at risk for glaucoma?* Retrieved from http://www.glaucoma.org/glaucoma/are-you-at-risk-for-glaucoma.php.

National Glaucoma Research. (2012). *Glaucoma statistics.* Retrieved from http://www.ahaf.org/glaucoma/about/understanding/facts.html.

Oron, Y., Zwecker-Lazar, I., Levy, D., Kreitler, S., & Roth Y. (2010). Cerumen removal: Comparison of cerumenolytic agents and effect on cognition among the elderly. *Archives of Gerontology and Geriatrics, 52*(2): 228–232. doi:10.1016/j.archger.2010.03.025

Sharts-Hopko, N., & Glynn-Milley, C. (2009). Primary open-angle glaucoma. *American Journal of Nursing, 109*(2): 40–47.

Chapter 1

Answers to NCLEX-PN® Questions

1. 4
2. 3
3. 1
4. 1, 2, and 4
5. 2
6. 2
7. 2
8. 4
9. 4
10. 1–3

Chapter 2

Answers to NCLEX-PN® Questions

1. 1
2. 2
3. 4
4. 4
5. 4
6. 1, 3, and 4
7. 2
8. 2
9. 3
10. 3

Chapter 3

Answers to NCLEX-PN® Questions

1. 3
2. 2
3. 1
4. 3
5. 1
6. 1
7. 1–4
8. 4
9. 4
10. 1

Chapter 4

Answers to NCLEX-PN® Questions

1. 3
2. 2
3. 3 and 4
4. 3
5. 2
6. 1–3
7. 2
8. 3
9. 1, 2, and 4
10. 3

Chapter 5

Answers to NCLEX-PN® Questions

1. 1
2. 3
3. 2

4. 1, 3, and 4
5. 3
6. 3
7. 4
8. 3
9. 2
10. 2

Chapter 6

Answers to NCLEX-PN® Questions

1. 1–3
2. 2
3. 2
4. 1
5. 3
6. 2
7. 2
8. 4
9. 3
10. 4

Chapter 7

Answers to NCLEX-PN® Questions

1. 3
2. 2
3. 4
4. 1
5. 2
6. 2
7. 3
8. 1
9. 3
10. 2

Chapter 8

Answers to NCLEX-PN® Questions

1. 4
2. 2
3. 4
4. 3
5. 1 and 2
6. 2
7. 3
8. 3
9. 4
10. 3

Answers to Case Study Questions

1. 3
2. 2–4
3. 4
4. 1–3

Chapter 9

Answers to NCLEX-PN® Questions

1. 4
2. 2

3. 3
4. 3
5. 2
6. 4
7. 1, 2, and 4
8. 2
9. 1
10. 1

Answers to Case Study Questions

1. 4
2. 4

Chapter 10

Answers to NCLEX-PN® Questions

1. 4
2. 3
3. 4
4. 1
5. 1
6. 2
7. 2
8. 3
9. 2 and 3
10. 3

Answers to Case Study Questions

1. 4
2. 2
3. 3
4. 1 and 3

Chapter 11

Answers to NCLEX-PN® Questions

1. 2
2. 1–4
3. 3
4. 3
5. 4
6. 1
7. 2
8. 3
9. 2
10. 3

Answers to Case Study Questions

1. 3
2. 1–4
3. 2
4. 3

Chapter 12

Answers to NCLEX-PN® Questions

1. 4
2. 2 and 3
3. 3

4. 3
5. 2
6. 2
7. 3
8. 1
9. 1–3
10. 3

Answers to Case Study Questions

1. 2
2. 1 and 4
3. 2
4. 3

Chapter 13

Answers to NCLEX-PN® Questions

1. 4
2. 3
3. 4
4. 1
5. 2
6. 3
7. 1, 2, and 4
8. 4
9. 3
10. 1

Answers to Case Study Questions

1. 3
2. 3
3. 3
4. 4

Chapter 14

Answers to NCLEX-PN® Questions

1. 4
2. 1
3. 1
4. 4
5. 3
6. 2 and 4
7. 3
8. 1
9. 1, 2, and 4
10. 4

Answers to Case Study Questions

1. 1, 2, and 4
2. 1
3. 1–3
4. 3

Chapter 15

Answers to NCLEX-PN® Questions

1. 4
2. 1, 2, and 4
3. 2

4. 3
5. 1
6. 2
7. 1
8. 2
9. 4
10. 3

Answers to Case Study Questions
1. 2
2. 3
3. 2
4. 4

Chapter 16

Answers to NCLEX-PN® Questions
1. 3
2. 3
3. 2
4. 3
5. 1
6. 1
7. 1, 2, and 4
8. 2
9. 3
10. 1–3

Answers to Case Study Questions
1. 2
2. 1
3. 3
4. 4

Chapter 17

Answers to NCLEX-PN® Questions
1. 3
2. 4
3. 2
4. 2
5. 3
6. 2
7. 2
8. 2 and 3
9. 4
10. 2

Answers to Case Study Questions
1. 3
2. 1
3. 4
4. 3

Chapter 18

Answers to NCLEX-PN® Questions
1. 3
2. 1
3. 2
4. 2
5. 4
6. 3

7. 2
8. 3
9. 4
10. 2

Answers to Case Study Questions
1. 3
2. 1
3. 1
4. 4

Chapter 19

Answers to NCLEX-PN® Questions
1. 2
2. 4
3. 4
4. 1
5. 2
6. 1, 2, and 4
7. 1
8. 1
9. 1
10. 3

Answers to Case Study Questions
1. 2
2. 2
3. 1
4. 3

Chapter 20

Answers to NCLEX-PN® Questions
1. 2
2. 1
3. 2
4. 2
5. 3
6. 1, 2, and 4
7. 4
8. 1
9. 3
10. 1–4

Answers to Case Study Questions
1. 2
2. 2
3. 1
4. 1

Chapter 21

Answers to NCLEX-PN® Questions
1. 2
2. 4
3. 2
4. 1–3
5. 1
6. 4
7. 2

8. 3
9. 2
10. 2

Answers to Case Study Questions
1. 4
2. 1
3. 4
4. 4

Chapter 22

Answers to NCLEX-PN® Questions
1. 3
2. 2
3. 2
4. 3
5. 1
6. 2
7. 1–3
8. 2
9. 2
10. 1

Answers to Case Study Questions
1. 4
2. 2
3. 3
4. 1

Chapter 23

Answers to NCLEX-PN® Questions
1. 4
2. 2
3. 3
4. 2
5. 1–4
6. 2
7. 3
8. 1
9. 4
10. 2

Answers to Case Study Questions
1. 4
2. 3
3. 2
4. 1

Chapter 24

Answers to NCLEX-PN® Questions
1. 3
2. 3
3. 3
4. 4
5. 2
6. 4
7. 1, 2, and 4
8. 4

9. 1
10. 4

Answers to Case Study Questions
1. 2
2. 1
3. 3
4. 2

Chapter 25

Answers to NCLEX-PN® Questions
1. 1, 2, and 4
2. 1 and 2
3. 4
4. 1
5. 3
6. 3
7. 2
8. 4
9. 4
10. 2

Answers to Case Study Questions
1. 4
2. 1
3. 3
4. 1, 3, and 4

Chapter 26

Answers to NCLEX-PN® Questions
1. 4
2. 2
3. 3
4. 1
5. 2
6. 1
7. 4
8. 1–4
9. 4
10. 4

Answers to Case Study Questions
1. 1
2. 2
3. 3
4. 1 and 3

Chapter 27

Answers to NCLEX-PN® Questions
1. 3
2. 4
3. 3
4. 1
5. 1 and 3
6. 4
7. 2–4
8. 2
9. 4
10. 1

Answers to Case Study Questions
1. 3
2. 3
3. 2
4. 1, 3, and 4

Chapter 28

Answers to NCLEX-PN® Questions
1. 3
2. 2
3. 1 and 4
4. 2
5. 2
6. 4
7. 2 and 4
8. 2
9. 3
10. 2

Answers to Case Study Questions
1. 3
2. 2
3. 2
4. 1

Chapter 29

Answers to NCLEX-PN® Questions
1. 1
2. 2
3. 1–3
4. 2
5. 2
6. 2
7. 1
8. 3
9. 2
10. 1

Answers to Case Study Questions
1. 4
2. 3
3. 1
4. 3

Chapter 30

Answers to NCLEX-PN® Questions
1. 3
2. 1 and 4

3. 1
4. 2
5. 1
6. 2
7. 2
8. 1
9. 1 and 2
10. 1

Answers to Case Study Questions
1. 1
2. 2 and 3
3. 1 and 2
4. 1

Chapter 31

Answers to NCLEX-PN® Questions
1. 3
2. 4
3. 1
4. 2
5. 3
6. 4
7. 2
8. 1–4
9. 3
10. 3

Answers to Case Study Questions
1. 2
2. 4
3. 1–4
4. 3

Chapter 32

Answers to NCLEX-PN® Questions
1. 1
2. 4
3. 3
4. 2
5. 2
6. 1 and 2
7. 3
8. 4
9. 1
10. 2 and 3

Answers to Case Study Questions
1. 3 and 4
2. 3

3. 3
4. 4

Chapter 33

Answers to NCLEX-PN® Questions
1. 1–3
2. 3
3. 2
4. 4
5. 3
6. 1
7. 2
8. 1–3
9. 4
10. 4

Answers to Case Study Questions
1. 1 and 2
2. 1, 2, and 4
3. 2–4
4. 1

Chapter 34

Answers to NCLEX-PN® Questions
1. 2
2. 1
3. 3
4. 2
5. 1–3
6. 2
7. 3
8. 4
9. 4
10. 4

Answers to Case Study Questions
1. 3
2. 4
3. 1 and 3
4. 2 and 4

Chapter 35

Answers to NCLEX-PN® Questions
1. 2
2. 4
3. 1
4. 3
5. 3
6. 1

7. 3
8. 3
9. 1 and 4
10. 4

Answers to Case Study Questions
1. 4
2. 1–4
3. 3
4. 4

Chapter 36

Answers to NCLEX-PN® Questions
1. 2
2. 4
3. 4
4. 1
5. 2
6. 1, 2, and 4
7. 2
8. 2
9. 1
10. 3

Answers to Case Study Questions
1. 2
2. 4
3. 2
4. 2–4

Chapter 37

Answers to NCLEX-PN® Questions
1. 2
2. 3
3. 1
4. 3
5. 1
6. 3
7. 1–3
8. 1
9. 3
10. 1

Answers to Case Study Questions
1. 3
2. 1
3. 1 and 3
4. 3

NOTE: The complete rationales and answers are located on the textbook's website.

APPENDIX C: Calculating Dosages

I. CALCULATING DOSAGE USING RATIOS AND PROPORTIONS

A. A *ratio* is used to express a relationship between two or more quantities. Ratios may be written using the following notations.

1:10 means 1 part of drug A to 10 parts of solution/solvent.

In drug calculations, ratios are usually expressed as a fraction:

$$\frac{1 \text{ part drug A}}{10 \text{ parts solution}} = \frac{1}{10}$$

A *proportion* shows the relationship between two ratios. It is a simple and effective means for calculating certain types of doses.

$$\frac{\text{Dose on hand}}{\text{Quantity on hand}} = \frac{\text{Desired dose}}{\text{Quantity desired } (X)}$$

Using cross-multiplication, we can write the same formula as follows:

$$\text{Quantity desired } (X) = \frac{\text{Desired dose} \times \text{Quantity on hand}}{\text{Dose on hand}}$$

Example 1: The healthcare provider orders erythromycin 500 mg. It is supplied in a liquid form containing 250 mg in 5 mL. How much drug should the nurse administer?

To calculate the dosage, use the formula:

$$\frac{\text{Dose on hand (250 mg)}}{\text{Quantity on hand (5 mL)}} = \frac{\text{Desired dose (500 mg)}}{\text{Quantity desired } (X)}$$

Then, cross-multiply:

$$250 \text{ mg} \times X = 5 \text{ mL} \times 500 \text{ mg}$$

Therefore, the dose to be administered is 10 mL.

B. The same proportion method can be used to solve solid dosage calculations.

Example 2: The healthcare provider orders methotrexate 20 mg/day. The methotrexate is available in 2.5-mg tablets. How many tablets should the nurse administer each day?

$$\frac{\text{Dose on hand (2.5 mg)}}{1 \text{ tablet}} = \frac{\text{Desired dose (20 mg)}}{\text{Quantity desired } (X \text{ tablets})}$$

Cross-multiplication gives:

$$2.5 \text{ mg } X = 20 \text{ mg} \times 1 \text{ tablet}$$

Therefore, the nurse should administer 8 tablets daily.

II. CALCULATING DOSAGE BY WEIGHT

Doses for pediatric patients are often calculated by using body weight. The nurse must use caution to convert between pounds and kilograms, as necessary (see Table 3.2 in Chapter 3, page 25). Use the formula:

Body weight (kg) × amount mg/kg = X mg of drug

Example 3: The healthcare provider orders 10 mg/kg of methsuximide for a client who weighs 90 kg. How much should be administered?

The patient should receive 900 mg of methsuximide.

Example 4: The healthcare provider orders 5 mg/kg/day of amiodarone. The patient weighs 110 pounds. How much of the drug should be administered daily?

Step 1: Convert pounds to kilograms.

$$110 \text{ lb} \times 1 \text{ kg}/2.2 \text{ lb} = 50 \text{ kg}$$

Step 2: Perform the drug calculation.

$$50 \text{ kg (body weight)} \times 5 \text{ mg/kg} = 250 \text{ mg}$$

The patient should receive 250 mg of amiodarone per day.

III. CALCULATING DOSAGE BY BODY SURFACE AREA

Many antineoplastic drugs and most pediatric doses are calculated using body surface area (BSA).

The formula for BSA in metric units is:

$$\text{BSA} = \sqrt{\frac{\text{weight (kg)} \times \text{height (cm)}}{3600}}$$

The formula for BSA in household units is

$$\text{BSA} = \sqrt{\frac{\text{weight (lb)} \times \text{height (inches)}}{3131}}$$

Example 5: The healthcare provider orders 10 mg/m² of an antibiotic for a child who is 2 feet tall and weighs 30 lb. How many milligrams should be administered?

Step 1: Calculate the BSA of the child.

$$\text{BSA} = \sqrt{\frac{30 \times 24}{3131}}$$

$$\text{BSA} = \sqrt{\frac{720}{3131}}$$

$$\text{BSA} = \sqrt{0.230} = 0.48 \text{ m}^2$$

Step 2: Calculate the drug amount.

$$10 \text{ mg/m}^2 \times 0.48 \text{ m}^2$$

The nurse should administer 4.8 mg of the antibiotic to the child.

IV. CALCULATING IV INFUSION RATES

Intravenous fluids are administered over time in units of mL/min or gtt/min (gtt = drops). The basic equation for IV drug calculations is as follows:

$$\frac{\text{mL of solution} \times \text{gtt/mL}}{\text{h of administration} \times 60 \text{ min/h}} = \frac{\text{gtt}}{\text{min}}$$

Example 6: The healthcare provider orders 1,000 mL of 5% normal saline to infuse over 6 hours. What is the flow rate?

$$\frac{1,000 \text{ mL} \times 10 \text{ gtt/mL}}{6 \text{ h} \times 60 \text{ min/h}} = \frac{28 \text{ gtt}}{\text{min}}$$

Other IV conversion formulas you may use include the following:

$$\text{mcg/kg/h} \rightarrow \text{mL/h}$$

$$\text{kg} \times \frac{\text{mcg/kg}}{\text{h}} \times \frac{\text{mg}}{1,000 \text{ mcg}} \times \frac{\text{mL}}{\text{mg}} = \frac{\text{mL}}{\text{h}}$$

$$\text{mcg/m}^2/\text{h} \rightarrow \text{mL/h}$$

$$\text{m}^2 \times \frac{\text{mcg/m}^2}{\text{h}} \times \frac{\text{mg}}{1,000 \text{ mcg}} \times \frac{\text{mL}}{\text{mg}} = \frac{\text{mL}}{\text{h}}$$

$$\text{mcg/kg/min} \rightarrow \text{gtt/min}$$

$$\text{kg} \times \frac{\text{mcg/kg}}{\text{min}} \times \frac{\text{mg}}{1,000 \text{ mcg}} \times \frac{\text{mL}}{\text{mg}} \times \frac{10 \text{ gtt}}{\text{mL}} = \frac{\text{gtt}}{\text{min}}$$

INDEX

Indexing style: Prototype drugs appear in **bold face**. Information in tables is denoted with a "*t*" after the page number. Information in figures is denoted with an "*f*" after the page number.

5-FU. *See* fluorouracil
5-HT (serotonin), 128
5-hydroxytryptamine (5-HT), 211
6-MP. *See* mercaptopurine

A

abacavir, 419*t*
abatacept, 576*t*
abciximab, 350*f*, 355*t*
Abilify. *See* aripiprazole
abiraterone, 444*t*
absence seizures, 183. *See also* petit mal
  seizures; seizure(s)
    succinimides treating, 191, 192*t*
absorption, 42*f*, 43
Abstral. *See* fentanyl
acamprosate calcium, 76
acarbose, 535*t*
Accupril. *See* quinapril
Accutane. *See* isotretinoin
ACE (angiotensin-converting enzyme), 274
ACE inhibitors. *See* angiotensin-converting
  enzyme (ACE) inhibitors
acebutolol, 100*t*
    clinical uses, 100
      angina, 306*t*
      dysrhythmias, 339*t*
      hypertension, 281*t*
    route and adult dose, 281*t*, 306*t*
Aceon. *See* perindopril
acetaminophen
    actions, 369*t*
    adverse effects, 369*t*
    black box warning, 369*t*
    clinical uses, 369*t*
      fever, 209*t*, 210
    Drug Prototype, 369*t*
    interactions, 369*t*
    route and adult dose, 209*t*
acetazolamide, 256, 257*t*, 603*t*
acetic acid and hydrocortisone, 607*t*
acetylcholine (Ach), 88, 160, 164
acetylcholinesterase (AchE), 165
acetylcholinesterase inhibitors
    adverse effects, 165
    for Alzheimer's disease, 164, 165*t*
    drugs classified as, 165*t*
acetylcysteine, 465
Acetylsalicylic acid. *See* **aspirin**
acid-base imbalances, 260, 260*f*, 260*t*
acidosis, 260, 260*f*, 260*t*
Aclovate. *See* alclometasone dipropionate
acne, 589–590, 590*t*
Acova. *See* argatroban
acquired resistance, 392, 392*f*

acrivastine, 460*t*
acromegaly, 516. *See also* growth hormone
  (GH)
Actemra. *See* tocilizumab
ACTH (adrenocorticotropic hormone), 513*f*,
  520, 521, 521*f*, 522
Acticin. *See* permethrin
Actifed Cold and Allergy, 461*t*
action potential, 189, 333
Actiq. *See* fentanyl
Activase. *See* **alteplase**
activated partial thromboplastin time
  (aPTT), 352
active immunity, 377, 378*f*
Activella. *See* ethinyl estradiol with norethindrone acetate
Actonel. *See* risedronate
Actos. *See* pioglitazone
Actron. *See* ketoprofen
Acuprin. *See* **aspirin**
acute dystonias, 148
acute glaucoma, 600*f*, 601. *See also* glaucoma
acute gouty arthritis, 577
acute promyelocytic leukemia (APL), 591*t*
acyclovir, 17*t*
    Drug Prototype, 425*t*
    route and adult dose, 424*t*
Adalat. *See* **nifedipine**
Adalat CC. *See* **nifedipine**
adalimumab, 576*t*
adapalene, 590*t*
adaptive body defenses, 375
ADD (attention deficit disorder), 78, 137
addiction, 16, 71. *See also* substance abuse
    agent or drug factors, 71
    drug, 80–81
    environmental factors, 71
    to opioids, 75
    user factors, 71
Addison's disease, 521
adefovir, 425
Adenocard. *See* adenosine
adenohypophysis. *See* anterior pituitary
adenoma(s), 432
Adenoscan. *See* adenosine
adenosine, 341*t*, 342
adenosine diphosphate (ADP) receptor
  blockers, 354, 355*t*
Aδ fibers, 199. *See also* sensory neurons
ADH (antidiuretic hormone; vasopressin), 270,
  514–515, 514*t*, 515*t*
ADHD (attention deficit hyperactivity disorder). *See* attention deficit hyperactivity
  disorder (ADHD)
adjuvant analgesics, 201

adjuvant chemotherapy, 433
ado-trastuzumab, 445*t*
adrenal atrophy, 521
adrenal disorders, 520–522
adrenal gland(s), 271*f*
Adrenalin. *See* **epinephrine**
adrenergic, 90, 97
adrenergic blockers (sympatholytics), 91
    actions, 99, 291*f*
    adverse effects, 282
    clinical uses, 99
      hypertension, 281–282, 281*t*
    drugs classified as, 91, 281*t*
    Nursing Process Focus, 101*t*
    Patients Need to Know, 102*t*
    prototypes of, 99
adrenergic drugs, 91, 97, 97*t*
    fight-or-flight symptoms of, 91
adrenocortical insufficiency, 521–522
adrenocorticotropic hormone (ACTH), 513*f*,
  520, 521, 521*f*, 522
adult-onset diabetes. *See* type 2 diabetes
  mellitus
Advicor, 242, 244
Advil. *See* **ibuprofen**
AEB (as evidenced by), 54
aerosol, 456
African Americans, antihypertension therapy
  in, 273
Afrin. *See* oxymetazoline
afterload, 289, 304
Aggrastat. *See* tirofiban
agonist(s), 47
agoraphobia, 107*t*
Agrylin. *See* anagrelide
akathisia, 147*t*, 148
Akineton. *See* biperiden
Albalon. *See* naphazoline
albendazole, 426*t*, 427
albuterol, 97*t*
    clinical uses, 97
      for asthma, 468*t*
      shock, 328
Alcaine. *See* proparacaine
alclometasone dipropionate, 592*t*
alcohol
    chronic consumption of, 75
    as CNS depressant, 75
    cross-tolerance, 73
    metabolism, 75
    overdose of, 75
    physical dependence and, 72
    physiological and psychological effects
      of, 73*t*
    withdrawal syndrome, 75

alcohol abuse, 499
Alcoholics Anonymous, 72, 75
"alcoholic" smell, 75
alcohol intoxication, 75
alcoholism, 75
alcohol sensitivity, 75
alcohol withdrawal syndrome, 75
Aldactone. *See* **spironolactone**
aldesleukin, 379, 379*t*
Aldomet. *See* methyldopa
aldosterone, 274, 520
alemtuzumab, 445*t*
alendronate
       Drug Prototype, 572*t*
       for osteoporosis, 571*t*
Aler-Dryl. *See* **diphenhydramine**
Aleve. *See* **naproxen sodium**
Alfenta. *See* alfentanil
alfentanil, 204, 226*t*, 228*t*
alfuzosin, 100*t*, 558*t*
alimentary canal, 478
alkaloids. *See* ergot alkaloids; vinca alkaloids
alkalosis, 260, 260*f*, 260*t*
alkylating agents, 437, 437*t*, 438*f*
alkylation, 435
Allerest. *See* naphazoline
Allergia-C. *See* **diphenhydramine**
allergic reaction, 22
       anaphylaxis and, 22
       signs of, 22
allergic rhinitis, 458, 459*f*
       H₁-receptor antagonists for. *See*
            H₁-receptor antagonists
       intranasal corticosteroids for, 462, 463*t*
allergy(ies), 459*t*
allopurinol
       Drug Prototype, 578*t*
       for gout and gouty arthritis, 577, 577*t*
almotriptan, 212*t*
aloe, 341*t*
aloe vera, 608*t*
       for skin conditions, 592*t*
alopecia, 436
Alora. *See* estradiol
alpha₂-adrenergic drugs, for glaucoma, 603, 603*t*
alpha-adrenergic blockers. *See* alpha blockers
alpha (α) blockers, 99, 281*t*. *See also*
       adrenergic blockers
Alphagan. *See* brimonidine tartrate
alpha (α) receptors, 90, 91*t*
alprazolam, 70, 74, 114*t*
Altace. *See* ramipril
alteplase
       actions, 357*t*
       adverse effects, 357*t*
       clinical uses, 357*t*
       Drug Prototype, 357*t*
       interactions, 357*t*
       route and adult dose, 312*t*
alternate healthcare systems, 60*t*
Altoprev. *See* lovastatin
altretamine, 445*t*
aluminum hydroxide, 482*t*
alveoli, 455
Alzheimer's disease, 164
       brain changes in, 164

causes, 164
characteristics, 164
drugs used for, 165*t*
ginkgo biloba use in, 167*t*
pharmacotherapy, 92, 165
symptoms, 164
Amanita muscaria, 90
amantadine
       clinical uses
            influenza, 424
            parkinsonism, 161*t*
       multiple sclerosis, 168*t*, 169
       route and adult dose, 424*t*
Amaryl. *See* glimepiride
ambenonium, 92*t*
Ambien. *See* **zolpidem**
amcinonide, 592*t*
amebiasis, 426
amenorrhea, 550
Amerge. *See* naratriptan
Americaine. *See* **benzocaine**
American Pharmaceutical Association
       (APhA), 5, 6*f*
American Psychiatric Association, 123
Amicar. *See* **aminocaproic acid**
Amidate. *See* etomidate
amides, 220–221, 221*t*, 222
amikacin, 399*t*
amiloride, 256*t*, 274*t*
aminocaproic acid
       actions, 358*t*
       adverse effects, 358*t*
       clinical uses, 357*t*, 358*t*
       Drug Prototype, 358*t*
       interactions, 358*t*
       route and adult dose, 357*t*
aminoglycosides, 399–400, 399*t*
aminopenicillins, 393
aminophylline, 468*t*
amiodarone
       actions, 341*t*
       adverse effects, 341*t*
       black box warning, 341*t*
       clinical uses, 341*t*
       Drug Prototype, 341*t*
       interactions, 341*t*
       route and adult dose, 340*t*
amitriptyline, 112*t*, 126*t*, 201
       clinical uses
            depression, 112, 126*t*
            migraine prophylaxis, 213, 213*t*
amitryptiline, 17*t*
amlodipine, 278*t*, 306*t*
amobarbital, 116*t*
       for sedation and insomnia, 116*t*
Amoeba, 389*f*
amoxapine, 126*t*
amoxicillin, 17*t*, 393, 394*t*
Amoxil. *See* amoxicillin
amphetamines, 70, 78, 202
       high doses of, 78
       physiological and psychological effects
            of, 73*t*
       withdrawal syndrome for, 78
amphotericin B, 414
       Drug Prototype, 416*t*
       interactions

with furosemide, 254*t*
with hydrochlorothiazide, 255*t*
with prednisone, 369*t*
route and adult dose, 415*t*
ampicillin, 393, 394*t*
Amrix. *See* **cyclobenzaprine**
amyloid plaques, 164
amyotrophic lateral sclerosis (ALS), 158*t*
Amytal. *See* amobarbital
Anacin. *See* **aspirin**
Anadrol. *See* oxymetholone
Anadrol-50. *See* oxymetholone
Anafranil. *See* clomipramine
anagrelide, 355*t*
anakinra, 381*t*, 576*t*
analgesics, 201
       adjuvant, 201
       categories of, 201
anaphylaxis/anaphylactic shock
       diagnosis, 320
       pathophysiology, 320*t*, 364
       pharmacotherapy, 326–328
       symptoms, 327*f*
Anaprox. *See* **naproxen sodium**
anastrozole, 444*t*
Anbesol. *See* **benzocaine**
Andro 100. *See* **testosterone**
Androderm. *See* **testosterone**
Androgel. *See* **testosterone**
androgens, 554, 555*t*
Android. *See* methyltestosterone
Anectine. *See* **succinylcholine**
anemia, 436*t*, 446
       iron-deficiency, 501, 501*t*
       megaloblastic (pernicious), 499
Anestacon. *See* **lidocaine**
anesthesia, 218. *See also* general anesthesia;
       local anesthesia
angina pectoris, 302–303, 303*t*, 347*t*
       Nursing Process Focus, 308*t*
       Patients Need to Know, 315*t*
       pharmacotherapy, 304–305
            beta blockers, 307
            mechanisms of action, 305*f*
            organic nitrates, 305–306, 306*t*
            ranolazine, 305
angioedema, 409*t*
Angiomax. *See* bivalirudin
angiotensin-converting enzyme (ACE), 274
angiotensin-converting enzyme (ACE)
       inhibitors
            actions, 272*f,* 291*f,* 294
            clinical uses
                 heart failure, 292, 293*t*
                 hypertension, 275*t*
                 myocardial infarction, 313
            drugs classified as, 275*t*
            Nursing Process Focus, 276–277*t*
            Patients Need to Know, 297*t*
angiotensin II, 274, 520
angiotensin-receptor blockers (ARB)
       actions, 272*f,* 294
       clinical uses, 275*t*
       drugs classified as, 275*t*
anidulafungin, 414, 415*t*
anorexia, 480
anorexiants, 491

Ansaid. *See* flurbiprofen
Antabuse. *See* disulfiram
antacids, 485
    drugs classified as, 482*t*
    interactions
        with aspirin, 208*t*
        with ciprofloxacin, 401*t*
        with haloperidol, 149*t*
        with isoniazid, 406*t*
        with levodopa, 163*t*
antagonism, 393
antagonists (blockers), 17
Antara. *See* fenofibrate
anterior pituitary, 511. *See also* pituitary gland
anthralin, 593*t*, 594
anthrax, 401
antibiotic, 390. *See also* anti-infectives
antibody(ies), 375
anticholinergics (cholinergic blockers), 91,
    94–95, 95*t*, 227
    adverse effects, 92, 163
    clinical uses, 95*t*, 228*t*
        asthma, 468–469, 468*t*
        parkinsonism, 163, 163*t*
    drugs classified as, 91, 163*t*, 228*t*, 468*t*
    interactions
        with procainamide, 339*t*
        with TCAs, 125
    Nursing Process Focus, 96*t*
    Patients Need to Know, 102*t*
anticipatory anxiety, 111
anticoagulants, 350
    actions, 350, 350*f*
    adverse effects, 350
    clinical uses, 312–313, 347*t*, 351*t*
    drugs classified as, 351*t*
    interactions
        with alteplase, 357*t*
        with aspirin, 208*t*
        with clopidogrel, 356*t*
        with gemfibrozil, 244*t*
        with hydrochlorothiazide, 255*t*
        with methylphenidate, 137*t*
        with tamoxifen, 444*t*
    Nursing Process Focus, 353–354*t*
    oral, 352
    parenteral, 350–352
    reversal, 350
anticonvulsants, 182. *See also* antiseizure
    drugs
antidepressants, 110, 125, 126–127*t*
    atypical antidepressants, 126–127*t*, 129
    clinical uses
        anxiety and insomnia, 111, 112*t*
        depression, 126–127*t*, 126*t*–127*t*
        monoamine oxidase inhibitors (MAOIs),
            127*t*, 132
    Nursing Process Focus, 130–131*t*
    Patients Need to Know, 139*t*
    primary classes of, 125, 126*t*
    selective serotonin reuptake inhibitors
        (SSRIs), 126*t*, 128–129
    tricyclic antidepressants (TCAs), 125, 126*t*
antidiarrheals, 489*t*
antidiuretic hormone (ADH; vasopressin), 270,
    514–515, 514*t*, 515*t*
antidysrhythmics
    actions, 335–336, 336*f*
    adverse effects, 336
    classes
        adenosine, 341*t*, 342
        beta-adrenergic blockers, 339, 339*t*
        calcium channel blockers, 341–342,
            341*t*
        digoxin, 341*t*, 342
        potassium channel blockers, 340, 340*t*
    classification, 336
    Nursing Process Focus, 336–337*t*
    sodium channel blockers, 338, 338*t*
antiemetics, 489, 490*t*, 492*t*
antiepileptic drugs (AED). *See* antiseizure drugs
antifibrinolytics. *See* hemostatics
antiflatulent, 485
antifungal drugs
    Nursing Process Focus, 417*t*
    Patients Need to Know, 427*t*
    systematic, 414–416, 415*t*
    topical and oral, 416–417, 417*t*
antigen(s), 326, 374
antihelminthics, 426, 426*t*
antihistamines, 95*t*
    interactions
        with atropine, 95*t*
anti-infectives, 390
    actions, 390–391, 391*f*
    allergic reactions, 409*t*
    bacterial resistance to, 391–392, 392*f*
    classifications, 390–391
        aminoglycosides, 399–400, 399*t*
        cephalosporins, 395–397, 396*t*
        fluoroquinolones, 400–401, 400*t*
        macrolides, 398–399, 398*t*
        miscellaneous antibacterial,
            403–404, 404*t*
        tetracyclines, 397–398, 397*t*
    Nursing Process Focus, 404*t*–405*t*
    Patients Need to Know, 409*t*
    prophylactic, 392
    selection of, 393
Antilirium. *See* physostigmine
antimalarials, 426*t*
antimetabolites, 439–440, 439*t*, 440*f*
antineoplastic drugs
    adverse effects, 435–436, 436*t*
    cell cycle and, 435–436, 435*f*
    classifications
        alkylating agents, 437, 437*t*, 438*f*
        antimetabolites, 439–440, 439*t*, 440*f*
        antitumor antibiotics, 440–441, 441*t*
        hormones and hormone antagonists,
            443, 443*t*–444*t*
        plant extracts, 442–*443*, 442*t*
        taxanes, 442, 442t
        topoisomerase inhibitors, 442, 442*t*
    dosing schedules and regimens, 435–436
    Nursing Process Focus, 447*t*–448*t*
    Patients Need to Know, 449*t*
antiobesity drugs, 491
antiplatelet drugs
    actions, 350, 354
    classes, 354
    clinical uses
        coagulation disorders, 354–356, 355*t*
        myocardial infarction, 312–313
    drugs classified as, 355*t*
    interactions
        with alteplase, 357*t*
        with clopidogrel, 356*t*
antiprotozoans, 426*t*, 427*t*
antipsychotics
    atypical (second generation), 146,
        151–153, 151*t*
    conventional (first-generation), 146–151,
        146*t*, 148*t*
    dopamine system stabilizers (DSSs) or
        third generation antipsychotics, 146, 154
    Patients Need to Know, 153*t*
antipyretics, 369–370
    goal of, 370
    marketing of, 370
    Patients Need to Know, 370*t*
antiretrovirals, 420
    for HIV-AIDS, 418–422, 419*t*
    Nursing Process Focus, 422–423*t*
antiseizure drugs, 182, 185*t*
    actions, 186
    adjunctive therapy and, 185
    clinical uses
        bipolar disorder, 135, 135*t*
        seizures, 181–196
    disadvantages of, 185
    discontinuation, 184
    drugs classified as
        barbiturates, 187*t*
        benzodiazepines, 187*t*
        GABA-related drugs, 186, 187*t*, 189
        hydantoins and related drugs, 189–190*t*
        succinimides, 184*t*
    FDA warnings, 184
    interactions
        with chlorpromazine, 147*t*
        with levodopa, 163*t*
        with oral contraceptives, 182, 185,
            188*t*, 190*t*, 190*t*
    Nursing Process Focus, 192–193*t*
    in pregnancy, 185
    pregnancy category, 182
antiseptics, urinary, 403
antispasmodic drugs
    centrally acting. *See* skeletal muscle
        relaxants
    direct-acting, 174*t*
antithrombin, recombinant, 351*t*
antithymocyte globulin, 381*t*
antitubercular drugs
    dosing regimens and schedules, 406–407*t*
    drugs classified as, 407*t*
    Nursing Process Focus, 407–408*t*
    for prophylaxis, 408
antitumor antibiotics, 440–441, 441*t*
antitussives, 457*f*, 465
antiviral drugs
    clinical uses
        herpesvirus infections, 423–424, 424*t*
        HIV-AIDS, 418–422, 419*t*
        influenza, 424, 424*t*
    Patients Need to Know, 427*t*
    strategies for use of, 418
Anturane. *See* sulfinpyrazone
anxiety, 106
    in Alzheimer's disease, 164, 166

anticipatory, 111
areas of brain responsible for, 108t
insomnia and, 109–110
management, 108–109
    antidepressants for, 111–113, 112t
    benzodiazepines for, 113–114, 114t
    nonbenzodiazepine, nonbarbiturate
      agents for, 117–119, 117t
    nonpharmacologic strategies for,
      108–109
    pharmacologic strategies for, 108–109
Nursing Process Focus, 115t
panic disorder, 106
Patients Need to Know, 119t
performance, 106
phobias, 106
situational, 106
treatment of, 110–111
anxiolytics, 109. *See also* anxiety, management
Apidra. *See* insulin glulisine
apixaban, 351t, 352
APL (acute promyelocytic leukemia), 591t
apomorphine, 161, 161t
apothecary system, 25
apraclonidine, 603t
Apresazide, 255
Apresoline. *See* **hydralazine**
aPTT (activated partial thromboplastin
    time), 352
Aquatensen. *See* methyclothiazide
aqueous humor, 599
Arava. *See* leflunomide
ARB (angiotensin-receptor blockers), 272f,
    275t, 294
Arduan. *See* pipecuronium
Aredia. *See* pamidronate
arformoterol, 468t
argatroban, 351, 351t
Aricept. *See* donepezil
aripiprazole, 146, 151t, 154
Aristocort. *See* triamcinolone acetonide
Aristospan. *See* triamcinolone
Arixtra. *See* fondaparinux
Armour Thyroid. *See* thyroid dessicated
arsenic trioxide, 445t
Artane. *See* trihexyphenidyl
artemether/lumefantrine, 426t
arthritis
    description, 574
    gouty, 577, 577t
    osteoarthritis, 574, 575
    rheumatoid, 575, 576t
articaine, 221t
ASA. *See* **aspirin**
ASAP order, 24t
Ascaris, 427
asenapine, 135t, 151t
Asendin. *See* amoxapine
Aspergillus, 389f, 414t
Aspergum. *See* **aspirin**
aspirin, 15, 15t
    actions, 208t, 350f, 355, 365t
    adverse effects, 208t, 366
    clinical uses, 208t
      as antiplatelet agent, 355, 355t
      fever, 370t
      myocardial infarction, 312

Drug Prototype, 208t
vs. ibuprofen, 47
interactions, 208t
    with alteplase, 357t
    with clopidogrel, 356t
    with methotrexate, 440t
    with spironolactone, 256t
    with valproic acid, 191t
    routes and adult dose, 209t, 355t, 365t
assessment phase of nursing process,
    52–53, 52f
asthma, 465
    characteristics, 465–466, 467f
    Nursing Process Focus, 469–470t
    pharmacotherapy, 467f
      anti-inflammatory drugs, 470t, 471
      bronchodilators, 467–469, 468t
    symptoms, 466
    triggers, 466t
Astramorph PF. *See* **morphine**
astringent effect, 31
Atacand. *See* candesartan
atazanavir, 419t
atenolol
    actions, 272f, 282, 309t
    adverse effects, 309t
    black box warning, 309t
    cardioselective effects of, 99
    clinical uses, 100t, 212t, 281t, 306t, 309t
      anxiety, 111, 117, 117t
    Drug Prototype, 309t
    interactions, 309t
    route and adult dose, 212t, 281t, 306t
atherosclerosis, 235, 302–303, 303f
Ativan. *See* lorazepam
atomoxetine, 137, 138t
atonic seizures, 183. *See also* drop attacks;
    seizure(s)
atopic dermatitis, 591
atorvastatin
    actions, 240t
    adverse effects, 240t
    clinical uses, 240t
    Drug Prototype, 240t
    interactions, 240t
    route and adult dose, 239t
atovaquone/proguanil, 426t
atracurium, 176t
atrial flutter, 333t
atrial tachycardia, 333t
atrioventricular bundle, 333
atrioventricular (AV) node, 333, 334f
Atromid-S. *See* clofibrate
Atro-Pen. *See* **atropine**
atropine, 95t, 227, 228t, 606t
    actions, 95t, 163
    adverse effects, 95t, 163
    clinical uses of, 95t
    Drug Prototype, 95t
    interactions, 95t
Atrovent. *See* ipratropium
ATryn. *See* antithrombin, recombinant
attention deficit disorder (ADD), 78, 137
attention deficit hyperactivity disorder
    (ADHD), 78, 136
    causes, 136
    Fast Facts, 136t

Patients Need to Know, 139t
pharmacotherapy
    CNS stimulants, 78, 137, 138t
    non-CNS stimulants, 137, 138t
symptoms, 136
atypical antidepressants
    adverse effects, 113
    clinical uses
      anxiety, 111, 112t
      depression, 126–127t
    drugs classified as, 129
atypical antipsychotics
    adverse effects, 152
    in Alzheimer's disease, 166
    discovery of, 146
    Nursing Process Focus, 153t
aura
    migraine, 211
    seizure, 183
Auralgan. *See* benzocaine and antipyrine
autoantibodies, 575
automaticity, 333
autonomic nervous system, 87
    drugs affecting functions of, 86–104
    parasympathetic nervous system, 87
    sympathetic nervous system, 87
    two primary neurotransmitters of, 88–91
Avage. *See* tazarotene
avanafil, 556t
Avandia. *See* rosiglitazone
Avapro. *See* irbesartan
AV (atrioventricular) bundle, 333
Aventyl. *See* nortriptyline
Avita. *See* **tretinoin**
AV (atrioventricular) node, 333, 334f
Avodart. *See* dutasteride
Avonex. *See* interferon beta-1a
Axert. *See* almotriptan
axitinib, 445t
Azasan. *See* azathioprine
azathioprine, 381t, 576t
azelaic acid, 590t
azelastine, 459t, 460
Azelex. *See* azelaic acid
azilsartan, 275t
azithromycin, 398t
Azopt. *See* brinzolamide
aztreonam, 404t
Azulfidine. *See* sulfasalazine

B

bacille calmette-guérin (BCG) vaccine,
    379, 379t
Bacillus anthracis, 390t, 401
baclofen, 170, 171t, 173
bacteria
    acquired resistance to anti-infectives,
      391–392, 392f
    characteristics, 389f
    classifications, 391–392, 392f
    common disease-causing, 390t
    descriptive methods, 390t
    infections caused by, 390t
bacteriocidal, 391
bacteriostatic, 391
balanced anesthesia, 224

Balnetar. *See* coal tar
Banflex. *See* orphenadrine
barbiturates, 74, 116–117
    clinical uses, 186
        sedation and insomnia, 116–117, 117*t*
        seizures, 186
    drugs classified as, 187*t*
    interactions
        with clopidogrel, 356*t*
        with lidocaine, 222*t*
        with prednisone, 369*t*
    physiological and psychological effects
        of, 73*t*
    tolerance, 114
    withdrawal syndrome, 78, 116
baroreceptors, 270, 271*f*
baseline data, 52
basiliximab, 381*t*
Bayer. *See* **aspirin**
B cell, 375
BCG (bacille calmette-guérin) vaccine, 379
beclomethasone
    inhaled, 470*t*
    intranasal, 463*t*
behavioral insomnia, 110. *See also* short-term
    insomnia
Benadryl. *See* **diphenhydramine**
Benadryl Allergy/Cold, 461*t*
benazepril, 275*t*
bendamustine, 437*t*
bendroflumethiazide and nadolol, 254*t*
Benemid. *See* probenecid
Benicar. *See* olmesartan
Benicar HCT, 255
benign prostatic hyperplasia (BPH), 556, 557,
    557*f*, 558*t*
benign tumors, 432
Bentyl. *See* dicyclomine
benzocaine
    Drug Prototype, 589*t*
    as local anesthetic, 221*t*, 222
    for sunburn and minor skin irritation, 589
benzocaine and antipyrine, 607*t*
benzodiazepines, 113–114
    abuse of, 74–75
    actions, 113–114
    adverse effects, 1113–114
    clinical uses
        as adjunct to anesthetics, 228*t*
        anxiety and insomnia, 113–114, 114*t*
        bipolar disorder, 135
        intravenous anesthetic, 226*t*
        muscle relaxation, 170
        seizures, 186
    drugs classified as, 110, 187*t*, 226*t*, 228*t*
    interactions
        with propofol, 227*t*
    introduction of, 113
    parenteral administration, 114
    Patients Need to Know, 119*t*
    physiological and psychological effects
        of, 73*t*
benzonatate, 465
benzoyl peroxide, 590, 590*t*
benztropine
    actions, 164*t*
    adverse effects, 164*t*

    clinical uses, 95*t*, 148, 164*t*
    Drug Prototype, 164*t*
    interactions, 164*t*
        with MAOIs, 164*t*
        with phenothiazines, 164*t*
        with procainamide, 164*t*
        with quinidine, 164*t*
        with tricyclic antidepressants, 164*t*
    route and adult dose, 163*t*
bepotastine, 605
Bepreve. *See* bepotastine
bepridil, 306*t*
beta-adrenergic agonists, 407, 460*t*
beta (β) blockers, 99. *See also* adrenergic
    blockers
    actions, 272*f*, 306*t*
    adverse effects, 307
    clinical uses
        angina and myocardial infarction, 305,
            306*t*, 307, 312
        anxiety, 111, 117, 117*t*
        dysrhythmias, 339, 339*t*
        glaucoma, 603, 603*t*
        heart failure, 295*t*, 296
        hypertension, 281*t*
        migraine prophylaxis, 212*t*
    drugs classified as, 99, 281*t*, 295*t*, 339*t*
    interactions, 149*t*
        with amiodarone, 341*t*
        with digoxin, 295*t*
        with dopamine, 326*t*
        with epinephrine, 327*t*
        with haloperidol, 149*t*
        with norepinephrine, 326*t*
        with propranolol, 340*t*
    Patients Need to Know, 343*t*
Betagan. *See* levobunolol
beta-lactamase, 393
beta-lactam ring, 393
betamethasone, 368*t*, 522*t*, 592*t*
betamethasone benzoate, 592*t*
betamethasone valerate, 592*t*
Betaoptic. *See* betaxolol
Betapace. *See* sotalol
Betapace AF. *See* sotalol
beta (β) receptors, 90, 91*t*
Betaseron. *See* interferon beta-1b
betaxolol, 281*t*, 603*t*
bethanechol, 228*t*, 229
    actions, 93*t*
    adverse effects, 93*t*
    clinical uses, 92*t*
    Drug Prototype, 93*t*
    interactions, 93*t*
        with ambenonium, 93*t*
        with epinephrine, 93*t*
        with neostigmine, 93*t*
        with quinidine, 93*t*
Betimol. *See* **timolol; timolol maleate**
bevacizumab, 445*t*
Bextra. *See* valdecoxib
bicalutamide, 444*t*
BiDil, 273, 283*t*, 295*t*
bile acid-binding agents
    actions, 243*f*
    adverse effects, 242
    drugs classified as, 239*t*

    Patients Need to Know, 245*t*
bile acids, 241
bimatoprost, 602
binding, 43
bioavailability, 15–16, 43
bioequivalence, 16
biologic response modifiers, 375, 379, 379*t*
biologics, 4
    characteristics of, 4*t*
    stages of approval for, 7–9
Biologics Control Act, 5, 6*f*
biologic therapies, 60*t*
bioterrorism, 9
    anthrax, 401
Bioterrorism Act, 6*f*
biotin (vitamin B$_7$), 498*t*
biotransformation, 43
biperiden, 163*t*
biphasic OC, 546, 546*t*
bipolar disorder, 133
    characteristics of, 134
    lithium for treating, 134–135
    pharmacotherapy, 135*t*
    symptoms of, 134
bisacodyl, 487*t*
bismuth salts, 489*t*
bisoprolol, 281*t*
bisphosphonates
    for osteoporosis, 571*t*, 572
    for Paget's disease, 574
bivalirudin, 351*t*
black box warning, 6, 111, 113, 129, 133, 137,
    203*t*, 205*t*, 228*t*, 277*t*, 292*t*, 309*t*, 326*t*, 339*t*,
    340*t*, 341*t*, 352*t*, 353*t*, 356*t*, 366*t*, 369*t*, 537*t*,
    547*t*, 551*t*, 552*t*, 553*t*, 554*t*, 571*t*, 591*t*
blackheads, 589
Blastomyces dermatitidis, 414*t*
bleomycin, 441*t*
Blocadren. *See* **timolol**
blockers (antagonists), 47. *See also* adrenergic
    blockers
    alpha, 99
    beta. *See* beta (β) blockers
blood-brain barrier, 43
blood glucose level, 529, 530*f*
blood-placental barrier, 43
blood pressure. *See also* hypertension
    control of, 269–271*f*, 270*f*
    diastolic, 267
    factors affecting, 269, 269*f*
    physiology, 267, 268*f*
    systolic, 267, 268*f*
blood products, 322, 323*t*
blood-testicular barrier, 43
blood thinners. *See* anticoagulants;
    antiplatelet drugs
blood volume, 269
bone deposition, 565
bone resorption, 565
Boniva. *See* ibandronate
boosters, 376
Borrelia burgdorferi, 390*t*
Botox. *See* onabotulinumtoxin A
botulinum toxin, 173, 174*f*
Bowman's capsule, 250
BPH (benign prostatic hyperplasia), 556, 557,
    557*f*, 558*t*

bradycardia, 282
bradykinesia, 148, 159
bradykinin, 208
brainstem, 107, 108t
brand name, 14, 15–16
breakthrough bleeding, 550
breastfeeding, medication use during, 44
Brethine. *See* terbutaline
Brevibloc. *See* esmolol
Brilinta. *See* ticagrelor
brimonidine tartrate, 603t
brinzolamide, 603t
broad-spectrum antibiotic, 393
broad-spectrum penicillins, 393
bromocriptine, 161, 161t, 515t, 536t
brompheniramine, 459t
bronchi, 455
bronchioles, 455
bronchoconstriction/bronchospasm, 466
bronchodilation, 467
bronchodilators
	for asthma, 467–469, 468t
	drugs classified as, 468t
	Nursing Process Focus, 469–470t
	Patients Need to Know, 472
buccal route, 26t, 27
budesonide, 463t, 470t
Bufferin. *See* **aspirin**
bumetanide, 252, 253t, 274t, 293t
Bumex. *See* bumetanide
bundle branches, 333, 334f
bupivacaine, 221t
bupivicaine, 221t
Buprenex. *See* buprenorphine
buprenorphine, 204t, 206
bupropion, 112t
	for bipolar disorder, 135
	for depression, 126t
	for nicotine withdrawal, 72
	smoking cessation and, 129
burns, 583–584. *See also* skin disorders
BuSpar. *See* buspirone
buspirone, 117–118, 117t
busulfan, 437t
butabarbital, 116t
butamben, 222
butenafine, 415t
Butisol. *See* butabarbital
butoconazole, 415t
butorphanol, 204t
Butrans. *See* buprenorphine
Byetta. *See* exenatide

C

cabazitaxel, 442t
CABG (coronary artery bypass graft)
	surgery, 304
Caduet, 244
Cafergot. *See* ergotamine with caffeine
caffeine, 78–79, 79t
	as CNS stimulant, 79
	content of common drugs, foods, and
		beverages, 79t
	diuretic effect of, 79
	physical effects of, 79
Calan. *See* **verapamil**

calcifediol, 565
Calciferol. *See* ergocalciferol
Calcijex. *See* **calcitriol**
calcipotriene, 593t, 594
Calcite-500. *See* calcium carbonate
calcitonin
	in calcium homeostasis, 565, 566f
	for osteoporosis, 570
	for Paget's disease, 574
calcitonin nasal spray, 574
calcitonin–salmon, 571t
calcitriol, 565
	Drug Prototype, 569
	route and adult dose, 568t
	in vitamin D activation, 565, 567f
calcium, 501t, 565, 566f. *See also*
	hypocalcemia
calcium acetate, 502t, 568t
calcium carbonate, 482t, 502t, 568t
calcium carbonate with magnesium
	hydroxide, 482t
calcium channel blockers (CCB), 132
	actions, 272f, 307, 309, 341–342, 341t
	adverse effects, 309, 342
	clinical uses
		angina and myocardial infarction, 305,
			306t, 307, 309
		dysrhythmias, 341, 341t
		hypertension, 278, 278t
		migraine prophylaxis, 212t
	drugs classified as, 278t
	interactions
		with dantrolene sodium, 175t
	Nursing Process Focus, 279–280t
	Patients Need to Know, 343t
calcium chloride, 568t
calcium citrate, 502t, 568t
calcium gluconate, 502t, 568t
calcium ion channels, 335, 336f
calcium lactate, 502t, 568t
calcium metabolism, 497
calcium phosphate tribasic, 568t
calcium polycarbophil, 487t
calcium salts
	Drug Prototype, 569t
	for osteomalacia and hypocalcemia, 566,
		567–568, 568t
calcium supplements
	interactions with phenytoin, 190t
Cal-Lac. *See* calcium lactate
Cambia. *See* diclofenac
camphorated opium tincture, 489t
Campral. *See* acamprosate calcium
CAM Therapy, 60–61, 60t
	See also Guide to Special Features
canagliflozin, 535
cancer, 431
	causes, 432
	characteristics, 431–432
	chemotherapy, 433–434, 434f. *See also*
		antineoplastic drugs
	incidence, 431
	metastases, 432f
	risk reduction methods, 433
candesartan, 275t, 293t, 294
Candida, 389f
Candida albicans, 414t

cannabinoids, 76
Cannabis sativa, 76
capecitabine, 439t
Capoten. *See* captopril
capsaicin, 173t
capsid, 417
capsules, 26t, 27
	guidelines for administering, 26t
	sustained-release, 27
captopril, 275t, 293t, 313
carbachol, 602t
carbamazepine, 185t, 190t, 201
	adverse effects, 189
	for mood disorders, 135, 135t
	for seizures, 185t, 189
	for trigeminal neuralgia, 189
carbamide peroxide, 607t
carbapenems, 404
carbenicillin, 393
carbidopa, 160
	actions and uses, 163t
	adverse effects, 163t
	Drug Prototype, 163t
	interactions, 163t
Carbocaine. *See* mepivacaine
carbonic anhydrase, 256
carbonic anhydrase inhibitors
	actions, 253f
	for glaucoma, 603, 603t
carboplatin, 437t
carboprost, 553t
carcinogens, 432
Cardene. *See* nicardipine
cardiac conduction pathway, 333–335, 334f
cardiac glycosides
	actions, 291f, 294
	for heart failure, 294, 295t
	interactions
		with succinylcholine, 228t
	Patients Need to Know, 297t
cardiac output, 269
cardiogenic shock, 320, 320t. *See also* shock
cardiotonic drugs. *See* inotropic drugs
Cardizem. *See* **diltiazem**
Cardura. *See* **doxazosin**
Cardura XL. *See* doxazosin XL
carisoprodol, 171t
carmustine, 437t
carnitine, 293t
carteolol, 100t, 603t
Cartia XT. *See* **diltiazem**
Cartrol. *See* carteolol
carvedilol
	actions, 291f, 296t
	adverse effects, 296t
	clinical uses, 100t
		heart failure, 296, 296t
		hypertension, 281t
	Drug Prototype, 296t
	interactions, 296t
	route and adult dose, 281t, 295t
caspofungin acetate, 414, 415t
castor oil, 487t
Cataflam. *See* diclofenac
Catapres. *See* clonidine
catecholamine O-methyl transferase
	(COMT), 128

catechol-O-methyl transferase (COMT) inhibitors, 162
cathartic, 486
catheter ablation, 336
cayenne *(Capsicum annum),* 173*t*
CBER (Center for Biologics Evaluation and Research), 5
CDC (Centers for Disease Control and Prevention), 9
CDER (Center for Drug Evaluation and Research), 5
cefaclor, 396*t*
cefadroxil, 396*t*
cefazolin, 396*t*
cefdinir, 396*t*
cefditoren, 396*t*
cefepime, 396*t*
cefixime, 396*t*
cefotaxime
    Drug Prototype, 396*t*
    route and adult dose, 396*t*
cefotetan, 396*t*
cefprozil, 396*t*
ceftriaxone, 396*t*
cefuroxime, 396*t*
Celebrex. *See* celecoxib
celecoxib, 8, 208, 209*t*, 365*t*, 366
Celestone. *See* betamethasone
Celexa. *See* citalopram
cell kill, 434, 434*f*
cell-mediated immunity, 375–376, 375*f*
Cenestin. *See* **estrogen, conjugated**
Center for Biologics Evaluation and Research (CBER), 5
Center for Drug Evaluation and Research (CDER), 5
Center for Food Safety and Applied Nutrition (CFSAN), 7
Centers for Disease Control and Prevention (CDC), 9
central nervous system (CNS), 87, 88*f*, 199, 200, 432
    cholinergic drugs and, 92
central nervous system (CNS) depressants
    abuse of, 74–76
    alcohol, 75–76
    for anxiety and sleep disorders, 110–111
    barbiturates, 74
    benzodiazepines, 74–75
    categorization of, 111
    opioids, 75
    Patients Need to Know, 119*t*
    sedatives and sedative-hypnotics, 74
    withdrawal syndrome, 111
central nervous system (CNS) stimulants
    abuse of, 78–79
    for ADHD, 137, 138*t*
    drugs classified as, 137, 138*t*
cephalexin, 396*t*
cephalosporins, 395–397, 396*t*
cerebral cortex, 107
cerebrovascular accident (stroke), 314–315, 347*t*
Cerebyx. *See* fosphenytoin
certolizumab pegol, 576*t*
Cervidil. *See* dinoprostone
Cetamide. *See* sulfacetamide sodium

cetirizine, 460*t*
cetuximab, 445*t*
cevimeline HCl, 92*t*
C fibers, 199
CFSAN (Center for Food Safety and Applied Nutrition), 7
chemical group name, 13, 14
chemical name, 14
chemoprophylaxis
    for cancer, 434
    for infections, 392
chemotherapy, cancer, 433–434, 434*f. See also* Antineoplastic Drugs
chest pain, 302–303, 303*t*
Childhood Vaccine Act, 6*f*, 7*t*
children
    AED use and development of, 184
    dorsogluteal site for, 36
    epilepsy in, 182
    febrile seizures and, 182
    vastus lateralis site for, 36
Chlamydia trachomatis, 390*t*
chlorambucil, 437*t*
chloramphenicol, 404*t*
chlordiazepoxide, 113, 114*t*
chloride, 501*t*
chloroethane, 221*t*
Chloromag. *See* magnesium chloride
chloroprocaine, 221*t*
chloroquine, 426, 426*t*
chlorothiazide, 254*t*, 274*t*
chlorpheniramine, 459*t*
chlorpromazine
    actions and uses, 147*t*
    adverse effects, 147*t*
    Drug Prototype, 147*t*
    interactions, 147*t*
        with kava, 147*t*
        with phenobarbital, 147*t*
        with St. John's wort, 147*t*
        with tricyclic antidepressants, 147*t*
    interaction with valproic acid, 191*t*
    introduction of, 143
    route and adult dose, 146*t*
chlorpropamide, 536*t*
chlorthalidone, 254, 254*t*, 274*t*
Chlor-Trimeton Allergy/Decongestant, 461*t*
chlorzoxazone, 171*t*
cholecalciferol, 565
cholesterol
    bad, 236
    biosynthesis and excretion, 238, 239*t*
    dietary, 235
    functions, 235
    good, 236
    laboratory values, 238*t*
    levels, 235*t*
    red yeast rice and, 238*t*
    total, 238*t*
cholestyramine
    actions, 240*t*
    adverse effects, 240*t*
    clinical uses, 240*t*
    Drug Prototype, 240*t*
    interactions, 240*t*
    Patients Need to Know, 245*t*
    route and adult dose, 239*t*

cholinergic, 90, 92
cholinergic drugs, 175
chondroitin sulfate, 578*t*
Chronic alcohol consumption, 75
chronic bronchitis, 471–472
chronic obstructive pulmonary disease (COPD), 471–472
chronic simple glaucoma, 600*f*, 601. *See also* glaucoma
Cialis. *See* tadalafil
ciclesonide, 463*t*, 470*t*
ciclopirox, 415*t*
cidofovir, 424*t*
ciliary body, 599
cilostazol, 355*t*
cimetidine, 482*t*
Cimzia. *See* certolizumab pegol
cinacalcet, 571*t*
CiproDex. *See* ciprofloxacin and dexamethasone
ciprofloxacin
    for anthrax exposure, 401
    Drug Prototype, 401*t*
    for ear infections, 607, 607*t*
    route and adult dose, 400*t*
ciprofloxacin and dexamethasone, 607*t*
ciprofloxacin and hydrocortisone, 607*t*
Cipro HC. *See* ciprofloxacin and hydrocortisone
cirrhosis, 75
cisatracurium, 176*t*
cisplatin, 437*t*
citalopram, 112*t*, 126*t*
Citracal. *See* calcium citrate
cladribine, 439*t*
clarithromycin, 398*t*, 485
Clearasil. *See* benzoyl peroxide
ClearEyes. *See* naphazoline
clemastine, 459*t*
Climara. *See* estradiol
clindamycin, 403, 404*t*
clinical depression, 111. *See also* major depressive disorder
clinical pharmacology, 7
clinical phase trials, 7–8
Clinoril. *See* sulindac
clobetasol, 592*t*
clocortolone, 592*t*
Cloderm. *See* clocortolone
clofarabine, 439*t*
clofibrate, 243
clomipramine, 112*t*, 125, 126*t*
clonazepam, 74, 114*t*
    for anxiety, 114*t*
    for muscle spasms, 170, 171*t*
    for seizures, 187*t*
clonic phase, tonic-clonic seizure, 183
clonic spasm, 169. *See also* muscle spasms
clonidine, 138*t*
    actions, 282
    clinical uses, 97*t*
        attention deficit-hyperactivity disorder, 138*t*
        hypertension, 281*t*
clopidogrel
    actions, 350*f*, 355*t*, 356*t*
    adverse effects, 356*t*
    black box warning, 356*t*

clinical uses, 356*t*
  myocardial infarction, 312
  stroke, 314
  Drug Prototype, 356*t*
  interactions, 356*t*
  route and adult dose, 355*t*
clorazepate, 114*t*, 187*t*, 188
closed-angle glaucoma, 600*f*, 601. *See also*
  glaucoma
closed comedones, 589
Clostridium botulinum, 173
clotrimazole, 415*t*
clotting factors, 347
cloves, for dental pain, 223*t*
cloxacillin, 393
clozapine, 151*t*, 152
  interactions with risperidone, 152*t*
Clozaril. *See* clozapine
CMV (cytomegalovirus), 423
CNS (central nervous system). *See* central
  nervous system (CNS)
coagulation, 347
coagulation cascade, 347, 348*f*
coagulation disorders, 347*t*
  incidence, 349*t*
  Patients Need to Know, 358*t*
coal tar, 593*t*, 594
co-analgesics. *See* adjuvant analgesics
cocaine, 70, 78
  Andean cultures and use of, 78
  history of uses, 78
  as local anesthetic, 222
  overdose of, 78
  physiological and psychological effects
    of, 73*t*
  as Schedule II drug, 78
  withdrawal syndrome for, 78
Coccidioides immitis, 414*t*
codeine, 204*t*, 465
coenzyme Q10, 242*t*
Cogentin. *See* benztropine
Cognex. *See* tacrine
cognitive-behavioral therapy, 125
Colace. *See* glycerin
colchicine, 577, 577*t*
Colcrys. *See* colchicine
colesevelam, 239*t*, 242
Colestid. *See* colestipol
colestipol, 239*t*
colloids, 323, 323*t*
combination drugs, 15
common cold
  antitussives for, 465
  decongestants for, 463–464, 464*t*
  expectorants for, 465
common collecting ducts, 250
Compazine. *See* prochlorperazine
competitive antagonists, 205
complement, 364*t*
complementary and alternative medicine
  (CAM), 60–61. *See also* herbal products;
  specialty supplements
    common characteristics of, 60
complementary and alternative medicine
  (CAM) therapy, 4, 57*t*
complex partial seizures, 183. *See also*
  seizure(s)

compliance, 22
Compoz Nighttime Sleep Aid. *See*
  diphenhydramine
Comprehensive Drug Abuse Prevention and
  Control Act, 16
COMT (catecholamine O-methyl
  transferase), 128
Comtan. *See* **entacapone**
Comvax, 377*t*
Concerta. *See* methylphenidate
congestive heart failure, 289. *See also* heart
  failure (HF)
conjugated estrogens with medroxyprogesterone, 551*t*
constipation, 486–487, 487*t*
contact dermatitis, 591
contractility, 289, 304
controlled substance, 16
Controlled Substances Act of 1970, 16
conventional antipsychotics
  adverse effects, 147*t*
  nonphenothiazines, 148*t*
  Nursing Process Focus, 149–151*t*
  phenothiazines and phenothiazine-like
    drugs, 146*t*
convulsions, 181. *See also* seizure(s)
Copaxone. *See* glatiramer
COPD (chronic obstructive pulmonary
  disease), 471–472
Cordarone. *See* **amiodarone**
Cordran. *See* flurandrenolide
Coreg. *See* **carvedilol**
Corgard. *See* nadolol
coronary arteries, 302
coronary artery bypass graft (CABG)
  surgery, 304
coronary heart disease, 302–303, 303*f*, 303*t*
corpora cavernosa, 555
corpus luteum, 544
corpus striatum, 160, 162*f*
Cortef. *See* **hydrocortisone**
corticosteroids
  for chemotherapy, 443
  clinical uses
    adrenocortical insufficiency, 521, 522*t*
    allergic rhinitis, 31, 461
    anaphylaxis, 328
    asthma, 470–471, 470*t*
    dermatitis, 591, 592*t*
    inflammation, 201, 365, 368,
      368*t*, 381
    inflammatory pain, 201
  control of, 520
  defined, 520
  drugs classified as
    inhaled, 470–471, 470*t*
    intranasal, 462, 463*t*
    oral, 471
    systemic, 522, 523–524*t*
    topical, 28, 591, 592*t*, 594
  inflammatory and immune responses,
    suppression, 522
corticotropin-releasing factor (CRF), 520
cortisone, 368*t*
Cortisporin. *See* polymyxin B, neomycin, and
  hydrocortisone
Cortizone. *See* **hydrocortisone**

Corvert. *See* ibutilide
Corzide. *See* bendroflumethiazide and nadolol
Coumadin. *See* **warfarin**
Cozaar. *See* losartan
cranberry, 251*t*, 353*t*
Crestor. *See* rosuvastatin
cretinism, 516
Crinone. *See* progesterone
Critical Path Initiative (FDA), 6*f*
Crohn's disease, 480
cromolyn, 471
  route and adult dose, 470*t*
cross-tolerance, 73
crotamiton, 587
crushing, tablets or capsules, 27
Cryptococcus neoformans, 414*t*
crystalloids, 323, 323*t*
crystamine. *See* **cyanocobalamin**
culture, 7
culture and sensitivity (C&S) testing, 393
Cushing's syndrome, 514*t*, 522
Cutar. *See* coal tar
Cutivate. *See* fluticasone propionate
Cuvposa. *See* glycopyrrolate
cyanocobalamin
  Drug Prototype, 499*t*
cyclic lipopeptides, 403–404
cyclizine, 490*t*
cyclobenzaprine
  actions and uses, 171*t*
  adverse effects, 171*t*
  Drug Prototype, 171*t*
  interactions, 171*t*
  route and adult dose, 171*t*
Cyclocort. *See* amcinonide
Cyclogyl. *See* cyclopentolate
cyclooxygenase, 208, 366
cyclooxygenase type 1 (COX-1), 208
cyclooxygenase type 2 (COX-2), 208
cyclopentolate, 95*t*, 606*t*
cyclophosphamide
  Drug Prototype, 438*t*
  route and adult dose, 437*t*
cycloplegia, 602
cycloplegic drugs, 605, 606*t*
Cycloset. *See* bromocriptine
cyclosporine
  Drug Prototype, 382*t*
  interactions, 398*t*
  for psoriasis, 593*t*, 594
  route and adult dose, 381*t*
Cymbalta. *See* duloxetine
cytarabine, 439*t*
cytokines, 375
cytomegalovirus (CMV), 423
Cytomel. *See* liothyronine
cytotoxic T cells, 375–376

D

dabigatran, 351, 351*t*
dacarbazine, 437*t*
dactinomycin, 441*t*
Dalmane. *See* flurazepam
dalteparin, 351*t*
danazol, 555*t*
d- and l-amphetamine racemic mixture, 137

Danocrine. *See* danazol
dantrolene
  actions, 175*t*
  adverse effects, 175*t*
  clinical uses, 175*t*
  Drug Prototype, 175*t*
  interactions, 175*t*
    with alcohol, 175*t*
    with antihistamines, 175*t*
    with verapamil, 175*t*
  route and adult dose, 174*t*
daptomycin, 403, 404*t*
darunavir, 419*t*
"date rape" drug. *See* ketamine
daunorubicin, 441*t*
daunorubicin liposomal, 441*t*
Daypro. *See* oxaprozin
Daytrana. *See* methylphenidate
DDAVP. *See* **desmopressin**
DEA (Drug Enforcement Administration), 16
Debrox. *See* carbamide peroxide
Decaspray. *See* dexamethasone
decongestants, 463–464, 464*t*
  in combination products, 461*t*
  Patients Need to Know, 472
deep vein thrombosis (DVT), 347*t*, 349
defecation, 486
deficient knowledge (drug teaching), 53
degarelix, 444*t*
dehydration, 273
Delatestryl. *See* testosterone enanthate
delavirdine, 419*t*
Delestrogen. *See* estradiol valerate
deltoid site, intramuscular injection, 36
delusions, 143
Demadex. *See* torsemide
demeclocycline, 397*t*
dementia, 164. *See also* Alzheimer's disease
  characteristics, 164
  gingko biloba use in, 167*t*
  Patients Need to Know, 176*t*
Demerol. *See* meperidine
demyelination, 167–168
denosumab, 571*t*
dental pain, cloves for, 223*t*
Depakene. *See* **valproic acid**
Depakote. *See* **valproic acid**
dependence, 16
  drugs causing, 16
  physical, 16, 17*t*
  psychological, 16, 17*t*
depolarization (blockers), 175, 335
depolarizing blockers, 175, 176*t*, 229. *See also*
  neuromuscular blocking drugs
Depo-Medrol. *See* methylprednisolone
Depo-Provera. *See* **medroxyprogesterone**
Depo-SubQ-Provera. *See*
  medroxyprogesterone
Depo-Testosterone. *See* testosterone cypionate
depression, 123
  in Alzheimer's disease, 164, 166
  biological, 123
  bipolar disorder and, 134
  clinical, 123
  management
    short-term psychotherapies, 124–125
    St. John's wort, 134*t*

Nursing Process Focus, 130–131*t*
  postpartum, 124
  psychotic, 124
  seasonal affective disorder (SAD), 124
  situational, 124
  situational and biological causes of, 123*t*
  symptoms of, 123
dermatitis, 591, 592*t*
Dermatop. *See* prednicarbate
dermis, 583
DES (diethylstilbestrol), 443*t*
desflurane, 225*t*
designer drugs, 70
desipramine, 112*t*, 126*t*
desirudin, 351, 351*t*
desloratadine, 460*t*
desmopressin
  for diabetes insipidus (DI), 515
  Drug Prototype, 514*t*
Desonate. *See* desonide
desonide, 592*t*
DesOwen. *See* desonide
desoximetasone, 592*t*
Detrol. *See* tolterodine
dexamethasone, 522*t*, 592*t*
  as antiemetic, 490*t*
  as antineoplastic agent, 443*t*
  route and adult dose, 368*t*
dexchlorpheniramine, 459*t*
Dexedrine. *See* dextroamphetamine
Dexferrum. *See* iron dextran
dexmethylphenidate, 138*t*
dextroamphetamine, 78, 137, 138*t*
dextromethorphan, 465
D.H.E. 45. *See* dihydroergotamine mesylate
DiaBeta. *See* glyburide
diabetes insipidus (DI), 514–515
diabetes mellitus (DM)
  causes, 529
  description, 529
  Patients Need to Know, 539*t*
  type 1. *See* type 1 diabetes mellitus
  type 2. *See* type 2 diabetes mellitus
diabetic ketoacidosis (DKA), 530
Diabinese. *See* chlorpropamide
diagnosis, medical, 53
diagnosis, nursing, 52*f*, 53, 54*t*
*Diagnostic and Statistical Manual of Mental
  Disorders,* 5th edition (DSM-5), 123
Diamox. *See* acetazolamide
diarrhea, 488–489, 489*t*
diastolic pressure, 267, 268*f*
diazepam, 72, 74, 185*t*
  actions and uses, 188*t*
  adverse effects, 113–114, 188*t*
  clinical uses, 185*t*
    alcohol withdrawal, 72
    anxiety, 114*t*
    intravenous anesthetic, 226*t*
    muscle spasms, 170, 171, 173
    seizures, 185*t*, 187*t*, 187*t*
  Drug Prototype, 188*t*
  interaction with omeprazole, 483*t*
  introduction of, 113
  route and adult dose, 187*t*
dibucaine, 221*t*
diclofenac, 209*t*, 365*t*

dicloxacillin, 394*t*
dicyclomine, 95*t*
didanosine, 419*t*
Didronel. *See* etidronate
diencephalon, 107, 108*t*
dietary fiber, 486
Dietary Reference Index (DRI), 498
Dietary Supplement and Nonprescription Drug
  Consumer Protection Act, 67
Dietary Supplement Health and Education Act
  (DSHEA) of 1994, 6*f*, 7, 66
  significant weaknesses of, 66
dietary supplements, 66. *See also* herbal
  products; specialty supplements
  defined, 66
  Dietary Supplement and Nonprescription
    Drug Consumer Protection Act and, 67
  DSHEA and, 66
  nonherbal. *See* specialty supplements
  regulation of, 66–67
  sales of, 60
diethylstilbestrol (DES), 443*t*
difenoxin with atropine, 489*t*
Differin. *See* adapalene
diflorasone, 592*t*
diflunisal, 209*t*, 365*t*
digestion, 478
digestive system, 478, 478*f*. *See also*
  gastrointestinal disorders
digoxin
  actions, 291*f*, 294, 295*t*
  adverse effects, 294, 295*t*
  clinical uses, 295*t*
    dysrhythmias, 341*t*
  Drug Prototype, 295*t*
  interactions, 295*t*
    with amiodarone, 341*t*
    with atorvastatin, 240*t*
    with carvedilol, 296*t*
    with cyclophosphamide, 438*t*
    with diltiazem, 309*t*
    with diuretics, 252
    with furosemide, 254*t*
    with heparin, 352*t*
    with hydrochlorothiazide, 255*t*
    with psyllium, 487*t*
    with spironolactone, 256*t*
    with vincristine, 443*t*
  route and adult dose, 295*t*, 325*t*, 341*t*
digoxin immune fab, 294
dihydroergotamine, 211
dihydroergotamine mesylate, 212*t*
Dilacor XR. *See* **diltiazem**
Dilantin. *See* **phenytoin**
Dilaudid. *See* hydromorphone
Dilocaine. *See* lidocaine
diltiazem
  actions, 309*t*
  adverse effects, 309*t*
  clinical uses
    angina, 306*t*
    dysrhythmias, 341*t*
  Drug Prototype, 309*t*
  interactions, 309*t*
  route and adult dose, 278*t*, 306*t*, 309*t*, 341*t*
dimenhydrinate, 459*t*, 489, 490*t*
Dimetapp Children's Cold and Allergy, 461*t*

dinoprostone, 553*t*

Diovan. *See* valsartan

Diovan HCT, 273

Diphedryl. *See* **diphenhydramine**

Diphenadryl. *See* **diphenhydramine**

diphenhydramine, 15, 15*t*
  for allergic reactions, 119
  clinical uses
    as antiemetic, 490*t*
    extrapyramidal symptoms, 160
    insomnia, 111, 117*t*
    parkinsonism, 163*t*
    shock, 328
  Drug Prototype, 460*t*
  route and adult dose, 459*t*

diphenoxylate with atropine
  Drug Prototype, 488*t*
  route and adult dose, 489*t*

diphtheria, tetanus, and pertussis vaccine, 377*t*

Dipivefrin HCl, 602, 602*t*

Diprivan. *See* **propofol**

Diprolene. *See* betamethasone

dipyridamole, 355*t*

dirithromycin, 398*t*

Disalcid. *See* salsalate

disease-modifying antirheumatic drugs (DMARDs), 575, 576*t*

disopyramide, 338*t*

disorganized behavior, 143

distal tubule, 250, 250*f*

distribution, 42*f*, 43

disulfiram, 75–76, 129*t*

diuretics, 252
  actions, 252, 269, 272*f*, 291*f*, 294
  adverse effects, 252, 273, 294
  classifications
    carbonic anhydrase inhibitors, 256–257, 257*t*
    loop diuretics, 252–253, 253*f*
    potassium-sparing diuretics. *See* potassium-sparing diuretics
  clinical uses, 252
    heart failure, 293*t*, 294
    hypertension, 273–274, 274*t*
  drugs classified as, 253*t*
  interactions
    with prazosin, 100*t*
  interventions
    with digoxin, 295*t*
    with prednisone, 369*t*
    with warfarin, 353*t*
  osmotic, 257
  Patients Need to Know, 257–258*t*, 262*t*, 297*t*

Diuril. *See* chlorothiazide

Divigel. *See* estradiol

DKA (diabetic ketoacidosis), 530

DMARDs (disease-modifying antirheumatic drugs), 575, 576*t*

dobutamine, 97, 97*t*, 325, 325*t*

Dobutrex. *See* dobutamine

docetaxel, 442*t*

docosanol, 424*t*

docusate, 487*t*

dofetilide, 340*t*

dolasetron, 490*t*

Dolgesic. *See* **ibuprofen**

Dolophine. *See* methadone

DOM (2,5 dimethoxy-4-methylamphetamine, "STP") drug, 77

donepezil
  actions, 167*t*
  adverse effects, 167*t*
  clinical uses, 92*t*, 167*t*
  Drug Prototype, 167*t*
  interactions, 167*t*
    with dexamethasone, 167*t*
    with phenobarbital, 167*t*
    with rifampin, 167*t*
  route and adult dose, 165*t*

dong quai, for premenstrual syndrome, 549*t*

dopamine
  actions, 326*t*
  adverse effects, 326*t*
  black box warning, 326*t*
  clinical uses, 97*t*
    shock, 325, 325*t*, 326*t*
  Drug Prototype, 326*t*
  interactions, 326*t*
    with isoflurane, 225*t*
  in neurodegenerative disorders, 160, 161, 162*f*
  route and adult dose, 325*t*
  in schizophrenia, 145*f*

dopamine blocker, 228*t*

dopamine partial agonists. *See* dopamine system stabilizers (DSS)

dopaminergic drugs, 160, 161*t*

dopamine system stabilizers (DSS), 146, 154

Dopastat. *See* **dopamine**

Doral. *See* quazepam

doripenem, 404*t*

dorsogluteal site, intramuscular injection, 36

dorzolamide, 603*t*

dose-response curve, 47

Dovonex. *See* calcipotriene

doxazosin, 558*t*
  actions, 282*t*
  adverse effects, 282*t*
  clinical uses, 99, 100*t*, 282*t*
    hypertension, 281*t*
  Drug Prototype, 282*t*
  interactions, 282*t*
  route and adult dose, 281*t*

doxazosin XL, 558*t*

doxepin, 112*t*, 126*t*

doxercalciferol, 568*t*

doxorubicin
  Drug Prototype, 441*t*
  interaction with vincristine, 443*t*
  route and adult dose, 441*t*

doxorubicin liposomal, 441*t*

doxycycline, 590, 590*t*
  actions, 397*t*
  clinical uses, 426*t*
  route and adult dose, 397*t*

doxylamine, 111, 117*t*

DPI (dry powder inhaler), 456

DRI. *See* Dietary Reference Index (DRI)

Drisdol. *See* ergocalciferol

dronedarone, 340*t*

drop attacks, 183. *See also* atonic seizures

droperidol, 225*t*, 227, 228*t*

drug action
  duration of, 46

onset of, 45
  termination of, 46

drug administration
  common abbreviations used to give directions about, 24*t*
  compliance with, 22–23
  enteral, 26*t*, 27–28
  health support staff responsibilities, 21
  nurse's responsibilities, 21–22
  parenteral, 32–39, 34–35*t*
  protocols and techniques, 25–26
  six rights, 22
  three checks, 22
  topical, 28–32, 30–31*t*

drug–drug interactions, 42, 46*f*

Drug Enforcement Administration (DEA), 16

drug forms, administration guidelines for, 26*t*, 30–31*t*, 34–35*t*

drug interaction, 42
  drug–drug interactions, 42, 46*f*
  food–drug interactions, 42, 46*f*

drug prototype. *See* Guide to Special Features

drug(s)
  antibiotics, 13
  anti-inflammatory, 13
  approval process, U.S., 7–9, 8*f*
  bioavailability of, 15
  brand name, 15–16
  chemical group name of, 14
  chemical name of, 14
  classification, 4
  combination, 15
  controlled substance, 16
  diuretic, 13
  efficacy of, 47, 48*f*
  FDA-unapproved uses of, 9
  generic name of, 14
  grapefruit juice and, 23
  half-life (t$_{1/2}$) of, 45
  labels, 7*f*
  names, 14–15
  off-label use of, 9
  pharmacologic classification, 13–14, 14*t*
  plasma half-life of, 45
  potency of, 47, 48*f*
  pregnancy categories, 17
  prodrugs, 43
  prototype, 13
  reactions to, 23
  regulation of, 5
  schedules, 16
  therapeutic classification, 13–14, 13*t*
  therapeutic range of, 45
  trade name of, 14

drug therapy
  factors influencing effectiveness of, 46*t*
  metabolism and, 43

DSS (dopamine system stabilizers), 146, 154

duloxetine, 112*t*, 126*t*
  for anxiety disorders, 112*t*
  for depression, 126*t*
  for generalized anxiety disorder, 129
  for neuropathic pain, 129

Durabolin. *See* nandrolone

Duragesic. *See* fentanyl

Duramorph. See **morphine**
duration of drug action, 46
dutasteride, 558*t*
DVT (deep vein thrombosis), 347*t*, 349
dwarfism, 515
Dyclone. See dyclonine
dyclonine, 221*t*
DynaCirc. See isradipine
Dyrenium. See triamterene
dysentery, 426
dysfunctional uterine bleeding, 549–550
dyslipidemia, 235
dysphoric symptoms, 134
dyspnea, 466
Dysport. See onabotulinumtoxin A
dysrhythmias, 332
    classification, 332–333
    diseases associated with, 333
    incidence, 332*t*
    nonpharmacologic therapy, 336
    Nursing Process Focus, 336–337*t*
    pathophysiology, 333–335
    Patients Need to Know, 343*t*
    pharmacotherapy
        adenosine, 341*t*, 342
        beta-blockers, 339, 339*t*. See also beta
            (β) blockers
        calcium channel blockers, 341–342,
            341t. See also calcium channel
            blockers (CCB)
        digoxin, 341*t*, 342
        potassium channel blockers, 340, 340*t*.
            See also potassium channel blockers
        sodium channel blockers, 338, 338*t*.
            See also sodium channel blockers
    symptoms, 332
dysrhythmic drugs, 201
dysthymic disorder, 124. See also depression
dystonias, 148, 172. See also spasticity
    with conventional antipsychotics, 148

E

ear, 606, 607*f*
ear disorders, 606–608, 607*t*
EC (emergency contraception), 547
ECG (electrocardiogram), 333, 334*f*
echinacea, 376
    interactions, 341, 440*t*
echothiophate iodide, 602, 602*t*
eclampsia, 183
econazole, 415*t*
Ecotrin. See **aspirin**
Ecstasy (MDMA), 77
ECT (electroconvulsive therapy), 125
ectopic foci/pacemakers, 335
eczema, 591, 592*t*
Edarbi. See azilsartan
Edecrin. See ethacrynic acid
edrophonium, 92*t*
Edular. See **zolpidem**
EEG (electroencephalogram), 181, 181*f*
efavirenz, 419*t*
Effexor. See venlafaxine
efficacy, of drugs, 5, 47, 48*f*
Elavil. See amitriptyline; amitryptiline
Eldepryl. See selegiline

electrocardiogram (ECG), 333, 334*f*
electroconvulsive therapy (ECT), 125
electroencephalogram (EEG), 181, 181*f*
electrolyte(s)
    defined, 258, 273
    imbalances, 258–259, 259*t*
Elestrin. See estradiol
eletriptan, 212*t*
elimination, 45. See also excretion
Elimite. See permethrin
Eliquis. See apixaban
Elitek. See rasburicase
Ella. See ulipristal
Elocon, ses mometasone furoate
embolus, 349
emergency contraception (EC), 547
emesis, 489
emetics, 490
emphysema, 472
Empirin. See **aspirin**
Empirin with Codeine No. 2, 205
Emsam. See selegiline
emtricitabine, 419*t*
enalapril
    actions, 277*t*
    adverse effects, 277*t*
    black box warning, 277*t*
    clinical uses, 277*t*
        heart failure, 293*t*
        hypertension, 275*t*
    Drug Prototype, 277*t*
    interactions, 277*t*
    route and adult dose, 275*t*, 293*t*
Enbrel. See etanercept
endocrine system, 511, 512*f*
endogenous opioids, 199–200
endometrial carcinoma, 550
Endometrin. See progesterone
endometriosis, 550
end-stage renal disease (ESRD), 251
Enduron. See methyclothiazide
enflurane, 225*t*
enfuvirtide, 419*t*, 420
Enjuvia. See **estrogen, conjugated**
enoxaparin, 351*t*
entacapone, 161, 161*t*, 162
    actions and uses, 163*t*
    adverse effects, 163*t*
    Drug Prototype, 163*t*
    interactions, 163*t*
    route and adult dose, 161*t*
enteral nutrition, 504–505, 504*f*
enteral route, 27
    buccal, 27, 28*f*
    nasogastric and gastrostomy tubes, 27*t*, 28
    sublingual, 27, 28*f*
    tablets and capsules, 27
enteric-coated tablets, 27
Enterobius, 427
Enterococci, 390*t*
enterohepatic recirculation, 44, 45*f*
enzalutamide, 444*t*
ephedra, 66, 133*t*
epidermis, 583
Epidermophyton floccosum, 414*t*
epidural anesthesia, 219*f*, 219*t*
epilepsy, 181. See also seizure(s)

classification of, 183–184
    Fast Facts, 182*t*
    idiopathic, 182
    ketogenic diet for, 188*t*
    Lennox-Gastaut syndrome (LGS), 191
    onset of, 183*t*
    symptoms of, 181
epileptic seizures, 183
    generalized, 183
    partial, 183
    special epileptic syndromes, 184
epinephrine, 90
    actions, 90*t*, 327*t*
    adverse effects, 282, 327*t*
    clinical uses, 97*t*, 98*t*
        in local anesthetics, 220
        shock, 325, 325*t*, 327*t*
    Drug Prototype, 327*t*
    interactions, 327*t*
        with isoflurane, 225*t*
    route and adult dose, 325, 325*t*
epirubicin, 441*t*
eplerenone, 256*t*, 274*t*, 293*t*
epoetin alfa
    in cancer chemotherapy, 252, 446
    Drug Prototype, 446*t*
eprosartan, 275*t*
EPS (extrapyramidal symptoms), 148, 160,
    166
Epsom salt. See magnesium sulfate
Epstein-Barr virus, 424
eptifibatide, 355*t*
Ercaf. See ergotamine with caffeine
erectile dysfunction, 555–556, 556*t*
ergocalciferol, 568*t*
Ergostat. See ergotamine tartrate
ergot alkaloids, 211
ergotamine tartrate, 211, 212*t*
ergotamine with caffeine, 212*t*
eribulin, 442*t*
erlotinib, 445*t*
ER (extended-release) medications, 27
ertapenem, 404, 404*t*
erythema, 584
erythromycin
    Drug Prototypes, 398*t*
    interactions
        with atorvastatin, 240*t*
        with valproic acid, 191*t*
    route and adult dose, 398*t*
erythropoietin, 252
Erythroxylon coca, 222
Escherichia coli, 390*t*
escitalopram
    actions, 113*t*
    adverse effects, 113*t*
    clinical uses, 113*t*
        for anxiety disorders, 112*t*
    Drug Prototype, 113*t*
escitalopram oxalate, 126*t*
Eskalith. See lithium
esmolol, 100*t*, 339*t*
esomeprazole, 482*t*
estazolam, 114*t*
esters, 220–222, 221*t*. See also local
    anesthetics
Estrace. See estradiol

Estraderm. *See* estradiol
estradiol, 550*t*
estradiol valerate, 550*t*
estradiol with norethindrone
    Drug Prototype, 547*t*
estradiol with norgestimate, 551*t*
estramustine, 437*t*
estrogen, conjugated
    Drug Prototype, 551*t*
    route and adult dose, 550*t*
estrogen-progestin oral contraceptives, 546*t*
    adverse effects, 546
    description, 546
    types, 546
estrogens
    interaction with phenytoin, 190*t*
    sex hormone, 544
estropipate, 550*t*
eszopiclone, 111, 117*t*, 119
etanercept, 576*t*
ethacrynic acid, 253*t*
ethambutol, 407*t*
ethinyl estradiol, 546, 590*t*. *See also* estrogen-progestin oral contraceptives
    clinical uses, 443*t*
ethinyl estradiol with norethindrone acetate, 551*t*
ethosuximide
    actions, 192*t*
    adverse effects, 192*t*
    clinical uses, 185*t*, 192*t*
    Drug Prototype, 192*t*
    interactions, 192*t*
        with valproic acid, 192*t*
    route and adult dose, 192*t*
ethotoin, 189*t*
Ethrane. *See* enflurane
ethyl alcohol. *See* alcohol
ethyl chloride, 221*t*
etidronate, 571*t*
etiologies, 53
etodolac, 209*t*, 365*t*
etomidate, 226*t*
etoposide, 442, 442*t*
etravirine, 419*t*
euphoria, 75, 76, 78
Eurax. *See* crotamiton
evaluation criteria, 54
evaluation phase, of nursing process, 52*f*, 56–57
evening primrose oil for pain, 211*t*
Evista. *See* **raloxifene**
Evithrom. *See* thrombin
Evoxac. *See* cevimeline HCl
Exalgo. *See* hydromorphone
excretion, 42*f*, 44. *See also* elimination
Exelon. *See* rivastigmine
exemestane, 444*t*
exenatide, 535*t*, 537
exercise-induced asthma, 466
expectorants, 457*f*, 465
Extavia. *See* interferon beta-1b
extended-release (ER) medications, 27
extended-spectrum penicillins, 393
external otitis, 606
extrapyramidal symptoms (EPS), 148, 160, 166

eye disorders
    glaucoma. *See* glaucoma
    minor conditions, 605, 606*t*
    Patients Need to Know, 608*t*
eye examination, 605, 606*t*
ezetimibe, 239*t*, 243*f*, 244
ezogabine, 187*t*

F

false neurotransmitter, 282
famciclovir, 424*t*
famotidine, 482*t*
Fanapt. *See* iloperidone
fasciculations, 175
Fast Facts. *See* Guide to Special Features
fat-soluble vitamin, 497–498. *See also* vitamin(s)
FDA (Food and Drug Administration). *See* Food and Drug Administration (FDA)
FDA Amendments Act, 6*f*
FDA Drug Modernization Act, 6*f*, 9
FDA Food Safety Modernization Act, 6*f*
febrile seizures, 182, 184
febuxostat, 577, 577*t*
Federal Bureau of Chemistry, 6*f*
felbamate, 190*t*, 191
Felbatol. *See* felbamate
Feldene. *See* piroxicam
felodipine, 278*t*
fenofibrate, 239*t*, 243
fenoprofen, 209*t*, 365*t*
fentanyl, 75
    as adjuncts to anesthesia, 228*t*
    adverse reactions, 204
    clinical uses, 203, 204*t*
    as intravenous anesthetic, 226*t*
Fentora. *See* fentanyl
Feosol. *See* **ferrous sulfate**
Feostat. *See* ferrous fumarate
Fergon. *See* ferrous gluconate
Ferranol. *See* ferrous fumarate
ferrous fumarate, 17*t*, 502*t*
ferrous gluconate, 502*t*
ferrous sulfate
    Drug Prototype, 501*t*
    route and adult dose, 502*t*
fesoterodine, 95*t*
feverfew, 208*t*, 352*t*, 353*t*, 357*t*, 366*t*
fexofenadine, 460*t*
fibric acid drugs, 239*t*, 243, 243*f*
Fibricor. *See* fenofibrate
fibrillation, 332
fibrin, 347
fibrinogen, 347
fibrinolysis, 349, 349*t*
field block (infiltration) anesthesia, 219*f*, 219*t*
fight-or-flight response, 87
filgrastim, 436, 446
filtrate, 250
Finacea. *See* azelaic acid
finasteride
    for benign prostatic hyperplasia, 558*t*
    Drug Prototype, 558*t*
Fioricet with Codeine, 205
Fiorinal, 205
first-degree burns, 583

first-dose phenomenon, 100*t*
first-pass effect (first-pass metabolism), 29, 31, 32, 33, 37, 43, 44*f*
fish oil, 244
flecainide, 201, 338*t*
Fleet Mineral Oil. *See* mineral oil
Flexeril. *See* **cyclobenzaprine**
Flomax. *See* tamsulosin
Florinef. *See* fludrocortisone
floxuridine, 439*t*
fluconazole, 414, 415*t*
flucytosine, 415*t*
fludarabine, 439*t*
fludrocortisone, 522*t*
fluid replacement drugs, 322–323, 323*t*
    blood products, 322, 323*t*
    colloids, 323, 323*t*
    crystalloids, 323, 323*t*
    Nursing Process Focus, 324*t*
flunisolide, 463*t*, 470*t*
flunitrazepam, 74
fluocinolone acetonide, 592*t*
fluocinonide, 592*t*
fluoroquinolones, 400–401, 400*t*
fluorouracil, 439*t*
fluoxetine, 17*t*
    anxiety, 112*t*
    clinical uses, 126*t*
        depression, 126*t*
fluoxymesterone, 443*t*, 555*t*
fluphenazine, 146*t*
flurandrenolide, 592*t*
flurazepam, 114*t*
flurbiprofen, 209*t*, 365*t*
flutamide, 444*t*
fluticasone
    Drug Prototype, 463*t*
    inhaled, 470*t*
    route and adult dose, 463*t*
fluticasone propionate, 592*t*
fluvastatin, 239*t*
fluvoxamine, 112*t*, 126*t*
Focalin. *See* dexmethylphenidate
Focalin-XR. *See* dexmethylphenidate
folic acid antagonists, 439*t*
folic acid/folate, 498*t*, 499
folic acid/folate (vitamin B9):
    chemical structure, 440*f*
    functions, 440*t*
follicle-stimulating hormone (FSH), 543
follicular cells, 516
fondaparinux, 351*t*
Food, Drug, and Cosmetic Act, 5, 6*f*, 7, 66
Food and Drug Administration (FDA), 5, 6*f*, 7, 8–9, 201, 238*t*
    antiseizure drug therapy related warnings issued by, 184
    black box warnings
        for antidepressants, 111, 113
    dietary supplement regulations, 66–67
    herbal products and dietary supplements, administration of, by, 7
    new drug approval process, 8–9
    restructuring of, 9
Food and Nutrition Board of the National Academy of Sciences, 498
food–drug interactions, 42, 46*f*

Foradil. *See* formoterol
Forane. *See* **isoflurane**
formoterol, 97*t*, 468*t*
formularies, 5
Fortamet. *See* **metformin**
Forteo. *See* teriparatide
Fortesta. *See* **testosterone**
Fortical. *See* calcitonin–salmon
Fosamax. *See* **alendronate**
fosamprenavir, 419*t*
foscarnet, 424*t*
fosfomycin, 402*t*
fosinopril, 275*t*, 293*t*
fosphenytoin, 189*t*
fosphenytoin sodium, 189, 189*t*
fospropofol, 226*t*
Fostex. *See* benzoyl peroxide
Fragmin. *See* dalteparin
Frova. *See* frovatriptan
frovatriptan, 212*t*
fungal infections, 413–414, 414*t*
fungi, 389*f*, 413, 414*t*
furosemide, 17*t*
    actions, 252, 253*f*, 254*t*, 291*f*
    adverse effects, 254*t*
    clinical uses, 254*t*
        heart failure, 293*t*
        hypertension, 274*t*
    Drug Prototype, 254*t*
    interactions, 254*t*
    route and adult dose, 253*t*, 274*t*, 293*t*

G

GABA (gamma-aminobutyric acid), 114
gabapentin, 185*t*, 187*t*, 201
    for multiple sclerosis, 168*t*, 169
    for seizures, 185*t*, 187*t*
Gabitril. *See* tiagabine
GAD (generalized anxiety disorder), 106
galantamine, 92, 92*t*, 165*t*
gamma-aminobutyric acid (GABA), 114
gamma-aminobutyric acid (GABA) receptor,
    116, 118, 186, 186*t*
    antiseizure drugs activating, 187*t*
ganciclovir, 424*t*
ganglia, 90
ganglionic blocking drugs, 175
garlic, 353*t*, 355*t*, 357*t*
gastroesophageal reflux disease (GERD), 480
gastrointestinal disorders, 477*t*
    constipation, 486–487, 487*t*
    diarrhea, 488–489, 489*t*
    nausea and vomiting, 489–490, 490*t*
    Nursing Process Focus, 487–488*t*
    pancreatic insufficiency, 492
    Patients Need to Know, 492
    peptic ulcer disease. *See* peptic ulcer
        disease
gastrointestinal (GI) tract, 457
gastrostomy tubes, 27*t*, 28
gatifloxacin, 400*t*
gefitinib, 445*t*
gemcitabine, 439*t*
gemfibrozil
    actions, 244*t*
    adverse effects, 244*t*

clinical uses, 243, 244*t*
    Drug Prototype, 244*t*
    interactions, 244*t*
    route and adult dose, 239*t*
gemifloxacin, 400*t*
gemtuzumab, 445*t*
general anesthesia, 218, 224. *See also* general
    anesthetics
    stages of, 224*t*
general anesthetics
    adjuncts, 227
    administration routes, 224
    inhaled
            gas. *See* **nitrous oxide**
            volatile liquid, 225*t*, 226
        intravenous, 226–227, 226*t*
            benzodiazepines, 226*t*
            etomidate, 226*t*
            fospropofol, 226*t*
            ketamine, 77, 226*t*
            opioids, 226*t*
            propofol, 226*t*
generalized anxiety disorder (GAD), 106
generalized seizures, 183. *See also* seizure(s)
    absence seizures, 183
    atonic seizures, 183
    tonic-clonic seizures, 183
generic drugs, 15–16
generic name, 14
Genotropin. *See* somatropin
Genpril. *See* **ibuprofen**
gentamicin
    Drug Prototypes, 400*t*
    route and adult dose, 399*t*
Geodon. *See* ziprasidone
GERD (gastroesophageal reflux
    disease), 480
ginger
    interactions, 352*t*, 353*t*, 357*t*
ginkgo biloba
    in dementia, 167*t*
    interactions, 352*t*, 353*t*, 357*t*
ginseng
    for cardiovascular disease, 314*t*
GI (gastrointestinal) tract, 457
glatiramer, 168–169, 168*t*
glaucoma, 600
    forms, 600*f*, 601
    Nursing Process Focus, 604–605*t*
    pharmacotherapy
        alpha₂-adrenergic drugs, 603, 603*t*
        beta-blocking drugs, 603, 603*t*
        carbonic-anhydrase inhibitors,
            603, 603*t*
        miotics, 602, 602*t*
        osmotic diuretics, 603*t*, 604
        prostaglandins, 601, 602, 602*t*
        sympathomimetics, 602, 602*t*
glimepiride, 536*t*
glioma(s), 432
glipizide, 536*t*
GLP-1 receptor, activation, 537
glucagon, 529
    hyperglycemic effect, 529
glucocorticoids, 520. *See* corticosteroids
    actions, 365, 368, 462
    adverse effects, 368

clinical uses
        allergic rhinitis, 462, 463*t*
        asthma, 470, 470*t*
    drugs classified as, 368*t*
        inhaled, 470*t*
        intranasal, 463*t*
    interactions
        with aspirin, 208*t*
        with corticosteroids, 254*t*
        with cyclophosphamide, 438*t*
        with phenytoin, 190*t*
        with warfarin, 353*t*
Glucophage. *See* **metformin**
Glucophage XR. *See* **metformin**
glucosamine sulfate, 578*t*
glucose, 529, 530*f*
Glucotrol. *See* glipizide
Glumetza. *See* **metformin**
glutamate, 165, 186, 189
glyburide, 536*t*
glyburide micronized, 536*t*
glycerin, 257*t*
glycoprotein IIb/IIIa, 356
glycoprotein IIb/IIIa blockers, 355*t*, 356
glycopyrrolate, 95*t*
Glynase. *See* glyburide micronized
Glyset. *See* miglitol
goal (outcome), 54
goldenseal, 395*t*
golimumab, 576*t*
gonadocorticoids, 521
gonadotropin-releasing hormone
    (GnRH), 543
goserelin, 444*t*
gout
    acute gouty arthritis, 577
    classification, 576
    description, 576
    pharmacotherapy, 577, 577*t*
gouty arthritis, 577
grand mal epilepsy, 183
grand mal seizures, 183
granisetron, 490*t*
grapefruit juice, drug interactions with,
    23, 240*t*
grape seed extract, 280*t*
Graves' disease, 516
green tea, 352*t*, 353*t*, 357*t*
griseofulvin, 415*t*
growth hormone (GH), 515–516
guaifenesin, 465

H

H⁺, K⁺-ATPase, 482
H₁-receptor antagonists (antihistamines), 458,
    460–461
    in combination products, 461*t*
    drugs classified as, 459–460*t*
    for insomnia, 117*t*
    interactions
        with dantrolene, 175*t*
        with heparin, 352*t*
    Nursing Process Focus, 461–462*t*
    onset and duration, 117*t*
    Patients Need to Know, 472
    prophylactic use, 460

H$_2$-receptor blockers:
actions, 483
adverse effects, 483
clinical uses, 483
drugs classified as, 482t
HAART (highly active antiretroviral therapy), 420
Haemophilus, 390t
Haemophilus influenza type B conjugate vaccine, 377t
halcinonide, 592t
Halcion. *See* triazolam
Haldol. *See* **haloperidol**
half-life (t$_{1/2}$), 45
hallucinations, 143, 144, 147
hallucinogens, 76–77, 202. *See also* psychedelics
physiological and psychological effects of, 73t
halobetasol, 592t
Halog. *See* halcinonide
haloperidol
actions and uses, 149t
adverse effects, 149t
Drug Prototype, 149t
interactions, 149t
with benztropine, 164t
with beta blockers, 149t
with levodopa, 149t, 163t
with lithium, 149t
with phenobarbital, 149t
with phenytoin, 149t
with rifampin, 149t
route and adult dose, 148t
Halotestin. *See* fluoxymesterone
halothane, interactions with dopamine, 326t
Haltran. *See* **ibuprofen**
hBNP (natriuretic peptide), 297
HDL (high-density lipoprotein), 236, 237f, 238t
headache
incidence, 199t
tension, 211
types, 211
healthcare practitioners, 3
health care providers, 3
biological and chemical attack, threat of, and, 9–10
CAM Therapy and, 4
Health Care Reform law, 6f
hearbal products
interactions with drugs
aspirin, 208t
heart
electrical conduction pathway, 333–335, 334f
function, 289, 290f, 291
heart block, 333t
heart failure (HF), 288
causes, 289
disorders associated with, 288t
incidence, 288t
nonpharmacologic therapy, 291–292
pathophysiology, 289, 290f, 291
Patients Need to Know, 297t
pharmacotherapy
ACE inhibitors, 292, 293t, 294
beta blockers, 295t, 296

cardiac glycosides, 294
diuretics, 293t, 294
mechanisms of action, 291f
phosphodiesterase inhibitors, 295t, 297
vasodilators, 295t, 296
signs and symptoms, 289, 290f
Hectorol. *See* doxercalciferol
Helicobacter pylori, 479, 485
helminths, 427, 427t
helper T cells, 375–376
Hemabate. *See* carboprost
hemoglobin, 501t
hemorrhagic stroke, 314
hemostasis, 347–348f
hemostatics, 350, 357, 357t
heparin
actions, 350f, 352t
administration, 33, 34t, 36
adverse effects, 352t
black box warning, 352t
clinical uses, 352t
Drug Prototype, 352t
interactions, 352t
LMWH, 351, 351t
low molecular weight heparin, 36, 351, 351t
route and adult dose, 351t
Safety Alert, 358t
hepatic portal circulation, 43
hepatitis A, 425
vaccine, 377t
hepatitis B, 425
hepatitis B vaccine
Drug Prototypes, 378t
schedule, 377t
hepatitis C, 425
herbal products, 61–65, 62t. *See also* CAM Therapy
allergic reactions and use of, 64
basic formulations of, 62
history of use, 61
interactions with drugs, 63–64
acetaminophen, 369t
alteplase, 357t
with amiodarone, 341t
aspirin, 208t
chlorpromazine, 147t
diazepam, 188t
haloperidol, 149t
heparin, 352t
imipramine, 129t
levodopa, 163t
lorazepam, 116t
morphine, 203t
phenelzine, 133t
phenytoin, 190t
risperidone, 152t
warfarin, 353t
zidovudine, 421t
popular, 62t
pregnant or lactating women and, 63–64
regulation of, 65–67
standardization, 62, 63t
herb–drug interactions, 64t
herb extracts, standardization of selected, 63t

herb(s), 61
heroin, 72, 73, 75, 78, 202, 205
herpes simplex viruses (HSVs), 423
herpesviruses, 423–424, 424t
high-density lipoprotein (HDL), 236, 237f, 238t
highly active antiretroviral therapy (HAART), 420
histamine, 363–364, 364t
Histoplasma capsulatum, 414t
histrelin, 444t
HIV (human immunodeficiency virus), 9, 418, 421f. *See also* HIV-AIDS
HIV-AIDS, 418–422, 419t
hives, 583
HMG-CoA reductase, 238
HMG-CoA reductase inhibitors (statins)
actions, 238, 243f
adverse effects, 240
drugs classified as, 239t
interactions
with gemfibrozil, 244t
Nursing Process Focus, 241t
Patients Need to Know, 245t
homatropine, 606t
hormone antagonists: as antineoplastic agents, 443, 443t–444t
hormone replacement therapy (HRT), 549, 550–551t
hormones. *See also* androgens; estrogens; specific hormone
clinical uses
as antineoplastic drugs, 443, 443t–444t
pituitary, 543
host flora, 393, 418
household system of measurement, 25, 25t
HSVs (herpes simplex viruses), 423
huffing, 70
Humalog. *See* insulin lispro
human immunodeficiency virus (HIV), 9, 418, 421f. *See also* HIV-AIDS
human papillomavirus vaccine, 377t
Humatrope. *See* somatropin
Humira. *See* adalimumab
humoral immunity, 375, 375f
Humulin N. *See* insulin isophane
Humulin R. *See* insulin; insulin regular
Huntington's chorea, 158t
Hybolin. *See* nandrolone
Hycodan. *See* hydrocodone
Hycort. *See* **hydrocortisone**
hydantoins and related drugs. *See also* antiseizure drugs
drugs classified as, 189–190t
Patients Need to Know, 194t
route and adult dose, 189–190t
for seizures, 189–190t
hydralazine
actions, 283t, 296
adverse effects, 283t
in African Americans, 273
clinical uses, 283t
Drug Prototype, 283t
interactions, 283t
route and adult dose, 283t
Hydramine. *See* **diphenhydramine**

hydrochlorothiazide, 17*t*
  actions, 253*f,* 255*t*
  adverse effects, 255*t*
  clinical uses, 255*t*
    heart failure, 293*t,* 296
    hypertension, 274*t*
  in combination of drugs, 255, 273
  Drug Prototype, 255*t*
  interactions, 255*t*
  route and adult dose, 254*t,* 274*t,* 293*t*
hydrocodone, 204*t,* 465
hydrocortisone
  Drug Prototype, 522*t*
  route and adult dose, 368*t*
  routes and adult dose, 522*t*
  topical, 592*t*
hydrocortisone valerate, 592*t*
Hydrocortone. *See* **hydrocortisone**
hydromorphone, 75, 204*t*
HydroURIL. *See* **hydrochlorothiazide**
hydroxychloroquine
  Drug Prototype, 575
  for helminth and protozoan infections, 426*t*
  for rheumatoid arthritis, 576*t*
hydroxyprogesterone, 553*t*
hydroxyzine, 490*t*
Hygroton. *See* chlorthalidone
hypercalcemia, 259*t,* 565
hyperchloremia, 259*t*
hypercholesterolemia, 235, 235*t*
hyperkalemia, 256, 259, 259*t,* 274
hyperlipidemia, 235
  laboratory values, 238*t*
  lifestyle changes for, 236–237
  pharmacotherapy
    bile-acid binding agents, 239*t,* 241–242
    combinations of drugs, 244
    diuretics, 273–274, 274*t*
    fibric acid agents, 239*t,* 242
    HMG-CoA reductase inhibitors, 238–240, 239*t*
    mechanisms of action, 274*f*
    niacin, 239*t,* 242
hypermagnesemia, 259*t*
hypernatremia, 259, 259*t*
hyperphosphatemia, 259*t*
hypersecretion of thyroid hormone, 516
hypertension, 266
  classification, 266*t*
  consequences of, 267, 267*t*
  grape seed extract for, 280*t*
  incidence, 267*t*
  nonpharmacologic therapy, 271–272
  pharmacotherapy
    adrenergic blockers, 281–282, 281*t*
    in African Americans, 273
    angiotensin-converting enzyme inhibitors, 274–275, 275*t*
    angiotensin-receptor blockers, 275*t*
    calcium channel blockers, 278, 278*t*
    initial, 266*t*
    Patients Need to Know, 284*t*
    selection of drugs, 272–273
    vasodilators, 282–283, 283*t*
  primary, 267
  secondary, 267
hypertensive emergency, 283

hypertriglyceridemia, 235
hyperuricemia, 577
hypervitaminosis, 499
hypnotics, 111
hypocalcemia, 259*t,* 565–566, 568*t*
hypochloremia, 259*t*
hypodermis, 583
hypoglycemia, insulin and, 532
hypogonadism, 554
hypokalemia, 259*t,* 260, 274
  with diuretic therapy, 252
hypomagnesemia, 259*t*
hyponatremia, 259, 259*t*
hypophosphatemia, 259*t*
hypothalamus, 271*f,* 511, 513*f*
hypothyroidism, 516
hypovolemic shock, 320, 320*t. See also* shock
Hytrin. *See* terazosin

I

I-131. *See* radioactive iodide
ibandronate, 571*t*
IBD (inflammatory bowel disease), 480
IB Pro. *See* **ibuprofen**
ibuprofen, 15, 15*t*
  adverse effects, 366
  vs. aspirin, 47
  clinical uses, 209*t,* 365*t,* 370*t*
  route and adult dose, 209*t,* 365*t*
ibutilide, 340*t*
ICDs (implantable cardioverter defibrillators), 336
icosapent, 239*t,* 244
idarubicin, 441*t*
idinavir, 419*t*
ID (intradermal) route, 33, 34*t*
IFNs (interferons), 379
ifosfamide, 437*t*
Ig (immunoglobulin), 375
illusions, 143
iloperidone, 151*t*
imatinib, 445*t*
Imdur. *See* isosorbide mononitrate
imipenem, 404
imipenem-cilastatin, 404*t*
imipramine, 201
  actions, 129*t*
  adverse effects, 129*t*
  anxiety, 112*t*
  clinical uses, 129*t*
    depression, 126*t*
    migraine prophylaxis, 213*t*
  Drug Prototype, 129*t*
  route and adult dose, 213*t*
Imitrex. *See* **sumatriptan**
immune response, 375
immunization (vaccination), 376
immunoglobulin (Ig), 375
immunomodulator, 374
immunostimulants, 168, 376
immunosuppressants, 380, 381*t*
Imodium. *See* loperamide
implantable cardioverter defibrillators (ICDs), 336
implementation phase, of nursing process, 52*f,* 55–56

impotence, 555. *See also* erectile dysfunction
IM (intramuscular) route, 34*t,* 36
Imuran. *See* azathioprine
inamrinone, 295*t*
Inapsine. *See* droperidol
incobotulinumtoxin A, 173, 174*t*
Increlex. *See* mecasermin
incretin enhancers, 535*t,* 537
incretin–glucose control mechanism, 537
incretins, 537
indapamide, 254, 254*t,* 274*t*
Inderal. *See* **propranolol**
Indocin. *See* indomethacin
indomethacin, 209*t*
infantile spasms, 184
infiltration (field block) anesthesia, 219*t*
inflammation, 363, 584
  clinical mediators of, 363–364, 364*t*
  pharmacotherapy
    goals, 365
    principles, 364–365
  steps in, 364*f*
inflammatory bowel disease (IBD), 480
infliximab, 576*t*
influenza
  antiviral drugs for, 424, 424*t*
  vaccine, 377*t*
inhalants
  abuse of, 70
  volatile, 70
  withdrawal from, 72
inhalation route, of drug administration, 456–457, 457*f,* 472*t*
innate body defenses, 374
Innohep. *See* tinzaparin
InnoPran XL. *See* **propranolol**
Inocor. *See* inamrinone
inotropic drugs, 325, 325*t*
inotropic effect, 289
INR (international normalized ratio), 352
insomnia, 109, 110
  anxiety and, 109–110
  barbiturates for, 116–117, 116*t*
  benzodiazepines for, 113–114, 114*t*
  Fast Facts, 110*t*
  long-term, 110
  nonbenzodiazepine, nonbarbiturate agents for, 117–118, 117*t*
  nonpharmacologic means of relieving, 110
  in older adults, 110*t*
  rebound, 110
  short-term or behavioral, 110
inspiration, 455
Inspra. *See* eplerenone
insulin, 529, 530*f*
  adverse effects, 531, 532
  hypoglycemia and, 532
  Nursing Process Focus, 533–534*t*
  types of, actions and administration, 531, 531*t*
insulin analogs, 531
insulin aspart, 531*t*
insulin-dependent diabetes mellitus. *See* type 1 diabetes mellitus
insulin detemir, 531*t*
insulin glargine, 531*t*
insulin glulisine, 531*t*

insulin isophane, 531*t*
insulin lispro, 531*t*
insulin pump, 531, 532*f*
insulin regular
    actions and administration, 531*t*
    Drug Prototype, 532*t*
insulin resistance, 534, 535
insulin(s)
    interactions
        with aspirin, 208*t*
        with carvedilol, 296*t*
        with furosemide, 254*t*
        with hydrochlorothiazide, 255*t*
    long-acting, administration, 33–34
Integrilin. *See* eptifibatide
interferon(s) (IFNs), 379, 380*t*
interferon alfa, 425
interferon alfa-2b, 379*t*
    Drug Prototype, 446*t*
    route and adult dose, 445*t*
interferon alfacon-1, 379*t*
interferon alfa-n3, 379*t*
interferon beta-1a, 168, 168*t,* 379*t*
interferon beta-1b, 168, 168*t,* 379*t*
interleukin(s), 379
intermittent infusion, 37
International Classification of Epileptic
    Seizures, 183
International Diabetes Federation, 529
international normalized ratio (INR), 352
International Union of Pure and Applied
    Chemistry (IUPAC), 14
interpersonal therapy, 124–125
intervention(s), 53
intracellular parasites, 418
intractable pain, 201
intradermal (ID) route, 33, 34*t*
intramuscular (IM) route, 34*t,* 36
intranasal corticosteroids, 462, 463*t*
intraocular pressure (IOP), 601
intravenous bolus (push) administration, 35*t,* 37
intravenous (IV) route, 35*t,* 37
intrinsic factor, 499*t*
Intropin. *See* **dopamine**
Invega. *See* paliperidone
Inversine. *See* mecamylamine
Invokana. *See* canagliflozin
iodine, 516
IOP (intraocular pressure), 601
Iopidine. *See* apraclonidine
ipratropium, 95*t*
    for asthma, 95*t,* 468*t*
    for nasal congestion, 464, 464*t*
Iprivask. *See* desirudin
irbesartan, 275*t*
irinotecan, 442, 442*t*
iron dextran, 502*t*
iron supplements, 501, 501*t,* 503*t*
islets of Langerhans, 529, 529*f*
Ismo. *See* isosorbide mononitrate
Ismotic. *See* isosorbide
Isocaine. *See* mepivacaine
isocarboxazid, 127*t*
isoflurane, 225*t*
    adverse effects, 225*t*
    clinical uses, 225*t*
    Drug Prototype, 225*t*

interactions
    with amino-glycosides, 225*t*
    with dopamine, 225*t*
    with epinephrine, 225*t*
    with levodopa, 225*t*
    with nitrous oxide, 225*t*
    with phenothiazine, 225*t*
    with systemic polymyxin, 225*t*
isoniazid
    Drug Prototype, 406*t*
    route and adult dose, 407*t*
isoproterenol, 97, 97*t*
Isoptin. *See* **verapamil**
Isopto Atropine. *See* **atropine**
Isopto Carpine. *See* pilocarpine
Isopto Homatropine. *See* homatropine
Isopto Hyoscine. *See* scopolamine
    hydrobromide
isosorbide, 603*t*
isosorbide dinitrate
    actions, 291*f,* 296, 306
    in African Americans, 273
    clinical uses
        angina, 306*t*
        heart failure, 295*t,* 296
    route and adult dose, 306*t*
isosorbide mononitrate, 306*t*
isotretinoin, 590*t*
isradipine, 278*t*
Isuprel. *See* isoproterenol
itraconazole, 414, 415*t*
IUPAC (International Union of Pure and
    Applied Chemistry), 14
ivermectin, 426*t,* 587
IV (intravenous) route, 35*t,* 37

J

Januvia. *See* sitagliptin
juvenile-onset diabetes. *See* type 1 diabetes
    mellitus
Juxtapid. *See* lomitapide

K

Kabikinase. *See* streptokinase
Kalcinate. *See* calcium gluconate
kanamycin, 399*t*
Kaon Tablets. *See* potassium gluconate
kappa receptors, 202, 202*f,* 202*t*
Kapvay. *See* clonidine
Kayexalate. *See* sodium polystyrene sulfate
KCl. *See* **potassium chloride**
Kenalog. *See* triamcinolone; triamcinolone
    acetonide
Keppra. *See* levetiracetam
keratinization, 589
keratolytic agents, 590
Kerlone. *See* betaxolol
Ketalar. *See* ketamine
ketamine, 77, 226*t,* 227
ketoacids, 530
ketoconazole, 414, 415*t*
ketoprofen, 209*t,* 365*t*
ketorolac, 209*t*
kidney(s)
    anatomy, 249–250, 249*f*
    functions, 249–250, 249*f,* 250*f*

Kineret. *See* anakinra
Klaron. *See* sulfacetamide sodium
Klebsiella pneumoniae, 390*t*
Klonopin. *See* clonazepam
K-Phos MF. *See* potassium/sodium phosphates
K-Phos neutral. *See* potassium/sodium
    phosphates
K-Phos original. *See* potassium/sodium
    phosphates
Krystexxa. *See* pegloticase
Kwell. *See* lindane
Kynamro. *See* mipomersan

L

labor, 552
Lacri-lube. *See* lanolin alcohol
LA (long-acting) medications, 27
Lamictal. *See* lamotrigine
lamivudine, 419*t,* 425
lamotrigine, 135*t,* 185*t,* 190*t*
    for bipolar disorder, 135, 135*t*
    for seizures, 185*t,* 190*t,* 191
lanolin alcohol, 606*t*
Lanoxicaps. *See* **digoxin**
Lanoxin. *See* **digoxin**
lanreotide, 515*t*
lansoprazole, 482*t*
Lantus. *See* insulin glargine
large-volume infusion, 37
Lasix. *See* **furosemide**
latanoprost
    Drug Prototype, 601*t*
    route and adult dose, 602*t*
laughing gas. *See* **nitrous oxide**
laxatives, 486–487, 487*t,* 492*t*
Lazanda. *See* fentanyl
L-carnitine, 66*f*
LDL (low-density lipoprotein), 236, 237*f,* 238*t*
leflunomide, 576*t*
lepirudin, 350*f,* 351, 351*t*
leprosy, 406
Lescol. *See* fluvastatin
letrozole, 444*t*
leukemia, 432
leukopenia, 436*t*
leukotriene modifiers, 470*t*
leukotriene(s), 364*t*
leuprolide, 444*t*
levalbuterol, 468*t*
levamisole, 445*t*
Levemir. *See* insulin detemir
levetiracetam, 185*t,* 190*t,* 191
Levitra. *See* vardenafil
levobunolol, 603*t*
levocetirizine, 460*t*
levodopa
    actions and uses, 163*t*
    adverse effects, 163*t*
    Drug Prototype, 163*t*
    interactions, 163*t*
        with atropine, 95*t*
        with diazepam, 188*t*
        with haloperidol, 149*t*
        with isoflurane, 225*t*
    for parkinsonism, 160, 161*t*
    route and adult dose, 161*t*

levodopa–carbidopa, 161*t*, 162, 176*t*
Levo-Dromoran. *See* levorphanol
levofloxacin, 400*t*
levonorgestrel, 547
Levophed. *See* **norepinephrine**
levorphanol, 204*t*
Levothroid. *See* **levothyroxine**
levothyroxine, 17*t*
levothyroxine
    Drug Prototype, 518*t*
    route and adult dose, 518*t*
Lexicaps. *See* **escitalopram**
Lexapro. *See* **escitalopram**
libido, 554
Librium. *See* chlordiazepoxide
lice, pharmacotherapy, 587
Lidex. *See* fluocinonide
lidocaine
    actions, 222*t*
    adverse effects, 222*t*
    clinical uses, 221*t*, 222, 222*t*
        dysrhythmias, 338*t*
    Drug Prototype, 222*t*
    epinephrine with, 220
    route and adult dose, 338*t*
Life Span Facts, *See* Guide to Special Features
limbic system, 107
linagliptin, 535*t*, 537
lincomycin, 404*t*
lindane, 587
linezolid, 403, 404*t*
liothyronine, 518*t*
liotrix, 518*t*
lipids, 235
    elevated levels, preventing, 236–237
    lipoproteins and, 236
    profile, 238*t*
    role of, in diet, 235
    types of, 235
Lipitor. *See* **atorvastatin**
lipoma(s), 432
lipoproteins, 236
    high-density, 236, 237*f*
    low-density, 236, 237*f*
    very low-density, 236, 237*f*
liposomes, 441*t*
liquid medications, 26*t*
Liquifilm. *See* polyvinyl alcohol
liraglutide, 535*t*, 537
lisinopril
    actions, 291*f*, 292*t*
    adverse effects, 292*t*
    black box warning, 292*t*
    clinical uses
        heart failure, 292*t*, 293*t*
        hypertension, 275*t*
        myocardial infarction, 313
    Drug Prototype, 292*t*
    interactions, 292*t*
    route and adult dose, 275*t*, 293*t*
lithium, 135*t*
    interactions
        with enalapril, 277*t*
        with furosemide, 254*t*
        with haloperidol, 149*t*
        with hydrochlorothiazide, 255*t*
        with sodium bicarbonate, 261*t*

monitoring, 134
    as mood stabilizer, 134–135, 135*t*
    toxicity, 134–135
    U.S. approval for, 134
lithium toxicity, 134–135
Livalo. *See* pitavastatin
liver fluke, 389*f*
LMWHs (low molecular weight heparins),
    351, 351*t*. *See also* **heparin**
local anesthesia, 218. *See also* local anesthetics
    Nursing Process Focus, 223*t*
    Patients Need to Know, 229*t*
    routes and methods, 218–219, 219*f*, 219*t*
local anesthetics
    actions, 220, 220*f*
    adverse effects, 222, 222*t*
    drugs classified as, 221*t*
Lodosyn. *See* **carbidopa**
Lofibra. *See* fenofibrate
lomitapide, 239*t*
lomustine, 437*t*
long-acting (LA) medications, 27
long-term insomnia, 110
Loniten. *See* minoxidil
loop (high ceiling) diuretics, 252–253,
    253*f*, 253*t*
loop of Henle, 250, 250*f*
loperamide, 17*t*, 488*t*, 489
Lopid. *See* **gemfibrozil**
lopinavir/ritonavir, 419*t*
Lopressor. *See* **metoprolol**
Lopressor HCT, 255
Lopurin. *See* **allopurinol**
loratadine, 460*t*
lorazepam
    actions, 116*t*
    adverse effects, 116*t*
    clinical uses, 116*t*
        as antiemetic, 490*t*
        anxiety, 114*t*
        intravenous anesthetic, 226*t*
        muscle spasms, 170, 171*t*
    digoxin toxicity and, 116*t*
    Drug Prototype, 116*t*
    seizures, 185*t*, 187*t*, 188
losartan, 275*t*
Lotensin. *See* benazepril
Lotrel, 273
Lovasa. *See* omega-3-acid ethyl esters
lovastatin, 239*t*
"love drug." *See* MDA (3,4-methylenedioxy-
    amphetamine)
Lovenox. *See* enoxaparin
low-density lipoprotein (LDL), 236, 237*f*, 238*t*
lower respiratory tract (LRT), 455
low molecular weight heparin, 36
low molecular weight heparins (LMWHs),
    351, 351*t*. *See also* **heparin**
loxapine, 148*t*
Loxitane. *See* loxapine
Lozol. *See* indapamide
LRT (lower respiratory tract), 455
LSD (lysergic acid diethylamide), 70,
    76–77, 77*f*
    effects of, 77
    street names of, 76
lubiprostone, 487*t*

lubricants, eye, 606*t*
Ludiomil. *See* maprotiline
Lugol's solution. *See* potassium iodide and
    iodine
lumefantrine/artemether, 426*t*
lumen, 269
Lumigan. *See* bimatoprost
Luminal. *See* **phenobarbital**
Lusedra. *See* fospropofol
luteinizing hormone (LH), 543
Luvox. *See* fluvoxamine
lymphocyte immune globulin, 381*t*
lymphocytes, 375
lymphoma(s), 432
Lyrica. *See* pregabalin
lysergic acid diethylamide (LSD), 70,
    76–77, 77*f*
    effects of, 77
    street names of, 76
Lysteda. *See* tranexamic acid

M

MAB (Monoclonal antibodies), 445
MAC (*Mycobacterium avium* complex), 406
macrolides, 398–399, 398*t*
magaldrate, 482*t*
Magnaprin. *See* **aspirin**
magnesium, 501*t*
magnesium chloride, 502*t*
magnesium hydroxide, 482*t*, 487*t*, 502*t*
magnesium hydroxide and aluminum
    hydroxide with simethicone, 482*t*
magnesium oxide, 502*t*
magnesium sulfate, 502*t*, 553*t*
Mag-Ox. *See* magnesium oxide
major depressive disorder, 123. *See also*
    depression
        criteria for diagnosis of, 124
        symptoms of, 124
        TCAs for, 125
major minerals (macrominerals), 499, 501*t*
Makena. *See* hydroxyprogesterone
malaria, 426
malathion, 587
malignant, 432
manic depression. *See* bipolar disorder
mannitol, 257, 257*t*, 603*t*
manual healing, 60*t*
MAO (monoamine oxidase), 128
MAOI (monoamine oxidase inhibitor),
    98*t*, 132
Maox. *See* magnesium oxide
maprotiline, 126*t*
MAR (medication administration record), 22,
    24, 25–26, 29, 37
maraviroc, 419*t*
Marcaine. *See* bupivicaine
margin of safety, 4
marijuana, 76, 202
    physical dependence or tolerance, 76
    physiological and psychological effects
        of, 73*t*
    street names of, 76
    symptom of use of, 76
masculinization, 554
mast cell(s), 363

mast cell stabilizer, 457*f*, 470*t*, 471
mastoiditis, 606
maturity-onset diabetes. *See* type 2 diabetes
  mellitus
Mavik. *See* trandolapril
Maxalt. *See* rizatriptan
Maxiflor. *See* diflorasone
MDA (3,4-methylenedioxyamphetamine), 77
MDIs (metered-dose inhalers), 456
MDMA (3,4-methylenedioxymethamphet-
  amine), 77
measles, mumps, and rubella (MMR) vaccine,
  376, 377*t*
measurement systems, 24–25
  apothecary system, 25, 25*t*
  household system, 25, 25*t*
  metric system, 24–25, 25*t*
Mebaral. *See* mephobarbital
mebendazole, 426*t*, 427
mecamylamine, 175
mecasermin, 515*t*
mechanism of action, 13. *See also* pharmacologic classification
mechlorethamine, 437*t*
meclizine, 490, 490*t*
medical diagnosis, 53
medication administration record (MAR), 22,
  24, 25–26, 29, 37
medication errors
  consequences of, 21
Medrol. *See* methylprednisolone
medroxyprogesterone
  clinical uses
    as antineoplastic agent, 444*t*
    with conjugated estrogens, 551*t*
  Drug Prototype, 552*t*
  route and adult dose, 551*t*
mefenamic acid, 209*t*
megaloblastic (pernicious) anemia, 499
megestrol, 444*t*
melanocytes, 583
melatonin receptor drugs, 117*t*
Mellaril. *See* thioridazine
meloxicam, 209*t*, 365*t*
melphalan, 437*t*
memantine, 165, 165*t*
memory B cells, 375
menopause, 124, 549
menorrhagia, 550
menstrual cycle, 124
meperidine, 204*t*
mephobarbital, 116*t*, 186, 187*t*
mepivacaine, 221*t*
mercaptopurine, 439*t*
meropenem, 404, 404*t*
mescaline, 77, 77*f*
Mestinon. *See* pyridostigmine
metabolic acidosis, 261*t*
metabolic alkalosis, 261*t*
metabolism, 42*f*, 43
  biotransformation reactions and, 43
  drug therapy and, 43
  prodrugs and, 43
Metadate. *See* methylphenidate
metaproterenol, 97*t*
metastasis, 432
metaxalone, 171*t*

metered-dose inhalers (MDIs), 456
metformin
  Drug Prototype, 537*t*
  for type 2 diabetes, 535*t*
methadone, 75, 204*t*
  as maintenance treatment, 75, 206
  for opioid withdrawal, 72, 206
  withdrawal from, 75
methamphetamine, 70, 74, 78, 137, 138*t*
methazolamide, 257*t*, 603*t*
methcathinone, 78
methenamine, 402*t*
Methergine. *See* methylergonovine
methicillin-resistant *Staphylococcus aureus*
  (MRSA), 392
methimazole, 518*t*
methocarbamol, 171*t*
methotrexate
  clinical uses, 381*t*
    psoriasis, 593*t*, 594
    rheumatoid arthritis, 576*t*
  Drug Prototype, 440*t*
  interactions
    with aspirin, 208*t*
    with vincristine, 443*t*
  route and adult dose, 381*t*, 439*t*
methscopolamine, 95*t*
methsuximide, 192*t*
methyclothiazide, 254*t*
methylcellulose, 487*t*
methyldopa, 97*t*
  actions, 281*t*
  for hypertension, 97*t*, 281*t*
methylergonovine, 553*t*
Methylin. *See* methylphenidate
methylparaben, 222
methylphenidate
  abuse of, 78
  actions, 137*t*
  adverse effects, 137*t*
  clinical uses, 78, 137*t*
    ADHD, 138*t*
  Drug Prototype, 137*t*
methylprednisolone, 522*t*
  as antiemetic, 490*t*
  for multiple sclerosis, 168*t*, 169
  route and adult dose, 368*t*
methyltestosterone, 555*t*
methysergide, 213*t*
metipranolol, 603*t*
metoclopramide, 486, 490*t*
metolazone, 254, 254*t*
metoprolol, 281*t*, 295*t*, 306*t*
  actions, 282
  clinical uses, 100*t*
    migraine prophylaxis, 212*t*
  interaction with diazepam, 188*t*
  route and adult dose, 212*t*
metric system of measurement, 24–25, 25*t*
MetroCream. *See* metronidazole
Metrogel. *See* **metronidazole**
metronidazole, 590*t*
  Drug Prototype, 427*t*
  for peptic ulcer disease, 485
  route and adult dose, 404*t*, 426*t*
Mevacor. *See* lovastatin
mexiletine, 201, 338*t*

Mexitil. *See* mexiletine
Miacalcin. *See* calcitonin–salmon
micafungin, 415*t*
Micardis. *See* telmisartan
miconazole, 415*t*
Micronase. *See* glyburide
Micronor. *See* norethindrone
Microsporum, 414*t*
microvilli, 478
Microzide. *See* **hydrochlorothiazide**
Midamor. *See* amiloride
midazolam, 74, 113
midazolam hydrochloride, 226*t*, 228*t*
midodrine, 97*t*
Midol. *See* **ibuprofen**
miglitol, 535*t*
migraine, 211
  incidence, 199*t*
  pharmacotherapy
    approach, 211
  prophylaxis, 211
    antiseizure drugs for, 212*t*
    beta-blockers for, 212*t*
    calcium channel blockers for, 212*t*
    methysergide for, 213*t*
    riboflavin for, 213*t*
    tricyclic antidepressants for, 213*t*
Migranal. *See* dihydroergotamine; dihydroergotamine mesylate
milk–alkali syndrome, 261*t*
Milk of Magnesia. *See* magnesium hydroxide
milrinone
  actions, 291*f*, 297*t*
  adverse effects, 297*t*
  clinical uses, 297*t*
  Drug Prototype, 297*t*
  interactions, 297*t*
  route and adult dose, 295*t*
mind–body interventions, 60*t*
mineralocorticoids, 520
mineral oil, 17*t*, 487*t*
minerals, 500–501, 501*t*
  for pharmacotherapy, 502*t*
minimum effective concentration, 45
minipills. *See* progestin-only OC
Minipress. *See* **prazosin**
Miniprin. *See* **aspirin**
Minocin. *See* minocycline
minocycline, 397*t*, 590*t*
minoxidil, 283*t*
miosis, 601
Miostat. *See* carbachol
miotics, 602, 602*t*
mipomersan, 239*t*
mirabegron, 97*t*
Mirapex. *See* pramipexole
mirtazapine, 112*t*, 127*t*, 129
misoprostol, 485
mitomycin, 441*t*
mitotane, 445*t*
mitotic inhibitors, 442
mitoxantrone
  for acute nonlymphocytic leukemia, 441*t*
  for multiple sclerosis, 168*t*, 169
mitral stenosis, 303*t*
Mivacron. *See* mivacurium
mivacurium, 176*t*, 228*t*, 229

MMR (measles, mumps, and rubella) vaccine, 376
Mobic. *See* meloxicam
modafinil, 168*t*, 169
moexipril, 275*t*
mometasone, 463*t*, 470*t*
mometasone furoate, 592*t*
Monascus purpureus, 238*t*
monoamine oxidase (MAO), 128
monoamine oxidase inhibitors (MAOIs), 98*t*, 132
　adverse effects, 113, 132
　clinical uses
　　anxiety, 112*t*
　　depression, 127*t*
　drugs classified as, 110, 125
　interactions, 113
　　with benztropine, 164*t*
　　with carvedilol, 296*t*
　　with diphenhydramine, 460*t*
　　with diphenoxylate with atropine, 488*t*
　　with dopamine, 326*t*
　　with epinephrine, 327*t*
　　with methylphenidate, 137*t*
　　with morphine, 203*t*
　　with phenylephrine, 98*t*
　　with propranolol, 340*t*
　　with sertraline, 133*t*
　　with sumatriptan, 213*t*
　Patients Need to Know, 139*t*
　serotonin syndrome and, 113
Monoclonal antibodies (MAB), 445
Monoket. *See* isosorbide mononitrate
monophasic OC, 546, 546*t*
Monopril. *See* fosinopril
montelukast, 470*t*
mood disorders, 123, 124, 125, 137. *See also* bipolar disorder; depression
　electroconvulsive therapy (ECT) and, 125
　perinatal, 124
mood stabilizers, 134, 135*t*. *See also* lithium
morphine
　actions, 203*t*
　adverse effects, 203*t*
　black box warning, 203*t*
　clinical uses, 203*t*, 204*t*
　Drug Prototype, 203*t*
　interactions
　　with monoamine oxidase inhibitors (MAOIs), 203*t*
　　with tricyclic antidepressants (TCAs), 203*t*
　route and adult dose, 204*t*
motion sickness, 461, 489
Motrin. *See* **ibuprofen**
Mountain Dew, 79*t*
moxifloxacin, 400*t*
MRSA (methicillin-resistant *Staphylococcus aureus*), 392
mucolytics, 457*f*, 465
Multaq. *See* dronedarone
multicellular parasites, 389*f*
multiple sclerosis, 158*t*, 167
　drugs for treating, 168*t*
　etiology of, 167–168
　relapsing-remitting MS (RRMS), 168
　symptoms of, 167–168

mu receptors, 202, 202*f*, 202*t*
Murine Plus. *See* tetrahydrozoline
Muro 128 5% ointment. *See* sodium chloride hypertonicity ointment
muromonab-CD3, 381*t*
muscarinic blockers, 94
muscarinic receptors, 90, 90*f*, 91*t*
muscle rigidity, 159
muscle spasms, 169
　causes, 169
　clonic spasms, 169
　etiology of, 169–170
　Fast Facts, 170*t*
　nonpharmacologic treatment, 169–170
　Nursing Process Focus, 172–173*t*
　Patients Need to Know, 176*t*
　pharmacotherapy, 170
　tonic spasm, 169
　treatment of, 169–170
mutations, 391
myasthenia gravis, 92*t*
　prednisone interactions in, 369*t*
Mycobacterium avium complex (MAC), 406
Mycobacterium bovis, 379
Mycobacterium leprae, 390*t*, 406
Mycobacterium tuberculosis, 390*t*, 406
mycophenolate, 381*t*
mycoses, 413, 414*t*
Mydfrin. *See* **phenylephrine**
Mydriacyl. *See* tropicamide
mydriasis, 601
mydriatic drugs, 605, 606*t*
Myobloc. *See* rimabotulinumtoxin B
myocardial infarction (MI), 303*t*, 310, 347*t*
　pathophysiology, 310, 311*f*
　pharmacotherapy
　　goals, 310
　　thrombolytics, 310, 312*t*. See also thrombolytics
　of symptoms and complications, 312–313
myocardial ischemia, 302
myoclonic seizures, 184
Myolin. *See* orphenadrine
Myrbetriq. *See* mirabegron
Mysoline. *See* primidone
Mytelase. *See* ambenonium
myxedema, 516

N

Na⁺ (sodium ions), 220, 220*f*
nabumetone, 209*t*, 365*t*
nadolol, 100*t*, 281*t*, 306*t*
nafcillin, 394*t*
naftifine, 415*t*
NaHCO₃. *See* **sodium bicarbonate**
nalbuphine, 204*t*
Nalfon. *See* fenoprofen
nalidixic acid, 400*t*, 402*t*
naloxone
　actions, 202, 205*t*
　adverse effects, 205*t*
　black box warning, 205*t*
　clinical uses, 204*t*, 205*t*
　Drug Prototype, 205*t*
　interactions, 205*t*
　route and adult dose, 205*t*

naltrexone, 204*t*
Namenda. *See* memantine
NANDA (North American Nursing Diagnosis Association), 53
nandrolone, 555*t*
naphazoline, 464*t*, 606*t*
Naprelan. *See* naproxen
Naprosyn. *See* **naproxen**
naproxen, 209*t*
　actions, 366*t*
　adverse effects, 366*t*
　black box warning, 366*t*
　clinical uses, 365*t*, 366*t*
　Drug Prototype, 366*t*
　interactions, 366*t*
　route and adult dose, 365*t*
naproxen sodium, 209*t*
　actions, 366*t*
　adverse effects, 366*t*
　black box warning, 366*t*
　clinical dose, 209*t*, 365*t*, 366*t*
　Drug Prototype, 366*t*
　interactions, 366*t*
　route and adult dose, 209*t*, 365*t*
naratriptan, 212*t*
Narcan. *See* naloxone
narcolepsy, 78
narcotics, 201–202
Nardil. *See* **phenelzine**
Naropin. *See* ropivacaine
narrow-spectrum antibiotic, 393
nasal administration, 30*t*, 31. *See also* transmucosal administration
nasogastric tubes, 26*t*, 28
Natazia. *See* quadriphasic OC
nateglinide, 536*t*
National Center for Complementary and Alternative Medicine (NCCAM), 7, 61
National Cholesterol Education Program (NCEP), 236, 237
National Formulary (NF), 5, 6*f*
National Institutes of Health, 236
Natrecor. *See* nesiritide
natriuretic peptide (hBNP), 297
Natural Alternatives, 4
natural alternative therapies, 4
　characteristics of, 4*t*
nausea and vomiting, 489–490, 490*t*
Navane. *See* thiothixene
NCCAM (National Center for Complementary and Alternative Medicine), 7, 61
NCEP (National Cholesterol Education Program), 236
NDA (new drug application), 6*f*, 7–8, 9
nebulizers, 456
nedocromil sodium, 470*t*, 471
nefazodone, 127*t*, 129
negative formulary, 16
negative symptoms, of schizophrenia, 144
Neisseria gonorrhoeae, 390*t*
Neisseria meningitidis, 390*t*
nelarabine, 439*t*
nelfinavir, 419*t*
Nembutal. *See* pentobarbital
neomycin, 399*t*
neoplasm, 432
neostigmine, 92, 92*t*

interactions
with bethanechol, 93*t*
Neo-Synephrine. *See* **phenylephrine**
nephron(s), 249–250, 250*f*
nephrotoxicity, 400
Neptazane. *See* methazolamide
nerve agents, 92
nervous system, 87, 88*f*
autonomic, 87
basic functions of, 87
central. *See* central nervous system (CNS)
peripheral. *See* peripheral nervous system (PNS)
somatic, 87
Nesacaine. *See* chloroprocaine
nesiritide, 295*t*, 297
neuroamidase inhibitors, 424
neurodegenerative diseases, 158*t*
Alzheimer's disease. *See* Alzheimer's disease
amyotrophic lateral sclerosis (ALS). *See* amyotrophic lateral sclerosis (ALS)
Fast Facts, 159*t*
Huntington's chorea. *See* Huntington's chorea
multiple sclerosis. *See* multiple sclerosis
Parkinson's disease. *See* Parkinson's disease
neurofibrillary tangles, 164
neurogenic shock, 320, 320*t*. *See also* shock
neurohypophysis. *See* posterior pituitary
neuroleptanalgesia, 227
neuroleptic malignant syndrome, 147*t*
neuroleptic(s), 146. *See also* antipsychotics
neuromuscular blocking drugs, 175, 176*t*
actions, 175
classification, 175
clinical uses, 175, 176*t*
as adjunct to anesthetics, 227, 228*t*
depolarizing blockers, 175, 176*t*
drugs classified as, 176*t*, 228*t*
nondepolarizing blockers, 175, 176*t*
Patients Need to Know, 176*t*
neuron, 88
postsynaptic, 88
presynaptic, 88
Neurontin. *See* gabapentin
neuropathic pain, 198
types of, 199*t*
neurotransmitter(s), 88, 91*t*
acetylcholine (Ach), 88, 91*t*
false, 282
norepinephrine (NE), 88, 91*t*
in pain transmission, 199–200, 200*f*
Neutra-Phos-K. *See* potassium/sodium phosphates
Neutrogena. *See* salicylic acid
nevirapine, 419*t*
new drug application (NDA), 6*f*, 7–8, 9
NF (National Formulary), 5, 6*f*
niacin (vitamin B₃), 498*t*
as lipid-lowering agent, 239*t*, 242, 245*t*
Niacor. *See* niacin (vitamin B₃)
Niaspan. *See* niacin (vitamin B₃)
nicardipine, 278*t*, 306*t*
nicotinamide, 242
nicotine, 90

cardiovascular effects of, 80
dependence, 80
effects, 80
nicotine replacement therapy (NRT) and, 72
Patients Need to Know, 80*t*
physiological and psychological effects of, 73*t*
symptoms of withdrawal of, 72
withdrawal syndrome, 72
nicotinic blocking drugs, 175
nicotinic receptors, 90, 90*f*
nifedipine, 553*t*
actions, 279*t*
adverse effects, 279*t*
clinical uses, 279*t*
angina, 306*t*
migraine prophylaxis, 212*t*
Drug Prototype, 279*t*
interactions, 279*t*
route and adult dose, 212*t*, 278*t*, 306*t*
nilutamide, 444*t*
Nimbex. *See* cisatracurium
nimodipine, 212*t*
Nimotop. *See* nimodipine
Nisocor. *See* nisoldipine
nisoldipine, 278*t*
Nitro-Bid. *See* **nitroglycerin**
Nitro-Dur. *See* **nitroglycerin**
nitrofurantoin, 402*t*, 487*t*
nitrogen mustards, 435
nitroglycerin
actions, 307*t*
adverse effects, 307*t*
clinical uses, 307*t*
angina, 306*t*
Drug Prototype, 307*t*
interactions, 307*t*
Nursing Process Focus, 308*t*
Patients Need to Know, 315*t*
route and adult dose, 306*t*
Nitropress. *See* nitroprusside
nitroprusside, 283, 283*t*
Nitrostat. *See* **nitroglycerin**
nitrous oxide
actions, 225*t*
adverse effects, 225*t*
clinical uses, 225*t*
Drug Prototype, 225*t*
interactions
with isoflurane, 225*t*
nits, 587
Nix. *See* permethrin
nizatidine, 482*t*
NMDA (*N*-methyl-D-aspartate) receptors, 165
N-methyl-D-aspartate (NMDA) receptors, 165
NNRTIs (nonnucleoside reverse transcriptase inhibitors), 419*t*, 420
nociceptor pain, 198, 210*f*
nodules, 589
Nolvadex. *See* **tamoxifen**
nonbenzodiazepine, nonbarbiturate CNS agents
for anxiety and insomnia, 117–118, 117*t*
drugs classified as, 110
noncompliance, 22–23, 53

nondepolarizing blockers, 175, 176*t*, 229. *See also* neuromuscular blocking drugs
nonnucleoside reverse transcriptase inhibitors (NNRTIs), 419*t*, 420
nonopioid analgesics
acetaminophen. *See* **acetaminophen**
centrally acting, 210
nonsteroidal anti-inflammatory drugs. *See* nonsteroidal anti-inflammatory drugs (NSAIDs)
nonphenothiazines
adverse effects, 148
drugs classified as, 146, 146*t*
Nursing Process Focus, 149–151*t*
route and adult dose, 148*t*
nonsteroidal anti-inflammatory drugs (NSAIDs), 8
actions, 208
adverse effects, 208
clinical uses, 208
drugs classified as
aspirin and salicylates, 209*t*, 365*t*, 366
ibuprofen and ibuprofen-like drugs, 209*t*, 365*t*, 366
selective COX-2 inhibitors, 209*t*, 210*f*, 365*t*, 366
interactions
with alteplase, 357*t*
with aspirin, 208*t*
with cefotaxime, 396*t*
with clopidogrel, 356*t*
with enalapril, 277*t*
with lisinopril, 292*t*
with methotrexate, 440*t*
with warfarin, 353*t*
and nociceptors, 200
Nursing Process Focus, 367*t*
Patients Need to Know, 383*t*
Patients Need to Know, 370*t*
usage statistics, 363*t*
Norcuron. *See* vecuronium
Norditropin. *See* somatropin
norepinephrine, 88, 90*f*, 91*t*
actions, 98*t*, 326*t*
adverse effects, 326*t*
black box warning, 326*t*
clinical uses, 98*t*
shock, 325, 326*t*
Drug Prototype, 326*t*
interactions, 326*t*
route and adult dose, 325*t*
norethindrone, 546, 551*t*. *See also* estrogen-progestin oral contraceptives
Norflex. *See* orphenadrine
norfloxacin, 400*t*
Norlutin. *See* norethindrone
normal serum albumin
actions, 323*t*
adverse effects, 323*t*
clinical uses, 323*t*
Drug Prototype, 323*t*
interactions, 323*t*
Norpace. *See* disopyramide
Norpramin. *See* desipramine
Nor-Q.D. *See* norethindrone
North American Nursing Diagnosis Association (NANDA), 53

nortriptyline, 112*t*, 126*t*, 201
Norvasc. *See* amlodipine
nosocomial infections, 392
Novantrone. *See* mitoxantrone
Novastan. *See* argatroban
Novocain. *See* procaine
Novolin N. *See* insulin isophane
Novolin R. *See* insulin regular
NovoLog. *See* insulin aspart
NPH. *See* insulin isophane
NRTIs (nucleotide reverse transcriptase
   inhibitors), 419*t*
Nubain. *See* nalbuphine
nucleoside reverse transcriptase inhibitors
   (NRTIs), 419*t*
Nupercainal. *See* dibucaine
Nuprin. *See* **ibuprofen**
nurse(s)
   diagnosis by, 53
   licensed practical nurse (LPN), 51
   licensed vocational nurse (LVN), 51
   registered nurse (RN), 51
   substance abuse in, 81
nursing diagnosis, 52*f*, 53, 54*t*
nursing process, 51–58
   assessment phase, 52–53, 52*f*
   diagnosis, 52*f*, 53, 54*t*
   evaluation phase, 52*f*, 56–57
   implementation phase, 52*f*, 55–56
   patient teaching in, 54, 55–56, 55*t*
   planning phase, 52*f*, 53–55
Nursing Process Focus. *See* Guide to Special
   Features
Nutropin. *See* somatropin
nystatin
   Drug Prototype, 416*t*
   route and adult dose, 415*t*
Nytol. *See* **diphenhydramine**

O

obesity, 529
objective data, 52
obsessive-compulsive disorder (OCD), 106
OC (oral contraceptives). *See* oral
   contraceptives (OC)
octreotide, 489*t*, 514*t*, 515*t*, 516
OcuClear. *See* oxymetazoline
Ocufen. *See* flurbiprofen
Ocupress. *See* carteolol
Ocusert. *See* pilocarpine
odansetron, 436
ofatumumab, 445*t*
off-label medications, 201
off-label use, of drugs, 9
ofloxacin, 400*t*
Ogen. *See* estropipate
olanzapine, 151*t*, 154, 166
older adults
   bleeding complications in, 352*t*
   blood pressure control in, 271*t*
   constipation in, 486*t*
   epilepsy in, 183*t*
   laxative misuse in, 486*t*
   medication-related sleep problems in, 110*t*
   tricyclic antidepressant use in, 125*t*
Oleptro. *See* trazodone

oligomenorrhea, 550
olmesartan, 275*t*
olopatadine, 460, 460*t*
omega-3-acid ethyl esters, 239*t*, 244
omega-3 fatty acids, 235, 237, 244, 534
omeprazole
   Drug Prototype, 483*t*
   route and adult dose, 482*t*
onabotulinumtoxin A, 173, 174*t*, 213, 213*t*
ondansetron, 229, 490*t*
   actions, 490*t*
   adverse effects, 490*t*
   Drug Prototype, 490*t*
   interactions, 490*t*
Onglyza. *See* saxagliptin
onset of drug action, 45
Onsolis. *See* fentanyl
Opana. *See* oxymorphone
open-angle glaucoma, 600*f*, 601. *See also*
   glaucoma
open comedones, 589
ophthalmic administration, 29, 29*f*, 30*t*
Ophthetic. *See* proparacaine
opiates, 201. *See also* opioid (narcotic) analgesics
   interactions with phenelzine, 133*t*
opioid agonists, 203
   with high effectiveness, 204*t*
   mixed agonist-antagonist, 204*t*
   with moderate effectiveness, 204*t*
opioid (narcotic) analgesics. *See also* narcotics
   abuse of, 70, 71, 73
   actions, 203
   clinical uses
      adjuncts to anesthesia, 228*t*
   drugs classified as
      agonists with high effectiveness, 204*t*
      agonists with moderate effectiveness,
         204*t*
      combination drugs, 205
      intravenous anesthetics, 226*t*
      mixed agonist-antagonist, 204*t*
   Nursing Process Focus, 206–207*t*
   Patients Need to Know, 214*t*
opioid antagonists, 205
opioid(s), 72, 75, 201. *See also* opioid
   (narcotic) analgesics
   acute intoxication, 205
   addiction to, 75
   adverse effects, 203
   effects of oral, 75
   endogenous, 199–200
   physiological and psychological effects
      of, 73*t*
   receptors, 202, 202*f*, 202*t*
   withdrawal from, 75
   withdrawal syndrome, 72
oprelvekin, 379, 446
OptiPranolol. *See* metipranolol
oral anticoagulants, 352. *See also* anticoagulants; **warfarin**
oral contraceptives (OC), 546–547
   adverse effects, 546
   alternative formulations, 547
   emergency contraception, 547
   estrogen–progestin, 546, 546*t*
   formulation types, 546, 546*t*

interactions
   with antiseizure drugs, 182, 185
   with diazepam, 188*t*
   with imipramine, 129*t*
   with phenytoin, 190*t*
   with tetracycline, 397*t*
   Nursing Process Focus, 548–549*t*
Oralet. *See* fentanyl
oral hypoglycemics
   interactions
      with aspirin, 208*t*
      with carvedilol, 296*t*
Orap. *See* pimozide
Orazinc. *See* zinc sulfate
Orencia. *See* abatacept
organic nitrates
   adverse effects, 307
   for angina, 305–306, 306*t*
   drugs classified as, 306*t*
   Patients Need to Know, 315*t*
organophosphate insecticides, 92
organ transplants, 380
Orinase. *See* tolbutamide
orlistat, 491
orphenadrine, 171*t*
orthostatic hypotension, 125, 132, 282
Orudis. *See* ketoprofen
Os-Cal. *See* calcium carbonate
oseltamivir, 424, 424*t*
Osmitrol. *See* mannitol
Osmoglyn. *See* glycerin
osmotic diuretics, 257
   clinical uses, 257
   drugs classified as, 257, 257*t*
   for glaucoma, 603*t*, 604
osteitis deformans. *See* Paget's disease
osteoarthritis (OA), 574, 575
osteoclasts, 565
osteomalacia
   cause of, 566
   description, 566
   pharmacotherapy
      calcium salts, 567–568, 568*t*
      vitamin D supplements, 567, 568, 568*t*
   signs and symptoms of, 567
osteoporosis, 501
   calcium metabolism in, 570*f*
   description, 569
   Nursing Process Focus, 572–573*t*
   pharmacotherapy
      bisphosphonates, 571*t*, 572
      calcitonin, 570
      selective estrogen-receptor modulators
         (SERMs), 570, 571*t*
   risk factors for, 569, 570
OTC (over-the-counter) drugs, 4–5, 7
otic administration, 30*t*, 31
otic preparations, 607*t*
otitis externa, 606
otitis interna, 606
otitis media, 606
ototoxicity, 400
outcome (goal), 54
overproductive oil glands, 589
over-the-counter (OTC) drugs, 4–5, 7
Ovide. *See* malathion
ovulation, 543

oxacillin, 393, 394*t*
oxaliplatin, 437*t*
Oxandrin. *See* oxandrolone
oxandrolone, 555*t*
oxaprozin, 209*t*, 365*t*
oxazepam, 114, 114*t*
oxazolidinones, 403
oxcarbazepine, 185*t*, 189, 190*t*
Oxecta. *See* oxycodone
oxiconazole, 415*t*
oxybutynin, 95*t*
oxycodone, 75, 215*t*
oxycodone terephthalate, 204*t*
OxyContin. *See* oxycodone
oxymetazoline, 606*t*
    clinical uses, 97*t*
    Drug Prototype, 464*t*
    route and adult dose, 464*t*
oxymetholone, 17*t*, 555*t*
oxymorphone, 204*t*
oxytocics, 552
oxytocin
    Drug Prototype, 553*t*
    for labor, 552
    route and adult dose, 553*t*

P

Pacerone. *See* **amiodarone**
paclitaxel, 442, 442*t*
Paget's disease, 573–574
pain, 198
    assessment, 198
    CAM Therapy, 211*t*
    classification, 198
    incidence, 199*t*
    mechanisms, 210*f*
    nonpharmacologic management, 200–201
    Patients Need to Know, 214*t*
    transmission, 199–200, 200*f*
pain-reducing drugs, 70
paliperidone, 151*t*
palliation, 433
Pamelor. *See* nortriptyline
pamidronate, 571*t*
Pamine. *See* methscopolamine
pancreas
    endocrine function, 529, 529*f*
    exocrine function, 529
pancreatic enzymes, 492
pancreatic insufficiency, 492
pancrelipase, 492
panic disorder, 106
    benzodiazepines for, 113
    characteristics of, 106
pantoprazole, 482*t*
pantothenic acid (vitamin B₅), 498*t*
papules, 589
Paraflex. *See* chlorzoxazone
parafollicular cells, 516
Parafon Forte. *See* chlorzoxazone
paranoia, 143
parasympathetic nervous system, 87
    activation of, 91
    effects of, 89*f*
    inhibition of, 91
    rest-and-digest response and, 87

parasympathomimetics (cholinergic drugs), 91
    actions, 92
    clinical uses
        as adjunct to anesthetics, 228*t*
    drugs classified as, 163, 163*t*, 228*t*
    Nursing Process Focus, 96*t*
    Patients Need to Know, 102*t*
parathyroid hormone (PTH), 565–566, 566*f*
Parcopa. *See* levodopa–carbidopa
Pardryl. *See* **diphenhydramine**
parenteral anticoagulants, 350–352
parenteral route, 32–39
    intradermal, 33, 34*t*
    intramuscular, 34*t*, 36
    intravenous, 35*t*, 37, 38*f*
    subcutaneous, 33–34, 34*t*
paricalcitol, 568*t*
parkinsonism, 147*t*, 148, 159. *See also* Parkinson's disease
Parkinson's disease, 158*t*, 159
    characteristics, 160
    extrapyramidal symptoms (EPS) in, 160
    incidence, 159
    Patients Need to Know, 176*t*
    pharmacotherapy, 163
        anticholinergics, 163, 163t. *See also* anticholinergics
        dopaminergic agents, 160–162, 161*t*
    symptoms, 159–160
        affective flattening, 160
        bradykinesia, 159
        muscle rigidity, 159
        postural instability, 160
        tremors, 159
Parlodel. *See* bromocriptine
Parnate. *See* tranylcypromine
paromomycin, 399*t*, 426*t*
paroxetine, 112*t*
    for anxiety disorders, 112*t*
    for depression, 126*t*
partial (focal) seizures, 183. *See also* seizure(s)
    complex partial seizures, 183
    simple partial seizures, 183
passive immunity, 376, 378*f*
pathogen(s), 389, 389*f*
    bacterial, 390*t*
    fungal, 414*t*
    protozoan, 425
    viruses, 417–418
pathogenicity, 389
pathophysiology, 3
patient adherence. *See* compliance
patient-controlled analgesia (PCA), 216
Patients Need to Know. *See* Guide to Special Features
patient teaching
    adult and, 55*t*
    children and, 55*t*
    implementation, 55–56
    in nursing process, 54, 55–56, 55*t*
    older adults and, 55*t*
    planning, 54
Paxil. *See* paroxetine
pazopanib, 445*t*
PCP (phencyclidine), 70, 77
peak plasma level, 46, 46*f*

PediaCare Children's Allergy. *See* **diphenhydramine**
pediculicides, 587
Pediculus, 587
Peganone. *See* ethotoin
pegaspargase, 445*t*
peginterferon, 425
peginterferon alfa-2a, 379*t*
PEG-L-asparaginase, 445*t*
pegloticase, 577, 577*t*
pegvisomant, 515*t*
pemetrexed, 439*t*
penciclovir, 424*t*
penicillinase, 393
    action of, 394*f*
penicillinase-resistant penicillins, 393
penicillin G benzathine, 394*t*
penicillin G procaine, 394*t*
penicillin G sodium/potassium
    Drug Prototype, 395*t*
    route and adult dose, 394*t*
penicillin(s), 17*t*
    actions, 393, 394*f*
    adverse effects, 395
    drugs classified as, 394*t*
    fixed-dose combinations, 395
    interactions
        with aspirin, 208*t*
        with cholestyramine, 240*t*
    Patients Need to Know, 409*t*
penicillin V, 394*t*
Pentalair. *See* cyclopentolate
pentamidine, 426*t*
pentazocine, 202, 204*t*
pentobarbital, 116*t*
pentostatin, 439*t*
pentoxifylline, 350*f*, 351*t*, 352
peptic ulcer disease, 479
    causes, 479, 479*f*
    natural defenses against, 479–480, 480*f*
    nonpharmacologic therapy, 481
    Nursing Process Focus, 484*t*
    Patients Need to Know, 492*f*
    pharmacotherapy, 481*f*, 485–486
        antacids, 482*t*, 485
        antibiotics, 485
        H₂-receptor blockers, 482*t*, 483
        proton-pump inhibitors, 482, 482*t*
    risk factors, 479
    symptoms, 479–480
Percocet, 205
Percocet-5. *See* oxycodone terephthalate
Percodan, 205
percutaneous transluminal coronary angioplasty (PTCA), 304
performance anxiety, 106
perfusion, 455
perindopril, 275*t*
peripheral edema, 289
peripheral nervous system (PNS), 87, 88*f*
    basic divisions of, 88*f*
    cholinergic drugs and, 92
peripheral resistance, 269
peristalsis, 478
permethrin, 587
    Drug Prototype, 587*t*
pernicious (megaloblastic) anemia, 499

perphenazine, 146*t*, 490*t*
Persantine. *See* dipyridamole
pertuzumab, 445*t*
petit mal epilepsy, 183
petit mal seizures, 183. *See also* absence
    seizures
pH, 260
pharmaceutics, 5
pharmacists, 5
pharmacodynamics, 46
pharmacokinetics, 42, 42*f*
pharmacologic classification, 13–14, 14*t*.
    See also mechanism of action
pharmacology, 3
pharmacopoeia, 5
pharmacotherapeutics, 3
pharmacotherapy
    common nursing diagnoses in, 54*t*
    diagnosis phase of the nursing process
        and, 53
pharmacy, 5
phencyclidine (PCP), 70, 77
phenelzine
    actions, 133*t*
    adverse effects, 133*t*
    anxiety disorders, 112*t*
    clinical uses, 133*t*
        depression, 127*t*
    Drug Prototype, 133*t*
    interactions
        with herbal supplements, 133*t*
        with meperidine, 133*t*
phenobarbital, 185*t*
    actions, 188*t*
    adverse effects, 188*t*
    antiseizure properties of, 186
    clinical uses, 188*t*
        route and adult dose, 187*t*
        sedation and insomnia, 116*t*
        seizures, 185*t*
    Drug Prototype, 188*t*
    interactions, 188*t*
        with aspirin, 208*t*
        with chlorpromazine, 147*t*
        with cyclophosphamide, 438*t*
        with donepezil, 167*t*
        with doxorubicin, 441*t*
        with haloperidol, 149*t*
        with valproic acid, 191*t*
phenothiazines and phenothiazine-like drugs
    adverse effects, 147*t*
    clinical uses
        as adjuncts to anesthesia, 228*t*
    drugs classified as, 146*t*
    interactions
        with atropine, 95*t*
        with benztropine, 164*t*
        with cyclobenzaprine, 171*t*
        with isoflurane, 225*t*
        with succinylcholine, 228*t*
    long-term use of, 148
    Nursing Process Focus, 149–151*t*
phentolamine, 100*t*
phenylephrine, 97, 97*t*, 606*t*
    actions, 98*t*
    adverse effects of, 98*t*
    clinical uses, 98*t*

    decongestant, 464*t*
    shock, 325, 325*t*
    Drug Prototype, 98*t*
    route and adult dose, 325*t*
Phenytek. *See* **phenytoin**
phenytoin, 185*t*
    actions, 190*t*
    adverse effects, 190*t*
    approved as a drug, 189*t*
    clinical uses, 190*t*
        dysrhythmias, 338*t*
        seizures, 185*t*
    Drug Prototype, 190*t*
    hematologic toxicities and, 189
    interactions, 190*t*
        with aspirin, 208*t*
        with calcium supplements, 190*t*
        with cyclophosphamide, 438*t*
        with diazepam, 188*t*
        with digoxin, 190*t*
        with donepezil, 167*t*
        with dopamine, 326*t*
        with doxorubicin, 441*t*
        with doxycycline, 190*t*
        with estrogens, 190*t*
        with ethosuximide, 192*t*
        with folic acid, 190*t*
        with furosemide, 190*t*
        with glucocorticoids, 190*t*
        with H2 antagonists, 190*t*
        with haloperidol, 149*t*
        with omeprazole, 483*t*
        with oral anticoagulants, 190*t*
        with oral contraceptives, 190*t*
        with oral theophylline, 190*t*
        with prednisone, 369*t*
        with valproic acid, 191*t*
        with vitamin D, 190*t*
    route and adult dose, 189*t*, 338*t*
phobias, 106
PhosLo. *See* calcium acetate
phosphodiesterase, 297
phosphodiesterase-5 (PDE-5) inhibitors, 556
phosphodiesterase inhibitors
    actions, 297
    drugs classified as, 295*t*
    for heart failure, 295*t*, 297
Phospholine iodide. *See* echothiophate iodide
phosphorus, 501*t*
photosensitivity, 398
physical dependence, 16, 17*t*, 72
physostigmine, 92, 92*t*
pill-rolling behavior, 159
pilocarpine, 92*t*, 602*t*
Pilopine. *See* pilocarpine
pimozide, 148*t*
pindolol, 281*t*
pioglitazone, 536*t*
pipecuronium, 176*t*
piperacillin, 393, 394*t*
piperacillin/tazobactam, 394*t*
pirbuterol, 468*t*
piroxicam, 209*t*, 365*t*
pitavastatin, 239*t*
Pitocin. *See* **oxytocin**
pituitary gland, 511, 513*f*
Plan B. *See* levonorgestrel

Plan B One Step. *See* levonorgestrel
planning phase, of nursing process, 52*f*, 53–55
plant extracts, 442–443, 442*t*
plaque, 235
    arterial, 302, 303*f*
Plaquenil. *See* **hydroxychloroquine**
plaques
    in psoriasis, 593
plasma cells, 375
plasma half-life, 45
plasmids, 392
plasmin, 349
plasminogen, 349
Plasmodium, 426
Plavix. *See* **clopidogrel**
Plendil. *See* felodipine
Pletal. *See* cilostazol
PMS (premenstrual syndrome), 550
pneumococcal 7-valent vaccine, 377*t*
pneumococcal polyvalent vaccine, 377*t*
Pneumococcus, 390*t*
Pneumocystis jiroveci, 414*t*
polarized, 335
poliovirus vaccine, 377*t*
Polocaine. *See* mepivacaine
polymyxin B, neomycin, and hydrocortisone,
    607*t*
polyvinyl alcohol, 606*t*
Ponstel. *See* mefenamic acid
Pontocaine. *See* tetracaine
posaconazole, 415*t*
positive feedback, 552
positive symptoms, of schizophrenia, 144
posterior pituitary, 511, 514, 515*t*. *See also*
    pituitary gland
postmarketing studies. *See* postmarketing
    surveillance
postmarketing surveillance, 8–9, 8*f*
postmenopausal bleeding, 550
postpartum depression, 124
postsynaptic neuron, 88
post-traumatic stress disorder (PTSD), 106,
    111
postural instability, 160
Posture. *See* calcium phosphate tribasic
potassium, 501*t*
potassium channel blockers, 340, 340*t*
potassium chloride, 17*t*, 502*t*
    actions, 260*t*
    adverse effects, 260*t*
    clinical uses, 260*t*
    Drug Prototype, 260*t*
    interactions, 260*t*
potassium gluconate, 17*t*
potassium imbalances. *See* hyperkalemia;
    hypokalemia
potassium iodide and iodine, 518*t*
potassium ion channels, 335, 336*f*
potassium/sodium phosphates, 502*t*
potassium-sparing diuretics, 255–256
    actions, 253*f*
    defined, 274
    drugs classified as, 256*t*
    interactions
        with enalapril, 277*t*
potency, of drugs, 47, 48*f*
Potiga. *See* ezogabine

PPIs (proton-pump inhibitors), 481*f*, 482, 482*t*
Pradaxa. *See* dabigatran
pralatrexate, 439*t*
pramipexole, 161–162, 161*t*
pramoxine, 221*t*
Prandin. *See* repaglinide
prasugrel, 355*t*, 356
Pravachol. *See* pravastatin
pravastatin, 239*t*
praziquantel, 426*t*
prazosin, 100*t*
   actions, 100*t*, 282
   adverse effects of, 100*t*
   clinical uses, 100*t*
     hypertension, 281*t*
   Drug Prototype, 100*t*
   interactions
     with antihypertensives, 100*t*
     with diuretics, 100*t*
   route and adult dose, 281*t*
preclinical investigation, 7, 8*f*
Precose. *See* acarbose
prednicarbate, 592*t*
prednisolone, 368*t*, 522*t*
prednisone
   actions, 369*t*
   adverse effects, 369*t*
   as antineoplastic agent, 444*t*
   clinical uses, 369*t*
   Drug Prototype, 369*t*
   interactions, 369*t*
     with vincristine, 443*t*
   route and adult dose, 368*t*, 522*t*
pre-eclampsia, 183
Prefest. *See* estradiol with norgestimate
pregabalin, 185*t*, 187*t*, 189, 201
pregnancy
   drug safety categories, 17
   herbal products and, 63–64
preload, 289, 304
Prelone. *See* prednisolone
Premarin. *See* **estrogen, conjugated**
premature atrial contractions, 333*t*
premature ventricular contractions (PVCs), 333*t*
premenstrual dysphoric disorder, 133*t*
premenstrual syndrome (PMS), 550
premenstrual syndrome, dong quai for, 549*t*
Premphase. *See* conjugated estrogens with medroxyprogesterone
Prempro. *See* conjugated estrogens with medroxyprogesterone
Prepidil. *See* dinoprostone
prescription drugs, 4, 5
Prescription Drug User Fee Act, 6*f*, 9
presynaptic neuron, 88
preterm labor, 552
Prialt. *See* ziconotide
prilocaine, 221*t*
primaquine, 426
primary adrenocortical insufficiency, 521
primary gout, 576. *See also* gout
primary hypertension, 267
primary hypogonadism, 554
primidone, 185*t*, 186, 187*t*
Prinivil. *See* **lisinopril**
Prinzmetal's (vasospastic) angina, 303, 309

prn order, 23
ProAmatine. *See* midodrine
Probalan. *See* probenecid
Pro-Banthine. *See* propantheline
probenecid, 577*t*
procainamide
   actions, 339*t*
   adverse effects, 339*t*
   black box warning, 339*t*
   clinical uses, 339
     dysrhythmias, 338*t*
   Drug Prototype, 339*t*
   interactions, 339*t*
     with atropine, 95*t*
     with benztropine, 164*t*
     with bethanechol, 93*t*
   route and adult dose, 338*t*
procaine, 221*t*, 222
procarbazine, 445*t*
Procardia. *See* **nifedipine**
Procardia XL. *See* **nifedipine**
Prochieve. *See* progesterone
prochlorperazine, 146*t*
   as antiemetic, 436, 490*t*
   as antipsychotic, 146*t*
   route and adult dose, 146*t*, 490*t*
prodrugs, 43
product name, 14
progesterone, 544, 551*t*
progestin-only OC, 546*t*, 547. *See also* estrogen-progestin oral contraceptives
proguanil/atovaquone, 426*t*
prolactin, 552
Prolia. *See* denosumab
Proloid. *See* thyroglobulin
promethazine
   as antiemetic, 490*t*
   as antihistamine, 459*t*
Prometrium. *See* progesterone
propafenone, 338*t*
propantheline, 95*t*
proparacaine, 221*t*, 222
Propine. *See* Dipivefrin HCl
Propionibacterium acnes, 589
propofol, 226*t*
   adverse effects, 227*t*
   clinical uses, 227*t*
   Drug Prototype, 227*t*
   interactions
     with benzodiazepines, 227*t*
     with opioids, 227*t*
propranolol
   actions, 340*t*
   adverse effects, 340*t*
   black box warning, 340*t*
   clinical uses, 100*t*, 340*t*
     angina, 306*t*
     anxiety, 111, 117*t*
     dysrhythmias, 339*t*
     hypertension, 281*t*
     migraine prophylaxis, 212*t*
   Drug Prototype, 340*t*
   interactions, 340*t*
   Patients Need to Know, 343*t*
   route and adult dose, 212*t*, 281*t*, 306*t*, 339*t*
proprietary name, 14

propylthiouracil, 513
   as an antihormone, 513
   Drug Prototype, 519*t*
   route and adult dose, 518*t*
Proquad, 377*t*
Proscar. *See* finasteride
prostaglandins, 208, 552
   for glaucoma, 601, 602, 602*t*
   in pain and inflammation, 210*f*, 364*t*
Prostigmin. *See* neostigmine
Prostin E$_2$. *See* dinoprostone
protamine sulfate, 350
protease inhibitors, 419*t*, 420
Proteus mirabilis, 390*t*
prothrombin, 347
prothrombin activator, 347
prothrombinase. *See* prothrombin activator
prothrombin time (PT), 352
proton-pump inhibitors (PPIs), 481*f*, 482, 482*t*
prototype drug, 13
   See also Drug Prototypes in Guide to Special Features
protozoan(s), 389*f*, 425, 427*t*
protriptyline, 126*t*, 213*t*
Proventil. *See* albuterol
Provera. *See* **medroxyprogesterone**
Provigil. *See* modafinil
provitamins, 497
proximal tubule, 250, 251, 253*f*
Prozac. *See* fluoxetine
pseudoephedrine, 97, 97*t*, 460*t*, 463, 464*t*
Pseudomonas aeruginosa, 390*t*
psilocybin, 76, 77*f*
psoralens, 594
psoriasis, 593–594, 593*t*
psychedelics, 76. *See also* hallucinogens
psychodynamic therapies, 125
psychological dependence, 16, 17*t*, 72
psychologically dependent individual, 16
psychomotor seizures, 183. *See also* complex partial seizures; seizure(s)
psychosis
   acute, 143
   chronic, 143
   Fast Facts, 144*t*
   incidence, 143
   pharmacotherapy, 146. *See also* antipsychotics
   signs and symptoms, 143
psychotic depression, 124
psyllium mucilloid
   Drug Prototype, 487*t*
   route and adult dose, 487*t*
PT (prothrombin time), 352
PTCA (percutaneous transluminal coronary angioplasty), 304
PTH (parathyroid hormone), 565–566, 566*f*
PTSD (post-traumatic stress disorder), 106, 111
PTU. *See* **propylthiouracil**
Public Health Service Act, 6*f*
pulmonary embolus, 347*t*
Pure Food and Drug Act of 1906, 5, 6*f*
purine(s), 439
purine analogs, 439*t*
Purkinje fibers, 333, 334*f*

pustules, 589
PUVA (psoralen plus ultraviolet light) therapy, 594
PVCs (premature ventricular contractions), 333t
P wave, 334f
pyrantel, 426t, 427
pyrazinamide, 407t
pyrethrin, 587
pyridostigmine, 92, 92t
pyridoxine (vitamin B₆), 498t
pyrimethamine, 426t
pyrimidine(s), 439
pyrimidine analogs, 439t

Q

QRS complex, 334f
quadriphasic OC, 546
quazepam, 114t
Questran. *See* **cholestyramine**
quetiapine, 135t, 151t
Quillivant XR. *See* methylphenidate
Quinamm. *See* quinine sulfate
quinapril, 275t, 293t
Quinidex. *See* quinidine sulfate
quinidine sulfate, 338, 338t
quinine sulfate, 175
quinupristin/dalfopristin, 403, 404t
Quiphile. *See* quinine sulfate

R

rabeprazole, 482t
rabeprazole sodium, 482t
radioactive iodide, 518t
raloxifene
    as antineoplastic agent, 444t
    Drug Prototype, 571
    for osteoporosis, 571t
raltegravir, 419t, 420
ramelteon, 111, 117t, 119
ramipril, 275t, 293t
Ranexa. *See* ranolazine
ranitidine, 17t
    Drug Prototype, 483t
    route and adult dose, 482t
ranolazine, 305, 306t
Rapaflo. *See* silodosin
RAS (reticular activating system), 107
rasburicase, 577, 577t
rate of elimination, 45–46
    drug responsiveness and, 45–46
Razadyne. *See* galantamine
RDA (recommended dietary allowances), 498–499, 498t
reabsorption, 250
Rebif. *See* interferon beta-1a
rebound congestion, 463
rebound insomnia, 110
receptor(s), 47
    cellular, 47f
receptor theory, 47
Reclast. *See* zoledronate
recommended dietary allowances (RDA), 498–499, 498t
Recothrom. *See* thrombin
rectal administration, 31t, 32

red-man syndrome, 403
reflex tachycardia, 270, 283, 326
Refludan. *See* lepirudin
regional anesthesia, 218–219, 219f, 219t
Regonol. *See* pyridostigmine
Relafen. *See* nabumetone
relapsing-remitting multiple sclerosis (RRMS), 168. *See also* multiple sclerosis
releasing hormones, 511
ReliOn N. *See* insulin isophane
Relpax. *See* eletriptan
Remeron. *See* mirtazapine
Remicade. *See* infliximab
remifentanil, 204, 226t, 228t
Reminyl. *See* galantamine
renal failure, 250t, 251–252
renin-angiotensin-aldosterone system (RAAS), 274–275
ReoPro. *See* abciximab
repaglinide, 536t
repetitive transcranial magnetic stimulation (rTMS), 125
Requip. *See* ropinirole
respiration, 455
respiratory acidosis, 261t
respiratory alkalosis, 261t
respiratory disorders
    allergic rhinitis. *See* allergic rhinitis
    chronic obstructive pulmonary disease, 471–472
    common cold. *See* common cold
respiratory system, 455–456, 456f, 457f
rest-and-digest response, 87
Restoril. *See* temazepam
restricted drugs, 16
Retavase. *See* **reteplase**
reteplase
    actions, 312t
    adverse effects, 312t
    clinical uses, 312t
    Drug Prototype, 312t
    interactions, 312t
    route and adult dose, 312t
reticular activating system (RAS), 107
reticular formation, 78, 107
    reticular activating system (RAS) and, 107
    stimulation of, 107
Retin-A. *See* **tretinoin**
retinoids, 590
reverse transcriptase, 420
ReVia. *See* naltrexone
rhabdomyolysis, 240
rheumatoid arthritis (RA), 575, 576t
rheumatoid factors, 575
Rheumatrex. *See* **methotrexate**
riboflavin, 213t
riboflavin (vitamin B₂), 498t
rickets. *See* osteomalacia
Rickettsia rickettsii, 390t
RID. *See* pyrethrin
Ridiprin. *See* **aspirin**
rifabutin, 407t
rifampin, 407t
rifapentine, 407t
rilpivirine, 419t
rimabotulinumtoxin B, 173, 174t
rimantadine, 424, 424t

Riomet. *See* **metformin**
risedronate, 571t
Risperdal. *See* **risperidone**
risperidone
    actions, 152t
    adverse effects, 152t
    clinical uses, 152t, 166
    Drug Prototype, 152t
    interactions, 152t
        with chamomile, 152t
        with valerian, 152t
    route and adult dose, 151t
Ritalin. *See* methylphenidate
ritonavir/lopinavir, 419t
Rituxan. *See* rituximab
rituximab, 445t, 576t
rivaroxaban, 351t, 352
rivastigmine, 92, 92t, 165, 165t
rizatriptan, 212t
Robaxin. *See* methocarbamol
Robinul. *See* glycopyrrolate
Rocaltrol. *See* **calcitriol**
rocuronium, 176t
rofecoxib, 8, 366
Rohypnol. *See* flunitrazepam
Rolaids. *See* calcium carbonate
ropinirole, 161–162, 161t
ropivacaine, 221t
rosacea, 589, 590, 590t
rosiglitazone, 536t
rosuvastatin, 239t, 240
rotavirus vaccine, 377t
roundworm, 389f, 427
routine orders, 24
Roxicet. *See* oxycodone terephthalate
rTMS (repetitive transcranial magnetic stimulation), 125
Rufen. *See* **ibuprofen**
Rythmol. *See* propafenone

S

Sabril. *See* vigabatrin
SAD (seasonal affective disorder), 124
Safety Alerts. *See* Guide to Special Features
Saizen. *See* somatropin
Salagen. *See* pilocarpine
Salax. *See* salicylic acid
salicylates, 209t
salicylic acid, 593t
salicylism, 366
salmeterol, 468t
    for asthma, 97t
Salmonella enteritidis, 390t
salsalate, 209t
Sandostatin. *See* octreotide
SA (sinoatrial) node, 333, 334f
Sansert. *See* methysergide
Saphris. *See* asenapine
saquinavir, 419t
Sarcoptes scabiei, 586
sargramostim, 379, 436
sarin, 92
saxagliptin, 535t, 537
scabicides, 587
scabies, 586
scheduled drugs, 16, 17t

Schedule I drugs, 16, 17*t*
Schedule II drugs, 16, 17*t*
Schedule V drugs, 16, 17*t*
Schedule I drugs, 16, 17*t*, 76. *See also* hallucinogens
Schedule II drugs, 16, 17*t*, 78
Schedule V drugs, 16, 17*t*
schizoaffective disorder, 144
schizophrenia, 143
    causes of, 145
    negative symptoms, 144
    pharmacotherapy for patients with, 146
    positive symptoms, 144
scinitinib, 445*t*
scopolamine, 95*t*, 489, 490*t*
scopolamine hydrobromide, 606*t*
seasonal affective disorder (SAD), 124
sea vegetables, 504*t*
seborrhea, 589
seborrheic dermatitis, 591
secobarbital, 116*t*
Seconal. *See* secobarbital
secondary adrenocortical insufficiency, 521
secondary gout, 576, 577. *See also* gout
secondary hypertension, 267
secondary hypogonadism, 554
second-degree burns, 583–584
secretion, tubular, 250*f*, 251
Sectral. *See* acebutolol
sedative-hypnotics, 74, 111
sedative(s), 74, 111. *See also* tranquilizers
    clinical uses
        for anxiety and insomnia, 117*t*
seizure(s), 181
    causes, 181, 182–183
    chronic depression and, 183
    classification, 183–184
    convulsions and, 181
    febrile, 182
    generalized seizures, 183
        absence seizures, 183
        atonic seizures, 183
        tonic-clonic seizures, 183
    impact on quality of life, 183
    infectious diseases and, 182
    ketogenic diet for, 188*t*
    metabolic disorders and, 182
    neoplastic disease and, 182
    partial (focal) seizures, 183
        complex partial seizures, 183
        simple partial seizures, 183
    pediatric disorders and, 182
    pharmacotherapy. *See also* antiseizure
    drugs
        goals, 186
        initiation of, 184
        selection of, 184
    in pregnancy, 182–183
    special epileptic syndromes, 184
        febrile seizures, 184
        myoclonic seizures, 184
    trauma and, 182
    vascular diseases and, 182
selective cox-2 inhibitors. *See also* nonsteroidal anti-inflammatory drugs (NSAIDs)
    actions, 210*f*
    drugs classified as, 209*t*, 365*t*, 366

selective estrogen-receptor modulators (SERM), 570, 571*t*
selective serotonin reuptake inhibitors (SSRIs), 126*t*, 128–129
    advantages of, 128
    adverse effects, 113, 128–129
    clinical uses
        anxiety disorders, 112*t*
        depression, 126*t*
    drugs classified as, 110, 125
    interactions
        with phenelzine, 133*t*
        with risperidone, 152*t*
        with sumatriptan, 213*t*
        with warfarin, 353*t*
    Patients Need to Know, 139*t*
    serotonin syndrome (SES) and, 129
selegiline, 127*t*, 161, 161*t*
selenium, 435*t*
senna, 487*t*
Senokot. *See* senna
Sensipar. *See* cinacalcet
Sensorcaaine. *See* bupivicaine
sensory neurons, 199
September 11, 2001, terrorist attacks, 9
septic shock, 320, 320*t*. *See also* shock
Septocaine. *See* articaine
Serevent. *See* salmeterol
SERM (selective estrogen-receptor modulators), 570, 571*t*
Seroquel. *See* quetiapine
Serostim. *See* somatropin
serotonin (5-HT), 128
serotonin-norepinephrine reuptake inhibitors (SNRIs), 129
    actions, 129*t*
    adverse effects, 113, 129*t*
    black box warning, 129*t*
    clinical uses
        anxiety, 112*t*
        depression, 129
    drugs classified as, 110
    generalized anxiety disorder and, 129
serotonin syndrome (SES), 129
sertaconazole, 415*t*
sertraline, 112*t*
    actions, 133*t*
    adverse effects, 133*t*
    clinical uses
        depression, 126*t*
    Drug Prototype, 132*t*
    interactions
        with digoxin, 133*t*
        with warfarin, 133*t*
sevoflurane, 225*t*
sex hormones, 544. *See also* estrogen; progesterone; **testosterone**
Sherley Amendment, 5, 6*f*
shock, 320
    classification, 320, 320*t*
    Fast Facts, 321
    initial treatment, 320–322, 322*f*
    Patients Need to Know, 328
    pharmacotherapy
        fluid replacement drugs, 322–323, 323*t*
    Nursing Process Focus, 324*t*

    inotropic drugs, 325, 325*t*
    vasoconstrictors, 324–325, 325*t*
    symptoms, 320, 321*f*
short stature, 515. *See also* growth hormone (GH)
short-term insomnia, 110. *See also* behavioral insomnia
short-term psychotherapies
    cognitive-behavioral therapy, 125
    interpersonal therapy, 124–125
sibutramine, 491
sildenafil
    administration, 24
    Drug Prototype, 556*t*
    for erectile dysfunction, 556, 556*t*
    interaction with nitroglycerin, 307*t*
Silenor. *See* doxepin
silodosin, 100*t*, 558*t*
silver sulfadiazine, 402*t*
Simcor, 242
simethicone, 482*t*, 485
simple partial seizures, 183. *See also* seizure(s)
Simponi. *See* golimumab
simvastatin, 239*t*
Sinequan. *See* doxepin
single order, 23
sinoatrial (SA) node, 333, 334*f*
sinus bradycardia, 333*t*
sinus rhythm, 333
sirolimus, 381*t*
sitagliptin, 535*t*, 537
situational anxiety, 106
situational depression, 124
six rights of drug administration, 22
Skelaxin. *See* metaxalone
skeletal muscle relaxants, 171*t*
Skelid. *See* tiludronate
skin disorders
    acne, 589–590, 590*t*
    parasites, 586–587
    Patients Need to Know, 594*t*
    psoriasis, 593–594, 593*t*
    rosacea, 589, 590, 590*t*
    sunburn and minor irritation, 588–589
Sklice. *See* ivermectin
Sloprin. *See* **aspirin**
Slow-Mag. *See* magnesium chloride
slow-release (SR) medications, 27
SL (sublingual) route, 26*t*, 27, 28*f*
smoking, 555
SNRIs (serotonin-norepinephrine reuptake inhibitors). *See* serotonin-norepinephrine reuptake inhibitors (SNRIs)
social anxiety disorder, 106
social phobia. *See* social anxiety disorder
sodium, 501*t*
sodium bicarbonate, 502*t*
    actions, 261*t*
    adverse effects, 261*t*
    clinical uses, 261*t*, 482*t*
    Drug Prototype, 261*t*
    interactions, 261*t*
    in local anesthetics, 220
sodium channel blockers, 220, 338, 338*t*
    interactions with lidocaine, 222*t*
sodium chloride, interaction with lithium, 134
sodium chloride hypertonicity ointment, 606*t*

sodium hydroxide, 220
sodium imbalances. *See* hypernatremia;
  hyponatremia
sodium ion channels, 335, 336*f*
sodium ions (Na+), 220, 220*f*
sodium oxybate, 74
sodium polystyrene sulfate, 259
Solorcaine. *See* **benzocaine**
Solu-Cortef. *See* **hydrocortisone**
Solu-Medrol. *See* methylprednisolone
Soma. *See* carisoprodol
somatic nervous system, 87, 88*f*
somatic pain, 198
somatotropin. *See* growth hormone (GH)
somatropin, 515*t*
Somatuline Depot. *See* lanreotide
Somavert. *See* pegvisomant
Sominex. *See* **diphenhydramine**
Sonata. *See* zaleplon
Sorine. *See* sotalol
sotalol, 100*t*, 340*t*
spasticity, 171
  causes, 172
  characteristics, 172
  nonpharmacologic therapy, 169
  Nursing Process Focus, 172–173*t*
  Patients Need to Know, 176*t*
  pharmacotherapy
    direct-acting antispasmodics, 174*f*
  signs and symptoms, 171
  treatment for, 172, 173
special epileptic syndromes, 184
  febrile seizures, 184
  myoclonic seizures, 184
specialty supplements, 65, 65*t. See also* Cam
  Therapy
    popular, 65*t*
    regulation of, 65–67
spectinomycin, 404*t*
"speedball." *See* heroin
spinal anesthesia, 219*f*, 219*t*
spiritual healing, 60*t*
Spiriva. *See* tiotropium
spironolactone
  actions, 253*f*, 256, 256*t*
  adverse effects, 256*t*
  clinical uses, 256*t*
    heart failure, 293*t*
    hypertension, 274*t*
  Drug Prototype, 256*t*
  interactions, 256*t*
    with aspirin, 208*t*
  route and adult dose, 293*t*
  routes and adult dose, 256*t*, 274*t*
Sporothrix schenckii, 414*t*
SR (slow-release) medications, 27
SSRIs (selective serotonin reuptake inhibitors).
  See selective serotonin reuptake inhibitors
  (SSRIs)
stable angina, 303
Stadol. *See* butorphanol
Stalevo. *See* **entacapone**
standing order, 24
Staphylococcus aureus, 390*t*
  methicillin-resistant, 392
Starlix. *See* nateglinide
stasis dermatitis, 591

statins. *See* HMG-CoA reductase inhibitors
  (statins)
STAT order, 23–24
status asthmaticus, 467
status epilepticus, 184
stavudine, 419*t*
steatorrhea, 492
Stendra. *See* avanafil
steroid(s), 236
St. John's wort
  interactions
    with anesthetics, 218*t*
    with chlorpromazine, 147*t*
    with cyclophosphamide, 438*t*
    with imipramine, 129*t*
    with isoflurane, 225*t*
    with sertraline, 133*t*
    with zidovudine, 421*t*
Strattera. *See* atomoxetine
stratum germinativum, 583
Streptococci, 390*t*
streptogramins, 403
streptokinase, 312*t*
streptomycin, 399*t*
streptozocin, 437*t*
Striant. *See* **testosterone**
Stroke, 314–315, 347*t*
subcutaneous layer, 583
subcutaneous (SC or SQ) route, 33–34, 34*t*
subjective data, 52
Sublimaze. *See* fentanyl
sublingual (SL) route, 26*t*, 27, 28*f*
Suboxone. *See* buprenorphine
substance abuse, 69–83
  chronic, 72
  classification, 70–71
  commonly abused substances, 71*t*
  in health care providers, 80–81
  opioids, 205
  in the U.S., 70
substance P, 199
substantia nigra, 160
succinimides. *See also* antiseizure drugs
  for absence seizures, 191–192
  drugs classified as, 185*t*
  Patients Need to Know, 194*t*
  route and adult dose, 192*t*
succinylcholine
  adverse effects, 176, 228*t*
  black box warning, 228*t*
  clinical uses, 176, 228*t*
    as adjuncts to anesthesia, 228*t*
  Drug Prototype, 228*t*
  interactions
    with aminoglycosides, 228*t*
    with cardiac glycosides, 228*t*
    with clindamycin, 228*t*
    with diazepam, 228*t*
    with furosemide, 228*t*
    with lidocaine, 228*t*
    with lithium, 228*t*
    with narcotics, 228*t*
    with phenothiazines oxytocin, 228*t*
    with promazine, 228*t*
    with quinidine, 228*t*
    with tacrine, 228*t*
    with thiazide diuretics, 228*t*

  route and adult dose, 176*t*
sucralfate, 485
Sudafed PE Nighttime Cold, 461*t*
Sudafed PE Sinus and Allergy, 461*t*
Sufenta. *See* sufentanil
sufentanil, 204, 226*t*, 228*t*
sulconazole, 415*t*
sulfacetamide sodium, 590*t*
sulfadiazine, 402*t*, 403
sulfadoxine–pyrimethamine, 402*t*, 403
sulfasalazine, 43, 402*t*, 576*t*
sulfinpyrazone, 577*t*
sulfisoxazole, 402*t*
sulfites, 222
sulfonamides
  actions, 401–402
  adverse effects, 403
  drugs classified as, 402*t*
  interactions
    with aspirin, 208*t*
    with furosemide, 254*t*
  Patients Need to Know, 409*t*
  resistance to, 402
  uses, 403
sulfur, 501*t*
sulindac, 209*t*
sumatriptan, 211
  actions, 213*t*
  adverse effects, 213*t*
  clinical uses, 212*t*, 213*t*
  Drug Prototype, 213*t*
  interactions, 213*t*
  route and adult dose, 212*t*
Sumycin. *See* **tetracycline**
sunburn, 588–589
sunitinib, 445*t*
superficial mycoses, 413
superinfections, 393
Suprane. *See* desflurane
supraventricular, 332
surface anesthesia. *See* regional anesthesia
surgical anesthesia, 224
Surmontil. *See* trimipramine
sustained-release capsules, 27
sustained-release tablets, 27
sympathetic nervous system, 87
  activation of, 91
  effects of, 89*f*
  fight-or-flight response and, 87
  inhibition of, 91
  norepinephrine (NE) and, 88
sympathomimetics (adrenergic drugs),
  91, 97*t*
  actions, 97
  clinical uses, 97*t*
    for asthma, 467
    glaucoma, 602, 602*t*
  drugs classified as, 91*t*, 468*t*
  effects of, 97
  Nursing Process Focus, 98–99*t*
  Patients Need to Know, 102*t*
Synalar. *See* fluocinolone acetonide
synapses, 88
synaptic cleft, 88
Synthroid. *See* **levothyroxine**
systemic mycoses, 413
systolic pressure, 267, 268*f*

T

$t_{1/2}$ (half-life), 45
tablets, 27
   enteric-coated, 27
   guidelines for administering, 26t
   orally disintegrating tablets (ODTs), 27
   sustained-release, 27
Tab-Profen. *See* **ibuprofen**
tacrine, 92, 92t, 165, 165t
tacrolimus, 381t
tadalafil, 556, 556t
tafluprost, 602t
Talwin. *See* pentazocine
Tambocor. *See* flecainide
tamoxifen, 443, 513
   Drug Prototype, 444t
   route and adult dose, 444t
tamsulosin, 100t, 558t
Tapazole. *See* methimazole
tapeworm, 389f
tardive dyskinesia, 147t, 148
Tasmar. *See* tolcapone
Tavist Allergy, 461t
taxanes, 442, 442t
tazarotene, 590t, 593t, 594
Tazorac. *See* tazarotene
T cells, 375
Tegretol. *See* carbamazepine
telavancin, 404t
telithromycin, 404t
telmisartan, 275t
temazepam, 74, 114t
Temovate. *See* clobetasol
temozolomide, 437t
temporal lobe seizures, 183. *See also* complex
   partial seizures; seizure(s)
TEN (toxic epidermal necrolysis), 583
tenecteplase, 312t
teniposide, 442, 442t
tenofovir, 419t
Tenormin. *See* **atenolol**
Tensilon. *See* edrophonium
tension headache, 211
teratogen, 17
terazosin, 100t, 281t, 558t
terbinafine, 415t
terbutaline, 97t, 553t
terconazole, 415t
teriparatide, 571t
termination of drug action, 46
Testim. *See* **testosterone**
testolactone, 444t
Testopel. *See* **testosterone**
testosterone
   androgen base, 544, 554
   buccal system, 554, 555t
   Drug Prototype, 554t
   for hypogonadism, 554, 555t
   implantable pellets, 554, 555t
   intramuscular, 554
   route and adult dose, 555t
   transdermal gel, 554, 555t
   transdermal patch, 554, 555t
testosterone cypionate, 555t
testosterone enanthate, 555t
Testred. *See* methyltestosterone

tetracaine, 221t
tetracycline, 397–398, 397t, 409t
   clinical uses
      acne, 590, 590t
      peptic ulcer disease, 485
   Drug Prototype, 397t
   interactions
      with heparin, 352t
      with sodium bicarbonate, 261t
   pregnancy category, 397, 397t
   route and adult dose, 397t
tetrahydrocannabinol (THC), 76
tetrahydrozoline, 464t, 606t
Teveten. *See* eprosartan
Thalitone. *See* chlorthalidone
THC (tetrahydrocannabinol), 76
theophylline, for asthma, 468t, 469
therapeutic classification, 13–14, 13t. *See also*
   therapeutic usefulness
therapeutic lifestyle changes
   for angina, 304
   for hyperlipidemia, 236–237
   for hypertension, 271–272
therapeutic range of drug, 45
therapeutics, 3
therapeutic usefulness, 13. *See also* therapeutic
   classification
thiamine (vitamin B₁), 498t
thiazide and thiazide-like diuretics
   actions, 253f
   adverse effects, 254
   drugs classified as, 254t
   interactions
      with cholestyramine, 240t
      with enalapril, 277t
thioguanine, 439t
thioridazine, 146t
thiotepa, 437t
thiothixene, 148t
third-degree burns, 584
three checks of drug administration, 22
thrombin, 347, 357, 357t
Thrombinar. *See* thrombin
thrombocytopenia, 436t
thromboembolic disorder, 349
thrombolytics, 350
   adverse effects, 310
   clinical uses, 356–357
      myocardial infarction, 310
      stroke, 314
   interactions
      with clopidogrel, 356t
   Nursing Process Focus, 313t
thrombophlebitis, 604
thrombotic stroke, 314
thrombus, 349
Thyrar. *See* thyroid dessicated
Thyro-block. *See* potassium iodide
   and iodine
thyroglobulin, 17t
thyroid dessicated, 518t
thyroid disorders, 514t, 516–519, 518t
thyroid gland
   anatomy, 512f
   feedback mechanisms, 517f
   function, 516
   pituitary gland and, 513f

thyroid-releasing hormone (TRH), 516
thyroid-stimulating hormone (TSH), 511, 513f
Thyroid USP. *See* thyroid dessicated
Thyrolar. *See* liotrix
thyroxine, 516
tiagabine, 185t, 187t
ticagrelor, 355t, 356
ticarcillin, 394t
Ticlid. *See* ticlopidine
ticlopidine, 355, 355t
tigecycline, 397t
Tikosyn. *See* dofetilide
tiludronate, 571t
timolol
   clinical uses, 100t, 212t
      glaucoma, 603t
      hypertension, 281t
   Drug Prototype, 604t
   route and adult dose, 212t, 281t
timolol maleate, 306t
Timoptic. *See* **timolol**
tinidazole, 426t
tinzaparin, 351t
tioconazole, 415t
tiotropium, 95t
tipranavir, 419t
tirofiban, 355t
tissue plasminogen activator (tPA), 349
titer, 376
tizanidine, 170, 171t
TNF (tumor necrosis factor), 375
TNKase. *See* tenecteplase
tobramycin, 399t
tocilizumab, 576t
tocolytics, 552
Tofranil. *See* **imipramine**
tolazamide, 536t
tolbutamide, 536t
tolcapone, 161–162, 161t
Tolectin. *See* tolmetin
tolerance, 73
   immunity and, 73
   marijuana and, 76
   resistance and, 73
Tolinase. *See* tolazamide
tolmetin, 209t, 365t
tolnaftate, 415t
tolterodine, 95t
tonic-clonic seizures, 183. *See also* grand mal
   seizures; seizure(s)
   clonic phase, 183
   hydantoin and related drugs for treating,
      189–190t
   status epilepticus and, 184
   tonic phase, 183
tonic phase, tonic-clonic seizure, 183
tonic spasm, 169. *See also* muscle spasms
tonometry, 601
Topamax. *See* topiramate
topical anesthesia, 219f, 219t
topical route, 28–29
   nasal, 30t, 31
   ophthalmic, 29, 29f, 30t
   otic, 30t, 31
   rectal suppositories, 31t, 32
   transdermal, 29, 30t
   vaginal, 30t, 31–32

Topicort. *See* desoximetasone
topiramate, 185*t*, 187*t*, 189, 191, 212*t*
topoisomerase inhibitors, 442, 442*t*
topotecan, 442, 442*t*
Toprol. *See* **metoprolol**
Toradol. *See* ketorolac
toremifene, 444*t*
torsemide, 252, 253*t*, 274*t*, 293*t*
total parenteral nutrition (TPN), 505
Toviaz. *See* fesoterodine
toxic concentration, 45
toxic epidermal necrolysis (TEN), 583
toxins, 389
toxoid vaccines, 376
tPA (tissue plasminogen activator), 349
TPN (total parenteral nutrition), 505
trabecular meshwork, 599
trace minerals, 499, 501*t*
trade name, 14
traditional therapeutic drugs, 4
    characteristics of, 4*t*
    stages of approval for, 7–9, 8*f*
Tradjenta. *See* linagliptin
tramadol, 209*t*, 210
trandolapril, 275*t*
tranexamic acid, 357, 357*t*
tranquilizer, 111
tranquilizers, 74. *See also* sedative(s)
transdermal administration, 29, 30*t*
transdermal testosterone gel, 554, 555*t*
transdermal testosterone patch, 554, 555*t*
transmucosal administration, 31. *See also* nasal
    administration
transplant rejection, 380
Tranxene. *See* clorazepate
tranylcypromine, 112*t*, 127*t*
trastuzumab, 445*t*
Travatan. *See* travoprost
travoprost, 602*t*
trazodone, 112*t*, 127*t*, 129
tremors, 159, 162*f*
Trental. *See* pentoxifylline
tretinoin
    clinical uses, 590*t*
    Drug Prototype, 591*t*
Trexall. *See* **methotrexate**
Trexan. *See* naltrexone
TRH (thyroid-releasing hormone), 516
triamcinolone, 522*t*
    inhaled, 470*t*
    intranasal, 463*t*
    for severe inflammation, 368*t*
triamcinolone acetonide, 592*t*
Triaminic Cold/Allergy, 461*t*
triamterene, 253*f*, 256*t*, 274*t*
triazolam, 74, 114*t*
Trichophyton, 414*t*
Tricor. *See* fenofibrate
tricyclic antidepressants (TCAS), 125, 126*t*
    actions, 125
    adverse effects, 113, 125
    amitriptyline, 201
    chemical structure, 125
    childhood enuresis (bed-wetting), treatment
        of, 125
    clinical uses
        anxiety disorders, 112*t*

chronic pain impluses, 201
    depression, 126*t*
    migraine prophylaxis, 213*t*
    neuropathic pain impluses, 201
    contraindications, 113
    drugs classified as, 110, 125
    half-life of, 125
    imipramine, 201
    interactions, 133*t*
        with atropine, 95*t*
        with benztropine, 164*t*
        with chlorpromazine, 147*t*
        with epinephrine, 327*t*
        with levodopa, 163*t*
        with morphine, 203*t*
        with norepinephrine, 326*t*
        with phenelzine, 133*t*
        with phenylephrine, 98*t*
    nortriptyline, 201
    Patients Need to Know, 139*t*
    pregnancy category, 113
trifluoperazine, 146*t*
trifluridine, 424*t*
triglycerides, 235, 236, 238*t*
trihexyphenidyl, 95, 95*t*, 163*t*
triiodothyronine, 516
trimethoprim-sulfamethoxazole
    Drug Prototype, 402*t*
    route and adult dose, 402*t*
trimipramine, 112*t*, 126*t*
Triostat. *See* liothyronine
triphasic OC, 546, 546*t*
triple therapy, 481
Triplix. *See* fenofibrate
triptans, 211
triptorelin, 444*t*
Tronothane. *See* pramoxine
Tropicacyl. *See* tropicamide
tropicamide, 606*t*
Trusopt. *See* dorzolamide
Trypanosoma, 389*f*
tube feeding, 504, 504*f. See also* enteral nutrition
tubercles, 406
tuberculin syringes (TB), 34
tuberculosis
    Nursing Process Focus, 407–408*t*
    pathophysiology, 406
    pharmacotherapy, 406, 407*t*
tubocurarine, 175, 176*t*, 228*t*
tubular secretion, 250*f*, 251
tumor, 432
tumor necrosis factor (TNF), 375
tumor suppressor genes, 432
Tums. *See* calcium carbonate
T wave, 334*f*
Twinrix, 377*t*
Tylenol. *See* **acetaminophen**
Tylenol Allergy Multisystem, 461*t*
Tylenol PM, 461*t*
Tylenol with Codeine, 205
type 1 diabetes mellitus
    description, 530
    pharmacotherapy. *See* insulin
    signs and symptoms, 530
type 2 diabetes mellitus
    description, 534
    insulin resistance, 534, 535

    Nursing Proces Focus, 538–539*t*
    pharmacotherapy, 535–536*t*, 535–537
        alpha-glucosidase inhibitors,
            535*t*, 536
        biguanide, 535*t*, 536
        incretin enhancers, 535*t*, 537
        meglitinides, 536, 536*t*
        sulfonylureas, 536, 536*t*
        thiazolidinediones, 536, 536*t*
tyramine, 132

U

ulcerative colitis, 480
ulipristal, 547
Uloric. *See* febuxostat
Ultane. *See* sevoflurane
Ultiva. *See* remifentanil
Ultram. *See* tramadol
Ultraprin. *See* **ibuprofen**
Ultravate. *See* halobetasol
ultraviolet A (UVA) phototherapy, 594
ultraviolet B (UVB) phototherapy, 594
undecylenic acid, 415*t*
undernutrition, 504
Uni-Buff. *See* **aspirin**
Unisom. *See* **diphenhydramine**
Uni-Tren. *See* **aspirin**
Univasc. *See* moexipril
unstable angina, 303
upper respiratory tract (URT), 455
urea, 257*t*
Ureaphil. *See* urea
Urecholine. *See* **bethanechol**
uric acid inhibitors, 577, 577*t*
uricosurics, 577, 577*t*
urinary antiseptics, 403
urinary system, 249–251, 249*f,* 250*f*
urinary tract infections (UTIs)
    hospital-acquired, 390*t*
urine, 250
Uro-KP neutral. *See* potassium/sodium
    phosphates
UroXatral. *See* alfuzosin
Uroxatral. *See* alfuzosin
URT (upper respiratory tract), 455
urticaria, 583
U.S. Department of Defense, 9
U.S. Department of Health and Human
    Services, 5, 6*f*
U.S. Department of Homeland Security, 9
U.S. Pharmacopoeia (USP), 5, 6*f*
*U.S. Pharmacopoeia-National Formulary
    (USP-NF),* 5, 6*f*
uterine stimulants and relaxants, 552, 553*t*
Uticort. *See* betamethasone benzoate

V

vaccination (immunization), 376
vaccine(s), 374, 376–378, 377*t*, 378*t*, 383*t*
    toxoid, 376
vaginal administration, 30*t*, 31–32
valacyclovir, 424*t*
valdecoxib, 8, 366
valerian, for anxiety and insomnia, 118*t*
Valisone. *See* betamethasone valerate

Valium. *See* **diazepam**
valproic acid, 201
  actions, 191*t*
  adverse effects, 191*t*
  clinical uses, 191*t*
    anxiety, 117*t*, 118
    bipolar disorder, 135*t*
    migraine prophylaxis, 212*t*
    seizures, 185*t*, 189, 190*t*
  Drug Prototype, 191*t*
  interactions, 191*t*
    with aspirin, 191*t*
    with chlorpromazine, 191*t*
    with cimetidine, 191*t*
    with clonazepam, 191*t*
    with diazepam, 188*t*
    with erythromycin, 191*t*
    with ethosuximide, 192*t*
    with felbamate, 191*t*
    with lamotrigine, 191*t*
    with phenytoin, 191*t*
    with rifampin, 191*t*
  route and adult dose, 190*t*, 212*t*
valsartan, 275*t*, 293*t*, 294
valvular heart disease, 347*t*
vancomycin
  clinical uses, 403, 404*t*
  Drug Prototype, 403*t*
  route and adult dose, 404*t*
vancomycin-resistant enterococci (VRE), 392
vardenafil, 556, 556*t*
varicella vaccine, 377*t*
varicella-zoster virus, 424
Vascepa. *See* icosapent
Vascor. *See* bepridil
vasoconstrictors, 324–325, 325*t*
vasodilators
  actions, 282–283, 295*t*, 296
  adverse effects, 296
  clinical uses
    heart failure, 295*t*, 296
    hypertension, 283, 283*t*
  drugs classified as, 283*t*, 295*t*
vasomotor center, 270, 271*f*
vasopressin (antidiuretic hormone), 270,
  514–515, 514*t*, 515*t*
vasospastic (Prinzmetal's) angina, 303, 309
Vasotec. *See* **enalapril**
vastus lateralis site, intramuscular injection, 36
vecuronium, 176*t*
venlafaxine, 112*t*, 127*t*, 129
ventilation, 455–456
Ventolin. *See* albuterol
ventricular flutter/fibrillation, 333*t*
ventricular tachycardia, 333*t*
ventrogluteal site, intramuscular injection,
  34*t*, 36
verapamil
  actions, 342*t*
  adverse effects, 342*t*
  clinical uses, 342*t*
    angina, 306*t*
    dysrhythmias, 341*t*
    migraine prophylaxis, 212*t*
  Drug Prototype, 342*t*
  interactions, 342*t*
    with clopidogrel, 356*t*

  with dantrolene, 175*t*
  with doxorubicin, 441*t*
  route and adult dose, 212*t*, 278*t*, 306*t*, 341*t*
Verdeso. *See* desonide
Versed. *See* midazolam; midazolam
  hydrochloride
vertigo, 461
very low-density lipoprotein (VLDL),
  236, 237*f*
Viagra. *See* **sildenafil**
Vibramycin. *See* doxycycline
Vicodin, 205
Victoza. *See* liraglutide
vigabatrin, 187*t*
Viibryd. *See* vilazodone
vilazodone, 126*t*
villi, 478
vinblastine, 442, 442*t*
vinca alkaloids, 442, 442*t*
vincristine, 442
  Drug Prototype, 443*t*
  route and adult dose, 442*t*
vincristine liposome, 442*t*
vinorelbine, 442*t*
Vioxx. *See* rofecoxib
virilization, 554
Virilon. *See* methyltestosterone
virulence, 389
virus(es), 389*f*, 417
visceral pain, 198
Visine. *See* tetrahydrozoline
Visine LR. *See* oxymetazoline
Visken. *See* pindolol
vismodegib, 445*t*
vitamin(s)
  accidental overdose of, 505*t*
  characteristics, 497
  classification, 497–498
  deficiency, 499
  description, 497
  fat-soluble, 497–498
  recommended dietary allowances (RDA),
    498–499, 498*t*
  water-soluble, 497
vitamin A, 498*t*
vitamin B₁ (thiamine), 498*t*
vitamin B₂. *See* riboflavin
vitamin B₂ (riboflavin), 498*t*
vitamin B₃ (niacin), 498*t*
vitamin B₅ (pantothenic acid), 498*t*
vitamin B₆ (pyridoxine), 498*t*
vitamin B₇ (biotin), 498*t*
vitamin B₉. *See* folic acid/folate
vitamin B₁₂
  deficiency, 498*t*, 499
  metabolism of, 500*f*
  recommended dietary allowance, 498*t*
vitamin C, 498*t*
vitamin D
  deficiency, 498*t*, 499
  functon, 498*t*
  interaction
    with phenobarbital, 188*t*
    with phenytoin, 190*t*
  pathway for activation and action, 567*f*
  recommended dietary allowance, 498*t*
  supplements

  drugs classified as, 568*t*
  for osteomalacia, 567, 568
vitamin E, 498*t*
vitamin K
  deficiency, 498*t*
  functions, 498*t*
  interactions with cholestyramine, 240*t*
  recommended dietary allowance, 498*t*
  for warfarin reversal, 350
Vivactil. *See* protriptyline
Vivatrol. *See* naltrexone
VLDL (very low-density lipoprotein),
  236, 237*f*
volatile inhalants, abuse of, 70
volatile liquid anesthetics. *See* general
  anesthetics, inhaled
Voltaren. *See* diclofenac
vomiting, 489–490, 490*t*
voriconazole, 415*t*
Vosol HC. *See* acetic acid and hydrocortisone
VoSpire. *See* albuterol
VRE (vancomycin-resistant enterococci), 392
Vytorin, 244

W

warfarin
  actions, 350*f*, 353*t*
  adverse effects, 353*t*
  black box warning, 353*t*
  clinical uses, 313, 352, 353*t*
  Drug Prototype, 353*t*
  interactions, 353*t*
    with acetaminophen, 369*t*
    with aspirin, 208*t*
    with ciprofloxacin, 401*t*
    with erythromycin, 398*t*
    with omeprazole, 483*t*
    with psyllium, 487*t*
    with sertraline, 133*t*
    with valproic acid, 191*t*
  route and adult dose, 351*t*
water-soluble vitamin, 497. *See also*
  vitamin(s)
weight loss, 491
Welchol. *See* colesevelam
Wellbutrin. *See* bupropion
Westcort. *See* hydrocortisone valerate
whiteheads, 589
withdrawal, 16
withdrawal syndromes, 72

X

Xalatan. *See* **latanoprost**
Xanax. *See* alprazolam
xanthines, 468*t*, 469
Xarelto. *See* rivaroxaban
Xeomin. *See* incobotulinumtoxin A
Xgen. *See* denosumab
XTC (MDMA), 77
Xylocaine. *See* **lidocaine**
xylometazoline, 464*t*
Xyrem. *See* sodium oxybate

Y

yeasts, 413

Z

zafirlukast, 470t
zaleplon, 111, 117t, 119
Zanaflex. *See* tizanidine
zanamivir, 424, 424t
Zantac. *See* penicillins; **ranitidine**
Zaroxolyn. *See* metolazone
Zebeta. *See* bisoprolol
Zelapar. *See* selegiline
Zemplar. *See* paricalcitol
Zemuron. *See* rocuronium
Zestoretic, 255, 273
Zestril. *See* **lisinopril**
Zetia. *See* ezetimibe
ziconotide, 209t, 210
zidovudine
    Drug Prototype, 421t

interactions
    with acyclovir, 425t
    with interferon alfa-2b, 446t
    route and adult dose, 419t
zileuton, 470t
Zincate. *See* zinc sulfate
zinc gluconate, 502t
zinc sulfate, 502t
Zioptan. *See* tafluprost
ziprasidone, 135t, 151t
Zipsor. *See* diclofenac
Zocor. *See* simvastatin
Zofran. *See* **ondansetron**
zoledronate, 571t
zoledronic acid, 571t
zoledronic acid (zoledronate sodium), 445t
Zollinger-Ellison syndrome, 482, 483t
zolmitriptan, 212t

Zoloft. *See* **sertraline**
zolpidem
    actions, 118t
    adverse effects, 118t
    clinical uses, 117t
    Drug Prototype, 118t
Zometa. *See* zoledronate
Zomig. *See* zolmitriptan
Zonegran. *See* zonisamide
zonisamide, 185t, 185t, 190t, 191
Zorbtive. *See* somatropin
Zorcaine. *See* articaine
Zorprin. *See* **aspirin**
Zovirax. *See* **acyclovir**
Zuplenz. *See* **ondansetron**
Zyban. *See* bupropion
Zyloprim. *See* **allopurinol**
Zyprexa. *See* olanzapine

GUIDE TO SPECIAL FEATURES

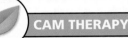 **CAM THERAPY**

Aloe Vera for Improving Eye and Ear Health, *p. 608, Ch. 37*

Aloe Vera for Skin Conditions, *p. 592, Ch. 36*

Carnitine and Heart Disease, *p. 293, Ch. 19*

Cayenne for Muscular Tension, *p. 173, Ch. 12*

Coenzyme Q10 for Heart Disease, *p. 242, Ch. 16*

Cranberry for Urinary System Health, *p. 251, Ch. 17*

Dong Quai for Premenstrual Syndrome, *p. 549, Ch. 34*

Echinacea for Boosting the Immune System, *p. 376, Ch. 25*

Evening Primrose Oil for Pain and Eczema, *p. 211, Ch. 14*

Garlic for Cardiovascular Health, *p. 355, Ch. 23*

Ginger for Nausea, *p. 491, Ch. 30*

Ginkgo biloba for Dementia, *p. 167, Ch. 12*

Ginseng and Cardiovascular Disease, *p. 314, Ch. 20*

Glucosamine and Chondroitin for Osteoarthritis, *p. 578, Ch. 35*

Grape Seed Extract for Hypertension, *p. 280, Ch. 18*

Medication Errors and Dietary Supplements, *p. 57, Ch. 5*

Milk Thistle for Liver Damage, *p. 74, Ch. 7*

Oil of Cloves for Dental Pain, *p. 223, Ch. 15*

Omega-3 Fatty Acids and Diabetes, *p. 534, Ch. 33*

Red Yeast Rice and Cholesterol, *p. 238, Ch. 16*

Sea Vegetables, *p. 504, Ch. 31*

Selenium's Role in Cancer Prevention, *p. 435, Ch. 28*

St. John's Wort for Depression, *p. 134, Ch. 10*

The Antibacterial Properties of Goldenseal, *p. 395, Ch. 26*

The Ketogenic Diet for Epilepsy, *p. 188, Ch. 13*

Valerian for Anxiety and Insomnia, *p. 118, Ch. 9*

Drug Prototype

acetaminophen, *p. 369, Ch. 24*

acyclovir, *p. 425, Ch. 27*

alendronate, *p. 572, Ch. 35*

allopurinol, *p. 578, Ch. 35*

alteplase, *p. 357, Ch. 23*

aminocaproic acid, *p. 358, Ch. 23*

amiodarone, *p. 341, Ch. 22*

amphotericin B, *p. 416, Ch. 27*

aspirin, *p. 208, Ch. 14*

atenolol, *p. 309, Ch. 20*

atorvastatin, *p. 240, Ch. 16*

atropine, *p. 95, Ch. 8*

benzocaine, *p. 589, Ch. 36*

benztropine, *p. 164, Ch. 12*

bethanechol, *p. 93, Ch. 8*

calcitriol, *p. 569, Ch. 35*

calcium salts, *p. 569, Ch. 35*

carbidopa, *p. 163, Ch. 12*

carvedilol, *p. 296, Ch. 19*

cefotaxime, *p. 396, Ch. 26*

chlorpromazine, *p. 147, Ch. 11*

cholestyramine, *p. 240, Ch. 16*

ciprofloxacin, *p. 401, Ch. 26*

clopidogrel, *p. 356, Ch. 23*

cromolyn, *p. 471, Ch. 29*

cyanocobalamin, *p. 499, Ch. 31*

cyclobenzaprine, *p. 171, Ch. 12*

cyclophosphamide, *p. 438, Ch. 28*

cyclosporine, *p. 382, Ch. 25*

dantrolene, *p. 175, Ch. 12*

desmopressin, *p. 514, Ch. 32*

diazepam, *p. 188, Ch. 13*

digoxin, *p. 295, Ch. 19*

diltiazem, *p. 309, Ch. 20*

diphenhydramine, *p. 460, Ch. 29*

diphenoxylate with atropine, *p. 488, Ch. 30*

donepezil, *p. 167, Ch. 12*

dopamine, *p. 326, Ch. 21*

doxazosin, *p. 282, Ch. 18*

doxorubicin, *p. 441, Ch. 28*

enalapril, *p. 277, Ch. 18*

entacapone, *p. 163, Ch. 12*

epinephrine, *p. 327, Ch. 21*

epoetin alfa, *p. 446, Ch. 28*

erythromycin, *p. 398, Ch. 26*

escitalopram, *p. 113, Ch. 9*

estradiol with norethindrone, *p. 547, Ch. 34*

estrogen, conjugated, *p. 551, Ch. 34*

ethosuximide, *p. 192, Ch. 13*

ferrous sulfate, *p. 501, Ch. 31*

finasteride, *p. 558, Ch. 34*

fluticasone, *p. 463, Ch. 29*

furosemide, *p. 254, Ch. 17*

gemfibrozil, *p. 244, Ch. 16*

gentamicin, *p. 400, Ch. 26*

haloperidol, *p. 149, Ch. 11*

heparin, *p. 352, Ch. 23*

hepatitis B vaccine, *p. 378, Ch. 25*

hydralazine, *p. 283, Ch. 18*

hydrochlorothiazide, *p. 255, Ch. 17*

hydrocortisone, *p. 522, Ch. 32*

hydroxychloroquine, *p. 575, Ch. 35*

imipramine, *p. 129, Ch. 10*

insulin regular, *p. 532, Ch. 33*

interferon alfa-2b (intron-A), *p. 380, Ch. 25*

interferon alfa-2b, *p. 446, Ch. 28*

isoflurane, *p. 225, Ch. 15*

isoniazid, *p. 406, Ch. 26*

latanoprost, *p. 601, Ch. 37*

levodopa, *p. 163, Ch. 12*

levothyroxine, *p. 518, Ch. 32*

lidocaine, *p. 222, Ch. 15*

lisinopril, *p. 292, Ch. 19*

lorazepam, *p. 116, Ch. 9*

medroxyprogesterone, *p. 552, Ch. 34*

metformin, *p. 537, Ch. 33*

methotrexate, *p. 440, Ch. 28*

methylphenidate, *p. 137, Ch. 10*

metronidazole, *p. 427, Ch. 27*

milrinone, *p. 297, Ch. 19*

morphine, *p. 203, Ch. 14*

naloxone, *p. 205, Ch. 14*

naproxen, *p. 366, Ch. 24*

naproxen sodium, *p. 366, Ch. 24*

nifedipine, *p. 279, Ch. 18*

nitroglycerin, *p. 307, Ch. 20*

nitrous oxide, *p. 225, Ch. 15*

norepinephrine, *p. 326, Ch. 21*

normal serum albumin, *p. 323, Ch. 21*

nystatin, *p. 416, Ch. 27*

omeprazole, *p. 483, Ch. 30*

ondansetron, *p. 490, Ch. 30*

oxymetazoline, *p. 464, Ch. 29*

oxytocin, *p. 553, Ch. 34*

penicillin G, *p. 395, Ch. 26*

permethrin, *p. 587, Ch. 36*

phenelzine, *p. 133, Ch. 10*

phenobarbital, *p. 188, Ch. 13*

phenylephrine, *p. 98, Ch. 8*

phenytoin, *p. 190, Ch. 13*

potassium chloride, *p. 260, Ch. 17*

prazosin, *p. 100, Ch. 8*

prednisone, *p. 369, Ch. 24*

procainamide, *p. 339, Ch. 22*

propranolol, *p. 340, Ch. 22*

propylthiouracil, *p. 519, Ch. 32*

psyllium mucilloid, *p. 487, Ch. 30*

raloxifene, *p. 571, Ch. 35*

ranitidine, *p. 483, Ch. 30*

reteplase, *p. 312, Ch. 20*

risperidone, *p. 152, Ch. 11*

sertraline, *p. 133, Ch. 10*

sildenafil, *p. 556, Ch. 34*

sodium bicarbonate, *p. 261, Ch. 17*

spironolactone, *p. 256, Ch. 17*

succinylcholine, *p. 228, Ch. 15*

sumatriptan, *p. 213, Ch. 14*

tamoxifen, *p. 444, Ch. 28*

testosterone, *p. 554, Ch. 34*

tetracycline, *p. 397, Ch. 26*

timolol, *p. 604, Ch. 37*

tretinoin, *p. 591, Ch. 36*

trimethoprim-sulfamethoxazole, *p. 402, Ch. 26*

valproic acid, *p. 191, Ch.13*

vancomycin, *p. 403, Ch. 26*

verapamil, *p. 342, Ch. 22*

vincristine, *p. 443, Ch. 28*

warfarin, *p. 353, Ch. 23*

zidovudine, *p. 421, Ch. 27*

zolpidem, *p. 118, Ch. 9*

Fast Facts

ADHD, *p. 136, Ch. 10*

Allergies, *p. 458, Ch. 29*

Alternative Therapies in America, *p. 61, Ch. 6*

Anesthesia and Anesthetics, *p. 218, Ch. 15*

Angina Pectoris and Coronary Heart Disease, *p. 304, Ch. 20*

Anxiety Disorders, *p. 107, Ch. 9*

Arthritis and Joint Disorders, *p. 575, Ch. 35*

Asthma, *p. 467, Ch. 29*

Bacterial Infections, *p. 388, Ch. 26*

Cancer, *p. 431, Ch. 28*

Clotting Disorders, *p. 349, Ch. 23*

Diabetes Mellitus, *p. 530, Ch. 33*

Dysrhythmias, *p. 332, Ch. 22*

Epilepsy, *p. 182, Ch. 13*

Fungal, Viral, and Parasitic Diseases, *p. 413, Ch. 27*

Gastrointestinal Tract Disorders, *p. 477, Ch. 30*

Glaucoma, *p. 600, Ch. 37*

Grapefruit Juice and Drug Interactions, *p. 23, Ch. 3*

Heart Failure, *p. 288, Ch. 19*

High Blood Cholesterol, *p. 235, Ch. 16*

Hypertension, *p. 267, Ch. 18*

Inflammatory Disorders, *p. 363, Ch. 24*

Insomnia, *p. 110, Ch. 9*

Muscle Spasms, *p. 170, Ch. 12*

Myocardial Infarction, *p. 310, Ch. 20*

Neurodegenerative Diseases, *p. 159, Ch. 12*

Pain, *p. 199, Ch. 14*

Potentially Fatal Drug Reactions, *p. 23, Ch. 3*

Psychosis, *p. 144, Ch. 11*

Renal Disorders, *p. 250, Ch. 17*

Shock, *p. 321, Ch. 21*

Skin Disorders, *p. 587, Ch. 36*

Stroke, *p. 315, Ch. 20*

Substance Abuse in the United States, *p. 70, Ch. 7*

Thyroid Disorders, *p. 517, Ch. 32*

Vaccines and Immune Disorders, *p. 374, Ch. 25*

Vitamins, Minerals, and Dietary Supplements, *p. 497, Ch. 31*

▶ Life Span Fact

Absorption of Food Diminishes with Age, *p. 499, Ch. 31*

ADHD in Children, *p. 137, Ch. 10*

Administering Ophthalmic Drugs to Children, *p. 29, Ch. 3*

Administering Otic Drugs to Children, *p. 31, Ch. 3*

Anticholinergic Side Effects in Older Adults, *p. 339, Ch. 22*

Bleeding Complications in Elderly Patients, *p. 352, Ch. 23*

Chewing and Swallowing Difficulties in Older Adults, *p. 504, Ch. 31*

Childhood Vaccine Act, *p. 7, Ch. 3*

Constipation in Older Adults, *p. 486, Ch. 30*

Crushing Medications for Children and Elderly Patients, *p. 27, Ch. 3*

Decrease in Bone Mass with Aging, *p. 500, Ch. 31*

Depression in Elderly Patients, *p. 124, Ch. 10*

Drug Compliance Among Elderly Patients, *p. 23, Ch. 3*

Drug Therapy in Older Adults, *p. 57, Ch. 5*

Effects of BPH, *p. 556, Ch. 34*

Elderly Patients May Need Vitamin D Supplements, *p. 499, Ch. 31*

Epilepsy in Youth and Elderly, *p. 183, Ch. 13*

Herbs and Dietary Supplements for Children, *p. 62, Ch. 6*

High Fever in Children, *p. 183, Ch. 13*

Laxative Misuse in Older Adults, *p. 486, Ch. 30*

Medication-Related Sleeping Problems in Elderly Patients, *p. 110, Ch. 9*

Older Adults at Particular Risk for Dehydration, *p. 274, Ch. 18*

Potassium Channel Blocker Side Effects in Older Adults, *p. 342, Ch. 22*

Potential Vitamin Deficiency in Infancy and Childhood, *p. 499, Ch. 31*

Reduced Metabolic Enzyme Activity in Very Young and Elderly Patients, *p. 44, Ch. 4*

TCA Use in Elderly Patients, *p. 125, Ch. 10*

Ventrogluteal Site for IM Injections in Children, *p. 36, Ch. 3*

Vitamin D Deficiency in Breastfed Infants, *p. 499, Ch. 31*

NURSING PROCESS FOCUS

Patients Receiving ACE Inhibitor Therapy, *p. 276, Ch. 18*

Patients Receiving Adrenergic Blocker Therapy, *p. 101, Ch. 8*

Patients Receiving Adrenergic Drug Therapy, *p. 98, Ch. 8*

Patients Receiving Antianxiety Therapy, *p. 115, Ch. 9*

Patients Receiving Antibacterial Therapy, *p. 404, Ch. 26*

Patients Receiving Anticoagulant and Antiplatelet Therapy, *p. 353, Ch. 23*

Patients Receiving Antidepressant Therapy, *p. 130, Ch. 10*

Patients Receiving Antidysrhythmic Drugs, *p. 336, Ch. 22*

Patients Receiving Antihistamine Therapy, *p. 461, Ch. 29*

Patients Receiving Antineoplastic Therapy, *p. 447, Ch. 28*

Patients Receiving Antiseizure Drug Therapy, *p. 192, Ch. 13*

Patients Receiving Antitubercular Drugs, *p. 407, Ch. 26*

Patients Receiving Atypical Antipsychotic Therapy, *p. 153, Ch. 11*

Patients Receiving Bronchodilators, *p. 469, Ch. 29*

Patients Receiving Calcium Channel Blocker Therapy, *p. 279, Ch. 18*

Patients Receiving Cholinergic Blocker (Anticholinergic) Therapy, *p. 96, Ch. 8*

Patients Receiving Direct- and Indirect-Acting Cholinergic Drug Therapy, *p. 93, Ch. 8*

Patients Receiving Diuretic Therapy, *p. 257, Ch.17*

Patients Receiving Drugs for Muscle Spasms or Spasticity, *p. 172, Ch. 12*

Patients Receiving Drug Therapy for Peptic Ulcer Disease, *p. 484, Ch. 30*

Patients Receiving Drug Therapy with HMG-CoA Reductase Inhibitors (Statins), *p. 241, Ch. 16*

Patients Receiving Immunosuppressants, *p. 382, Ch. 25*

Patients Receiving Insulin Therapy, *p. 533, Ch. 33*

Patients Receiving Intravenous Fluid Therapy, *p. 324, Ch. 21*

Patients Receiving Iron Supplements, *p. 503, Ch. 31*

Patients Receiving Laxative Therapy, *p. 487, Ch. 30*

Patients Receiving Local Anesthesia, *p. 223, Ch. 15*

Patients Receiving NSAID Therapy, *p. 367, Ch. 24*

Patients Receiving Opioids, *p. 206, Ch. 14*

Patients Receiving Oral Contraceptive Therapy, *p. 548, Ch. 34*

Patients Receiving Organic Nitrate Therapy, *p. 308, Ch. 20*

Patients Receiving Pharmacotheraphy for HIV-AIDS, *p. 422, Ch. 27*

Patients Receiving Pharmacotherapy for Glaucoma, *p. 604, Ch. 37*

Patients Receiving Pharmacotherapy for Lice or Mite Infestation, *p. 588, Ch. 36*

Patients Receiving Pharmacotherapy for Osteoporosis, *p. 572, Ch. 35*

Patients Receiving Pharmacotherapy for Type 2 Diabetes, *p. 538, Ch. 33*

Patients Receiving Phenothiazines and Nonphenothiazine Therapy, *p. 149, Ch. 11*

Patients Receiving Superficial Antifungal Therapy, *p. 417, Ch. 27*

Patients Receiving Systemic Corticosteroid Therapy, *p. 523, Ch. 32*

Patients Receiving Thrombolytic Therapy, *p. 313, Ch. 20*

Patients Receiving Thyroid Hormone Replacement, *p. 519, Ch. 32*

PATIENTS NEED TO KNOW

Antidepressants, *p. 139, Ch. 10*

Antiseizure Medications, *p. 194, Ch. 13*

Anxiolytics and CNS Depressants, *p. 119, Ch. 9*

Autonomic Medications, *p. 102, Ch. 8*

Bacterial Infections, *p. 409, Ch. 26*

Bone or Joint Disorders, *p. 578, Ch. 35*

Cancer, *p. 449, Ch. 28*

Coagulation Disorders, *p. 358, Ch. 23*

Digestive Disorders, *p. 492, Ch. 30*

Drugs for Fluid, Acid–Base, and Electrolyte Disorders, *p. 262, Ch. 17*

Drugs for Pain, *p. 315, Ch. 20*

Dysrhythmias, *p.343, Ch. 22*

Endocrine Disorders, *p. 524, Ch. 32*

Eye and Ear Disorders, *p. 608, Ch. 37*

Fungal, Viral, or Parasitic Infections, *p. 427, Ch. 27*

Heart Failure, *p. 297, Ch. 19*

Hypertension, *p. 284, Ch. 18*

Immune Disorders, *p. 383, Ch. 25*

Inflammatory Disorders, *p. 370, Ch. 24*

Lipid Disorders, *p. 245, Ch. 16*

Local Anesthetic Medications, *p. 229, Ch. 15*

Medications with Abuse Potential, *p. 80, Ch. 7*

Neuromuscular System Disorders, *p. 176, Ch. 12*

Pain Medications, *p. 214, Ch. 14*

Psychoses and Degenerative Diseases of the Nervous System, *p. 154, Ch. 11*

Pulmonary Disorders, *p. 472, Ch. 29*

Reproductive Disorders, *p. 558, Ch. 34*

Shock, *p. 328, Ch. 21*

Skin Disorders, *p. 594, Ch. 36*

Taking Medications, *p. 39, Ch. 3*

Treatment for Diabetes Mellitus, *p. 539, Ch. 33*

Vitamins, Minerals, or Nutritional Supplements, *p. 505, Ch. 31*

SAFETY ALERT

Accidental Overdose of Vitamins and Other Medications, *p. 505, Ch. 31*

Allergic Reactions and Antibiotics, *p. 409. Ch. 26*

Drug-to-Food Interactions, *p. 284, Ch. 18*

Expiration Dates on Multidose Vials, *p. 539, Ch. 33*

Interpreting Physician Orders, *p. 119. Ch. 9*

Medication Administration Error–Mistaken Patient Identity, *p. 37, Ch. 3*

Medication Label Confusion: Heparin, *p. 358. Ch. 23*

Soundalike Drug Names, *p. 579, Ch. 35*

LISA MATTIN